Fundamentals of
Nursing

Concepts, Process
and Practice

**Barbara Kozier, Glenora Erb,
Audrey Berman, Shirlee Snyder,
Richard Lake and Sharon Harvey**

Harlow, England • London • New York • Boston • San Francisco • Toronto
Sydney • Tokyo • Singapore • Hong Kong • Seoul • Taipei • New Delhi
Cape Town • Madrid • Mexico City • Amsterdam • Munich • Paris • Milan

PEARSON EDUCATION
NURSING&HEALTH

FIRST FOR HEALTH

Pearson Education Limited
Edinburgh Gate
Harlow
Essex CM20 2JE
England

and Associated Companies throughout the world

Visit us on the World Wide Web at:
www.pearsoned.co.uk

First published 2008

ISBN: 978-0-13-197653-5

British Library Cataloguing-in-Publication Data
A catalogue record for this book is available from the British Library

10 9 8 7 6 5 4 3 2 1
11 10 09 08

Typeset in 9.5/12pt Minion by 35
Printed and bound by Rotolito Lombarda, Italy

The publisher's policy is to use paper manufactured from sustainable forests.

Fundamentals of
Nursing

Visit the *Fundamentals of Nursing* Companion Website at
www.pearsoned.co.uk/kozier to find valuable **student**
learning material including:

+ Multiple choice questions to help test your learning
+ Links to relevant sites on the web
+ Additional case studies
+ Extra assessment tools and care plans for core topics

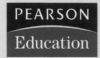

Brief contents

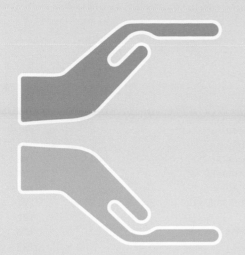

Contents

Supporting resources

Visit www.pearsoned.co.uk/kozier to find valuable online resources

Companion Website for students
+ Multiple choice questions to help test your learning
+ Links to relevant sites on the web
+ Additional case studies
+ Extra assessment tools and care plans for core topics

Also: The Companion Website provides the following features:

+ Search tool to help locate specific items of content
+ E-mail results and profile tools to send results of quizzes to instructors
+ Online help and support to assist with website usage and troubleshooting

For more information please contact your local Pearson Education sales representative or visit www.pearsoned.co.uk/kozier

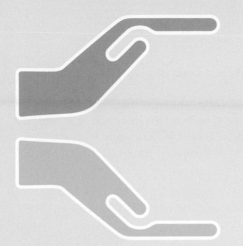
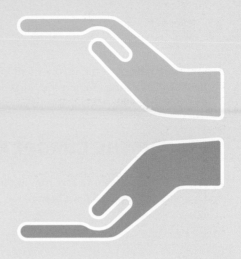

Preface

INTRODUCTION

Nursing is a difficult concept to define despite the fact that thousands of people experience nursing in some shape or form. We all know it's important, yet it's a concept that is often misunderstood. However, according to the Royal College of Nursing (2003) the purpose of nursing is easier to define and the RCN identifies six key purposes: 'to promote and maintain health, to care for people when their health is compromised, to assist recovery, to facilitate independence, to meet needs and to improve/maintain well-being/quality of life'.

However you define nursing, it involves a number of key components; evidence-based decision making, competent clinical skills, efficient management, teaching, effective use of advancing technology and effective interpersonal skills, but ultimately it involves working with individuals, groups and families to improve the quality of life. All of which will be discussed in this book.

THE AIM OF THIS BOOK

The aim of this book is to explore the underpinning knowledge required to care for an individual whether they are an adult or child, or have physical or mental health problems.

The text aims to be:

+ *Current and evidence-based*: up-to-date references have been used to support current nursing practices.
+ *Comprehensive* in its coverage of the significant concepts within nursing.
+ *Practical and clinically based*: clinical procedures are clearly explained using step-by-step guides with illustrations.
+ *European* in the examples used.

WHO SHOULD USE THIS BOOK?

This book has been designed as a study guide to support adult, child and mental health student nurses at undergraduate level particularly those on the Common Foundation Programme. However, students on other programmes such as Access to Health and Social Care may also find this book useful.

DISTINCTIVE FEATURES

+ **Learning outcomes** are included in all chapters and set objectives for the student when reading the particular chapter.
+ **Case studies** are included in all chapters and are suitable for personal reflection or group discussion. The case studies are short, current and serve as an illustration of the issues raised in the chapter.
+ **Research notes** consider current research on a particular subject and serve as an illustration of research used in evidence-based practice.
+ **Critical reflections** are included in all chapters and are linked to the case study presented at the beginning of each chapter. The aim of these is to allow the student to reflect on the case study and answer pertinent questions about the issues raised in it.
+ **Chapter highlights** are included in all chapters and summarise the main ideas discussed in the chapter.
+ **References** are included at the ends of all chapters and allow the student to search for the primary texts used to write the chapter. Some chapters also have **guidance and further information** sections at the end to cover legal aspects.
+ **Clinical anecdotes** are actual comments made by student nurses and qualified nurses and aim to provide the view points of real individuals within clinical practice.
+ **Procedures** are included in all clinical chapters. Clinical procedures are discussed using a step-by-step approach and are based on the stages of the nursing process: assessment, planning, implementation and education. Rationale is provided for aspects within the procedures based on current clinical evidence.
+ **Clinical alerts** are used in clinical chapters to highlight particular areas of practice that need to be taken into account when caring for an individual or group.
+ **Teaching: Patient care** boxes are used to discuss particular issues relating to teaching individuals or groups.
+ **Lifespan considerations** are used, where appropriate, to highlight alternatives to practice when caring for infants, children and/or older adults.
+ **Community care considerations** provide information related to caring for an individual in the home care setting, including communication with the patient and

multi-disciplinary team, involvement of carers and suggestions for alternatives for practice as indicated by the home care environment.

NEW FOR THE EUROPEAN EDITION

Although we have aimed to stay true to the original American text a number of changes have been made.

+ The book has been visually redesigned to emphasise key features.
+ There is an emphasis on European nursing practice.
+ Each chapter begins with a case study and links with the critical reflection at the end of the chapter.
+ There are new pedagogical features such as clinical anecdotes.

Acknowledgements

We are grateful to the following for permission to reproduce copyright material:

Line illustrations and tables:

Figure 1.3 © Bettman/CORBIS; Figures 2.2 and 2.3 from *A Theory for Nursing: Systems, Concepts, Processes*, Delmar (King, I. 1981); Figure 2.4 from Neuman, Betty and Fawcett, Jacqueline, *Neuman Systems Model, The*, 4th Edition, © 2002, pg 15, reprinted by permission of Pearson Education, Inc., Upper Saddle River, NJ; Figure 3.2 from the Nursing and Midwifery Council's website at www.nmc-uk.org/aFrameDisplay.aspx?DocumentID=1679; Figure 3.4 from *Legal Aspects of Nursing*, Pearson Education, © Pearson Education (Dimmond, B. 2005); Figure 5.1 from *Wellness: Concepts and Applications*, 6th edn, The McGraw-Hill Companies, © The McGraw-Hill Companies, Inc. (Anspaugh, D. J., Hamrich, M. H. and Rosato, F. D. 2003); Table 5.1 from Spector, Rachael E., *Cultural Diversity in Health and Illness*, 5th Edition, © 2000, pg 100, reprinted by permission of Pearson Education, Inc., Upper Saddle River, NJ; Figure 5.4 reprinted with permission, from the *Wellness Workbook*, 3rd edn, by John W. Travis, MD and Regina Sara Ryan, Celestial Arts, Berkeley, CA © 1981, 1988, 2004 by John W. Travis. www.wellnessworkbook.com; Figure 5.8 from *Psychology of Human Behaviour*, 5th edn, Wadsworths, a subdivision of Thomson Learning (Kalish, R. A. 1983); Figure 6.4 adapted from Edline, G., Golanty, E. and Brown, K. M., *Health and Wellness: A Holistic Approach*, 7th edn, 2002, Jones and Bartlett Publishers, Sudbury, MA. www.jbpub.com, reprinted with permission; Table 6.9 from Fontaine, Karen Lee, *Mental Health Nursing*, 5th Edition, © 2003, pgs 11–12, reprinted by permission of Pearson Education, Inc., Upper Saddle River, NJ; Figure 7.2 from 'Knowledge and control in health promotion: a test case for social policy and social theory', in *The Sociology of Health Service*, edited by J. Gabe, M. Calnan and M. Bury, Routledge (Beattie, A. 1991); Figure 7.3 from 'Healthstyle: A Self-test', University of Florida, Institute of Food and Agricultural Sciences (UF/IFAS) (Bobroff, L. B. 1999); Figure 7.4 adapted from 'A stage planning programme model for health education/health promotion practice', in *Journal of Advanced Nursing*, Blackwell Publishing (Whitehead, D. 2001); Figures 8.1, 8.2, 8.3 and 8.4 adapted from *The ACP Guide to the Structure of the NHS in the United Kingdom*, Association of Clinical Pathologists (Galloway, M. 2005), we thank Dr. M. J. Galloway and the Association of Clinical Pathologists for allowing us to reproduce this material; Table 9.10 from *NANDA Nursing Diagnosis: Definitions and Classifications, 2007–2008*, NANDA International (NANDA I 2007); Table 9.5 and Figure 9.7 from Wilkinson, Judith M., *Nursing Process and Critical Thinking*, 3rd Edition, © 2001, pg 436, reprinted by permission of Pearson Education, Inc., Upper Saddle River, NJ; Figures 12.1, 12.3, 12.4, 12.6, 12.7, 12.8, 12.9, 12.10, 12.11, 12.12, 12.13, 12.16, 12.17, 12.18, 12.19, 12.20, 12.21, 12.25, 12.27, 12.28, 12.29, 12.30, 12.31 and 12.32 are manual handling illustrations © EDGE Services (2006) reproduced by kind permission of EDGE Services – The Manual Handling Training Co. Ltd (01904 677853) sourced from People Handling & Risk Assessment Key Trainer's Certificate course materials; Figure 12.15 from Health and Safety Executive, © Crown copyright material is reproduced with the permission of the Controller of the HMSO; Figure 12.43 provided courtesy of the University of North Carolina at Chapel Hill School of Nursing: Illustration by Jean LeCluyse; Figure 15.1 adapted from *Fever and the Regulation of Body Temperature*, Charles C. Thomas (DuBois, E. F. 1948); Figure 15.2 (figure 25.25, p. 953) from *Human Anatomy and Physiology*, 4th edn, by Elaine N. Marieb, copyright © 1998 by the Benjamin/Cummings Publishing Company, reprinted by permission of Pearson Education, Inc.; Figures 17.1 and 17.2 and Table 17.1 from R. Hogston and P. M. Simpson (eds), *Foundations of Nursing Practice: Making the Difference*, 2002, Palgrave Macmillan, reproduced with permission of Palgrave Macmillan; Figure 17.3, The 'Malnutrition Universal Screening Tool' ('MUST') is reproduced here with the kind permission of BAPEN (British Association for Parenteral and Enteral Nutrition), for further information on MUST see www.bapen.org.uk; Table 18.2 from *Nelson Textbook of Pediatrics*, R.E. Behman, p. 107, copyright Elsevier (1992); Figure 18.14(a) courtesy of and © Becton, Dickinson and Company; Figures 20.5, 20.7, 20.8, 20.9 and 20.10 courtesy of C.R. Bard, Inc., all trademarks used are trademarks and/or registered trademarks of C.R. Bard, Inc. or an affiliate; Figure 21.4 from Welsh Chief Pharmacists; Figure 21.64 from MABIS DMI Healthcare; Figure 21.66 property of TMI, used under permission from TMI; Figure 22.6 from *Cancer Pain Relief*, 2nd edn, World Health Organization (WHO 1996); Figures 25.3, 25.4, 25.15 and 25.17 from *Immediate Life Support Manual*,

2nd edn (Resuscitation Council UK 2006); Figures 25.1, 25.5, 25.12 and 25.13 are reproduced with kind permission by Michael Scott and the Resuscitation Council (UK).

Photographs:

Figure 1.1(a) Rex Features: Everett Collection; Figure 1.4 Nils Jorgensen; Figures 1.5(a), 1.6, 6.2, 8.1, 12.2, 16.36(a) and (b), 17.9(a) and (b), 18.21, 21.12, 21.17, 24.10 Wellcome Images; Figure 1.5(b) Mediscan; Figure 1.5(c) Gregory Hale; Figure1.5(d) James King-Holmes; Figure 1.5(e) John Cole; Figures 2(b) and (c) Granada International; Figure 8.2 NHS Direct; Figures 11.2, 11.3, 13.26, 14.11, 14.12, 15.11, 15.12, 15.21(1) and (b), 15.22, 16.9, 16.11, 16.20, 16.23, 18.17, 18.18, 19.9, 19.12, 21.8, 21.14, 24.4, 24.5 and 24.6, photographer Elena Dorfman; Figure 11.5 Science Photo Library Ltd; Figure 12.22 ME Design Ltd; Figures 12.23 and 12.35 Phil-e-slide patient handling system, Ergo Ike Ltd. www.phil-e-slide-uk.com; Figures 12.24(a) and (b) Hoist and Shower Chair Company Ltd; Figures 12.26(a) and (b), 12.34, 12.37, 12.40, Dumas; Figure 12.41 ARJO MED AB Ltd; Figures 13.1, 13.2, 13.11, 13.27, 14.8, 15.13, 15.34, 16.8, 16.11, 16.24, 16.29, 16.33, 16.34, 21.23, 21.24, 21.46, 21.53, 21.54, 21.57, 22.10, 23.47 and 24.12, photographer Jenny Thomas; Figure 13.30 from David Parker/Science Photo Library; Figure 15.7 Art Directors and TRIP photo Library: Helene Rogers; Figure 14.5 from Ease Seating Systems; Figure 14.6 from Hill-Rom, courtesy of Hill-Rom Services, Inc., reprinted with permission, all rights reserved; Figure 14.7, Therapulse® II, courtesy of KCI Licensing, Inc. 9/2007; Figures 15.35 and 15.36 from Nonin Medical Inc.; Figure 16.21 from Smiths Medical International; Figures 16(a) and (b) Air Products and Chemicals 2007; Figure 17.16 from Abbott Nutrition, Abbott Laboratories Ltd, used with permission; Figure 18.12 Paul Graggs; Figure 18.14(a) Courtesy and © Becton, Dickinson and Company; Figure 21.64 from MABIS DMI Healthcare; Figure 21.67 Saturn Stills; Figure 24.1 Homecraft Rolyan Ltd, www.Independentliving.co.uk; Figure 24.15 C. Greenhill; Figure 21.43 Geoff Tompkinson; Figure 24.7 AJ Photo 659; Figure 24.12 MYCO Medical; Figure 24.16 Mike Devlin; Figures 25.1, 25.5, 25.6, 25.7, 25.7, 25.8, 25.9, 25.10(a) and (b), 25.11(a) and (b), 25.14, reproduced with kind permission by Michael Scott and the Resuscitation Council (UK); Figures 25.5 and 25.6 SECA Ltd. UK Medical Scales and Weighing Systems; Figure 26.7 Marsden Weighing Machine Group Ltd; Figure 26.8 Josh Sher; Figure 26.9 Sotiris Zafeiris; Figure 26.10 (H) from American Academy of Dermatology, reprinted with permission from the American Academy of Dermatology, all rights reserved; Figure 26.16 Scot Camazine.

All other images © Pearson Education.

Text:

Research Note, p. 11, from 'Why women and men choose nursing', *Nursing and Health Care Perspectives*, (22)1, National League for Nursing (Broghn, S. 2001); Box 4.1, p. 45, from *ICN Code of Ethics for Nurses*, copyright © 2006 by ICN – International Council of Nurses, 3, Place Jean-Marteau, 1201 Geneva, Switzerland; Box 4.2, p. 45, and Box 12.6, p. 230, from *Code of Professional Conduct: Standards for Conduct, Performance and Ethics*, Nursing and Midwifery Council (NMC 2004); Lifespan Considerations, p. 61, from *Gerontological Nursing Care*, S. R. Tyson, 'Elders: Issues that influence the health and well-being of elders', p. 9, copyright Elsevier, 1999; Box 5.6, p. 71, from *Toward a Psychology of Being*, 2nd edn, Van Nostrand Reinhold (Maslow, A. H. 1968), reprinted with permission of John Wiley & Sons, Inc.; Box 8.6, p. 132, from R. Baggot, *Health and Health Care in Britain*, 2004, Palgrave Macmillan, reproduced with permission of Palgrave Macmillan; Box 9.3, p. 151, from *Interviewing: Principles and Practices*, 10th edn, The McGraw-Hill Companies, © The McGraw-Hill Companies, Inc. (Stewart, C. J. and Cash, Jr, W. B. 2002); Box 9.4, p. 152, from *Getting Too Close (or Too Far) for Comfort*, http://travel.boston.com/columns/sl/030502_close.html, Smarter Travel Media (O'Carroll, E. 2001), reprinted with permission from Smarter Travel Media LLC (www.smartertravel.com); Box 12.5, p. 229, from *Simple Guide to the Lifting Operations and Lifting Equipment Regulations 1998*, Health and Safety Executive (HSE 1998), © Crown copyright material is reproduced with the permission of the Controller of the HMSO; p. 234, from *Don't Take Pain Lying Down* at www.welshbacks.com, Welsh Backs (Welsh Backs 2006); Box 17.1, p. 417, from 'Know how: nutritional assessment', *Nursing Times*, (94)8, Emap Healthcare (Walters, E. 1998), copyright Emap Public Sector 2007, reproduced by permission of Nursing Times; Box 18.1, p. 438, from R. Hogston and P. M. Simpson (eds), *Foundations of Nursing Practice: Making the Difference*, 2002, Palgrave Macmillan, reproduced with permission of Palgrave Macmillan; Practice Guidelines, p. 462, from 'Getting a line on central vascular access devices', *Nursing*, 32(4), Wolters Kluwer Health (Masoorli, S. and Angeles, T. 2002); Box 22.2, p. 582, from 'Undertreated pain: could it land you in court?', *Nursing*, 32, Wolters Kluwer Health (LaDuke, S. 2002).

In some instances we have been unable to trace the owners of copyright material, and we would appreciate any information that would enable us to do so.

Guided Tour of the book

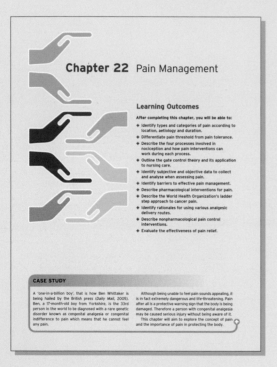

Chapter 22 Pain Management

Learning Outcomes

After completing this chapter, you will be able to:

+ Identify types and categories of pain according to location, aetiology and duration.
+ Differentiate pain threshold from pain tolerance.
+ Describe the four processes involved in nociception and how pain interventions can work during each process.
+ Outline the gate control theory and its application to nursing care.
+ Identify subjective and objective data to collect and analyse when assessing pain.
+ Identify barriers to effective pain management.
+ Describe pharmacological interventions for pain.
+ Describe the World Health Organization's ladder step approach to cancer pain.
+ Identify rationales for using various analgesic delivery routes.
+ Describe nonpharmacological pain control interventions.
+ Evaluate the effectiveness of pain relief.

CASE STUDY

A 'one-in-a-billion boy', that is how Ben Whittaker is being hailed by the British press (*Daily Mail*, 2005). Ben, a 17-month-old boy from Yorkshire, is the 33rd person in the world to be diagnosed with a rare genetic disorder known as congenital analgesia or congenital indifference to pain which means that he cannot feel any pain.

Although being unable to feel pain sounds appealing, it is in fact extremely dangerous and life-threatening. Pain after all is a protective warning sign that the body is being damaged. Therefore a person with congenital analgesia may be caused serious injury without being aware of it. This chapter will aim to explore the concept of pain and the importance of pain in protecting the body.

Learning Outcomes - set your objectives when reading the chapter.

Case Studies - can be used for your own personal reflection or group discussion. They are short, current, and illustrate the issues raised in the chapter.

Research Notes - consider current research on a particular subject and serve as an illustration of research used in evidence-based practice.

---

362   **CHAPTER 15** VITAL SIGNS

RESEARCH NOTE

How Long Should a Patient Lie and Stand When Taking Orthostatic Blood Pressures?

Lack of agreement within the research literature and in their own institution regarding the technique for measuring orthostatic blood pressures led these authors (Lance *et al.*, 2000) to conduct this study. Thirty-five normal participants exercised, had their pulse and blood pressure measured when rested, then had pulse, blood pressure and dizziness measured when standing. The variables were the length of time required for resting to produce baseline values and the minimum time standing to return indications of blood pressure drop or dizziness.

The results of the study showed that 10 minutes of resting were needed for baseline values. This was longer than the five-minute departmental standard and shorter than the 15-minute nursing unit practice. Pulse, blood pressure and dizziness readings taken immediately upon standing and at two minutes were sufficient. Measurements taken after longer periods of standing did not show significant differences from the two-minute readings.

Implications

The authors acknowledged that their results could not be easily extrapolated to the broader population since their participants were healthy, young (under 25 years old) adults. However, they felt secure enough with their results to implement the standard in their institution while recommending further study on patients with higher risk of orthostatic variations. The article is clear and well written and would easily permit replication of the research. Nurses should pursue the investigation of similar clinical practices that are unstudied or have conflicting results in the published literature.

Note: From 'Comparison of Different Methods of Obtaining Orthostatic Vital Signs,' by R. Lance et al., 2000, Clinical Nursing Research, 9, pp. 479–491.

+ Assist the patient to slowly sit or stand. Support the patient in case of faintness.
+ After one minute in the upright position, recheck the pulse and blood pressure in the same sites as previously.
+ Record the results. A rise in pulse of 40 beats per minute or a drop in blood pressure of 30 mm Hg indicates abnormal orthostatic vital signs.

Assessing Blood Pressure

Blood pressure is measured with a *blood pressure cuff*, a *sphygmomanometer* and a *stethoscope*. The blood pressure cuff consists of a rubber bag that can be inflated with air. It is called the *bladder* (see Figure 15-25). It is covered with cloth and has two tubes attached to it. One tube connects to a rubber bulb that inflates the bladder. When turned counterclockwise, a small valve on the side of this bulb releases the air in the bladder. When the valve is tightened (turned clockwise), air pumped into the bladder remains there.

The other tube is attached to a sphygmomanometer. The sphygmomanometer indicates the pressure of the air within the bladder. There are two types of sphygmomanometers: *aneroid* and *mercury* (see Figure 15-26). The aneroid sphygmomanometer is a calibrated dial with a needle that points to the calibrations.

The mercury sphygmomanometer is a calibrated cylinder filled with mercury. The pressure is indicated at the point to

Figure 15-25 *A*, A blood pressure cuff and bulb; *B*, the bladder inside the cuff.

which the rounded curve of the **meniscus** (the crescent-shaped dome) rises (see Figure 15-27). The blood pressure reading should be made with the eye at the level of the rounded curve in order to be accurate.

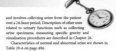

Clinical Anecdotes – actual comments made by students and qualified nurses provide the viewpoints of real individuals within clinical practice.

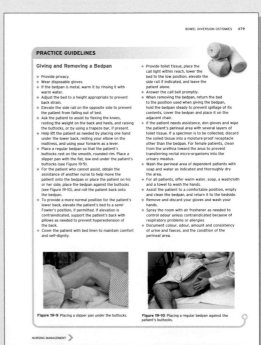

Practice Guidelines – contain instant-access summaries of clinical dos and don'ts.

Step-by-Step Procedures – are included in all clinical chapters. Clinical procedures are discussed using a step-by-step approach. Rationale is provided for aspects within the procedures based on current clinical evidence.

WOUND HEALING   313

dead tissue debris and dead and living bacteria. Purulent exudates vary in colour, some acquiring tinges of blue, green or yellow. The colour may depend on the causative organism.

Haemorrhagic exudate consists of large amounts of red blood cells, indicating damage to capillaries that is severe enough to allow the escape of red blood cells from plasma. This type of exudate is frequently seen in open wounds.

> **CLINICAL ALERT**
>
> *A bright haemorrhagic exudate indicates fresh bleeding, whereas dark sanguineous exudate denotes older bleeding.*

Mixed types of exudates are often observed. A *haemoserous* (consisting of clear and blood-tinged drainage) exudate is commonly seen in surgical incisions.

Complications of Wound Healing

Several untoward events can occur to interfere with the healing of a wound. These include excessive bleeding, infection and dehiscence.

Haemorrhage

Some escape of blood from a wound is normal. **Haemorrhage** (massive bleeding), however, is abnormal. It may be caused by a dislodged clot, a slipped stitch or erosion of a blood vessel, for example.

Internal haemorrhage may be detected by swelling or distention in the area of the wound and, possibly, by the presence of blood in a surgical drain. Some patients will have a **haematoma**, a localised collection of blood underneath the skin that may appear as a reddish blue swelling (bruise). A large haematoma may be dangerous in that it places pressure on blood vessels and can thus obstruct blood flow.

The risk of haemorrhage is greatest during the first 48 hours after surgery. Haemorrhage is an emergency; the nurse should apply pressure dressings to the area and monitor the patient's vital signs. Medical advice should be sought immediately as the patient may need to be taken to theatre for surgical intervention.

Infection

Colonisation is the presence of micro-organisms without illness or reaction. Most if not all wounds are contaminated as the skin is surrounded by micro-organisms. These micro-organisms compete with the new cells in the wound for oxygen and nutrition and as a result can delay wound healing. If these micro-organisms multiply excessively or invade tissues, infection can result. If a wound and surrounding tissues become infected there are generally a few tell-tale signs including:

♦ pain,
♦ change in the colour of the wound bed,
♦ malodorous (offensive smelling) exudate,
♦ heat,
♦ swelling.

If infection is suspected the nurse should swab the wound and send it for culture and sensitivity. This test will identify the micro-organism and suggest a drug that the micro-organism is sensitive to. Severe infection causes fever and elevated white blood cell count. Patients who are immunosuppressed are especially susceptible to wound infections.

A wound can be infected with micro-organisms at the time of injury, during surgery or postoperatively. Wounds that occur as a result of injury (e.g. bullet and knife wounds) are most likely to be contaminated at the time of injury. Surgery involving the intestines can also result in infection from the micro-organisms inside the intestine.

Dehiscence

Dehiscence is the partial or total rupturing of a sutured wound. Dehiscence usually involves an abdominal wound in which the layers below the skin also separate. A number of factors, including obesity, poor nutrition, multiple trauma, failure of suturing, excessive coughing, vomiting and dehydration, heighten a patient's risk of wound dehiscence. Wound infection can be the cause of the wound dehiscing (Tobon *et al.* 2005).

Dehiscence may be preceded by sudden straining, such as coughing or sneezing. It is not unusual for a patient to feel that 'something has given away'. When dehiscence occurs, the wound should be quickly supported by large sterile dressings, the patient should be placed in a bed in a position that puts as little pressure on the wound as possible. The surgeon must be notified because immediate surgical repair of the area may be necessary.

Factors Affecting Wound Healing

Characteristics of the individual such as age, nutritional status, lifestyle and medications influence the speed of wound healing.

Developmental Considerations

Healthy children and adults often heal more quickly than older people, who are more likely to have chronic diseases that hinder healing. For example, reduced liver function can impair the synthesis of blood clotting factors. Box 14-2 on page 314 lists factors inhibiting wound healing in older adults.

Nutrition

Wound healing places additional demands on the body. Patients with wounds require a diet rich in protein, carbohydrates, lipids, vitamins A and C and minerals, such as iron, zinc and copper (Anderson, 2005). Malnourished patients may require time to improve their nutritional status before surgery, if this is possible.

Clinical Alerts – are used in clinical chapters to highlight particular areas of practice that need to be taken into account when caring for an individual or group.

---

570   **CHAPTER 21**   ADMINISTRATION OF MEDICATION

are holding chambers into which the medication is fired and from which the patient inhales, so that the dose is not lost by exhalation. *Teaching: patient care* provides instructions for

patients about using an MDI. Newer breath-activated MDIs are being produced in which inhalation triggers the release of a pre-measured dose of medication.

> **TEACHING: PATIENT CARE**
>
> **Using a Metered-dose Inhaler**
> ♦ Make sure the canister is firmly and fully inserted into the inhaler.
> ♦ Remove the mouthpiece cap and, holding the inhaler upright, shake the inhaler vigorously for 3–5 seconds to mix the medication evenly.
> ♦ Exhale comfortably (as in a normal full breath).
> ♦ Hold the canister upside down.
> ♦ Put the mouthpiece far enough into the mouth with its opening toward the throat. Close the lips tightly around the mouthpiece. An MDI with a spacer or extender is always placed in the mouth (see Figure 21-67).
>
> **Administering the Medication**
> ♦ Press down once on the MDI canister (which releases the dose) and inhale slowly and deeply through the mouth.
> ♦ Hold your breath for 10 seconds. *This allows the aerosol to reach deeper airways.*
> ♦ Remove the inhaler from or away from the mouth.
> ♦ Exhale slowly through pursed lips. *Controlled exhalation keeps the small airways open during exhalation.*
> ♦ Repeat the inhalation if ordered. Wait 20–30 seconds between inhalations of bronchodilator medications so *the first inhalation has a chance to work and the subsequent dose reaches deeper into the lungs.*
> ♦ After the inhalation is completed, rinse mouth with tap water to remove any remaining medication and reduce irritation and risk of infection.
> ♦ Clean the MDI mouthpiece after each use. Use mild soap and water, rinse it, and let it air dry before replacing it on the device.
> ♦ Store the canister at room temperature. Avoid extremes of temperature.
>
>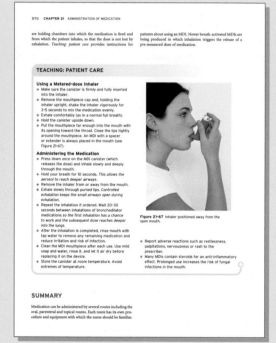
> **Figure 21-67** Inhaler positioned away from the open mouth.
>
> ♦ Report adverse reactions such as restlessness, palpitations, nervousness or rash to the prescriber.
> ♦ Many MDIs contain steroids for an anti-inflammatory effect. Prolonged use increases the risk of fungal infections in the mouth.

SUMMARY

Medication can be administered by several routes including the oral, parenteral and topical routes. Each route has its own procedure and equipment with which the nurse should be familiar.

Teaching: Patient Care - discuss particular issues relating to teaching individuals or groups.

---

722   **CHAPTER 26**   PHYSICAL ASSESSMENT AND DIAGNOSTIC TESTING

> **LIFESPAN CONSIDERATIONS**
>
> **Assessing the Neurological System**
>
> **Infants**
> ♦ Reflexes commonly tested in newborns include the rooting reflex – when the baby's cheek is touched, the head turns toward that side; palmar grasp – the baby's fingers curl around an object; tonic neck reflex – when the baby is supine and the head is turned to one side, the arm and leg on that side extend while those on the opposite side flex (fencing position). Most of these disappear by six months of age.
>
> **Children**
> ♦ Present the procedures as games whenever possible.
> ♦ Positive Babinski reflex is abnormal after the child ambulates or at age two.
> ♦ Note the child's ability to understand and follow directions.
> ♦ Assess immediate recall or recent memory by using names of cartoon characters. Normal recall in children is one less than age in years.
> ♦ Assess for signs of hyperactivity or abnormally short attention span.
>
> ♦ Should be able to walk backward by age two, balance on one foot for five seconds by age four, heel-toe walk by age five, and heel-toe walk backward by age six.
> ♦ Romberg test is appropriate over age three.
>
> **Older Adults**
> ♦ A full neurological assessment can be lengthy. Conduct in several sessions if indicated and cease the tests if the patient is noticeably fatigued.
> ♦ A decline in mental status is not a normal result of ageing. Changes are more the result of physical or psychological disorders (e.g. fever, fluid and electrolyte imbalances, medications). Acute, abrupt-onset mental status changes are usually caused by delirium. These changes are often reversible with treatment. Chronic subtle insidious mental health changes are usually caused by dementia and are usually irreversible.
> ♦ Intelligence and learning ability are unaltered with age. Many factors, however, inhibit learning (e.g. anxiety, illness, pain, cultural barrier).
> ♦ Short-term memory is often less efficient. Long-term memory is usually unaltered.
> ♦ As a person ages, reflex responses may become less intense.

> **CLINICAL ANECDOTE**
>
> I honestly didn't realise how important assessing a patient's neurological status was until I went on placement last week. A lady was admitted via her GP after having a severe headache for over a week. She had deteriorated at home and had become quite confused. On admission we could not get much information from her as she was in so much pain and was quite agitated. The information we did have came from her husband and her GP. We checked her vital signs which appeared stable and her Glasgow Coma Scale was 12. We informed the doctors of our assessment and decided that we needed to keep a close eye on her by assessing her neurological status every half hour. The next time she was assessed her GCS had dropped to 10 so we informed the doctors who decided to send her straight to theatre for investigation. It turned out that she had a subarachnoid haemorrhage and would have died if we had not picked up her deterioration.
>
> *Sarah Roberts, student nurse*

NECK

Examination of the neck includes the muscles, lymph nodes, trachea, thyroid gland, carotid arteries and jugular veins (Figure 26-35).

One of the most common reasons for examining the neck is to assess the lymph nodes for size, shape, mobility and tenderness.

Lymph nodes occur throughout the body however chains of lymph nodes can be found in the neck, armpits and groin. Lymph nodes play an important part in a patient's immune system as lymph and lymph nodes contain lymphocytes and antibodies that fight off infection (see Table 26-6). As a result, if there is systemic or localised infection the lymph nodes can become swollen and tender. Also some forms of cancer, such as Hodgkin's

Lifespan Considerations – highlight alternatives to practice when caring for infants, children and/or older adults.

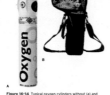

Community Care Considerations - provide information related to caring for an individual in the community setting, including communication with the patient and multidisciplinary team, involvement of carers, and suggestions for alternatives for practice as indicated by the community environment.

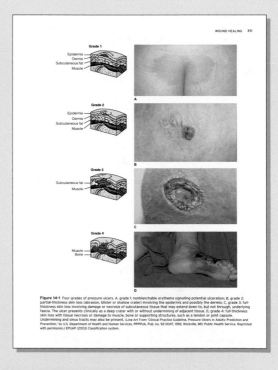

Photographs – bring the theory to life, showing you what you can expect to see in a clinical setting.

Critical Reflections – are linked to the case study presented at the beginning of the chapter. They allow you to reflect on the case study and think more critically about the issues raised.

Chapter Highlights – summarise the main ideas discussed in the chapter. Ideal for reference and quick revision.

References – are included in all chapters and allow you to see the evidence base for the material covered within each chapter

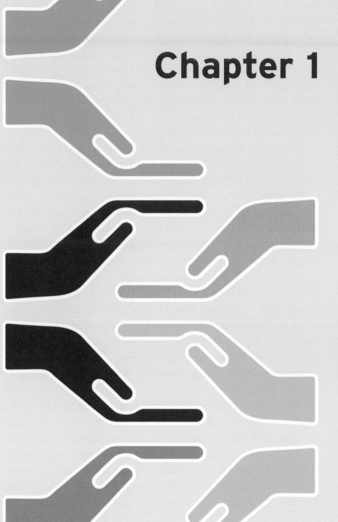

Chapter 1

Historical and Current Nursing Practice

Learning Outcomes

After completing this chapter, you will be able to:

+ Discuss historical and contemporary factors influencing the development of nursing.
+ Identify the essential aspects of nursing.
+ Identify the three main areas within the scope of nursing practice.
+ Identify the potential settings for nursing practice.
+ Discuss the organisation of nursing work.
+ Describe the roles of nurses.
+ Discuss the criteria of a profession.
+ Describe factors that could influence current nursing practice.
+ Discuss nurse education in the UK.
+ Discuss the importance of research in nursing.

CASE STUDY

Nurses are 'too posh to wash' and 'too clever to care'. These are the media headlines that faced the public in 2004 when the Royal College of Nursing (RCN) Congress broached the idea that the caring component of nursing should be devolved to healthcare assistants so that nurses could concentrate on treatment and more technical tasks. However 95% of nurses who voted in the Congress agreed that the caring role should not be delegated in this way.

Nursing does involve the 'basics' or 'fundamentals' of care but this should not be seen as a negative. Imagine caring for a person who is unable to care for their most basic human needs such as going to the toilet. Imagine the humiliation that person would feel having to rely on you to meet those needs. Some may say that this is unskilled work but nurses may miss important and subtle clues that can aid in the treatment and diagnosis of the patient by not doing such tasks. Nursing is more than the task itself, it is about holistically assessing and caring for the patient, which requires skill and professionalism.

After reading this chapter you will be able to reflect on the nursing role in providing healthcare, the way care is organised and how nursing is classified as a profession.

STEREOTYPES OF NURSES

Battleaxe, bimbo or angel, is this how the public perceives nurses? Well according to a Mori Poll commissioned by the RCN in 1984, this was indeed how the public perceived nurses, with one in ten people (10%) seeing nurses as having sex appeal (Payne, 2000). However a similar poll in 1999 showed that this perception of nurses has changed with only 6% of the public viewing nurses as having sex appeal (Payne, 2000). Despite this fact, the poll also showed that in the public's eyes the most famous nurses were Florence Nightingale, the Crimean war nurse, Hattie Jacques' 'matron' character and Barbara Windsor's 'saucy' character, both from the 'Carry On' films (see Figure 1-1).

Since Florence Nightingale's era nursing has been inextricably linked with the female gender and although the perception that to be a good nurse you must be female has lessened in the public's eyes (Payne, 2000), it is a perception that is hard to shake off particularly when you consider the famous nurses highlighted by the public in the 1999 RCN poll (Payne, 2000).

In order to find out where these stereotypes of nurses come from, we must delve into the history of nursing.

THE HISTORY OF NURSING

It's hard to say when the art of nursing began, but if we think about it logically there have always been illnesses and wounds that need tending, so it is fair to say that probably nursing has been around long before written records began. In fact the first written reference to nursing care can be found in the *Old Testament* where midwives cared for expectant mothers in their own homes. Other than this there are very few records of nursing pre-Christianity. However it is interesting to note that medical history can be traced back over the past 6,000 years.

For centuries after the birth of Jesus Christ, the Roman Empire ruled most of Europe. During this time, physicians moved from being slaves to high ranking Roman citizens, and nursing was finally considered as a vocation worthy of Roman ladies rather than female slaves.

It was also during this time that the first organised hospitals or *valetudinaria* were erected. These were built for Rome's most precious asset, its soldiers. Roman soldiers injured in battle needed to be placed somewhere where they could recover in readiness for their next battle as they were essential to the continuation of the Roman Empire.

In AD 335 Emperor Constantine ordered that Christianity be the official religion of the Roman Empire. It was during this time that some of the earliest nurses are recorded. Saint Helena, a British Princess and mother of Emperor Constantine, set up the first hospital in Jerusalem. While Fabiola, a high-ranking woman, gave up all her worldly goods in order to nurse. It seemed fashionable for high ranking females within the Roman Empire to give up everything in order to nurse others. Indeed early religious values, such as self-denial, spiritual calling and devotion to duty and hard work, have dominated nursing throughout its history. Nurses' commitment to these values often resulted in exploitation and few monetary rewards. For some time, nurses themselves believed it was inappropriate to expect economic gain from their 'calling'.

It was probably during these early Roman times that nursing became a predominantly female vocation, possibly as a result of the nurturing and caring roles already undertaken by the women of the household. However, women were not always the sole providers of nursing care. For instance, during the Crusades several orders of knights were formed, including the Knights of Saint John of Jerusalem (also known as the Knights Hospitalers), the Teutonic Knights and the Knights of Saint Lazarus (see Figure 1-2), all of which provided nursing care to their sick and injured comrades. During these times, hospitals were built throughout Europe providing care to people with leprosy, syphilis and chronic skin conditions.

It appears that throughout history, war has played an important part in the development of the nurses' role. None

(a)

(b)

(c)

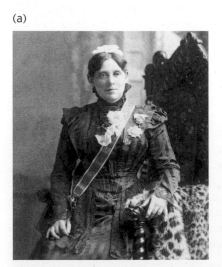
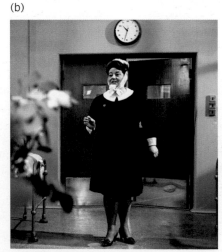
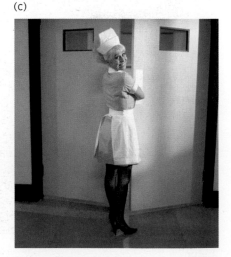

Figure 1-1 Public perception of nurses: (a) Florence Nightingale; (b) Hattie Jacques; (c) Barbara Windsor.

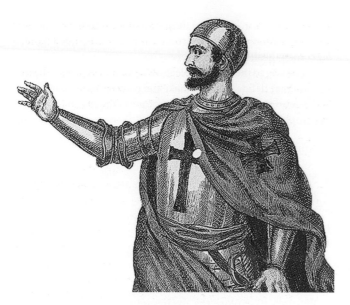

Figure 1-2 The Knights of Saint Lazarus.

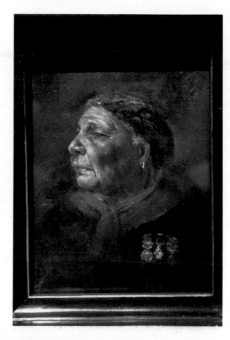

Figure 1-4 Mary Seacole.

more so than the Crimean War (1854–1856), where British soldiers were dying from cholera and malaria soon after arriving in Turkey. The inadequacy of care given to soldiers led to a public outcry in Great Britain resulting in Florence Nightingale, a resident lady superintendent of a hospital for invalid women in London, volunteering her nursing services. The British Government eventually gave permission for Florence Nightingale to take 38 nurses to Turkey in a bid to treat those soldiers suffering as a result of these two diseases (see Figure 1-3).

One other nurse, Mary Seacole, a Jamaican born nurse, also sought permission to care for the soldiers struck down by cholera and malaria in Turkey as she was incensed by the inadequacy of the care these soldiers were receiving (see Figure 1-4). However she was refused permission on at least four occasions. Mary Seacole was shocked by this, believing that the decisions were based on racial discrimination. As a

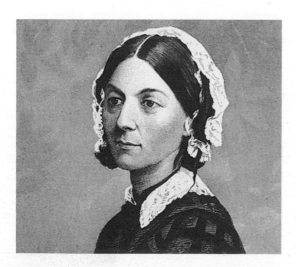

Figure 1-3 Florence Nightingale, founder of modern nursing (© Bettman/CORBIS).

result she decided to travel to Turkey herself, and set up a British hotel at her own cost. Here she cared for and fed British soldiers. Mary Seacole was a brave soul, often going into the actual battlefields to provide essential nursing care to those who needed it.

After the Crimean War both Mary Seacole and Florence Nightingale arrived back in the UK as national heroines and were awarded several medals for their bravery during the war. Florence Nightingale's legacy led to a transformation in military hospitals by improving sanitation practices such as handwashing and also led to the establishment of the Nightingale Fund for the training of nurses, which continues today in the Florence Nightingale School of Nursing and Midwifery in King's College in London.

Florence was also instrumental in shaping the image of the nursing profession. Society now viewed nurses as *Guardian Angels* or *Angels of Mercy*. After Nightingale brought respectability to the nursing profession, nurses were viewed as noble, compassionate, moral, religious, dedicated and self-sacrificing; a view that encouraged middle class women into the profession.

It is not only the Crimean War that led to the development of the nursing profession. During the First World War the Queen Alexandra's Imperial Military Nursing Services (QAIMNS) provided a 50,000-strong nursing workforce to the army. Many of these nurses worked near the front line in field hospitals' theatres. Again in the Second World War the QAIMNS were mobilised to provide nursing care at the front line under the charge of the Matron-in-Chief.

Following the Second World War the Army Medical Services, which included the QAIMNS, were reorganised and in 1949 the Queen Alexandra's Royal Army Nursing Corps was formed. Currently, military nurses from the Corps now serve on the front line across the world and also staff Ministry of Defence Hospital Units within the UK.

As a result of these wars the image of the nurse as heroine emerged. However, other perhaps more damaging perceptions of nurses have also emerged since the early 19th century. One such image is that of the *doctor's handmaiden*. This image evolved when women had yet to obtain the right to vote, when family structures were largely paternalistic and when the medical profession portrayed increasing use of scientific knowledge that, at that time, was viewed as a male domain.

Despite some of these lingering perceptions of nurses, society's views do appear to be changing. Indeed the public is taking a more positive view of nurses as being hardworking and trustworthy. Sarah Mullally, the Department of Health's Chief Nursing Officer (1999–2004), also aimed to improve the image of nurses within society, envisaging society's view of nurses as being 'knowledgeable and skilled, yet . . . caring and compassionate' (Mullally, 2004: 17).

In order to continue improving the public's perception of nursing as a profession, the public needs to be made aware of nurses' current roles and responsibilities within healthcare. In order to do this we need to explore what current nursing practice involves.

CURRENT NURSING PRACTICE

Nursing is and continues to be an ever-evolving practice that is hard to define. However a number of definitions of nursing have been suggested. Over 100 years ago, Florence Nightingale defined nursing as 'the act of utilising the environment of the patient to assist him in his recovery' (Nightingale, 1969). Nightingale considered a clean, well-ventilated and quiet environment essential for recovery.

On the other hand, Virginia Henderson, one of the first modern nurses to define nursing wrote, 'the unique function of the nurse is to assist the individual, sick or well, in the performance of those activities contributing to health or its recovery (or to peaceful death) that he would perform unaided if he had the necessary strength, will, or knowledge, and to do this in such a way as to help him gain independence as rapidly as possible' (Henderson, 1966: 3). Like Nightingale, Henderson described nursing in relation to the patient and the patient's environment. Unlike Nightingale, Henderson saw the nurse as concerned with both healthy and ill individuals, acknowledged that nurses interact with patients even when recovery may not be feasible, and mentioned the teaching and advocacy roles of the nurse.

In 2003, the Royal College of Nursing published a position statement 'Defining Nursing' (RCN, 2003). It states that the purpose of nursing 'is to promote health, healing, growth and development, and to prevent disease, illness, injury and disability' (RCN, 2003: 3). In the latter half of the 20th century, a number of nurse theorists developed their own theoretical definitions of nursing. Theoretical definitions are important because they go beyond simplistic common definitions. They describe what nursing is and the interrelationship among nurses, nursing, the patient, the environment and the intended patient outcome – health.

According to the Royal College of Nursing (2003), the characteristics that define nursing make the profession unique. Many of the definitions of nursing have common themes that describe its complexity:

+ Nursing is caring.
+ Nursing is an art.
+ Nursing is a science.
+ Nursing is patient centred.
+ Nursing is holistic.
+ Nursing is adaptive.
+ Nursing is concerned with health education, health promotion and prevention of ill health.
+ Nursing is evidence based.

Research to explore the meaning of caring in nursing has been increasing and has gone down a number of avenues. This has led to a number of theories on caring in nursing being presented. McCance *et al.* (1999) review a number of these theories, noting a number of similarities and differences between the theories. Most of the theories of caring in nursing they present are grounded in humanism, some of them being less abstract than others. Watson's Theory of Human Care is one such theory that has its origins in humanism and can be easily applied to nursing practice. Watson (1985, cited in McCance *et al.*, 1999) clearly defines caring as 'a value and an attitude that has become a will, an intention or a commitment, that manifests itself in concrete acts' (p. 1390) – as such, caring is an integral part of the role of nursing.

In order to have a clear understanding of nursing we also need to consider the recipients of nursing and the scope of nursing practice.

Recipients of Nursing

The recipients of nursing are sometimes called consumers, service users, patients or clients depending on the situation.

The terms **consumer** and **service user** are similar in that they refer to an individual, a group of people or a community that uses a healthcare service or commodity. Therefore a **patient** is said to be a consumer or service user. However the term patient usually implies that the person is waiting for or undergoing medical treatment and care. The word *patient* comes from a Latin word meaning 'to suffer' or 'to bear'. Traditionally, the person receiving healthcare has been called a patient. Usually, people become patients when they seek assistance because of illness or for surgery. Some nurses believe that the word *patient* implies passive acceptance of the decisions and care of health professionals. Additionally, with the emphasis on health promotion and prevention of illness, many recipients of nursing care are not ill. Moreover, nurses interact with family members and significant others to provide support, information and comfort in addition to caring for the patient.

For these reasons, some nurses refer to recipients of healthcare as *clients*. A **client** is a person who engages the advice or services of another who is qualified to provide this service. The term *client* presents the receivers of healthcare as collaborators in the care, that is, as people who are also responsible for their own health. Thus, the health status of a client is the responsibility of the individual in collaboration with health professionals.

Scope of Nursing

Nurses provide care to a number of different parties, namely individual patients, families and communities as a whole. This nursing care usually involves a combination of the following areas: promoting health and preventing illness, restoring health and care of the dying.

Promoting Health and Preventing Illness

The World Health Organization's (1948) definition of health is 'a state of complete physical, mental and social well-being and not merely the absence of disease or infirmity', which implies engaging in attitudes and behaviour that enhance the quality of life and feelings of well-being. Nurses promote wellness in patients who are healthy or ill. This may involve individual and community activities to enhance healthy lifestyles, such as improving nutrition and physical fitness, immunisations, preventing drug and alcohol misuse, restricting smoking, and preventing accidents and injury in the home and workplace. See Chapter 7 for details.

Restoring Health

Restoring health focuses on the ill patient and it extends from early detection of disease through helping the patient during the recovery period. Nursing activities include the following:

+ Providing direct care to the ill person, such as administering medications, baths and specific procedures and treatments.
+ Performing diagnostic and assessment procedures, such as measuring blood pressure and examining faeces for occult blood.
+ Consulting with other healthcare professionals about patient problems.
+ Teaching patients techniques that aid recovery following illness, such as exercises that will accelerate recovery after a stroke.
+ Rehabilitating patients to their optimal functional level following physical or mental illness, injury or drug addiction.

Care of the Dying

This area of nursing practice involves comforting and caring for people of all ages who are dying. It includes helping patients live as comfortably as possible until death and helping to support those coping with death. Nurses carrying out these activities work in homes, hospitals and extended care facilities such as *hospices*, which are specifically designed to care for dying patients and their families.

Settings of Nursing

There are many settings for nursing within the UK. Many nurses work in hospitals, but increasingly they work in patients' homes, long-term care, hospices, nursing homes, residential homes and general practitioner surgeries, among others (see Figure 1-5 on page 6).

Nurses have different degrees of nursing autonomy and responsibility in these different settings but have many roles in common including providing care, education and support, acting as advocates and agents of change, and helping to determine health policies that affect their patients.

The Organisation of Nursing Work

According to Thomas and Bond (1990) nursing work within the hospital setting is organised into three broad categories: functional, team and primary nursing.

Functional Nursing

This mode of organising nursing work is based purely on task allocation. The ward manager delegates tasks to individual nurses who have the skills to perform these tasks, but any decision making or responsibility lies with the ward manager.

Team Nursing

This mode of organising nursing work revolves around a team. The team leader coordinates the care provided and the responsibility and decision making lies with the team leader, resulting in the ward manager having less involvement and accountability for the care provided. This form of organising nursing work is the most common (Adams, 1998).

Primary Nursing

This involves the allocation of individual nurses to individual patients. It allows the nurse to assess, plan, implement and evaluate the care they provide to the patient and as a consequence the nurse has full responsibility and accountability for the care provided. This way of organising workload requires a team that can provide effective evidence-based care that is cost effective. The nurses need to have excellent clinical skills, communication skills and be experts in that particular field of nursing.

All three forms of organising nursing workload are found in clinical practice today. However there is a move away from functional nursing as this may not provide individualised holistic care to the patient. Primary nursing for many is the gold standard; however, it is labour intensive as it requires a core of expert nurses within the team, which is often lacking in some clinical environments. Each of these forms of organising workload requires a nurse who is able to adapt and perform numerous roles and functions.

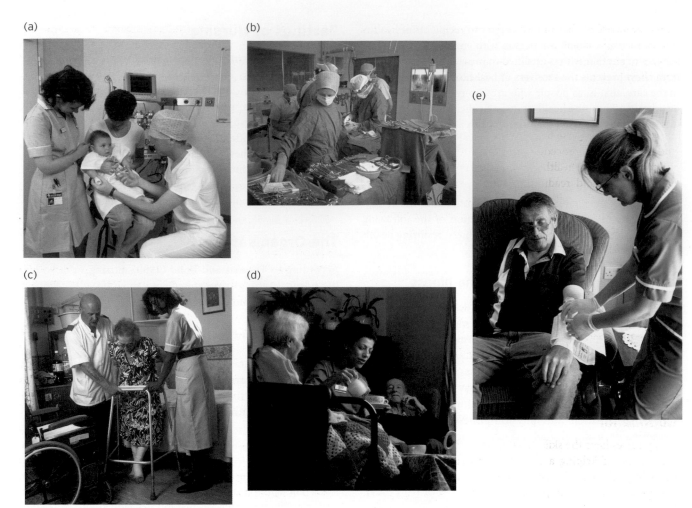

Figure 1-5 Nurses practise in a variety of settings.

Community nursing, however, is organised differently. Nurses care either for patients in a particular geographical area or for patients on a general practitioner's list. Geographical nursing is the most common way of organising nursing care in the community according to the White Paper 'The New NHS' (DOH, 1997). This White Paper proposed the development of Primary Care Groups in England and Local Care Groups in Wales that are geographically based. This means that community nurses are no longer linked to one general practitioner's practice but serve the community, which allows for sharing and pooling of resources and therefore is beneficial for patients.

ROLES AND FUNCTIONS OF THE NURSE

Nurses assume a number of roles when they provide care to patients, often carrying out these roles concurrently, not exclusively of one another. The roles required at a specific time depend on the needs of the patient and aspects of the particular environment.

Caregiver

The **caregiver** role has traditionally included those activities that assist the patient physically and psychologically while preserving the patient's dignity. The nurse may be required to provide a continuum of care from total nursing care for dependent patients to the supportive-educative care provided to patients who need assistance in attaining their highest possible level of health and wellness. Caregiving encompasses the physical, psychosocial, developmental, cultural and spiritual levels. The nursing process provides nurses with a framework for providing care (see Chapter 8) which they may provide themselves or delegate to others (e.g. healthcare assistants).

Communicator

Communication is integral to all nursing roles. Nurses communicate with a range of people; the patient, other healthcare professionals and support staff to name a few.

In the role of **communicator**, nurses identify patient problems and then communicate these verbally or in writing to other members of the multidisciplinary team. The quality of a nurse's communication is an important factor in nursing care. The nurse must be able to communicate effectively and accurately in order for a patient's healthcare needs to be met.

Teacher

As a **teacher**, the nurse helps patients learn about their health and the healthcare procedures they need to perform to restore or maintain their health. The nurse assesses the patient's learning needs and readiness to learn, sets specific learning goals in conjunction with the patient, enacts teaching strategies and measures learning. Nurses also teach other members of the multidisciplinary team, including support staff, in order to share expert knowledge.

Advocate

Advocacy is a key role for the nurse. The nurse has a duty to protect the patient and their human rights. The nurse may represent the patient's needs and wishes to other health professionals, such as relaying the patient's wish for information to medical staff. They also assist patients in exercising their rights and help them speak up for themselves (see Chapter 4).

Counsellor

Some nurses have the skills to counsel patients. **Counselling** is the process of helping a patient to recognise and cope with stressful psychological or social problems, to develop improved interpersonal relationships and to promote personal growth. It involves providing emotional, intellectual and psychological support to patients.

Leader

A **leader** influences others to work together to accomplish a specific goal. The leader role can be employed at different levels: individual patient, family, groups of patients, colleagues or the community. Effective leadership is a learned process requiring an understanding of the needs and goals that motivate people, the knowledge to apply the leadership skills and the interpersonal skills to influence others.

Manager

The nurse manages the nursing care of individuals, families and communities. The nurse-**manager** also delegates nursing activities to support staff and other nurses, and supervises and evaluates their performance. Managing requires knowledge about organisational structure and dynamics, authority and accountability, leadership, change theory, advocacy, delegation, and supervision and evaluation.

Evidence-Based Practitioner

In order to provide individualised, holistic care that is based on the most recent evidence nurses need to refer to current research. However in order to use research as a means of improving the care they provide they need to (a) understand the process and language of research, (b) have an awareness of issues relating to protecting the rights of human subjects (ethics), (c) recognise areas within care that need further investigation and research, and (d) be a discriminating user of research findings.

The Reflective Practitioner

Reflection within nursing is used as a means of articulating and developing knowledge embedded within practice (Benner *et al.*, 1996) and has been promoted as a way of enhancing learning since Dewey's (1933) writings. Boud *et al.* (1985) suggests that 'reflection in the context of learning is a generic term for those intellectual and affective activities in which individuals engage to explore their experiences in order to lead to new understanding and appreciations' (p. 19). Schon (1983) agrees stating that reflection is a means of uncovering the complex epistemology of practice. Atkins and Murphy (1993) suggest that reflection consists of three key stages, the first of which is the identification of uncomfortable feelings or thoughts, which is followed by a critical analysis of these feelings, leading to new perspectives being uncovered. However this model can be criticised as focusing on negative experiences, indeed Belenky *et al.* (1986) suggest that positive thoughts and feelings can also lead to critical reflective evaluation and thereby promote self-awareness. In order to structure the reflective process nurses are encouraged to use reflective diaries or journals and also to implement a reflective framework.

Expanded Career Roles

Nurses are fulfilling expanded career roles, such as those of nurse practitioner, clinical nurse specialist, nurse educator and nurse researcher, all of which allow greater independence and autonomy (see *Box 1-1* on page 8).

As nursing changes so do the roles and functions of the nurse. Indeed the above roles and functions aid the recognition of nursing as a profession.

CRITERIA OF A PROFESSION

Nursing is a profession. Where a **profession** is defined as an occupation that requires extensive education or a calling that requires special knowledge, skill and preparation, a profession is generally distinguished from other kinds of occupations by: (a) its requirement of prolonged, specialised training; (b) a body of knowledge based on research; (c) autonomy; and (d) a regulatory professional body.

Specialised Education

Specialised education is an important aspect of professional status. In modern times, the trend in education for the

BOX 1-1 Selected Expanded Career Roles for Nurses

Nurse Practitioner

The RCN (2005) defines a nurse practitioner (see Figure 1-6) as 'a registered nurse who has undertaken a specific course of study of at least first degree (Honours)' who sees patients with undiagnosed health problems; is autonomous; has decision-making and problem-solving skills; has advanced nursing skills which should include health education and counselling; has the authority to admit, discharge and refer patients; and is an effective leader and consultant.

Clinical Nurse Specialist

A clinical nurse specialist (CNS) is a nurse who has a relevant specialist qualification and is deemed by the employer to be competent to work in the speciality (UKCC, 1996). Miller (1995) states that a CNS has five main roles: clinical expert; researcher; consultant; teacher; and change agent.

Nurse Researcher

Nurse researchers investigate nursing problems to improve nursing care and to refine and expand nursing knowledge. They are employed in academic institutions, teaching hospitals and research centres. Nurse researchers usually have advanced education at masters or doctoral level.

Nurse Manager

The nurse administrator manages patient care, including the delivery of nursing services. The administrator may have a middle management position, such as head nurse or supervisor, or a more senior management position, such as director of nursing services. The functions of nurse managers include budgeting, staffing, and planning programmes. The educational preparation for nurse managers' positions is at least a degree in nursing and frequently a masters or doctoral degree.

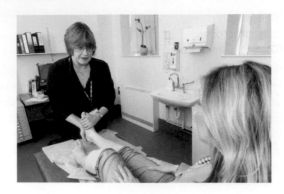

Figure 1-6 A nurse practitioner.

Nurse Educator

Nurse educators are employed in nursing programmes in higher education institutions. The nurse educator usually has a first degree, masters or doctoral degree and frequently has expertise in a particular area of practice.

Nurse Consultant

The role of the nurse consultant is to enhance the quality of healthcare provision and to ensure that professional leadership is strengthened. Some of these posts require cross boundary and interprofessional working. A nurse consultant will usually have to perform skills that are complex and show a breadth of expertise over and above that of a clinical nurse specialist.

Nurse Lead

This is a nurse who provides direction and leadership to all nurses and allied healthcare professionals involved in a particular speciality. These are relatively new posts that have their basis in leadership and management of care services.

---

professions has shifted toward higher education. Within the UK there are three means of entry into registered nursing: the undergraduate diploma in nursing, the undergraduate degree in nursing and the postgraduate diploma in nursing, which are discussed in detail later in this chapter.

Body of Knowledge Based on Research

Nursing relies on a range of knowledge from different disciplines including biology, sociology and psychology. The creation of a body of knowledge that is distinct to nursing is vital to establish nursing as a profession. According to Aggleton and

Chalmers (1986) for nursing to develop autonomous practices it must establish its own research base. From this research, nursing theories and conceptual frameworks are developed that contribute to nursing's knowledge base.

Autonomy

A profession is autonomous if it regulates itself and sets standards for its members. If nursing is to have professional status, it must function autonomously in the formation of policy and in the control of its activity. By defining its scope of practice, describing its particular functions and roles, and determining its goals and responsibility in healthcare delivery, the Nursing

BOX 1-2 The Nine Regulators Responsible for Healthcare Professionals in the UK

+ General Chiropractic Council (GCC) regulates chiropractors
+ General Dental Council (GDC) regulates dentists, dental hygienists and dental therapists
+ General Medical Council (GMC) regulates doctors
+ General Optical Council (GOC) regulates dispensing opticians and optometrists
+ General Osteopathic Council (GOsC) regulates osteopaths

+ Health Professions Council (HPC) regulates 13 professions
+ Nursing and Midwifery Council (NMC) regulates nurses, midwives and specialist community public health nurses
+ Pharmaceutical Society of Northern Ireland (PSNI) regulates pharmacists
+ Royal Pharmaceutical Society of Great Britain (RPSGB) regulates pharmacists

and Midwifery Council (NMC) provides nurses with autonomy to practise within their particular expertise (see Chapter 4 for Autonomy).

Regulating Professional Body

The Nursing and Midwifery Council is the nursing and midwifery professional regulating body that was created by an Act of Parliament in 2002 to protect the public by ensuring that high standards of care are provided to patients by nurses and midwives. It replaced the UK Central Council (UKCC). In order to achieve its aims the NMC maintains a register of all qualified nurses, midwives and specialist community public health nurses. It sets standards for practice, education and professional conduct and provides advice for nurses and midwives. It also considers allegations of misconduct or unfitness due to ill health.

The NMC is part of the Council for Healthcare Regulatory Excellence (CHRE), which was set up in April 2003 by the National Health Service Reform and Health Care Professions Act 2002. The CHRE is funded by the Department of Health and must answer to the UK Parliament. It covers the nine regulators currently responsible for healthcare professions throughout the UK (see *Box 1-2*).

As a regulating body for the profession, the NMC sets out standards for nurses' conduct in and out of practice.

The NMC Code of Professional Conduct: Standards for Conduct, Performance and Ethics

The purpose of this document is to 'inform the professions of the standard of professional conduct required of them in the exercise of their professional accountability and practice' (NMC, 2004a: 4) and to inform the general public and other professionals of the standard of conduct that they should expect from a registered practitioner.

The Code of Professional Conduct (NMC, 2004a) states that the nurse, midwife or specialist community public health nurse must: protect and support the health of the patient; protect and support the health of the community; act in such a way as to

maintain the trust and confidence the general public has in the profession; and uphold and enhance the reputation of the profession.

Although nursing is strictly controlled by its regulating body, the NMC, a number of factors influence current nursing practice.

FACTORS INFLUENCING CURRENT NURSING PRACTICE

To understand nursing as it is practised today and as it will be practised tomorrow requires an understanding of some of the social forces currently influencing this profession. These forces usually affect the entire healthcare system, and nursing, as a major component of that system, cannot avoid the effects.

Agenda for Change

In a bid to change the much disliked grading system for nurses, midwives and public health nurses, and as part of the modernisation of the National Health Service (NHS), the Agenda for Change pay strategy was developed (Benton, 2003) and successfully completed in November 2002. This is the biggest change that the NHS has seen for many years. Its aim is to ensure fair pay and a clearer system for career progression, paying NHS staff according to their skills and knowledge (Benton, 2003). However there are claims that the Agenda for Change is underfunded by £24 millon causing nursing redundancies across the country (The Politics Show Wales, BBC1, 2006).

Consumer Demands

Consumers of nursing services (the public) have become an increasingly effective force in changing nursing practice. On the whole, people are better educated and have more knowledge about health and illness than in the past. Consumers also have become more aware of others' needs for care. The ethical and moral issues raised by poverty and neglect have made people more vocal about the needs of minority groups and the poor.

The public's concepts of health and nursing have also changed. Most now believe that health is a right of all people, not just a privilege of the rich. Also the patient/client has become an active participant in making decisions about the health and nursing care they receive. This is encouraged as the media emphasise that individuals must assume responsibility for their own health by obtaining a physical examination regularly, checking for the seven danger signals of cancer, and maintaining their mental well-being by balancing work and recreation. Interest in health and nursing services is therefore greater than ever. Furthermore, many people now want more than freedom from disease – they want energy, vitality, and a feeling of wellness.

Family Structure

New family structures are influencing the need for and provision of nursing services. More people are living away from the extended family and the nuclear family, and the family breadwinner is no longer necessarily the man. Today, many single men and women bring up children, and in many two-parent families both parents work. It is also common for young parents to live at great distances from their own parents. These young families need support and frequently access social services and childcare centres.

Indeed the image of the family is no longer two parents with children, particularly as the number of divorces granted in England and Wales reached 155,052 between 2004 and 2005 compared with 27,224 in 1961 (Office for National Statistics, 2005). One of the consequences of such a divorce rate is the increase in lone parents. Hinchliff *et al.* (1993) suggest that lone parent families are much more likely to be hit by poverty and as a consequence more likely to have poorer health, which impacts on nursing services.

Information and Telecommunications

The Internet has already impacted on healthcare, with more and more patients becoming well informed about their health concerns. No longer the sole provider of health information, doctors and nurses may need to interpret Internet sources of information to patients and their families. Because not all Internet-based information is accurate, nurses need to become information brokers so they can help people to access high-quality, valid websites; interpret the information; and then help patients evaluate the information and determine if it is useful to them. Clark (2000) predicts that the difference between the future novice and expert nurse will be in knowing where to look for information and how to use it.

Telecommunications is the transmission of information from one site to another, using equipment to transmit information in the form of signs, signals, words or pictures by cable, radio or other systems (Chaffee, 1999: 27). NHS Direct is a national clinical service that utilises telecommunications to provide nurse led help and advice for patients over the telephone and Internet. It is available to patients 24 hours a day seven days a week.

Legislation

Legislation about nursing practice and health matters affects both the public and nursing. Legislation related to nursing is discussed in Chapter 3. Changes in legislation relating to health also affect nursing. For example, the **Hospital Complaints Procedure Act (1985)** resulted in each health authority establishing a complaints procedure. This Act was reviewed by Professor Alan Wilson who found that the system for dealing with complaints relating to health services confusing and bureaucratic. In 1996, a new complaints procedure was implemented nationwide. Since nurses are at the front line of healthcare, they need to be aware of the three stages of the new complaints procedure and its place within everyday nursing practice.

Ultimately, nurses should be aware of the limits that the law puts upon them as 'ignorance of the law is no defence' (Dimond, 2002: 4). See Chapter 3 for further discussion regarding the legal aspects of nursing.

Demography

Demography is the study of population, including statistics about distribution by age and place of residence, mortality (death) and morbidity (incidence of disease). From demographic data, the needs of the population for nursing services can be assessed. For example:

+ The total population in the UK is increasing (Office for National Statistics, 2006). The proportion of elderly people has also increased, creating an increased need for nursing services for this group.
+ The population is shifting from rural to urban settings. This shift signals an increased need for nursing relating to problems caused by pollution and by the effects on the environment of high concentrations of people. Thus, most nursing services are now provided in urban settings.
+ Mortality and morbidity studies reveal the presence of risk factors. Many of these risk factors (e.g. smoking) are major causes of death and disease that can be prevented through changes in lifestyle. The nurse's role in assessing risk factors and helping patients make healthy lifestyle changes is discussed in Chapter 6.

Nursing Associations

Professional nursing associations have provided leadership that affects many areas of nursing. There are a number of different nursing associations that represent and support nurses within the UK. The International Council of Nurses (ICN) was established in 1899. Nurses from Great Britain, the USA and Canada were among the founding members.

The ICN provides an organisation through which member national associations can work together with the aim of representing nursing worldwide, advancing the profession and influencing health policy. The five core values of the ICN are visionary leadership, inclusiveness, flexibility, partnership and achievement (ICN, n.d.). The official journal of the ICN is the *International Nursing Review*.

The Royal College of Nurses (RCN) is a member of the International Council of Nurses and aims to promote excellence in practice and shape health policies in the UK. In 2003, the RCN published its first strategic plan that lays out its aims for the organisation as well as nursing as a whole. The strategic plan states that it aims to represent 'the interests of nurses and nursing and be their voice locally, nationally and internationally' (RCN, 2003: 3) and influence the government to implement policies that improve patient care and to build upon the value of nurses, healthcare assistants and nursing students (RCN, 2003).

Student nurses, along with registered nurses, can become members of the RCN and automatically become members of the Association of Nursing Students (ANS). Together with the universities' student union (the NUS) the ANS aims to ensure the rights of the students are upheld and that they have a forum in which their voices can be heard.

Nurse Unions

The main nurse unions within the UK are the Royal College of Nursing (RCN) and Unison. As well as being a professional body for nursing, the RCN is also a trade union for nurses, midwives, healthcare support workers (nursing auxiliaries) and nursing students, and has over 370,000 members. Its members in general work within healthcare of some sort. However Unison, the largest trade union in the UK with over 1.3 million members, deals with people working in any public service, such as the NHS, local authorities, schools and colleges, as well as utility providers such as electricity companies.

Nurses are advised to join a nurse union as membership generally includes indemnity insurance, an insurance that protects the member from personal claims against them by patients, colleagues or member of the public. Nurse unions also represent nurses locally, nationally and internationally, fighting for better pay and conditions and providing help and advice on a range of nursing issues including legal advice. The RCN also offers further education for nurses and is instrumental in the development of a number of clinical guidelines such as 'Cervical Screening: RCN Guidance for Good Practice' published in 2006.

One of the most important criteria for a profession is a body of knowledge as stated earlier. Nurse education is key to the development of the individual nurse and to the development of the profession as a whole.

RESEARCH NOTE

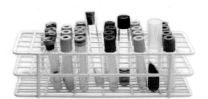

Why Women and Men Choose Nursing

Using grounded theory methodology, a study by Boughn (2001) revisited data from two previous studies to compare and contrast why women and men selected nursing. The analysis of the data focused on three main constructs: caring, power and practical motivations.

The subjects included 12 males and 16 females who were enrolled in the same nursing programme. Each of the four class levels was represented. Except for two men and two women, all subjects were under 23 years of age and single.

Both female and male subjects expressed that the desire to care for others motivated their decision to become a nurse. Likewise both sexes indicated a strong interest in power and empowerment for themselves by expressing such statements as desiring to be the best or advancing to a management position. A difference did exist between the two groups, however, in the desire to empower others. The female subjects were more interested in empowering others while the male subjects were more interested in empowering the profession and themselves as professionals. Another difference between the two groups concerned the third construct: practical motivation or expectations regarding salary and working conditions. The men clearly chose nursing based on financial expectations while only one of the female subjects mentioned finance as a motivating factor in choosing nursing as a profession.

Implications

Both male and female nursing students were motivated by the desire to care for others. The differences in the focus of power and empowerment could complement each other. The author discusses that caring theory points out that caring for self is needed in order to care for others. Male and female nurses need to incorporate both values into their thinking. Salary and working conditions have been and continue to be chronic complaints among nurses. The author suggests that female nursing students be socialised to become assertive and proactive, and subsequently to expect financial rewards and favourable working conditions.

Note: From 'Why Women and Men Choose Nursing' by S. Boughn (2001) in *Nursing and Health Care Perspectives*, 22(1), 14–19. Reprinted with permission from the National League for Nursing.

NURSE EDUCATION

Pre-registration Nurse Education

Pre-registration nurse education has adopted many guises over the past two decades. It is broadly described as post-compulsory education, which means that it takes place after compulsory education and has the purpose of providing a nursing workforce that is fit for practice and purpose (UKCC, 1999).

Nurse education is a relative newcomer to higher education. Until the early 1990s the majority of student nurses undertook a hospital-based apprentice style course of nurse education. They were considered part of the workforce and were paid a salary. However, higher education institutions such as the University of Edinburgh have been offering pre-registration degree courses for nurses since 1960 (Weir, 1996). In the late 1980s nurse education was reformed and the Project 2000 (P2K) curriculum developed. This form of nurse education was university-based and students who embarked on this course were supernumerary and in receipt of a bursary or training allowance. If successful, students would qualify with a university diploma or degree as well as registration on to the appropriate part of the UK Central Council for Nursing, Midwifery and Health Visiting (UKCC) register. The course was made up of 18 months of a Common Foundation Programme followed by an 18-month Branch Programme, leading to registration as an adult nurse, child nurse, mental health nurse or learning disability nurse.

This form of nurse education reduced the amount of clinical experience student nurses were exposed to, but concentrated on the social sciences such as sociology and psychology. However, concerns were raised by clinical staff about the lack of clinical skills shown by students and newly qualified nurses. This resulted in the UKCC setting up a Commission for Nursing and Midwifery Education, which recommended in 1999 that there should be more emphasis on the development of competency in clinical skills within pre-registration nursing and midwifery programmes.

The recommendations set out by the UKCC were broadly accepted by the nursing profession and a new curriculum was developed, colloquially known as 'Fitness for Practice'. This course has a one-year Common Foundation Programme followed by a two-year Branch Programme with students receiving a bursary for the duration of the course. However there is a shortened (two-year) pre-registration programme for graduates who have achieved an undergraduate degree in a health-related discipline. It remains to be seen if the recommendation made in 1999 will result in nurses who are indeed fit for practice and purpose.

Entry onto Register

The NMC sets out clear criteria for entry onto its register, which includes evidence of course completion, a declaration of good health and good character along with a declaration of any police cautions or criminal convictions. The NMC currently recognises both the Diploma in Nursing and Degree in Nursing, which are both made up of 2,300 hours of practice and 2,300 hours of theory. The Higher Education Institution informs the NMC that the minimum hours have been met and that the applicant has indeed completed the course.

The Nursing and Midwifery Order states that the applicant has to declare that they are in good health and have good character in order to protect the public. The Order also states that the NMC requires evidence of good health and good character so that the NMC Registrar is satisfied that the applicant is capable of safe and effective practice. This has been included in the entry requirements following 'a number of high profile cases involving the health and character of doctors and nurses' (NMC, 2004b).

Post-registration Nurse Education: Continuing Professional Development

Continuing professional development (CPD) refers to formalised education that is designed to enhance the knowledge and skills of practitioners. The NMC requires that each nurse must maintain their professional knowledge and competence (NMC, 2004b) and as such continuing professional development plays a major role in maintaining this requirement. Also nurses are required to show that they have met the Post-Registration Education and Practice (PREP) standards in order to maintain their registration. Currently nurses have to undertake at least five days of learning activity relevant to their profession during a three-year period.

Continuing education and professional development is the responsibility of each practising nurse. Constant updating and growth are essential to keep abreast of scientific and technological change and changes within the nursing profession. A variety of educational and healthcare institutions conduct continuing education programmes. They are usually designed to meet one or more of the following needs: (a) to keep nurses abreast of new techniques and knowledge; (b) to help nurses attain expertise in a specialised area of practice, such as intensive care nursing; and (c) to provide nurses with information essential to nursing practice, for example, knowledge about the legal aspects of nursing. Post-registration nurse education currently comes in a number of formats, for example level 2 or 3 modules, first degrees, masters degrees and doctoral programmes.

Many post-registration nurse education programmes require the nurse to understand, apply, participate and initiate research as a means of improving and informing practice.

NURSING RESEARCH

Today, nurses are actively generating, publishing and applying research in practice to improve patient care and enhance the nursing scientific knowledge base. Although the focus for all nurses is use of research findings, in practice the degree of participation in research depends on the nurse's educational level, position, experience and practical environment.

As early as 1854, Florence Nightingale demonstrated the importance of research in the delivery of nursing care. When Nightingale arrived in the Crimea in November 1854, she found the military hospital barracks overcrowded, filthy, rat and flea infested, and lacking in food, drugs and essential medical supplies. As a result of these conditions, men died from starvation and diseases such as dysentery, cholera and typhus (Woodham-Smith, 1950: 151–167). By systematically collecting, organising and reporting data, Nightingale was able to institute sanitary reforms and significantly reduce mortality rates from contagious disease.

Clark and Hockey (1989) state that nurses have in the past depended upon other disciplines for the study of their own profession. However, the concept of research has been embraced within nursing curricula particularly since the integration of nurse education into higher education.

Nursing organisations such as the RCN have been crucial in supporting nursing research, promoting and developing nursing research within the UK (Parahoo, 1997). In 1995 the RCN and the London School of Hygiene and Tropical Medicine joined forces to form the Centre for Policy in Nursing Research and currently the RCN has an Institute of Research that aims to raise the profile of research in nursing by providing funding and resources.

Approaches to Nursing Research

There are two major approaches to investigating diverse phenomena in nursing research. These approaches originate from different philosophical perspectives and use different methods for the collection and analysis of data.

Quantitative Research

Quantitative research progresses through systematic, logical steps according to a specific plan to collect numerical informa- tion, often under conditions of considerable control, which is then analysed using statistical procedures. The quantitative approach is most frequently associated with positivism or logical positivism, a philosophical doctrine that emphasises the rational and the scientific (Polit and Hungler, 1999: 10). Quantitative research is often viewed as 'hard' science and uses deductive reasoning and the measurable attributes of human experience.

The following is an example of a research question that lends itself to a quantitative approach: What are the differential effects of continuous versus intermittent application of negative pressure on tracheal tissue during endotracheal suctioning?

Qualitative Research

The qualitative approach is often associated with naturalistic inquiry, which explores the subjective and complex experiences of human beings. Qualitative research investigates 'the human experience as it is lived through careful collection and analysis of narrative, subjective materials' (Polit and Hungler, 1999: 13). Data collection and its analysis occur concurrently. Using the inductive method, data are analysed by identifying themes and patterns to develop a theory or framework that helps explain the processes under observation (Polit and Hungler, 1999: 14). The qualitative approach would be appropriate for the following types of research questions:

+ What is the nature of the bereavement process in spouses of patients with terminal cancer?
+ What is the nature of coping and adjustment after a radical prostatectomy?
+ What is the process of family caregiving for elderly family relatives with Alzheimer's dementia as experienced by the caregiver?

Box 1-3 gives examples of some nursing research studies.

BOX 1-3 Examples of Nursing Studies

+ Fader *et al.* (2004) conducted a quantitative study to determine the effects of absorbent pads on the pressure relieving properties of 'standard' and pressure management mattresses and found that there were indeed substantial adverse effects on pressure distribution properties of mattresses when absorbent incontinence pads were used.
+ Hopia *et al.* (2004) conducted a qualitative study to describe how nurses promoted the health of families of children with chronic conditions and found that the nurses used a number of different strategies to promote health.
+ Hellstrom *et al.* (2004) performed a quantitative research project that explored the quality of life and symptoms among older people.

+ Clover *et al.* (2004) conducted a qualitative study to explore patients' understanding of their discussions about end-of-life care with nurses in a palliative care setting.
+ Black and Ford (2004) performed a study to examine the relationships among mother's resilience, family health promotion and mother's health promoting lifestyle practices in single parent families led by adolescent mothers.
+ Letterstal *et al.* (2004) conducted a quantitative study that aimed to evaluate the effects of structured written pre-operative information on patients' post-operative psychological and physical well-being after surgery for abdominal aortic aneurysm.

CRITICAL REFLECTION

Let us revisit the case study on page 2. Now that you have read this chapter, think about the nurse's role in healthcare. Is nursing a profession that should devolve the caring element to healthcare assistants? Is it more important for the profession to move into more technical areas or is the current scope of nursing practice adequate?

CHAPTER HIGHLIGHTS

+ Historical perspectives of nursing practice reveal recurring themes or influencing factors. For example, women have traditionally cared for others, but often in subservient roles. Religious orders left an imprint on nursing by instilling such values as compassion, devotion to duty and hard work. Wars created an increased need for nurses and medical specialties. Societal attitudes have influenced nursing's image. Visionary leaders have made notable contributions to improving the status of nursing.

+ The scope of nursing practice includes promoting wellness, preventing illness, restoring health and care of the dying.

+ Nurse practice is guided by legislation and it is the nurses' responsibility for knowing the law that governs their practice.

+ Standards of clinical nursing practice provide criteria against which the effectiveness of nursing care and professional performance behaviours can be evaluated.

+ Every nurse may function in a variety of roles that are not exclusive of one another; in reality, they often occur together and serve to clarify the nurse's activities. These roles include caregiver, communicator, teacher, advocate, counsellor, leader, manager and research consumer.

+ With advanced education and experience, nurses can fulfil advanced practice roles such as clinical nurse specialist, nurse practitioner educator, manager and researcher.

+ A desired goal of nursing is professionalism, which needs specialised education; a unique body of knowledge based on research; autonomy; and a regulating professional body.

+ Current nursing practice is influenced by Agenda for Change, consumer demand, family structure, science and technology, information and telecommunications, legislation, demographic and social changes, nursing shortages and the work of nursing associations.

+ Participation in the activities of nursing associations enhances the growth of involved individuals and helps nurses collectively influence policies that affect nursing practice.

REFERENCES

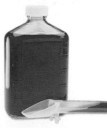

Adams, A. (1998) 'Nursing organisational practice and its relationship with other features of ward organisation and job satisfaction', *Journal of Advanced Nursing*, 27(6), 1212–1222.

Aggleton, P. and Chalmers, H. (1986) 'Nursing research, nursing theory and the nursing process', *Journal of Advanced Nursing*, 11, 197–202.

Atkins, S. and Murphy, K. (1993) 'Reflection: a review of the literature', *Journal of Advanced Nursing*, 18, 1188–1192.

Belenky, M., Clinchy, B., Goldbergre, N. and Tarule, J. (1986) *Women's ways of knowing: The development of self, voice and mind*, New York: Basic Books.

Benner, P., Tanner, C. and Chesla, C. (1996) *Expertise in nursing practice: Caring, clinical judgement and ethics*, New York: Springer.

Benton, D. (2003) 'Agenda for Change: job evaluation', *Nursing Standard*, 17(36), 39–42.

Black, C. and Ford, M. (2004) 'Adolescent mothers: resilience, family health work and health promoting practices', *Journal of Advanced Nursing*, 48(4), 351–360.

Boughn, S. (2001) 'Why Women and Men Choose Nursing', *Nursing and Health Care Perspectives*, 22(1), 14–19.

Boud, D., Keogh, T. and Walker, D. (1985) *Reflection, turning experience into learning*, Worcester: Billing & Son.

Chaffee, M. (1999) 'A telehealth odyssey', *American Journal of Nursing*, 99(7), 27–32.

Clark, D.J. (2000) 'Old wine in new bottles: Delivering nursing in the 21st century', *Journal of Nursing Scholarship*, 32(1), 11–15.

Clark, J.M. and Hockey, L. (1989) *Further research for nursing*, London: Scutari.

Clover, A., Brown, J., McErlain, P. and Vandenberg, B. (2004) 'Patient approaches to clinical conversations in the palliative care setting', *Journal of Advanced Nursing*, 48(4), 333–341.

Dewey, J. (1933) *How we think*, Boston: D.C. Heath.

Dimond, B. (2002) *Legal aspects of nursing* (3rd edn), London: Longman.

DOH (1997) *The new NHS – Modern, dependable*, London: The Stationery Office.

Fader, M., Bain, D. and Cottenden, A. (2004) 'The effects of absorbent incontinence pads on pressure management mattresses', *Journal of Advanced Nursing*, 48(6), 569.

Hopia, H., Paavilainen, E. and Astedt-Kurki, P. (2004) 'Promoting health for families of children with chronic conditions', *Journal of Advanced Nursing*, 48(6), 575.

Hellstrom, Y., Persson, G. and Hallberg, I. (2004) 'Quality of life and symptoms among older people living at home', *Journal of Advanced Nursing*, 48(6), 584–593.

Henderson, V. (1966) *The nature of nursing: A definition and its implications for practice, research and education*, New York: Macmillan.

Hinchliff, S.M., Norman, S.E. and Schober, J.E. (1993) *Nursing practice and health care*, London: Edward Arnold.

International Council of Nurses (n.d.) 'About the International Council of Nurses'. Available from http://www.icn.ch/abouticn.htm. (Accessed 29 April 2005.)

Letterstal, A., Sandstrom, V., Olofsson, P. and Forsberg, C. (2004) 'Post-operative mobilisation of patients with abdominal aortic aneurysm', *Journal of Advanced Nursing*, 48(6), 560–568.

McCance, T.V., McKenna, H.P. and Boore, J.R.P. (1999) 'Caring: theoretical perspectives of relevance to nursing', *Journal of Advanced Nursing*, 30(6), 1388–1395.

Miller, L. (1995) 'The clinical nurse specialist: a way forward?', *Journal of Advanced Nursing*, 22, 494–501.

Mullally, S. (2004) 'The shape of things to come', *Nursing Standard*, 18(17), 16–17.

Nightingale, F. (1969) *Notes on nursing: What it is, and what it is not*, New York: Dover (original work published 1860).

NMC – Nursing and Midwifery Council (2004a) *The NMC code of professional conduct: Standards for conduct, performance and ethics*, London: NMC.

Nursing and Midwifery Council (2004b) *NMC guidance: requirements for evidence of good health and good character*, London: NMC.

Office for National Statistics (2005) *Divorces*, Newport: Office for National Statistics. Available from http://www.statistics.gov.uk/cci/nugget.asp?id=170. (Accessed on 17 April 2007.)

Office for National Statistics (2006) *Population Estimates*, Newport: Office for National Statistics. Available from http://www.statistics.gov.uk/cci/nugget.asp?id=6. (Accessed on 17 April 2007.)

Parahoo, K. (1997) *Nursing research: Principles, process and issues*, Basingstoke: Macmillan Press.

Payne, D. (2000) 'New Year, new image', *Nursing Times*, 96(1), 14–15.

Polit, D.F. and Hungler, B.P. (1999) *Nursing research: Principles and methods*, Philadelphia: Lippincott.

RCN (2003) *Defining nursing*, London: RCN.

RCN (2005) *Nurse practitioner – a RCN guide to the nurse practitioner role, competencies and programme approval*, London: RCN.

Schon, D. (1983) *The reflective practitioner*, London: Temple Smith.

The Politics Show Wales (2006) BBC 1, 5 May.

Thomas, L. and Bond, S. (1990) 'Towards defining the organisation of nursing care in hospital wards: an empirical study', *Journal of Advanced Nursing*, 15(9), 1106–1112.

UKCC (1996) *Registrar's Letter 7/1996 The Council's Standards for Education following PREP. Transitional arrangements – Specialist practitioner title/specialist qualification*, London: UKCC.

UKCC (1999) *Fitness for practice: The UKCC Commission for Nursing and Midwifery Education*, London: UKCC.

Weir, R. (1996) *A Leap in the Dark: The origins and development of the Department of Nursing Studies at the University of Edinburgh*, London: Book Factory.

Woodham-Smith, C. (1950) *Florence Nightingale*, London: Constable & Co.

World Health Organization (1948) *Constitution of the World Health Organization Basic Documents*, Geneva: WHO.

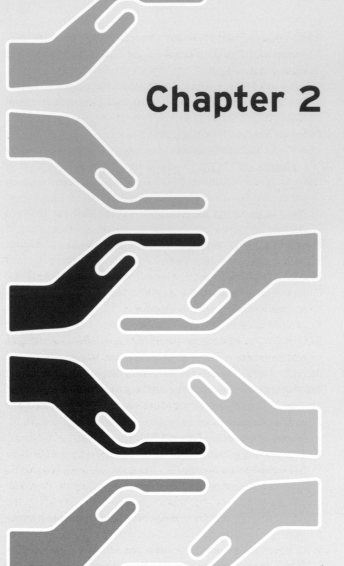

Chapter 2

Nursing Models, Theories and Care Pathways

Learning Outcomes

After completing this chapter, you will be able to:

+ Define the terms nursing model, care pathway, concept, conceptual framework and theory, for nursing.

+ Identify the purposes of nursing theory in nursing education, research and clinical practice.

+ Identify the components of the metaparadigm for nursing.

+ Describe the major purpose of theory in the social sciences and practice disciplines.

+ Identify one positive and one negative effect of using theory to understand clinical practice.

CASE STUDY

Janine is 24 years old and has been admitted to your ward from the emergency admissions unit with an acute jaundice. You begin by completing the admission documentation paperwork and selecting an appropriate model with which to assess the patient. As you assess Janine thoughts are surging through your head as to what may be the cause of the jaundice. Aspects of anatomy, physiology and pathology are coming to your thoughts as you develop a theory for the cause of this illness. As you consider the patient's feelings regarding her

appearance, theories of psychology and sociology are applied.

After assessing the patient for her unique nursing needs you begin planning the patient's care using the care pathway recently introduced into your clinical area for this illness. With the aid of both the model and the care pathway the patient's nursing needs are identified and planned for.

After reading this chapter you will be able to discuss the role of nursing models in the caring for patients such as Janine.

INTRODUCTION

Nursing like all disciplines has its own unique knowledge base on which both the profession and nursing interventions are founded. This body of knowledge is an essential building block of nursing practice and may sometimes be referred to as the science of nursing. For many, this knowledge base can be difficult to identify clearly, with many students and practitioners struggling to understand the key fundamental concepts and terms. Although difficult to understand, nurses need to become familiar with and recognise these key elements of the profession that help to inform nursing practice.

INTRODUCTION TO THEORIES IN OTHER DISCIPLINES

A **theory** may be defined as a hypothesis or system of ideas that is proposed to explain a given phenomenon or idea. A theory can often be considered as a major, very well articulated idea about something important to a particular individual or group. There have been many influential theories proposed in the 20th century including Marx's theory of alienation, Freud's theory of the unconscious, Darwin's theory of evolution and Einstein's theory of relativity. Although these are not theories of nursing they do in some way influence nursing theory and practice. Marx's theory of alienation can be considered in a social context and is important to nursing; as nurses need an awareness of social systems and sociology in their practice. Freud's theory of the unconscious is a psychological theory and relates to nursing as nurses need an awareness of psychology in their practice. Darwin's theory of evolution may be considered a proposal for charting the development of the human race and relates to the biological aspects of nursing practice. Einstein's theory of relativity can be linked to nursing as some important diagnostic tests, including some radiological diagnostic procedures, have utilised this theory in their development.

Most university students are introduced to the major theories in their disciplines as a basis on which to build their knowledge. The extent to which theories build on or modify previous theories varies with the discipline, as does the importance of theory in the discipline. Undergraduate music and art students often take some courses in theory, for example how an instrument works, how sound is produced or colours mixed to make another colour. But these students generally focus on creating art or performing music. Management students study management theories, but the relationship between the theory of management and the practice of management is not as strong or clear as the relationship between the theory of physics and the practice of physics. This is because the practice of physics *is* theory and research, whereas the practice of management, teaching, nursing, art, music, law, clinical psychology and pastoral care is something else entirely. The term **practice discipline** is used for fields of study in which the central focus is performance of a professional role (nursing, teaching, management, music). Practice disciplines are differentiated from the disciplines that have research and theory development as their central focus, for example, chemistry and biological sciences. In the practice disciplines, the main function of theory (and research) is to provide a basis and to aid in understanding the discipline's focus.

Context for Theory Development in Nursing

In the 19th century, Florence Nightingale thought that the people of Great Britain needed to know more about how to maintain healthy homes and to care for sick family members. Nightingale's *Notes on Nursing: What It Is, and What It Is Not* (1969) was our first textbook on home care and community health. However, the audience for that text was the public at large, not a separate discipline or profession. To Nightingale, the knowledge required to provide good nursing was neither unique nor specialised. Rather, Nightingale viewed nursing as a central human activity grounded in observation, reason and commonsense health practices. However she considered that the key fundamental components required for the practice of nursing included education and understanding of the discipline by the individual.

Nursing within the UK and Europe in the late 1980s and early 1990s began to move into institutions of higher education from the more traditional fragmented hospital schools of nursing. During this time, disciplines seeking to establish themselves in universities had to demonstrate something that Nightingale had not envisioned for nursing – a unique body of theoretical knowledge.

The biological and technological sciences were often seen as role models for this purpose. Theories in the biological sciences provided a foundation and direction for research. Research in these disciplines often produced tangible results: knowledge that could be used in our efforts to control nature, disease and threats to health.

The term *practice discipline* was not in common use until the very end of the 20th century. Disciplines without a strong theory and research base were referred to as 'soft', a negative comparison with the 'hard' biological sciences where clear examples could be made. Many of the soft disciplines attempted to emulate the sciences, so theory and scientific research became a more important part of academic life, both in the practice disciplines and in the humanities.

Whereas theories in the biological sciences provide a suitable framework for productive research, theories serve a different purpose in the social sciences and practice disciplines such as nursing. In these disciplines, theories work like lenses through which we may interpret things like market forces, industrial efficiency, the human mind, pain and suffering. Their usefulness comes from helping us interpret phenomena from unique perspectives, building new understandings, relationships and possibilities.

Defining Terms

Theoretical models and systems often use terms that can be difficult to understand but these terms are often used as part of the framework of the theory. **Concepts** are often called the building blocks of theories or the ideas on which it is based. Concepts can be hard to define because the definition has to include everything that makes up that theory. Concepts are easier to understand by example. For example, the theory of the chain of infection, used to minimise the spread of disease, is made up of a number of concepts. These include that an infective organism (bacteria or virus) is present, needs a host (someone or something to breed on or in), needs a mode of transport (someone's unclean hands) and a new host such as another person. However, theories are not always built like houses out of block-like concepts. Freud's theory of the unconscious, considered by some to be important in the understanding of how the human mind functions, not only required some new concepts it required a completely new model. Freud needed a model for the mind that could bring a host of human experiences (or concepts or phenomena) together under one mental roof: dreams, wishes, decisions, behaviours, feelings, anxieties, sexuality. Freud's theory of the mind included three new concepts: the ego, the id and the superego. It would not be right to say that Freud's theory of the unconscious evolved out of these concepts. Rather, these new concepts helped him create a model in which his larger idea, the unconscious, might be understood.

A **conceptual framework**, however, is a group of related ideas, statements or concepts. Freud's structure of the mind (id, ego, superego) could be considered a conceptual framework or model. The term **conceptual model** is often used interchangeably with conceptual framework, and sometimes with **grand theories**, those that consider a broad range of the significant relationships among the concepts of a discipline.

No scientific theory is purely objective, because each is developed in cultures and expressed in language. Theories offer ways of looking at or conceptualising the central interests of a discipline. In the biological and chemical sciences, theories are often expressed in mathematical terms. In the social and behavioural sciences such as psychology, theories attempt to explain relationships between concepts. Although it is helpful when these theories are presented in clear, specific, non-ambiguous language, they are most often presented in books that in turn generate other books of critique and explanation. This can make it very difficult for a student of a new discipline to understand and appreciate the theories and building blocks of the discipline.

A **paradigm** is another building block of theory; it refers to a pattern of shared understandings and assumptions about reality and the world. Paradigms include our notions of reality that are largely unconscious or taken for granted. For example it is common knowledge that concrete when set is hard and if you fall on it an individual could be injured. This fact is based upon either experience of falling onto concrete as a child or seeing someone who has been injured in a fall. Every time a person walks past concrete it is not a conscious thought that it is hard and you could be injured if you fall, the fact is taken for granted.

THE METAPARADIGM FOR NURSING

In the late 20th century, much of the theoretical work in nursing focused on developing relationships with four major concepts: person, environment, health and nursing. Because these four concepts can be superimposed on almost any work in nursing, they are sometimes collectively referred to as a **metaparadigm** for nursing, or key concepts of all theories. The term originates from two Greek words: *meta*, meaning 'with' and *paradigm*, meaning 'pattern'.

Nursing theorists consider the following four concepts to be central to nursing.

1. **Patient**, the recipient of nursing care (includes individuals, families, groups and communities).
2. **Environment**, the internal and external surroundings that affect the patient. This includes people in the physical environment, such as families, friends and significant others.
3. **Health**, the degree of wellness or well-being that the patient experiences.
4. **Nursing**, the attributes, characteristics and actions of the nurse providing care on behalf of, or in conjunction with, the patient.

The work of nurse theorists reflects a wide range of ideas about people, health, values and the world. Each nurse theorist's definitions of these four major concepts vary in accordance with scientific and philosophical orientation, experience in nursing and the effects of that experience on the theorist's view of nursing. A single metaparadigm or basis of nursing may be impossible given the variety of world views expressed in nursing models.

Nursing theories fall into one of two paradigms or building blocks. One view reflects prevailing understandings in medicine and the healthcare system. The other view reflects emerging understandings in transpersonal psychology. **Transpersonal psychology** is the extension of psychological studies into consciousness, spiritual inquiry, body–mind relationships and transformation; simply the psychology of health and human potential.

It is important to remember that any organised approach to understanding the world – including theories, social practices and people – can both illuminate and obscure what is of central importance to nurses.

PURPOSES OF NURSING THEORY

Direct links exist among theory, education, research and clinical practice.

In Education

Because nursing theory is used primarily to establish the profession's place in the university, it is not surprising that nursing theory has become more firmly established in academia than in clinical practice. In the 1970s and 1980s, many nursing programmes identified the major concepts in one or two nursing models, organised these concepts into a conceptual framework and then attempted to organise the entire curriculum around that framework. The unique language in these models was typically introduced into programme objectives, course objectives, course descriptions and clinical performance criteria used to assess students. The purpose was to define the central meanings of the profession and to gain status alongside other established professions.

In Research

Nurse scholars have repeatedly insisted that nursing research identifies the philosophical assumptions or theoretical frameworks on which it is based. That is because all thinking, writing, and speaking is based on previous assumptions about people and the world. New theoretical perspectives provide an essential framework by identifying gaps in the way we approach specific fields of study such as symptom management or quality of life. Different theoretical perspectives can also help generate new ideas, research questions and interpretations.

Grand theories only occasionally direct nursing research. Nursing research is more often informed by **midlevel theories** that focus on the exploration of concepts such as pain, self-esteem and learning. Qualitative research in nursing and the social sciences can also be based on theories from philosophy or the social sciences such as psychology and sociology. The term **critical theory** is used in academia to describe theories that help describe how social structures affect a wide variety of human experiences from art to social practices. In nursing, critical theory helps explain how structures such as race, gender, sexual orientation and economic class affect patient experiences and health outcomes.

In Clinical Practice

Where nursing theory has been utilised in a clinical setting, its main contribution has been the facilitation of reflection, questioning and thinking about what nurses do. An increasing body of theoretical scholarship in nursing has been outside the framework of the formal theories. Benner (2000) and MacIntyre (2001) argue that formalistic theories are too often superimposed on the life-worlds of patients, overshadowing core values of the profession and our patients' humanity. Family theorists and critical theorists have encouraged the profession to move the focus from individuals to families and social structures. Debates about the role of theory in nursing practice provide evidence that nursing is maturing, both as an academic discipline and as a clinical profession.

OVERVIEW OF SELECTED NURSING THEORIES/MODELS

The theories discussed in this chapter can be categorised as philosophies, conceptual frameworks or grand theories, or midlevel theories (Tomey and Alligood, 1998). A **philosophy** is often an early effort to define nursing phenomena and serves as the basis for later theoretical formulations of theory. Examples of philosophies are those of Nightingale, Henderson and Watson. Conceptual models/grand theories include those of Orem, Roper, Logan and Tierney, Rogers, Roy, and King; whereas midlevel theorists are Peplau, Leininger, Parse and Neuman. Only brief summaries of the author's philosophy, central theme and basic assumptions are included here.

Nightingale's Environmental Theory

Florence Nightingale, often considered the first nurse theorist, defined nursing more than 100 years ago as 'the act of utilising the environment of the patient to assist him in his recovery' (Nightingale, 1969). She linked health with five environmental factors: (1) pure or fresh air, (2) pure water, (3) efficient drainage, (4) cleanliness and (5) light, especially direct sunlight. Deficiencies in these five factors produced lack of health or illness.

These environmental factors attain significance when one considers that sanitation conditions in the hospitals of the mid-1800s were extremely poor and that women working in the hospitals were often unreliable, uneducated and incompetent to care for the ill. In addition to those factors, Nightingale also stressed the importance of keeping the patient warm, maintaining a noise-free environment, and attending to the patient's diet in terms of assessing intake, nutritional value, timeliness of the food and its effect on the person.

Nightingale set the stage for further work in the development of nursing theories. Her general concepts about ventilation, cleanliness, quiet, warmth and diet remain integral parts of nursing and healthcare today.

Peplau's Interpersonal Relations Model

Hildegard Peplau, a psychiatric nurse, introduced her interpersonal concepts in 1952 as one of the first models of psychiatric nursing care. Central to Peplau's theory is the use of a therapeutic relationship between the nurse and the patient.

Nurses enter into a personal relationship with an individual when a need is present. The nurse–patient relationship evolves in four phases:

1. *Orientation.* During this phase, the patient seeks help, and the nurse assists the patient to understand the problem and the extent of the need for help.
2. *Identification.* During this phase, the patient assumes a posture of dependence, interdependence or independence in relation to the nurse (relatedness). The nurse's focus is to assure the person that the nurse understands the interpersonal meaning of the patient's situation.

3. *Exploitation.* In this phase, the patient derives full value from what the nurse offers through the relationship. The patient uses available services based on self-interest and needs. Power shifts from the nurse to the patient.
4. *Resolution.* In this final phase, old needs and goals are put aside and new ones adopted. Once older needs are resolved, newer and more mature ones emerge.

To help patients fulfil their needs, nurses assume many roles: stranger, teacher, resource person, surrogate, leader and counsellor. Peplau's model continues to be used by clinicians when working with individuals who have psychological problems.

Henderson's Definition of Nursing

In 1966, Virginia Henderson's definition of the unique function of nursing was a major stepping stone in the emergence of nursing as a discipline separate from medicine. Virginia Henderson has been described as the *first lady of nursing*. An accomplished author, avid researcher and a visionary, she is considered by many to be the most important nursing figure in the 20th century. Like Nightingale, Henderson described nursing in relation to the patient and the patient's environment. Unlike Nightingale, Henderson saw the nurse as concerned with both healthy and ill individuals, acknowledged that nurses interact with patients even when recovery may not be feasible, and mentioned the teaching and advocacy roles of the nurse.

Henderson (1966) conceptualised the nurse's role as assisting sick or healthy individuals to gain independence in meeting 14 fundamental needs:

1. Breathing normally
2. Eating and drinking adequately
3. Eliminating body wastes
4. Moving and maintaining a desirable position
5. Sleeping and resting
6. Selecting suitable clothes
7. Maintaining body temperature within normal range by adjusting clothing and modifying the environment
8. Keeping the body clean and well groomed to protect the integument
9. Avoiding dangers in the environment and avoiding injuring others
10. Communicating with others in expressing emotions, needs, fears or opinions
11. Worshipping according to one's faith
12. Working in such a way that one feels a sense of accomplishment
13. Playing or participating in various forms of recreation
14. Learning, discovering or satisfying the curiosity that leads to normal development and health, and using available health facilities.

Henderson has published many works and continues to be cited in current nursing literature. Her emphasis on the importance of nursing's independence from, and interdependence with, other healthcare disciplines is well recognised.

Rogers Science of Unitary Human Beings

The concept of Unitary Health Care emerged from the dynamic and innovative work of the nursing academic Professor Martha E. Rogers during the 1950s to 1970 in New York. She created the conceptual healthcare system that became known throughout the world as the Science of Unitary Human Beings. It contains complex conceptualisations relating to multiple scientific disciplines (e.g. Einstein's theory of relativity; and many other disciplines, such as anthropology, psychology, sociology, astronomy, religion, philosophy, history, biology and literature).

Rogers views the person as an irreducible whole, the whole being greater than the sum of its parts. *Whole* is differentiated from *holistic*, the latter often being used to mean only the sum of all parts. She states that humans are dynamic energy fields in continuous exchange with environmental fields, both of which are infinite. The 'human field image' perspective surpasses that of the physical body. Both human and environmental fields are characterised by pattern, a universe of open systems, and four dimensionality. According to Rogers (1970), unitary man:

+ is an irreducible, four-dimensional energy field identified by pattern;
+ manifests characteristics different from the sum of the parts;
+ interacts continuously and creatively with the environment;
+ behaves as a totality;
+ as a sentient being, participates creatively in change.

Nurses applying Rogers theory in practice (a) focus on the person's wholeness, (b) seek to promote symphonic interaction between the two energy fields (human and environment) to strengthen the coherence and integrity of the person, (c) coordinate the human field with the rhythmicities of the environmental field, and (d) direct and redirect patterns of interaction between the two energy fields to promote maximum health potential.

Nurses' use of noncontact therapeutic touch is based on the concept of human energy fields. The qualities of the field vary from person to person and are affected by pain and illness. Although the field is infinite, realistically it is most clearly 'felt' within several feet of the body. Nurses trained in noncontact therapeutic touch claim they can assess and feel the energy field and manipulate it to enhance the healing process of people who are ill or injured.

Orem's General Theory of Nursing

Dorothea Orem's theory, first published in 1971, includes three related concepts: self-care, self-care deficit and nursing systems. Orem was a nurse academic and pioneer in the development of distinctive nursing knowledge. Self-care theory is based on four concepts: self-care, self-care agency, self-care requisites and therapeutic self-care demand. Self-care refers to those activities an individual performs independently throughout life to promote and maintain personal well-being. Self-care agency is the individual's ability to perform self-care activities.

It consists of two agents: a self-care agent (an individual who performs self-care independently) and a dependent care agent (a person other than the individual who provides the care). Most adults care for themselves, whereas infants and people weakened by illness or disability require assistance with self-care activities.

Self-care requisites, also called self-care needs, are measures or actions taken to provide self-care. There are three categories of self-care requisites:

1. Universal requisites are common to all people. They include maintaining intake and elimination of air, water and food; balancing rest, solitude and social interaction; preventing hazards to life and well-being; and promoting normal human functioning.
2. Developmental requisites result from maturation or are associated with conditions or events, such as adjusting to a change in body image or to the loss of a spouse.
3. Health deviation requisites result from illness, injury or disease, or its treatment. They include actions such as seeking healthcare assistance, carrying out prescribed therapies, and learning to live with the effects of illness or treatment.

Therapeutic self-care demand refers to all self-care activities required to meet existing self-care requisites, or in other words, actions to maintain health and well-being (see Figure 2-1).

Self-care deficit results when self-care agency is not adequate to meet the known self-care demand. Orem's self-care deficit theory explains not only when nursing is needed but also how people can be assisted through five methods of helping: acting or doing for, guiding, teaching, supporting, and providing an environment that promotes the individual's abilities to meet current and future demands.

Orem identifies three types of nursing systems:

1. Wholly compensatory systems are required for individuals who are unable to control and monitor their environment and process information.
2. Partly compensatory systems are designed for individuals who are unable to perform some, but not all, self-care activities.
3. Supportive-educative (developmental) systems are designed for persons who need to learn to perform self-care measures and need assistance to do so.

The methods of helping discussed for self-care deficit can be used in each nursing system.

Roper, Logan and Tierney's Activities of Living Model

The foundations for this model were developed and published in several books by three nurse academics during the 1980s including *The Elements of Nursing* (Roper *et al.*, 1980), *Learning to Use the Nursing Process* (Roper *et al.*, 1981) and *Using a Model of Nursing* (Roper *et al.*, 1983). The basis of the model developed from the theories of the psychologist Maslow (1954) and his hierarchy of biological needs; indeed this hierarchy and the work of Roper *et al.* to a degree supports Henderson's notion of 14 universal needs. This model now used extensively with the UK has evolved from these beginnings.

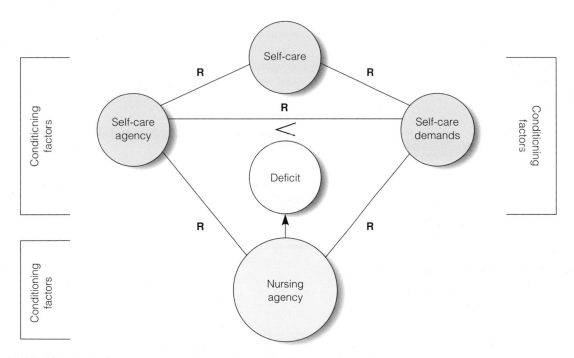

Figure 2-1 The major components of Orem's self-care deficit theory. R indicates a relationship between components; < indicates a current or potential deficit where nursing would be required. (*Note*: From *Nursing Concepts of Practice*, 6th edn (p. 491), by D.E. Orem *et al.*, 2001, St. Louis, MO: Mosby. Reprinted with permission from Elsevier Science.)

BOX 2-1 Activities of Living

1. MAINTAINING A SAFE ENVIRONMENT
2. COMMUNICATING
3. BREATHING
4. EATING AND DRINKING
5. ELIMINATING
6. PERSONAL CLEANSING AND DRESSING
7. CONTROLLING BODY TEMPERATURE
8. MOBILISING
9. WORKING AND PLAYING
10. EXPRESSING SEXUALITY
11. SLEEPING
12. DYING

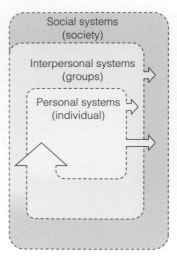

Figure 2-2 King's conceptual framework for nursing: dynamic interacting systems. (*Note*: From *A Theory for Nursing: Systems, Concepts, Process* (p. 11), by I.M. King, 1981, Albany, NY: Delmar. Copyright Imogene M. King. Used with permission.)

The Roper–Logan–Tierney (RLT) model has 12 activities of living centrally at its core, each activity is linked closely with either biological, social or psychological needs required for health (see *Box 2-1*).

The 12 activities are a means by which to assess the patient and identify any deficit in their care needs. Once identified an intervention to assist the patient along their path of recovery may be implemented.

In addition to the 12 core activities of living considered within the model, three behaviour traits are also identified: preventing, comforting and seeking. These refer to the mainten-ance and restoration of health aspects of the model, and the strategies which may be used to correct any health deficits.

King's Goal Attainment Theory

Imogene King's theory of goal attainment (1981) was derived from her conceptual framework (see Figure 2-2). King a nurse academic from the USA developed a framework that demon-strates the relationship of operational systems (individuals), interpersonal systems (groups such as nurse-patient), and social systems (such as educational system, healthcare system). She selected 15 concepts from the nursing literature (self, role, perception, communication, interaction, transaction, growth and development, stress, time, personal space, organisation, status, power, authority and decision making) as essential knowledge for use by nurses.

Ten of the concepts in the framework were selected (self, role, perception, communication, interaction, transaction, growth and development, stress, time and personal space) as essential knowledge for use by nurses in concrete nursing situ-ations. Within this theory, a transaction process model was designed (see Figure 2-3). This process describes the nature of and standard for nurse–patient interactions that leads to

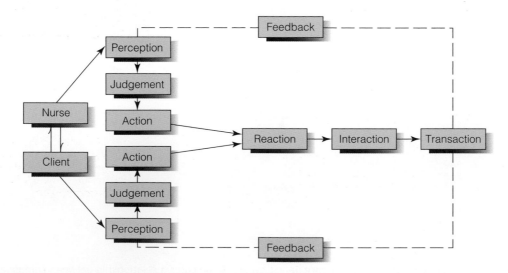

Figure 2-3 King's model of transactions. (*Note*: From *A Theory for Nursing: Systems, Concepts, Process* (p. 145), by I.M. King, 1981, Albany, NY: Delmar. Copyright Imogene M. King. Reprinted with permission.)

goal attainment – that nurses purposefully interact and mutually set, explore and agree to means to achieve goals. Goal attainment represents outcomes. When this information is recorded in the patient record, nurses have data that represent evidence-based nursing practice.

King's theory offers insight into nurses' interactions with individuals and groups within the environment. It highlights the importance of a patient's participation in decisions that influence care and focuses on both the process of nurse–patient interaction and the outcomes of care.

Neuman's Systems Model

Betty Neuman (Neuman and Fawcett, 2002), a community health nurse and clinical psychologist, developed a model based on the individual's relationship to stress, the reaction to it, and reconstitution factors that are dynamic in nature. Reconstitution is the state of adaptation to stressors.

Neuman views the patient as an open system consisting of a basic structure or central core of energy resources (physiological, psychological, sociocultural, developmental and spiritual) surrounded by two concentric boundaries or rings referred to as lines of resistance (see Figure 2-4). The lines of resistance represent internal factors that help the patient defend against a stressor; one example is an increase in the body's leukocyte

count to combat an infection. Outside the lines of resistance are two lines of defence. The inner or normal line of defence, depicted as a solid line, represents the person's state of equilibrium or the state of adaptation developed and maintained over time and considered normal for that person. The flexible line of defence, depicted as a broken line, is dynamic and can be rapidly altered over a short period of time. It is a protective buffer that prevents stressors from penetrating the normal line of defence. Certain variables (e.g. sleep deprivation) can create rapid changes in the flexible line of defence.

Neuman categorises stressors as intra-personal stressors, those that occur within the individual (e.g. an infection); interpersonal stressors, those that occur between individuals (e.g. unrealistic role expectations); and extrapersonal stressors, those that occur outside the person (e.g. financial concerns). The individual's reaction to stressors depends on the strength of the lines of defence. When the lines of defence fail, the resulting reaction depends on the strength of the lines of resistance. As part of the reaction, a person's system can adapt to a stressor, an effect known as reconstitution.

Nursing interventions focus on retaining or maintaining system stability. These interventions are carried out on three preventive levels: primary, secondary and tertiary:

+ Primary prevention focuses on protecting the normal line of defence and strengthening the flexible line of defence.

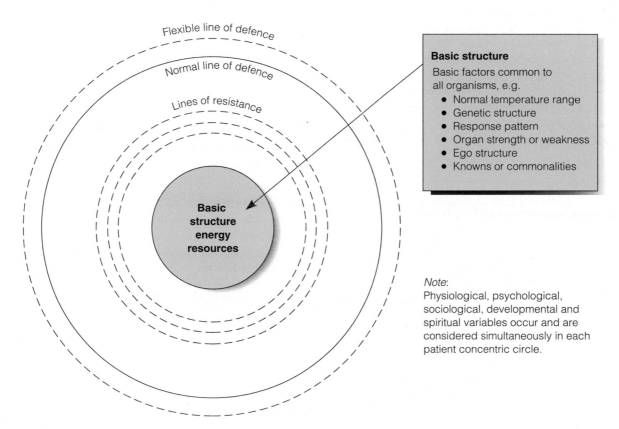

Figure 2-4 Neuman's patient system. (*Note*: From Neuman, Betty; Fawcett, Jacqueline, *Neuman Systems Model, The*, 4th Edition, © 2002, pg 15. Reprinted by permission of Pearson Education Inc., Upper Saddle River, NJ.

✦ Secondary prevention focuses on strengthening internal lines of resistance, reducing the reaction and increasing resistance factors.

✦ Tertiary prevention focuses on readaptation and stability and protects reconstitution or return to wellness following treatment.

Betty Neuman's model of nursing is applicable to a variety of nursing practice settings involving individuals, families, groups and communities.

Roy's Adaptation Model

Sister Callista Roy (1997), an eminent nurse theorist and professor of nursing, defines adaptation as 'the process and outcome whereby the thinking and feeling person uses conscious awareness and choice to create human and environmental integration' (p. 44).

Roy's work focuses on the increasing complexity of person and environment self-organisation, and on the relationship between and among persons, universe, and what can be considered a supreme being or God. Her philosophical assumptions have been refined using major characteristics of 'creation spirituality' – a view that 'persons and the earth are one, and that they are in God and of God' (Roy, 1997: 46).

Roy focuses on the individual as a biopsychosocial adaptive system that employs a feedback cycle of input (stimuli), throughput (control processes) and output (behaviours or adaptive responses). Both the individual and the environment are sources of stimuli that require modification to promote adaptation, an ongoing purposive response. Adaptive responses contribute to health, which she defines as the process of being and becoming integrated; ineffective or maladaptive responses do not contribute to health. Each person's adaptation level is unique and constantly changing.

Individuals respond to needs (stimuli) in one of four modes:

1. The physiological mode involves the body's basic physiological needs and ways of adapting with regard to fluid and electrolytes, activity and rest, circulation and oxygen, nutrition and elimination, protection, the senses, and neurological and endocrine function.
2. The self-concept mode includes two components: the physical self, which involves sensation and body image, and the personal self, which involves self-ideal, self-consistency and the moral-ethical self.
3. The role function mode is determined by the need for social integrity and refers to the performance of duties based on given positions within society.
4. The interdependence mode involves one's relations with significant others and support systems that provide help, affection and attention.

The goal of Callista Roy's model is to enhance life processes through adaptation in the four adaptive modes.

Leininger's Cultural Care Diversity and Universality Theory

Madeleine Leininger, a well-known nurse anthropologist, put her views on transcultural nursing in print in the 1970s and then in 1991 published her book *Culture Care Diversity and Universality: A Theory of Nursing*.

Leininger states that care is the essence of nursing and the dominant, distinctive and unifying feature of nursing. She emphasises that human caring, although a universal phenomenon, varies among cultures in its expressions, processes and patterns; it is largely culturally derived. Leininger produced the Sunrise model to depict her theory of cultural care diversity and universality. This model emphasises that health and care are influenced by elements of the social structure, such as technology, religious and philosophical factors, kinship and social systems, cultural values, political and legal factors, economic factors and educational factors. These social factors are addressed within environmental contexts, language expressions and ethnohistory. Each of these systems is part of the social structure of any society; healthcare expressions, patterns and practices are also integral parts of these aspects of social structure (Leininger and McFarland, 2002). In order for nurses to assist people of diverse cultures, Leininger presents three intervention modes:

1. Culture care preservation and maintenance
2. Culture care accommodation, negotiation, or both
3. Culture care restructuring and repatterning.

Watson's Human Caring Theory

Jean Watson (1979), a distinguished professor of nursing from the USA, believes the practice of caring is central to nursing; it is the unifying focus for practice. Her major assumptions about caring are shown in *Box 2-2*. Nursing interventions relating to human care are referred to as *carative factors*, a guide Watson refers to as the 'Core of Nursing'. Watson outlines the following 10 factors:

1. Forming a humanistic-altruistic system of values
2. Instilling faith and hope
3. Cultivating sensitivity to one's self and others
4. Developing a helping-trust (human care) relationship
5. Promoting and accepting the expression of positive and negative feelings
6. Systematically using the scientific problem-solving method for decision making
7. Promoting interpersonal teaching–learning
8. Providing a supportive, protective or corrective mental, physical, sociocultural and spiritual environment
9. Assisting with the gratification of human needs
10. Allowing for existential-phenomenological forces (aspects from outside the individual or their area of control).

Watson's theory of human caring has received worldwide recognition as a major force in redefining nursing as a caring-healing health model.

BOX 2-2 Watson's Assumptions of Caring

+ Human caring in nursing is not just an emotion, concern, attitude or benevolent desire. Caring connotes a personal response.
+ Caring is an intersubjective human process and is the moral ideal of nursing.
+ Caring can be effectively demonstrated only interpersonally.
+ Effective caring promotes health and individual or family growth.
+ Caring promotes health more than does curing.
+ Caring responses accept a person not only as they are now, but also for what the person may become.
+ A caring environment offers the development of potential while allowing the person to choose the best action for the self at a given point in time.
+ Caring occasions involve action and choice by nurse and patient. If the caring occasion is transpersonal, the limits of openness expand, as do human capacities.
+ The most abstract characteristic of a caring person is that the person is somehow responsive to another person as a unique individual, perceives the other's feelings and sets one person apart from another.
+ Human caring involves values, a will and a commitment to care, knowledge, caring actions and consequences.
+ The ideal and value of caring is a starting point, a stance and an attitude that has to become a will, an intention, a commitment and a conscious judgement that manifests itself in concrete acts.

Note: From J. Watson, personal communication, 22 September 2002.

Parse's Human Becoming Theory

Parse (1995), a member of the American academy of nursing and professor of nursing, proposes three assumptions about *human becoming*:

1. Human becoming is freely choosing personal meaning in situations in the inter-subjective process of relating value priorities.
2. Human becoming is co-creating rhythmic patterns or relating in mutual process with the universe.
3. Human becoming is cotranscending multidimensionally (finding unique ways of living in many aspecs of life), with the emerging possibles.

These three assumptions focus on meaning, rhythmicity and cotranscendence (finding unique ways of living).

+ Meaning arises from a person's interrelationship with the world and refers to happenings to which the person attaches varying degrees of significance.
+ Rhythmicity is the movement toward greater diversity.
+ Cotranscendence is the process of reaching out beyond the self.

Parse's model of human becoming emphasises how individuals choose and bear responsibility for patterns of personal health. Parse contends that the patient, not the nurse, is the authority figure and decision maker. The nurse's role involves helping individuals and families in choosing the possibilities for changing the health process. Specifically, the nurse's role consists of illuminating meaning (uncovering what was and what will be), synchronising rhythms (leading through discussion to recognise harmony), and mobilising transcendence (dreaming of possibilities and planning to reach them).

The Parse nurse uses 'true presence' in the nurse–patient process. 'In true presence the nurse's whole being is immersed with the patient as the other illuminates the meanings of his or her situation and moves beyond the moment' (Parse, 1994: 18).

CRITIQUE OF NURSING THEORY

Several nurse scholars have developed strong critiques of 20th century nursing theories, choosing to ground their work in philosophy or the social sciences (Benner, 2000; Munhall, 2001). The best theories in philosophy and the social sciences are often used in the humanities for the insights and perspectives that can be brought to literature and art. So far, other disciplines have not discovered a sufficiently unique or interesting perspective on the human condition in nursing theories.

Nursing scholars continue to debate whether grounding our research in the best theories from other disciplines is good or bad. Some think this detracts from the development of nursing as a separate discipline; others argue that nursing research becomes more relevant when informed by scholarship that addresses larger social concerns.

Theory can be used to broaden our perspectives in nursing and facilitate the altruistic (showing unselfish concern for the welfare of others), and humanistic values of the profession. At the same time, rational and predictive theory can produce language and social practices that are superimposed onto the lives of vulnerable patients and violence to the fragility of human dignity. As a lens in which to view the world through, theory can either illuminate or obscure. As a tool, theory can either liberate or enslave.

NURSING PROCESS, CARE AND FRAMEWORKS

Models and theories of nursing may be seen as part of the nursing process in order to assess and manage the care of the patient. The nursing process was proposed by Yura and

Walsh (1967) with the publication of *The Nursing Process*. They suggested that nursing should develop a problem-solving approach in which the nurse and patient undertake four steps of care;

1. Identify together problems and causes requiring intervention.
2. Make plans that remedy the problems identified.
3. Take the steps necessary to alleviate the problems.
4. Reflect upon what has happened.

The four stages are really summarised as: assessment, planning, implementation and evaluation. The assessment and goal planning stage of the nursing process are linked closely to the use of nursing models. A patient can be assessed efficiently with an appropriate nursing model in order to identify care deficits and allow for realistic goal setting to be performed. The model used for patient assessment and goal planning can also be used for evaluation in order to see if the goals have been met in full. (See Chapter 9 – The Nursing Process.)

Care Pathways

Care pathways have been developed over a number of years since the 1990s, as a means of assisting healthcare professionals, managers and administrators to deliver high quality, evidence-based, cost effective care. The integrated care pathway is both a tool and a concept that incorporates locally agreed protocols that are evidence-based; patient centred and form part of everyday practice for individual patients in a specified group.

Care pathways have the aim of:

+ targeting the right patient group;
+ undertaking the correct interventions for that patient group agreed locally;
+ placing the interventions in the appropriate order;
+ ensuring the intervention occurs in the appropriate environment;
+ ensuring that all interventions have a positive patient outcome.

It is important to remember though that it is rare that a single care pathway will cover the full span of a patient's journey through a clinical care area. The patient journey may comprise aspects of a different care pathway for each phase of the patient journey such as an assessment and admission phase, a set of interventions and the discharge phase. Care pathways should amalgamate all aspects of care and treatment from members of the multidisciplinary team and have an agreed time frame for achievement of agreed outcomes.

Care pathways may have several component parts including:

+ multidisciplinary, multi-agency, clinical and administrative activities,
+ evidence-based, locally agreed, best practice,
+ local and national standards (linked to national service frameworks),
+ variance tracking,

+ tests, charts, assessments, diagrams, letters, forms, information leaflets, satisfaction questionnaires, etc.,
+ scales for measurement of clinical effectiveness,
+ outcomes,
+ freehand notes,
+ 'space' to add activities or comments to a standard individual care plan to individualise care for a particular patient,
+ problem, plan, goal and notes or a similar structured free-hand area (a multidisciplinary template for recording and variance tracking an individual patient's problems, goals, plans and freehand notes).

It is important to remember though that a care pathway is **not**:

+ a protocol
+ a flow chart of events
+ a care map
+ a process map
+ a decision tree
+ a guideline
+ a care plan.

Care pathways are also known by many different names including:

+ Anticipated Recovery Pathways
+ Multidisciplinary Pathways of Care
+ Care Protocols
+ Critical Care Pathways
+ Pathways of Care
+ Care Packages
+ Collaborative Care Pathways
+ Care Maps
+ Care Profiles.

Since 1992, care pathways have been developed and implemented across many healthcare settings in the UK including community, primary, acute, private, independent, mental health and the NHS. Care pathways are also used throughout international healthcare systems including those of Germany, Belgium, the Netherlands, Australia, New Zealand, Canada and the USA.

National Service Frameworks

National Service Frameworks (NSFs) have been developed in the UK by the Department of Health, the Scottish Health Department and the Welsh Assembly to address the high priority illnesses. The conditions with the highest mortality rates such as cancer and coronary heart disease are addressed, as well as common conditions such as mental health problems and diabetes. National service frameworks are also identified for key patient groups including children and young people.

The main functions of NSFs are to set clear requirements for care that are based upon the best available evidence for treatments and service that work most effectively for patients. They also offer strategies and support for organisations and agencies to achieve these. NSFs are developed in partnership with healthcare professionals, patients, carers, health service managers, voluntary agencies and other experts in the area of the framework. Currently there are NSFs for:

+ cancer
+ children
+ coronary heart disease

+ diabetes
+ long-term conditions
+ mental health
+ older people
+ renal services.

These frameworks can be accessed electronically via the National Electronic Library for Health.

CRITICAL REFLECTION

Let us revisit the case study on page 16. Now that you have read this chapter, what concepts are present in this case? Which nursing model would you use to assess Janine's nursing needs? What nursing needs might Janine have?

CHAPTER HIGHLIGHTS

+ In the natural biological sciences, the main function of theory is to guide research. In the practice disciplines such as nursing, the main function of theory (and research) is to provide new possibilities for understanding the discipline's focus.
+ To Nightingale, the knowledge required to provide good nursing was neither unique nor specialised. Rather, Nightingale viewed nursing as a central human activity grounded in observation, reason and commonsense health practices.
+ During the latter half of the 20th century, disciplines seeking to establish themselves in universities had to demonstrate something that Nightingale had not envisioned for nursing – a unique body of theoretical knowledge.
+ Theories articulate significant relationships between concepts in order to point to something larger, such as gravity, the unconscious or the experience of pain.
+ Paradigms include our notions of reality that are largely unconscious or taken for granted. Most theories reflect the dominant paradigm of a culture, although some may grow out of a developing rival paradigm.
+ In the late 20th century, much of the theoretical work in nursing focused on articulating relationships

between four major concepts: person, environment, health and nursing. Because these four concepts can be superimposed on almost any work in nursing, they are sometimes collectively referred to as a 'metaparadigm' for nursing.
+ It is important to remember that any organised approach to understanding the world – including theories, social practices and people – can both illuminate and obscure what is of central importance to nurses.
+ Debates about the role of theory in nursing practice provide evidence that nursing is maturing, both as an academic discipline and a clinical profession.
+ Models of nursing can guide the care patients receive as a means of assessment linking with the nursing process and key nursing theories.
+ Care pathways can assist all parties responsible for patient care to deliver high quality, evidence-based, cost-effective care.
+ National service frameworks have been developed in the UK by the Department of Health to address high priority illnesses, common conditions and key patient groups.

REFERENCES

Benner, P. (2000) 'The roles of embodiment, emotion and life-world for rationality and agency in nursing practice', *Nursing Philosophy*, 1(1), 5–19.

Henderson, V.A. (1966) *The nature of nursing: A definition and its implications for practice, research, and education*, Riverside, NJ: Macmillan.

King, I.M. (1981) *A theory for nursing: Systems, concepts, process*, Albany, NY: Delmar.

Leininger, M.M. (Edn) (1991) *Culture care diversity and universality: A theory of nursing*, New York: National League for Nursing Press.

Leininger, M. and McFarland, M.R. (2002) *Culture care diversity and universality: A theory of nursing* (3rd edn), New York: McGraw-Hill.

MacIntyre, R.C. (2001) 'Interpretive analysis', in P. Munhall (Edn), *Nursing research: A qualitative perspective* (3rd edn, pp. 439–466), Boston: Jones and Bartlett.

Maslow, A. (1954) *Motivation and Personality*, New York: Harper.

Munhall, P.L. (Edn) (2001) *Nursing research: A qualitative perspective* (3rd edn), Boston: Jones and Bartlett.

Neuman, B. and Fawcett, J. (2002) *The Neuman systems model* (4th edn), Upper Saddle River, NJ: Prentice Hall.

Nightingale, F. (1969) *Notes on nursing: What it is, and what it is not*, New York: Dover. (Original work published in 1860.)

Orem, D.E. (1971) *Nursing: Concepts of practice*, Hightstown, NJ: McGraw-Hill.

Orem, D.E., Taylor, S.G. and Renpenning, K.M. (2001) *Nursing: Concepts of practice* (6th edn), St. Louis, MO: Mosby.

Parse, R.R. (1994) 'Quality of life: Sciencing and living the art of human becoming', *Nursing Science Quarterly*, 7(1), 16–21.

Parse, R.R. (Edn) (1995) *Illumination: The human becoming theory in practice and research*, New York: National League for Nursing Press.

Rogers, M.E. (1970) *An introduction to the theoretical basis of nursing*, Philadelphia: F.A. Davis.

Roper, N., Logan, W. and Tierney, A. (1980) *The Elements of Nursing*, Edinburgh: Churchill Livingstone.

Roper, N., Logan, W. and Tierney, A. (1981) *Learning to Use the Process of Nursing*, Edinburgh: Churchill Livingstone.

Roper, N., Logan, W. and Tierney, A. (1983) *Using a Model for Nursing*, Edinburgh: Churchill Livingstone.

Roy, C. (1997) 'Future of the Roy model: Challenge to redefine adaptation', *Nursing Science Quarterly*, 10(1), 42–48.

Tomey, A.M. and Alligood, M.R. (1998) *Nursing theorists and their work* (4th edn), St. Louis, MO: Mosby.

Watson, J. (1979) *Nursing: The philosophy and science of caring*, Boston: Little, Brown.

Yura, H. and Walsh, M. (1967) *The Nursing process*, Norwalk, CT: Appleton–Century-Crofts.

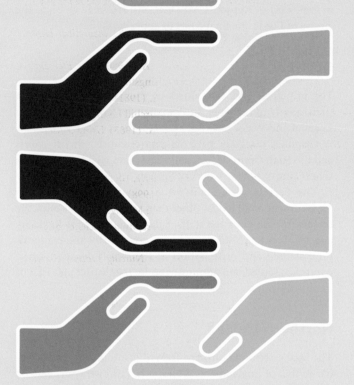

Chapter 3 Legal Aspects of Nursing

Learning Outcomes

After completing this chapter, you will be able to:

+ Discuss the development of nursing as a profession.

+ Discuss factors relating to the regulation of the nursing profession.

+ List four areas of accountability affecting nursing.

+ State how legislation influences healthcare practice.

+ Discuss factors affecting consent or refusal of treatment including age and mental state.

+ List two pieces of legislation governing the access to and storage of medical records.

CASE STUDY

Dianne is admitted to an acute medical ward with a chest infection secondary to advanced cancer and a progressive degenerative neurological disease. Her family discusses during admission that she has been having a course of experimental chemotherapy. As further discussions and assessments take place while Dianne is admitted it also becomes apparent that due to the chronic health problems she is no longer able to make informed decisions about her treatment. Her daughter, who states she is the next of kin, shows the registered nurse a sealed envelope and states that it contains an advanced directive/living will that Dianne made before her condition deteriorated.

Due to her illness a decision needs to be made whether to treat the infection aggressively or keep Dianne 'comfortable' with pain relief. Her family want no active treatment but the medical staff believe she could live another few months if treated.

After reading this chapter you will be able to discuss the legislation that influences healthcare and the effects this will have on Dianne's care.

OVERVIEW OF THE BRITISH LEGAL SYSTEM AND COMMON LEGAL TERMS

The British legal system varies slightly between the four countries that comprise the UK. Although the UK is effectively one state, England and Wales, Scotland and Northern Ireland all have their own legal systems, with some variations in law, organisation and practice. However, a large amount of modern legislation applies throughout the UK. Law may be divided into **criminal law** and **civil law**; the latter regulates the conduct of people in ordinary relations with one another. The distinction between the two branches of the law is reflected in the procedures used, the courts in which cases can be heard and the actions they may take.

The legal system of the UK comprises a historic body of systems known as **common law**, Parliamentary and European Community legislation. Parliamentary and European Community legislation frequently applies throughout the UK but may only apply to one specific country such as the Government of Wales Act 2006. (This Act allowed additional law-making powers to the Welsh Assembly.) **Common law**, which is based on custom and interpreted in court cases by judges, has never been precisely defined. It forms the basis of the law except when superseded by parliamentary legislation or an Act. An **Act of Parliament** or **Act** is law enacted by the government. The starting point of an Act of Parliament is often a formal written proposal known as a **White Paper**, which if accepted will be prepared in the form of a proposed law known as a **Bill**. The Bill will then be introduced into the House of Commons or House of Lords for debate and possible enactment as an Act.

European Community law, deriving from the UK's membership of the European Union, is confined mainly to economic and social matters; in certain circumstances it takes precedence over domestic law. It is normally applied by the domestic courts, but the most authoritative rulings are given by the European Court.

The Courts

Criminal Courts

Summary or less serious offences, which make up the vast majority of criminal cases, are tried in England and Wales by unpaid lay magistrates – justices of the peace (JPs), although in areas with a heavy workload there are a number of full-time, stipendiary (paid) magistrates. More serious offences are tried by the Crown Court, presided over by a judge sitting with a jury of citizens randomly picked from the local electoral register. The Crown Court sits at about 90 centres in England and Wales and is presided over by High Court judges, full-time 'circuit judges' and part-time recorders.

Appeals from the magistrates' courts go before the Crown Court or the High Court. Appeals from the Crown Court are made to the Court of Appeal (Criminal Division). The House of Lords is the final appeal court in all cases within the UK.

Civil Courts

Magistrates' courts have limited civil powers but county courts have a wider jurisdiction; and cases are normally tried by judges sitting alone. The judges of the High Court consider civil cases, some criminal cases and also deal with the appeals. The High Court sits at the Royal Courts of Justice in London or at 26 district registries. Appeals from the High Court are heard in the Court of Appeal (Civil Division), and may go on to the House of Lords, the final court of appeal.

Scotland

The principles and procedures of the Scottish legal system (particularly in civil law) differ in many respects from those of England and Wales.

Criminal cases are tried in district courts, sheriff courts and the High Court of Justiciary. The main civil courts are the sheriff courts and the Court of Session.

The Secretary of State for Scotland recommends the appointment of all judges other than the most senior ones. He or she also appoints the staff of the High Court of Justiciary and the Court of Session, and is responsible for the composition, staffing and organisation of the sheriff courts. District courts are staffed and administered by the district and islands local authorities.

Northern Ireland

The legal system of Northern Ireland is in many respects similar to that of England and Wales. It has its own court system: the superior courts are the Court of Appeal, the High Court and the Crown Court, which together comprise the Supreme Court of Judicature. A number of arrangements differ from those in England and Wales. A major example is that those accused of terrorist-type offences are tried in non-jury courts to avoid any intimidation of jurors.

NURSING AS A PROFESSION

Nursing in the UK is a legally regulated healthcare profession with a regulatory body that registrants are accountable to. The Nursing and Midwifery Council (NMC) which has been established by an Act of Parliament, maintains the professional register of practitioners who are able to use the legally protected title Registered Nurse, Registered Midwife or Specialist Community Public Health Nurse.

The establishment of regulation within nursing is a process that has developed since the mid-19th century, when at that time there was no formal education for nurses. *Box 3-1* charts the time line of regulation within nursing.

BOX 3-1 Establishment of Nursing Regulation since the mid-19th Century

1840 – Sisterhoods formed to improve standards of care offered to the sick and vulnerable. These sisterhoods were formed in a similar manner to catholic nursing orders in continental Europe.

1848 – St. Johns House Anglican sisterhood formed in London.

1854-56 – Fund established by public subscription to enable Florence Nightingale to establish a nursing training school.

1860 – Nightingale School of Nursing established in St. Thomas's Hospital, London.

1860 onwards – Other hospitals, workhouses and institutions established schools of nursing with Superintendents who had often been trained at the Nightingale School.

1887 – Queens Institute of District Nursing formed for the care of the sick and poor in their homes.

1919 – Nurses Registration Act established the General Nursing Council to regulate proposed nurse training and nurses.

1943 – Nurses Act established a roll of assistant nurses in response to nurse shortages.

1948 – National Health Service established, which took over running of hospitals and schools of nursing attached to hospitals.

1979 – Following the recommendations of the Briggs Report the Nursing, Midwives and Health Visitors Act recommended the establishment of the UK Central Council for Nursing, Midwifery and Health Visiting (UKCC) as the regulatory body.

1983 – The UKCC was formally established with National Boards in England, Wales, Scotland and Northern Ireland to maintain standards for education and monitor training records.

2002 – The UKCC was replaced by the Nursing Midwifery Council and the National Boards were abolished.

THE NURSING AND MIDWIFERY COUNCIL

The role of the Nursing Midwifery Council (NMC) reaches far beyond that of an organisation that maintains a register of practitioners. The formal constitution of the NMC states the council shall consist of:

+ 12 members who are appointed by the council on being elected under the election scheme (registrant members). That is one member from each of the three professions and from each of the four UK countries are elected to the council by all those with effective registration.
+ 11 members who are appointed by the Privy Council (lay members/non healthcare professionals) – The Privy Council comprises of all Cabinet Ministers and a number of Junior Ministers.
+ 12 members appointed by the council on being elected under the election scheme (alternative members); elected in the same manner as registrant members. If a registrant member is unable to attend a council meeting, their corresponding alternate member may attend and vote in their place.

The NMC register is divided into two sub-parts – sub-part 1 for all level 1 nurses and sub-part 2 for all level 2 nurses. The level of nurse refers to the educational programme the individual practitioner has studied and completed. Those nurses referred to as level 2 have undertaken a two-year enrolled nurse education programme (no longer offered in the UK), whereas a level 1 registered practitioner has taken and completed a three- or four-year education programme (see Table 3-1 on page 32).

The Registration entry code relates to how the practitioner is recorded on the register. All level 1 and 2 nurses usually write their qualification as RN after their name, whereas all those on other parts of the register write their qualification as the registration entry code appears.

Additionally, practitioners registered with the NMC may also record additional qualifications relating to prescribing or specialist practice. See *Box 3-2*.

BOX 3-2 Additional Recorded Qualifications

Prescribing
+ Community Practitioner Nurse Prescriber
+ Nurse Independent Prescriber
+ Nurse Independent/Supplementary Prescriber

Specialist Practitioner - Adult Nursing
+ Specialist Practitioner - Mental Health
+ Specialist Practitioner - Children's Nursing
+ Specialist Practitioner - Learning Disability Nurse
+ Specialist Practitioner - General Practice Nursing
+ Specialist Practitioner - Community Mental Health Nursing
+ Specialist Practitioner - Community Learning Disabilities Nursing
+ Specialist Practitioner - Community Children's Nursing
+ Specialist Practitioner - District Nursing

Table 3-1 Parts of the NMC Nursing Register

Sub-part 1: Level 1 Nurse		Sub-part 2: Level 2 Nurse (Formerly enrolled nurses)	
Field of practice	Registration entry code	Field of practice	Registration entry code
Adult	RN1, RNA	Adult	RN2
Mental Health	RN3, RNMH	Mental Health	RN4
Learning Disabilities	RN5, RNLD	Learning Disabilities	RN6
Children	RN8, RNC	General	RN7
		Fever	RN9

Midwives part of the register

Field of practice	Registration entry code
Midwifery	RM

Specialist community public health nurses part of the register

Field of practice	Registration entry code
Specialist Community Public Health Nursing - HV (1)	RHV
Specialist Community Public Health Nursing - SN (2)	RSN
Specialist Community Public Health Nursing - OH (3)	ROH
Specialist Community Public Health Nursing - FHN (4)	RFHN

THE ROLE OF THE NURSING AND MIDWIFERY COUNCIL

The role of the NMC includes the setting of standards for nurse education, the conduct and performance of nurses and midwives and ensures the maintenance of those standards. In order to maintain these standards the NMC publishes guidance documents and advice that is reviewed on a regular basis. This advice and guidance includes the core documents of:

+ Code of Professional Conduct: standards for conduct performance and ethics – see *Box 3-3*,
+ guidelines for the administration of medicines,
+ guidelines for records and record keeping.

These documents are considered a fundamental part of the practice of a registered nurse. If any nurse deviates from the standards set by the NMC then they may be requested to appear before one of the council's three practice committees. The practice committees comprise of:

+ the Investigating Committee,
+ the Conduct and Competence Committee,
+ the Health Committee.

In order to maintain registration all nurses must re-register every three years and have completed at least 35 hours of continuing professional development (PREP) and practised as a registered nurse for at least 450 hours in this three-year period. Each nurse registrant must also sign a form in order to declare they are medically fit to practise as a registered practitioner.

BOX 3-3 The NMC Code of Professional Conduct: Standards for Conduct, Performance and Ethics

As a registered nurse, midwife or specialist community public health nurse, you are personally accountable for your practice. In caring for patients and clients you must:

+ Respect the patient or client as an individual
+ Obtain consent before you give any treatment or care
+ Protect confidential information
+ Cooperate with others in the team
+ Maintain your professional knowledge and competence
+ Be trustworthy
+ Act to identify and minimise risk to patient and clients.

These are the shared values of all the UK healthcare regulatory bodies.

Source: NMC.

ACCOUNTABILITY

Nurses as healthcare professionals are therefore accountable for their actions and omissions within four areas:

1. To the public in the format of criminal law and the criminal courts.

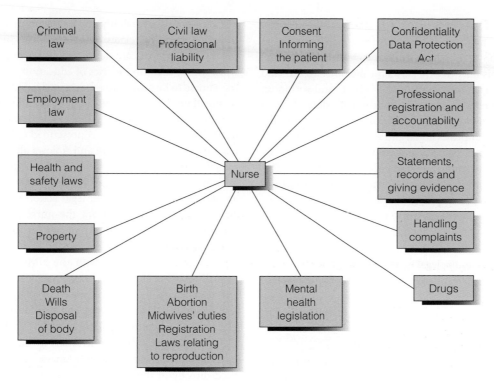

Figure 3-1 Areas that concern the nurse.

Source: From Dimmond, B. (2005) *Legal Aspects of Nursing* (4th edn). Harlow: Pearson. Copyright © Pearson Education Ltd 2005.

2. Professionally to the NMC via the Code of Conduct and NMC Conduct and Competence Committee.

3. Accountability to the patient via civil law and the civil courts.

4. Accountability to the employer via the contract of employment and via employment tribunals.

Employment tribunals are judicial legal bodies established to resolve disputes between employers and employees over employment rights. Many areas of law therefore affect nursing practice on a daily basis (see Figure 3.1).

HUMAN RIGHTS ACT 1998

Nursing practice is affected by many pieces of legislation and some directly affect the care that certain patients or groups of patients may receive. The Human Rights Act 1998 has the potential to affect significantly clinical practice and management of specific groups of patients. This Act was developed to allow UK citizens to make legal complaints if they believed their human rights were being breached. The UK was a signatory to the 1950 European Convention for the Protection of Human Rights and Fundamental Freedoms. If a citizen considered their rights had been breached then the only legal path available in the past would be directly to the European Court of Human Rights in Strasbourg. This course of action could take over five years to reach a conclusion. In order to address this unfair imbalance and ensure the protection of human rights

the Act was made law in October 2000. This now allows legal action to be brought against a public authority or organisation exercising public functions for a breach of the 1950 Convention.

The right to life is considered by article 2(1) of the Act, which states: 'everyone's right to life shall be protected by law. No one shall be deprived of his life intentionally save in the execution of a sentence of a court following his conviction for a crime for which a penalty is provided in law'. However within article 3 it is stated: 'no one should be subjected to inhuman or degrading treatment or punishment'.

It may be argued that in accordance with article 2 all patients have a right to life and therefore aggressive management of symptoms to improve potential outcome. This was argued in a legal case in 2000 when parents challenged a not for resuscitation order for their severely disabled baby. The courts upheld the order – this was neither a breach of articles 2 or 3 by allowing full palliative care (pain relief and nutritional support only) and allowing the baby to die with dignity (*National Health Service Trust A v D and Others* (2000)).

Arguably some aggressive forms of treatment could be considered to be inhuman or degrading for the individual who has a diminished capacity or understanding to make a decision. Examples of this could include chemotherapy where the patient loses their hair and their appearance can be affected, and drugs that cause incontinence as a side effect. This too may be considered to be degrading to the individual receiving the treatment but no challenges have yet been made to this in law.

DUTY OF CARE

The nurse does however have a duty of care to respond to all patient needs. This duty of care exists for the nurse to care and manage their patient to the best of their ability and within set local and national policies. It may be argued that a duty of care is fundamental to nursing practice and failure to respond to the duty of care is both unprofessional and immoral. The best interests of the patients can, on occasions, appear a grey area, but the nurse must always be guided by best practice and the law. This guidance may be from the NMC as the professional regulatory body in addition to the employer via policies and procedures.

Like all other employees the nurse is governed by the Health and Safety at Work Act 1974. Before 1974 approximately eight million employees in the UK had no legal safety protection at work. The Act provides the legal framework to promote, stimulate and encourage high standards of health and safety in places of work. It protects employees and the public from work activities. Everyone has a duty to comply with the Act, including employers, employees, trainees, the self-employed, manufacturers, suppliers, designers and importers of work equipment.

This legislation places a general duty to 'ensure so far as is reasonably practicable the health, safety and welfare at work of all their employees'.

Employers must comply with the Act to:

+ Provide and maintain safety equipment and safe systems of work such as moving and handling equipment.
+ Ensure materials used are properly stored, handled, used and transported including clinical waste and sharps.
+ Provide information, training, instruction and supervision. Ensure all staff are aware of instructions provided by manufacturers and suppliers of equipment.
+ Provide a safe place of employment.
+ Provide a safe working environment.
+ Provide a written safety policy/risk assessment.
+ Look after health and safety of others including public/patients.
+ Talk to safety representatives.

Employers are forbidden to charge their employees for any measures which they are required to provide in the interests of health and safety. An example is personal protective equipment, which in the case of nursing and healthcare includes uniforms and infection control equipment such as gloves and aprons.

Employees also have specific responsibilities to take care of their own health and safety and that of other persons. All employees must cooperate with their employers to comply with the legislation and also not interfere with anything provided in the interest of health and safety.

LIABILITY FOR ACTS OR OMISSIONS

All members of staff in a healthcare setting are protected by vicarious liability if an incident occurs potentially affecting the nurse in terms of liability for prosecution or a civil action. **Vicarious liability** relates to the employers being accountable for the standard of care delivered by the employee when they work within their boundaries of education and skill. Therefore for a nurse to be protected by vicarious liability they must work within their level of competence, education and skill. As an example, Nurse X gives a patient a medication that they have never had before, checks it is prescribed correctly, the patient has no allergies to the drug and follows all local policies. The patient has an allergic reaction to the drug and the family attempts to take legal action against Nurse X. As the nurse is an employee of the hospital, legal action would be instigated against the employer and not the nurse as employee as she acted in accordance with all policies, procedures and guidelines. Therefore the nurse is protected by vicarious liability.

This links very closely with the NMC Code of Conduct regarding acts or omissions on the part of the nurse. All incidents and deficits should be reported to comply with the Health and Safety at Work Act 1974 and the Control of Substances Hazardous to Health Regulations 2002 (COSHH).

COSHH help protect individuals in the workplace against health risks from hazardous substances. The substances may be used directly in the work (e.g. cleaning chemicals or medications such as chemotherapy) or may arise from work activities (e.g. clinical waste products).

COSHH requires that:

+ assessment of the risks involved with any hazardous activity should be performed;
+ decisions are made regarding what precautions are needed;
+ risks are prevented or controlled;
+ control measures should be maintained;
+ monitoring exposure and health surveillance, where necessary, such as exposure to latex and latex allergies should be performed;
+ informing, instructing and training employees about the risks and precautions needed should be undertaken.

Risk management will depend on a number of factors, such as the hazard presented by the substance, how it is used, how exposure is controlled, and the degree and extent of exposure. All healthcare environments should have a written COSHH policy available to all staff.

Any incidents involving accidents should be reported in accordance with RIDDOR. RIDDOR is an abbreviation for the Reporting of Injuries, Diseases and Dangerous Occurrences Regulations 1995. The regulations came into force on 1 April 1996. **RIDDOR** developed from the Health and Safety at Work Act 1974 with the requirement of immediate reporting to the enforcing authority in cases of any accident connected with work; or an employee involving a major injury; or a member of the public being killed or hospitalised.

The Act applies to all work activities with the reporting of accidents and ill health at work being the main legal requirement as described by RIDDOR. The information enables the enforcing authorities such as the Health and Safety Executive (HSE) to identify where and how risks arise and to investigate serious accidents. In a clinical area therefore accidents (an occurrence that affects the health of an individual), incidents (such as failure of a piece of equipment which may have affected health or well-being) or a 'near miss' (an incident that nearly resulted in adverse affects to any individual), should all have report forms completed as necessary in accordance with local policy.

On the whole a reportable accident, dangerous occurrence or case of disease under RIDDOR is comparatively rare in a health setting. However, in order to comply with the Act the following incidents have to be reported:

+ deaths
+ major injuries
+ accidents resulting in three days off work
+ certain infectious diseases
+ dangerous occurrences.

Reportable major injuries as described by RIDDOR include:

+ fracture other than to fingers, thumbs or toes;
+ amputation;
+ dislocation of the shoulder, hip, knee or spine;
+ loss of sight – temporary or permanent;
+ chemical or hot metal burn to the eye or any penetrating injury to the eye;
+ injury resulting from an electric shock or electrical burn;
+ any other injury requiring admittance to hospital for more than 24 hours;
+ acute illness requiring medical treatment, or loss of consciousness arising from absorption of any substance by inhalation, ingestion or through the skin.

The reporting of accidents and incidents is a statutory requirement and protects both the employee and the service user.

A further fundamental legal consideration in clinical practice is consent.

CONSENT

Consent to treatment is a fundamental aspect of patient management, and not only applies to procedures but information given to the patient to make consent valid and informed. For consent to be valid and informed the patient should be made aware of all the facts relating to their care and treatment, both positive and negative. All risks and potential for harm should be explained to the patient in a form of communication they understand. It is also essential that the patient understands the implications of treatment or withholding treatment fully. Communication difficulties may arise on occasions with patients from another ethnic background when the first language is not English or those who are culturally deaf. The culturally deaf community is comprised of people who are culturally deaf as opposed to those who are deaf from the medical, audiological or pathological perspective. That is to say they are born deaf and have never had any hearing; frequently

their main mode of communication is sign language. The information should be given to the patient in a form of communication they understand and if using an interpreter the interpreter should, as far as possible, be experienced in communicating information of this nature.

Consent may be summarised as an informed decision-making process where risks have been explained to the patient, as well as the benefits of the treatment.

Consent may be given by an individual as either verbal consent for everyday procedures such as recording vital signs or in a written form when an invasive procedure is involved. The Department of Health has produced guidelines for consent for both examination and treatment in addition to good practice to gain consent and standard consent forms.

Issues relating to consent arise when the patient is not considered mentally competent to make a decision due to illness or age. If a patient is considered not to be competent psychologically to make an informed consent decision for treatment or otherwise then it is the responsibility of the next of kin to give consent. The next of kin is the patient's closest living blood relative or individual previously identified by the patient as their next of kin. If this is not possible or there is a disagreement with the next of kin it may be up to the courts to decide what is in the best interests of the patient. An exception to this is emergency treatment where consent would be difficult or time consuming to obtain and therefore affect the condition of the patient. In this emergency situation consent does not have to be obtained but all actions must be based on best practice and be in the best interests of the patient, with all members of the healthcare team agreeing.

Young People and Consent

Consent procedure for those under the age of 18 varies depending upon the age of the child. Section 8 of the Family Law Reform Act 1969 states that a child of 16 or 17 can give valid consent to treatment. This treatment can be defined widely and includes both consent to procedures and nursing care. If the child is unable to give consent themselves then it would be the responsibility of the next of kin or court to make a decision on behalf of the child. A decision made by the court would involve consideration of the Children Act 1989.

The main aims of the Act are:

+ to bring together private and public law relating to children in one framework;
+ to achieve a better balance between protecting children and enabling parents to challenge state intervention;
+ to encourage greater partnership between statutory authorities and parents;
+ to promote the use of voluntary arrangements;
+ to restructure the framework of the courts to facilitate the management of family proceedings.

Two of the main principles of the act relate to the concept of parental responsibility replacing parental rights; with children having the ability to be parties separate from their parents in legal proceedings. A child under the age of 16 should have their feelings regarding treatment taken into account in accordance with the Children Act 1989. Sections of the Act state that if the child has sufficient understanding then the child's consent should be given before they agree to medical or physical examination. It is ultimately the decision of the parent or legal guardian to give consent for the treatment of children. This principle is based on the term **Gillick competence**, which is based upon a legal test case.

The rights of parents regarding medical matters concerning their children are subject to the ruling of the House of Lords in the case *Gillick v West Norfolk and Wisbech Area Health Authority* [1985] 3 All ER 402 (HL). The case concerned a teenage girl's right to consent to medical treatment (access to contraceptive medication) without the parents' knowledge. The case was heard in the House of Lords by three of the Law Lords; Lord Fraser, Lord Scarman and Lord Bridge. Lord Fraser stated that the degree of parental control varied according to the child's understanding and intelligence, and Lord Scarman further suggested that parental rights only existed so long as they were needed to protect the property and person of the child. That is to say, protect the child from any potential or actual harm. He said:

> As a matter of law the parental right to determine whether or not their minor child below the age of 16 will have medical treatment terminates if and when the child achieves sufficient understanding and intelligence to enable him to understand fully what is proposed.

Case law has developed following this legal precedence and supports the term Gillick competence. Gillick competence is an individual test that needs to be applied on a case-by-case basis and relates to a particular child, their treatment and the ability of the child to understand the treatment and give informed consent. There have been cases where a 17-year-old has been found insufficiently competent to refuse medical treatment, while in other cases much younger children have been deemed sufficiently competent. In addition, where a child is 16 or 17 either parent or child can consent to treatment independently (though neither can override the other or exercise a veto). The court can, however, override the wishes of both where treatment is vital to the child's welfare. Examples of this can include the live saving treatment of a child with blood products when an objection may be made on the grounds of religious or cultural belief. The principle being that the treatment can save and improve quality of life.

Attempts by healthcare professionals to further clarify the law have been specifically discouraged by the courts. It has become a matter for the healthcare professional to decide whether a child under 16 is **Gillick competent**. Individual healthcare facilities issue guidelines and policies relating to this important aspect.

A further anomaly was provided by the Access to Health Records Act 1990, which allows a child under 16 deemed Gillick competent by a doctor to veto the parent's access to medical information held by that doctor, even though the parent can consent to treatment that the child cannot refuse.

The result is that a doctor, if they judge the child to be Gillick competent, can only disclose information to the parent with the child's consent, regardless of parental responsibility. An example of this is the prescription of contraceptive medication to a child under the age of 16.

MENTAL HEALTH ACT 1983

A person may also be deemed to be competent or otherwise to give consent in accordance with the Mental Health Act 1983, which covers the assessment, treatment and rights of people with a mental health condition. Many people receive specialist mental healthcare and treatment in the community. However, some people can experience severe mental health problems that require admission to hospital for assessment and treatment.

Individuals can only be detained if the strict criteria laid down in the Act are met and the person must be suffering from a mental disorder as defined by the Act. An application for assessment or treatment must be supported in writing by two registered medical practitioners. The recommendation must include a statement about why assessment and/or treatment are necessary, and why other methods of dealing with the patient are not appropriate.

Most people who receive treatment in hospitals or psychiatric units for mental health conditions are there on a voluntary basis and have the same rights as people receiving treatment for physical illnesses. However, a small number of patients may need to be compulsorily detained under a section of the Mental Health Act.

The Act defines who is involved in the decision regarding compulsory admission or detention, and the individual's or their nearest relative's right of appeal against such a decision.

Approved social workers are involved in the process and are specially trained in both mental health and the law relating to it. They are appointed by local authorities to interview and assess people and can make an application for admission where they consider that detention is the most appropriate way of providing care and treatment.

The Act gives certain rights to the nearest relative, which can be used to protect the patient's interests. Usually, the nearest relative is the older of the two people who occur highest in the following list, regardless of gender:

+ husband or wife (or same-sex partner)
+ daughter or son
+ father or mother
+ brother or sister
+ grandfather or grandmother
+ aunt or uncle
+ nephew or niece.

The nearest relative has the right to:

+ make application for compulsory assessment or treatment of the patient;

BOX 3-4 Other Sections of the Mental Health Act

Section 5

Section 5(2) relates to a doctor's holding power. It can only be used on persons who are informally (willingly) admitted to a hospital, but who then change their mind and wish to leave. It can be implemented following a (usually brief) assessment by the Residential Medical Officer or his deputy, which, in effect, means any hospital doctor, including psychiatrists but also those based on medical or surgical wards. It lasts up to 72 hours, during which time a further assessment may result in either discharge from the section or detention under section 2 or section 3.

Section 5(4) is a similar holding power that can be used for the same group of persons as those that may be detained under section 5(2) (as above). It is implemented by a registered mental nurse (RMN). It lasts up to six hours and is usually promptly converted to a section 5(2) order upon an assessment by a doctor.

Sections 135 and 136

Section 135 is a magistrates' order. It can be applied for by an Approved Social Worker in the best interests of a person who is thought to be mentally disordered, but who is refusing to allow mental health professionals into their residence for the purposes of a Mental Health Act assessment. Section 135 gives police officers the right to enter the property and to take the person to a 'place of safety', which is locally defined and is usually either a police station or a psychiatric hospital ward.

Section 136 is a similar order that allows a police officer to take a person whom they consider to be mentally disordered to a 'place of safety'. Once a person subject to section 135 or section 136 is at a place of safety, they are further assessed and, in some cases, a section 2 or section 3 order implemented.

- be consulted and challenge decisions made by the approved social worker;
- discharge the patient;
- apply to a mental health tribunal on behalf of the patient;
- receive written information about the patient's treatment unless the patient objects.

The appointment of the nearest relative can only be changed by a county court. The nearest relative's power of discharge can be overruled by the doctor who is responsible for the patient's treatment.

The most common civil sections of the Act under which patients are compulsorily admitted to a hospital are:

- section 2: admission to hospital for up to 28 days for assessment;
- section 3: admission to hospital for up to six months for treatment;
- section 4: admission on an emergency basis for up to 72 hours.

Illnesses that would warrant admission under the Mental Health Act are discussed in Chapter 10.

Less commonly used sections governing the emergency management of patients include those detailed in *Box 3-4*.

ADVANCED DIRECTIVES

Living wills or advanced directives are recognised as common law, which is law made and interpreted by judges as there is currently no Act of Parliament or central government law regarding these. The document is a signed and witnessed state-

ment that enables the patient to specify their wishes should they become incapable of making a decision relating to management of their medical care and treatment. In 1992, the Appeal Court indicated that when an informed and competent patient has made an anticipatory choice (a decision in advance prior to any serious deterioration in medical condition), which is 'clearly established and applicable in the circumstances' doctors would be bound by it. This view was confirmed by later cases (*Airedale NHS Trust v Bland* (1993) 1 All ER 859 and *Re C* (1994) 1 All ER 819). In these cases, legal discussion revolved around the legally binding nature of an informed refusal of specific treatment.

A clear example of a document that would be legally binding at common law is a directive prior to any treatment drawn up by Jehovah's Witnesses declining blood in all circumstances and releasing the treatment provider from liability for the consequences. Documents that are equally specific would also be binding. A healthcare professional who knowingly acted in disregard of such a competent advance refusal would be likely to be held guilty of assault. Conversely, a healthcare professional who acts in good faith in accordance with an apparently valid advance statement would not be considered negligent. The Law Commission, which is an independent body set up by Parliament to review and recommend reform of the law in England and Wales, has published draft legislation designed to clarify this situation. It proposes that patients should not be able to refuse 'basic care' and hygiene through an advance statement although they can legally refuse specific medical procedures.

Healthcare professionals should, of course, respect any general statement of a patient's wishes and feelings. A document outlining such factors will be helpful in achieving medical decisions that reflect the long-held values of people who are now mentally incapacitated. Such a document may also be called an advance statement or living will but if it lacks specific decisions regarding the drafter's intention regarding treatment it would be unlikely to have the same force of law as a specific refusal. People who wish to make a general statement may support that by nominating a proxy to speak for them about specific aspects of treatment.

The courts have also made it clear that patients can authorise or refuse treatments but cannot make legally-enforceable demands about specific treatments they want to receive. Nor can healthcare professionals be required to act contrary to the law and so, for example, a current or advance request for active euthanasia would be invalid.

ACCESS TO HEALTH RECORDS AND THE DATA PROTECTION ACT

All patients have a right to access their medical records under two pieces of legislation, the Data Protection Act 1998 and the Access to Health Records Act 1990.

The Data Protection Act 1998 governs access to the health records of living people. It became effective from 1 March 2000, and superseded the Data Protection Act 1984 and the Access to Health Records Act 1990. However the Access to Health Records Act 1990 still governs access to the health records of deceased people. The Data Protection Act 1998 gives every living person the right to apply for access to their health records.

For the purposes of the legislation a health record is defined in the Data Protection Act 1998 as a record consisting of information about the physical or mental health or condition of an identifiable individual made by or on behalf of a health professional in connection with the care of that individual. A health record can be recorded in a computerised form, in a manual form or a mixture of both. Health records may include such things as hand-written clinical notes, letters to and from other health professionals, laboratory reports, radiographs and other imaging records (e.g. X-rays and not just X-ray reports), printouts from monitoring equipment, photographs, videos and tape-recordings of telephone conversations.

The Data Protection Act 1998 is not confined to health records held for the purposes of the NHS. It applies equally to the private health sector and to health professionals' private practice records. It also applies to the records of employers who hold information relating to the physical or mental health of their employees, if the record has been made by or on behalf of a health professional in connection with the care of the employee. Individuals have a right to apply for access to records irrespective of when they were compiled. Whereas the Access to Health Records Act 1990 did not provide individuals with a statutory legal right of access to records compiled prior to November 1991, under the Data Protection Act 1998 there is no such limitation.

Individuals are entitled to apply for access to their total health record as it stands at the time the request was received.

The information provided may, however, take account of any amendment or deletion that is made to the record in the period between the request having been received and dealt with. Any amendment or deletion that would have been made regardless of the receipt of the request is not considered, so for example if a set of records were due to be destroyed then there is no right of access to that portion of the record.

The responsibility for dealing with a subject access request lies with the 'data controller'. A data controller is defined in the Data Protection Act 1998 as a person who (either alone or jointly or in common with other persons) determines the purposes for which, and the manner in which, any personal data about an individual are, or are to be, processed. The data controller in a hospital, for example, could be the medical records department manager or their nominated deputy. On receiving a request in writing from a data subject or their representative, the data controller should log the application and immediately examine it to confirm its validity as part of best practice. This is very important as patients have a right to have their personal health information kept confidential.

In accordance with the Data Protection Act 1998 there are certain circumstances in which the record holder may withhold information. Access may be denied, or limited, where the data controller judges that information in the records would cause serious harm to the physical or mental health or condition of the patient, or any other person, or where giving access would disclose information relating to or provided by a third person who had not consented to the disclosure. An example could be where a relative of friend had given information about the behaviour pattern of a mental health patient on admission without the knowledge of the patient. Data controllers must be prepared to justify decisions to withhold information.

If a patient feels information recorded on their health record is incorrect then they should firstly make an informal approach to the health professional concerned to discuss the situation in an attempt to have the records amended. If this avenue is unsuccessful then they may pursue a complaint under the NHS complaints procedure in an attempt to have the information corrected or erased.

Access to health records for children may be permitted to any person with parental responsibility and can therefore apply to access to a child's health record. For the purposes of the legislation parental responsibility for a child is defined in the Children Act 1989 as 'all the rights, duties, powers, responsibilities and authority which by law a parent of a child has in relation to the child and his property'. Although not defined specifically, responsibilities therefore would include:

+ safeguarding and promoting a child's health, development and welfare;
+ financially supporting the child;
+ maintaining direct and regular contact with the child.

Access to a child's health record may be refused as the child grows older and gains sufficient understanding – they will be able to make decisions about their own life. Where a child is considered capable of making decisions about their medical treatment, the consent of the child must be sought before a person with parental responsibility can be given access. Where, in the view of the appropriate health professional, the child patient is not capable of understanding the nature of the application, the holder of the record is entitled to deny access if it were not felt to be in the patient's best interests.

Nursing has evolved into a unique, clearly identified and regulated profession that is governed by legislation and the NMC. As a registered professional, the nurse is accountable in a range of spheres and has a duty of care to provide a professional service in accordance with best practice and the law.

It is essential that the nurse has a fundamental awareness of issues relating to employment legislation such as the Health and Safety at Work Act 1974 and COSHH. In addition the nurse must be confidently aware of the laws relating to consent of patients of all ages, data protection, advanced directives and the Mental Health Act.

CRITICAL REFLECTION

Let us revisit the case study on page 29. Now that you have read this chapter what must the nurse consider and ensure when examining the advanced directive?

Does consent have to be given before Dianne receives treatment for her infection? Who is the nurse accountable to in this situation?

CHAPTER HIGHLIGHTS

+ Nurse regulation has developed from 1840 to the present day and is now regulated in the UK by the NMC.
+ The role of the NMC not only consists of nurse regulation but protection of the public via the publication of standards for practitioners.
+ Nurses are accountable to the public, their employers and the profession of nursing.
+ The Human Rights Act 1998 ensures that all patients have the right to life and treatment with dignity.
+ Nurses have a duty of care to patients via the NMC and their employer via the Health and Safety at Work Act 1974.

+ All employees in the health sector have to be aware of the COSHH Regulations 2002 and RIDDOR Regulations 1995 when considering their work practices.
+ All patients must give consent to treatment and special consideration should be given to children in accordance with the Children Act 1989 and Gillick competence.
+ The Mental Health Act 1983 considers the assessment, treatment and rights of people with a mental health condition.
+ The Data Protection Act 1998 and the Access to Health Records Act 1990 establish guidelines for the storage and management of information relating to patients, including health records.

GUIDANCE

For the full texts of Acts and Regulations mentioned in this chapter see www.legislation.hmso.gov.uk.

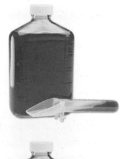

REFERENCE

Dimmond, B. (2005) *Legal aspects of nursing* (4th edn), Harlow: Pearson.

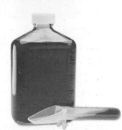

Chapter 4

Professional and Ethical Aspects of Nursing

Learning Outcomes

After completing this chapter, you will be able to:

+ Explain how cognitive development, values, moral frameworks and codes of ethics affect moral decisions.

+ Explain how nurses use knowledge of values transmission and values clarification to make ethical decisions and facilitate ethical decision making by patients.

+ When presented with an ethical situation, identify the moral issues and principles involved.

+ Explain the uses and limitations of professional codes of ethics.

+ Discuss common ethical issues currently facing healthcare professionals.

+ Describe ways in which nurses can enhance their ethical decision making and practice.

+ Discuss the advocacy role of the nurse.

CASE STUDY

Britain has the highest teenage pregnancy rate in Europe. In a bid to tackle this problem the Royal College of Nursing (RCN) has proposed that school nurses should be able to provide emergency contraception to teenagers as young as 11 years of age without consulting parents. However the anti-abortion charity Life stated that this would make nurses 'agents of the sex industry'.

Nurses face many moral and professional dilemmas in practice. This chapter will consider professional and ethical aspects of nursing.

INTRODUCTION

Within the unique nurse–patient relationship nurses face a multitude of ethical dilemmas. Nurses deal with intimate and fundamental human events such as birth, death and suffering. They are the ones who are there to support and advocate for patients and families facing difficult choices. As a result, nurses consider the morality of their own actions when they face the many ethical issues that surround such sensitive areas.

The present cost-driven environment of nursing care tends to give highest priority to business values. Inadequate staffing and inadequate provision of resources create new moral problems and intensify old ones, making it more critical than ever for nurses to make sound moral decisions. Therefore, nurses need to (a) develop sensitivity to the ethical dimensions of nursing practice, (b) examine their own and their patients' values, (c) understand how values influence their decisions, and (d) think ahead about the kinds of moral problems they are likely to face. This chapter explores the influences of values and moral frameworks on the ethical dimensions of nursing practice and on the nurse's role as a patient advocate.

VALUES

Values are our personal beliefs and attitudes about a person, object, idea or action. Values are important because they influence decisions and actions, including nurses' ethical decision making. Even though they may be unspoken and perhaps even unconsciously held, questions of value underlie all moral dilemmas. Of course, not all values are moral values. For example, people hold values about work, family, religion, politics, money and relationships, to name just a few. Values are often taken for granted. In the same way that people are not aware of their breathing, they usually do not think about their values; they simply accept them and act on them.

A **value set** is the small group of values held by an individual. People organise their set of values internally along a continuum from most important to least important, forming a **value system**. Value systems are basic to a way of life, give direction to life and form the basis of behaviour – especially behaviour that is based on decisions or choices.

Beliefs and attitudes are related to, but not identical to, values. People have many different beliefs and attitudes, but only a small number of values. **Beliefs** (or opinions) are assumptions that the individual accepts as being true. They are based more on faith than fact and may or may not be true. Beliefs do not necessarily involve values. For example, the statement 'I believe if I study hard I will get a good grade' expresses a belief that does not involve a value. While statements such as 'Good grades are really important to me. I believe I must study hard to obtain good grades' involves both a belief and a value.

Attitudes are the individual's way of thinking, behaving and feeling. Attitudes can be positive, negative or neutral to a particular person, object and action, and tend to develop and continue over time, whereas a belief may last only briefly.

Attitudes are often judged as bad or good, positive or negative, whereas beliefs are judged as correct or incorrect. Attitudes have thinking and behavioural aspects, but feelings are an especially important component because they vary so greatly among individuals. For example, some patients may feel strongly about their need for privacy, whereas others may dismiss it as unimportant.

Values Transmission

Values are learned through observation and experience. As a result, they are heavily influenced by a person's sociocultural environment – that is, by traditions, cultural, ethnic and religious groups; and by family and peer groups. For example, if a parent consistently demonstrates honesty in dealing with others, the child will probably begin to value honesty.

Personal Values

Although people derive values from society and their individual subgroups, they internalise some or all of these values and perceive them as **personal values**. People need societal values to feel accepted, and they need personal values to have a sense of individuality.

Professional Values

Nurses' **professional values** are acquired during socialisation into nursing from codes of ethics, nursing experiences, teachers and peers. Waters (2005) states that the core fixed values of nursing are:

+ compassion
+ teamwork
+ versatility
+ making a difference.

The Nursing and Midwifery Council (NMC) further clarifies these values (see *Box 4-2* on page 45).

Values, whether personal or professional, can be developed. Indeed there is an expectation that nurses as part of their personal and professional development identify and examine their own values in a process of **values clarification**. A principle of values clarification is that no one set of values is right for everyone. When people can identify their values, they can retain or change them and thus act on the basis of freely chosen, rather than unconscious, values. Values clarification promotes personal growth by fostering awareness, empathy and insight. Therefore, it is an important step for nurses to take in dealing with ethical problems.

Clarifying the Nurse's Values

Nurses and student nurses need to examine the values they hold about life, death, health and illness. One strategy for gaining awareness of personal values is to consider one's attitudes about specific issues such as termination of pregnancy or euthanasia, asking: 'Can I accept this, or live with this?', 'Why does this bother me?', 'What would I do or want done in this situation?'

Table 4-1 Behaviours that May Indicate Unclear Values

Behaviour	Example
Ignoring a health professional's advice	A patient with heart disease who values hard work ignores advice to exercise regularly.
Inconsistent communication or behaviour	A pregnant woman says she wants a healthy baby, but continues to drink alcohol and smoke tobacco.
Numerous admissions to a health agency for the same problem	A middle-aged, obese woman repeatedly seeks help for back pain but does not lose weight.
Confusion or uncertainty about which course of action to take	A woman wants to obtain a job to meet financial obligations, but also wants to stay at home to care for an ailing husband.

Clarifying Patient Values

To plan effective care, nurses need to identify patients' values as they influence and relate to their particular health problem. A patient's personal values can have an impact on the perception of their health problem: for example, a patient with failing eyesight will probably place a high value on the ability to see or a patient with chronic pain will value comfort. Normally, people take such things for granted. When patients hold unclear or conflicting values that are detrimental to their health, the nurse may find it difficult to manage the patient. This may require the nurse to ask the patient to identify and examine their values and aid development of these values. Table 4-1 provides some examples of behaviours that may require the nurse to clarify the patient's personal values.

The following process may help patients clarify their values.

1. *List alternatives.* Make sure that the patient is aware of all alternative actions. Ask 'Are you considering other courses of action? Tell me about them.'
2. *Examine possible consequences of choices.* Make sure the patient has thought about possible results of each action. Ask: 'What do you think you will gain from doing that?', 'What benefits do you foresee from doing that?'
3. *Choose freely.* To determine whether the patient chose freely, ask 'Did you have any say in that decision?', 'Do you have a choice?'
4. *Feel good about the choice.* To determine how the patient feels, ask 'How do you feel about that decision (or action)?' Because some patients may not feel satisfied with their decision, a more sensitive question may be 'Some people feel good after a decision is made; others feel bad. How do you feel?'
5. *Affirm the choice.* Ask 'What will you say to others (family, friends) about this?'
6. *Act on the choice.* To determine whether the patient is prepared to act on the decisions, ask, for example, 'Will it be difficult to tell your wife about this?'
7. *Act with a pattern.* To determine whether the patient consistently behaves in a certain way, ask 'How many times have you done that before?' or 'Would you act that way again?'

When implementing these seven steps to clarify values, the nurse assists the patient to think each question through, but does not impose personal values. The nurse offers an opinion only when the patient asks for it – and then only with care.

MORALITY AND ETHICS

Ethics has several meanings, some of which are quite ambiguous. It can be defined as a set of values that define right and wrong or a guide to decisions relating to moral duty and obligations. Ethics are generally perceived as a set of standards that encompass the norms of a community.

Bioethics, on the other hand, are the ethics as applied to life (e.g. to decisions about termination of pregnancy or euthanasia), while, **nursing ethics** refers to ethical issues that occur in nursing practice. The NMC 'Code of Professional Conduct' (2004) holds nurses accountable for their ethical conduct.

Morality (or morals) is similar to ethics and many use the terms interchangeably. **Morality** usually refers to private, personal standards of what is right and wrong in conduct, character and attitude. Sometimes the first clue to the moral nature of a situation is an aroused conscience or an awareness of feelings such as guilt, hope or shame. Another indicator is the tendency to respond to the situation with words such as *ought, should, right, wrong, good* and *bad*. Moral issues are concerned with important social values and norms; they are not about trivial things.

Nurses should distinguish between morality and law. Laws do reflect the moral values of a society, and they offer guidance in determining what is moral. However, an action can be legal but not moral. For example, an order for full resuscitation of a dying patient is legal, but one could still question whether the act is moral. On the other hand, an action can be moral but illegal. For example, if a child at home stops breathing, it is moral but not legal to exceed the speed limit when driving to the hospital. Legal aspects of nursing practice are covered in Chapter 3.

Nurses should also distinguish between morality and religion, although the two concepts are related. For example, according to some religious beliefs, women should undergo procedures such as female circumcision that may cause physical mutilation. Other religions or groups may consider this practice to be a violation of human rights (Sala and Manara, 2001).

> ## CLINICAL ALERT
>
> *Confucian religious beliefs do not consider a foetus a human being. However, Buddhists believe the foetus is a form of life. Thus, Chinese people vary in their views on termination of pregnancy depending on religious affiliation.*

Moral Development

Ethical decisions require nurses to think and reason before making a decision. Reasoning is a cognitive function and is, therefore, developmental. Individual moral or ethical values develop over time. **Moral development**, the process of learning to tell the difference between right and wrong and of learning what ought and ought not to be done, is a complex process that begins in childhood and continues throughout life.

Theories of moral development attempt to answer questions such as:

+ How does a person become moral?
+ What factors influence the way a person behaves in a moral situation?

Two well-known theorists of moral development are Lawrence Kohlberg (1969) and Carol Gilligan (1982). Kohlberg's theory emphasises rights and formal reasoning; Gilligan's theory emphasises care and responsibility, although it points out that people use the concepts of both theorists in their moral reasoning.

Moral Frameworks

Some nurses believe that ethics has very little to do with their practice. However when faced with the situation when one patient needs a bedpan and another's intravenous infusion pump is alarming, who does the nurse go to first? The nurse is faced with an ethical dilemma and a decision needs to be made but what does the nurse base her decision on. Such decisions can be based on one of two ethical models: (1) consequences (teleology) or (2) principles and duty (deontology).

Consequence-based (teleological) theories look to the consequences of an action in judging whether that action is right or wrong. **Utilitarianism**, one form of teleology, views a good act as one that brings the most good and the least harm for the greatest number of people. This approach is often used in making decisions about the funding and delivery of healthcare. For example, some trusts are reluctant to prescribe expensive drugs such as Herceptin (a treatment for breast cancer) as they feel that the money spent on one person could treat three patients requiring operations such as knee or hip replacements.

Principles-based (deontological) theories argue that there are basic duties and obligations with which people should conform. This means that the action is not judged on its consequence but is judged on whether it agrees with moral principles. For example, is it morally right to sterilise a mentally handicapped teenager to prevent her from conceiving? In deontologist eyes the act of sterilising the teenager would be morally wrong as there is no health reason for the sterilisation and the procedure infringes her human rights.

A moral model or framework guides moral decisions, but does not determine the outcome. This can be illustrated by imagining a situation in which a frail, elderly patient has insisted that he does not want further surgery, but the family and surgeon insist. Two nurses have each decided that they will not help with preparations for surgery and that they will work through proper channels to try to prevent it. Using consequence-based reasoning, Nurse A thinks, 'Surgery will cause him more suffering; he probably will not survive it anyway; and the family may even feel guilty later.' While Nurse B, using principles-based reasoning, thinks, 'This violates the principle of autonomy. This man has a right to decide what happens to his body.'

Moral Principles

Applying these models or frameworks in everyday practice would involve a deep knowledge of the models and their intricacies. Therefore, in order for individuals to work with these models or frameworks, moral principles have been established. Moral principles are statements about broad, general, philosophical concepts such as autonomy and justice. They provide the foundation for **moral rules**, which are specific prescriptions for actions. For example, the rule 'People should not lie' is based on the moral principle of respect for persons (autonomy).

Autonomy refers to the right to make one's own decisions. Nurses who follow this principle recognise that each patient is unique, has the right to be what that person is, and has the right to choose personal goals.

Honouring the principle of autonomy means that the nurse respects a patient's right to make decisions even when those choices seem to the nurse not to be in the patient's best interest. It also means treating others with consideration. In a healthcare setting this principle is violated, for example, when a nurse disregards patients' subjective accounts of their symptoms (e.g. pain). Finally, respect for autonomy means that people should not be treated as an impersonal source of knowledge or training. This principle comes into play, for example, in the requirement that patients provide informed consent before tests, procedures, research or being a teaching subject, can be carried out (see Chapter 3).

Nonmaleficence is duty to 'do no harm'. Although this would seem to be a simple principle to follow, in reality it is complex. Harm can mean intentionally causing harm, placing someone at risk of harm and unintentionally causing harm. In nursing, intentional harm is never acceptable. However, placing a person at risk of harm has many facets. A patient may be at risk of harm as a known consequence of a nursing intervention that is intended to be helpful. For example, a patient may react adversely to a medication. Unintentional harm occurs when the risk could not have been anticipated. For example, while trying to catch a patient who is falling, the nurse grips the patient tightly enough to cause bruises to the patient's arm.

Beneficence means 'doing good'. Nurses are obligated to do good, that is, to implement actions that benefit patients and their support persons. However, doing good can also pose a risk of doing harm. For example, a nurse may advise a patient about a strenuous exercise programme to improve general health, but should not do so if the patient is at risk of a heart attack.

Justice is often referred to as fairness. Nurses often face decisions in which a sense of justice should prevail. For example, a nurse making home visits finds one patient tearful and depressed, and knows she could help by staying for 30 more minutes to talk. However, that would take time from her next patient, who is a diabetic and needs a great deal of teaching and observation. The nurse will need to weigh the facts carefully in order to divide her time justly among her patients.

Fidelity means to be faithful to agreements and promises. By virtue of their standing, nurses have responsibilities to patients, employers, government and society, as well as to themselves. Nurses often make promises such as 'I'll be right back with your pain medication' or 'I'll find out for you.' Patients take such promises seriously, and so should nurses.

Veracity refers to telling the truth. Although this seems straightforward, in practice choices are not always clear. Should a nurse tell the truth when it is known that it will cause harm? Does a nurse tell a lie when it is known that the lie will relieve anxiety and fear? Lying to sick or dying people is rarely justified. The loss of trust in the nurse and the anxiety caused by not knowing the truth, for example, usually outweigh any benefits derived from lying.

Nurses must also have professional accountability and responsibility. According to *The Code of Professional Conduct* (NMC, 2004), nurses are personally accountable for their practice, which the NMC defines as being answerable for any actions or omissions that the nurse might make. On the other hand, **responsibility** refers to the accountability or liability associated with the duties undertaken by the nurse. Thus, the ethical nurse is able to explain the rationale behind every action and recognises the standards to which they will be held accountable.

NURSING ETHICS

In the past, nurses looked on ethical decision making as the doctor's responsibility. However, no one profession is responsible for ethical decisions, nor does expertise in one discipline such as medicine or nursing necessarily make a person an expert in ethics. As situations become more complex, input from all caregivers becomes increasingly important.

Indeed there is an increasing awareness of the importance of ethical issues in healthcare and as such **clinical ethical committees** have been developed. Currently only a handful of

NHS Trusts within the UK have such committees. The role of the clinical ethical committee is to:

+ provide ethical input into policy making and development of guidelines for practice;
+ facilitate ethics education for healthcare professionals;
+ provide ethical advice on specific ethical dilemmas.

The committees are made up of doctors from different specialities including mental health, public health and general practice, nurses, social workers, therapists such as physiotherapists, professionals with backgrounds in religion, philosophy and law, and usually a member of the Trust board and representatives of the public.

Ethical committees ensure that the relevant facts of a case are brought out, provide a forum in which diverse views can be expressed, provide support for caregivers, and can reduce the Trust's legal risks.

Codes of Ethics in Nursing

A **code of ethics** is a formal statement of a group's ideals and values. It is a set of ethical principles that (a) is shared by members of the group, (b) reflects their moral judgements over time, and (c) serves as a standard for their professional actions. Codes of ethics usually have higher requirements than legal standards, and they are never lower than the legal standards of the profession. Nurses are responsible for being familiar with the code that governs their practice.

International and national nursing associations have established codes of ethics. The International Council of Nurses (ICN) first adopted a code of ethics in 1953 and the most recent revisions are shown in *Box 4-1*. The Nursing and Midwifery Council has recently updated the 'Code of Professional Conduct' to encompass not only professional conduct and performance but also ethics. For a summary of the current version see *Box 4-2*.

Nursing codes of ethics have the following purposes:

1. Inform the public about the minimum standards of the profession and help them understand professional nursing conduct.
2. Provide a sign of the profession's commitment to the public it serves.
3. Outline the major ethical considerations of the profession.
4. Provide ethical standards for professional behaviour.
5. Guide the profession in self-regulation.
6. Remind nurses of the special responsibility they assume when caring for the sick.

Making Ethical Decisions

Ethical dilemmas differ from problems. Problems can be solved whereas ethical dilemmas require a choice to be made. Responsible ethical reasoning is rational and systematic and should be based on ethical principles and codes rather than on emotions, intuition, fixed policies or precedent (that is, an earlier similar occurrence).

BOX 4-1 International Council of Nurses Code of Ethics

Preamble

Nurses have four fundamental responsibilities: to promote health, to prevent illness, to restore health and to alleviate suffering. The need for nursing is universal.

Inherent in nursing is respect for human rights, including the right to life, to dignity and to be treated with respect. Nursing care is unrestricted by considerations of age, colour, creed, culture, disability or illness, gender, nationality, politics, race or social status.

Nurses render health services to the individual, the family and the community and coordinate their services with those of related groups.

The Code

The *ICN Code of Ethics for Nurses* has four principal elements that outline the standards of ethical conduct.

Elements of the Code

1. **Nurses and people**

   The nurse's primary professional responsibility is to people requiring nursing care.

   In providing care, the nurse promotes an environment in which the human rights, values, customs and spiritual beliefs of the individual, family and community are respected.

   The nurse ensures that the individual receives sufficient information on which to base consent for care and related treatment.

   The nurse holds in confidence personal information and uses judgement in sharing this information.

   The nurse shares with society the responsibility for initiating and supporting action to meet the health and social needs of the public, in particular those of vulnerable populations.

The nurse also shares responsibility to sustain and protect the natural environment from depletion, pollution, degradation and destruction.

2. **Nurses and practice**

   The nurse carries personal responsibility and accountability for nursing practice, and for maintaining competence by continual learning.

   The nurse maintains a standard of personal health such that the ability to provide care is not compromised.

   The nurse uses judgement regarding individual competence when accepting and delegating responsibility.

   The nurse at all times maintains standards of personal conduct that reflect well on the profession and enhance public confidence.

   The nurse, in providing care, ensures that use of technology and scientific advances are compatible with the safety, dignity and rights of people.

3. **Nurses and the profession**

   The nurse assumes the major role in determining and implementing acceptable standards of clinical nursing practice, management, research and education.

   The nurse is active in developing a core of research-based professional knowledge.

   The nurse, acting through the professional organisation, participates in creating and maintaining equitable social and economic working conditions in nursing.

4. **Nurses and co-workers**

   The nurse sustains a cooperative relationship with co-workers in nursing and other fields.

   The nurse takes appropriate action to safeguard individuals when their care is endangered by a co-worker or any other person.

Note: From *ICN Code of Ethics for Nurses*, International Council of Nurses, 2000, Geneva: Imprimeries Populaires. Reprinted with permission. Copyright © 2006 by ICN-International Council of Nurses, 3 place Jean-Marteau, 1201 Geneva, Switzerland.

BOX 4-2 The NMC Code of Professional Conduct: Standards for Conduct, Performance and Ethics (2004)

As a registered nurse, midwife or specialist community public health nurse, you are personally accountable for your practice. In caring for patients and clients, you must:

+ Respect the patient or client as an individual
+ Obtain consent before you give any treatment or care

+ Protect confidential information
+ Cooperate with others in the team
+ Maintain professional knowledge and competence
+ Be trustworthy
+ Act to identify and minimise risk to patients and clients.

Note: From Nursing and Midwifery Council (2004) *Code of Professional Conduct: Standards for Conduct, Performance and Ethics*, Nursing and Midwifery Council, London.

BOX 4-3 Examples of Nurses' Obligations in Ethical Decisions

+ Maximise the patient's well-being.
+ Balance the patient's need for autonomy with family members' responsibilities for the patient's well-being.
+ Support each family member and enhance the family support system.
+ Carry out hospital policies.
+ Protect other patients' well-being.
+ Protect the nurse's own standards of care.

A good decision is one that is in the patient's best interest and at the same time preserves the integrity of all involved. Nurses have ethical obligations to their patients, to their employers and to other healthcare professionals. Therefore, nurses must weigh competing factors when making ethical decisions (see *Box 4-3* for some examples). Although ethical reasoning is principle-based and has the patient's well-being at heart, being involved in ethical problems and dilemmas is stressful for the nurse. The nurse may feel torn between obligations to the patient, the family and the employer. What is in the patient's best interest may be contrary to the nurse's personal belief system. In settings in which ethical issues arise frequently, nurses should establish support systems such as clinical supervision, counselling and debriefing sessions to allow expression of their feelings.

Many nursing problems are not moral problems at all, but simply questions of good nursing practice. An important first step in ethical decision making is to determine whether a moral situation exists. The following criteria may be used:

+ A difficult choice exists between actions that conflict with the needs of one or more persons.
+ Moral principles or frameworks exist that can be used to provide some justification for the action.
+ The choice is guided by a process of weighing reasons.
+ The decision must be freely and consciously chosen.
+ The choice is affected by personal feelings and by the particular context of the situation.

Although the nurse's input is important, in reality several people are usually involved in making an ethical decision. Therefore, collaboration, communication and compromise are important skills for health professionals. When nurses do not have the autonomy to act on their moral or ethical choices, compromise becomes essential.

CLINICAL ALERT

Ethical behaviour is contextual – what is an ethical action or decision in one situation may not be ethical in a different situation.

Strategies to Enhance Ethical Decisions and Practice

Several strategies help nurses overcome possible organisational and social constraints that may hinder the ethical practice of nursing and create moral distress for nurses. You as a nurse should do the following:

+ Become aware of your own values and the ethical aspects of nursing.
+ Be familiar with nursing codes of ethics.
+ Respect the values, opinions and responsibilities of other healthcare professionals that may be different from your own.
+ Strive for collaborative practice in which nurses function effectively in cooperation with other healthcare professionals.

SPECIFIC ETHICAL ISSUES

Some of the ethical problems the nurse encounters most frequently are issues in the care of patients undergoing termination of pregnancy, organ transplantation, end-of-life decisions and breaches of patient confidentiality.

Termination of Pregnancy

Termination of pregnancy is a highly publicised issue about which many people feel very strongly. Debate continues, pitting the principle of sanctity of life against the principle of autonomy and the woman's right to control her own body. This is an especially volatile issue because no public consensus has yet been reached.

Under the Abortion Act 1967 nurses have the right to refuse to assist with an termination of pregnancy if doing so violates their religious or moral principles. However, nurses have no right to impose their values on a patient. Nursing codes of ethics support patients' rights to information and counselling in making decisions.

Organ Transplantation

Organs for transplantation may come from living donors or from donors who have just died. Ethical issues related to organ transplantation include allocation of organs, selling of body parts, involvement of children as potential donors, consent, clear definition of death, and conflicts of interest between potential donors and recipients. In some situations, a person's religious belief may also present conflict. For example, certain religions forbid the mutilation of the body, even for the benefit of another person.

End-of-Life Issues

The increase in technological advances and the growing number of older adults have expanded the ethical dilemmas faced by healthcare professionals. Providing patients, who are at the end of life, with information and professional assistance, as well as the highest quality of care and caring, is of the utmost importance. Some of the most frequent disturbing ethical problems for nurses involve issues that arise around death and dying. These include euthanasia, assisted suicide, termination of life-sustaining treatment, and withdrawing or withholding of food and fluids.

Euthanasia and Assisted Suicide

Euthanasia, a Greek word meaning 'good death', is popularly known as 'mercy killing', **Active euthanasia** involves actions to directly bring about the patient's death, with or without patient consent. An example of this would be the administration of a lethal medication to end the patient's suffering. Regardless of the caregiver's intent, active euthanasia is forbidden by law and can result in criminal charges of murder.

Active euthanasia includes **assisted suicide**, or giving patients the means to kill themselves if they request it (e.g. providing pills or a weapon). Some countries have laws permitting assisted suicide for patients who are severely ill, near death and who wish to kill themselves. In any case, the nurse should recall that legality and morality are not one and the same. Determining whether an action is legal is only one aspect of deciding whether it is ethical. The questions of suicide and assisted suicide are still controversial in our society.

Passive euthanasia involves the withdrawal of extraordinary means of life support, such as removing a ventilator or withholding special attempts to resuscitate a patient (e.g. do not resuscitate orders).

Withdrawing or Withholding Food and Fluids

It is generally accepted that providing food and fluids is part of ordinary nursing practice and, therefore, a moral duty. However, when food and fluids are administered by tube to a dying patient, or are given over a long period of time to an unconscious patient who is not expected to improve, then some consider it to be an extraordinary, or heroic, measure. A nurse is morally obligated to withhold food and fluids (or any treatment) if it is determined to be more harmful to administer them than to withhold them. The nurse must also honour competent patients' refusal of food and fluids.

Confidentiality

In keeping with the principle of autonomy, nurses are obligated to respect patients' privacy and confidentiality. Patients must be able to trust that nurses will reveal details of their situations only as appropriate and will communicate only the information necessary to provide for their healthcare. Computerised patient records make sensitive data accessible to more people and emphasise issues of confidentiality. Nurses should help develop and follow security measures and policies to ensure appropriate use of patient data. For example, nurses should not give their system security codes to unauthorised persons to allow access to computer files.

ADVOCACY

When people are ill, they are frequently unable to assert their rights as they would if they were healthy. An **advocate** is one who expresses and defends the cause of another. A **patient advocate** is an advocate for patients' rights. The healthcare system is complex and many patients are too ill to deal with it. If they are to be kept from 'falling through the cracks', patients need an advocate to cut through the layers of bureaucracy and help them get what they require. Values basic to patient advocacy are shown in *Box 4-4*. Patients may also advocate for themselves. Today, patients are seeking more self-determination and control over their own bodies when they are ill.

If a patient lacks decision-making capacity, is legally incompetent or is a minor, these rights can be exercised on the patient's behalf by a designated individual. It is important, however, for the nurse to remember that patient control over health decisions is a Western view. In other countries and societies, such decisions may normally be made by the head of the family or another member of the community. The nurse must ascertain the patient's and family's views and honour their traditions regarding the locus of decision making.

The Advocate's Role

The overall goal of the patient advocate is to protect patients' rights. An advocate informs patients about their rights and provides them with the information they need to make informed decisions.

An advocate supports patients in their decisions, giving them full or at least mutual responsibility in decision making when they are capable of it. The advocate must be careful to remain objective and not convey approval or disapproval of the patient's choices. Advocacy requires accepting and respecting the patient's right to decide, even if the nurse believes the decision to be wrong.

In mediating, the advocate directly intervenes on the patient's behalf, often by influencing others. An example of acting on behalf of a patient is asking a doctor to review with the patient the reasons for and the expected duration of therapy because the patient says he always forgets to ask the doctor.

BOX 4-4 Values Basic to Patient Advocacy

+ The patient is a holistic, autonomous being who has the right to make choices and decisions.
+ Patients have the right to expect a nurse-patient relationship that is based on shared respect, trust, collaboration in solving problems related to health and healthcare needs, and consideration of their thoughts and feelings.
+ It is the nurse's responsibility to ensure the patient has access to healthcare services that meet health needs.

Advocacy in the Community Setting

Although the goals of advocacy remain the same, caring for a person at home poses unique concerns for the nurse advocate. For example, while in the hospital, people may operate from the values of the hospital and the healthcare professionals. When they are at home they tend to operate from their own personal values, and may revert to old habits and ways of doing things that may not be beneficial to their health. The nurse may see this as noncompliance; nevertheless, patient autonomy must be respected.

Professional and Public Advocacy

Nurses who function responsibly as professional and public advocates are in a position to effect change. To act as an advocate in this arena, the nurse needs an understanding of the ethical issues in nursing and healthcare, as well as knowledge of the laws and regulations that affect nursing practice and the health of society (see Chapter 3).

Being an effective patient advocate involves the following:

+ being assertive;
+ recognising that the rights and values of patients and families must take precedence when they conflict with those of healthcare providers;
+ being aware that conflicts may arise over issues that require consultation, confrontation or negotiation between the nurse and administrative personnel, or between the nurse and doctor;
+ working with community agencies and lay practitioners;
+ knowing that advocacy may require political action – communicating a patient's healthcare needs to government and other officials who have the authority to do something about these needs.

CRITICAL REFLECTION

Let us revisit the case study on page 40. Now that you have read this chapter do you think that children as young as 12 should be given emergency contraception without consulting their parents? What are your own personal values with regard to this matter? Would you say these values are based on consequence or duty? Would these values affect your ability to make decisions about whether to offer teenagers contraception?

CHAPTER HIGHLIGHTS

+ Values give direction and meaning to life and guide a person's behaviour.
+ Values are freely chosen, prized and cherished, affirmed to others, and consistently incorporated into one's behaviour.
+ Values clarification is a process in which people identify, examine and develop their own values.
+ Nursing ethics refers to the moral problems that arise in nursing practice and to ethical decisions that nurses make.
+ Morality refers to what is right and wrong in conduct, character or attitude.
+ Moral issues are those that arouse conscience, are concerned with important values and norms, and evoke words such as *good, bad, right, wrong, should* and *ought.*
+ Three common moral frameworks (approaches) are consequence-based (teleologic), principles-based (deontologic) and relationships-based (caring-based) theories.

+ Moral principles (e.g. autonomy, beneficence, nonmaleficence, justice, fidelity and veracity) are broad, general philosophical concepts that can be used to make and explain moral choices.
+ A professional code of ethics is a formal statement of a group's ideals and values that serves as a standard and guideline for the group's professional actions and informs the public of its commitment.
+ Nurses' ethical decisions are influenced by their moral theories and principles, levels of cognitive development, personal and professional values, and nursing codes of ethics.
+ The goal of ethical reasoning, in the context of nursing, is to reach a mutual, peaceful agreement that is in the best interests of the patient; reaching the agreement may require compromise.
+ Nurses are responsible for determining their own actions and for supporting patients who are making

- moral decisions or for whom decisions are being made by others.
- Nurses can enhance their ethical practice and patient advocacy by clarifying their own values, understanding the values of other healthcare professionals, and becoming familiar with nursing codes of ethics.
- Patient advocacy involves concern for and actions on behalf of another person or organisation in order to bring about change.
- The functions of the advocacy role are to inform, support and mediate.

REFERENCES

Gilligan, C. (1982) *In a different voice*. Cambridge, MA: Harvard University Press.

International Council of Nurses (2000) *ICN code for nurses: Ethical concepts applied to nursing*, Geneva: Imprimeries Populaires.

Kohlberg, L. (1969) 'Stage and sequence: The cognitive-developmental approach to socialisation', in D.A. Goslin (Edn), *Handbook of socialisation theory and research* (pp. 347–480), Chicago: Rand McNally.

NMC (2004) *Code of Professional Conduct – standards for conduct performance and ethics*, London: NMC.

Sala, R. and Manara, D. (2001) 'Nurses and requests for female genital mutilation: Cultural rights versus human rights', *Nursing Ethics*, 8, 247–258.

Waters, A. (2005) 'Nursing is the most emotionally rewarding career', *Nursing Standard*, 19(30), 22–28.

Chapter 5 Health, Wellness and Illness

Learning Outcomes

After completing this chapter, you will be able to:

+ Differentiate health, wellness and well-being.
+ Describe five dimensions of wellness.
+ Identify factors affecting health status, beliefs and practices.
+ Differentiate illness from disease and acute illness from chronic illness.
+ Identify Parsons' four aspects of the sick role.
+ Describe the effects of illness on individuals' and family members' roles and functions.
+ Explain the relationship of individuality and holism to nursing practice.
+ Give four main characteristics of homoeostatic mechanisms.
+ Identify common risk factors regarding family health.
+ Identify theoretical frameworks used in individual and family health promotion.
+ Identify various types of communities.

CASE STUDY

David is 50 years old and has been admitted to your care. Sarah, his daughter, asks you to explain why her father, who has been recently diagnosed with Chronic Obstructive Pulmonary Disease (COPD), which is a chronic condition, has been admitted with an acute infection. Although he has this chronic illness he normally feels fit and well and cannot understand why he feels so unwell at the moment.

As you discuss with Sarah you discover that David is not taking his prescribed medications as he does not believe in taking tablets. As you explain the differences between chronic and acute illness, you also explain the need to adhere to prescribed medications by using health belief models.

After reading this chapter you will be able to differentiate between health, wellness and illness and be able to understand the impact chronic diseases like COPD can have on a person's well-being.

INTRODUCTION

Nurses need to clarify their understanding of health and wellness because their definitions largely determine the scope and nature of nursing practice. As individuals we all have a unique outlook on the world of health determined by our own life experiences and those of healthcare. Patients' health beliefs also influence nurses' health practices. Some people think of health and wellness (or well-being) as the same thing or, at the very least, as accompanying one another. However, health may not always accompany well-being: a person who has a terminal illness may have a sense of well-being; conversely, another person may lack a sense of well-being yet be in a state of good health. For many years the concept of disease was the measure by which health was monitored. In the late 19th century the 'how' of disease (pathogenesis) was the major concern of health professionals. Currently the emphasis on health and wellness is increasing.

CONCEPTS OF HEALTH, WELLNESS AND WELL-BEING

Health, wellness and well-being have many definitions and interpretations. The nurse should be familiar with the most common aspects of the concepts and consider how they may be individualised with specific patients.

Health

There is no consensus about any definition of health. There is knowledge of how to attain a certain level of health, but health itself cannot be measured as this is subjective to the individual.

Traditionally **health** has been defined in terms of the presence or absence of disease. Nightingale defined health as a state of being well and using every power the individual possesses to the fullest extent (Nightingale, 1969). The World Health Organization (WHO) takes a more holistic view of health. Its constitution defines health as 'a state of complete physical, mental, and social well-being, and not merely the absence of disease or infirmity' (WHO, 1948). This definition:

+ Reflects concern for the individual as a total person functioning physically, psychologically and socially. Mental processes determine people's relationship with their physical and social surroundings, their attitudes about life and their interaction with others.
+ Places health in the context of environment. People's lives, and therefore their health, are affected by everything they interact with – not only environmental influences such as climate and the availability of nutritious food, comfortable shelter, clean air to breathe and pure water to drink, but also other people, including family, lovers, employers, co-workers, friends and associates of various kinds.
+ Equates health with productive and creative living. It focuses on the living state rather than on categories of disease that may cause illness or death.

Health has also been defined in terms of role and performance. Talcott Parsons (1951), an eminent sociologist and creator of the concept 'sick role', conceptualised health as the ability to maintain normal roles. Parsons utilised social concepts of norms to construct a theoretical view of individuals who are sick, hence the 'sick role'.

The Ottowa Charter (published in 1986) was developed during the first international conference on health promotion. It suggests health is seen as 'the extent to which an individual or group is able, on the one hand, to identify and to realise aspirations and satisfy needs, and on the other, to change or cope with the environment. Health is therefore seen as a resource for everyday life, not the objective of living; it is a positive concept, encompassing social and personal resources as well as physical capacities.'

In the past few decades a number of health professionals, including nurse theorists, have provided definitions of health and wellness.

Personal Definitions of Health

Health is a highly individual perception. Consider the following examples of individuals who would probably say they are healthy even though they have physical impairments that some would consider an illness:

+ Paul, a 12-year-old with diabetes, needs injectable insulin each morning. He plays on the school football team and is a member of the local theatre group.
+ Daniel, age 24, is paralysed from the waist down and needs a wheelchair for mobility. He is taking computing at a local college and uses a specially designed car for transportation.
+ Heather, age 72, takes antihypertensive medications to treat high blood pressure. She swims once a week is a member of the neighbourhood gardening club, makes handicrafts for a church, and travels internationally on holiday two months each year.

Most people define and describe health as the following:

+ being free from symptoms of disease and pain as much as possible;
+ being able to be active and to do what they want or must;
+ being in good spirits most of the time.

These characteristics indicate that health is not something that a person achieves suddenly at a specific time. It is an ongoing process – a way of life – through which a person develops and encourages every aspect of the body, mind and feelings to interrelate harmoniously as much as possible.

Many factors affect individual definitions of health. Definitions vary according to an individual's previous experiences, expectations of self, age and sociocultural influences.

Nurses should be aware of their own personal definitions of health and should appreciate that other people have their own individual definitions as well. A person's definition of health influences behaviour related to health and illness. By understanding patients' perceptions of health and illness, nurses can

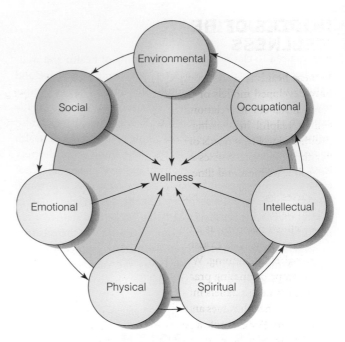

Figure 5-1 The seven components of wellness. (From
Wellness: Concepts and Applications, 6th edn (p. 4), by D.J. Anspaugh,
M.H. Hamrick and F.D. Rosato, copyright 2003, New York: McGraw-
Hill. Reprinted by permission.)

provide more meaningful assistance to help them regain or attain
a state of health. For aid in developing a personal definition of
health, see *Box 5-1*.

Wellness and Well-being

Wellness is a state of well-being – feeling fully fit and ready
for life. Basic concepts of wellness include self-responsibility;
an ultimate goal to achieve in life; a dynamic ever-developing,
growing process; daily decision making in the areas of nutrition, stress management, physical fitness, preventive healthcare, emotional health and other aspects of health; and, most
importantly, the whole being of the individual.

Anspaugh *et al.* (2003: 3–7) propose seven components of
wellness (see Figure 5-1). To realise optimal health and wellness, people must deal with the factors within each component:

+ *Physical.* The ability to carry out daily tasks, achieve fitness
  (e.g. pulmonary, cardiovascular, gastrointestinal), maintain adequate nutrition and proper body fat, avoid abusing
  drugs and alcohol or using tobacco products, and generally
  to practise positive lifestyle habits.
+ *Social.* The ability to interact successfully with people and
  within the environment of which each person is a part, to
  develop and maintain intimacy with significant others, and
  to develop respect and tolerance for those with different
  opinions and beliefs.

+ *Emotional.* The ability to manage stress and to express emotions appropriately. Emotional wellness involves the ability
  to recognise, accept and express feelings, and to accept one's
  limitations.
+ *Intellectual.* The ability to learn and use information effectively for personal, family and career development. Intellectual
  wellness involves striving for continued growth and learning
  to deal with new challenges effectively.
+ *Spiritual.* The belief in some force (nature, science, religion
  or a higher power) that serves to unite human beings and
  provide meaning and purpose to life. It includes a person's
  own morals, values and ethics.
+ *Occupational.* The ability to achieve a balance between
  work and leisure time. A person's beliefs about education,
  employment and home influence personal satisfaction and
  relationships with others.
+ *Environmental.* The ability to promote health measures
  that improve the standard of living and quality of life in the
  community. This includes influences such as food, water
  and air.

The seven components overlap to some extent, and factors
in one component often directly affect factors in another. For
example, a person who learns to control daily stress levels from
a physiological perspective is also helping to maintain the emotional stamina needed to cope with a crisis. Wellness involves
working on all aspects of the model.

'**Well-being** is a subjective perception of vitality and feeling
well . . . can be described objectively, experienced, and measured
. . . and can be plotted on a continuum' (Hood and Leddy, 2002:
264). It is a component of health.

MODELS OF HEALTH AND WELLNESS

Because health is such a complex concept, various researchers have developed models or paradigms to explain health and in some instances its relationship to illness or injury. Models can be helpful in assisting health professionals to meet the health and wellness needs of individuals to formulate a plan of health promotion. Nurses need to clarify their understanding of health, wellness and illness for the following reasons:

+ Nurses' definitions of health largely determine the scope and nature of nursing practice. For example, when health is defined narrowly as a physiological phenomenon, nurses confine themselves to assisting patients to regain normal physiological functioning. When health is defined more broadly, the scope of nursing practice increases correspondingly.

+ People's health beliefs influence their health practices. Thus a nurse's health values and practices may differ from those of a patient. For example a patient may believe that it is appropriate to put butter on a burn whereas the nurse is aware from scientific research that this can be harmful. Nurses need to ensure that a plan of care developed for an individual relates to the patient's conception of health. Otherwise the patient may fail to respond to a healthcare regimen.

Models of health developed from clinical practice and psychology include the clinical model, the role performance model, the adaptive model, the eudemonistic model, the agent–host–environment model and health–illness continua.

Clinical Model

The narrowest interpretation of health occurs in the clinical model. People are viewed as physiological systems with related functions, and health is identified by the absence of signs and symptoms of disease or injury. To laypeople it is considered the state of not being 'sick'. In this model the opposite of health is disease or injury.

Many medical practitioners use the clinical model in their focus on the relief of signs and symptoms of disease and elimination of malfunction and pain. When these signs and symptoms are no longer present, the medical practitioner considers the individual's health restored.

Role Performance Model

Health is defined in terms of the individual's ability to fulfil societal roles, that is, to perform work. According to this model, people who can fulfil their roles are healthy even if they appear clinically ill. For example, a man who works all day at his job as expected is healthy even though an x-ray film of his lung indicates a tumour.

It is assumed in this model that sickness is the inability to perform one's work. A problem with this model is the assumption that a person's most important role is the work role. People usually fulfil several roles (e.g. mother, daughter, friend), and certain individuals may consider nonwork roles paramount in their lives.

Adaptive Model

The focus of the adaptive model is adaptation. In the adaptive model, health is a creative process; disease is a failure in adaptation, or maladaption. The aim of treatment is to restore the ability of the person to adapt, that is, to cope. According to this model, extreme good health is flexible adaptation to the environment and interaction with the environment to maximum advantage. Roy's adaptation model of nursing (Roy, 1999) views the person as an adaptive system (see Chapter 2). The focus of this model is stability, although there is also an element of growth and change.

Murray and Zentner (2001) indicate this growth and change in their definition of health: 'a state of well-being in which the person is able to use purposeful, adaptive responses and processes, physically, mentally, emotionally, spiritually and socially, in response to internal and external stimuli (stressors) in order to maintain relative stability and comfort and to strive for personal objectives and cultural goals'.

Eudemonistic Model

Eudemonism is a system of ethics that evaluates actions in terms of their capacity to produce happiness. The eudemonistic model incorporates a comprehensive view of health. Health is seen as a condition of actualisation or realisation of a person's psychological potential. Actualisation is the top of the fully developed personality, described by Abraham Maslow. In this model the highest aspiration of people is fulfilment and complete development, which is actualisation. Illness, in this model, is a condition that prevents self-actualisation.

Pender, a nurse theorist, includes stabilising and actualising tendencies in her definition of health: 'Health is the actualisation of inherent and acquired human potential through goal-directed behaviour, competent self-care, and satisfying relationships with others while adjustments are made as needed to maintain structural integrity and harmony with relevant environments' (Pender *et al.*, 2002: 22).

Agent–Host–Environment Model

The agent–host–environment model of health and illness also called the ecologic model, originated in the community health work of Leavell and Clark (1965) and has been expanded into a general theory of the multiple causes of disease. The model is used primarily in predicting illness rather than in promoting wellness, although identification of risk factors that result from the interactions of agent, host and environment are helpful in promoting and maintaining health. The model has three dynamic interactive elements (see Figure 5-2 on page 54):

1. *Agent.* Any environmental factor or stressor (biological, chemical, mechanical, physical or psychosocial) that by

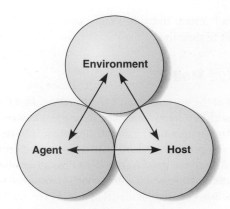

Figure 5-2 The agent-host-environment triangle.

its presence or absence (e.g. lack of essential nutrients) can lead to illness or disease.

2. *Host.* Person(s) who may or may not be at risk of acquiring a disease. Family history, age and lifestyle habits influence the host's reaction.

3. *Environment.* All factors external to the host that may or may not predispose the person to the development of disease. Physical environment includes climate, living conditions, sound (noise) levels and economic level. Social environment includes interactions with others and life events, such as the death of a spouse.

Because each of the agent–host–environment factors constantly interacts with the others, health is an ever-changing state. When the variables are in balance, health is maintained; when variables are not in balance, disease occurs.

Health-Illness Continua

Health–illness continua (graduated scales) can be used to measure a person's perceived level of wellness. Health and illness or disease can be viewed as the opposite ends of a health continuum. From a high level of health a person's condition can move through good health, normal health, poor health and extremely poor health, eventually to death. People move back and forth within this continuum day by day. There is no distinct boundary across which people move from health to illness or from illness back to health. How people perceive themselves and how others see them in terms of health and illness will also affect their placement on the continuum. The ranges in which people can be thought of as healthy or ill are considerable.

Dunn's High-level Wellness Grid

Dunn (1959) describes a health grid in which a health axis and an environmental axis intersect. The grid demonstrates the interaction of the environment with the illness–wellness continuum (see Figure 5-3). The health axis extends from peak wellness to death, and the environmental axis extends from very favourable to very unfavourable. The intersection of the two axes forms four quadrants of health and wellness:

1. *High-level wellness in a favourable environment.* An example is a person who implements healthy lifestyle behaviours and has the biological, psychological, social, spiritual and economic resources to support this lifestyle.

2. *Emergent high-level wellness in an unfavourable environment.* An example is a woman who has the knowledge to implement healthy lifestyle practices but does not implement adequate

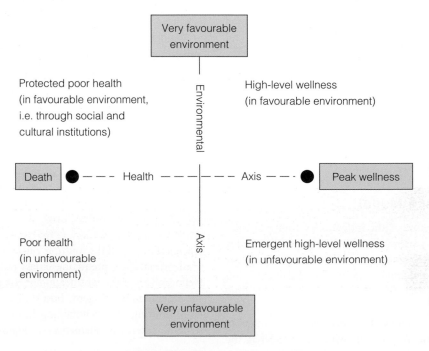

Figure 5-3 Dunn's health grid: its axes and quadrants. (From 'High-Level Wellness for Man and Society,' by H.L. Dunn, 1959, *American Journal of Public Health, 49*, p. 788. Reprinted with permission of American Public Health Association.)

self-care practices because of family responsibilities, job demands or other factors.

3. *Protected poor health in a favourable environment.* An example is an ill person (e.g. one with multiple fractures or severe hypertension) whose needs are met by the healthcare system and who has access to appropriate medications, diet and healthcare instruction.

4. *Poor health in an unfavourable environment.* An example is a young child who is starving in a drought-stricken country.

In his book about high-level wellness in the individual, Dunn (1973) explores the concept of wellness as it relates to family, community, environment and society. He believes that family wellness enhances wellness in individuals. In a well family that offers trust, love and support, the individual does not have to expend energy to meet basic needs and can move forward on the wellness continuum. By providing effective sanitation and safe water, disposing of sewage safely, and preserving beauty and wildlife, the community enhances both family and individual wellness. Environmental wellness is related to the premise that humans must be at peace with and guard the environment. Societal wellness is significant because the status of the larger, social group affects the status of smaller groups. Dunn believes that social wellness must be considered on a worldwide basis.

Travis's Illness-Wellness Continuum

The illness–wellness continuum (Figure 5-4) developed by Travis ranges from high-level wellness to premature death (Travis and Ryan, 2001). The model illustrates two arrows pointing in opposite directions and joined at a neutral point. Movement to the right of the neutral point indicates increasing levels of health and well-being for an individual. This is achieved in three steps: (a) awareness, (b) education and (c) growth. In contrast, movement to the left of the neutral point indicates progressively decreasing levels of health. Travis and Ryan believe it is possible to be physically ill and at the same time oriented toward wellness, or be physically healthy and at the same time function from an illness mentality.

The model also compares the traditional treatment model with the wellness model. The former can help an individual move from the left only to the neutral point, where symptoms of the illness are alleviated. For example, a man with hypertension who takes an antihypertensive medication to reduce blood pressure and relieve any associated symptoms moves to the neutral point. However, wellness-oriented measures such as reducing weight or ceasing to smoke are needed to move the person beyond the neutral point to a higher level of wellness. Note that wellness interventions can be initiated at any point on the continuum. Thus, both the wellness model and treatment model can work together.

A newer model, the 4+ model of wellness (Baldwin and Conger, 2001), consists of the four domains of the inner self – physical, spiritual, emotional and intellectual – plus the elements of the outer systems (environment, culture, nutrition, safety and many other elements). The nurse assesses the inner self for strengths and excesses, sources of nurturing and of depletion, and the interactions between the inner self and the outer systems. This model is useful when working with individuals, families or communities.

There are many models of health and wellness, as has been discussed, which can be applied to clinical practice and patient management. No one model will meet all situations but aspects of several models may need to be considered when exploring the health beliefs of any individual.

VARIABLES INFLUENCING HEALTH STATUS, BELIEFS AND PRACTICES

Many variables influence a person's health status, beliefs and behaviours or practices. *Box 5-2* on page 56 differentiates health status, beliefs and behaviours or practices. These factors may or may not be under conscious control. People can usually control their health behaviours and can choose healthy or unhealthy activities. In contrast, people have little or no choice over their genetic makeup, age, sex, culture and sometimes their geographical environments.

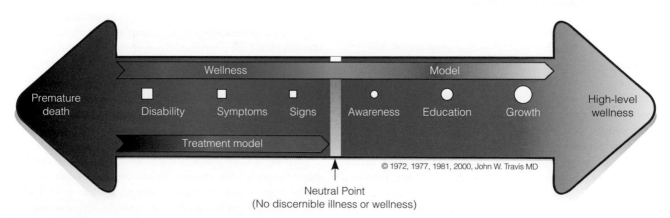

Figure 5-4 Illness-wellness continuum. (Reprinted with permission, *Wellness Workbook*, 3rd edn, by John W. Travis, MD and Regina Sara Ryan, Celestial Arts, Berkeley, CA © 1981, 1988, 2004 by John W. Travis, MD. www.wellnessworkbook.com.)

BOX 5-2 Differentiating Health Status, Beliefs and Behaviours

+ **Health status.** State of health of an individual at a given time. A report of health status may include anxiety, depression or acute illness and thus describe the individual's problem in general. Health status can also describe such specifics as pulse rate and body temperature.

+ **Health beliefs.** Concepts about health that an individual believes true. Such beliefs may or may not be founded on fact. An example of a culturally related health belief is the belief that health and illness are closely associated with the amount and quality of blood in the body. For example, some cultures say that 'high blood', meaning too much blood in the body, causes headaches and dizziness.

+ **Health behaviours.** The actions people take to understand their health state, maintain an optimal state of health, prevent illness and injury, and reach their maximum physical and mental potential. Behaviours such as eating wisely, exercising, paying attention to signs of illness, following treatment advice, avoiding known health hazards such as smoking, taking time for rest and relaxation, and managing one's time effectively are all examples.

Health behaviour is intended to prevent illness or disease or to provide for early detection of disease. Nurses preparing a care plan with an individual need to consider the person's health beliefs before they suggest a change in health behaviours.

Internal Variables

Internal variables include biological, psychological and cognitive dimensions. They are often described as nonmodifiable variables because, for the most part, they cannot be changed. However, when internal variables are linked to health problems, the nurse must be even more diligent about working with the patient to influence external variables (such as exercise and diet) that may assist in health promotion and prevention of illness. Regular health exams and appropriate screening for early detection of health problems become even more important.

Biological Dimension

Genetic makeup, sex, age and developmental level all significantly influence a person's health.

Genetic makeup influences biological characteristics, innate temperament, activity level and intellectual potential. It has been related to susceptibility to specific disease, such as diabetes and breast cancer. In some cases, genetic predisposition for health or illness is enhanced when parents are from the same ethnic genetic pool. For example, people of African heritage have a higher incidence of sickle-cell anemia and hypertension than the general population but may be less susceptible to malaria.

Sex influences the distribution of disease. Certain acquired and genetic diseases are more common in one sex than in the other. Disorders more common among females include osteoporosis and autoimmune disease such as rheumatoid arthritis. Those more common among males are stomach ulcers, abdominal hernias and respiratory diseases.

Age is also a significant factor. The distribution of disease varies with age. For example, arteriosclerotic heart disease is common in middle-aged males but occurs infrequently in younger people; such communicable diseases as whooping cough and measles are common in children but rare in older adults, who have acquired immunity to them.

Psychological developmental level has a major impact on health status. Consider these examples:

+ Infants lack physiological and psychological maturity so their defences against disease are lower during the first years of life.
+ Toddlers who are learning to walk are more prone to falls and injury.
+ Adolescents who need to conform to peers are more prone to risk-taking behaviour and subsequent injury.
+ Declining physical and sensory-perceptual abilities limit the ability of older adults to respond to environmental hazards and stressors.

Psychological Dimension

Psychological (emotional) factors influencing health include mind–body interactions and self-concept, which will now be discussed individually.

Mind–body interactions can affect health status positively or negatively. Emotional responses to stress affect body function. For example, a student who is extremely anxious before an exam may experience urinary frequency and diarrhoea. A person worried about the outcome of surgery or about the behaviour of a teenager may chain-smoke. Prolonged emotional distress may increase susceptibility to organic disease or precipitate it. Emotional distress may influence the immune system through the central nervous system and endocrine alterations. Alterations in the immune system are related to the incidence of infections, cancer and autoimmune diseases.

Increasing attention is being given to the mind's ability to direct the body's functioning. Relaxation, meditation and biofeedback techniques are gaining wider recognition by individuals and healthcare professionals. For example, women often use relaxation techniques to decrease pain during childbirth. Other people may learn biofeedback skills to reduce hypertension.

Emotional reactions also occur in response to body conditions. For example, a person diagnosed with a terminal illness may experience fear and depression. *Self-concept* is how a person feels about self (self-esteem) and perceives the physical self (body image), needs, roles and abilities. Self-concept affects how people view and handle situations. Such attitudes can affect health practices, responses to stress and illness, and the times when treatment is sought. An example is the anorexic woman who deprives herself of needed nutrients because she believes she is too fat even though she is well below an acceptable weight level. Self-perceptions are also associated with a person's definition of health. For example, a 75-year-old man who can no longer move large objects as he was accustomed to do may need to examine and redefine his concept of health in view of his age and abilities, as he is no longer able to perform tasks in the same way.

Cognitive Dimension

Cognitive or intellectual factors influencing health include lifestyle choices and spiritual and religious beliefs.

Lifestyle refers to a person's general way of living, including living conditions and individual patterns of behaviour that are influenced by sociocultural factors and personal characteristics. In brief, lifestyle is often considered as behaviour and activities over which people have control. Lifestyle choices may have positive or negative effects on health. Practices that have potentially negative effects on health are often referred to as **risk factors**. For example, overeating, getting insufficient exercise and being overweight are closely related to the incidence of heart disease, arteriosclerosis, diabetes and hypertension. Tobacco use is clearly implicated in lung cancer, emphysema and cardiovascular diseases. See *Box 5-3* for examples of healthy lifestyle choices.

Spiritual and religious beliefs can significantly affect health behaviour. For example, Jehovah's Witnesses oppose blood transfusions. Likewise some fundamentalists believe that a serious illness is a punishment from God, for example if a child is born with a learning disability the parents may believe that they are being punished for a sin they have committed. Some religious groups are strict vegetarians; and Orthodox Jews perform circumcision on the eighth day of a male baby's life.

BOX 5-3 Examples of Healthy Lifestyle Choices

+ Regular exercise
+ Weight control
+ Avoidance of saturated fats
+ Alcohol and smoking avoidance
+ Bike helmet use
+ Immunisation updates
+ Regular dental checkups
+ Regular health maintenance visits for screening examinations or tests

---

External Variables

External variables affecting health include the physical environment, standards of living, family and cultural beliefs, and social support networks.

Environment

People are becoming increasingly aware of their environment and how it affects their health and level of wellness. Geographical location determines climate and climate affects health. For instance, malaria and malaria-related conditions occur more frequently in tropical rather than temperate climates. Pollution of the water, air and soil affects the health of cells. Pollution can occur naturally (e.g. lightning-caused fires produce smoke, which pollutes the air). Other substances in the environment, such as asbestos used in older buildings for insulation, are considered carcinogenic (i.e. they cause cancer). Cigarette smoke is hazardous to one's health, with rates of cancer higher among smokers and those who live or work near smokers.

Another environmental hazard is radiation. Two sources of radiation that can be hazardous to health are machines such as pipeline scanning machines and drugs that emit radiation used for bone density scanning. The improper use of x-rays, for example, can harm many of the body's organs. Another common source of radiation is the sun's ultraviolet rays. Light-skinned people are more susceptible to the harmful effects of the sun than are dark-skinned people.

An environmental hazard that is receiving increasing media attention is an increase in the 'greenhouse effect'. The glass roof of a greenhouse permits the sun's radiation to penetrate, but the resulting heat does not escape back through the glass. Carbon dioxide in the earth's atmosphere acts like the glass roof of a greenhouse, and as carbon dioxide levels increase due to industrial and vehicle emissions, the surface temperature of the earth may also be increasing. This as a consequence means hotter summers affecting those with respiratory illness and disease more usually seen in tropical climates emerging in the more temperate regions of the world.

Other sources of environmental contamination are pesticides and chemicals used to control weeds and plant diseases. These contaminants can be found in some animals and plants that are subsequently ingested by people from the skin of fruit and vegetables. In excessive levels, they are harmful to health.

Standards of Living

An individual's standard of living (reflecting occupation, income and education) is related to health, morbidity and mortality. Hygiene, food habits and the propensity to seek healthcare advice and follow health regimens vary among high-income and low-income groups.

Research by sociologists has concluded low-income families often define health in terms of work; if people can work they are healthy. They tend to be fatalistic and believe that illness is not preventable. Because their present problems are so great and all efforts are exerted toward survival, an orientation to the future may be lacking.

The environmental conditions of poverty-stricken areas also have a bearing on overall health. Slum neighbourhoods are overcrowded and in a state of deterioration. Sanitation services tend to be inadequate. Many streets are strewn with rubbish and rats overrun alleys. Fires and crime are constant threats. Recreational facilities are almost nonexistent, forcing children to play in streets and alleys. This is a problem seen frequently in the more deprived inner city areas and is a problem that has occurred for many years despite government intervention.

Occupational roles also predispose people to certain illnesses. For instance, some industrial workers may be exposed to carcinogenic agents, such as road workers with tar have an increased risk of developing bladder cancer. More affluent people may fulfil stressful social or occupational roles that predispose them to stress-related diseases such as lawyers have an increased risk of high blood pressure and stroke. Such roles may also encourage overeating or social use of drugs or alcohol.

Family and Cultural Beliefs

The family passes on patterns of daily living and lifestyles to offspring. For example, a man who was abused as a child may physically abuse his child. Physical or emotional abuse may cause long-term health problems. Emotional health depends on a social environment that is free of excessive tension and does not isolate the person from others. A climate of open communication, sharing and love fosters the fulfilment of the person's optimum potential.

People of certain cultures may perceive home remedies or complimentary therapies as superior and more dependable than traditional healthcare practices. For example, a person of Chinese origin may prefer to use herbal remedies and acupuncture to treat pain rather than analgesic medications. Cultural rules, values and beliefs give people a sense of being stable and able to predict outcomes.

Social Support Networks

Having a support network (family, friends or a confidant) and job satisfaction helps people avoid illness. Support people also help the person confirm that illness exists by observing symptoms such as pale skin or a rash. People with inadequate support networks sometimes allow themselves to become increasingly ill before confirming the illness and seeking therapy. Support people also provide the stimulus for an ill person to become well again (Hurdle, 2001).

HEALTH BELIEF MODELS

Several theories or models of health beliefs and behaviours have been developed by nurse theorists, psychologists and sociologists to help determine whether an individual is likely to participate in disease prevention and health-promotion activities. These models can be useful tools in developing programmes for helping people change to healthier lifestyles and develop a more positive attitude toward preventive health measures.

Health Locus of Control Model

Locus of control (LOC) is a concept from social learning theory (the theory of how we learn to interact socially with the world), that nurses can use to determine whether patients are likely to take action regarding health, that is, whether patients believe that their health status is under their own or others' control. People who believe that they have a major influence on their own health status – that health is largely self-determined – are called *internals*. People who exercise internal control are more likely than others to take the initiative on their own healthcare, be more knowledgeable about their health, and adhere to prescribed healthcare regimens such as taking medication, making and keeping appointments with physicians, maintaining diets and giving up smoking. By contrast, people who believe their health is largely controlled by outside forces (e.g. chance or powerful others) are referred to as *externals*.

Research has shown that locus of control plays a role in patients' choices about health behaviours. In some cases, externals demonstrate better compliance to medical regimes (e.g. Wong and White, 2002) while in others, internals with appropriate support systems have better compliance (Murphy *et al.*, 2001).

Locus of control is a measurable concept that can be used to predict which people are most likely to change their behaviour. Many measurement instruments are available to assess LOC. One widely used example is the Multidimensional Health Locus of Control (MHLC) Scale (Wallston *et al.*, 1978). Nurses can use LOC results to plan internal reinforcement training if necessary in order to improve patient efforts toward better health.

Rosenstock's and Becker's Health Belief Models

In the 1950s Rosenstock (1974) proposed a health belief model (HBM) intended to predict which individuals would or would not use such preventive measures as screening for early detection of cancer. Becker (1974) modified the health belief model to include these components: individual perceptions, modifying factors and variables likely to affect initiating action. The health belief model (see Figure 5-5) is based on motivational theory. Rosenstock (1974) assumed that good health is an objective common to all people. Becker added 'positive health motivation' as a consideration.

Individual Perceptions

Individual perceptions include the following:

+ *Perceived susceptibility*. A family history of a certain disorder, such as diabetes or heart disease, may make the individual feel at high risk.
+ *Perceived seriousness*. The question here is this: In the perception of the individual, does the illness cause death or have serious consequences? Concern about the spread of acquired immune deficiency syndrome (AIDS) reflects the general public's perception of the seriousness of this illness, many are concerned regarding its spread so it is considered a serious illness.

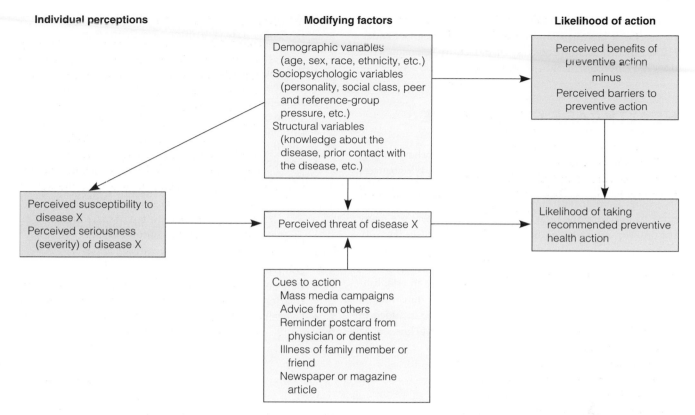

Figure 5-5 The health belief model. (From 'Selected Psychosocial Models and Correlates of Individual Health-Related Behaviors,' by M.H. Becker *et al.*, 1977, *Medical Care*, *15*(5 Suppl.), pp. 27-46. Reprinted with permission.)

+ *Perceived threat.* According to Becker (1974), perceived susceptibility and perceived seriousness combine to determine the total perceived threat of an illness to a specific individual. For example, a person who perceives that many individuals in the community have AIDS may not necessarily perceive a threat of the disease; if the person is a drug addict or a homosexual, however, the perceived threat of illness is likely to increase because the susceptibility is combined with seriousness.

Modifying Factors

Factors that modify a person's perceptions include the following:

+ *Demographic variables.* Demographic variables include age, sex, race and ethnicity. An infant, for example, does not perceive the importance of a healthy diet; an adolescent may perceive peer approval as more important than family approval and as a consequence may participate in hazardous activities or adopt unhealthy eating and sleeping patterns.
+ *Socio psychological variables.* Social pressure or influence from peers or other reference groups (e.g. self-help or vocational groups) may encourage preventive health behaviours even when individual motivation is low. Expectations of others may motivate people, for example, not to drive a car after drinking alcohol to prevent accidents or death.
+ *Structural variables.* Knowledge about the target disease and prior contact with it are structural variables that are

presumed to influence preventive behaviour. Becker (1974) found higher compliance rates with prescribed treatments among mothers whose children had frequent ear infections and occurrences of asthma. A rationale for this may be the mothers could see a visible improvement in their child following treatment.

+ *Cues to action or treatment.* Cues can be either internal or external. Internal cues include feelings of fatigue, uncomfortable symptoms, or thoughts about the condition of an ill person who is close.

Likelihood of Action

The likelihood of a person's taking recommended preventive health action depends on the perceived benefits of the action minus the perceived barriers to the action.

+ *Perceived benefits of the action.* Examples include refraining from smoking to prevent lung cancer and eating nutritious foods and avoiding snacks to avoid weight gain.
+ *Perceived barriers to action.* Examples include cost, inconvenience, unpleasantness and lifestyle changes.

Nurses play a major role in helping patients implement healthy behaviours. They help patients monitor health, they supply anticipatory guidance and they impart knowledge about health. Nurses can also reduce barriers to action (e.g. by minimising inconvenience or discomfort) and can support positive actions.

Pender *et al.* (2002) have modified this health belief model to develop a health-promotion model. According to Pender, HBM explains health-protecting or preventive behaviours but does not emphasise health-promoting behaviours.

HEALTHCARE COMPLIANCE

Compliance is the extent to which an individual's behaviour (e.g. taking medications, following diets or making lifestyle changes) coincides with medical or health advice. Degree of compliance may range from disregarding every aspect of the recommendations to following the total therapeutic plan. There are many reasons why some people adhere and others do not (see *Box 5-4*).

To enhance compliance, nurses need to ensure that the patient is able to perform the prescribed therapy, understands the necessary instructions, is a willing participant in establishing goals of therapy, and values the planned outcomes of behaviour changes. Examples of questions to be included in assessment are found in the *Assessment interview* below.

BOX 5-4 Factors Influencing Compliance

+ Patient motivation to become well
+ Degree of lifestyle change necessary
+ Perceived severity of the healthcare problem
+ Value placed on reducing the threat of illness
+ Difficulty in understanding and performing specific behaviours
+ Degree of inconvenience of the illness itself or of the treatment plans
+ Beliefs that the prescribed therapy or treatment will or will not help
+ Complexity, side effects and duration of the proposed treatment plan
+ Specific cultural heritage that may make compliance difficult
+ Degree of satisfaction and quality and type of relationship with the healthcare providers
+ Overall cost of prescribed treatment

ASSESSMENT INTERVIEW

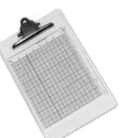

Determining the Risk for Medication Noncompliance

+ Are you having side effects from any of your medication?
+ Do you think your medications are helping?
+ Do you have 'tools' to remind you to take your medication? Examples could be an alarm, patient medication box with times on it or environmental cues (television/radio news).
+ Is there someone at home who helps you with your medications?

+ How many times per day are your medications prescribed?
+ How many tablets do you take every day?
+ Are there any special storage requirements for your medications?
+ How much do your medication requirements interfere with your lifestyle?
+ How well are you able to follow special dosing requirements?
+ How many doses of your medications have you missed over the past three days?

When a nurse identifies noncompliance, it is important to take the following steps:

+ *Establish why the patient is not following the treatment plan.* Depending on the reason, the nurse can provide information, correct misconceptions, attempt to decrease expense or suggest counselling if psychological problems are interfering with compliance. It is also essential that the nurse reevaluate the suitability of the health advice provided. In situations where the patient's cultural beliefs or age conflict with planned therapies, the nurse needs to consider ways to redevelop and restructure care that will preserve and accommodate the patient's practices.
+ *Demonstrate caring.* Show sincere concern about the patient's problems and decisions and at the same time accept the patient's right to a course of action. For example, a nurse might tell a patient who is not taking his cardiac medication,

'I can appreciate how you feel about this, but I am very concerned about your heart.'
+ *Encourage healthy behaviours through positive reinforcement.* If the man who is not taking his cardiac medication is walking every day, the nurse might say, 'You are really doing well with your walking.'
+ *Use aids to reinforce teaching.* For instance, the nurse can leave pamphlets for the patient to read later or make a 'tablet calendar', a paper with the date and number of tablets to be taken.
+ *Establish a therapeutic relationship of freedom, mutual understanding and mutual responsibility with the patient and support persons.* By providing knowledge, skills and information, the nurse gives patients control over their health and establishes a cooperative relationship, which results in greater compliance.

Aspects influencing patients of varying ages are found in *Lifespan considerations.*

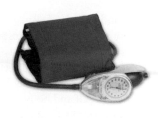

LIFESPAN CONSIDERATIONS

Children

Several causes of noncompliance are specific to teenagers. It is important for the nurse to consider these when working with adolescents, because they:

+ don't consider the consequences of their actions;
+ are in the early stages of problem solving;
+ assert independence by rejecting adult values;
+ conform to their peers and don't like being 'different';
+ focus on self-concept and body image;
+ live in the 'here and now';
+ may regress developmentally at times of stress or illness;
+ may be unable to distinguish benefits from disadvantages.

Note: From 'Rebels with a Cause: When Adolescents Won't Follow Medical Advice,' by M.E. Muscari, 1998, *American Journal of Nursing*, 98(12), pp. 26-31. Adapted with permission.

Older Adults

Issues that influence the health and well-being of older adults include:

+ lifestyle choices and individual responsibility for health maintenance;
+ availability of home- and community-based services to maximise independence;
+ alternative/complimentary therapies;
+ housing and home modifications to accommodate the physical aspects of ageing;
+ affordable and accessible transportation;
+ preventive nursing and medical care;
+ available mental health services;
+ the care giving crisis (caring for an elderly/sick relative with little external support) that overburdens some family and informal caregivers.

Note: From *Gerontological Nursing Care*, by S.R. Tyson, 'Elders: Issues That Influence the Health and Well-Being of Elders,' p. 9, copyright 1999, with permission from Elsevier.

Other factors affecting older adults' compliance include:

+ forgetfulness,
+ dementia,
+ feeling that they have lived their life and it is time for life to end.

When considering health it is also necessary to consider illness and disease that affects normal health patterns.

ILLNESS AND DISEASE

Illness is a highly personal state in which the person's physical, emotional, intellectual, social, developmental or spiritual functioning is thought to be diminished. It is not synonymous with disease and may or may not be related to disease. An individual could have a disease, for example, a growth in the stomach, and not feel ill. Similarly a person can feel ill, that is, feel uncomfortable, yet have no discernible disease. Illness is highly subjective; only the individual person can say he or she is ill.

Disease can be described as an alteration in body functions resulting in a reduction of capacities or a shortening of the normal life span. Traditionally intervention by physicians has the goal of eliminating or ameliorating disease processes. Today multiple factors are considered to interact in causing disease and determining an individual's response to treatment.

The causation of a disease is called its **aetiology**. A description of the aetiology of a disease includes the identification of all causal factors that act together to bring about the particular disease. For example, the tubercle bacillus is designated as the biological agent of tuberculosis. However, other aetiological factors, such as age, nutritional status and even occupation, are involved in the development of tuberculosis and influence the course of infection. There are many diseases for which the cause is unknown (e.g. multiple sclerosis).

Nurses have traditionally taken a holistic view of people and base their practice on the multiple-causation theory of health problems.

There are many ways to classify illness and disease; one of the most common is as acute or chronic. **Acute illness** is typically characterised by severe symptoms of relatively short duration. The symptoms often appear abruptly and subside quickly and, depending on the cause, may or may not require intervention by healthcare professionals. Some acute illnesses are serious (e.g. appendicitis may require surgical intervention), but many acute illnesses, such as colds, subside without medical intervention or with the help of over-the-counter medications. Following an acute illness, most people return to their normal level of wellness.

A **chronic illness** is one that lasts for an extended period, usually six months or longer, and often for the person's life. Chronic illnesses usually have a slow onset and often have periods of **remission**, when the symptoms disappear, and **exacerbation**, when the symptoms reappear.

Examples of chronic illnesses are arthritis, heart and lung diseases such as chronic obstructive pulmonary disease and diabetes mellitus. Nurses are involved in caring for chronically ill individuals of all ages in all types of settings – homes, nursing homes, hospitals, clinics and other institutions. Care needs to be focused on promoting the highest level possible of independence, sense of control and wellness. Patients often need to modify their activities of daily living, social relationships and perception of self and body image. In addition, many must learn how to live with increasing physical limitations and discomfort.

Illness Behaviours

Illness behaviour is a coping mechanism, involves ways individuals describe, monitor and interpret their symptoms, take remedial actions and use the healthcare system. How people behave when they are ill is highly individualised and affected by many variables, such as age, sex, occupation, socioeconomic status, religion, ethnic origin, psychological stability, personality, education and modes of coping.

Parsons (1979), a sociologist, described four aspects of the sick role which is an illness behaviour:

1. Patients are not held responsible for their condition.
2. Patients are excused from certain social roles and tasks.
3. Patients are obliged to try to get well as quickly as possible.
4. Patients or their families are obliged to seek competent help.

Suchman (1979) expanded on this to describe five stages of illness: symptoms, sick role, medical care contact, dependent patient role, and recovery or rehabilitation. Not all patients progress through each stage. For example, the patient who experiences a sudden heart attack is taken to the emergency department and immediately enters stages 3 and 4, medical care contact and dependent patient role. Other patients may progress through only the first two stages and then recover. The work of both Parsons and Suchman enable the healthcare professional to understand better the illness experience of the patient. Details of Suchman's five stages are as follows.

Stage 1 Symptom Experiences

At this stage the person comes to believe something is wrong. Either someone significant mentions that the person looks unwell, or they experience some symptoms such as pain, rash, cough, fever or bleeding. Stage 1 has three aspects:

+ the physical experience of symptoms;
+ the cognitive aspect (the interpretation of the symptoms in terms that have some meaning to the person);
+ the emotional response (e.g. fear or anxiety).

During this stage, the ill person usually consults others about the symptoms or feelings, validating with a spouse or support people that the symptoms are real. At this stage the sick person may try home remedies. If self-management is ineffective, the individual enters the next stage.

Stage 2 Assumption of the Sick Role

The individual now accepts the sick role and seeks confirmation from family and friends. Often people continue with self-treatment and delay contact with healthcare professionals as long as possible. During this stage people may be excused from normal duties and role expectations. Emotional responses such as withdrawal, anxiety, fear and depression are not uncommon depending on the severity of the illness, perceived degree of disability and anticipated duration of the illness. When symptoms of illness persist or increase, the person is motivated to seek professional help.

Stage 3 Medical Care Contact

Sick people seek the advice of a health professional either on their own initiative or at the urging of significant others. When people seek professional advice they are really asking for three types of information:

+ validation of real illness;
+ explanation of the symptoms in understandable terms;
+ reassurance that they will be all right or prediction of what the outcome will be.

The health professional may determine that the patient does not have an illness or that an illness is present and may even be life threatening. The patient may accept or deny the diagnosis. If the diagnosis is accepted, the patient usually follows the prescribed treatment plan. If the diagnosis is not accepted, the patient may seek the advice of other healthcare professionals or quasi-practitioners who will provide a diagnosis that fits the patient's perceptions.

Stage 4 Dependent Patient Role

After accepting the illness and seeking treatment, the patient becomes dependent on the professional for help. People vary greatly in the degree of ease with which they can give up their independence, particularly in relation to life and death. Role obligations – such as those of wage earner, father, mother, student, rugby team member or choir member – complicate the decision to give up independence.

Most people accept their dependence on the physician, although they retain varying degrees of control over their own lives. For example, some people request precise information about their disease and treatment, and they delay the decision to accept treatment until they have all this information. Others prefer that the physician proceed with treatment and do not request additional information.

For some patients illness may meet dependence needs that have never been met and thus provide satisfaction. Other people have minimal dependence needs and do everything possible to return to independent functioning. A few may even try to maintain independence to the detriment of their recovery.

Stage 5 Recovery or Rehabilitation

During this stage the patient is expected to relinquish the dependent role and resume former roles and responsibilities. For people with an acute illness, their time as an ill person is generally short and recovery is usually rapid. Thus most find it relatively easy to return to their former lifestyles. People who have long-term illnesses and must adjust their lifestyles may find recovery more difficult. For patients with a permanent disability, this final stage may require therapy to learn how to make major adjustments in functioning.

Effects of Illness

Illness brings about changes in both the involved individual and in the family. The changes vary depending on the nature, severity and duration of the illness, attitudes associated with the illness by the patient and others, the financial demands, the lifestyle changes incurred, adjustments to usual roles, and so on.

Impact on the Patient

Ill patients may experience behavioural and emotional changes, changes in self-concept and body image, and lifestyle changes. Behavioural and emotional changes associated with short-term illness are generally mild and short lived. The individual, for example, may become irritable and lack the energy or desire to interact in the usual fashion with family members or friends. More acute responses are likely with severe, life-threatening, chronic or disabling illness. Anxiety, fear, anger, withdrawal, denial, a sense of hopelessness and feelings of powerlessness are all common responses to severe or disabling illness. For example, a patient experiencing a heart attack fears for his life and the financial burden it may place on his family. Another patient informed about a diagnosis of cancer or AIDS or crippling neurological disease may, over time, experience episodes of denial, anger, fear and hopelessness.

Certain illnesses can also change the patient's body image or physical appearance, especially if there is severe scarring or loss of a limb or special sense organ. The patient's self-esteem and self-concept may also be affected. Many factors can play a part in low self-esteem and a disturbance in self-concept: loss of body parts and function, pain, disfigurement, dependence on others, unemployment, financial problems, inability to participate in social functions, strained relationships with others and spiritual distress. Nurses need to help patients express their thoughts and feelings, and to provide care that helps the patient effectively cope with change.

Ill individuals are also vulnerable to loss of **autonomy**, the state of being independent and self-directed without outside control. Family interactions may change so that the patient may no longer be involved in making family decisions or even decisions about their own healthcare. Nurses need to support the patient's right to self-determination and autonomy as much as possible by providing them with sufficient information to participate in decision-making processes and to maintain a feeling of being in control.

Illness also often necessitates a change in lifestyle. In addition to participating in treatments and taking medications, the ill person may need to change diet, activity and exercise, and rest and sleep patterns.

Nurses can help patients adjust their lifestyles by these means:

+ providing explanations about necessary adjustments;
+ making arrangements wherever possible to accommodate the patient's lifestyle;
+ encouraging other healthcare professionals to become aware of the person's lifestyle practices and to support healthy aspects of that lifestyle;
+ reinforcing desirable changes in practices with a view to making them a permanent part of the patient's lifestyle.

Impact on the Family

A person's illness affects not only the person who is ill but also the family or significant others. The kind of effect and its extent depend chiefly on three factors: (a) the member of the family who is ill, (b) the seriousness and length of the illness, and (c) the cultural and social customs the family follows.

The changes that can occur in the family include the following:

+ role changes;
+ task reassignments and increased demands on time;
+ increased stress due to anxiety about the outcome of the illness for the patient and conflict about unaccustomed responsibilities;
+ financial problems;
+ loneliness as a result of separation and pending loss;
+ change in social customs.

Nurses assess and plan healthcare for three types of patients: the individual, the family and the community. Care of the individual is enhanced when the nurse understands the concepts of individuality, holism, homoeostasis, human needs and systems theory. The beliefs and values of each person and the support he or she receives come in large part from the family and are reinforced by the community. Thus an understanding of family dynamics and the context of the community assists the nurse in planning care. When a family is the patient, the nurse determines the health status of the family and its individual members, the level of family functioning, family interaction patterns, and family strengths and weaknesses. When a community is the patient, the nurse determines what environmental problems are present, for example, pollution, poor sanitation, waste disposal, incidence of crime, housing conditions, and so on, and intervenes to promote healthful living and prevent health problems.

INDIVIDUAL HEALTH

Dimensions of individuality include the person's total character, self-identity and perceptions. The person's total character encompasses behaviours, emotional state, attitudes, values, motives, abilities, habits and appearances. The person's self-identity encompasses perception of self as a separate and distinct entity alone and in interactions with others. The person's perceptions encompass the way the person interprets the environment or situation, directly affecting how the person thinks, feels and acts in any given situation.

Concept of Individuality

To help patients attain, maintain or regain an optimal level of health, nurses need to consider them as individuals. Each individual is a unique being who is different from every other human being, with a different combination of genetics, life experiences and environmental interactions.

When providing care, nurses need to focus on the patient within both a total care and an individualised care context. In the total care context, the nurse considers all the principles and areas that apply when taking care of any patient of that age and condition. In the individualised care context, the nurse becomes acquainted with the patient as an individual, referring to the total care principles and using those principles that apply to this person at this time. For example, a nurse who is advising the mother of a preschooler understands that the child's desire to explore his world is a developmental stage that all preschoolers experience. However, the preschooler diagnosed with attention deficit hyperactivity disorder (ADHD) may have an increased risk of accidents and injuries when interacting with his environment, due to his impulsivity and poor self-control.

Although the individual is important when considering the experience of the patient he or she needs to be viewed as a whole and not as a set of symptoms or a disease.

Concept of Holism

Nurses are concerned with the individual as a whole, complete or holistic person, not as an assembly of parts and processes. When applied in nursing, the concept of **holism** emphasises that nurses must keep the whole person in mind and strive to understand how one area of concern relates to the whole person. The nurse must also consider the relationship of the individual to the external environment and to others. For example, in helping a man who is grieving over the death of his spouse, the nurse explores the impact of the loss on the whole person (i.e. on the man's appetite, rest and sleep pattern, energy level, sense of well-being, mood, usual activities, family relationships, and relationships with others). Nursing interventions are directed toward restoring overall harmony, so they depend on the man's sense of purpose and meaning of his life.

But in order to understand the patient holistically the nurse needs to be able to understand the patient's symptoms and their physiological affect.

Concept of Homoeostasis

The concept of **homoeostasis** was first introduced by Cannon (1939) a physiologist to describe the relative constancy of the internal processes of the body, such as blood oxygen and carbon dioxide levels, blood pressure, body temperature, blood glucose, and fluid and electrolyte balance. To Cannon, the word *homoeostasis* did not imply something stagnant, set or immobile; it meant a condition that might vary but remained relatively constant. Cannon viewed the human being as

separate from the external environment and constantly endeavouring to maintain physiological **equilibrium**, or balance, through adaptation to that environment. Homoeostasis, then, is the tendency of the body to maintain a state of balance or equilibrium while continually changing.

Physiological Homoeostasis

Physiological homoeostasis means that the internal environment of the body is relatively stable and constant. All cells of the body require a relatively constant environment to function; thus the body's internal environment must be maintained within narrow limits. Homoeostatic mechanisms have four main characteristics:

1. They are self-regulating.
2. They are compensatory.
3. They tend to be regulated by negative feedback systems.
4. They may require several feedback mechanisms to correct only one physiological imbalance.

Self-regulation means that homoeostatic mechanisms come into play automatically in the healthy person. However, if a person is ill, or if a respiratory organ such as a lung is injured, the homoeostatic mechanisms may not be able to respond to the stimulus as they would normally. Homoeostatic mechanisms are **compensatory** (counterbalancing) because they tend to counteract conditions that are abnormal for the person. An example is a sudden drop in air temperature. The compensatory mechanisms are that the peripheral blood vessels constrict, thereby diverting most of the blood internally; and increased muscular activity and shivering occur to create heat. Through these mechanisms the body temperature remains stable despite the cold.

Homoeostasis occurs within the physiological **system**, a set of interacting identifiable parts or components. The fundamental components of a system are matter, energy and communication. Without any one of these, a system does not exist. The individual is a human system with matter (the body), energy (chemical or thermal) and communication (e.g. the nervous system). The **boundary** of a system, such as the skin in the human system, is a real or imaginary line that differentiates one system from another system or a system from its environment.

There are two general types of systems: closed and open. A **closed system** does not exchange energy, matter or information with its environment; it receives no input from the environment and gives no output to the environment. An example of a closed system is a chemical reaction that takes place in a test tube. In reality, outside the laboratory, no closed systems exist. In an **open system**, energy, matter and information move into and out of the system through the system boundary. All living systems, such as plants, animals, people, families and communities, are open systems, since their survival depends on a continuous exchange of energy. They are, therefore, in a constant state of change.

An open system depends on the quality and quantity of its input, output and feedback. **Input** consists of information, material or energy that enters the system. After the input is

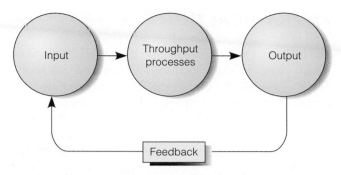

Figure 5-6 An open system with a feedback mechanism.

absorbed by the system, it is processed in a way useful to the system. This transformation is called **throughput**. For example, food is input to the digestive system; it is digested (throughput) so that it can be used by the body. **Output** from a system is energy, matter or information given out by the system as a result of its processes. Output from the digestive system includes caloric energy, nutrients, urine and faeces.

Feedback is the mechanism by which some of the output of a system is returned to the system as input. Feedback enables a system to regulate itself by redirecting the output of a system back into the system as input, thus forming a feedback loop (see Figure 5-6). This input influences the behaviour of the system and its future output. **Negative feedback** inhibits change; **positive feedback** stimulates change. Most biological systems are controlled by negative feedback to bring the system back to stability. This type of feedback system senses and counteracts any deviations from normal. The deviations may be greater or less than the normal level or range. For example, an increase in the production of parathyroid hormone is stimulated by a drop in blood calcium, but when additional parathyroid hormone raises the level of blood calcium, the hormone's production is then inhibited (see Figure 5-7).

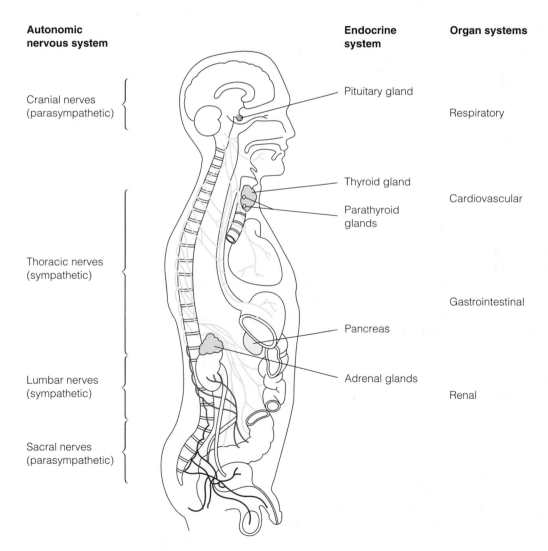

Figure 5-7 The homoeostatic regulators of the body: autonomic nervous system, endocrine system and specific organ systems.

With hypoxia (shortage of oxygen), the concentration of red blood cells increases and the heart rate becomes faster to transport the blood and available oxygen around the body adequately. People interact with the environment by adjusting themselves to it or adjusting it to themselves. This premise directs the nurse to look at environmental factors influencing the system and to plan nursing interventions to help the patient maintain homoeostasis. For example, the individual who is experiencing severe anxiety may be taught a variety of stress management techniques.

Feedback mechanisms are also found within family and community systems. In the family system, parents provide feedback to children to regulate behaviour. In the community, laws, rules and regulations control the behaviour of citizens.

Psychological Homoeostasis

The term **psychological homoeostasis** refers to emotional or psychological balance or a state of mental well-being. It is maintained by a variety of mechanisms. Each person has certain psychological needs, such as the need for love, security and self-esteem, which must be met to maintain psychological homoeostasis. When one or more of these needs is not met or is threatened, certain coping mechanisms are activated to protect the person and provide psychological homoeostasis.

Psychological homoeostasis is acquired or learned through the experience of living and interacting with others. In addition, societal norms and culture influence behaviour. Some prerequisites for a person to develop psychological homoeostasis can be summarised as follows:

+ A stable physical environment in which the person feels safe and secure. For example, the basic needs for food, shelter and clothing must be met consistently from birth onward.
+ A stable psychological environment from infancy onward, so that feelings of trust and love develop. Growing children and adolescents also need kind but firm and consistent discipline, encouragement and support to be their own unique selves.
+ A social environment that includes adults who are healthy role models. Children learn the customs and values of society from these individuals.
+ A life experience that provides satisfactions. Throughout life, people encounter many frustrations. People deal with these better if enough satisfying experiences have occurred to counterbalance the frustrating ones.

Assessing the Health of Individuals

A thorough assessment of the individual's health status is basic to health promotion. Components of this assessment are the health history and physical examination, physical fitness assessment, lifestyle assessment, health risk appraisal, health beliefs review and life-stress review.

FAMILY HEALTH

The **family** is a basic unit of society. It consists of those individuals, male or female, youth or adult, legally or not legally related, genetically or not genetically related, who are considered by the others to represent the significant persons in their lives. In the nursing profession, interest in the family unit and its impact on the health, values and productivity of individual family members is expressed by **family-centred nursing**: nursing that considers the health of the family as a unit in addition to the health of individual family members.

Functions of the Family

The economic resources needed by the family are secured by adult members. The family protects the physical health of its members by providing adequate nutrition and healthcare services. Nutritional and lifestyle practices of the family also directly affect the developing health attitudes and lifestyle practices of the children.

In addition to providing an environment conducive to physical growth and health, the family creates an atmosphere that influences the cognitive and the psychosocial growth of its members. Children and adults in healthy, functional families receive support, understanding and encouragement as they progress through predictable developmental stages, as they move in or out of the family unit, and as they establish new family units. In families where members are physically and emotionally nurtured, individuals are challenged to achieve their potential in the family unit. As individual needs are met, family members are able to reach out to others in the family and the community, and to society.

Families from different cultures are an integral part of a country's rich heritage. Each family has values and beliefs that are unique to their culture of origin and that shape the family's structure, methods of interaction, healthcare practices and coping mechanisms. These factors interact to influence the health of families. Families of a particular culture may cluster to form mutual support systems and to preserve their heritage; however, this practice may isolate them from the larger society.

Types of Families in Today's Society

Families consist of persons (structure) and their responsibilities within the family (roles). A family structure of parents and their offspring is known as the **nuclear family**. The relatives of nuclear families, such as grandparents or aunts and uncles, compose the **extended family**. In some families, members of the extended family live with the nuclear family. Although members of the extended family may live in different areas, they may be a source of emotional or financial support for the family.

Traditional Family

The traditional Western family is viewed as an autonomous unit in which both parents reside in the home with their children, the mother often assuming the nurturing role and the father providing the necessary economic resources. In today's society both males and females are less bound to traditional role patterns. For example, fathers are more likely to be involved with the household activities, their children and family life.

Two-career Family

In two-career (or dual-career) families, both partners are employed. They may or may not have children. Two-career families have steadily increased since the 1960s because of increased career opportunities for women, a desire to increase their standard of living and economic necessity. Finding good-quality, affordable childcare is one of the many stresses faced by working parents.

Single-parent Family

There are 1.8 million lone parent families in Britain. There are many reasons for single parenthood, including death of a spouse, separation, divorce, birth of a child to an unmarried woman, or adoption of a child by a single man or woman (Economic and Social Research Council, 2006). The stresses of single parenthood are many: childcare concerns, financial concerns, role overload and fatigue in managing daily tasks, and social isolation.

Adolescent Family

A growing proportion of infants are born each year to adolescent parents. These young parents are often developmentally, physically, emotionally and financially ill prepared to undertake the responsibility of parenthood. Adolescent pregnancies frequently interrupt or stop formal education. Children born to an adolescent are often at greater risk of health and social problems, and they have few role models to assist in breaking out of the cycle of poverty.

Foster Family

Children who can no longer live with their birth parents may require placement with a family that has agreed to include them temporarily. The legal agreement between the foster family and the court to care for the child includes the expectations of the foster parents and the financial compensation they will receive. A family (with or without its own children) may house more than one foster child at a time or different children over many years. Hopefully, at some time the fostered child can return to the birth parent(s) or be legally and permanently adopted by other parents.

Blended Family

Existing family units who join together to form new families are known as *blended*, *step* or *reconstituted families*. Family integration requires time and effort. Stresses occur as blended families get acquainted with each other, respect differences and establish new patterns of behaviour.

Intragenerational Family

In some cultures, and as people live longer, more than two generations may live together. Children may continue to live with their parents even after having their own children or the grandparents may move in with their grown children's families after some years of living apart. In other situations, a generation is skipped or missing; that is, grandparents live with and care for their grandchildren but the children's parents are not a part of this family. Many life events and choices can lead to this type of family.

Cohabiting Family

Cohabiting (or communal) families consist of unrelated individuals or families who live under one roof. Reasons for cohabiting may be a need for companionship, a desire to achieve a sense of family, testing a relationship or commitment, or sharing expenses and household management. Cohabiting families illustrate the flexibility and creativity of the family unit in adapting to individual challenges and changing societal needs.

Homosexual Family

Homosexual adults may form gay and lesbian families based on the same goals of caring and commitment seen in heterosexual relationships. Children raised in these family units develop sex role orientations and behaviours similar to children in the general population. The greater danger to children in these families is the prejudice and ridicule expressed by others in society.

Single Adults Living Alone

Individuals who live by themselves represent a significant portion of today's society. Singles include young self-supporting adults who have recently left the nuclear family as well as older adults living alone. Older adults may find themselves single through divorce, separation or the death of a spouse.

In order to manage the nursing care of a patient the nurse needs a good awareness of health, illness and family structures. This management needs to be in the context of the nursing process.

NURSING MANAGEMENT

ASSESSING

Health Beliefs

To promote health, the nurse must understand the health beliefs of individuals and families. Health beliefs may reflect a lack of information or misinformation about health or disease. They may also include folklore and practices from different cultures. Because of the many advances in medicine and healthcare during the last few decades, patients may have outdated information about health, illness, treatment and prevention. The nurse is frequently in a position to give information or correct misconceptions. This function is an important component of the nursing care plan.

Family Communication Patterns

The effectiveness of family communication determines the family's ability to function as a cooperative, growth-producing unit. Messages are constantly being communicated among family members, both verbally and nonverbally. The information transmitted influences how members work together, fulfil their assigned roles in the family, incorporate family values and develop skills to function in society. Intrafamily communication plays a significant role in the development of self-esteem, which is necessary for the growth of personality.

Families that communicate effectively transmit messages clearly. Members are free to express their feelings without fear of jeopardising their standing in the family. Family members support one another and have the ability to listen, empathise and reach out to one another in times of crisis. When the needs of family members are met, they are more able to reach out to meet the needs of others in society.

When patterns of communication among family members are dysfunctional, messages are often communicated unclearly. Verbal communication may be incongruent with nonverbal messages. Power struggles may be evidenced by hostility, anger or silence. Members may be cautious in expressing their feelings because they cannot predict how others in the family will respond. When family communication is impaired, the growth of individual members is stunted. Members often turn to other systems to seek personal validation and gratification.

The nurse needs to observe intrafamily communication patterns closely. Nurses should pay special attention to who does the talking for the family, which members are silent, how disagreements are handled, and how well the members listen to one another and encourage the participation of others. Nonverbal communication is important because it gives valuable clues about what people are feeling.

Family Coping Mechanisms

Family coping mechanisms are the behaviours families use to deal with stress or changes imposed from either within or without. Coping mechanisms can be viewed as an active method of problem solving developed to meet life's challenges. The coping mechanisms families and individuals develop reflect their individual resourcefulness. Families may use coping patterns rather consistently over time or may change their coping strategies when new demands are made on the family. The success of a family largely depends on how well it copes with the stresses it experiences.

Nurses working with families realise the importance of assessing coping mechanisms as a way of determining how families relate to stress. Also important are the resources available to the family. Internal resources, such as knowledge, skills, effective communication patterns and a sense of mutuality and purpose within the family, assist in the problem-solving process. In addition, external support systems promote coping and adaptation. These external systems may be extended family, friends, religious affiliations, healthcare professionals or social services. The development of social support systems is particularly valuable today because many families, due to stress, mobility or poverty, are isolated from the resources that would traditionally have helped them cope.

Poverty and social isolation may be a factor contributing to the increase in family violence in recent years. Statistics are not accurate, because many cases remain unreported. Family violence includes abuse between intimate partners, child abuse and elder abuse, and may include physical, mental and verbal abuse, as well as neglect. Early symptoms are evident in burns, cuts, fractures and even death. Later manifestations often seen are depression, alcohol and substance abuse, and suicide attempts. Nurses should be alert to the symptoms of family violence and take appropriate measures to report it and obtain resources for the family.

Risk for Health Problems

Risk assessment helps the nurse identify individuals and groups at higher risk than the general population of developing specific health problems, such as stroke, diabetes and lung cancer. The vulnerability of family units to health problems may be based on the maturity level of individual family members, heredity or genetic factors, sex or race, sociological factors and lifestyle practices.

Maturity Factors

Families with members at both ends of the age continuum are at risk of developing health problems. Families entering childbearing and child-rearing phases experience many changes in roles, responsibilities and expectations. The many, often conflicting, demands on the family cause stress and fatigue, which may impede growth of individual family members and the functioning of the group as a unit. Adolescent mothers, because of their developmental level and lack of knowledge about parenthood, and single-parent families, because of role overload experienced by the head of the household, are more likely to develop health problems. Many elderly persons feel a lack of purpose and decreased self-esteem. These feelings in turn reduce their motivation to engage in health-promoting behaviours, such as exercise or community and family involvement.

Hereditary Factors

Persons born into families with a history of certain diseases, such as diabetes or cardiovascular disease, are at greater risk of developing these conditions. A detailed family health history, including genetically transmitted disorders, is crucial to the identification of persons and families at risk. These data are used not only to monitor the health of individual family members but also to recommend modifications in health practices that potentially reduce the risk, minimise the consequences or postpone the development of genetically related conditions.

Gender or Race

Some family units or family members may be at risk of developing a disease by reason of sex or race. Males, for example, are at greater risk of having cardiovascular disease at an earlier age than females, and females are at greater risk of developing osteoporosis, particularly after menopause. Although it is sometimes difficult to separate genetic factors from cultural factors, certain risk factors seem to be related to race. Sickle-cell anemia, for example, is a hereditary disease limited to people of African descent and Tay-Sachs is a neurodegenerative disease that occurs primarily in descendants of Eastern European Jews.

Sociological Factors

Poverty is a major problem that affects not only the family but also the community and society. Poverty is a real concern among the rising number of single-parent families, and as the number of these families increases, poverty will affect a large number of growing children.

When ill, the poor are likely to put off seeking services until the illness reaches an advanced state and requires longer or more complex treatment. Although the health of the people of industrialised nations has improved significantly during the past century, this progress has not benefited all segments of society, particularly the poor.

Lifestyle Factors

Many diseases are preventable, the effects of some diseases can be minimised or the onset of disease can be delayed through lifestyle modifications. Certain cancers, cardiovascular disease, adult-onset diabetes and tooth decay are among the lifestyle diseases. The incidence of lung cancer, for example, would be greatly reduced if people stopped smoking. Good nutrition, dental hygiene and use of fluoride – in the water supply, in toothpaste, as a topical application or as supplements – have been shown to reduce dental decay. Other important lifestyle considerations are exercise, stress management and rest. Today health professionals have the knowledge to prevent or minimise the effects of some of the main causes of disease, disability and death. The challenge is to disseminate information about prevention and to motivate families to make lifestyle changes prior to the onset of illness.

PLANNING

Being sensitive to cultural differences such as the practices of ethnic groups is important in assessment and planning care. Knowing who makes most of the decisions in the family, especially in healthcare, helps the nurse know to whom to direct questions in order to obtain information and also to whom to give instructions. The extended family unit is found in many cultures and there may be a difference in health beliefs and health practices within the family. Older members of the family may use their traditional practices, while younger members may have had more exposure to modern practices. Building a trusting relationship with these families is the first step toward planning more effective care by being able to talk to them about their beliefs and practices.

Nursing needs to focus on assisting the family to plan realistic goals/outcomes and strategies that enhance family functioning, such as improving communication skills, identifying and utilising support systems, and developing and rehearsing parenting skills. For families who are functioning well, anticipatory guidance may assist them in preparing for predictable developmental transitions that occur in the life of families.

The Family Experiencing a Health Crisis

Illness of a family member is a crisis that affects the entire family system. The family is disrupted as members abandon their usual activities and focus their energy on restoring family equilibrium. Roles and responsibilities previously assumed by the ill person are delegated to other family members, or those functions may remain undone for the duration of the illness. The family experiences anxiety because members are concerned about the sick person and the resolution of the illness. This anxiety is compounded by additional responsibilities when there is less time or motivation to complete the normal tasks of daily living. See *Box 5-5* on page 70 for some factors that determine the impact of illness on the family unit.

The family's ability to deal with the stress of illness depends on the members' coping skills. Families with good communication skills are better able to discuss how they feel about the illness and how it affects family functioning. They can plan for the future and are flexible in adapting these plans as the

BOX 5-5 Factors Determining the Impact of Illness on the Family

+ The nature of the illness, which can range from minor to life threatening
+ The duration of the illness, which ranges from short term to long term
+ The residual effects of the illness, including none to permanent disability
+ The meaning of the illness to the family and its significance to family systems
+ The financial impact of the illness, which is influenced by factors such as insurance and ability of the ill member to return to work
+ The effect of the illness on future family functioning (for instance, previous patterns may be restored or new patterns may be established)

situation changes. An established social support network provides strength, encouragement and services to the family during the illness. During health crises, families need to realise that it is a strength, not a sign of weakness, to turn to others for support. Nurses can be part of the support system for families, or they can identify other sources of support in the community.

During a crisis, families are often drawn together by a common purpose. In this time of closeness, family members have the opportunity to reaffirm personal and family values and their commitment to one another. Indeed, illness may provide a unique opportunity for family growth.

The Nurse's Role with Families Experiencing Illness

Nurses committed to family-centred care involve both the ailing individual and the family in the nursing process. Through their interaction with families, nurses can give support and information. Nurses make sure that not only the individual but also each family member understands the disease, its management and the effect of these two factors on family functioning. The nurse also assesses the family's readiness and ability to provide continued care and supervision at home when warranted. After carefully planned instruction and practice, families are given an opportunity to demonstrate their ability to provide care under the supportive guidance of the nurse. When the care indicated is beyond the capability of the family, nurses work with families to identify available resources that are socially and financially acceptable.

In helping families reintegrate the ill person into the home, nurses use data gathered during family assessment to identify family resources and deficits. By formulating mutually acceptable goals for reintegration, nurses help families cope with the realities of the illness and the changes it may have brought about, which may include new roles and functions of family members or the need to provide continued medical care to the ill or recovering person. Working together, nurses and families can create environments that restore or reorganise family functioning during illness and throughout the recovery process.

Death of a Family Member

The death of a family member often has a profound effect on the family. The structure of the family is altered, and this change may in turn affect how it functions as a unit. Individual members experience a sense of loss. They grieve for the lost person and for the family that once was. Family disorganisation may occur. However, as the family begins to recover, a new sense of normalcy develops, the family reintegrates its roles and functions, and it comes to grips with the reality of the situation. This painful blow takes time to heal.

After the death of a member, families may need counselling to deal with their feelings and to talk about the person who died. They may also want to talk about their fears and hopes for the future. At this time, families often derive comfort from their religious beliefs and their spiritual advisers. Support groups are also available for families experiencing the pain of death. It is often difficult for nurses to deal with grieving families because the nurses also feel the loss and feel inadequate in knowing what to say or do. By understanding the effect death has on families, nurses can help families resolve their grief and move ahead with life.

IMPLEMENTING AND EVALUATING

Nursing interventions are based on the medical diagnoses and selected goals or outcomes. In evaluating the success of the family care plan, the nurse assesses for the presence of the indicators identified for the chosen outcomes. If the indicators are present, it is likely that the outcome has been achieved. If the indicators or outcomes are partially or not met, all aspects of the family situation must be re-examined: Have the intervention activities been carried out? Are the indicators and outcomes appropriate? Is the nursing diagnosis proper? Has the medical condition or diagnosis changed?

Recognition of individual and family strengths helps to maintain wellness and also directs behaviour in crises situations. If a plan of care has to be modified to be more effective, these strengths should be identified and utilised.

APPLYING THEORETICAL FRAMEWORKS TO INDIVIDUALS AND FAMILIES

A variety of theoretical frameworks provide the nurse with a holistic overview of health promotion for the individual and families across the life span. Major theoretical frameworks that nurses use in promoting the health of the individual and family are needs theories, developmental stage theories, systems theories and structural–functional theories.

Needs Theories

In needs theories, human needs are ranked on an ascending scale according to how essential the needs are for survival. Abraham Maslow (1970), perhaps the most renowned needs theorist, ranks human needs on five levels (see Figure 5-8 and Box 5-6). The five levels in ascending order are as follows:

1. *Physiological needs.* Needs such as air, food, water, shelter, rest, sleep, activity and temperature maintenance are crucial for survival.
2. *Safety and security needs.* The need for safety has both physical and psychological aspects. The person needs to feel safe, both in the physical environment and in relationships.
3. *Love and belonging needs.* The third level of needs includes giving and receiving affection, attaining a place in a group and maintaining the feeling of belonging.
4. *Self-esteem needs.* The individual needs both self-esteem (i.e. feelings of independence, competence and self-respect) and esteem from others (i.e. recognition, respect and appreciation).
5. *Self-actualisation.* When the need for self-esteem is satisfied, the individual strives for self-actualisation, the innate need to develop one's maximum potential and realise one's abilities and qualities.

BOX 5-6 Maslow's Characteristics of a Self-Actualised Person

+ Is realistic, sees life clearly and is objective about his or her observations
+ Judges people correctly
+ Has superior perception, is more decisive
+ Has clear notion of right and wrong
+ Is usually accurate in predicting future events
+ Understands art, music, politics and philosophy
+ Possesses humility, listens to others carefully
+ Is dedicated to some work, task, duty or vocation
+ Is highly creative, flexible, spontaneous, courageous and willing to make mistakes
+ Is open to new ideas
+ Is self-confident and has self-respect
+ Has low degree of self-conflict; personality is integrated
+ Respects self, does not need fame, possesses a feeling of self-control
+ Is highly independent, desires privacy
+ Can appear remote and detached
+ Is friendly, loving and governed more by inner directives than by society
+ Can make decisions contrary to popular opinion
+ Is problem centred rather than self-centred
+ Accepts the world for what it is

Note: From *Toward a Psychology of Being*, 2nd edn, by A.H. Maslow, copyright 1968, NY: Van Nostrand Reinhold. This material is used by permission of John Wiley and Sons, Inc.

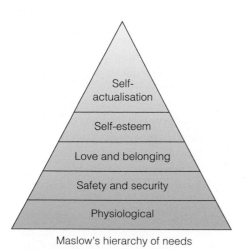

Maslow's hierarchy of needs

Maslow's hierarchy of needs, as adapted by Kalish

Figure 5-8 Maslow's needs. (From *Psychology of Human Behavior*, 5th edn by R.A. Kalish, copyright 1983. Reprinted with permission of Wadsworth, a division of Thomson Learning: www.thomsonrights.com. Fax 800-730-2215.)

Kalish's Hierarchy of Needs

Richard Kalish (1983) has adapted Maslow's hierarchy of needs into six levels rather than five. He suggests an additional category between the physiological needs and the safety and security needs. This category, referred to as *stimulation needs*, includes sex, activity, exploration, manipulation and novelty. Kalish emphasises that children need to explore and manipulate their environments to achieve optimal growth and development. He notes that adults, too, often seek novel adventures or stimulating experiences before considering their safety or security needs.

Characteristics of Basic Needs

All people have the same basic needs; however, each person's needs and the ways in which they react to those needs are influenced by the culture with which the person identifies. For example, professional achievement, independent functioning and privacy may be important in one culture or subculture and unimportant in another.

+ People meet their own needs relative to their own priorities. For example, a poor mother might give up her share of food so that her child might have sufficient food to live.
+ Although basic needs generally must be met, some needs can be deferred. An example is the need for independence, which an ill person can defer until well.
+ Failure to meet needs results in one or more homoeostatic imbalances, which can eventually result in illness.
+ A need can make itself felt by either external or internal stimuli. An example is the need for food. A person may experience hunger as a result of physiological processes (internal stimulation) or as a result of seeing a beautiful cake (external stimulation).
+ A person who perceives a need can respond in several ways to meet it. The choice of response is largely a result of learned experiences, lifestyle and the values of the culture. For example, one woman who comes home from work feeling tired may meet the need for relaxation by walking around the park while another takes a quick nap. Many people's food choices at mealtimes and snack times are based on past experiences, lifestyle and culture.
+ Needs are interrelated. Some needs cannot be met unless related needs are also met. The need for hydration can be influenced by the need for elimination of urine. Likewise, the need for security can be markedly altered if the need for oxygen is threatened by a respiratory obstruction.

Needs can be satisfied in healthy and unhealthy ways. Ways of meeting basic needs are considered healthy when they are not harmful to others or to self, conform to the individual's sociocultural values, and are within the law. Conversely, unhealthy behaviour may be harmful to others or to self, does not conform to the individual's sociocultural values or is not within the law. People who satisfy their basic needs appropriately are healthier, happier and more effective than those whose needs are frustrated.

Throughout their lifetime, individuals strive to meet needs. A person's perception of a need and his or her response to satisfy a need may be influenced by ethnocultural standards, by external and internal stimuli (e.g. hunger), and by self-determined priorities (e.g. stopping smoking). Positive factors that affect the satisfying of needs are an individual's healthy position on the wellness–illness continuum, the presence of supportive relationships, a good self-concept, and the satisfactory achievement of developmental stages. For example, if an infant achieves the developmental task of learning to trust, then the basic needs of feeling loved and secure are readily resolved.

Knowledge of the theoretical bases of human needs assists nurses in responding therapeutically to a patient's behaviours and in understanding themselves and their own responses to needs. Human needs serve as a framework for assessing behaviours, assigning priorities to desired outcomes and planning nursing interventions. For example, an adult with poor self-esteem would have difficulty accomplishing self-actualisation. Therefore, nursing interventions would focus on increasing the patient's self-esteem.

Developmental Stage Theories

Developmental stage theories of psychology related to individuals categorise a person's behaviours or tasks into approximate age ranges or in terms that describe the features of an age group. The age ranges of the stages do not take into account individual differences; however, the categories do describe characteristics associated with the majority of individuals at periods when distinctive developmental changes occur and with the specific tasks that must be accomplished. Because human development is highly complex and multifaceted, developmental stage theories describe only one aspect of development, such as cognitive, psychosexual, psychosocial, moral and faith development. Stage theories emphasise a definite, predictable sequence of development that is orderly and continuous. Each stage is affected by those stages preceding it and affects those stages that follow. For example, an adolescent who is unable to establish a stable sense of personal identity may have difficulty in later developmental stages with adult roles and career aspirations.

Developmental stage theories allow nurses to describe typical behaviours of an individual within a certain age group, explain the significance of those behaviours, predict behaviours that might occur in a given situation and provide a rationale to control behavioural manifestations. Individuals can be compared with a representative group of people at the same point in time or compared at different points in time. During care, the nurse's knowledge of stage theories can be used in parental and patient education, counselling, and anticipatory guidance.

Developmental stage theories view families as ever changing and growing. Crucial, yet predictable, tasks occur at each level or stage of development. Achievement of tasks appropriate at one level is a prerequisite for successfully achieving the tasks expected at the next level. A major task of the family, from a developmental perspective, is to create an environment where the family can master critical developmental tasks. This ensures orderly progression through the stages of the family life cycle.

Systems Theories

The basic concepts of general systems theory were proposed in the 1950s. One of its major proponents, Ludwig von Bertalanffy (1969) introduced systems theory as a universal theory that could be applied to many fields of study. Nurses are increasingly using systems theory to understand not only biological systems but also systems in families, communities, and nursing and healthcare. General systems theory provides a way of examining interrelationships and deriving principles.

Systems may be complex and the systems components are often studied as **subsystems**. For family systems, the subsystems would be individuals. Looking back up the hierarchy, the systems above other systems are referred to as **suprasystems** – the family is the suprasystem of the individual. See Figure 5-9 for a hierarchy of the human system.

The biological system can be subdivided into the neurological, musculoskeletal, respiratory, circulatory, gastrointestinal and urinary subsystems, among others. Each subsystem can in turn be subdivided. For example, the urinary system consists of the kidneys, the ureters and the bladder; the circulatory system consists of the heart and the blood vessels; the neurological system consists of the brain, the spinal cord and the nerves. The biological system can also be subdivided into categories of needs or functional health patterns or activities of daily living, such as nutrition and hydration, sleep/rest, activity/exercise, elimination, and so on.

The psychological and social systems consist of subsystems that include thinking, feeling and interaction patterns. Names of the psychological and social subsystems vary considerably according to individual nurse theorists. For example, Johnson (1980) describes the human system in terms of behaviours and lists the psychological subsystems as attachment-affiliative, dependence, achievement and aggressive.

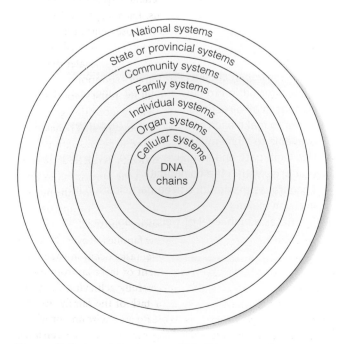

Figure 5-9 A common system hierarchy.

The interrelatedness of all the parts of a system is the basis for nursing's holistic view of the patient. A tumour of the liver affects the whole individual, that is, the person may be nauseated, tired, anxious, and so on. A psychological problem such as stress or anxiety may also manifest itself by physiological symptoms, such as sleeplessness, nausea or changes in cardiac function.

The family unit can also be viewed as a system. Its members are interdependent, working toward specific purposes and goals. Families, as open systems, are continually interacting with and influenced by other systems in the community. Boundaries regulate the input from other systems that interact with the family system; they also regulate output from the family system to the community or to society. Boundaries protect the family from the demands and influences of other systems. Families are likely to welcome input from without, encourage individual members to adapt beliefs and practices to meet the changing demands of society, seek out healthcare information and use community resources.

Structural-Functional Theory

The structural–functional theory, as the name implies, focuses on family structure and function. The structural component of the theory addresses the membership of the family and the relationships among family members. Intrafamily relationships are complex because of the numerous relationships that exist within the family structure: mother–daughter, brother–sister, spouse–partner, and so on. These relationships are constantly evolving as children mature and leave the family nest and adults age and become more dependent on others to meet their daily needs.

The functional aspect of the theory examines the effects of intrafamily relationships on the family system, as well as their effects on other systems. Some of the main functions of the family include developing a sense of family purpose and affiliation, adding and socialising new members, and providing and distributing care and services to members. A healthy family organises its members and resources in meeting family goals; it functions in harmony, working toward shared goals.

Nurses generally use a combination of theoretical frameworks in promoting the health of individuals and families. For example, the nurse may provide education for the mother of a toddler who is struggling to accomplish the developmental stage of autonomy described by Erikson (1963). Simultaneously, the nurse may provide guidance for the same family in its stressful transition period between developmental stages as their older school-age child becomes an adolescent.

COMMUNITY HEALTH

Increasingly those requiring healthcare are being managed in the community. A **community** is a collection of people who share some attribute of their lives. It may be that they live in the same locale, attend a particular church or even share a

---

BOX 5-7 Five Main Functions of a Community

1. *Production, distribution and consumption of goods and services.* These are the means by which the community provides for the economic needs of its members. This function includes not only the supplying of food and clothing but also the provision of water, electricity, police and fire protection, and the disposal of refuse.
2. *Socialisation.* Socialisation refers to the process of transmitting values, knowledge, culture and skills to others. Communities usually contain a number of established institutions for socialisation: families, churches, schools, media, voluntary and social organisations, and so on.
3. *Social control.* Social control refers to the way in which order is maintained in a community. Laws are enforced by the police; public health

regulations are implemented to protect people from certain diseases. Social control is also exerted through the family, church and schools.
4. *Social interparticipation.* Social interparticipation refers to community activities that are designed to meet people's needs for companionship. Families and churches have traditionally met this need; however, many public and private organisations also serve this function.
5. *Mutual support.* Mutual support refers to the community's ability to provide resources at a time of illness or disaster. Although the family is usually relied on to fulfil this function, health and social services may be necessary to augment the family's assistance if help is required over an extended period.

---

particular interest such as gardening. Groups that constitute a community because of common member interests are often referred to as a *community of interest* (e.g. religious and cultural groups). A community can also be defined as a social system in which the members interact formally or informally and form networks that operate for the benefit of all people in the community. Five of the main functions of a community are described in *Box 5-7*. In community health, the community may be viewed as having a common health problem, such as a high incidence of infant mortality or of tuberculosis, HIV infection, or another communicable disease. *Box 5-8* lists the characteristics of a healthy community. **Community health nursing** focuses on promoting and preserving the health of population groups.

BOX 5-8 Ten Characteristics of a Healthy Community

A Healthy Community
+ Is one in which members have a high degree of awareness of being a community
+ Uses its natural resources while taking steps to conserve them for future generations
+ Openly recognises the existence of subgroups and welcomes their participation in community affairs
+ Is prepared to meet crises
+ Is a problem-solving community; it identifies, analyses and organises to meet its own needs

+ Possesses open channels of communication that allow information to flow among all subgroups of citizens in all directions
+ Seeks to make each of its systems' resources available to all members
+ Has legitimate and effective ways to settle disputes that arise within the community
+ Encourages maximum citizen participation in decision making
+ Promotes a high level of wellness among all its members

NURSING MANAGEMENT

ASSESSING

Several community assessment frameworks have been devised which can be utilised to identify community health needs and target health interventions where they are required. As an example, Anderson and McFarlane (2000) identify eight subsystems of the community for analysis. The subsystems are illustrated around a core, which consists of the people and their characteristics, values, history and beliefs. The first stage in assessment is to learn about the people in the community. Figure 5-10 shows some of the major components of the community core. Surrounding the core are the eight subsystems. *Box 5-9* on page 76 shows major aspects of a community assessment and *Box 5-10* on page 76 shows sources of community data.

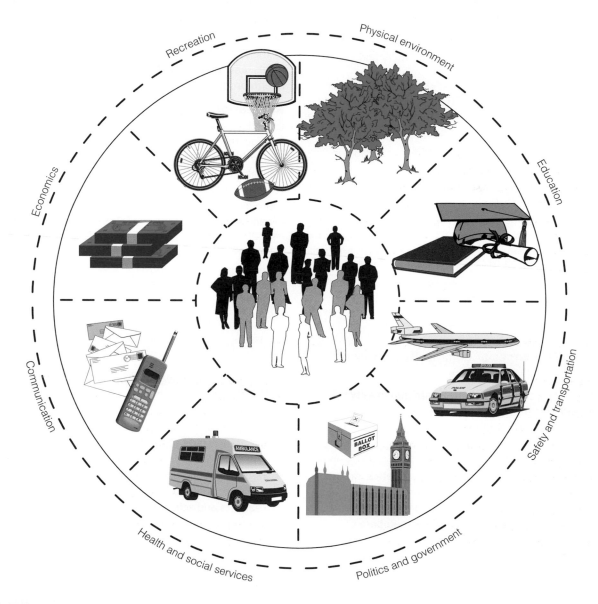

Figure 5-10 The community assessment wheel, the assessment segment of the community-as-partner model. (*Note*: From *Community as Partner: Theory and Practice in Nursing*, 3rd edn (p. 166), by E.T. Anderson and J. McFarlane, 2000, Philadelphia: Lippincott Williams and Wilkins.)

BOX 5-9 Major Aspects of a Community Assessment

Physical Environment

Consider the natural boundaries, size and population density; types of dwellings; and incidence of crime, vandalism and substance abuse.

Education

Consider educational facilities; existing school health facilities; type and amount of health services handled by the school; school lunch programmes; extracurricular sports, libraries and counselling services; continuing education or extended education programmes; and extent of parental involvement in the schools.

Safety and Transportation

Consider emergency service provision and sanitation services; sources of water and its treatment; quality of the air; waste disposal service; availability and safety of public transportation.

Politics and Government

Consider kind of local government; organisations active in the community; influential people in the community; issues that have recently appeared in the local press; and the average election turnout.

Health and Social Services

Consider existing hospitals, healthcare facilities and healthcare services; number, type and routine caseloads of community health professionals; geographic, economic and cultural accessibility to healthcare services; sources of health information; level of immunisation among children and adults; life expectancy in the community; availability of home healthcare and long-term care services; availability of transportation service to all major health facilities.

Communication

Consider local newspapers; radio and TV stations, postal services, Internet access and telephone services; frequency of public forums; and presence of informal bulletin boards.

Economics

Consider the main industries and occupations; percentage of the population employed or attending school; income levels and quality and type of housing; occupational health programmes; major employers in the community.

Recreation

Consider recreational facilities in the community and outside the community; theatre and cinemas; number and types of church and religious services; number and utilisation of playgrounds, pools, parks and sports facilities; level of participation in various church programmes; number and types of social committees, organisations and clubs available.

Note: From *Community as Partner: Theory and Practice in Nursing,* 3rd edn (pp. 168–170), by E.T. Anderson and J. McFarlane, 2000, Philadelphia: Lippincott Williams and Wilkins. Adapted with permission.

BOX 5-10 Sources of Community Assessment Data

+ Ordinance survey maps to locate community boundaries, roads, places of worship, schools, parks, hospitals, and so on
+ Local census data for population composition and characteristics
+ Local authority for employment statistics, major industries and primary occupations
+ Local health board for location of health facilities, occupational health programmes, numbers of health professionals, and so on
+ Local authority or telephone book for location of social, recreational and health organisations, committees and facilities
+ Public, college and university libraries for local social and cultural research reports

+ Health facility administrators for information about employee caseloads, prevalent types of problems and dominant needs
+ Recreational directors for programmes provided and participation levels
+ Police department for incidence of crime, vandalism and drug addiction
+ Teachers and school nurses for incidence of children's health problems and information on facilities and services to maintain and promote health
+ Local newspapers for community activities related to health and wellness, such as health lectures or health fairs
+ Online computer services that may provide access to public documents related to community health

PLANNING AND IMPLEMENTING

Planning community health may be oriented toward improved crisis management, disease prevention, health maintenance or health promotion. The responsibility for planning at the community level is usually broadly based. The exact resources and skills of members of the community often depend on the size of the community. A broadly based planning group is most likely to create a plan that is acceptable to members of the community. Also, people who are involved in planning become educated about the problems, the resources and the interrelationships within the system.

When setting priorities, health planners must work with consumers, interest groups, or other involved persons to prioritise health problems. It is important to take into consideration the values and interests of community members, the severity of the problems, and the resources available to identify and act on the problems. Because any plan is likely to result in change, members of the planning group should understand and use planned change theory.

EVALUATING

In community health, evaluation determines whether the planned interventions have led to the achievement of the established goals and objectives; for example, was the immunisation rate of preschool children improved? Because community health is usually a collaborative process between health providers, community leaders, politicians and consumers, all may be involved in the evaluation process. Often the community health nurse is the agent of evaluation, collecting and assessing the data that determine the effectiveness of implemented programmes.

CULTURE AND CULTURAL CARE NURSING

To provide quality care, nurses must become informed about and sensitive to the culturally diverse subjective meanings of **health**, illness, caring and healing practices.

Culture can be defined as the nonphysical traits, such as values, beliefs, attitudes and customs, that are shared by a group of people and passed from one generation to the next (Spector, 2000). Culture also defines how health is perceived; how healthcare information is received; how rights and protections are exercised; what is considered to be a health problem and how symptoms and concerns about the health problem are expressed; who should provide treatment and how; and what kind of treatment should be given. **Cultural care nursing** is a concept that describes the provision of nursing care across cultural boundaries and that takes into account the context in which the patient lives and the situations in which the patient's health problems arise. It is comprised of both content and process and is essential to the delivery of quality healthcare to all patients.

Nurses must be aware that, although people from a given group share certain beliefs, values and experiences, often there is also widespread intra-group diversity. Major differences within groups may be due to such factors as age, gender, level of education, socioeconomic status and area of origin in the home country (rural or urban). Such factors influence the patient's beliefs about health and illness, practices, help-seeking behaviours and expectations of nurses. For these reasons, effort must be made and care taken to avoid the stereotyping of people from a specific group.

Cultural Care Nursing

Cultural care is professional nursing care that is culturally sensitive, culturally appropriate and culturally competent respecting the patients individuality. Cultural care nursing is critical to meeting the complex nursing care needs of a given person, family and community. It is the provision of nursing care across cultural boundaries and takes into account the context in which the patient lives as well as the situations in which the patient's health problems arise.

+ **Culturally sensitive** implies that the nurse possesses some basic knowledge of and constructive attitudes toward the health traditions observed among the diverse cultural groups found in the setting in which they are practising.
+ **Culturally appropriate** implies that the nurse applies the underlying background knowledge that must be possessed to provide a given patient with the best possible healthcare.
+ **Culturally competent** implies that within the delivered care the nurse understands and attends to the total context of the patient's situation and uses a complex combination of knowledge, attitudes and skills.

Countless conflicts in the healthcare setting can be predicated on cultural misunderstandings. Although many of these misunderstandings are related to universal situations, such as verbal and nonverbal language misunderstandings, the conventions of courtesy, sequencing of interactions, phasing of interactions, objectivity, and so forth, many cultural misunderstandings are unique to the delivery of nursing care. Cultural sensitivity is essential and it demands that nurses be able to assess and interpret a given patient's health beliefs and practices, and cultural needs.

CONCEPTS RELATED TO CULTURAL CARE NURSING

All groups of people face issues in adapting to their environment: providing nutrition and shelter, caring for and educating children, dividing labour, developing social organisation, controlling disease and maintaining health. Humans adapt to varying environments by developing cultural solutions to meet these needs. Culture is a universal experience, but no two cultures are exactly alike. Cultural patterns are learned, and it is important for nurses to note that members of a particular group may not share identical cultural experiences. Thus, each member of a cultural group will be somewhat different from their own cultural counterparts.

Subculture

Large cultural groups often have cultural subgroups or sub-systems. A **subculture** is usually composed of people who have a distinct identity and yet are related to a larger cultural group. A subcultural group generally shares ethnic origin, occupation or physical characteristics with the larger cultural group. Examples of cultural subgroups include occupational groups (e.g. nurses), societal groups (e.g. feminists) and ethnic groups.

Bicultural

Bicultural is used to describe a person who crosses two cultures, lifestyles and sets of values (Giger and Davidhizar, 1999). For example, a young man whose father is Asian and whose mother is British may honour his traditional heritage while also being influenced by his mother's cultural values.

Diversity

Diversity refers to the fact or state of being different. Many factors account for diversity: race, gender, sexual orientation, culture, ethnicity, socioeconomic status, educational attainment, religious affiliation, and so on. Diversity therefore occurs not only between cultural groups but also within a cultural group.

Assimilation

Assimilation is the process by which an individual develops a new cultural identity. Assimilation means becoming like the members of the dominant culture. The process of assimilation encompasses various aspects, such as behavioural, marital, identification and civic. The underlying assumption is that the person from a given cultural group loses their original cultural identity to acquire the new one. In fact, because this is a conscious effort, it is not always possible, and the process may cause severe stress and anxiety. Assimilation can also be described as a collection of subprocesses: a process of inclusion through which a person gradually ceases to conform to any standard of life that differs from the dominant group standards

and, at the same time, a process through which the person learns to conform to all the dominant group standards. The process of assimilation is considered complete when the foreigner is fully merged into the dominant cultural group (McLemore *et al.*, 2001).

The concepts of assimilation and acculturation are complex and sensitive. The dominant society expects that all immigrants are in the process of acculturation and assimilation and that the world view that we share as nurses is commonly shared by our patients. Because we live in a society with many cultures, however, many variations of health beliefs and practices exist. Several other factors for cultural consideration include race, prejudice, stereotyping, discrimination and culture shock.

Race

Race is the classification of people according to shared biological characteristics, genetic markers or features. People of the same race have common characteristics such as skin colour, bone structure, facial features, hair texture and blood type. Different ethnic groups can belong to the same race and different cultures can be found within one ethnic group. It is important to understand that not all people of the same race have the same culture. Culture should not be confused with either race or ethnic group.

Prejudice

Prejudice is a negative belief or preference that is generalised about a group and that leads to 'prejudgement'. Prejudice occurs because either the person making the judgement does not understand the given person or his or her heritage, or the person making the judgement generalises an experience of one individual from a culture to all members of that group.

Stereotyping

Stereotyping is assuming that all members of a culture or ethnic group are alike. For example, a nurse may assume that all Italians verbally express pain loudly or that all Chinese people like rice. Stereotyping may be based on generalisations founded in research or it may be unrelated to reality. For example, research indicates that most Italians are likely to express pain verbally; however, a specific Italian patient may not do so. Stereotyping that is unrelated to reality is frequently an outcome of racism or discrimination. Nurses need to realise that not all people of a specific group have the same health beliefs, practices and values. It is therefore essential to identify a specific patient's beliefs, needs and values rather than assuming they are the same as those attributable to the larger group.

Discrimination

Discrimination, the differential treatment of individuals or groups based on categories such as race, ethnicity, gender, social class or exceptionality, occurs when a person acts on prejudice and denies another person one or more of the fundamental rights.

Culture Shock

Culture shock is a disorder that occurs in response to transition from one cultural setting to another. A person's former behaviour patterns are ineffective in such a setting, and basic cues for social behaviour are absent (Spector, 2000). This phenomena may occur when one moves from one geographic location to another or when a person immigrates to a new country. It may occur when a person is admitted into a hospital and has to adapt to a foreign situation. Expressions of culture shock may range from silence and immobility to agitation, rage or fury.

Ethnicity

Cultural background is a fundamental component of one's **ethnic** background or ethnicity, a group within the social system that claims to possess variable traits such as a common religion or language. The term *ethnic* has for some time aroused strongly negative feelings and often is rejected by the general population.

Religion

The third major component of a person's heritage is religion. Although the word has many definitions, **religion** may be considered a system of beliefs, practices and ethical values about divine or superhuman power or powers worshipped as the creator(s) and ruler(s) of the universe. The practice of religion is revealed in numerous cults, sects, denominations and churches. Ethnicity and religion are clearly related, and one's religion quite often is determined by one's ethnic group. Religion gives a person a frame of reference and a perspective with which to organise information. Religious teachings *vis-à-vis* health help to present a meaningful philosophy and system of practices within a system of social controls having specific values, norms and ethics. These are related to health in that compliance to a religious code is conducive to spiritual harmony. Illness is sometimes seen as the punishment for the violation of religious codes and morals. It is not possible to isolate the aspects of culture, religion and ethnicity that shape a person's world view. Each is part of the other and all three are united within the person.

Socialisation

Socialisation is the process of being raised within a culture and acquiring the characteristics of that group. Education – be it primary school, secondary school, college or nursing – is a form of socialisation. In addition, many people who have been socialised in cultures wherein traditional healthcare resources are used may prefer to use this type of care even when residing within a cultural setting with modern healthcare resources available.

HEALTH TRADITIONS AND HEALTH BELIEFS

The Health Traditions Model

The health traditions model is predicated on the concept of holistic health and describes what people do from a traditional perspective to maintain, protect and restore health. Imagine health as a complex, interrelated, threefold phenomenon, that is, the balance of all aspects of the person – the body, mind and spirit.

Interrelated Aspects

+ The body includes all physical aspects, such as genetic inheritance, body chemistry, gender, age, nutrition and physical condition.
+ The mind includes cognitive processes, such as thoughts, memories and knowledge of such emotional processes as feelings, defences and self-esteem.
+ The spiritual facet includes both positive and negative learned spiritual practices and teachings, dreams, symbols, stories; protecting forces; and metaphysical or native forces.

These aspects are in constant flux and change over time, yet each is completely related to the others and also related to the context of the person. The context includes the person's family, culture, work, community, history and environment (Spector, 2000).

The health traditions model (see Table 5-1 on page 80) consists of nine interrelated facets, represented by the following:

1. *Traditional methods of maintaining health* – physical, mental and spiritual – include following a proper diet and wearing proper clothing, concentrating and using the mind, and practising one's religion.
2. *Traditional methods of protecting health* – physical, mental and spiritual – include wearing protective objects, such as amulets, avoiding people who may cause trouble and placing religious objects in the home.
3. *Traditional methods of restoring health* – physical, mental and spiritual – include the use of herbal remedies, exorcism and healing rituals.

Three Views of Health Beliefs

Andrews and Boyle (2002) describe three views of health beliefs: magico-religious, scientific and holistic. In the **magico-religious health belief view**, health and illness are controlled by supernatural forces. The patient may believe that illness is the result of 'being bad' or opposing God's will. Getting well is also viewed as dependent on God's will. The patient may make statements such as 'If it is God's will, I will recover' or 'What did I do wrong to be punished with cancer?' Some cultures believe that magic can cause illness. A sorcerer or witch may put a spell or hex on the patient. Some people view illness as possession by an evil spirit. Although these beliefs are not supported by empirical evidence, patients who believe that

Table 5-1 The Nine Interrelated Facets of Health (Physical, Mental and Spiritual) and Personal Methods of Maintaining Health, Protecting Health and Restoring Health

	Physical	Mental	Spiritual
Maintain health	Proper clothing	Concentration	Religious worship
	Proper diet	Social and family support systems	Prayer
	Exercise/rest	Hobbies	Meditation
Protect health	Special foods and food combination	Avoid certain people who can cause illness	Religious customs
	Symbolic clothing	Family activities	Superstitions
			Wearing amulets and other symbolic objects to prevent the 'Evil Eye' or defray other sources of harm
Restore health	Homoeopathic remedies	Relaxation	Religious rituals, special prayers
	Liniments	Exorcism	Meditation
	Herbal teas	Curanderos and other traditional healers	Traditional healings
	Special foods	Nerve teas	Exorcism
	Massage		
	Acupuncture/moxibustion		

Note: From Spector, Rachel E., *Cultural Diversity in Health and Illness*, 5th Edition, © 2000, pg 100. Reprinted by permission of Pearson Education Inc., Upper Saddle River, NJ.

such things can cause illness may in fact become ill as a result. Such illnesses may require magical treatments in addition to scientific treatments. For example, a man who experiences gastric distress, headaches and hypertension after being told that a spell has been placed on him may recover only if the spell is removed by the culture's healer.

The **scientific or biomedical health belief** is based on the belief that life and life processes are controlled by physical and biochemical processes that can be manipulated by humans (Andrews and Boyle, 2002). The patient with this view will believe that illness is caused by germs, viruses, bacteria or a breakdown of the human machine, the body. This patient will expect a pill, treatment or surgery to cure health problems.

The **holistic health belief** holds that the forces of nature must be maintained in balance or harmony. Human life is one aspect of nature that must be in harmony with the rest of nature. When the natural balance or harmony is disturbed, illness results.

The concept of *yin* and *yang* in the Chinese culture and the hot–cold theory of illness in many Spanish cultures are examples of holistic health beliefs. When a Chinese patient has a *yin* illness or a 'cold' illness, the treatment may include a *yang* or 'hot' food (e.g. hot tea). For example, a Chinese patient who has been diagnosed with cancer, a *yin* disease, will want to eat cultural foods that have *yang* properties.

What is considered hot or cold varies considerably across cultures. In many cultures, the mother who has just delivered a baby should be offered warm or hot foods and kept warm with blankets because childbirth is seen as a 'cold' condition.

Conventional scientific thought recommends cooling the body to reduce a fever. The patient may have cool compresses applied to the forehead, the axillae or the groin. Galanti (1997) states that many cultures believe that the best way to treat a fever is to 'sweat it out'. Patients from these cultures may want to cover up with several blankets, take hot baths and drink hot beverages. The nurse must keep in mind that a treatment strategy that is consistent with the patient's beliefs may have a better chance of being successful.

Folk medicine

Sociocultural forces, such as politics, economics, geography, religion and the predominant healthcare system, influence the patient's health status and healthcare behaviour. For example, people who have limited access to scientific healthcare may turn to folk medicine or folk healing. **Folk medicine** is defined as those beliefs and practices relating to illness prevention and healing that derive from cultural traditions rather than from modern medicine's scientific base. Many students can recall special teas or 'cures' used by older family members to prevent or treat colds, fevers, indigestion and other common health problems. People also continue to use chicken soup as a treatment for influenza (the 'flu').

Why do individuals use these nontraditional folk healing methods? Folk medicine, in contrast to biomedical healthcare, is thought to be more humanistic. The consultation and treatment takes place in the community of the recipient, frequently in the home of the healer. It is less expensive than scientific or biomedical care because the health problem is identified primarily through conversation with the patient and the family. The healer often prepares the treatments, for example, teas to be ingested, poultices to be applied, or charms or amulets to be worn. A frequent component of treatment is some ritual practice on the part of the healer or the patient to cause healing to occur. Because folk healing is more culturally based, it is often more comfortable and less frightening for the patient.

It is important for the nurse to obtain information about folk or family healing practices that may have been used before the patient decided to seek traditional medical treatment. Often patients are reluctant to share home remedies with healthcare professionals for fear of being laughed at or rebuked.

COMMUNICATION STYLE

Communication and culture are closely interconnected. Through communication, culture is transmitted from one generation to the next, and knowledge about culture is transmitted within the group and to those outside the group. Communicating with patients of various ethnic and cultural backgrounds is critical to providing culturally competent nursing care. There can be cultural variations in both verbal and nonverbal communication.

Verbal Communication

The most obvious cultural difference is in verbal communication: vocabulary, grammatical structure, voice qualities, intonation, rhythm, speed, pronunciation and silence. In the UK, the dominant language is English; however, in some areas traditional dialect like Welsh and Gaelic are spoken. Even when English is spoken the nurse may still encounter language differences because English words can have different meanings in different English-speaking cultures/areas.

Initiating verbal communication may be influenced by cultural values. The busy nurse may want to complete nursing admission assessments quickly. The patient, however, may be offended when the nurse immediately asks personal questions. In some cultures, it is believed that social courtesies should be established before business or personal topics are discussed. Discussing general topics can convey that the nurse is interested in the patient and has time for them. This enables the nurse to develop a rapport before progressing to discussion that is more personal.

Verbal communication becomes even more difficult when an interaction involves people who speak different languages (see the *Practice guidelines* below). Both patients and health professionals experience frustration when they are unable to communicate verbally with each other.

For the patient whose language is not the same as that of the healthcare provider, an intermediary may be necessary. A **translator** converts written material (such as patient education pamphlets) from one language into another. An **interpreter** is 'an individual who mediates spoken communication between people speaking different languages without adding, omitting, distorting meaning or editorialising. A true interpreter has demonstrated ethical and interpreting skills and the knowledge and expertise required to function in a healthcare situation. In some hospitals a language line may be used, which is a 24-hour a day interpretation line. The nurse is able to have a three-way conference call with the patient and interpreter, in order to discuss clinical care. A language line aims to have an interpreter available on a phone within a few minutes of a request being made and covers all major international languages. Many hospitals that are located in culturally diverse communities have translators available on staff or maintain a list of employees who are fluent in other languages. Embassies, consulates, ethnic churches (e.g. Russian Orthodox, Greek Orthodox), and ethnic clubs may also be able to provide interpreters. However, asking a family member or other non-professional to interpret can create difficulties. Cultural rules often dictate who can discuss what with whom. Guidelines for using an interpreter are shown in the *Practice guidelines* on page 82.

PRACTICE GUIDELINES

Verbal Communication with Patients Who Have Limited Knowledge of English

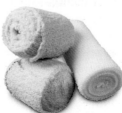

+ Avoid slang words, medical terminology and abbreviations.
+ Augment spoken conversation with gestures or pictures to increase the patient's understanding.
+ Speak slowly, in a respectful manner, and at a normal volume. Speaking loudly does not help the patient understand and may be offensive.
+ Frequently check the patient's understanding of what is being communicated. Be wary of interpreting a patient smiling and nodding to mean that they understand; the patient may only be trying to please the nurse and not understand what is being said.

Nurses and other healthcare providers must remember that patients for whom English is a second language may lose command of their English when they are in stressful situations. Patients who have used English comfortably for years in social and business communication may forget and revert back to their primary language when they are ill or distressed. It is important for the nurse to assure the patient that this is normal and to promote behaviours to facilitate verbal communication.

Nonverbal Communication

To communicate effectively with culturally diverse patients, the nurse needs to be aware of two aspects of nonverbal communication behaviours: what nonverbal behaviours mean to the patient and what specific nonverbal behaviours mean in the patient's culture. Before assigning meaning to nonverbal behaviour, the nurse must consider the possibility that the behaviour may have a different meaning for the patient and the family. To provide safe and effective care, nurses who work with specific cultural groups should learn more about cultural behaviour and communication patterns within these cultures.

PRACTICE GUIDELINES

Using an Interpreter

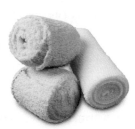

+ Avoid asking a member of the patient's family, especially a child or spouse, to act as interpreter. The patient, not wishing family members to know about his or her problem, may not provide complete or accurate information.
+ Be aware of gender and age differences; it is preferable to use an interpreter of the same gender as the patient to avoid embarrassment and faulty translation of sexual matters.
+ Avoid an interpreter who is politically or socially incompatible with the patient. For example, a Bosnian Serb may not be the best interpreter for a Muslim, even if he speaks the language, due to cultural differences.
+ Address the questions to the patient, not to the interpreter.
+ Ask the interpreter to translate as closely as possible the words used by the nurse.
+ Speak slowly and distinctly. Do not use metaphors, for example, 'Does it swell like a grapefruit?' or 'Is the pain stabbing like a knife?'
+ Observe the facial expressions and body language that the patient assumes when listening and talking to the interpreter.

Nonverbal communication can include the use of silence, touch, eye movement, facial expressions and body posture. Some cultures are quite comfortable with long periods of silence, whereas others consider it appropriate to speak before the other person has finished talking. Many people value silence and view it as essential to understanding a person's needs or use silence to preserve privacy. Some cultures view silence as a sign of respect, whereas to other people silence may indicate agreement.

Touching involves learned behaviours that can have both positive and negative meanings. In the American culture, a firm handshake is a recognised form of greeting that conveys character and strength. In some European cultures, greetings may include a kiss on one or both cheeks. In some societies, touch is considered magical and because of the belief that the soul can leave the body on physical contact, casual touching is forbidden. In some Asian cultures (e.g. people from India, Sri Lanka, Thailand and Laos), only certain older adults are permitted to touch the heads of others, and children are never patted on the head. Nurses should therefore touch a patient's head only with permission.

Cultures dictate what forms of touch are appropriate for individuals of the same sex and opposite sex. In many cultures, for example, a kiss is not appropriate for a public greeting between persons of the opposite sex, even those who are family members; however, a kiss on the cheek is acceptable as a greeting among individuals of the same sex. The nurse should watch interaction among patients and families for cues to the appropriate degree of touch in that culture.

Facial expression can also vary between cultures. Giger and Davidhizar (1999) state that Italian, Jewish, African and Spanish-speaking persons are more likely to smile readily and use facial expression to communicate feelings, whereas Irish, English and Northern European people tend to have less facial expression and are less open in their response, especially to strangers. Facial expressions can also convey a meaning opposite to what is felt or understood.

Eye movement during communication has cultural foundations. In Western cultures, direct eye contact is regarded as important and generally shows that the other is attentive and listening. It conveys self-confidence, openness, interest and honesty. Lack of eye contact may be interpreted as secretiveness, shyness, guilt, lack of interest, or even a sign of mental illness. However, other cultures may view eye contact as impolite or an invasion of privacy. In the China Hmong culture, continuous direct eye contact is considered rude, but intermittent eye contact is acceptable. The nurse should not misinterpret the character of the patient who avoids eye contact.

Body posture and hand gestures are also culturally learned. For example, the V sign means victory in some cultures, but it is an offensive gesture in other cultures. Communication is an essential part of establishing a relationship with a patient and his or her family. It is also important for developing effective working relationships with healthcare colleagues. To enhance their practice, nurses can observe the communication patterns of patients and colleagues and be aware of their own communication behaviours.

Space Orientation

Space is a relative concept that includes the individual, the body, the surrounding environment and objects within that environment. The relationship between the individual's own body and objects and persons within space is learned and is influenced by culture. For example, in nomadic societies, space is not owned; it is occupied temporarily until the tribe moves on. In Western societies people tend to be more territorial, as reflected in phrases such as 'This is my space' or 'Get out of my space.' In Western cultures, spatial distances are defined as the intimate zone, the personal zone and the social and public zones. The size of these areas may vary with the specific culture. Nurses move through all three zones as they provide care for patients. The nurse needs to be aware of the patient's response to movement toward the patient. The patient may physically withdraw or back away if the nurse is perceived as being too close. The nurse will need to explain to the patient why there is a need to be close to the patient. To assess the lungs with a stethoscope, for example, the nurse needs to move into the patient's intimate space. The nurse should first explain the procedure and await permission to continue.

Patients who reside in long-term care facilities, or who are hospitalised for an extended time, may want to personalise their space. They may want to arrange their room differently or control the placement of objects on their bedside cabinet or over-bed table. The nurse should be responsive to patients' needs to have some control over their space. When there are no medical contraindications, patients should be permitted and encouraged to have objects of personal significance. Having personal and cultural items in one's environment can increase self-esteem by promoting not only one's individuality but also one's cultural identity. Of course, the nurse should caution the patient about responsibility for loss of personal items.

Nutritional Patterns

Nutrition is essential when considering health and healing from illness or disease. Most cultures have staple foods, that is, foods that are plentiful or readily accessible in the environment. For example, the staple food for Asians is rice; of Italians, pasta; and of Eastern Europeans, wheat. Even patients who have been in the USA or UK for several generations often continue to eat the foods of their cultural homeland.

The way food is prepared and served is also related to cultural practices. For example, some Asian cultures prefer steamed rice; others prefer boiled rice. Southern Asians from India prepare unleavened bread from wheat flour rather than the leavened bread of Western culture.

Food-related cultural behaviours can include whether to breastfeed or bottle-feed infants, and when to introduce solid foods to them. Food can also be considered part of the remedy for illness. Foods classified as 'hot' foods or foods that are hot in temperature may be used to treat illnesses that are classified as 'cold' illnesses. For example, corn meal (a 'hot' food) may be used to treat arthritis (a 'cold' illness). Each culture group defines what it considers to be hot and cold entities.

Religious practice associated with specific cultures also affects diet. Some Roman Catholics avoid meat on certain days, such as Ash Wednesday and Good Friday, and some Protestant faiths prohibit meat, tea, coffee or alcohol. Both Orthodox Judaism and Islam prohibit the ingestion of pork or pork products. Orthodox Jews observe kosher customs, eating certain foods only if they have been inspected by a rabbi and prepared according to dietary laws. For example, the eating of milk products and meat products at the same meal is prohibited. Some Buddhists, Hindus and Sikhs are strict vegetarians. The nurse must be sensitive to such religious dietary practices.

CRITICAL REFLECTION

Let us revisit the case study on page 50. Now that you have read this chapter what is the difference between an acute and chronic illness? Which health belief models could you use in your explanation? How may David define health, wellness and illness? What external environmental factors could affect David and his health?

CHAPTER HIGHLIGHTS

+ Nurses need to clarify their understanding of health because their definitions of health largely determine the scope and nature of nursing practice. Likewise, people's health beliefs influence their health practices.

+ The perspective from which health is viewed has changed; instead of absence of disease, health has come to mean a high level of wellness or the fulfilment of one's maximum potential for physical, psychosocial and spiritual functioning.

+ Most people describe health as freedom from symptoms of disease, the ability to be active and a state of being in good spirits.

+ Because notions of health are highly individual, the nurse must determine a patient's perception of health in order to provide meaningful assistance. This involves well-developed communication skills. Nurses need to be aware of their own personal definitions of health.

+ Internal variables include biological, psychological and cognitive dimensions. The biological dimension includes genetic makeup, sex, age and developmental level. The psychological dimension includes mind–body interactions and self-concept. The cognitive dimension includes lifestyle choices and spiritual and religious beliefs.

+ External variables influencing health are physical environment, standards of living, family and cultural beliefs, and social support networks.

+ Nurses can enhance healthcare compliance by identifying the reasons for noncompliance if it occurs, demonstrating caring, using positive reinforcement to encourage healthy behaviours, using aids to reinforce teaching, and establishing a therapeutic relationship of freedom, mutual understanding and mutual responsibility with the patient and support persons.

+ Illness is usually associated with disease but may occur independently of it. Illness is a highly personal state in which the person feels unhealthy or ill. Disease alters body functions and results in a reduction of capacities or a shortened life span.

+ Various theorists have described stages and aspects of illness. Parsons describes four aspects of the sick role. Suchman outlines five stages of illness: symptom experience, assumption of the sick role, medical care contact, dependent patient role, and recovery or rehabilitation.

+ Nursing involves viewing the patient as an individual and in a holistic way.

+ To ensure holistic healthcare, the nurse considers all components of health (health promotion, health maintenance, health education and illness prevention, and restorative-rehabilitative care) and recognises that disturbance in one part of a person affects the whole being.

+ Homoeostasis is the tendency of the body to maintain a state of relative balance or constancy in response to a changing internal and external environment.

+ Homoeostatic mechanisms regulate hormone secretion, fluid and electrolyte levels, the functions of body viscera, and metabolic processes that provide energy for the body.

+ Psychological homoeostasis, or emotional well-being, is acquired or learned through the experience of living and interacting with others.

+ The family is the basic unit of society.

+ The family plays an important role in forming the health beliefs and practices of its members.

+ Family-centred nursing addresses the health of the family as a unit, as well as the health of family members.

+ Maslow's hierarchy of human needs consists of five categories: physiological (survival) needs, safety needs, love and belonging needs, self-esteem needs and self-actualisation needs.

+ A community is a collection of people who share some attribute of their lives.

+ For community assessment, eight subsystems proposed by Anderson and McFarlane (2000) can be used: physical environment, education, safety and transportation, politics and government, health and social services, communication, economics and recreation.

REFERENCES

Anderson, E.T. and McFarlane, J. (2000) *Community as partner: Theory and practice in nursing* (3rd edn), Philadelphia: Lippincott Williams and Wilkins.

Andrews, M.M. and Boyle, J.S. (2002) *Transcultural concepts in nursing care* (4th edn), Philadelphia: Lippincott Williams and Wilkins.

Anspaugh, D.J., Hamrick, M. and Rosato, F.D. (2003) *Wellness: Concepts and applications* (5th edn), New York: McGraw-Hill.

Baldwin, J.H. and Conger, C.O. (2001) 'Health promotion and wellness', in K.S. Lundy and S. Janes (Eds), *Community health nursing: Caring for the public's health* (pp. 286–307), Boston: Jones and Bartlett.

Becker, M.H. (Ed.) (1974) *The health belief model and personal health behavior*, Thorofare, NJ: Charles B. Slack.

Becker, M.H. Haefner, D.P., Kasl, S.V., Kirscht, J.P., Maiman, L.A. and Rosenstock, I.M. (1977) 'Selected psychosocial models and correlates of individual health-related behaviors', *Medical Care*, 15(5 Suppl.), 27–46.

Cannon, W.B. (1939) *The wisdom of the body* (2nd edn), New York: Norton.

Dunn, H.L. (1959) 'High-level wellness in man and society', *American Journal of Public Health*, 48, 786.

Dunn, H.L. (1973) *High-level wellness* (7th edn), Arlington, VA: Beatty.

Economic and Social Resource Council (2006). www.esrc.ac.uk. (Accessed March 2006.)

Erikson, E. (1963) *Childhood and society* (2nd edn), New York: Norton.

Galanti, G. (1997) *Caring for patients from different cultures: Case studies from American hospitals* (2nd edn), Philadelphia: University of Pennsylvania Press.

Giger, J.N. and Davidhizar, R. (1999) *Transcultural nursing: Assessment and intervention* (3rd edn), St. Louis, MO: Mosby.

Hood, L. and Leddy, S.K. (2002) *Leddy and Pepper's conceptual basis of professional nursing* (5th edn), Philadelphia: Lippincott Williams and Wilkins.

Hurdle, D.E. (2001) 'Social support: A critical factor in women's health and health promotion', *Health and Social Work*, 26(2), 72–79.

Johnson, D.E. (1980) 'The behavioral system model for nursing', in J.P. Riehl and C. Roy (Eds), *Conceptual models for nursing practice* (2nd edn, pp. 207–216), New York: Appleton-Century-Crofts.

Kalish, R.A. (1983) *The psychology of human behavior* (5th edn), Monterey, CA: Brooks/Cole.

Leavell, H.R. and Clark, E.G. (1965) *Preventive medicine for the doctor in his community* (3rd edn), New York: McGraw-Hill.

Maslow, A.H. (1968) *Toward a psychology of being* (2nd edn), New York: John Wiley and Sons.

Maslow, A.H. (1970) *Motivation and personality* (2nd edn), New York: Harper and Row.

McLemore, S., Romo, H.D. and Baker, S.G. (2001) *Racial and ethnic relations in America* (6th edn), Needham Heights, MA: Allyn and Bacon.

Murphy, P.A., Prewitt, T.E., Bote, E., West, B. and Iber, F.L. (2001) 'Internal locus of control and social support associated with some dietary changes by elderly participants in a diet intervention trial', *Journal of the American Dietetic Association*, 101, 203–208.

Murray, R.B. and Zentner, J.P. (2001) *Health assessment promotion strategies through the life span* (7th edn), Upper Saddle River, NJ: Prentice Hall.

Muscari, M.E. (1998) 'Rebels with a cause: When adolescents won't follow medical advice', *American Journal of Nursing*, 98(12), 26–31.

Nightingale, F. (1969) *Notes on nursing: What it is, and what it is not*, New York: Dover Books. (Original work published in 1860.)

Parsons, T. (1951) *The social system*, Glencoe, IL: Free Press.

Parsons, T. (1979) 'Definitions of health and illness in the light of American values and social structure', in E.G. Jaco (Ed.), *Patients, physicians, and illness* (3rd edn), New York: Free Press.

Pender, N.J., Murdaugh, C.L. and Parsons, M.J. (2002) *Health promotion in nursing practice* (4th edn), Upper Saddle River, NJ: Prentice Hall.

Rosenstock, I.M. (1974) 'Historical origins of the health belief model', in M.H. Becker (Edn), *The health belief model and personal health behavior*, Thorofare, NJ: Charles B. Slack.

Roy, C. (1999) *The Roy adaptation model* (2nd edn), Upper Saddle River, NJ: Prentice Hall.

Suchman, E.A. (1979) 'Stages of illness and medical care', in E.G. Jaco (Ed.), *Patients, physicians, and illness* (3rd edn), New York: Free Press.

Spector, R.E. (2000) *Cultural diversity in health and illness* (5th edn), Upper Saddle River, NJ: Prentice Hall.

Travis, J.W. and Ryan, R.S. (2001) *Simply well*, Berkeley, CA: Ten Speed Press.

Tyson, S.R. (1999) *Gerontological nursing care. 'Elders: Issues that influence the health and well-being of elders'*, Philadelphia: W.B. Saunders.

von Bertalanffy, L. (1969) *General system theory*, New York: George Braziller.

Wallston, K.A., Wallston, B.S. and DeVellis, R. (1978, Spring) 'Development of the Multidimensional Locus of Control (MHLC) scales', *Health Education Monographs*, 6, 160–170.

Wong, V.K. and White, M.A. (2002) Family dynamics and health locus of control in adults with ostomies. *Journal of WOCN*, 29(1), 37–44.

World Health Organization (1948) *Preamble to the constitution of the World Health Organization as adopted by the International Health Conference. New York, 19–22 June 1946; signed on 22 July 1946 by the representatives of 61 States* (Official Records of the World Health Organization, no. 2, p. 100) and entered into force on 7 April 1948.

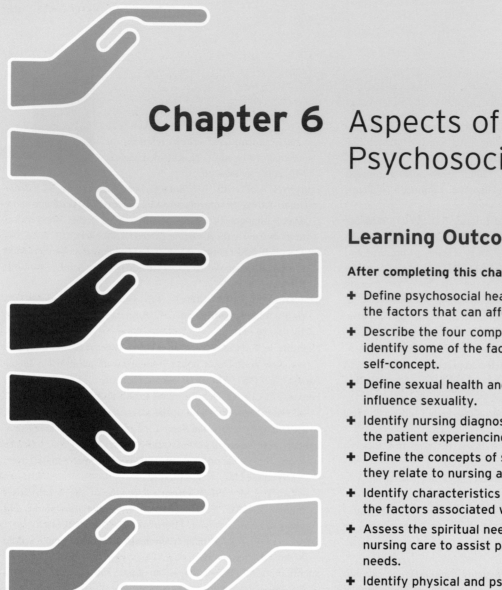

Chapter 6 Aspects of Psychosocial Health

Learning Outcomes

After completing this chapter, you will be able to:

+ Define psychosocial health and describe some of the factors that can affect it.

+ Describe the four components of self-concept and identify some of the factors that could affect self-concept.

+ Define sexual health and identify factors that influence sexuality.

+ Identify nursing diagnoses and interventions for the patient experiencing sexuality problems.

+ Define the concepts of spirituality and religion as they relate to nursing and healthcare.

+ Identify characteristics of spiritual well-being and the factors associated with spiritual distress.

+ Assess the spiritual needs of patients and plan nursing care to assist patients with spiritual needs.

+ Identify physical and psychological indicators of stress.

+ Differentiate four levels of anxiety.

+ Identify behaviours related to specific ego defence mechanisms.

+ Discuss types of coping and coping strategies.

+ Identify essential aspects of assessing a patient's stress and coping patterns and plan appropriate interventions to help the patient manage stress.

CASE STUDY

Terry is a 32-year-old married man who was in a serious road traffic accident a month ago. He was in intensive care for three weeks on a ventilator but now is on a surgical ward. During the car accident Terry severely injured his pelvis and had to have one of his testes removed. While you are caring for Terry, he comments, 'I might as well die right now because I'm not going to get well.' His wife has also expressed concern over the possibility of never having children although Terry has not discussed this matter with you.

After reading this chapter you will understand the importance of managing this patient's psychosocial health.

INTRODUCTION

Psychosocial health is basically how we see life and our experiences and is fundamental in a person's general well-being, encompassing mental, emotional, social, sexual and spiritual aspects of health. A psychosocially healthy individual is more likely to appreciate life and have what is considered a 'good quality of life'.

The roots of the term psychosocial health lie in the World Health Organization's (1948) definition of health which states that health is a 'state of complete physical, mental and social well-being and not merely the absence of disease and infirmity' (p. 1).

Psychosocial health is affected by a number of factors, some internal and others external. External influences are those parts of our life experiences that we have little or no control over, for instance our family and where we grow up. Research studies in this area have found that children who grow up in a happy family have more chances of becoming a successful adult while children who grow up in families with violence, negative behaviours, drug abuse, emotional and physical abuse are more likely to have difficulties dealing with life, experiencing possible depression (Randolph and Dykman, 1998) and physical illnesses such as coronary heart disease (Rozanski *et al.*, 2005).

In fact, the government have recently recognised this area as so problematic it has initiated a pilot project in Leeds Teaching Hospitals NHS Trust to identify tomorrow's anti-social children before they are even born, colloquially termed 'foetal Asbos' (BBC News, 2006). As part of this project, midwives have been charged with identifying unborn children who are likely to be exposed to risk factors such as domestic violence, alcohol abuse, drug abuse and poor education in a bid to put supporting interventions in place for the parents. These interventions are aimed at improving the parents' self-concept; increasing confidence; reducing social and psychological isolation and encouraging the parents to take control of their lives.

The internal factors associated with psychosocial health are equally as important as the external factors; however they are harder to see as they are inside the person. Internal factors such as self-concept, hereditary traits, physical health status, physical fitness level, hormonal functioning, and mental, social, sexual, spiritual and emotional health all have an impact on the individual's psychosocial health.

Self concept is one of the key aspects of balanced psychosocial health and can be said to be the mental image of oneself. A person is not born with a self-concept; rather, it is learned as a result of social interactions with others (see Chapter 9). A positive self-concept is essential to a person's mental and physical health. Individuals with a positive self-concept are better able to develop and maintain relationships and avoid psychological and physical illness. Also a person with a strong self-concept is usually better able to accept and adapt to change.

Self-concept involves all of the self-perceptions, that is, appearance, values and beliefs that influence behaviour and that are referred to when using the words *I* or *me*. Self-concept is a complex idea that influences:

+ how we think, talk and act;
+ how we see and treat other people;
+ the choices that we make;
+ our ability to give and receive love;
+ our ability to take action and to change things.

Nurses have a responsibility not only to identify people with a negative self-concept, but also to identify the possible causes in order to help people develop a more positive view of themselves and their lives. Individuals who have a poor self-concept may express feelings of worthlessness, self-dislike or even self-hatred, and may feel sad or hopeless and lack energy to perform even the simplest of tasks.

Although it is important that the nurse identifies patients with possible negative self-concepts, it is equally important that the nurse also recognises the different dimensions of himself or herself; his or her individual attitudes, beliefs and conflicts. Nurses who feel positive about themselves are more likely to help patients meet their needs.

In order to recognise these dimensions require **self-awareness**; the realisation that one exists. It is the concept that an individual exists separate to others with private thoughts, feelings, attitudes and beliefs. Becoming self aware is an active process that requires time and energy and is never complete. It requires introspection, looking inward, which is encouraged in the form of reflection within nursing and other healthcare disciplines. Reflection lets the nurse gain insight into the self, recognising individual strengths and weaknesses and allows for personal and professional development. Once the nurse has developed a clear understanding and awareness of self, he or she can respect and avoid projecting his or her own beliefs onto others.

COMPONENTS OF SELF-CONCEPT

Self-concept is generally composed of four components: personal identity, body image, role performance and self-esteem. Developing a positive self-concept requires balancing each of these four components.

Personal Identity

Personal identity is a person's conscious sense of individuality and is often viewed in terms of name, age, sex, race, occupation, marital status and education. However personal identity is far more than this, it includes our beliefs and values, personality and character. For instance, is the person outgoing, friendly, reserved, generous or selfish? Personal identity thus encompasses both the tangible and factual, such as name and sex, and the intangible, such as values and beliefs. Identity is what distinguishes self from others.

One key component of a person's identity is their **sexuality**. Sex is central to who we are, to our emotional well-being, and to the quality of our lives. All people have the potential to positively experience and pleasurably express their sexuality. One does not have to be in a relationship to be sexual. The idea that you need another person to feel sexual is both disempowering and untrue.

As nurses it is important to remember that patients do not leave their sexuality behind when they enter the healthcare system – their sexuality is always a part of them. Thus when providing holistic care, nurses have a responsibility to allow patients to express their sexuality.

Sexuality and spirituality are important aspects of a person's identity and therefore are explored in more detail later in this chapter.

Body Image

Body image is the perception of one's physical appearance: size, appearance and functioning of the body and its parts. Body image is more than what the person sees in the mirror but is linked to their sense of personal identity, their self-esteem and perceived acceptance by others.

For many body image encompasses more than just their body but includes what some may consider trivial aspects of a person's appearance such as clothing, makeup, hairstyle and jewellery (see Figure 6-1). However it also encompasses more crucial aspects such as hairpieces, artificial limbs and dentures, as well as devices required for functioning, such as wheelchairs, canes and eyeglasses.

If a person's body image closely resembles one's body ideal, the individual is more likely to think positively about the physical and nonphysical components of the self. However, perception of the ideal body is influenced by a number of factors; none more influential than the media. We are constantly bombarded with women and men with 'perfect bodies' in the media. Indeed society has now set its standards that females should be extraordinarily thin and for many this is an unrealistic goal. The obvious discrepancy between the actual body and the ideal body portrayed in the media can result in a negative body image which impacts on self-esteem, personal identity and role performance. The person with a negative body image may become socially isolated, may not be able to look or touch their body and may express feelings of helplessness, hopelessness, powerlessness and vulnerability, and may exhibit self-destructive behaviour such as over- or under-eating or suicide attempts.

Role Performance

Throughout life people undergo numerous role changes and may hold more than one role at any point in time, for example husband, parent, brother, son, employee and friend. A **role** is a set of expectations according to a person's social position, while **role performance** relates to the ways in which the person in a particular role behaves. Expectations, or standards

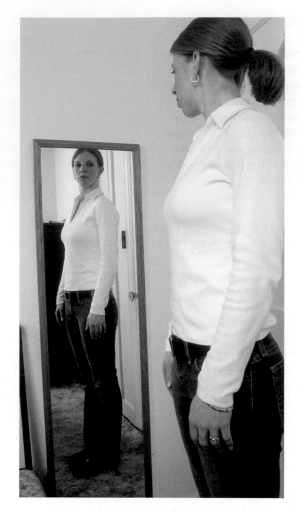

Figure 6-1 Body image is the sum of a person's conscious and unconscious attitudes about his or her body.

of behaviour of a role, are set by society, a cultural group or a smaller group to which a person belongs. If the person meets these expectations they are said to have mastered the role. Failure to master a role creates frustration and feelings of inadequacy, often with consequent lowered self-esteem.

Self-esteem

Self-esteem or self-worth is a person's emotional self image and is based on the person's own standards and performances. A high self-esteem means that a person appreciates themselves and their own personal worth. However there are two types of self-esteem: global and specific. **Global self-esteem** is how much one likes one's self as a whole. **Specific self-esteem** is how much one approves of a certain part of oneself. Global self-esteem is influenced by specific self-esteem. For example, if a man values his looks, then how he looks will strongly affect his global self-esteem. By contrast, if a man places little value on his cooking skills, then how well or badly he cooks will have little influence on his global self-esteem.

Self-esteem is not a static entity but in fact changes from day to day and moment to moment. In fact the foundations for self-esteem are established during early life and change according to life experiences, personal changes such as relationship breakdown and bereavement and affect many of the decisions that are made in life. People frequently focus on their negative aspects and spend less time on their positive aspects, but self-esteem is like a garden – it needs to be tended regularly to keep it in order. It is important therefore that the person considers their strengths as well as their weaknesses.

FACTORS THAT AFFECT SELF-CONCEPT

A positive self-concept is a delicate 'creature' even for the strongest of individuals. Many factors affect a person's self-concept including development, family, stress and illness.

As an individual develops, the factors that affect the self-concept change. For example, an infant requires a supportive, caring environment, while a child requires freedom to explore and learn. However, in order for a positive self-concept to development it requires the balanced social environment. If a child is nurtured in a supportive family environment, given encouragement and allowed to develop normally they are more likely to develop a positive self-concept and have a higher self-esteem than a child who is criticised, chastised and under-valued in the family environment.

Stress also has an impact on the development of positive self-concept. Indeed stress can actually help to strengthen self-concept particularly if the individual copes with the stress successfully. However, if the individual is exposed to excessive stress negative self-concept can result, causing maladaptive responses to the situation including substance abuse, withdrawal and anxiety.

Illness and trauma can also affect self-concept. For example, a woman who has undergone a mastectomy (removal of a breast) may see herself as less attractive, less of a female and ultimately may feel a loss of her sexuality. This loss may affect how she acts and values herself. A person's response to stress and illness is individual – some may accept the stress while others may deny it and withdraw from society often resulting in depression. Stress will also be considered later in this chapter.

SEXUALITY

The expression of sexuality is, as stated earlier, fundamental to a positive self-concept. **Sex** is the term most commonly used to identify male or female status. The more appropriate and descriptive term, however, is **gender**. The term *sex* is also used to describe sexual behaviour in general such as 'When is the last time you had sex?' **Sexuality** on the other hand includes how a person feels about their body, interest in sexual activity, the need for touch and the ability to engage in satisfying sexual activity.

Sexual health, however, is a difficult concept to define. Nevertheless the World Health Organization attempted to define **sexual health** in 1975 as 'the integration of the somatic, emotional, intellectual, and social aspects of sexual being, in ways that are positively enriching and that enhance personality, communication, and love' (p. 6). For most people though, sexual health is a phenomenon that is only considered when it is impaired or absent.

Because sexuality and sexual functioning are aspects of health and well-being, they are a part of nursing care and need to be assessed. When doing so, nurses should assess the patients nonjudgementally, encouraging them to discuss their concerns and offer suggestions to assist the return of intimacy and sexual function.

Patients are often hesitant to introduce the topic of sex with healthcare professionals as they may be too embarrassed, however it is the nurses responsibility to raise the topic in order to holistically care for the patient.

Nurses require six basic skills to help patients in the area of sexuality:

1. Self-knowledge and comfort with their own sexuality.
2. Acceptance of sexuality as an important area for nursing intervention and a willingness to work with patients expressing their sexuality in a variety of ways.
3. Knowledge of sexual growth and development throughout the life cycle.
4. Knowledge of basic sexuality, including how certain health problems and treatments may affect sexuality and sexual function and which interventions facilitate sexual expression and functioning.
5. Therapeutic communication skills.
6. Ability to recognise the need of the patient and family members to have the topic of sexuality introduced not only in written or audiovisual materials but also in a verbal discussion.

Development of Sexuality

The development of sexuality begins with conception and continues throughout the life span. Every society develops expectations about acceptable forms of sexual expression. Table 6-1 on page 90 outlines characteristics of sexual development through the life span, with nursing interventions and teaching guidelines for each developmental stage.

Sexuality, as it is developing in the human is affected by a number of factors: culture, religious values, personal ethics, health status and medications (see Table 6-3 on page 91).

In order to improve sexual health the nurse can implement a number of strategies: sex education, teaching self-examination, promoting responsible sexual behaviour and counselling for altered sexual function.

Table 6-1 Sexual Development throughout Life

Stage	Characteristics	Nursing interventions and teaching guidelines
Infancy Birth to 18 months	Given gender assignment of male or female. Differentiates self from others gradually. External genitals are sensitive to touch. Male infants have penile erections; females, vaginal lubrication.	Self-manipulation of the genitals is normal. Caregivers need to recognise these behaviours as common in children.
Toddler 1-3 years	Continues to develop gender identity. Able to identify own gender.	Body exploration and genital fondling is normal. Use names for body parts. Children from single-parent homes should have contact with adults of both sexes.
Preschooler 4-5 years	Becomes increasingly aware of self. Explores own and playmates' body parts. Learns correct names for body parts. Learns to control feelings and behaviour. Focuses love on parent of the other sex.	Answer questions about 'where babies come from' honestly and simply. Parental overreaction to exploration of genitals and masturbation can lead to feelings that sex is 'bad'.
School age 6-12 years	Has strong identification with parent of same gender. Tends to have friends of the same gender. Has increasing awareness of self. Increased modesty, desire for privacy. Continues self-stimulating behaviour. Learns the role and concepts of own gender as part of the total self-concept. At about 8 or 9 years becomes concerned about specific sex behaviours and often approaches parents with explicit concerns about sexuality and reproduction.	Provide parents and children with opportunities to express their concerns and ask questions regarding sex. Answer all questions with factual data and perhaps follow up with appropriate books and other material. Advise parents to discuss basic information about sexual intercourse, menstruation and reproduction with children at about 10 years of age. Give children reading material and then discuss it with them.
Adolescence 12-18 years	Primary and secondary sex characteristics develop. Females usually begin menstruating. Develops relationships with interested partners. Masturbation is common. May participate in sexual activity. Sexually transmitted infections are the most common bacterial infections among adolescents.	Adolescents require information about body changes. Peer groups have great importance at this time and assist in forming gender roles. Dating helps adolescents prepare for adult roles. Parents influence values and beliefs regarding behaviour. Teenagers require information about contraceptive measures and precautions to take in regard to STDs (see Table 6-2 for clinical signs of sexually transmitted diseases).
Young adulthood 18-40 years	Sexual activity is common. Establishes own lifestyle and values. Many couples share financial obligations and household tasks.	Young adults often require information about measures to prevent unwanted pregnancies (i.e. abstinence or contraceptive devices). Require information to prevent STDs. Regular communication is required to understand partner's sexual needs and to work through problems and stresses.
Middle adulthood 40-65 years	Men and women experience decreased hormone production. The menopause occurs in women, usually anywhere between 40 and 55 years. The climacteric occurs gradually in men. Quality rather than the number of sexual experiences becomes important. Individuals establish independent moral and ethical standards.	Women and men may need help to adjust to new roles. People may require counselling to help them re-evaluate and direct their energies. Encourage couples to look at the positive aspects of this time of life.
Late adulthood 65 years and over	Interest in sexual activity often continues. Sexual activity may be less frequent. Women's vaginal secretions diminish, and breasts atrophy. Men produce fewer sperm and need more time to achieve an erection and to ejaculate.	Older adults often continue to be sexually active. Couples may require counselling about adapting their affection and sexual needs to physical limitations.

Table 6-2 Clinical Signs of Sexually Transmitted Diseases

Disease	Male	Female
Gonorrhoea	Painful urination; urethritis with watery white discharge, which may become purulent.	May be asymptomatic; or vaginal discharge, pain and urinary frequency may be present.
Syphilis	Chancre (ulcer), usually on glans penis, which is painless and heals in 4-6 weeks; secondary symptoms – skin eruptions, low-grade fever, inflammation of lymph glands – in 6 weeks to 6 months after chancre heals.	Chancre (ulcer) on cervix or other genital areas, which heals in 4-6 weeks; symptoms same as for male.
Genital warts (condyloma acuminatum)	The infection is caused by the human papilloma virus (HPV). Single lesions or clusters of lesions growing beneath or on the foreskin, at external meatus, or on the glans penis. On dry skin areas, lesions are hard and yellow-grey. On moist areas, lesions are pink or red and soft with a cauliflower-like appearance.	Certain strains of HPV have been linked to cervical cancer. Lesions appear at the bottom part of the vaginal opening, on the perineum, the vaginal lips, inner walls of the vagina, and the cervix.
Chlamydial urethritis	Urinary frequency; watery, mucoid urethral discharge.	Commonly a carrier; vaginal discharge, dysuria, urinary frequency.
Trichomoniasis	Slight itching; moisture on top of penis; slight, early morning urethral discharge. Many males are asymptomatic.	Itching and redness of vulva and skin inside thighs; copious watery, frothy vaginal discharge.
Candidiasis	Itching, irritation, discharge, plaque of cheesy material under foreskin.	Red and excoriated vulva; intense itching of vaginal and vulvar tissues; thick, white, cheesy or curd-like discharge.
Acquired immune deficiency syndrome (AIDS)	Symptoms can appear anytime from several months to several years after acquiring the virus. The person has reduced immunity to other diseases. Symptoms include any of the following for which there is no other explanation: persistent heavy night sweats; extreme fatigue; severe weight loss; enlarged lymph glands in neck, axillae or groin; persistent diarrhoea; skin rashes; blurred vision or chronic headache; harsh, dry cough; thick grey-white coating on tongue or throat.	
Herpes genitalis (herpes simplex of the genitals)	Primary herpes involves the presence of painful sores or large, discrete vesicles that last for weeks; vesicles rupture. Recurrent herpes is itchy rather than painful; it lasts for a few hours to 10 days.	

Table 6-3 Factors Influencing Sexuality

Factor	Examples	Nursing considerations
Culture	Culture influences the sexual nature of dress, rules about marriage, monogamy, polygamy, pre-marital sexual intercourse and homosexuality. Male and female roles may vary according to culture. There may also be specific sex practices such as female circumcision and genital mutilation.	Patients may differ in their approaches to sexuality; therefore nurses must be aware of and consider cultural factors when approaching sexual issues in healthcare.
Religious values	Religion can influence sexual expression. It often provides guidelines for sexual behaviour. Some religions may consider the following unnatural or against the rules: sexual contact other than male-female, virginity before marriage, unwed motherhood, abortion, pre-marital sex and homosexuality.	Nurses should be aware that religious values can affect sexual expression and practices and should consider these during the assessment process.
Personal ethics	Personal ethics is integral to religion; however ethical thought and approaches to sexuality can be viewed separately. What one person considers perverted or unnatural may be perfectly normal to another, for example, masturbation, oral intercourse and cross dressing.	Nurses, when working with couples may need to consider each of the individual's personal ethics about sexual practices and expressions.
Health status	Sexual health is based on healthy bodies, emotions and minds. Many physical health factors can affect sexual health such as heart disease, hysterectomies, prostate cancer, diabetes mellitus, spinal cord injury and depression.	A thorough physical assessment could help to highlight potential health problems that could affect the expression of sexuality and ultimately sexual health.
Medications	Many prescription and non-prescription medications could affect sexual functioning (see Table 6-4 on page 92)	It is important that when discussing medication with patients the possible sexual side effects are considered.

Table 6-4 Effects of Medications on Sexual Function

Medication	Possible effects*
Alcohol	Moderate amounts: increased sexual functioning; chronic use: decreased sexual desire, orgasmic dysfunction and impotence
Alpha-blockers	Inability to ejaculate
Amphetamines	Increased sex drive, delayed orgasm
Amyl nitrate	Reported enhanced orgasm; vasodilation, fainting
Anabolic steroids	Decreased sex drive, shrinking of testicles and infertility in men
Antianxiety agents	Decreased sexual desire; orgasmic dysfunction in women; delayed ejaculation
Anticonvulsants	Decreased sexual desire; reduced sexual response
Antidepressants	Decreased sexual desire; orgasmic delay or dysfunction in women; delayed or failed ejaculation; painful erection
Antihistamines	Decreased vaginal lubrication; decreased desire
Antihypertensives	Decreased sexual desire; erectile failure; ejaculation dysfunction
Antipsychotics	Decreased sexual desire; orgasmic dysfunction in women; delayed ejaculation; ejaculatory failure
Barbiturates	In low doses, increased sexual pleasure; in large doses, decreased sexual desire, orgasmic dysfunction and impotence
Beta-blockers	Decreased sexual desire
Cardiotonics	Decreased sexual desire
Cocaine	Increased intensity of sexual experience; with chronic use, decreased sexual desire and sexual dysfunction
Diuretics	Decreased vaginal lubrication; decreased sexual desire; erectile dysfunction
Marijuana	As above for cocaine, but prolonged use reduces testosterone levels and reduces sperm production
Narcotics	Inhibited sexual desire and response; erectile and ejaculatory dysfunctions

*Nurses and patients must familiarise themselves with the specific medication prescribed or used, because effects vary in each category of drug.

Sex Education

Nurses can assist patients to understand their anatomies and how their bodies function. For example, understanding the anatomy of the genitals may help women learn how their bodies respond to sexual stimulation. Both men and women need to learn the kind of stimulation that is pleasing and causes arousal. The importance of open communication between partners should also be encouraged. Women may also benefit from learning Kegel exercises. These exercises involve contraction and relaxation of the pubococcygeal muscle, the muscle that contracts when a person prevents urine flow. The benefits of Kegel exercises include increased pelvic floor muscle tone; increased vaginal lubrication during sexual arousal; increased sensation during intercourse; increased genital sensitivity; stronger gripping of the base of the penis; earlier postpartum recovery of the pelvic floor muscle; and increased flexibility of episiotomy scars (Berman and Berman, 2001). The steps to perform Kegel exercises are discussed in Chapter 20 because these exercises are also used in bladder retraining.

Details about physiological changes associated with age and health status should be discussed. For example, the nurse needs to discuss the effects of puberty, pregnancy, menopause and the male climacteric on sexual function. When patients experience illness or surgery that alters sexual function, the nurse needs to discuss effects of treatment (e.g. medications) and any changes that need to be undertaken to ensure safe sex (e.g. position changes or a safe time to resume sexual intercourse after a heart attack).

When considering the difficult questions that children ask about sex, parents often need assistance to learn ways to answer these questions. They may need to know what information they should give to the child and at what age. Parents should be aware that although they may feel they are the primary educators with regard to sex and sexuality, children may get information about these subjects from other sources such as their friends, books, television, teachers, etc.

Although there is an increasing awareness today of sexuality and sexual functioning, some people still hold certain myths and misconceptions about sexuality. Many of these are handed down in families and are part of the beliefs in a particular culture. It is highly important that nurses learn about the beliefs patients hold and provide up-to-date information. Table 6-5 lists some common sexual myths and misconceptions.

Teaching Self-examination

Monthly breast self-examination (BSE) for women and monthly testicular self-examination (TSE) for men can play

Table 6-5 Common Sexual Misconceptions

Misconception	Fact
Nearly all men over 70 years old have erectile dysfunction.	Sexual ability is not lost due to age. Changes may be due to disease or medication.
Masturbation causes certain mental instabilities.	Masturbation is a common and healthy behaviour.
Sexual activity weakens a person.	There is no evidence that sexual activity weakens a person.
Women who have experienced orgasm are more likely to become pregnant.	Conceiving is not related to experiencing orgasm.
Nice girls shouldn't feel entitled to their own sexual satisfaction.	As women become more comfortable with their own sexuality, they advocate for their own sexual fulfilment.
A large penis provides greater sexual satisfaction to women than a small penis.	There is no evidence that a large penis provides greater satisfaction.
Alcohol is a sexual stimulant.	Alcohol is a relaxant and central nervous system depressant. Chronic alcoholism is associated with erectile dysfunction.
Intercourse during menstruation is dangerous (i.e. it will cause vaginal tissue damage).	There is no physiological basis for abstinence during menses.
The face-to-face coital position is the moral or proper one.	The position that offers the most pleasure and is acceptable to both partners is the correct one.

an important role in early detection of disease resulting in a greater chance of cure and less complex treatment. Patients need to be assured that most lumps discovered are not cancerous, but that it is essential that all lumps or other detected abnormalities be checked by the patient's general practitioner for accurate diagnosis and possible referral.

Responsible Sexual Behaviour

Responsible sexual behaviour involves the prevention of sexually transmitted diseases and the prevention of unwanted pregnancy.

STD Prevention

The prevention of STDs is an essential part of sexual health teaching (see Figure 6-2). Note that *Trichomonas* and *Candida* infections can also be acquired nonsexually. Increases in these diseases are due to two factors: (a) changing sexual morality that has permitted increased sexual activity and (b) an increase in the number of sexual partners. Because the term *sexually transmitted disease* elicits feelings of guilt, shame and fear, people frequently do not seek medical help as early as they should. Patients need education about these diseases, preventive measures and early treatment. Many STDs can be treated quickly and effectively. Others may have serious consequences. For example, women may develop pelvic inflammatory disease (PID) resulting in damage to the reproductive structures and possible infertility. AIDS has no cure. The anxiety about AIDS transmission has caused many individuals to alter their sexual behaviour, such as using a condom during intercourse.

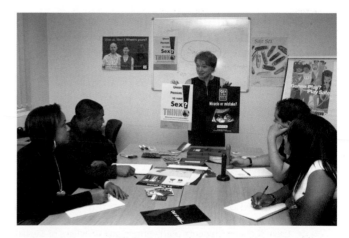

Figure 6-2 Adolescents require age-appropriate teaching about sexuality and STDs. (Will Hart/PhotoEdit.)

Table 6-2, earlier in this chapter, lists common signs of STDs for which people should seek medical care.

Prevention of Unwanted Pregnancies

Prevention of unwanted pregnancies must be addressed not only with adolescents but also with couples who are planning the time of their first birth and want to space children and limit family size. Nurses need to be familiar with various contraceptive methods and their advantages, disadvantages, contraindications, effectiveness, safety and cost (see Figure 6-3 on page 94). It is beyond the scope of this text to discuss contraceptives in detail but the various methods are outlined in *Box 6-1* on page 94.

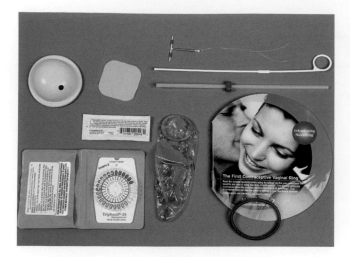

Figure 6-3 Methods of contraception.

> **BOX 6-1** Methods of Contraception
>
> + Abstinence
> + Withdrawal of the penis before ejaculation (coitus interruptus)
> + Fertility awareness (identification of the days of the month when conception could take place and abstaining during that time)
> + Mechanical barriers: vaginal diaphragm, cervical cap, condom
> + Chemical barriers: insertion of spermicidal foams, creams, jellies or suppositories into the vagina before intercourse
> + Intrauterine devices (IUDs)
> + Hormonal: oral contraceptives (birth control pills), subdermal implants of synthetic progestin
> + Surgical sterilisation: tubal ligation and vasectomy

RESEARCH NOTE

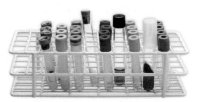

What Are College Students' Perceptions and Practices of Sexual Activities in Sexual Encounters?

An exploratory study of 84 college students examined the understanding college students have of safer sexual encounters that include ideas about what constitutes 'safe' sex, expectations for sexual activities and planning for sexual encounters (von Sadovszky et al., 2002). Analysis of three open- and closed-ended questions about sexual activities revealed no significant difference between expectations regarding sexual activities among participants who had risky and safer encounters. Planning of an encounter was not related to safer sexual activities and what constitutes safer sexual activities was generally misunderstood. Participants believed risky encounters to be safer because of the use of a condom only during vaginal sex, the use of hormone-based birth control pills or because of the belief that no sex had occurred during oral sex.

Implications

Nurses need to assess the patients' knowledge and beliefs about sexual activities related to STDs and unwanted pregnancy.

Note: From 'College Students' Perceptions and Practices of Sexual Activities in Sexual Encounters,' by V. von Sadovszky, M. Keller, and K. McKinney, 2002, *Journal of Nursing Scholarship*, 34, pp. 133-138.

Counselling for Altered Sexual Function

One technique nurses can use to help patients with altered sexual function is the PLISSIT model, developed by Annon (1974) for this purpose. The model involves four progressive levels represented by the acronym PLISSIT:

P   Permission giving
LI Limited information
S   Specific suggestions
IT Intensive therapy

At each level, the nurse provides additional guidance and information to the patient and therefore requires more specialised and specific knowledge and skill. All professional nurses should be able to function at the first three levels.

Permission Giving

Patients may feel that they need permission to be sexual beings, to ask questions, to show affection and to express themselves sexually. Giving permission means that the nurse by attitude or word lets the patient know that sexual thoughts, fantasies and behaviours between informed consenting adults are allowed. Giving permission begins when the nurse acknowledges the patient's spoken and unspoken sexual concerns and conveys the attitude that sexual concerns and needs are important to health and recovery.

For example, the nurse might ask a patient recuperating from a heart attack the following questions:

+ 'Now that you're recovering and you've had some time to sort out your feelings, have you thought about how your heart attack might alter your sex life?'
+ 'Have you and your partner discussed how you both feel about it?'

Limited Information

Patients need accurate but concise information. The nurse might explain what is normal; how some medical conditions, treatments, injuries or surgeries may affect sexuality and sexual functioning; or how ageing may affect sexuality and functioning.

Continuing with the preceding example, the nurse shares information and informs the patient about how the heart attack might affect the patient's sex life, including the following:

+ 'Your heart attack will not alter your capacity for sexual response. Most people can resume intercourse in four to six weeks, but this should be confirmed by your doctor.'
+ 'Many patients who have suffered a heart attack fear sexual intercourse because of increased heart and respiratory rates associated with it. However, your treatment and rehabilitation will build your tolerance for physical activity and therefore sexual activity.'

Many patients recovering after childbirth, for example, or specific illness or disease (e.g. heart attack) need instruction about safe sexual activities and the effects that therapy may have on sexual functioning. The following topics need to be considered:

+ when sexual activity is safe;
+ specific sexual activities that are unsafe and why;
+ adaptations needed for resuming a satisfactory sexual life;
+ the side effects of prescribed medications on sexual functioning and the need to notify the physician of possible dose or medication adjustment should problems develop.

Specific Suggestions

At this level, the nurse requires specialised knowledge and skill about how sexuality and functioning may be affected by a disease process or therapy and what interventions might be effective. The nurse offers suggestions to help the patient adapt sexual activity to promote optimal functioning, such as what measures might be used to alleviate vaginal dryness, safe positions for intercourse following a total hip replacement, safe and unsafe sexual practices following a heart attack, and ways to handle ostomy appliances, Foley catheters, casts or other devices (e.g. prostheses) during sexual activity. Similarly, nurses on a cardiac unit need specialised knowledge about sexual readjustment during cardiac rehabilitation, and nurses working with patients with spinal cord injuries need information about the sexual consequences of spinal injuries at various levels.

Using the example of the patient recuperating from a heart attack, the nurse may offer the following suggestion:

+ 'Many people express concern about the stress of certain positions for intercourse, but you may use whatever position is comfortable for you and your partner, or try side-lying or partner-on-top positions.'

Intensive Therapy

Intensive therapy, provided by a clinical nurse specialist or sex therapist, is used when the first three levels of counselling are ineffective. It may involve such issues as sexual motivation, marriage or self-concept.

Discussing sexuality can be difficult for nurses as they are almost viewed as taboo subject areas or subjects that illicit feelings of embarrassment or inadequacy. Despite these feelings, both nurses and patients, agree that sexuality cannot be ignored as it is an integral part of holistic care.

Spiritual nursing care suffers similar problems. In fact, many nurses feel spirituality is a concept that is meaningless within their care (Golberg, 1998). However Golberg (1998) states that nurses do not realise they are providing spiritual care by just being with the patient or giving hope to a patient who has been given some terrible news.

SPIRITUALITY

Holistic nursing care provides care not only for the physical body and mind but also for the patient's spirit. But what is a person's spirit? Anne Fry, a senior lecturer in mental health nursing in the University of Western Sydney and leading expert in spirituality and mental health nursing, believes that humans are spiritual beings and argues that 'spirituality is a profound and central aspect of the existence of many people' (Fry, 1997: 5). Dr Aru Narayanasamy, a Senior Health Lecturer at the University of Nottingham, concurs stating that spirituality is 'the essence of our being and it gives meaning and purpose to our existence' (Narayanasamy, 2004).

According to many researchers spirituality is important to well-being and health (Larson *et al.*, 1992; Cohen *et al.*, 2000); therefore meeting spiritual needs may decrease suffering and improve physical and mental well-being. However there is evidence to suggest that the practice of spiritual care by nurses is often infrequent. Some believe that this is due to the notion that spiritual care should be performed by pastoral teams or chaplains. However it is the nurse that is ideally placed to support and comfort the patient and their loved ones who are in spiritual distress.

Spiritual care demands a trusting nurse–patient relationship, one which involves sensitivity, empathy and understanding of the patient's spiritual needs. It is important for nurses to develop a broad concept of spirituality and understand their own spiritual beliefs and needs. Within this multi-cultural, multi-faith society, nurses cannot rely solely on their own spiritual practices, but need to be aware of the array of religious traditions and spiritual expressions to which their patients may subscribe.

Spirituality Described

Spirituality, faith and religion are separate entities, yet the words are often used interchangeably. The word *spiritual* derives from the Latin word *spiritus*, which means 'to blow' or 'to breathe', and has come to connote that which gives life or essence to being human. **Spirituality** generally involves a belief in a relationship with some higher power, creative force, divine being or infinite source of energy. For example, a person may believe in 'God', 'Allah', the 'Great Spirit' or a 'Higher Power'.

Spiritual Needs

Spiritual needs are those needs that evolve from the person's spiritual being. Spiritual needs may include religious needs but are more likely to relate to emotional feelings and thoughts. These needs are often brought forward by an illness or other health crisis. For example, patients faced with a life threatening illness may express a need to understand why this has happened to them. Spiritual needs are as individual as physical needs and can range from the need for love to a need for exploration of the meaning of life. (*Box 6-2* lists other examples of spiritual needs.) Nurses need to be sensitive to indications of the patient's spiritual needs and respond appropriately, as discussed later.

Spiritual Well-being

Spiritual health, or **spiritual well-being**, can be defined as a state of feeling 'generally alive, purposeful and fulfilled' (Ellison, 1983: 332). Indeed spiritual health and well-being is integral to general health and well-being. Spiritual well-being can be described in terms of a number of characteristics (see *Box 6-3*).

Spiritual health and well-being can be enhanced in many ways. Some people focus on developing their inner self through meditation, relaxation or prayer, while others choose to express their spirituality with others by entering into loving relationships, serving others (e.g. through charity work), participation in religious services or by expressing compassion, empathy, forgiveness and hope.

BOX 6-2 Examples of Spiritual Needs

+ Need for love
+ Need for hope
+ Need for trust
+ Need for forgiveness
+ Need to be respected and valued
+ Need for dignity
+ Need for meaning to the fullness of life
+ Need for values
+ Need for creativity
+ Need to connect with a God or Higher Power, or a Being greater than oneself
+ Need to belong to a community

BOX 6-3 Characteristics Indicative of Spiritual Well-Being

+ Sense of inner peace
+ Compassion for others
+ Reverence for life
+ Gratitude
+ Appreciation of both unity and diversity
+ Humour
+ Wisdom
+ Generosity
+ Ability to transcend the self
+ Capacity for unconditional love

Note: From *Spiritual Dimensions of Nursing Practice*, by V.B. Carson, 1989, Philadelphia: Saunders. Reprinted with permission from Elsevier.

Spiritual Distress

Spiritual distress refers to an unresolved spiritual or religious conflict and doubt which challenges spiritual well-being. A number of factors can cause spiritual distress including pain, loss of limb, miscarriage or stillbirth, and bereavement.

In order to assess spiritual distress in a patient, the nurse needs to recognise signs of spiritual distress. Kenny (1999) defines a number of the characteristics of spiritual distress:

+ unable to accept self,
+ description of somatic complaints,
+ cues about relationships with others,
+ cues about guilt and forgiveness,
+ cues about religious/spiritual needs,
+ inadequate coping,
+ despair/hopelessness,
+ fear,
+ depression,
+ helplessness,
+ anorexia,
+ silence,
+ bitterness.

Not all patients who are spiritually distressed will experience these feelings; therefore the nurse must understand the patient's individual spiritual needs and indicators in order to identify spiritual distress.

SPIRITUAL PRACTICES AFFECTING NURSING CARE

According to Kenneth Pargament (1997), a leading researcher of religious beliefs and health, some patients use religious practices such as prayer as a means of coping with illness. Many of the practices can impact on the care provided to them by

Table 6-6 Spiritual Practices Affecting Nursing Care

Religion	Beliefs/practices
Protestant	Worship of one God and his son Jesus Christ. Religious practices vary according to denomination but may include prayer. Protestants have two sacraments: ✚ Baptism – spiritual cleansing and rebirth usually performed on infants. ✚ Eucharist – ritual of the church in which bread and wine is transformed into the body and blood of Christ. **Death and bereavement**: cremation common, organ donation increasing, bereavement less ritualised than other religions. **Abortion and birth control**: generally accepted however some church teachings prohibit. If a miscarriage occurs some will wish to have the foetus/child baptised/christened. **Diet**: varies according to denomination and personal preference. **Specific nursing considerations**: there are usually no specific objections to nursing or medical treatments.
Roman Catholic	Worship of one God revealed to the world by Jesus Christ. Human life is seen as a sacred gift of God. Roman Catholics have seven sacraments: ✚ Baptism – spiritual cleansing and rebirth usually performed on infants. ✚ Eucharist – ritual of the church in which bread and wine is transformed into the body and blood of Christ. ✚ Confirmation – rite of initiation into full membership of the church. ✚ Penance – confession of sins to an ordained priest. ✚ Extreme Unction – anointing of the sick by a priest. ✚ Ordination – the process where a clergy becomes authorised to perform religious rituals and ceremonies. ✚ Matrimony – marriage. **Death and bereavement**: if there is a danger of death, a priest should be called immediately. The priest may also help console those recently bereaved. **Abortion and birth control**: forbids direct abortion and birth control. **Diet**: abstinence from meat and meat products on Ash Wednesday and Good Friday. **Religious objects**: rosaries are the most common. **Specific nursing considerations**: usually do not have any objections to nursing or medical treatments however some Catholics do have an issue with the origins of some vaccines especially those that which have been derived from aborted foetuses.
Hinduism	Doctrine of Transmigration. They believe in a universal eternal soul Brahman but also worship Ram, Shiva, Lakshmi and Hanuman. Hindus believe in a cycle of birth, death and rebirth governed by Karma. **Death and bereavement**: if the family wish, when death occurs, inform the Hindu priest (Brahmin). The family may wish to read from the Bhagavad Gita during last offices. The family may want to stay with the patient during last offices. The patient's family may also ask for the patient to be placed on the floor. Post-mortems are deemed as disrespectful. **Abortion and birth control**: generally opposed to abortion unless the mother's life is at risk. Hindus may use birth control. **Diet**: most are strict vegetarians. The cow is considered sacred therefore even those who eat other meat definitely do not eat beef. **Specific nursing considerations**: Hindus should be nursed in single-sex wards where possible. Also female patients usually will need to be nursed by female nurses. Men will usually be reluctant to be nursed by female staff. As most Hindus are vegetarians it is important that they are not prescribed drugs that contain animal products especially beef derivatives. Hindu women are expected to keep their legs, breasts and upper arms covered at all times.
Jehovah's Witnesses	A Christian-based religious movement that believes in one God who was revealed by Jesus Christ. **Death and bereavement**: family may wish to be present during last offices either to pray or read from the Bible. **Abortion and birth control**: Jehovah's Witnesses believe that life is sacred therefore abortion is considered wrong. They also avoid surrogate motherhood, donation of sperm, eggs and embryos. **Diet**: Jehovah's Witnesses avoid eating meat that has not been properly bled as they feel it is wrong to consume blood. **Specific nursing considerations**: blood transfusions violate God's laws and therefore are not allowed.
Judaism	Jews believe that there is one God with whom they have a covenant. **Death and bereavement**: after death 8 minutes are required to elapse before the body is moved. Usually close relatives with deal with the patient after death however the patient must not be washed. The rabbi may be required. The body is watched until burial which usually takes place within 24 hours of death. Post-mortems are permitted if they are legally required. Organ donation is encouraged. Cremation is forbidden.

Table 6-6 *(continued)*

Religion	Beliefs/practices
	Abortion and birth control: abortion is allowed for serious reasons. Contraception is allowed. **Diet**: acceptable food is called Kosher. Pork and shellfish is not permitted to be eaten. Orthodox Jews will need to wash before and after food. **Specific nursing considerations**: Jews have strict guidelines regarding modesty so should be nursed in single-sex bays.
Islam (Muslim)	Muslims believe in Allah, their God and must be able to practise the Five Pillars of Islam which are faith, prayer, charity, fasting and pilgrimage. **Death and bereavement**: Muslims believe in resurrection so care of the dead body is important. Non-Muslims are not permitted to touch the patient's body with bare hands but must wear gloves. The patient's head should be turned to face Mecca which is south east in the UK. The body should be covered completely with a white cloth and the arms, legs straightened. The body is usually washed by a family member of the same sex. Post-mortems are not allowed unless there is a legal requirement. In the case of organ donation, it is permitted as long as the organ is immediately given to another Muslim. Muslims are usually buried rather than cremated within 24 hours of death. **Abortion and birth control**: family planning is frowned upon as Allah decides when a Muslim is blessed with children. **Diet**: Halal foods are those foods that Allah has stated is good to eat. Alcohol, blood, bloody meat, pork and shellfish are not considered to be Halal foods. Muslims fast during Ramadan. **Specific nursing considerations**: women and men are not encouraged to mix freely so therefore should be nursed in single-sex wards. Muslim women may become distressed if asked to wear a hospital gown. During Ramadan no food, liquid or medication may be taken.
Sikhism	Sikhs believe in one God. **Death and bereavement**: healthcare staff should not touch the Sikh's body with ungloved hands. Post-mortem is allowed. Organ donation is accepted. Burial or cremation is accepted. **Abortion and birth control**: birth control is allowed under certain circumstances. Abortion though is not allowed. If miscarriage or stillbirth occurs do not offer a lock of the child's hair as a Sikh's hair is sacred. **Diet**: alcohol is not permitted. Some Sikhs may not eat meat while others do eat some meat. Beef and pork are not permitted. Some older Sikhs may fast. **Specific nursing considerations**: if possible Sikhs should be placed in single-sex wards. Drugs that contain alcohol will be taken as long as the drug is not meant to intoxicate the patient.

the nurse. Therefore, within our multi-cultural and multi-faith society, the nurse should be aware of the spiritual practices of, at least, the major religions followed within the UK (see Table 6-6 on page 97).

SPIRITUAL HEALTH AND THE NURSING PROCESS

The nursing process, which includes assessing, diagnosing, planning, implementing and evaluating, can be applied to the area of spiritual health as it is key to the health of the individual. Assessment of a patient's spiritual beliefs and practices are usually obtained by talking to the patient and family. However the nurse can also establish some information about the patient by observation of the patient's behaviour, mood and verbalisations.

Although the nurse will continually be assessing, the initial spiritual assessment is best taken at the end of the assessment process, or following the psychosocial assessment, after the nurse has developed a relationship with the patient and/or support person. A nurse who has demonstrated sensitivity and

personal warmth, earning some rapport, will be more successful during a spiritual assessment.

Once a spiritual assessment has been made, the goal for spiritual care should be in line with the patient's own practices and beliefs and not what the nurse thinks the goals should be. The goal of spiritual care will usually be to maintain or restore spiritual well-being. Once the goal of spiritual care has been established the nurse needs to plan appropriate care for the patient, identifying interventions that will help the patient to achieve the overall goal of spiritual care.

Planning in relation to spiritual needs should be designed to do one or more of the following:

+ Help the patient fulfil religious obligations.
+ Help the patient draw on and use inner resources more effectively to meet the present situation.
+ Help the patient maintain or establish a dynamic, personal relationship with a supreme being in the face of unpleasant circumstances.
+ Help the patient find meaning in existence and the present situation.

+ Promote a sense of hope.
+ Provide spiritual resources otherwise unavailable.

Interventions to maintain or restore spiritual well-being may include:

+ being available to the patient, sometimes known as *presencing*;
+ supporting religious and spiritual practices such as assisting patients with prayer;
+ referring patients to spiritual or religious leaders;
+ being there in a way that is meaningful to another person.

Regardless of the interventions implemented to maintain or restore spiritual well-being in the person, it is important that evaluation of these interventions takes place. Evaluation of care provided is usually judged by seeing if the goal of spiritual care has been achieved. This can be done by talking with the patient and observing any improvements in mood, attitude and behaviour. If the nurse finds that the goal of spiritual care has not been achieved a new plan of care should be discussed with the patient.

Failure to meet a person's physical, psychological or social needs can lead to stress. When considering psychosocial health if key aspects, such as spiritual health or sexual health, are not considered within nursing care this can lead to the individual feeling 'stressed' which in turn can lead to a delay in healing or recovering from an illness.

STRESS

Stress to most people is something that we deal with and accept. Everyone at some point in their lives will suffer with stress. Parents refer to the stress of raising children, working people talk of the stress of their jobs, and students at all levels talk of the stress of school. Stress can result from both positive and negative experiences. For example, a bride preparing for her wedding, a graduate preparing to start a new job, and a husband concerned about caring for his wife and family following a diagnosis of cancer, all experience stress reactions.

The concept of stress is important because it provides a way of understanding the person as a being who responds in totality (mind, body and spirit) to a variety of changes that take place in daily life.

Concept of Stress

Stress is a physiological or psychological response to a **stressor**, event or stimulus, beyond what is needed to accomplish a task. When a person faces stressors, responses are referred to as *coping strategies*, *coping responses* or *coping mechanisms*.

Sources of Stress

There are many sources of stress. They can be broadly classified as internal or external stressors. *Internal stressors* originate

Table 6-7 Stressors throughout Life

Developmental stage	Stressors
Child	Beginning school Establishing peer relationships Coping with peer competition
Adolescent	Accepting changing body Developing relationships involving sexual attraction Achieving independence Choosing a career
Young adult	Getting married Leaving home Managing a home Getting started in an occupation Continuing one's education Rearing children
Middle adult	Accepting physical changes of ageing Maintaining social status and standard of living Helping teenage children to become independent Adjusting to ageing parents
Older adult	Accepting decreasing physical abilities and health Adjusting to retirement and reduced income Adjusting to death of spouse and friends

within a person, for example, cancer or feelings of depression, while *external stressors* originate outside the individual, for example, a move to another city, a death in the family or pressure from peers. Table 6-7 provides examples of both internal and external stressors.

The degree to which any of these events affects the person will depend on the individual's developmental stage. For example, the death of a parent may be more stressful for a 12-year-old than for a 40-year-old.

Effects of Stress

Stress can affect an individual physically, emotionally, socially and spiritually. Usually the effects are mixed, because stress affects the whole person. Physically, stress can threaten a person's physical well-being. Emotionally, stress can produce negative feelings about the self. Socially, stress can alter a person's relationships with others. Spiritually, stress can challenge one's beliefs and values. Many illnesses have been linked to stress (see Figure 6-4 on page 100).

Indicators of Stress

Stress in an individual can have physical and psychological indicators which the nurse should be aware of.

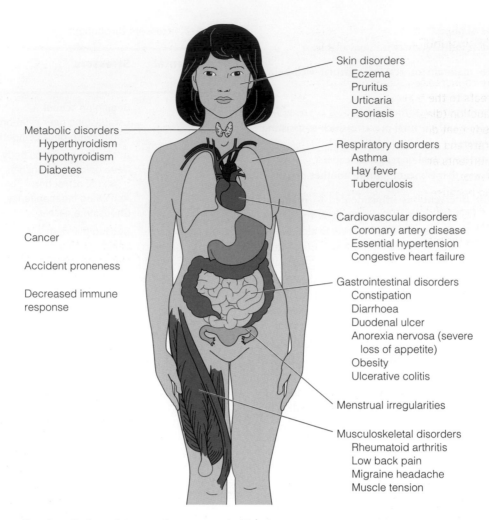

Metabolic disorders
Hyperthyroidism
Hypothyroidism
Diabetes

Cancer

Accident proneness

Decreased immune
response

Skin disorders
Eczema
Pruritus
Urticaria
Psoriasis

Respiratory disorders
Asthma
Hay fever
Tuberculosis

Cardiovascular disorders
Coronary artery disease
Essential hypertension
Congestive heart failure

Gastrointestinal disorders
Constipation
Diarrhoea
Duodenal ulcer
Anorexia nervosa (severe
loss of appetite)
Obesity
Ulcerative colitis

Menstrual irregularities

Musculoskeletal disorders
Rheumatoid arthritis
Low back pain
Migraine headache
Muscle tension

Figure 6-4 Some disorders that can be caused or aggravated by stress. (From *Health and Wellness: A Holistic Approach*, 7th edn (p. 44), by G. Edline, E. Golanty, and K.M. Brown, 2002, Boston: Jones and Barlett. Adapted with permission.)

Physical Indicators

Responses to stress vary from person to person, and depend on the perception of the stressor. The physical signs and symptoms of stress result from the activation of the sympathetic and neuroendocrine systems of the body. *Box 6-4* lists some of the physical indicators of stress.

Psychological Indicators

Psychological manifestations of stress include anxiety, fear, anger, depression and defence mechanisms. Some of these manifestations can be helpful depending on the situation and the length of time they are experienced.

Anxiety. This is a feeling of unease or helplessness within a situation and differs from fear as the source of the anxiety may not be identifiable. **Anxiety** may be manifested on four levels:

1. Mild anxiety – this is generally good and is tolerated by most people. It increases perception, learning and productivity in most people.

2. Moderate anxiety – some people cope with short periods of moderate anxiety however it can produce feelings of tension, nervousness or concern.

3. Severe anxiety – this is an all consuming form of anxiety that can debilitate the individual and requires some form of intervention.

4. Panic – an overpowering, frightening level of anxiety causing the person to lose control. It is less frequently experienced than other levels of anxiety. The perception of a panicked person can be affected to the degree that the person distorts events.

Table 6-8 lists indicators of these levels.

Fear. This is an emotion or feeling of apprehension aroused by impending or seeming danger, pain or other perceived threat. The **fear** may be in response to something that has already occurred, in response to an immediate or current threat, or in response to something the person believes will happen. The object of fear may or may not be based in reality. For example, a student nurse at the beginning of their training

BOX 6-4 Physical Indicators of Stress

+ Pupils dilate to increase visual perception when serious threats to the body arise.
+ Sweat production (diaphoresis) increases to control elevated body heat due to increased metabolism.
+ The heart rate and cardiac output increase to transport nutrients and by-products of metabolism more efficiently.
+ Skin is pallid because of constriction of peripheral blood vessels, an effect of norepinephrine (noradrenaline).
+ Sodium and water retention increase due to release of mineralocorticoids, which results in increased blood volume.

+ The rate and depth of respirations increase because of dilation of the bronchioles, promoting hyperventilation.
+ Urinary output decreases.
+ The mouth may be dry.
+ Peristalsis of the intestines decreases, resulting in possible constipation and flatus.
+ For serious threats, mental alertness improves.
+ Muscle tension increases to prepare for rapid motor activity or defence.
+ Blood sugar increases because of release of glucocorticoids and gluconeogenesis.

Table 6-8 Indicators of Levels of Anxiety

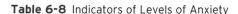

Category	Level of anxiety			
	Mild	**Moderate**	**Severe**	**Panic**
Verbalisation	Increased questioning	Voice tremors and pitch changes	Communication difficult to understand	Communication may change, and may not be understandable
Motor activity changes	Mild restlessness Sleeplessness	Tremors, facial twitches and shakiness Increased muscle tension	Increased motor activity, inability to relax Fearful facial expression	Increased motor activity, agitation Unpredictable responses
Perception and attention changes	Feelings of increased arousal and alertness Uses learning to adapt	Narrowed focus of attention Able to focus but selectively inattentive Learning slightly impaired	Inability to focus or concentrate Easily distracted Learning severely impaired	Trembling, poor motor coordination Perception distorted or exaggerated Unable to learn or function
Respiratory and circulatory changes	None	Slightly increased respiratory and heart rates	Tachycardia, hyperventilation	Dyspnoea, palpitations, choking, chest pain or pressure
Other changes	None (e.g. 'butterflies in the stomach')	Mild gastric symptoms	Headache, dizziness, nausea Paresthesia, sweating	Feeling of impending doom

Note: From *Nursing Diagnosis: Application to Clinical Practice*, 9th edn, by L.J. Carpenito, 2001, Philadelphia: Lippincott; *Mental Health Nursing*, 5th edn (p. 273), by K.L. Fontaine and J.S. Fletcher, 2003, Upper Saddle River, NJ: Pearson Education, Inc.

may fear their first experience within a hospital or community placement. They may fear that the patient will not want to be cared for by the student or that the student may inadvertently harm the patient.

Anger. This is a word that is commonly used for a range of emotions and usually results in a feeling of animosity or strong displeasure. People may feel guilty when they feel **anger** because they have been taught that to feel angry is wrong. However, anger may not always be negative; in fact if anger

with a situation or person is expressed in a nonalienating manner it could be considered a positive emotion that is beneficial to a situation.

A verbal expression of anger can be considered a signal to others of one's internal psychological discomfort. Anger differs from other negative behaviours associated with anger such as hostility (a sign of overt antagonism), aggression (an unprovoked or hostile action) and violence (an exertion of physical force to injure or abuse). However anger can lead to these destructive behaviours if it persists.

Depression. This is a common reaction to events that seem overwhelming or negative. **Depression**, an extreme feeling of sadness, despair, dejection, lack of worth or emptiness, affects millions of people in the UK each year. The signs and symptoms of depression and the severity of the problem vary with the patient and the significance of the precipitating event. Emotional symptoms can include feelings of tiredness, sadness, emptiness or numbness. Behavioural signs of depression include irritability, inability to concentrate, difficulty making decisions, loss of sexual desire, crying, sleep disturbance and social withdrawal. Physical signs of depression may include loss of appetite, weight loss, constipation, headache and dizziness. Many people experience short periods of depression in response to overwhelming stressful events, such as the death of a loved one or loss of a job; prolonged depression, however, is a cause for concern and may require treatment.

Defence Mechanisms. These are psychological adaptive mechanisms or, in the words of Sigmund Freud (1946), mental mechanisms that develop as the personality attempts to defend itself, establish compromises among conflicting impulses and allay inner tensions. **Defence mechanisms** are the unconscious mind working to protect the person from anxiety. They can be considered precursors to conscious cognitive coping mechanisms that will ultimately solve the problem. Like some verbal and motor responses, defence mechanisms release tension. Table 6-9 describes these mechanisms and lists examples of their adaptive and maladaptive use.

Table 6-9 Defence Mechanisms

Defence mechanism	Example(s)	Use/purpose
Compensation Covering up weaknesses by emphasising a more desirable trait or by overachievement in a more comfortable area.	A high school student too small to play football becomes the star long-distance runner for the track team.	Allows a person to overcome weakness and achieve success.
Denial An attempt to screen or ignore unacceptable realities by refusing to acknowledge them.	A woman, though told her father has metastatic cancer, continues to plan a family reunion 18 months in advance.	Temporarily isolates a person from the full impact of a traumatic situation.
Displacement The transferring or discharging of emotional reactions from one object or person to another object or person.	A husband and wife are fighting, and the husband becomes so angry he hits a door instead of his wife.	Allows for feelings to be expressed through or to less dangerous objects or people.
Identification An attempt to manage anxiety by imitating the behaviour of someone feared or respected.	A new graduate suddenly left in charge emulates her faculty role model.	Helps a person avoid self-devaluation.
Intellectualisation A mechanism by which an emotional response that normally would accompany an uncomfortable or painful incident is evaded by the use of rational explanations that remove from the incident any personal significance and feelings.	The pain over a parent's sudden death is reduced by saying, 'He wouldn't have wanted to live with a disability.'	Protects a person from pain and traumatic events.
Introjection A form of identification that allows for the acceptance of others' norms and values into oneself, even when contrary to one's previous assumptions.	A 7-year-old tells his little sister, 'Don't talk to strangers.' He has introjected this value from the instructions of parents and teachers.	Helps a person avoid social retaliation and punishment; particularly important for the child's development of superego.
Minimisation Not acknowledging the significance of one's behaviour.	A person says, 'Don't believe everything my wife tells you. I wasn't so drunk I couldn't drive.'	Allows a person to decrease responsibility for own behaviour.
Projection A process in which blame is attached to others or the environment for unacceptable desires, thoughts, shortcomings and mistakes.	A mother is told her child must repeat a year in school, and she blames this on the teacher's poor instruction. A husband forgets to pay a bill and blames his wife for not giving it to him earlier.	Allows a person to deny the existence of shortcomings and mistakes; protects self-image.
Rationalisation Justification of certain behaviours by faulty logic and ascribing motives that are socially acceptable but did not in fact inspire the behaviour.	A mother spanks her toddler too hard and says it was all right because he couldn't feel it through the nappies anyway.	Helps a person cope with the inability to meet goals or certain standards.
Reaction formation A mechanism that causes people to act exactly opposite to the way they feel.	An executive resents his bosses for calling in a consulting firm to make recommendations for change in his department but verbalises complete support of the idea and is exceedingly polite and cooperative.	Aids in reinforcing repression by allowing feelings to be acted out in a more acceptable way.

Table 6-9 *(continued)*

Defence mechanism	Example(s)	Use/purpose
Regression Resorting to an earlier, more comfortable level of functioning that is characteristically less demanding and responsible.	An adult throws a temper tantrum when she does not get her own way. A critically ill patient allows the nurse to bathe and feed him.	Allows a person to return to a point in development when nurturing and dependency were needed and accepted with comfort.
Repression An unconscious mechanism by which threatening thoughts, feelings and desires are kept from becoming conscious; the repressed material is denied entry into consciousness.	A teenager, seeing his best friend killed in a car accident, becomes amnesic about the circumstances surrounding the accident.	Protects a person from a traumatic experience until he or she has the resources to cope.
Sublimation Displacement of energy associated with more primitive sexual or aggressive drives into socially acceptable activities.	A person with excessive sexual drives invests psychic energy into a well-defined religious value system.	Protects a person from behaving in irrational, impulsive ways.
Substitution The replacement of a highly valued, unacceptable or unavailable object by a less valuable, acceptable or available object.	A woman wants to marry a man exactly like her dead father and settles for someone who looks a little bit like him.	Helps a person achieve goals and minimises frustration and disappointment.
Undoing An action or words designed to cancel some disapproved thoughts, impulses or acts in which the person relieves guilt by making reparation.	A father spanks his child and the next evening brings home a present for him. A teacher writes an exam that is far too easy, then constructs a grading curve that makes it difficult to earn a high grade.	Allows a person to appease guilty feelings and atone for mistakes.

Note: From Fontaine, Karen Lee, *Mental Health Nursing*, 5th Edition, © 2003, pgs 11–12. Reprinted by permission of Pearson Education Inc., Upper Saddle River, NJ.

Coping

Coping may be described as dealing with problems and situations, or contending with them successfully. A **coping strategy (coping mechanism)** is an innate or acquired way of responding to a changing environment or specific problem or situation. According to Folkman and Lazarus (1991), coping is 'the cognitive and behavioural effort to manage specific external and/or internal demands that are appraised as taxing or exceeding the resources of the person' (p. 210).

Two types of coping strategies have been described: problem-focused and emotion-focused coping. *Problem-focused coping* refers to efforts to improve a situation by making changes or taking some action. *Emotion-focused coping* includes thoughts and actions that relieve emotional distress. Emotion-focused coping does not improve the situation, but the person often feels better.

Coping strategies are also viewed as long term or short term. *Long-term coping strategies* can be constructive and realistic. For example, in certain situations talking with others about the problem and trying to find out more about the situation are long-term strategies.

Other long-term strategies include those that involve a change in lifestyle patterns such as eating a healthy diet, exercising regularly, balancing leisure time with working, or using problem solving in decision making instead of anger or other nonconstructive responses.

Short-term coping strategies can reduce stress to a tolerable limit temporarily but are in the end ineffective ways to deal with reality. They may even have a destructive or detrimental effect on the person. Examples of short-term strategies are using alcoholic beverages or drugs, daydreaming and fantasising, relying on the belief that everything will work out and giving in to others to avoid anger.

Coping strategies vary among individuals and are often related to the individual's perception of the stressful event. Three approaches to coping with stress are to alter the stressor, adapt to the stressor or avoid the stressor. A person's coping strategies often change with a reappraisal of a situation. There is never only one way to cope. Some people choose avoidance; others confront a situation as a means of coping. Still others seek information or rely on religious beliefs as a means of coping.

Coping can be adaptive or maladaptive. *Adaptive coping* helps the person to deal effectively with stressful events and minimises distress associated with them. *Maladaptive coping* can result in unnecessary distress for the person and others associated with the person or stressful event. In nursing literature, effective and ineffective coping are often differentiated. *Effective coping* results in adaptation; *ineffective coping* results in maladaptation. Although the coping behaviour may not always seem appropriate, the nurse needs to remember that coping is always purposeful.

Table 6-10 Examples of the Effects of Stress on Basic Human Needs

Needs	Example
Physiological	Altered elimination pattern Change in appetite Altered sleep pattern
Safety and security	Expresses nervousness and feelings of being threatened Focuses on stressors, inattention to safety measures
Love and belonging	Isolated and withdrawn Becomes overly dependent Blames others for own problems
Self-esteem	Fails to socialise with others Becomes a workaholic Draws attention to self
Self-actualisation	Preoccupied with own problems Shows lack of control Unable to accept reality

The effectiveness of an individual's coping is influenced by a number of factors, including:

+ the number, duration and intensity of the stressors;
+ past experiences of the individual;
+ support systems available to the individual;
+ personal qualities of the person.

If the duration of the stressors is extended beyond the coping powers of the individual, that person becomes exhausted and may develop increased susceptibility to health problems including mental illness. As coping strategies or defence mechanisms (see Table 6-9) become ineffective, the individual may find they have problems in relationships, work and may have difficulties with meeting their own basic human needs (see Table 6-10).

Stress Management

Stress can be destructive for the individual therefore it needs to be managed. Indeed stress can lead an individual to turn to prescription and non-prescription medication, illegal drugs, alcohol and tobacco in a bid to relieve the stress. When we think about stress management, we naturally think of eliminating the stress in an individual's life. But how dull would life be if all stress was removed from that life. Remember not all stress is negative. Therefore stress management not only looks at teaching individuals ways of coping with the negative effects of stress levels but also aims to look at the more positive attributes of stress.

Stress management can be complex for some patients therefore the inexperienced nurse may need to consider referring the patient on to a more experienced colleague. If the nurse feels able to manage the individual's stress they must first fully assess the patient to identify the individual's current health status, physical and psychological, positive and negative stressors and level of stress and anxiety. It may also be necessary in some cases to include the patient's significant others in order to ascertain particular problems.

Once a full assessment of the patient has been completed, the nurse should plan an individualised stress management package for the patient, and in collaboration with the patient and their family. The goal for the stress management programme should be agreed with the patient. Involvement of the patient at this point is vital to ensure the patient concords with the plan and feels in control.

The overall patient goals for an individual experiencing stress may be to:

+ decrease or resolve anxiety;
+ increase ability to manage or cope with stressful events or circumstances;
+ improve role performance.

Once the goal of the stress management programme is established, the individual programme can be designed. There are many ways in which negative stress can be alleviated and the positive effects of stress enhanced. These include:

+ identifying the source of stress,
+ lifestyle changes such as exercise, diet, rest and sleep,
+ promoting ways of minimising anxiety,
+ relaxation,
+ prayer,
+ art therapy,
+ music therapy,
+ massage.

Stress is highly individual; a situation that may be a major stressor to one person may not be to another. Likewise some methods that help to reduce stress in one person will be totally ineffective for another. A nurse who is sensitive to patients' needs and reactions can choose those methods of intervention that will be most effective for each individual.

Identifying the Source of Stress

The cause of stress cannot always be identified. In fact for the person experiencing chronic stress, it is unlikely to go away unless they are able to identify the sources of the stress. Identifying the source of the stress will allow the individual with help and support to work out the cause of their stress and take steps to manage these situations and their stress levels.

Exercise

Regular exercise promotes both physical and emotional health. Physical benefits include improved muscle tone, increased cardiopulmonary function and weight control. Psychological benefits include relief of tension, a feeling of well-being and relaxation. In general, health guidelines recommend exercise at least three times a week for 30 to 45 minutes.

Diet

Optimal nutrition is essential for health and in increasing the body's resistance to stress. To minimise the negative effects of stress (e.g. irritability, hyperactivity, anxiety), people need to avoid excesses of caffeine, salt, sugar and fat, and deficiencies in vitamins and minerals.

Rest and Sleep

Rest and sleep restore the body's energy levels and are an essential aspect of stress management. To ensure adequate rest and sleep, patients may need help to attain comfort (such as pain management) and to learn techniques that promote peace of mind and relaxation.

Minimising Anxiety

Whenever nurses carry out a procedure they take measures to minimise patients' anxiety and stress. For example, nurses encourage patients to take deep breaths before an injection, explain procedures before they are implemented including sensations likely to be experienced during the procedure, administer a massage to help the patient relax, and offer support to patients and families during times of illness. The nurse recognises that quick action may be necessary to avoid the contagious nature of anxiety. That is, the anxious feeling of one person tends to make others around him or her also anxious. This can include family members, other patients nearby, or healthcare providers. General guidelines for helping patients who are stressed and feeling anxious are outlined in *Box 6-5*.

Relaxation

Several relaxation techniques can be used to quieten the mind, release tension and counteract the fight or flight responses. Nurses can teach these techniques to patients. Nurses should also encourage patients to use these techniques when they encounter stressful health situations. Examples of these situations are (a) during childbirth, (b) postoperatively to cope with pain and (c) before and during a painful procedure. Many clinical areas have relaxation tapes available that the patient can borrow. Some patients make their own recordings. Specific relaxation techniques include:

+ breathing exercises,
+ massage,
+ progressive relaxation,
+ imagery,
+ biofeedback,
+ yoga,
+ meditation,
+ therapeutic touch,
+ music therapy,
+ humour and laughter.

Stress Management for Nurses

Nurses, like patients, are susceptible to experiencing anxiety and stress. Nursing practice involves many stressors related to both patients and the work environment – understaffing, increasing severity of patient illnesses, adjusting to various work shifts, being expected to assume responsibilities for which

---

BOX 6-5 Minimising Stress and Anxiety

+ Listen attentively; try to understand the patient's perspective on the situation.
+ Provide an atmosphere of warmth and trust; convey a sense of caring and empathy.
+ Determine if it is appropriate to encourage patients' participation in the plan of care; give them choices about some aspects of care but do not overwhelm them with choices.
+ Stay with patients as needed to promote safety and feelings of security and to reduce fear.
+ Control the environment to minimise additional stressors such as reducing noise, limiting the number of persons in the room and providing care by the same nurse as much as possible.
+ Implement suicide precautions if indicated.
+ Communicate in short, clear sentences.
+ Help patients to:
  • determine situations that precipitate anxiety and identify signs of anxiety;

  • verbalise feelings, perceptions and fears as appropriate (some cultures discourage the expression of feelings);
  • identify personal strengths;
  • recognise usual coping patterns and differentiate positive from negative coping mechanisms;
  • identify new strategies for managing stress (e.g. exercise, massage, progressive relaxation);
  • identify available support systems.
+ Teach patients about:
  • the importance of adequate exercise, a balanced diet, and rest and sleep to energise the body and enhance coping abilities;
  • support groups available such as Alcoholics Anonymous, Weight Watchers or Overeaters Anonymous, and parenting and child abuse support groups;
  • educational programmes available such as time management, assertiveness training and meditation groups.

LIFESPAN CONSIDERATIONS

Middle-Aged Adults

Middle-aged adults are often called the 'sandwich generation'. They find themselves caring for children and grandchildren and often caring for ageing parents at the same time. When these activities become time and energy consuming, there is often not enough time left for attention to self. Nurses need to be aware of this and assist in suggesting resources and effective planning to ease the strain.

Older Adult

Older adult experience many losses and changes in their lives. They may be incremental and, over time, become stressful and possibly overwhelming. Changes in health, decreased functional ability and independence, need for relocation, loss of family and friends, and becoming a caregiver for a spouse or friend are a few of the stresses often experienced by older adults. Many of them have survived significant challenges in their earlier lives and have learned effective coping skills. Nurses can help them plan, evaluate their strategies, and learn new strategies, if needed. Informal and formal social supports are very important in learning to successfully live with these changes and stress.

Some effective coping methods for older adult are exercise, learning different relaxation techniques, participation in activities, adequate nutrition and rest, and engaging in expressive creative activities, such as art, music and writing. Referral to community resources and supports should be done when appropriate. It is most important to see older adults as unique individuals, with unique past experiences and very specific needs as they get older.

one is not prepared, inadequate support from supervisors and colleagues, caring for dying patients, and so on. Although most nurses cope effectively with the physical and emotional demands of nursing, in some situations nurses become overwhelmed and develop **burnout**, a complex syndrome of behaviours. The nurse with burnout manifests physical and emotional depletion, a negative attitude and self-concept, and feelings of helplessness and hopelessness.

Nurses can prevent burnout by using the techniques to manage stress discussed for patients. Nurses must first recognise their stress and become attuned to such responses as feelings of being overwhelmed, fatigue, angry outbursts, physical illness, and increases in coffee drinking, smoking or alcohol intake. Once attuned to stress and personal reactions, it is necessary to identify which situations produce the most pronounced reactions so that steps may be taken to reduce the stress. Suggestions include:

+ Plan a daily relaxation programme with meaningful quiet times to reduce tension (e.g. read, listen to music, soak in a tub or meditate).
+ Establish a regular exercise programme to direct energy outward.
+ Study assertiveness techniques to overcome feelings of powerlessness in relationships with others. Learn to say no.

+ Learn to accept failures – your own and others – and make it a constructive learning experience. Recognise that most people do the best they can. Learn to ask for help, to share your feelings with colleagues and to support your colleagues in times of need.
+ Accept what cannot be changed. There are certain limitations in every situation. Get involved in constructive change efforts if organisational policies and procedures cause stress.
+ Develop collegial support groups to deal with feelings and anxieties generated in the work setting.
+ Participate in professional organisations to address workplace issues.
+ Seek counselling, if indicated, to help clarify concerns.

As with all management plans the interventions implemented should be evaluated. The goal of the programme needs to be revisited and the care evaluated. If outcomes are not achieved, the nurse, patient and family, if appropriate, need to explore the reasons before modifying the care plan.

Psychosocial health is key to the well-being of an individual and therefore should be an integral part of the holistic management of a patient. Patients who are holistically cared for are said to recover quicker. Nurses need to broaden their concerns beyond the physical care of the patient as failure to meet psychosocial care needs can have disastrous results for the patient, as demonstrated in this chapter.

CRITICAL REFLECTION

Let us revisit the case study on page 86. Now that you have read this chapter what information would lead you to believe that Terry may be spiritually distressed? How would a spiritual assessment be of benefit to Terry? Do you approach Terry about his wife's concerns? If so, how would you do this? How would sexual health assessment benefit Terry and his wife?

CHAPTER HIGHLIGHTS

+ Psychosocial health is fundamental to a person's general well-being.
+ A positive self-concept is essential to a person's physical and psychological well-being.
+ Individuals who grow up in families whose members value each other are likely to feel good about themselves.
+ Factors affecting self-concept include development, family and culture, stressors, resources, history of success and failure, and illness.
+ The nurse assesses four areas of self-concept: personal identity, body image, self-esteem and role performance.
+ Sexuality is important in developing self-identity, interpersonal relationships, intimacy and love.
+ In its broad sense, sexuality involves all aspects of being and behaving.
+ The components that contribute to the development of sexuality are numerous; both biological and psychological components exist at all ages.
+ Factors that affect sexuality include developmental level, culture, religious values, personal ethics, disease processes and medications.
+ Nursing interventions focus largely on teaching patients about sexual function and sexuality, responsible sexual behaviour that includes the prevention of STDs and unwanted pregnancies, and self-examination of the breasts and testicles.
+ Counselling patients with altered sexual functions can be facilitated by using the PLISSIT model: permission giving (P), limited information (LI) and specific suggestions (SS). Intensive therapy (IT) requires intervention by clinical nurse specialists or sex therapists.
+ To implement spiritual care, nurses need to be skilled in establishing a trusting nurse-patient relationship.

+ Patients have a right to receive care that respects their individual spiritual and religious values.
+ Because spiritual beliefs and practices are highly personal, nurses must respect the rights of people to hold their own spiritual beliefs and to communicate or not these to others.
+ Nurses need to be aware of their own spiritual beliefs in order to be comfortable assisting others.
+ The spiritual needs of patients and support persons often come into focus at a time of illness. Spiritual beliefs can help people accept illness and plan for what lies ahead.
+ Spiritual distress refers to a disturbance in or a challenge to a person's belief or value system that provides strength, hope and meaning to life. Possible factors in spiritual distress include physiological problems, treatment-related concerns and situational concerns. Spiritual distress may be reflected in a number of behaviours, including depression, anxiety, verbalisations of unworthiness and fear of death.
+ Nursing interventions that promote spiritual well-being include offering one's presence, supporting the patient's religious practices and referring the patient to a religious counsellor.
+ Stress is a state of physiological and psychological tension that affects the whole person – physically, emotionally, intellectually, socially and spiritually.
+ There are physical and psychological indicators of stress. Physical indicators are the result of increased activity of the sympathetic and neuroendocrine systems.
+ Common psychological indicators are anxiety, fear, anger and depression. Anxiety, the most common response, has four levels: mild, moderate, severe and panic.

+ Coping strategies to deal with stress vary significantly among individuals. Strategies may be problem focused or emotion focused, long term or short term, and effective or ineffective.

+ The effectiveness of individual coping depends on the number, duration and intensity of the stressors; past experience; support systems available; and the personal qualities of the person.

+ Prolonged stress and ineffective coping interfere with the meeting of basic needs and can affect physical and mental health.

+ Nursing assessment of a patient experiencing stress involves a patient history to identify perceptions of and duration of stressors and coping strategies, and also a physical examination for physical indicators of stress.

+ Nursing interventions for patients who are stressed are aimed at encouraging health promotion strategies (exercise, healthy diet and adequate rest), minimising anxiety, mediating anger, teaching about specific relaxation techniques, and implementing crisis interventions as needed.

+ Because nursing practice involves many stressors related to both patients and the work environment, nurses are susceptible to anxiety and burnout. Like patients, they need to implement stress reduction measures.

REFERENCES

Annon, J. (1974) *The behavioral treatment of sexual problems. Vol. 1. Brief therapy*, New York: Harper and Row.

BBC News (2006) *'Problem families' scheme set out*, London: BBC. Available from http://news.bbc.co.uk/1/hi/uk_politics/5312928.stm.(Accessed on 20 December 2006.)

Berman, J. and Berman, L. (2001) *For women only*, New York: Henry Holt and Company.

Carpenito, L.J. (2001) *Nursing diagnosis: Application to clinical practice* (9th edn), Philadelphia: Lippincott.

Carson, V.B. (1989) *Spiritual dimensions of nursing practice*, Philadelphia: Saunders.

Cohen, M., Headley, J. and Sherwood, G.W. (2000) 'Spirituality and bone marrow transplantation: when faith is stronger than fear', *International Journal for Human Caring* 4(2): 41–48.

Edline, G., Golanty, E. and Brown, K.M. (2002) *Health and wellness: A holistic approach* (7th edn), Boston: Jones and Bartlett.

Ellison, C.W. (1983) 'Spiritual well-being: Conceptualisation and measurement', *Journal of Psychology and Theology*, 11, 330–340.

Folkman, S. and Lazarus, R.S. (1991) 'Coping and emotion', in A. Monat and R.S. Lazarus (Eds), *Stress and coping* (3rd edn), New York: Columbia University Press.

Fontaine, K.L. and Fletcher, J.S. (2003) *Mental health nursing* (5th edn), Upper Saddle River, NJ: Pearson Education, Inc.

Freud, S. (1946) *The ego and the mechanisms of defence*, New York: International Universities Press.

Fry, A.J. (1997) 'Spirituality: Connectedness through being and doing', in S. Ronaldson (Edn) *Spirituality: The heart of nursing*, Melbourne: Alismed Publications.

Golberg, B. (1998) 'Connection: An exploration of spirituality in nursing care', *Journal of Advanced Nursing*, 27, 836–842.

Kenny, G. (1999) 'Assessing children's spirituality: what is the way forward?', *British Journal of Nursing*, 8(1), 28–32.

Larson, D.B., Sherrill, K.A., Lyons, J.S., Craigie, F.C., Thielman, S., Greenword, A. and Larson, S.S. (1992) 'Associations between dimensions of religious commitment and mental health reported in the American Journal of Mental Health and Archives of General Psychiatry: 1978–1989', *American Journal of Psychiatry*, 149: 557–559.

Narayanasamy, A. (2004) 'Commentary to: MacLaren's article: a kaleidoscope of understandings: spiritual nursing in a multi-faith society', *Journal of Advanced Nursing*, 45(5), 457–464.

Pargament, K.I. (1997) *The psychology of religion and coping*, New York: Guilford.

Randolph, J.J. and Dykman, B.M. (1998) 'Perceptions of parenting and depression-proneness in the Offspring: Dysfunctional attitudes as a mediating mechanism', *Cognitive Therapy and Research*, 22(4), 377–400.

Rozanski, A., Blumenthal, J.A., Davidson, K.W., Saab, P.G. and Kubansky, L. (2005) 'The epidemiology, pathophysiology and management of psychosocial risk factors in cardiac practice: The emerging field of behavioural cardiology', *Journal of the American College of Cardiology*, 45(5), 637–651.

Von Sadovszky, V., Keller, M. and McKinney, K. (2002) 'College students' perceptions and practices of sexual activity in sexual encounters', *Journal of Nursing Scholarship*, 34, 133–138.

World Health Organization (1948) *Constitution of the World Health Organization: Basic Documents*, Geneva: WHO.

World Health Organization (1975) *Education and treatment in human sexuality: The training of health professionals*, Geneva: WHO.

Chapter 7 Health Promotion

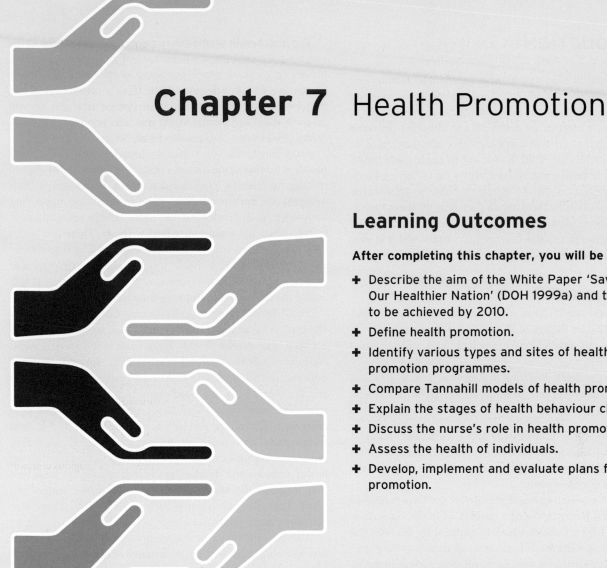

Learning Outcomes

After completing this chapter, you will be able to:

+ Describe the aim of the White Paper 'Saving Lives: Our Healthier Nation' (DOH 1999a) and the targets to be achieved by 2010.

+ Define health promotion.

+ Identify various types and sites of health promotion programmes.

+ Compare Tannahill models of health promotion.

+ Explain the stages of health behaviour change.

+ Discuss the nurse's role in health promotion.

+ Assess the health of individuals.

+ Develop, implement and evaluate plans for health promotion.

CASE STUDY

Childhood obesity is on the increase according to the Parliamentary Office of Science and Technology (2003). A recent case of an eight-year-old who weighed over 14 stone hit the headlines with discussions about whether this child should be put into care in order to protect him. However social services and child protection experts decided that he could stay with his parents but that he must follow a diet and exercise regime to reduce his weight.

According to the BMA (2007), there are currently around a million obese children under the age of 16 in the UK. Childhood obesity can lead to childhood type II diabetes, early puberty in girls and in the future can lead to heart disease, osteoarthritis and some cancers.

This chapter will aim to demonstrate the importance of health promotion in nursing and outline health promotion models that can be used to tackle health issues such as obesity.

INTRODUCTION

Health promotion is an important component of nursing and is the responsibility of all healthcare professionals working in clinical practice and the government alike, particularly as the UK faces a number of health issues, some minor, some debilitating and some that carry high mortality rates such as coronary heart disease (CHD). In a bid to tackle these health issues the government published a White Paper 'Saving Lives: Our Healthier Nation' (DOH, 1999a) that aims to improve the health of the nation by focusing on four priority areas: coronary heart disease and stroke, cancer, accidents and mental health. The strategy sets out four specific targets, which it aims to achieve by the year 2010:

+ to reduce the death rate of cancer in people under the age of 75 years by at least 20%;
+ to reduce the death rate of coronary heart disease and stroke in people under the age of 75 years by at least 40%;
+ to reduce the death rate from suicide and undetermined injury by 20%;
+ to reduce the death rate from accidents by at least 20% and to reduce the rate of serious injury from accidents by at least 10%.

By implementing this strategy the government hopes to bring new emphasis to the promotion of health and prevention of ill health. It not only aims to save lives but also improve the quality of life for the nation.

As part of promoting healthy lifestyles the Department of Health (DOH) has introduced a number of initiatives including Healthy Living Centres which are funded by the National Lottery and target the most disadvantaged sectors of the population, offering advice on a range of subjects such as housing, benefits, healthy eating and exercise (DOH, 1999b). The DOH has, in response to the increase in childhood obesity, begun a National Child Measurement Programme for children aged five and 11 that involves measuring and recording their height and weight (DOH, 2007).

Nursing is fundamental to the effective delivery of a number of these initiatives. Whitehead (2001a) states that the main health-related activity that nurses are involved in is giving health information which, according to Downie *et al.* (1996), is the most common health promotion method adopted. By providing information and health education to patients nurses aim to influence patients to change their lifestyle.

DEFINING HEALTH PROMOTION

According to Kemm and Close (1995) health promotion is any activity that intends to prevent disease or promote health. Health promotion is a process that enables individuals to control and change their lifestyles so that their health is improved. It is an activity that is done with and for people rather than done on or to them.

The term **health promotion** has been around since the 1970s and is used to encompass a plethora of strategies to improve the person's overall health including health education, illness prevention and health protection. Health promotion is not just focused on the prevention of disease but also on the person's social and mental health and revolves around a philosophy of wholeness, wellness and well-being.

According to the World Health Organization (WHO, 1998) health education comprises of 'consciously constructed opportunities for learning involving some form of communication designed to improve health literacy, including improving knowledge and developing life skills which are conducive to individual and community health' (p. 4). Therefore health education is considered to be more wide-ranging than merely the communication of risk factors but also the development of skills such as self-awareness and decision making that will enable the individual to improve their health.

The FRESH (Focusing Resources on Effective School Health) programme (2000), developed by a partnership between the World Health Organization (WHO), United Nations Children's Fund (UNICEF), United Nations Educational, Scientific and Cultural Organization (UNESCO) and the World Bank, is a good example of a skills-based health education programme. The target population for this programme is school age children across the world and it aims to promote knowledge about diseases/illnesses including symptoms, transmission and risk factors as well as considering health attitudes and developing the individual's life skills that may improve the health of school age children around the world. It tackles health issues such as HIV/AIDS prevention, early pregnancy and tobacco and substance abuse.

Alternatively, illness or disease prevention is seen as 'measures not only to prevent the occurrence of disease, such as risk factor reduction, but also to arrest its progress and reduce its consequences once established' (WHO, 1998: 4). According to Naidoo and Wills (2000), senior lecturers in health promotion and illness prevention can be divided into three categories:

+ Primary prevention that seeks to avoid the onset of disease by detecting those groups that are at increased risk of developing disease and providing them with information, advice and counselling (e.g. immunisation).
+ Secondary prevention that aims to shorten the episodes of illness and prevent progression of the disease (e.g. providing education healthy eating for diabetic patients).
+ Tertiary prevention that aims to limit the effects and complications of the illness or disease process (e.g. rehabilitation for cardiac patients).

Health promotion is a priority for many healthcare professionals including nurses and is written into many of their job descriptions. In particular, community nurses, health visitors and community psychiatric nurses have a defined role in promoting the health of their patients/patients and fostering effective working relationships with them while the patient is in their own home. However there are many different sites in which health promotion can take place.

SITES FOR HEALTH-PROMOTION ACTIVITIES

Health-promotion programmes are found in many settings. Programmes and activities may be offered to individuals and families in the home or in the community setting and at schools, hospitals or in the workplace. Some health promotion programmes are aimed at the individual while others are aimed at groups, with the latter being more efficient but maybe not the most effective as it can be difficult to ascertain if members of the group have understood what has been discussed. However many people prefer the group approach, find it more motivating and enjoy the socialising and support.

LIFESPAN CONSIDERATIONS

Health-Promotion Topics

Infants
+ Breastfeeding
+ Immunisations
+ Parenting skills for new parents

Children
+ Nutrition
+ Dental checkups
+ Immunisations
+ Safety promotion and injury control

Adolescents
+ Bullying - which can impact on psychological and physical health
+ Drugs
+ Peer group influences
+ Self-concept and body image
+ Nutrition and weight control

+ Alcohol abuse
+ Physical fitness
+ Personal safety
+ Smoking cessation
+ Sex education

Older Adults
+ Dental/oral health
+ Exercise
+ Health screening recommendations
+ Hearing aid use
+ Immunisations
+ Medication instruction
+ Mental health
+ Malnutrition
+ Exercise
+ Preventive health services
+ Safety precautions
+ Smoking cessation
+ Weight control

Community based programmes are frequently offered. The type of programme depends on the current health concerns and may include health promotion, specific protection and screening for early detection of disease (see the Lifespan Considerations above for different health promotion topics). For example, there is a national policy set out by the DOH to offer influenza immunisation to specific at-risk groups within the community. Influenza, or 'flu', is a highly contagious acute viral infection that affects people of all ages. The signs and symptoms of the disease are fever, headache, aching muscles and a cough or other respiratory symptoms which most people recover from. However, for certain groups of people (see *Box 7-1*) it can cause serious illness and even death. Flu epidemics occur mainly in the winter months and can result in widespread disruption to healthcare and other services. As a result of the devastating effects both on the individual and healthcare services the DOH health protection programme was developed.

School health-promotion programmes may serve as a foundation for children of all ages to gain basic knowledge about lifestyle and health issues. The school is the centre of the community; therefore by promoting health to school children it is thought that the health promotion message will reach the whole community. The school nurse may teach programmes about basic nutrition, dental care, drug and alcohol abuse, domestic violence and issues related to sexuality and pregnancy. Classroom teachers may include health-related topics in their lesson plans, for example, the way the normal heart functions or the need for clean air and water in the environment.

Worksite programmes for health promotion have developed out of the need for businesses to control the rising cost of

BOX 7-1 'At Risk' Groups Offered Influenza Immunisation

+ All those aged 65 years or over
+ All those aged six months and over with the following health problems:
  • chronic respiratory disease including asthma
  • chronic heart disease
  • chronic renal disease
  • chronic liver disease
  • diabetes
  • Immunosuppression (e.g. splenic dysfunction and HIV infection).

healthcare and employee absenteeism. Many industries feel that both employers and employees benefit from healthy lifestyles and behaviours. The convenience of the workplace setting makes these programmes particularly attractive to many adults who would otherwise not be aware of them or motivated to attend them. Health promotion programmes may be held in the company cafeteria so that employees can watch a film or attend a discussion group during their lunch break. Workplace programmes may be aimed at specific populations, such as accident prevention for the machine worker or back care programmes for individuals involved in heavy lifting; programmes to screen for high blood pressure; or health enhancement programmes, such as fitness information and relaxation techniques. Benefits to the worker may include an increased feeling of well-being, fitness, weight control and decreased stress. Benefits to the employer may include an increase in employee motivation and productivity, an increase in employee morale, a decrease in absenteeism and a lower rate of employee turnover, all of which may decrease business and healthcare costs (Mills, 2005).

Although it is important to consider the setting for health promotion it is equally important to adopt the most appropriate approach to health promotion.

APPROACHES TO HEALTH PROMOTION

According to Ewles and Simnet (1995) there are five approaches to health promotion:

1. **Medical approach**, which focuses on disease and the biological and medical explanations of health ignoring the impact of social and environmental dimensions on health.
2. **Behavioural change approach**, which encourages individuals to adopt healthy behaviours such as exercise.
3. **Educational approach**, which is the provision of information and education to allow the individual to make informed decisions.
4. **Empowerment approach**, which helps individuals to identify their own health concerns and needs.
5. **Social change approach**, which involves lobbying and policy planning. This approach focuses on the socioeconomic environment in determining health such as low income.

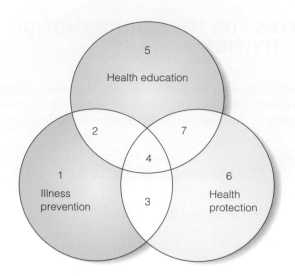

Figure 7-1 Tannahill's Model of Health Promotion (1985). (From Naidoo J. and Wills J. (2001) *'Health Studies: An Introduction'*, Palgrave, Basingstoke.)

Ewles and Simnet (1999) do not guide nurses to use a particular approach for health promotion. Jones (2000) suggests that more than one approach may be used in effective health promotion. Indeed the Cardiovascular Health Strategy Group (1999) recommends that healthcare professionals use both an individualistic- and population-based approach to health promotion.

HEALTH PROMOTION MODELS

In order to provide structure for health promotion a number of health promotion models have been developed. These provide the underlying theoretical perspectives of health promotion and provide a framework for action.

One of the better known descriptive models of health promotion is Tannahill's model that describes health promotion as three interlinked circles that include health education, prevention and protection (see Figure 7-1). However as the circles interlink there are overlaps (see *Box 7-2*).

Despite the simplicity of this model, it has many critics, some of which believe that it ignores the social and economic roots of ill health as it does not consider why the individual

---

BOX 7-2 Dimensions of Health Promotion as indicated in Tannahill's Model of Health Promotion

+ Preventive services, e.g. immunisation or cervical screening
+ Preventive health education, e.g. smoking advice
+ Preventive health protection, e.g. fluoridation of water
+ Health education for preventive health protection, e.g. seat belt campaigns

+ Health education, e.g. building lifeskills with groups such as exercise programmes
+ Health protection, e.g. implementing a workplace no-smoking policy
+ Health education aimed at health protection, e.g. campaigning for protective legislation

Source: Adapted from Naidoo J. and Wills J. (2001) *Health Studies: An Introduction*, Palgrave, Basingstoke.

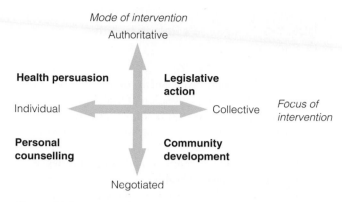

Figure 7-2 Beattie's Model of Health Promotion (1991) (From Naidoo J. and Wills J. (2000) *'Health Promotion: Foundations for Practice'* Bailliere Tindall.)

or community has behaviours that could lead to ill health. However, many argue that this model highlights the fact that it is difficult to change health behaviours using only one approach and that approaches need to complement one another. Indeed many aspects of health promotion practice overlap one another (Naidoo and Wills, 2001).

Beattie's model (see Figure 7-2), however, allows empowerment of the individual and the community and highlights the values and moral principles that underpin health promotion. This model allows the healthcare professional to consider the roots of ill-health such as income, poverty, housing, etc. It shows the importance of partnership between the individual, the healthcare professional and the government.

The advantages of Beattie's model is that it allows the healthcare professional to question the actions used to deliver change and where a particular health promotion initiative fits into the overall strategy.

STAGES OF HEALTH BEHAVIOUR CHANGE

It is important to note that any model for health promotion activity needs to be underpinned by the patient's intention to change behaviour. For instance, in recent years there has been increased awareness of the links between diseases such as coronary heart disease (CHD) and particular lifestyle activities such as smoking and poor diet. However people apparently still find it difficult to engage in health promoting behaviours such as eating a low fat diet.

In order to understand some of the factors that can influence the individual's decisions there is a need to consider Ajzen's (1991) Model of Planned Behaviour. Icek Ajzen, a professor in psychology, developed this model in order to explain how behaviour can be changed in three steps:

+ step 1 – the individual's attitude, determined by their beliefs about consequences;
+ step 2 – the expectations of others;

+ step 3 – the individual's perceived control and belief in their ability to change.

In order to change behaviour the individual must recognise the health benefit of making the change and also the consequence of not changing the behaviour (step 1). For example, an individual considering the incorporation of exercise into their life may think 'taking exercise will improve my health and being healthier would be good'.

However some individuals may need outside influences in order to feel the need to change (step 2). For example an individual considering incorporating exercise into their life may be more inclined to do so if they think 'my doctor thinks I should exercise more and what she thinks is important to me'.

Some individuals may feel that there are barriers to changing their behaviours and therefore may feel unable to change (step 3). For example an individual considering incorporating exercise into their life may feel 'I don't have the facilities to exercise and this will make exercising difficult'.

In order to develop an effective health promotion programme it is vital that the healthcare professional establishes the individual's attitude and beliefs toward changing their behaviour and establishing their individual perceived obstruction to changing their behaviour (e.g. themselves, others or outside barriers or loci of control).

The Nurse's Role in Health Promotion

Individuals and communities who seek to increase their responsibility for personal health and self-care require health education. The trend toward health promotion has created the opportunity for nurses to strengthen the profession's influence on health promotion, disseminate information that promotes an educated public, and assist individuals and communities to change long-standing health behaviours.

A variety of programmes can be used for the promotion of health, including (a) information dissemination, (b) health risk appraisal and wellness assessment, (c) lifestyle and behaviour change, and (d) environmental control programmes.

Information dissemination is the most basic type of health-promotion programme. This method makes use of a variety of media to offer information to the public about the risk of particular lifestyle choices and personal behaviour, as well as the benefits of changing that behaviour and improving the quality of life. Leaflets, posters, brochures, newspaper features, books and health fairs all offer opportunities for the dissemination of health-promotion information. Alcohol and drug abuse, driving under the influence of alcohol, hypertension and the need for immunisations are some of the topics frequently discussed. Information dissemination is a useful strategy for raising the level of knowledge and awareness of individuals and groups about health habits.

When planning information dissemination, it is important to consider factors such as cultural factors and different age groups. Knowing the best place and method to distribute information will increase the effectiveness. For example, some people who may be at risk from coronary heart disease may not go to their GP, therefore some GP practices have decided to do health assessments at shopping centres in a bid to identify and encourage people to adopt healthier lifestyles. This provides a stepping stone for providing information and suggesting resources for special needs – all done in a nonthreatening environment.

Lifestyle and behaviour change programmes require the participation of the individual and are geared toward enhancing the quality of life and extending the life span. Individuals generally consider lifestyle changes after they have been informed of the need to change their health behaviour and have become aware of the potential benefits of the change. Many programmes are available to the public, both on a group and individual basis, some of which address stress management, nutrition awareness, weight control, smoking cessation and exercise.

Health-promotion activities, such as the variety of programmes previously discussed, involve collaborative relationships with both patients and healthcare professionals. The role of the nurse is to work *with* people, not *for* them – that is, to act as a facilitator of the process of assessing, evaluating and understanding health. The nurse may act as advocate, consultant, teacher or coordinator of services. For examples of the nurse's role in health promotion, see *Box 7-3*.

These roles allow the nurse to work with individuals of all age groups and diverse family units or to concentrate on a specific population, such as new parents, school-age children or older adults. In any case, the nursing process is a basic tool for the nurse in a health-promotion role. Although the process

BOX 7-3 The Nurse's Role in Health Promotion

+ Facilitate patient involvement in the assessment, implementation and evaluation of health goals.
+ Educate patients on ways of enhancing fitness, improving nutrition, managing stress and enhancing relationships.
+ Assist individuals, families and communities to increase their levels of health.
+ Assist patients, families and communities to develop and choose healthier options.
+ Reinforce good health behaviours.
+ Advocate community changes that promote a healthy environment.

is the same, the nurse emphasises teaching the patient (who can be either an individual or a family unit) self-care responsibilities.

THE NURSING PROCESS AND HEALTH PROMOTION

A key aspect of planning an effective health promotion strategy for an individual is a thorough assessment of the individual's health status.

NURSING MANAGEMENT

ASSESSING

Components of this assessment need to include information about the patient's past medical history, a physical examination, lifestyle assessment, social support review, health risk assessment, health beliefs review and life stress review.

Health History and Physical Examination

Information about the patient's past medical history along with a physical examination can detect any existing health problems. For example, patients may present with symptoms that may seem nonspecific, such as tiredness and weight loss, however symptoms such as these may be indicative of underlying disease such as type 2 diabetes. Physical examination, including blood tests and a detailed assessment of the patient's health history, can uncover diseases such as type 2 diabetes which if undetected and untreated could lead to the development of serious health problems such as stroke or heart attack.

Type 2 diabetes is also known as maturity onset, or non-insulin dependent diabetes. It develops mainly in people older than 40 (but can occur in younger people). Currently in the UK about three in 100 people aged over 40, and about 10 in 100 people aged over 65, have type 2 diabetes. It is more common in people who are overweight or obese. It also tends to run in families.

Lifestyle Assessment

Lifestyle assessment focuses on the personal lifestyle and habits of the patient as they affect health. Categories of lifestyle generally assessed are physical activity, nutritional information, stress management and such habits as smoking, alcohol consumption and drug use. Other categories may be included. The goals of lifestyle assessment tools are to provide the following:

+ an opportunity for patients to assess the impact of their present lifestyle on their health;
+ a basis for decisions related to changing behaviours and lifestyle.

Several tools are available to assess lifestyle. A form for self-assessment of lifestyle is shown in Figure 7-3.

Healthstyle: A Self-Test

Everyone wants good health. But many of us don't know how to be as healthy as possible. Health experts describe *lifestyle* as one of the most important factors affecting our health. In fact, it is estimated that 7 of the 10 leading causes of death could be reduced through common-sense changes in lifestyle. The first step in a healthier lifestyle is thinking about what we are doing now.

This brief self-test, developed by the Public Health Service, will let you know how well you are doing to stay healthy. The behaviors included in the test are recommended for most adult Americans. Some behaviors may not apply to persons with certain chronic diseases or handicaps, or to pregnant women. Such persons may need special advice from their doctor or other health care provider.

Cigarette Smoking

If you never smoke, enter a score of 10 for this section and go to the next section on *Alcohol and Drugs*.

	Almost Always	Sometimes	Almost Never
1. I avoid smoking cigarettes.	2	1	0
2. I smoke only low tar and nicotine cigarettes OR I smoke a pipe or cigars.	2	1	0

Smoking Score: ___

Alcohol and Drugs

	Almost Always	Sometimes	Almost Never
1. I avoid drinking alcoholic beverages or I drink no more than 1 or 2 drinks a day.	4	1	0
2. I avoid using alcohol or other drugs (especially illegal drugs) as a way of handling stressful situations or the problems.	2	1	0
3. I am careful not to drink alcohol when taking certain medicines (for example, medicine for sleeping, pain, colds, and allergies) or when pregnant.	2	1	0
4. I read and follow the label directions when using prescribed and over-the-counter drugs.	2	1	0

Alcohol and Drugs Score: ___

Eating Habits

	Almost Always	Sometimes	Almost Never
1. I eat a variety of foods each day, such as fruits and vegetables; whole grain breads and cereals; lean meats; dairy products; dry peas; beans; nuts and seeds.	4	1	0
2. I limit the amount of fat, saturated fat, and cholesterol I eat (including fat on meats, eggs, butter, cream, shortenings, and organ meats such as liver).	2	1	0
3. I limit the amount of salt I eat by cooking with only small amounts, not adding salt at the table, and avoiding salty snacks.	2	1	0
4. I avoid eating too much sugar (especially frequent snacks of sticky candy or soft drinks).	2	1	0

Eating Habits Score: ___

Exercise/Fitness

	Almost Always	Sometimes	Almost Never
1. I do vigorous exercises for 20–30 minutes a day at least 3 times a week (examples include jogging, swimming, brisk walking, bicycling).	4	2	0
2. I do exercises that enhance my muscle tone for 15–30 minutes at least 3 times a week (examples include using weight machines or free weights, yoga and calisthenics).	3	1	0
3. I use part of my leisure time participating in individual, family, or team activities that increase my level of fitness (such as gardening, dancing, bowling, golf, baseball).	3	1	0

Exercise/Fitness Score: ___

Stress Control

	Almost Always	Sometimes	Almost Never
1. I have a job or do other work that I enjoy.	2	1	0
2. I find it easy to relax and express my feelings freely.	2	1	0
3. I recognize early, and prepare for, events or situations likely to be stressful for me.	2	1	0
4. I have close friends, relatives, or others whom I can talk to about personal matters and call on for help when needed.	2	1	0
5. I participate in group activities (such as religious worship and community organizations) and/or have hobbies that I enjoy.	2	1	0

Stress Control Score: ___

Safety

	Almost Always	Sometimes	Almost Never
1. I wear a seat belt while riding in a car.	2	1	0
2. I avoid driving while under the influence of alcohol and other drugs.	2	1	0
3. I obey traffic rules and the speed limit when driving.	2	1	0
4. I am careful when using potentially harmful products or substances (such as household cleaners, poisons, and electrical devices).	2	1	0
5. I avoid smoking in bed.	2	1	0

Safety Score: ___

(continued)

Figure 7-3 Healthstyle: A Self-Test (*Note:* From 'Healthstyle: A Self-Test,' by L.B. Bobroff, 1999, University of Florida, Institute of Food and Agricultural Sciences (UF/IFAS). Retrieved 23 March 2003, from http://edis.ifas.ufl.edu/BODY_HE778. Copyright 1999 by UF/IFAS. Reprinted with permission.)

Your Lifestyle Scores

After you have figured your scores for each of the six sections, circle the number in each column that matches your score for that section of the test. Remember: There is no total score for this self-test. Think about each section separately. You are identifying aspects of your lifestyle that you an improve in order to be healthier. So let's see what your scores reveal.

What Your Score Means to You (By Section)

Scores of 9 and 10

Excellent! Your answers show that you are aware of the importance of this area to your health. More important, you are putting your knowledge to work for you by practicing good health habits. As long as you continue to do so, this area should not pose a serious health risk. It's likely that you are setting an example for the rest of your family and friends to follow. Since you got a very high test score on this part of the test, you may want to consider other areas where your scores indicate room for improvement.

Scores of 6 to 8

Your health practices in this area are good, but there is room for improvement. Look again at the items you answered with a 'Sometimes' or 'Almost Never.' What changes can you make to improve your score? Even a small change can help you achieve better health.

Scores of 3 to 5

Your health risks are showing. Would you like more information about the risks you are facing? Do you want to know why it is important for you to change these behaviours? Perhaps you need help in deciding how to make the changes you desire. In either case, help is available.

Scores of 0 to 2

Obviously, you were concerned enough about your health to take this test. But your answers show that you may be taking serious risks with your health. Perhaps you were not aware of the risks and what to do about them. You can easily get the information and help you need to reduce your health risks and have a healthier lifestyle if you wish. The next step is up to you.

YOU CAN START RIGHT NOW

The test you just completed included many suggestions to help you reduce your risk of disease and premature death. Here are some of the most significant:

Avoid cigarettes.

Cigarette smoking is the single most important preventable cause of illness and early death. It is especially risky for pregnant women and their unborn babies. Persons who stop smoking reduce their risk of getting heart disease and cancer. So if you're a cigarette smoker, think twice before lighting that next cigarette. If you choose to continue smoking, try decreasing the number of cigarettes you smoke and switching to a low tar and nicotine brand.

Follow sensible drinking habits.

Alcohol produces changes in mood and behaviour. Most people who drink are able to control their intake of alcohol and to avoid undesired, and often harmful, effects. Heavy, regular use of alcohol can lead to cirrhosis of the liver, a leading cause of death. Also, statistics clearly show that mixing drinking and driving is often the cause of fatal or crippling accidents. So, if you drink, do it wisely and in moderation.

Use care in taking drugs.

Today's greater use of drugs – both legal and illegal – is one of our most serious health risks. Even some drugs prescribed by your doctor can be dangerous if taken when drinking alcohol or before driving. Use prescription drugs as directed and discard out-dated medications. Excessive or continued use of tranquilizers (or 'pep pills') can cause physical and mental problems. Using or experimenting with illicit drugs such as marijuana, heroin, cocaine, and other street drugs may lead to a number of damaging effects or even death.

Eat sensibly.

Your eating habits are related to risk for high blood pressure, heart disease, and many forms of cancer. Good eating habits mean holding down the amount of fat (especially saturated fat), cholesterol, sugar, and salt in your diet. Include a wide variety of plant foods like whole grain foods, beans, nuts, fresh fruits, and vegetables in your daily diet. They contain nutrients as well as protective factors that may reduce your risk of chronic diseases. You'll feel better.

Exercise regularly.

Almost everyone can benefit from exercise – and there's some form of exercise almost everyone can do. (If you have any doubt, check first with your doctor). Usually as little as 20–30 minutes of vigorous exercise a day three times a week will help you have a healthier heart, tone up sagging muscles, and sleep better. Think about how these changes can improve the way you feel.

Learn how to handle stress.

Stress is a normal part of living. The causes of stress can be good (like a promotion on the job) or bad (loss of a spouse). Properly handled, stress does not need to be a problem. But unhealthy responses to stress – such as driving too fast, drinking too much, or prolonged anger or grief – can cause a variety of physical and mental problems. Even on a very busy day, find a few minutes to slow down and relax. Talking over a problem with someone you trust can often help you find a satisfactory solution. Learn to distinguish between things that are 'worth fighting about' and things that are less important.

Be safety conscious.

Think 'safety first' at home, at work, at school, at play, and on the highway. Buckle seat belts and place young children in child restraint seats. Children under 12 should sit in the back seat. Obey traffic rules. Keep poisons and weapons out of the reach of children, and follow label directions for care and use. Keep emergency numbers by your telephone – when the unexpected happens, you'll be prepared.

Figure 7.3 (*continued*)

Social Support Review

Understanding the social context in which a person lives and works is important in health promotion. Individuals and groups can provide comfort, assistance, encouragement and information. Social support fosters successful coping and promotes satisfying and effective living (Pender *et al.*, 2002: 238).

Social support contributes to health by creating an environment that encourages healthy behaviours, promotes self-esteem and wellness, and provides feedback that the person's actions will lead to desirable outcomes. Examples of social support include family, peer support groups, religious support systems (e.g. churches) and self-help groups (e.g. Weight Watchers).

According to Pender *et al.* (2002), authors of *Health Promotion in Nursing Practice*, the nurse begins a social support review by asking the patient to do a number of tasks:

+ List individuals who provide personal support.
+ Indicate the relationship of each person (e.g. family member, fellow worker or colleague, social acquaintance).
+ Identify which individuals have been a source of support for five or more years.

This assessment allows the nurse and patient to discuss and evaluate the adequacy of their social support together and, if necessary, plan options for enhancing the support system.

Health Risk Assessment

A **health risk assessment (HRA)** is an assessment and educational tool that indicates an individual's risk for disease or injury. The individual's general health, lifestyle behaviours and demographic data are considered and compared to national data. The HRA includes a summary of the person's health risks and lifestyle behaviours with educational suggestions on how to reduce the risk. Specific HRAs exist such as the cardiovascular risk assessment that has been developed in response to the National Service Framework for Coronary Heart Disease (DOH, 2001). The National Service Framework demands that every primary care team identify all patients with coronary heart disease and using a health risk assessment tool such as 'Risk', a computer program designed to assess a wide range of risk factors associated with coronary heart disease, can aid this process (Squire, 2002).

Many HRA instruments are available today in paper-and-pencil as well as computerised forms. Recently, HRAs have begun to reflect a broader approach to health and health promotion. For instance, occupational health nurses can identify risk factors and subsequently plan interventions aimed at decreasing illness, absenteeism and disability.

Health Beliefs Review

Patients' health beliefs need to be clarified, particularly those beliefs that determine how they perceive control of their own health. Assessment of patients' health beliefs provides the nurse with an indication of how much the patient believes they can influence or control health through personal behaviours.

Several individuals have a strong belief in fate: 'Whatever will be, will be.' If people hold this belief, they do not feel that they can do anything to change the course of their disease. For example, educating diabetic patients about lifestyle changes such as diet and exercise would be made more problematic if the person believes they have no control over the outcome. In order to make changes in behaviour or lifestyle the individual needs to be motivated and ready to make those changes. Therefore a review of the individual's health beliefs is key to effective health promotion.

Life Stress Review

There is abundant literature about the impact of stress on mental and physical well-being. A variety of stress-related instruments have been found in the literature. For example, Holmes and Rahe (1967: 213) developed a Social Readjustment Rating Scale, a tool that assigns numerical values to life events (see *Box 7-4* on page 118). Studies have shown that a high score is associated with the increased possibility of illness in an individual.

PLANNING

Health-promotion plans are crucial to health improvement and need to be developed according to the needs, desires and priorities of the individual. The patient needs to be active in this process, deciding on health-promotion goals, the activities or interventions to achieve those goals, the frequency and duration of the activities, and the method of evaluation. During the planning process the nurse acts as a resource person rather than as an adviser or counsellor. The nurse provides information when asked, emphasises the importance of small steps to behavioural change, and reviews the patient's goals and plans to make sure they are realistic, measurable and acceptable to the patient.

Steps in Planning

According to Whitehead (2001b), a senior lecturer at the University of Plymouth, in order for health promotion to be effective it needs to be systematically planned. As a result he developed a flowchart that maps the planning process (see Figure 7-4 on page 119).

This model describes two approaches to health promotion: the empowerment approach, which usually focuses on the individual and their ability to take control in sometimes difficult situations in which the nurse acts as facilitator and advocate; while the preventive approach is generally derived from medical science and focuses on disease prevention.

1. *Identify the health promotion approach to be adopted.* The nurse will decide the approach that is most appropriate to the individual based on a number of factors including personality and resources. According to Whitehead (2001b) the most common approach adopted is the preventive approach; however it is noted that many nurses are trying to break free from this framework to adopt more empowering approaches.

BOX 7-4 Life-Change Index

Life event	Impact score	Life event	Impact score
Death of spouse	100	Change in living conditions	20
Divorce	60	Change in personal habits	20
Menopause	60	Trouble with boss	20
Separation from a living partner	60	Change in work hours or conditions	15
Prison sentence	60	Moving to new residence	15
Death of close family member	60	Presently in pre-menstrual period	15
Personal injury or illness	45	Change in schools	15
Marriage	45	Change in religious activities	15
Termination of employment or sacked	45	Change in social activities (more or less than before)	15
Marital reconciliation	40	Minor financial loan	10
Retirement	40	Change in number of family get-togethers	10
Change in health of family member	40	Holiday	10
Work more than 40 hours per week	35	Christmas approaching	10
Pregnancy	35	Minor violation of the law	5
Sex difficulties	35		
Gain of a new family member	35		
Business or work role change	35		
Change in financial state	35		
Death of a close friend	30		
Change in number of arguments with spouse or partner	30		
Mortgage or loan for a major purpose	25		
Default in paying mortgage or loan	25		
Sleep less than 8 hours per night	25		
Change in responsibilities in work	25		
Trouble with in-laws or children	25		
Outstanding personal achievement	25		
Spouse begins or stops work	20		
Begin or end school	20		

Life change units	Likelihood of illness in near future
300+	About 80%
150–299	About 50%
Less than 150	About 30%

The higher your life change score, the harder you have to work to get yourself back into a state of good health.

Source: Holmes and Rahe (1967).

2. *Identify the individual's health needs*
- *Empowerment approach:* These needs are established from the individual. This means that the individual will be assisted to decide their own health needs. For example, the individual may identify the need to stop smoking to improve their health.
- *Preventive approach:* The needs will be identified from current established or 'expert-driven' needs and resources. For example the individual may be entered onto a smoking cessation programme as smoking is known to be a risk factor for a number of diseases including cardiovascular diseases.

3. *Establish a health programme*
- *Empowerment approach:* The health promotion programme is based on the nature of the health need, the individual's expressed wishes and is developed *with* the individual *not for* the individual. The individual is seen as an active part of this process, which is developed in collaboration with the individual and other appropriate

agencies, for example dieticians for nutritional education for the obese. The programme often involves education, improving the individual's self-esteem and empowering the individual to make informed choices about their health.
- *Preventive approach:* A health promotion programme is offered to the individual based on disease or illness management and risk reduction/prevention. These types of programmes tend to address the physical but do not consider societal, economic and environmental factors as they often focus on the disease or biological or medical problem rather than the socioeconomic or environmental dimensions of health.

4. *Evaluate the effectiveness of the programme*
- *Empowerment approach:* The developed health promotion programme is evaluated not only by the nurse and other agencies but also by the individual. At this stage the nurse, in collaboration with the individual, may redefine or reset objectives if requested.

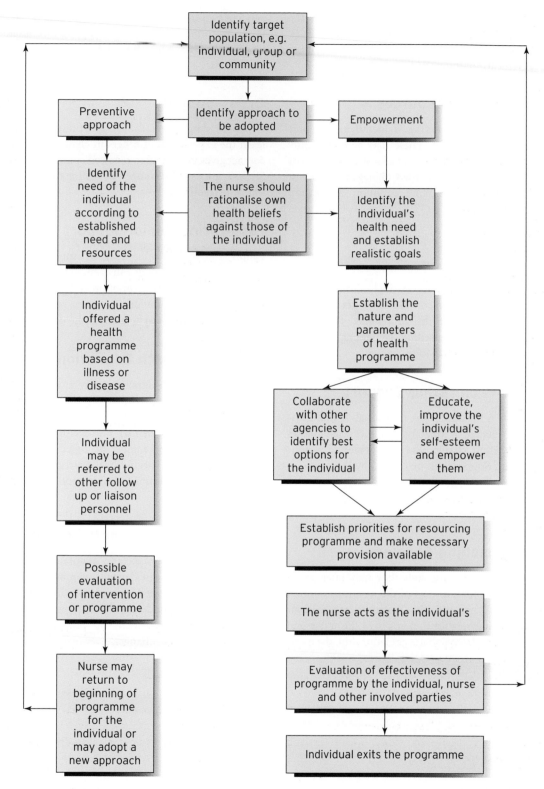

Figure 7-4 Planning Health Promotion.

Source: Adapted from Whitehead, D. (2001b) 'A stage planning programme model for health education/health promotion practice', *Journal of Advanced Nursing*, 36(2), 311-320.

- *Preventive approach:* There may be evaluation of the programme either by the nurse or by the individual. The evaluation is based on short-term behaviour change and/or modification of illness/disease status.

Exploring Available Resources

Another essential aspect of planning is identifying support resources available to the patient. These may be community resources, such as a fitness programme at a local gymnasium or educational programmes, such as stress management, breast self-examination, nutrition, smoking cessation and health lectures.

IMPLEMENTING

When developing a plan for promoting the health of an individual or group it is important to consider the types of nursing interventions needed to assist the individual. These may include providing support, counselling, facilitating, teaching, consulting and encouraging behaviour change.

Providing and Facilitating Support

A major nursing role is to support the individual. A vital component of lifestyle change is ongoing support that focuses on the desired behaviour change and is provided in a non-judgemental manner. Support can be offered by the nurse on an individual basis or in a group setting. The nurse can also facilitate the development of support networks for the patient, such as family members and friends.

Individual Counselling Sessions

If the nurse has the appropriate skills they may offer counselling sessions to individuals as part of the health promotion plan or if the individual has difficulties with the interventions or plan. The counselling relationship requires the nurse and individual to share ideas. In this sharing relationship, the nurse acts as a facilitator, promoting the individual's decision making in regard to the health promotion plan. Counselling may also be offered over the telephone but this may not be suitable for all patients.

Group Support

Group sessions provide an opportunity for participants to learn the experiences of others in changing behaviour. Group contact gives individuals a renewed commitment to their goals. Sessions are usually arranged according to the group needs and available resources.

Facilitating Social Support

Family and friends often play an important part in health promotion plans as they can facilitate or impede the efforts directed toward health promotion and prevention. The nurse's role is to assist the individual to assess, modify and develop the social support necessary to achieve the desired change.

Providing Health Education

Health education programmes on a variety of topics discussed earlier can be provided to groups, individuals or communities. Group programmes need to be planned carefully before they are implemented. The decision to establish a health promotion programme must be based on the health needs of the people; also, specific health promotion goals must be set. After the programme is implemented, outcomes must be evaluated.

Encouraging Behaviour Change

Whether people will make and maintain changes to improve health or prevent disease depends on many interrelated factors. To help patients succeed in implementing behaviour changes, the nurse needs to understand the stages of change and effective interventions that focus on progressing the individual through the stages of change.

CRITICAL REFLECTION

Let us revisit the case study on page 109. Now that you have read this chapter how would you tackle the problem of childhood obesity? How could you as the nurse promote behaviour change in this type of family?

CHAPTER HIGHLIGHTS

+ Health promotion is not just focused on the prevention of disease but also the person's social and mental health and revolves around a philosophy of wholeness, wellness and well-being.
+ Tannahill's model describes health promotion as three interlinked circles that include health education, prevention and protection.
+ Beattie's analytical model of health promotion highlights the values and moral principles that underpin health promotion.
+ The nurse's role in health promotion is to act as a facilitator of the process of assessing, evaluating and understanding health. It is the opportunity for nurses to strengthen the profession's influence on health promotion, disseminate information that promotes an educated public, and assist individuals and communities to change long-standing adverse health behaviours.

+ A complete and accurate assessment of the individual's health status is basic to health promotion. Lifestyle assessment tools give patients the opportunity to assess the impact of their present lifestyle behaviours on their health and to make decisions about specific lifestyle changes.
+ Health-promotion plans need to be developed according to the needs, desires and priorities of the patient.
+ The nurse acts as a resource person, provides ongoing support, and supplies additional information and education in a nonjudgemental manner in order to help individuals change their lifestyles or health behaviours.
+ During the evaluation phase of the health-promotion process, the nurse assists patients in determining whether they will continue with the plan, reorder priorities or revise the plan.

REFERENCES

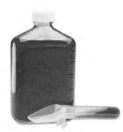

Ajzen, I. (1991) 'The theory of planned behaviour', *Organizational Behaviour and Human Decision Processes*, 50, 179–211.

British Medical Association (2007) *Childhood obesity*. London: BMA. Available from http://www.bma.org.uk/ap.nsf/Content/ChildObesity?OpenDocumentandHighlight=2,childhood,obesity. (Accessed on 20 April 2007.)

Cardiovascular Health Strategy Group (1999) *Building healthier hearts: The report of the Cardiovascular Health Strategy Group*, Dublin: The Stationery Office.

Department of Health (2007) *Supporting healthy lifestyles: The National Child Measurement Programme*, London: DOH. Available from http://www.dh.gov.uk/en/Policyandguidance/Healthandsocialcaretopics/Healthy. (Accessed on 20 April 2007.)

Department of Health (2001) *National Service Framework for Coronary Heart Disease: Executive Summary*, London: DOH.

Department of Health (1999a) *'Saving lives: Our healthier nation'* White Paper and 'Reducing health inequalities: an action report', London: DOH. Available from http://www.dh.gov.uk/en/Publicationsandstatistics/Lettersandcirculars/LocalAuthorityCirculars/AllLocalAuthority/DH_4004292. (Accessed on 20 April 2007.)

Department of Health (1999b) *Healthy Living Centres*. London: DOH. Available from http://www.dh.gov.uk/en/Publicationsandstatistics/Lettersandcirculars/Healthservicecirculars/DH_4004550. (Accessed on 20 April 2007.)

Downie, R.S., Tannahill, C. and Tannahill, A. (2nd edn) (1996) *Health promotion: Models and values*, Oxford: Oxford University Press.

Ewles, L. and Simnet, I. (1995) *Promoting health*, London: Scutari.

Ewles, L. and Simnet, I. (1999) *Promoting health: A practical guide.* Edinburgh: Bailliere Tindall.

Holmes, T.H. and Rahe, T.H. (1967) 'The social readjustment rating scale', *Journal of Psychosomatic Research*, 11(8), 213–218.

Jones, L. (2000) 'What is health?' in J. Katz, A. Peberdy, J. Douglas, (Eds) *Promoting health knowledge and practice*, London: Macmillan.

Kemm, J. and Close, A. (1995) *Health promotion: Theory and practice*, London: Macmillan Press.

Mills, P.R. (2005) 'The development of a new corporate specific health risk measurement instrument, and its use in investigating the relationship between health and well-being and employee productivity', *Environmental Health: A Global Access Science Source* 4, 1. Available from http://www.ehjournal.net/content/pdf/1476-069X-4-1.pdf. (Accessed on 21 April 2007.)

Naidoo, J. and Wills, J. (2000) *Health promotion: Foundations for practice* (2nd edn), London: Bailliere Tindall.

Naidoo, J. and Wills, J. (2001) *Health studies: An introduction*, Basingstoke: Palgrave.

Parliamentary Office of Science and Technology (2003) 'Childhood Obesity', *Postnote*, September 2003, No. 205, 1–4. Available from www.parliament.uk/post/pu205.pdf.

Pender, N.J., Murdaugh, C.L. and Parsons, M.A. (2002) *Health promotion in nursing practice* (4th edn). Upper Saddle River, NJ: Prentice Hall.

Squire, T. (2002) 'Easy risk assessment to meet NSF targets', *Practice Nursing*, 13(10), 444–446.

WHO (1998) *Health for all for the 21st century*, Geneva: WHO.

Whitehead, D. (2001a) 'Health education, behavioural change and social psychology: Nursing's contribution to health promotion', *Journal of Advanced Nursing*, 34(6), 822–832.

Whitehead, D. (2001b) 'A stage planning programme model for health education/health promotion practice', *Journal of Advanced Nursing*, 36(2), 311–320.

Chapter 8

Healthcare Delivery: Settings and Process

Learning Outcomes

After completing this chapter, you will be able to:

+ Differentiate primary, secondary and tertiary healthcare services.

+ Describe the functions and purposes of the healthcare services outlined in this chapter.

+ Identify the roles of various healthcare professionals.

+ Describe the factors that affect healthcare delivery.

+ Discuss the different frameworks for the delivery of effective nursing care.

CASE STUDY

In 2006, the government stated that the NHS budget deficit had reached £512 million which was more than double that in 2005. This resulted in over 12,000 jobs being cut, wards closed and operations delayed as the National Health Service (NHS) struggled to recover from these losses. Some feel that the cause of this deficit is due to poor management within the trusts (BBC News, 2006).

After reading this chapter, you will be able to reflect on the NHS as it was in 1948 compared to the new modernised NHS. You will also be able to discuss the different types of healthcare professionals and healthcare settings available to patients.

INTRODUCTION

Society today is presenting the healthcare system with an ever increasing burden. The population is ageing, with almost a fifth of the UK population aged over 65. Technological advances mean that almost 31% of the adult population are classed as leading sedentary lifestyles and one survey (DOH/FSA, 2000) found that one in five children ate no fruit and most young people over the age of seven years are physically inactive. This along with lifestyle factors such as smoking lead to 100,000 deaths per year, alcohol-related diseases accounting for 28,000 premature deaths and approximately 13,000 people dying as a result of accidents. Today's healthcare system needs to be robust to cope with these patients.

Traditionally the majority healthcare needs have been met by the NHS. However the strain on the NHS is overwhelming. In a bid to meet the ever-growing needs of the population and to modernise healthcare delivery in the UK, government ministers are planning a huge shake-up of current healthcare delivery systems. For example the reform 'Commissioning a Patient Led NHS' aims to reorganise local healthcare bodies so that private firms can provide services such as district nursing and podiatry to patients in the community. Such reforms aim to improve patient care, save money and raise morale within the NHS.

This and other NHS reforms are moving healthcare from the traditional hospital-based care to more diverse healthcare settings such as the home, clinics and GP surgeries. This chapter will explore the different settings for healthcare and the diverse processes involved in delivering these services.

THE NATIONAL HEALTH SERVICE

We tend to take the NHS for granted. But just think what healthcare was like before the NHS – a luxury that only a few could afford. Life in the 1930s and 1940s was tough especially during the Second World War. Infectious diseases such as tuberculosis, diphtheria and polio were rife and infant mortality was at an all time high with one in 20 infants dying before they reached a year old.

Healthcare was generally free to workers who were on lower pay through National Health Insurance but this did not cover their wives or their children. Also workers who earned a little more were unable to access free healthcare. This meant that many went without medical treatment or relied on dubious home remedies. Some doctors and hospitals, such as the Royal Free Hospital in London, however did give their services for free to those poorer patients. Despite these efforts to provide medical care to patients it was recognised that there needed to be a fairer way of delivering healthcare in the UK.

The NHS was the result of decades of reports and campaigns to improve healthcare in the UK and began with the Dawson Report in 1920, which recommended a comprehensive healthcare system for the UK. In 1926 the Royal Commission on National Health Insurance was developed, which brought about the idea of publicly funded healthcare. Then during the Second World War the Emergency Medical Services sped up the process of a unified healthcare system. In 1941 the government commissioned an independent inquiry into healthcare across the UK and found that healthcare provision varied vastly. Then in 1942 the Beveridge report into social care identified a national health service as one of three essential elements for a viable social security system.

On 5 July 1948 the NHS was introduced and transformed the lives of millions of people almost instantly. However its first few years were difficult. In post-war Britain, food was still being rationed, building materials, fuel and housing were in short supply. This along with the fact that all those who were unable to afford healthcare in the past and now wanted access to its free medical care meant that the new NHS was put under extreme pressure.

It became apparent that the need far exceeded what was estimated, including the cost. The concept of the NHS was that medical care was free at the point of delivery but in 1952 a small charge for prescriptions was introduced as a means of recouping some of the costs. Despite these and other problems that have faced the NHS through the years it has been heralded as a success that has changed the lives of many within the UK.

The NHS today is somewhat different with more advanced medical procedures, coping with an increasing and ageing population and the advent of information technology. However the concept of the NHS remains the same: to provide healthcare free at the point of delivery.

The primary purpose of the NHS is to provide care to the ill and injured and it is structured with this in mind. However, with increasing awareness of health promotion, illness prevention and levels of wellness, there is a drive for healthcare systems and the role of nurses to change.

Within the four countries of the UK – England, Wales, Scotland and Northern Ireland – there are significant differences in how the NHS is operated and structured (see *Boxes 8-1* and *8-2*, *Boxes 8-3* and *8-4* on page 126). However the fundamental philosophy to provide essential services free at the point of delivery is the same throughout.

The NHS is the fourth largest employer in the world, currently employing 1.3 million, and is a key public service and the basis for the welfare state within the UK. It is an ever-evolving entity that is structured and managed by the UK government. Up until now the NHS has taken many guises, being structured by different reforms, White Papers and plans. In 2001, The NHS Plan (see *Box 8-5* on page 126), a government vision for the future NHS, outlined a number of targets and initiatives to be implemented within the NHS to improve its performance. Some of these reforms were new while others were earlier commitments reworked. Despite these reforms the main principles of the NHS have been sustained including the principle that care should be free at the point of delivery.

BOX 8-1 Structure of the NHS in England (April 2005)

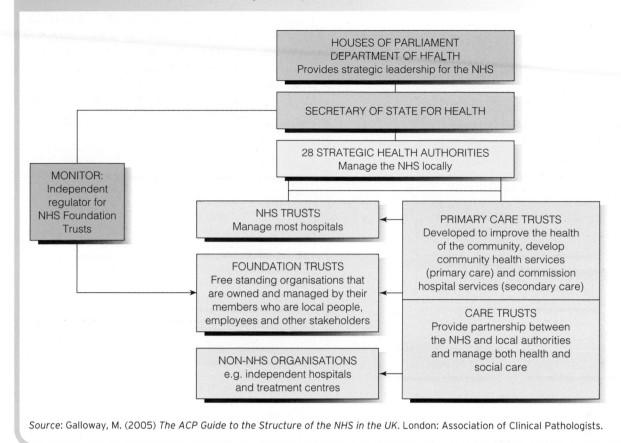

HOUSES OF PARLIAMENT
DEPARTMENT OF HEALTH
Provides strategic leadership for the NHS

SECRETARY OF STATE FOR HEALTH

28 STRATEGIC HEALTH AUTHORITIES
Manage the NHS locally

MONITOR:
Independent regulator for NHS Foundation Trusts

NHS TRUSTS
Manage most hospitals

PRIMARY CARE TRUSTS
Developed to improve the health of the community, develop community health services (primary care) and commission hospital services (secondary care)

FOUNDATION TRUSTS
Free standing organisations that are owned and managed by their members who are local people, employees and other stakeholders

CARE TRUSTS
Provide partnership between the NHS and local authorities and manage both health and social care

NON-NHS ORGANISATIONS
e.g. independent hospitals and treatment centres

Source: Galloway, M. (2005) *The ACP Guide to the Structure of the NHS in the UK*. London: Association of Clinical Pathologists.

BOX 8-2 Structure of the NHS in Wales (April 2005)

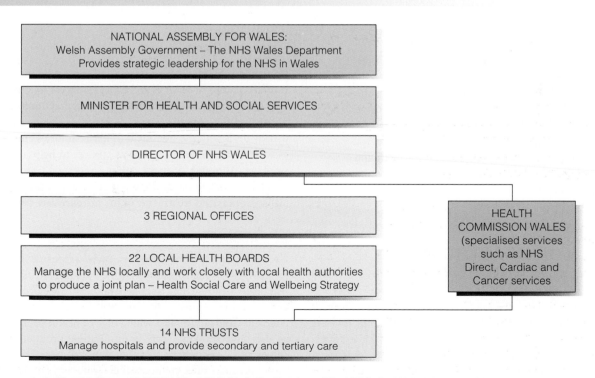

NATIONAL ASSEMBLY FOR WALES:
Welsh Assembly Government – The NHS Wales Department
Provides strategic leadership for the NHS in Wales

MINISTER FOR HEALTH AND SOCIAL SERVICES

DIRECTOR OF NHS WALES

3 REGIONAL OFFICES

HEALTH COMMISSION WALES (specialised services such as NHS Direct, Cardiac and Cancer services

22 LOCAL HEALTH BOARDS
Manage the NHS locally and work closely with local health authorities to produce a joint plan – Health Social Care and Wellbeing Strategy

14 NHS TRUSTS
Manage hospitals and provide secondary and tertiary care

Source: adapted from Galloway, M. (2005) *The ACP Guide to the Structure of the NHS in the UK*. London: Association of Clinical Pathologists.

BOX 8-3 Structure of the NHS in Scotland (April 2005)

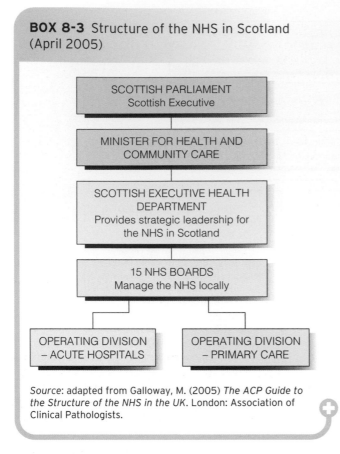

Source: adapted from Galloway, M. (2005) *The ACP Guide to the Structure of the NHS in the UK*. London: Association of Clinical Pathologists.

BOX 8-4 Structure of the NHS in Northern Ireland (April 2005)

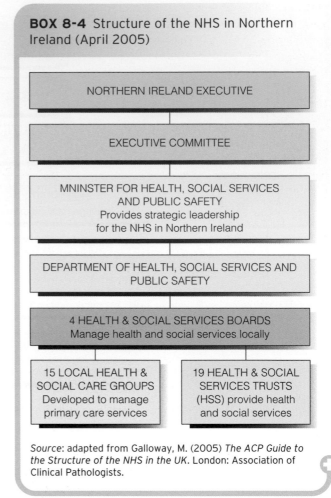

Source: adapted from Galloway, M. (2005) *The ACP Guide to the Structure of the NHS in the UK*. London: Association of Clinical Pathologists.

BOX 8-5 The Key Components of the NHS Plan

+ Investment in NHS facilities, e.g. the plan for 100 new hospitals by 2010
+ Investment in staff, e.g. 7,500 more consultants and 20,000 more nurses
+ Setting of national standards and regular inspections
+ A pooling of resources between the NHS and social services to provide a more comprehensive service to patients

TYPES OF HEALTHCARE AGENCIES AND SERVICES

Healthcare services in the UK are both varied and numerous and available in different settings. Some healthcare providers offer a number of different services to patients; for example, a hospital may provide acute inpatient services, outpatient clinics and accident and emergency services. Patients may be seen by any number and type of providers depending on their healthcare needs.

Primary Care

Primary care is usually the first point of contact for most people. It offers a range of services and provides access to a number of healthcare professionals, including general practitioners (GPs), nurses, dentists, pharmacists and opticians. The care provided usually deals with the treatment of minor injuries and illnesses as well as preventive care, such as services to help people stop smoking. Although primary care is concerned primarily with general healthcare needs there is a drive to provide more specialist services and treatments in the primary care setting.

GP Practices

General practitioners (GPs) provide extensive healthcare services within the community which are free of charge. They primarily diagnose and treat general healthcare problems; for example, minor infections. However they also provide health education and advice on a wide range of health problems such as diet and smoking; run immunisation programmes; and sometimes carry out simple surgical procedures.

GP practices offer an increasingly wide range of services and treatments which are provided by a team of healthcare professionals including doctors, nurses, health visitors, midwives, physiotherapists and occupational therapists. However, if the team of healthcare professionals are unable to deal with a particular healthcare need they will usually refer the patient to a hospital for tests or treatment, or to a consultant who has specialist knowledge.

Dentists

Dentists provide routine and specialist care for teeth and gums and are mainly found within dental practices. The care provided includes routine check-ups and treatments such as fillings, extractions and fitting dentures. However dentists, like GP practices, also provide preventive care, advising people how to care for their teeth and gums.

Dental practices can provide care for both private and NHS patients with most practices taking both types of patients. However, in recent years more and more dental practices are only providing care to private patients as a result of bureaucracy and insufficient funds to maintain NHS-funded dentists. This has obviously put an increasing financial strain on many individual patients.

Dentists can also be found in Community Dental Services whose aim is to care for children and adults with special needs. Specialist dental care is usually performed by hospital dentists or the new dentists with special interests (DwSis) at other dental surgeries.

Opticians

These generally carry out eye sight examinations and prescribe and fit spectacles. There are three types of eye specialist available: ophthalmic medical practitioners who are qualified doctors specialising in diseases and abnormalities of the eyes; optometrists (or ophthalmic opticians) are trained to recognise diseases and abnormalities associated with the eye such as diabetes and glaucoma; and dispensing opticians who fit and supply spectacles that have been prescribed by an optometrist.

Pharmacists

Pharmacists or chemists supply prescription and 'over the counter' medicines and healthcare advice to patients. They are expert in the pharmacology of medicines and therefore have a key role in patient care. They can be found in the community in pharmacies, or in hospitals, and dispense both prescription-only medications and over-the-counter medications. Many pharmacists also offer health checks to the community such as monitoring of diabetes and high blood pressure.

NHS Walk-in Centres

Walk-in Centres are a relatively new concept that provides quick and easy access to health advice and treatment for minor illnesses and injuries without the need for appointments. They were developed by the government in 1999/2000 as part of the provision for unscheduled healthcare. Currently there are 66 Walk-in Centres in England situated in convenient locations such as high streets, train stations or near Accident and Emergency

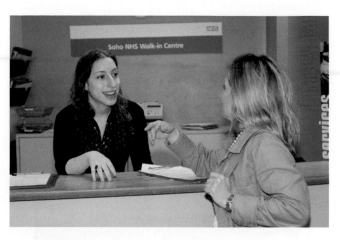

Figure 8-1 A Walk-in Centre.

(A&E) departments. They are normally run by experienced nurses and are open seven days a week (see Figure 8-1).

NHS Direct

This is a 24-hour, nurse-led service that provides confidential health advice over the telephone. The service provides information on local health services (e.g. doctors, dentists), what to do if an individual becomes ill, self-help groups and support organisations. NHS Direct also offers a range of health information and advice with its online service and has also launched NHS Direct Interactive digital TV, which aims to make health advice available through satellite television, again making it increasing more accessible to the community (see Figure 8-2 on page 128).

Secondary Care

Secondary care or acute care is the care provided in or by hospitals (NHS Trusts) and usually encompasses both elective care and emergency care. Elective care are those procedures that are seen as not urgent, not compulsory, routine or planned, while emergency care is care that is needed to maintain life or prevent further damage.

Ambulance Trusts

These are local organisations who are responsible for responding to 999 calls (emergency calls), transporting patients to or from hospitals and day care services and providing out-of-hours care.

In order to effectively and efficiently manage emergency (999) calls they are prioritised into three categories by personnel in a control room. Category A are deemed as life threatening; Category B are serious but not immediately life threatening; and Category C are nonurgent conditions. Once categorised, an appropriate team of emergency care providers are sent to the patient. The team will then assess the patient and decide whether they need to be transported to hospital. Ambulance crews are expert in the provision of pre-hospital emergency care in a range of situations such as cardiac arrests and road traffic accidents.

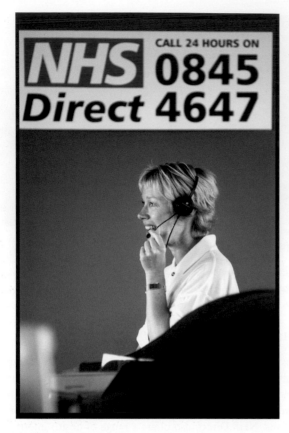

Figure 8-2 NHS Direct.

For patients who do not need to be treated in hospital the ambulance crew may treat the patient at the scene or give healthcare advice and referrals to other healthcare professionals or settings including NHS Direct or Walk-in Centres.

NHS Trusts

Hospitals in the NHS are managed by NHS Trusts who ensure the provision of high-quality healthcare and that hospitals spend their money efficiently. NHS Trusts provide a wide range of services and treatments to patients and employ most of the NHS workforce.

NHS hospitals vary in size and are generally classified according to the service they provide. General hospitals offer elective and emergency care to patients with a variety of conditions. Other hospitals offer only specialty services, such as psychiatric or paediatric care. Hospitals can be further described as acute care or chronic (long-term) care. An acute care hospital provides assistance to patients who are acutely ill or whose illness and need for hospitalisation are relatively short term, for example, two days. Long-term care hospitals provide services for longer periods, sometimes for years or the remainder of the patient's life.

Elective care takes place as a result of referral from primary care (i.e. GP) and includes treatments such as hip replacements or kidney dialysis. Elective care includes inpatient treatment as well as day case treatment and outpatient consultation.

Increasingly, the drive is to move to more day case treatment. In particular day surgery, where patients are treated and can go home on the same day, is increasingly successful, particularly as there have been increases in the number of procedures that can be done as day surgery. The benefits of such services are that patients are able to recover at home, resulting in less disruption to their work and home life and decreased hospital costs.

As a result of reforms in the NHS, **NHS Foundation Trusts** have been developed as a means of modernising the NHS and allowing trusts more freedom to run their own services. The plan is that trusts will be released from government control making them more responsive to the needs of their patients. The trusts are run by local managers, staff and members of the public and are accountable to the local community rather than the Secretary of State. However only the highest performing NHS hospitals/trusts can apply for this status and as a result it is speculated that a two-tier healthcare system is being formed.

Mental Health Trusts

These trusts offer a range of services to patients with mental health problems including psychological therapy and specialist care for people with severe mental health. However, these days less severe mental health problems such as depression and stress can be treated by the GP and a number of services are offered in the community such as family support, counselling and psychological therapies.

Care Trusts

These trusts combine NHS and social care in a single organisational structure. Social care is difficult to define but is generally perceived as services provided to older adults in their own homes or in care homes. Social care can be provided by local authorities or by the independent sector and provide services such as help with washing, dressing and shopping.

The benefits of combining the NHS and social care is that patients do not have to find their way around two different systems of care in order to meet their needs. The trusts offer a range of services that provide care for patients with complex needs. For example an older person may suffer a fall and fracture the neck of the femur (head of the thigh bone) and will require urgent hospital care followed by intermediate care to get them back on their feet and then longer-term care to support them in their own home.

Occupational Health Clinics

Occupational health clinics are gaining in importance within the delivery of healthcare. They provide healthcare to employees, usually within the workplace. Employee health has long been recognised as important to productivity. Today, more companies recognise the value of healthy employees with some encouraging healthy lifestyles by providing exercise facilities and coordinating health-promotion activities.

Worker safety has always been a concern of occupational health nurses. Today, nursing functions in industrial healthcare include work safety and health education, and annual employee health screening. Other functions may include screening for such health problems as hypertension and obesity, caring for employees following injury and counselling.

Residential and Nursing Homes

At times some people find it difficult to look after themselves in their own home. This could be the result of an accident or sudden illness or could happen gradually. Some people may be able to stay in their own home with help from family, friends, social services and the NHS. For example a older adult who is unable to cook or clean may receive home care provided by social services. However some people find it difficult to stay in their home as a result of their condition or their inability to cope. As a result they may take the decision to move into a care home.

Currently there are two types of care home available: residential homes that provide meals and personal care; and nursing home that must have qualified nurses on the premises. Some individuals who express the wish to move to a care home are able to make their own arrangements while others who are not in a position to make this decision are assessed by social services in order to work out their needs. From this assessment, a decision is made on the type of care home most appropriate to meet those needs.

The cost of moving into a residential or nursing home is substantial and may be met by social services, the NHS or by the individual. Social services assessment of an individual's needs will also include a financial assessment. Currently, if an individual has more than £20,500 capital they will have to meet the full cost of the care. However if they have less than £12,500 they will not have to pay for the care provided and the cost will be covered by the local council. If, however, an individual's stay is arranged by the NHS, for example following a long illness, the costs of care will be met by the NHS.

Rehabilitation Centres

Rehabilitation centres in the UK are usually managed by the NHS or the private sector and tend to be specialist units. However, because rehabilitation ideally starts the moment the patient enters the healthcare system, nurses who are employed on paediatric, psychiatric or surgical units of hospitals also help to rehabilitate patients. Rehabilitation centres play an important role in assisting patients to restore their health and recuperate. Drug and alcohol rehabilitation centres, for example, help free patients of drug and alcohol dependence and assist them to re-enter the community and function to the best of their ability. However there are rehabilitation centres throughout the UK for patients following cerebrovascular accidents (CVA or stroke) and brain injuries. Today, the concept of rehabilitation is applied to all illness and injury (physical and mental). Nurses in the rehabilitation setting coordinate patient

activities and ensure that patients are complying with their treatments. This type of nursing often requires specialised skills and knowledge.

Home Care Agencies

Home care provides a range of care interventions, including assistance with personal care such as washing and dressing, assistance going to bed and getting out of bed and/or a range of practical domestic tasks. The aim of home care is to support the individual in their own home thereby easing the pressure both on the NHS and care homes.

Home care services are provided by a number of different organisations including voluntary organisations, private organisations, non-profit making organisations and social services. In order to find out the sort of help needed by an individual a health and social care assessment is completed by social services. This assessment also includes a financial assessment in order to work out the level of payment required for the care provided.

TYPES OF HEALTHCARE SERVICES

Three types of healthcare services are often described in correlation with levels of disease prevention: (a) primary prevention, which involves implementing strategies to improve health and prevent illness, (b) secondary prevention, which is concerned with the diagnosis and treatment of illness and disease, and (c) tertiary prevention, which involves rehabilitation and health restoration.

Primary Prevention – Health Improvement and Illness Prevention

When the NHS was established in 1948, one of its main principles was to improve health and prevent disease and not just treat those who are ill. However, much of the healthcare provided within the NHS is aimed at diagnosis and treatment of ill health.

Primary prevention is concerned with identifying factors that can affect health and educating people about these factors in order for those individuals to make lifestyle changes. In 2004, the Government issued a White Paper 'Choosing Health, Making Healthier Choices Easier' in a bid to improve the health of the nation. This report outlines the main health issues faced by the population and identifies strategies to tackle these. According to the report, the main priorities are to tackle health inequalities, reduction in the number of people who smoke, obesity, improving sexual health, improving mental health and encouraging sensible levels of alcohol consumption. The proposed strategy for tackling these problems involves raising awareness of health risks and implementing campaigns to educate people to make healthier lifestyle choices. The main principle of this document is emphasising the important role individuals play in maintaining their own health.

Illness prevention programmes may be directed at the patient or the community and involve such practices as providing immunisations, identifying risk factors for illnesses, and helping people take measures to prevent these illnesses from occurring. Illness prevention also includes environmental programmes that can reduce the incidence of illness or disability. For example, steps to decrease air pollution include requiring inspection of car exhaust systems to ensure acceptable levels of fumes. Environmental protective measures are frequently legislated by governments and lobbied for by citizens groups.

Primary prevention also involves the early detection of disease. This is accomplished through routine screening of the population and focused screening of those at increased risk of developing certain conditions. Examples of early detection services include the new bowel cancer screening programme introduced in 2006 for men and women aged 60–69 years and mammograms (an x-ray of the breast) for women aged 50 years and over.

Secondary Prevention - Diagnosis and Treatment

In the past, the largest segment of the healthcare services has been dedicated to the diagnosis and treatment of illness. Hospitals and general practitioner (GP) services have been instrumental in offering these complex services. Hospitals continue to focus significant resources on patients requiring emergency, intensive and round-the-clock acute care.

Tertiary Prevention - Rehabilitation, Health Restoration and Palliative Care

Tertiary prevention implements strategies to minimise further deterioration of an individual who is already ill or minimise the symptoms of that disease process, for example, providing kidney dialysis for a person whose kidneys do not function or insulin to a person who has Type 1 Diabetes mellitus (insulin dependent diabetes). Tertiary prevention is made up of rehabilitation, health restoration and palliative care. Rehabilitation is a process of restoring ill or injured people to optimum and functional levels of wellness, for example cardiac rehabilitation is a process by which patients with cardiac disease are supported and encouraged to achieve and maintain physical and psychosocial health in partnership with healthcare professionals. The goal of rehabilitation is to help people move to their previous level of health (i.e. to their previous capabilities) or to the highest level they are capable of given their current health status. Rehabilitation may begin in the hospital, but will eventually lead patients back into the community for further treatment and follow-up once health has been restored.

Sometimes, people cannot be returned to health. A growing field of nursing and healthcare services is that of palliative care – providing comfort and treatment for symptoms. End-of-life care may be conducted in many settings including the home.

PROVIDERS OF HEALTHCARE

The providers of healthcare, also referred to as the healthcare team or health professionals, are health personnel from different disciplines who coordinate their skills to assist patients and those who support them. Their mutual goal is to restore a patient's health and promote wellness. The choice of personnel for a particular patient depends on the needs of the patient. Health teams commonly include the nurse and some or all of the personnel that follow.

Nurse

The role of the nurse varies with the needs of the patient, the nurse's credentials, and the type of employment setting. A registered nurse (RN) assesses a patient's health status, identifies health problems and develops and coordinates care. As nursing roles have expanded, new dimensions for nursing practice have been established. Nurses can pursue a variety of practice specialties (e.g. critical care, mental health and oncology). Nurse practitioners and clinical nurse specialists have the appropriate education and advanced knowledge to provide direct specialist patient care.

Dentist

Dentists diagnose and treat dental problems. Dentists are also actively involved in preventive measures to maintain healthy oral structures (e.g. teeth and gums). Many hospitals, especially long-term care facilities, have dentists on their staff.

Dietician

When dietary and nutritional services are required, the dietician or nutritionist may be a member of a health team. A registered dietician has specialist knowledge about the diets required to maintain health and to treat disease. Dieticians in hospitals generally are concerned with therapeutic diets, may design special diets to meet the nutritional needs of individual patients, and supervise the preparation of meals to ensure that patients receive the proper diet.

Occupational Therapist

An occupational therapist (OT) assists patients with an impaired function to gain the skills to perform activities of daily living. For example, an occupational therapist might teach a man with severe arthritis in his arms and hands how to adjust his kitchen utensils so that he can continue to cook. The occupational therapist teaches skills that are therapeutic and at the same time provide some fulfilment. For example, weaving is a recreational activity but also exercises the arthritic man's arms and hands.

Technologists

Laboratory technologists, radiological technologists and pathologists are just three kinds of technologists in the expanding field of medical technology. *Pathologists* examine specimens such as urine, faeces, blood and discharges from wounds to provide exact information that facilitates the medical diagnosis and the prescription of a therapeutic regimen. The radiologist assists with a wide variety of x-ray film procedures, from simple chest radiography to more complex fluoroscopy. These technologists have highly specialised skills and knowledge important to patient care.

Pharmacist

A pharmacist prepares and dispenses pharmaceuticals in hospital and community settings. The role of the pharmacist in monitoring and evaluating the actions and effects of medications on patients is becoming increasingly prominent. A pharmacy assistant works in the pharmacy under the direction of the pharmacist.

Physiotherapist

Physiotherapists assist patients with musculoskeletal problems. Physiotherapists treat movement dysfunctions by means of heat, water, exercise, massage and electric current. Their functions include assessing patient mobility and strength, providing therapeutic measures (e.g. exercises and heat applications to improve mobility and strength) and teaching new skills (e.g. how to walk with an artificial leg). Some physiotherapists provide their services in hospitals; however, independent practitioners establish offices in communities and serve patients either at the office or in the home. Physiotherapy assistants also work with physiotherapists and patients.

Doctor

The doctor is responsible for medical diagnosis and for determining the treatment required by a person who has a disease or injury. Their role has traditionally been the treatment of disease and trauma (injury) but many doctors are now including health promotion and disease prevention in their practice. Some doctors are surgeons, oncologists, orthopaedists, paediatricians or psychiatrists.

Podiatrist

Podiatrists, previously known as chiropodists, diagnose and treat foot conditions. They may work within a hospital or privately.

Social Worker

A social worker counsels patients and support people to overcome their social problems, such as finances, marital difficulties and adoption of children. It is not unusual for health problems to produce problems in living and vice versa. For example, an elderly woman who lives alone and has a stroke resulting in impaired walking may find it impossible to continue to live in her third-floor apartment. Finding a more suitable living arrangement can be the responsibility of the social worker if the patient has no support network in place.

Spiritual Support Person

Chaplains, pastors, rabbis, priests and other religious or spiritual advisers serve as part of the healthcare team by attending to the spiritual needs of patients. In most facilities, local clergy volunteer their services on a regular or on-call basis. They usually offer regularly scheduled religious services. The nurse is often instrumental in identifying the patient's desire for spiritual support and notifying the appropriate person.

Healthcare Support Workers

Healthcare support workers are healthcare staff who assume delegated aspects of patient care. These tasks include bathing, assisting with feeding, and collecting specimens.

It is important to note that there can be significant overlaps among those providers who can perform certain healthcare activities. For example, a doctor, a nurse or a physiotherapist may be responsible for assisting a person with breathing problems.

FACTORS AFFECTING HEALTHCARE DELIVERY

Today's healthcare users have greater knowledge about their health than in previous years and they are increasingly influencing healthcare delivery. Formerly, people expected a doctor to make decisions about their care but today patients are no longer passive recipients of healthcare but actively participate in their own healthcare, with many aware of how lifestyle affects health. However it is not just the individual that affect the healthcare delivery system.

Increasing Number of Older Adults

By the year 2026 it is estimated that one fifth of the adult population in the UK will be over the age of 65 (Office for National Statistics, 2002). Chronic illnesses and disability are prevalent among this group who frequently require health and social care support.

The ageing population has changed the look of the NHS. Older adults are the main users of health and social care services but their needs have not always been met. However in 2001, the National Service Framework (NSF) for older people was introduced in a bid to ensure that high-quality integrated health and social care is provided to older adults. It outlines a ten-year programme aimed at improving health and social care services for the older adult (see *Box 8-6* on page 132).

BOX 8-6 The National Service Framework for Older People's Eight Service Standards

+ *Age discrimination:* health and social care should be provided based on need rather than age.
+ *Person-centred care:* the older person should be enabled to make choices. Health and social care should be integrated to provide an efficient and effective service for the older person.
+ *Intermediate care:* if older people have complex health and social needs and are being cared for outside the hospital environment the health and social care services should be coordinated to provide a package of care to support them in the community.
+ *General hospital care for older people:* this should be delivered by skilled and specialist staff.
+ *Stroke prevention:* to prevent stroke the NHS needs to work in partnership with relevant agencies.
+ *Falls:* Falls and fractures need to be prevented with the NHS working in partnership with councils.
+ *Older people with mental health problems:* older people should have access to integrated mental health services.
+ *The promotion of active, healthy life in older people:* this should be promoted through co-ordinated programmes led by the NHS and in partnership with councils.

Source: Baggott, R. (2004) *Health and Healthcare in Britain.* Basingstoke, Palgrave Macmillan.

Advances in Technology

Scientific knowledge and technology related to healthcare are rapidly increasing. Improved diagnostic procedures and sophisticated equipment permit early recognition of diseases that might otherwise have remained undetected. New antibiotics and medications are continually being manufactured to treat infections and multiple drug-resistant organisms. Surgical procedures involving the heart, lungs and liver that were nonexistent 20 years ago are common today. Laser and microscopic procedures streamline the treatment of diseases that required surgery in the past.

Computers, bedside charting and the ability to store and retrieve large volumes of information in databases are commonplace in healthcare organisations. In addition, as a result of the Internet and World Wide Web, patients now have access to medical information similar to that of healthcare providers (although not all websites provide accurate information!).

These discoveries have changed the profile of the patient. Patients are now more likely to be treated in the community, utilising resources, technology and treatments outside the hospital. For example, years ago a person having cataract surgery had to remain in bed in the hospital for 10 days; today, most cataract removals are performed on an outpatient basis in outpatient surgery centres. These technological advances and specialised treatments and procedures may come, unfortunately, with a high price tag.

Social and Economic Factors

Social and economic status has a profound impact on health. Social class particularly has an influence on the individual's health status. According to many sociologists life expectancy varies considerably between social classes (Hattersley, 1997; Smith and Harding, 1997). According to Professor George Davey Smith, who conducted research into social status and health (DOH, 2002), people who are in the lower social classes (Social Class III–V, see *Box 8-7*) are at increased risk of having cardiovascular disease, including heart disease and stroke, than those who were in higher social classes (Social Class I–II). In particular the National Heart Forum, a leading alliance of over 40 national organisations working to reduce the risk of coronary heart disease in the UK, have found that men in Social Class V are three times more likely to suffer from coronary heart disease than those men in Social Class I (National Heart Forum, 1998).

The British Medical Association (BMA), a voluntary professional association for doctors, published *Growing Up in Britain*, a report focusing on health inequalities among infants and children. It found that infant mortality rates were lower in Social Class I and II compared with those in Social Class IV and V (BMA, 1999).

There are many theories why social class should influence health in this way. One such theory is that social class differences in health arise from social selection (Stern, 1983). This means that healthy people tend to move up the social classes whereas unhealthy people tend to stay in the lower social classes (IV and V). In other words the individual's health status produces social inequalities.

BOX 8-7 Registrar General's Classification of Social Class

SOCIAL CLASS I	Professional occupations
SOCIAL CLASS II	Managerial and technical occupations
SOCIAL CLASS III (N)	Skilled occupations, nonmanual
SOCIAL CLASS III (M)	Skilled occupation, manual
SOCIAL CLASS IV	Partly-skilled occupations
SOCIAL CLASS V	Unskilled occupations

Women's Health

Women's health and feminism have been instrumental in changing healthcare practices. For example, birthing centres were developed over 50 years ago in order to provide relaxed, unhurried environment for delivering babies. Until recently, women's health issues focused on the reproductive aspects of health, disregarding many healthcare concerns that are unique to women. For example, until recently heart disease was seen as a male disease but in 2004 coronary heart disease was responsible for the death of 47,287 women in the UK (BHF 2007). Changes are occurring in the provision of healthcare for women with an increased awareness of the impact of multiple roles, for example mother, wife and career person, on the woman's health (Waldron, 1998, cited in United Nations, 1998).

Access to Health Services

Access to healthcare services is essential to the maintenance of good health. However it is not just access to any healthcare but to good quality healthcare that is essential. A number of factors impede such access, including financial barriers, geographic considerations and social class. For patients living in rural areas this may mean that they have to travel long distances for treatment. For example, coronary heart bypass surgery, a surgical treatment for coronary heart disease, is only offered in two hospitals in South Wales. This means that patients living in North Wales have to travel to Liverpool for this type of surgery.

There is also the issue that some treatments are available on the NHS in some parts of the country but not in others, otherwise known as the 'postcode lottery' of healthcare services. One such example is the 'Herceptin postcode lottery' where the drug was offered to breast cancer patients in some areas but not to those in other areas.

Demographic Changes

The characteristics of the population of the UK are every evolving. There are certain points in the individual's life that makes them more prone to health problems. Accidents and injuries are the most likely cause of death in younger people, while cancers and circulatory diseases usually afflict the older age groups.

Despite people living longer, the prevalence of chronic illness and disability is still high. This means that although life expectancy has increased this is usually plagued by ill health or disability.

Healthcare delivery is dependent on a number of factors including its setting and factors such as population demographics. However effective healthcare delivery is also dependent on appropriate frameworks for the delivery of that care. Frameworks of care are basically ways in which effective and efficient health and nursing care is delivered to patients.

FRAMEWORKS FOR CARE

A number of frameworks exist for the delivery of effective nursing care. It is important to note that the setting and population served is considered when choosing the type of framework used to provide nursing care.

Case Management

Case management describes a range of models that provide holistic nursing care for patients. Holistic nursing care is caring for the whole person and includes caring for the physical, psychological, spiritual, sexual and social aspects of the person. Case management allows the nurse to focus on the patient and their family and emphasises empowerment rather than dependence on the nurse or the healthcare system.

Generally, case management involves multidisciplinary teams that assume collaborative responsibility for planning and assessing needs, and coordinating, implementing and evaluating care for groups of patients from preadmission to discharge or transfer and recuperation. Case management usually involves an experienced nurse working with a patient and their family. The aim of case management is for the patient to receive all the necessary health and social care services to promote the patient's health and oversee any illnesses they may have.

In order to track the patient's progress, case managers or nurses will often use **integrated care pathways**. An integrated care pathway is an interdisciplinary (or multidisciplinary) plan or tool that specifies interdisciplinary assessments, interventions, treatments and outcomes for health-related conditions across a time line.

Team Nursing

Team nursing is the delivery of individualised nursing care to patients by a team led by a professional nurse. A nursing team consists of registered nurses, student nurses and support staff (e.g. healthcare support workers). This team is responsible for providing coordinated nursing care to a group of patients. It is difficult to say when team nursing developed but it is one of the earliest forms of organised nursing care.

The registered nurse retains responsibility and authority for patient care but delegates appropriate tasks to the other team members. Proponents of this model believe the team approach increases the efficiency of the registered nurse. Opponents state that inpatients' high acuity of illness leaves little to be delegated.

Primary Nursing

Primary nursing is a system in which one nurse is responsible for total care of a number of patients 24 hours a day, 7 days a week. It is a method of providing comprehensive, individualised and consistent care.

Primary nursing uses the nurse's clinical knowledge and management skills. The primary nurse assesses and prioritises each patient's needs, develops and implements a plan of care with the patient, and evaluates the effectiveness of care. Other nurses and support workers provide some care, but the primary nurse coordinates it and communicates information about the patient's health to other nurses and other health professionals. Primary nursing encompasses all aspects of the professional role, including teaching, advocacy, decision making and continuity of care. The primary nurse is the first-line manager of the patient's care with all its inherent accountabilities and responsibilities.

Healthcare delivery is a complex phenomenon. Effective delivery of healthcare depends on a number of factors including the setting it is provided in, for example a GP practice, and the population served, for example the patient's age, sex and social class. Nurses delivering healthcare to patients need to be aware of the factors affecting their practice in order to organise the way in which the nursing care is delivered.

CRITICAL REFLECTION

Let us revisit the case study on page 123. Now that you have read this chapter how does the modern NHS differ from the NHS established in 1948? How can the NHS be made more efficient in today's society? What can nurses do to improve the situation?

CHAPTER HIGHLIGHTS

+ Healthcare delivery services can be categorised as primary, secondary or tertiary and, generally, they can also be grouped by the type of service: (1) health promotion and illness prevention, (2) diagnosis and treatment and (3) rehabilitation.
+ Hospitals provide a wide variety of services on an inpatient and outpatient basis.
+ Various providers of healthcare coordinate their skills to assist a patient. Their mutual goal is to restore a patient's health and promote wellness.

+ The many factors affecting healthcare delivery include the increasing number of elderly people, advances in knowledge and technology, socioeconomics, increased emphasis on women's health, access to healthcare and demographic changes.
+ There are a number of frameworks for patient healthcare, including case management and primary nursing.

REFERENCES

Baggott, R. (2004) *Health and healthcare in Britain*, Basingstoke: Palgrave Macmillan.

BBC News (2006) 'Managers Blamed for NHS Deficits', BBC News 24, 10 July. Available from http://news.bbc.co.uk.

British Heart Foundation (BHF) (2007) *Women and heart attacks*, London: BHF. Available from http://www.bhf.org.uk/Doubtkills/what_to_wook_out_form/women_heart_attacks.asp.

British Medical Association (BMA) (1999) *Growing up in Britain*, London: BMA.

Department of Health (DOH) and Food Standards Agency (FSA) (2000) *Vol 1: Report of the Diet and Nutrition Survey. National Diet and Nutrition Survey: Young people aged 4–18 years*, London: The Stationery Office.

Department of Health (DOH) (2001) *National Service Framework for Older People*, London: DOH.

Department of Health (DOH) (2002) *SE6: Social status in early life, social mobility, health behaviours and CVD mortality risk*, London: DOH.

Department of Health (DOH) (2004) *Choosing health: Making healthy choices easier*. London: DOH.

Galloway, M. (2005) *The ACP guide to the structure of the NHS in the UK*, London: Association of Clinical Pathologists.

Hattersley, L. (1997) 'Expectations of Life by Social Class', in F. Drever and M. Whitehead (Eds), *Health inequalities series DS. 15*, London: TSO.

National Heart Forum (1998) *Social inequalities in heart disease*, London: The Stationery Office.

Office for National Statistics (2002) *Social trends 2000*, London: The Stationery Office.

Smith, J. and Harding, S. (1997) 'Mortality of men and women using alternative social classification', in F. Drever and M. Whitehead (Eds) *Health inequalities series DS. 15*, London: TSO.

Stern, J. (1983) 'Social mobility and the interpretation of social class mortality differentials', *Journal of Social Policy*, 12(1), 27–49.

Waldron, I. (1998) 'Sex, differences in infant and early childhood mortality: major causes of death and possible biological causes', in United Nations (1998) *Too young to die: Genes or gender?*, New York: United Nations Population Division.

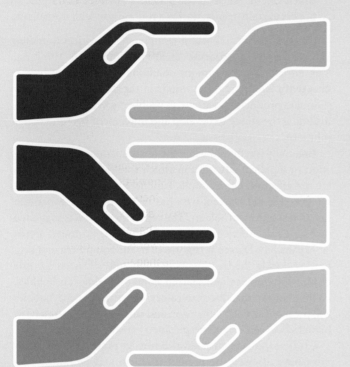

Chapter 9 The Nursing Process

Learning Outcomes

After completing this chapter, you will be able to:

+ Discuss the term critical thinking and how this relates to nursing decision making and the nursing process.

+ Describe the phases of the nursing process.

+ Identify major characteristics of the nursing process.

+ Identify the purpose of assessing.

+ Compare closed and open-ended questions, providing examples and listing advantages and disadvantages of each.

+ Contrast various frameworks used for nursing assessment.

+ Identify the components of a nursing diagnosis.

+ Compare nursing diagnoses, medical diagnoses and collaborative problems.

+ Compare and contrast initial planning, ongoing planning and discharge planning.

+ Identify activities that occur in the planning process.

+ Explain how standards of care and preprinted care plans can be individualised and used in creating a comprehensive nursing care plan.

+ Identify guidelines for writing goals/desired outcomes.

+ Discuss the five activities of the implementing phase.

+ Describe five components of the evaluation process.

+ Differentiate quality improvement from quality assurance.

CASE STUDY

Mrs. L. is a 74-year-old lady with a history of irritable bowel syndrome that causes frequent diarrhoea and rectal bleeding. Her husband died from bowel cancer. It is mid-November when she comes to your clinical area complaining about 'not feeling good, abdominal ache and some rectal bleeding'. You conclude she is having a reoccurrence of her intestinal problem.

After reading this chapter you will be able to devise a plan of care for her using the nursing process.

CRITICAL THINKING

The nursing process is a systematic, patient-centred method for structuring the delivery of nursing care. The nursing process entails gathering and analysing information in order to identify patient strengths and potential or actual health problems, developing and continually reviewing a plan of nursing interventions to achieve mutually agreed outcomes. At every stage of the process, the nurse works closely with the patient to individualise care and build a relationship of mutual regard and trust.

In order to practise safely, nurses need to think in a critical manner about all the activities and interventions they undertake. Without critical thinking and a reflection on previous performance an intervention can just become another task being performed automatically. This can endanger the safety of patients and potentially lead to an adverse incident causing harm or even death to the patient. Critical thinking is therefore essential to safe, competent, skilful nursing practice. In order to understand the nursing process it is first necessary to consider critical thinking.

The amount of knowledge that nurses must use and the continuing rapid growth of this knowledge prevent nurses from being effective practitioners if they attempt to function with only the information acquired in education or outlined in books. Decisions that nurses must make about patient care and about the distribution of limited resources force them to think and act in areas where there are neither clear answers nor standard procedures, and where conflicting forces turn decision making into a complex process. Nurses therefore need to embrace the attitudes that promote critical thinking and master critical-thinking skills in order to process and evaluate both previously learned and new information.

Nurses use critical-thinking skills in a variety of ways:

+ *Nurses use knowledge from other subjects and fields.* Because nurses deal holistically with human responses, they must draw meaningful information from other subject areas (i.e. make interdisciplinary connections) in order to understand the meaning of patient data and to plan effective interventions. Nursing students take courses in the biological and social sciences and in the humanities so that they can acquire a strong foundation on which to build their nursing knowledge and skill. For example, the nurse might use knowledge from nutrition, physiology and physics to promote wound healing and prevent further injury to a patient with a pressure ulcer.
+ *Nurses deal with change in stressful environments.* Nurses work in rapidly changing situations. Treatments, medications and technology change constantly, and a patient's condition may change from minute to minute. Routine actions may therefore not be adequate to deal with the situation at hand. Familiarity with the routine for giving medications, for example, does not help the nurse deal with a patient who is frightened of injections or with one who does not wish to take a medication. When unexpected situations arise, critical thinking enables the nurse to recognise important cues, respond quickly and adapt interventions to meet specific patient needs.
+ *Nurses make important decisions.* During the course of a workday, nurses make vital decisions of many kinds. These decisions often determine the well-being of patients and even their very survival, so it is important that the decisions be sound. Nurses use critical thinking to collect and interpret the information needed to make decisions. Nurses must, for example, use good judgement to decide which observations must be reported to another practitioner immediately and which can be noted in the patient record for other practitioners to address later, during a routine visit with the patient.

Creativity is an important component of critical thinking. When nurses incorporate creativity into their thinking, they are able to find unique solutions to unique problems. **Creativity** is thinking that results in the development of new ideas and products. Creativity in problem solving and decision making is the ability to develop and implement new and better solutions.

Creativity is required when the nurse encounters a new situation or a patient situation in which traditional interventions are not effective. For example, Pauline, a child nurse, is caring for five-year-old Darren, who has ineffective chest expansion due to respiratory problems. The physiotherapist has suggested incentive spirometry (a treatment device that promotes alveolar expansion). Darren is frightened by the equipment and tires quickly during the treatments. Pauline offers Darren a bottle of blowing bubbles and Darren enjoys blowing the bubbles. Pauline knows that the respiratory effort in blowing bubbles will promote alveolar expansion and suggests that Darren blow bubbles between incentive spirometry treatments.

Creative thinkers must have knowledge of the problem. They must have assessed the present problem and be knowledgeable about the underlying facts and principles that apply. For example, in the previous situation, Pauline knows the anatomy and physiology of respiratory function and is aware of the purpose of incentive spirometry. She also understands paediatric growth and development. In trying to assist Darren, she builds on her knowledge and comes up with a creative solution. Using creativity, nurses:

+ generate many ideas rapidly;
+ are generally flexible and natural; that is, they are able to change viewpoints or directions in thinking rapidly and easily;
+ create original solutions to problems;
+ tend to be independent and self-confident, even when under pressure;
+ demonstrate individuality.

SKILLS IN CRITICAL THINKING

Complex mental processes such as analysis, problem solving and decision making require the use of cognitive critical-thinking skills. These skills include critical analysis, inductive and

BOX 9-1 Socratic Questions

Questions about the question (or problem)
+ Is this question clear, understandable and correctly identified?
+ Is this question important?
+ Could this question be broken down into smaller parts?
+ How might an experienced nurse state this question?

Questions about assumptions
+ You seem to be assuming ____; is that so?
+ What could you assume instead? Why?
+ Does this assumption always hold true?

Questions about point of view
+ You seem to be using the perspective of ____. Why?
+ What would someone who disagrees with your perspective say?
+ can you see this any other way?

Questions about evidence and reasons
+ What evidence do you have for that?
+ Is there any reason to doubt that evidence?
+ How do you know?
+ What would change your mind?

Questions about Implications and consequences
+ What effect would that have?
+ What is the probability that will actually happen?
+ What are the alternatives?
+ What are the implications of that?

and ideas and discard superfluous information and ideas. The questions are not sequential steps; rather, they are a set of criteria for judging an idea. Not all questions will need to be applied to every situation, but one should be aware of all the questions in order to choose those questions appropriate to a given situation. Socrates (born about 470 BC) was a Greek philosopher who developed the Socratic method of posing a question and seeking an answer. *Box 9-1* lists Socratic questions which can be used in critical analysis. **Socratic questioning** is a technique one can use to look beneath the surface, recognise and examine assumptions, search for inconsistencies, examine multiple points of view and differentiate what one knows from what one merely believes. Nurses can employ Socratic questioning when listening to an end-of-shift report/handover, reviewing a presenting history or progress notes, planning care or discussing a patient's care with colleagues.

Two other critical thinking skills are inductive and deductive reasoning. In **inductive reasoning**, generalisations are formed from a set of facts or observations. When viewed together, certain bits of information suggest a particular interpretation. For example, the nurse who observes that a patient has dry skin, poor turgor (skin elasticity), sunken eyes and dark amber urine may make the generalisation that the patient appears dehydrated. **Deductive reasoning**, by contrast, is reasoning from the general to the specific. The nurse starts with a conceptual framework – for example, Maslow's hierarchy of needs or a self-care framework – and makes descriptive interpretations of the patient's condition in relation to that framework. For example, the nurse who uses the needs framework might categorise data and define the patient's problem in terms of elimination, nutrition or protection needs.

In a more simplistic example, inductive reasoning is like looking at the pieces of a jigsaw puzzle and attempting to describe the whole (without seeing a picture of the completed puzzle). As the puzzler puts more and more pieces together, the whole picture becomes clearer. In deductive reasoning, the puzzler sees the whole picture (from the box cover) and puts the puzzle together by organising the pieces into border pieces, colours or some other grouping.

In critical thinking, the nurse also differentiates statements of fact, inference, judgement and opinion. Table 9-1 shows how these may be applied to a patient. Evaluating the credibility of

deductive reasoning, making valid inferences, differentiating facts from opinions, evaluating the credibility of information sources, clarifying concepts and recognising assumptions.

Critical analysis is the application of a set of questions to a particular situation or idea to determine essential information

Table 9-1 Differentiating Types of Statements

Statement	Description	Example
Facts	Can be verified through investigation	Blood pressure is affected by blood volume.
Inferences	Conclusions drawn from the facts, going beyond facts to make a statement about something not currently known	If blood volume is decreased (e.g. in haemorrhagic shock), the blood pressure will drop.
Judgements	Evaluation of facts or information that reflect values or other criteria; a type of opinion	It is harmful to the patient's health if the blood pressure drops too low.
Opinions	Beliefs formed over time and include judgements that may fit facts or be in error	Nursing intervention can assist in maintaining the patient's blood pressure within normal limits.

information sources is an important step in critical thinking. Unfortunately, we cannot always believe what we read or are told. The nurse may need to ascertain the accuracy of information by checking other documents, with other informants or making a valued judgement.

Concepts are ideas or views representing things in the real world and their meanings, such as very hot water can cause a burn. Each person has developed their conceptualisations based on experience, input from others, study and other activities. To clearly comprehend a patient situation, the nurse and the patient must agree on the meaning of concept terms. For example, if the patient says to the nurse, 'I think I have a tumour,' the nurse needs to clarify what this word means to the patient – the medical definition of tumour (a solid mass) or the common lay meaning of cancer – before responding.

APPLYING CRITICAL THINKING TO NURSING PRACTICE

Nurses function effectively some part of every day without thinking critically. Many small decisions are based primarily on habit with minimal thinking involved; examples include selecting what clothes to wear, choosing which route to take to work and deciding what to eat for lunch. Psychomotor skills in nursing often involve minimal thinking, such as operating a familiar piece of equipment. But the higher order skills of critical thinking are put into play as soon as a new idea is encountered or a less-than-routine decision must be made.

The **nursing process** is a systematic, rational method of planning and providing individualised nursing care utilising all aspects of critical thinking and problem solving.

Problem Solving

In **problem solving**, the nurse obtains information that clarifies the nature of the problem and suggests possible solutions. The nurse then carefully evaluates the possible solutions and chooses the best one to implement. The situation is carefully monitored over time to ensure its initial and continued effectiveness. The nurse does not discard the other solutions but holds them in reserve in the event that the first solution is not effective. The nurse may also encounter a similar problem in a different patient situation where an alternative solution is determined to be the most effective. Therefore, problem solving for one situation contributes to the nurse's body of knowledge for problem solving in similar situations.

There are various approaches to problem solving. Commonly used are trial and error, intuition, the research process and the scientific/modified scientific method.

Trial and Error

One way to solve problems is through trial and error, in which a number of approaches are tried until a solution is found. However, without considering alternatives systematically, one cannot know why the solution works. Trial-and-error methods in nursing care can be dangerous because the patient might suffer harm if an approach is inappropriate. However, nurses often use trial and error in the home setting where, due to logistics, equipment and patient lifestyle, hospital procedures cannot work as effectively (e.g. there may be no stand from which to hang a bottle of enteral feed or no electricity to plug in a pump device).

Intuition

Intuition is the understanding or learning of things without the conscious use of reasoning. It is also known as sixth sense, hunch, instinct, feeling or suspicion. As a problem-solving approach, intuition is viewed by some people as a form of guessing and, as such, an inappropriate basis for nursing decisions. However, others view intuition as an essential and legitimate aspect of clinical judgement acquired through knowledge and experience. The nurse must first have the knowledge base necessary to practise in the clinical area and then use that knowledge in clinical practice. Clinical experience allows the nurse to recognise cues and patterns and begin to reach correct conclusions.

Experience is important in improving intuition because the rapidity of the judgement depends on the nurse having seen similar patient situations many times before. Sometimes nurses use the words 'I had a feeling' to describe the critical-thinking element of considering evidence. These nurses are able to judge quickly which evidence is most important and to act on that limited evidence. Nurses in critical care often pay closer attention than usual to a patient when they sense that the patient's condition could change suddenly. Benner (1984), a nurse theorist, has looked at this form of critical thinking/intuition extensively in her now classical work, *Novice to expert*.

Although the intuitive method of problem solving is gaining recognition as part of nursing practice, it is not recommended for novices or students, however, because they usually lack the knowledge base and clinical experience on which to make a valid judgement.

Research Process and Scientific/Modified Scientific Method

The research process is a formalised, logical, systematic approach to solving problems. The classic scientific method is most useful when the researcher is working in a controlled situation such as a laboratory. Health professionals, often working with people in uncontrolled situations, require a modified approach to the scientific method for solving problems. For example, unlike experiments with animals, the effects of diet on health are complicated by a person's race, lifestyle and personal preferences. The person is able to choose what they eat whereas an animal on the whole will eat what it is given.

Table 9-2 compares the research process or scientific method with the modified scientific method. Critical thinking is important in all problem-solving processes as the nurse evaluates all potential solutions to a given problem and makes a decision to select the most appropriate solution for that situation.

Table 9-2 Comparison between the Research Process and the Modified Scientific Method

Research process (scientific method)	Modified scientific method
State a research question or problem.	Define the problem.
Define the purpose of or the rationale for the study.	
Review related literature.	Gather information.
Formulate hypotheses and defining variables.	Analyse the information.
Select a method to test hypotheses.	Develop solutions.
Select a population, sample and setting.	
Conduct a pilot study.	Make a decision.
Collect the data.	Implement the decision.
Analyse the data.	Evaluate the decision.
Communicate conclusions and implications.	

Decision Making

Nurses make decisions in the course of solving problems, for example, in each step of the nursing process. Decision making, however, is also used in situations that do not involve problem solving. Nurses make value decisions (e.g. to keep patient information confidential); time management decisions (e.g. taking clean linen to the patient bedside the same time as the medication in order to save steps); scheduling decisions (e.g. to assist the patient with hygiene needs before visiting hours); and priority decisions (e.g. which interventions are most urgent and which can be delegated or delayed until another time).

Decision making is a critical-thinking process for choosing the best actions to meet a desired goal. Nurses must make decisions and assist patients to make decisions. When faced with several patient needs at the same time, the nurse must prioritise and decide which need to action first. The nurse may (a) look at advantages and disadvantages of each option, (b) apply Maslow's hierarchy of needs (see Chapter 5), (c) consider which interventions can be delegated to others or (d) use another priority-setting framework. When a patient is trying to make a decision about what course of treatment to follow, the nurse may need to provide information or resources the patient can use in making a decision. Nurses must make decisions in their own personal and professional lives. For example, the nurse must decide whether to work in a hospital or community setting, whether to join a professional association/union and whether to carry individual personal professional liability insurance.

There are sequential steps to the decision-making process:

1. *Identify the purpose.* The nurse identifies why a decision is needed and what needs to be determined.
2. *Set the criteria.* When the nurse sets the criteria for decision making, three questions must be answered: What is the desired outcome? What needs to be preserved? and What needs to be avoided? For example, for a patient with pain, the criteria would be as follows:
   - What needs to be achieved? Relief of pain.
   - What needs to be preserved? Physical functioning, cognitive functioning, psychologic functioning, patient comfort.
   - What needs to be avoided? Central nervous system depression, respiratory depression, nausea.
3. *Weight the criteria.* In this step, the decision maker sets priorities or ranks activities or services in order of importance from least important to most important as they relate to the specific situation. Because the weighting is specific to the situation, an activity may be ranked as most important in one situation and of less importance in another situation. For example, if a patient with pain has terminal cancer, pain relief may be more important than avoiding the side effects of the pain medication.
4. *Seek alternatives.* The decision maker identifies all possible ways to meet the criteria. In clinical situations, the alternatives may be selected from a range of nursing interventions or patient care strategies. Pain may be treated with oral or parenteral (injectable) medications, as needed or on a schedule, or without pharmacological intervention at all, instead using complementary alternative modalities (CAM), such as relaxation or distraction therapies.
5. *Examine alternatives.* The nurse analyses the alternatives to ensure that there is an objective rationale in relation to the established criteria for choosing one strategy over another. For pain that results from a procedure (such as removal of a foreign object), CAM may not be strong enough relief and oral medication may be effective but act too slowly, so an intravenous narcotic or inhaled analgesic (such as analgesic gas/entonox) may be the better choice.
6. *Project.* The nurse applies creative thinking and scepticism to determine what might go wrong as a result of a decision and develops plans to prevent, minimise or overcome any problems. If the intravenous narcotic is selected, what safety procedures need to be in place, for example, a narcotic antidote and supplemental oxygen being available promptly.
7. *Implement.* The decision plan is placed into action. The pain treatment is begun.
8. *Evaluate the outcome.* As with all nursing care, in evaluating, the nurse determines the effectiveness of the plan and whether the initial purpose was achieved. How does the patient rate the level of pain following the procedure?

Table 9-3 Comparison between the Nursing Process and the Decision-Making Process

Nursing process	Decision-making process*
Assess	Identify the purpose
Diagnose	
Plan	Set the criteria
	Weight the criteria
	Seek alternatives
	Examine alternatives
	Project
Implement	Implement
Evaluate	Evaluate the outcome

*The decision-making process parallels the nursing process but is also used during each step of the process.

The decision-making process and the nursing process share similarities and the nurse uses decision making in all steps of the nursing process. Table 9-3 compares these processes.

CLINICAL ANECDOTE

Aida, a third-year student nurse: 'I always thought throughout my nurse education in the first and second year that reflection and reflective practice was a waste of time. I often used to think why keep a reflective journal and diary? Now that I look back to the entries I made in my first and second year I can see how my skills and understanding have developed as a nurse. If anyone were to ask me as they start their nurse education, is it worth keeping a reflective diary and looking at their practice after a shift, I would say definitely. I can see my development fully now and how theory applies to practice.'

DEVELOPING CRITICAL-THINKING ATTITUDES AND SKILLS

After gaining an idea of what it means to think critically, solve problems and make decisions, nurses need to become aware of their own thinking style and abilities. Acquiring critical-thinking skills and a critical attitude then becomes a matter of practice. Critical thinking is not an 'either-or' phenomenon; people develop and use it more or less effectively along a continuum. Some people make better evaluations than others; some people believe information from nearly any source; and still others seldom believe anything without carefully evaluating the credibility of the information. Critical thinking is not easy. Solving problems and making decisions is risky. Sometimes the outcome is not what was desired. With effort, however, everyone can achieve some level of critical thinking to become an effective problem solver and decision maker.

Self-assessment

The nurse should reflect on some of the attitudes that facilitate critical thinking, attitudes such as curiosity, fair-mindedness, humility, courage and perseverance. A nurse might benefit from a rigorous personal assessment to determine which attitudes they already possess and which need to be cultivated. This could also be done with a partner or as a group as part of a clinical supervision programme. The nurse first determines which attitudes are held strongly and form a base for thinking, and which are held minimally or not at all. The nurse also needs to reflect on situations where they made decisions that were later regretted and analyses thinking processes and attitudes or asks a trusted colleague to assess them. This will aid in personal growth and the development of skills. Identifying weak or vulnerable skills and attitudes is also important – models of reflection and reflective practice may assist this process.

Tolerating Dissonance and Ambiguity

The nurse needs to take deliberate efforts to cultivate critical-thinking attitudes. For example, to develop fair-mindedness, one could deliberately seek out information that is in opposition to one's own views; this provides practice in understanding and learning to be open to other viewpoints. An example of this may be the use or nonuse of blood products for a patient with a religious objection, several alternative strategies could be used as an alternative such as cell salvage process. Cell salvage is a process of collecting blood from wound drains, 'cleaning it' with a specialist process and re-infusing it into the patient.

It is a human tendency to seek out information that corresponds to one's previously held beliefs and to ignore evidence that may contradict cherished ideas. This perspective is true for both the nurse and the patient. Older adults may have great difficulty accepting the pervasiveness of technology or that people do not stay in hospital as long as they did in the late 20th century or that having a diagnosis of cancer does not always mean that one is going to die. On the other hand, older adults have a wealth of knowledge and experience, and often know better than the healthcare provider what will work well and be acceptable to them. Examples of these could be 'folk lore' or alternative health treatments that have not been fully evaluated by the scientific community. To improve clinical practice nurses should increase their tolerance for ideas that contradict previously held beliefs and should practise suspending judgement.

Suspending judgement means tolerating ambiguity for a time. If an issue is complex, it may not be resolved quickly or neatly, and judgement should be postponed. For a while, the nurse will need to say, 'I don't know' and be comfortable with that answer until more is known. Although postponing judgement may not be feasible in emergency situations where fast action is required, it is usually feasible in other situations.

Seeking Situations Where Good Thinking Is Practised

Nurses will find it valuable to attend conferences/symposia/courses in clinical or educational settings that support open examination of all sides of issues and respect for opposing viewpoints. Cultivating a questioning attitude, using either Socratic questioning or another technique, is vital. Nurses need to review the standards for evaluating thinking and apply them to their own thinking. If nurses are aware of their own thinking – while they are doing the thinking – they can detect thinking errors in judgement.

Creating Environments that Support Critical Thinking

A nurse cannot develop or maintain critical-thinking attitudes in a vacuum. Nurses in leadership positions must be particularly aware of the climate for thinking that they establish, and they must actively create a stimulating environment that encourages differences of opinion and fair examination of ideas and options. In order to deliver culturally competent care nurses must embrace exploration of the perspectives of persons from different ages, cultures, religions, socioeconomic levels and family structures. As leaders, nurses should encourage colleagues to examine evidence carefully before they come to conclusions, and to avoid 'group think', the tendency to defer unthinkingly to the will of the group.

LIFESPAN CONSIDERATIONS

Older adults

While it is important to include patients in decision making and planning nursing care, it is especially difficult to do this when working with patients with impaired cognitive abilities, such as Alzheimer's disease. The goal should be to allow them to have as much control and input as possible, while keeping things simple and direct so they may be understood. Older adults with thought disorders, such as dementia, are usually unable to perform multiple tasks or even to think of more than one step at a time.

Presenting and discussing issues at their level helps to maintain respect and dignity and allows them to participate in their own care for as long as possible. Multiple stimuli should be avoided when making decisions in this patient group, for example discussing care options during meal times which may lead to increased confusion and disorientation.

ASSESSMENT AS PART OF THE NURSING PROCESS

Hall originated the term *nursing process* in 1955 in a lecture entitled 'The quality of nursing care', delivered in New Jersey, USA and Johnson (1959), Orlando (1961) and Wiedenbach (1963) were among the first nurse theorists to use it to refer to a series of phases describing the process of nursing. Since then, various nurses have described the process of nursing and organised the phases in different ways.

The purpose of the nursing process is to identify patients' health status and actual or potential healthcare problems or needs, to establish plans to meet the identified needs, and to deliver specific nursing interventions to meet those needs. The patient may be an individual, a family or a group.

See Figure 9-1 on page 142 for an illustration of the nursing process in action.

Phases of the Nursing Process

Although nursing theorists may use different terms to describe the phases of the nursing process, the activities of the nurse using the process are similar. For example, *diagnosing* may also be called *analysis*, and *implementing* may be called *intervention* or *intervening*.

An overview of the five-phase nursing process is shown in Table 9-4 on page 143. Each of the five phases is discussed in depth later in the chapter. The phases of the nursing process are not discrete entities but overlapping, continuing subprocesses (see Figure 9-2 on page 144). For example, assessing, which may be considered the first phase of the nursing process, is also carried out during the implementing and evaluating phases. This occurs, for instance, when, while actually administering medications (implementing), the nurse continuously notes the patient's skin colour, level of consciousness, and so on.

Each phase of the nursing process affects the others; they are closely interrelated. For example, if inadequate data is obtained during assessing, the nursing diagnoses will be incomplete or incorrect; inaccuracy will also be reflected in the planning, implementing and evaluating phases.

Characteristics of the Nursing Process

The nursing process has unique characteristics that enable responsiveness to the changing health status of the patient.

The nursing process is a systematic, rational method of planning and providing nursing care. Its goal is to identify a patient's healthcare status, and actual or potential health problems, to establish plans to meet the identified needs, and to deliver specific nursing interventions to address those needs.

The nursing process is cyclical; that is, its components follow a logical sequence, but more than one component may be involved at one time. At the end of the first cycle, care may be terminated if goals are achieved, the cycle may continue with reassessment or the plan of care may be modified.

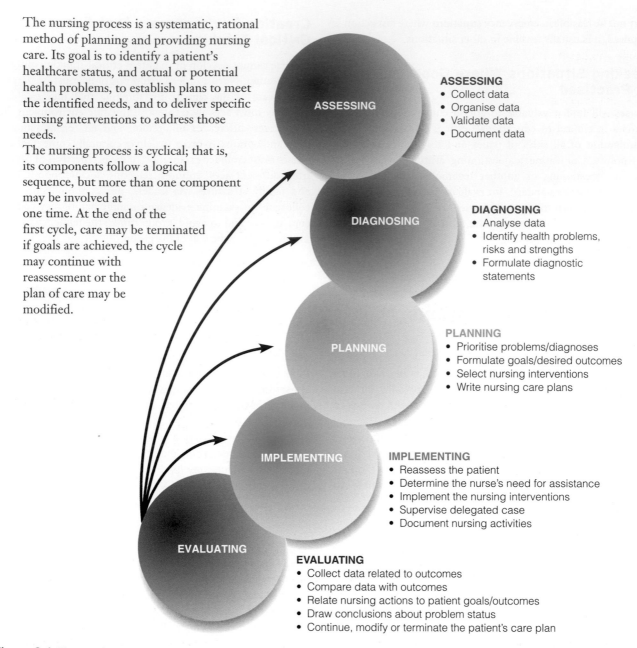

ASSESSING
- Collect data
- Organise data
- Validate data
- Document data

DIAGNOSING
- Analyse data
- Identify health problems, risks and strengths
- Formulate diagnostic statements

PLANNING
- Prioritise problems/diagnoses
- Formulate goals/desired outcomes
- Select nursing interventions
- Write nursing care plans

IMPLEMENTING
- Reassess the patient
- Determine the nurse's need for assistance
- Implement the nursing interventions
- Supervise delegated case
- Document nursing activities

EVALUATING
- Collect data related to outcomes
- Compare data with outcomes
- Relate nursing actions to patient goals/outcomes
- Draw conclusions about problem status
- Continue, modify or terminate the patient's care plan

Figure 9-1 The nursing process in action.

These characteristics include its cyclic and dynamic nature, patient centredness, focus on problem solving and decision making, interpersonal and collaborative style, universal applicability and use of critical thinking.

✚ Data from each phase provides input into the next phase. Findings from evaluating feed back into assessing. Hence, the nursing process is a regularly repeated event or sequence of events (a cycle) that is continuously changing (dynamic) rather than staying the same (static).

✚ The nursing process is patient centred. The nurse organises the plan of care according to patient problems rather than

nursing goals. In the assessment phase, the nurse collects data to determine the patient's habits, routines and needs, enabling the nurse to incorporate patient routines into the care plan as much as possible.

✚ The nursing process is an adaptation of problem solving and systems theory. It can be viewed as parallel to but separate from the process used by doctors (the medical process). Both processes (a) begin with data gathering and analysis, (b) base action (intervention or treatment) on a problem statement (nursing diagnosis or medical diagnosis) and (c) include an evaluative component. However, the medical process focuses on physiologic systems and the disease

Table 9-4 Overview of the Nursing Process

Phase and description	Purpose	Activities
Assessing Collecting, organising, validating and documenting patient data	To establish a database/ collection of baseline information about the patient response to health concerns or illness and the ability to manage healthcare needs	Establish a database: ✚ Obtain a nursing health history. ✚ Conduct a physical assessment. ✚ Review patient records. ✚ Review nursing literature. ✚ Consult support persons/multidisciplinary team. Update data as needed. Organise data. Validate data. Communicate/document data.
Diagnosing Analysing and synthesising data	To identify patient strengths and health problems that can be prevented or resolved by collaborative and independent nursing interventions. To develop a list of nursing and collaborative problems	Interpret and analyse data. ✚ Compare data against standards. ✚ Cluster or group data (generate tentative hypotheses). ✚ Identify gaps and inconsistencies. Determine patient strengths, risks, diagnoses and problems. Formulate nursing diagnoses and collaborative problem statements. Document nursing diagnoses on the care plan.
Planning Determining how to prevent, reduce or resolve the identified patient problems; how to support patient strengths; and how to implement nursing interventions in an organised, individualised and goal-directed manner	To develop an individualised care plan that specifies patient goals/desired outcomes, and related nursing interventions	Set priorities and goals/outcomes in collaboration with patient. Write goals/desired outcomes. Select nursing strategies/interventions. Consult other health professionals. Write nursing care plan. Communicate care plan to relevant healthcare providers/multidisciplinary team.
Implementing Carrying out the planned nursing interventions	To assist the patient to meet desired goals/outcomes; promote wellness; prevent illness and disease; restore health; and facilitate coping with altered functioning	Reassess the patient to update the care plan. Determine need for nursing assistance. Perform planned nursing interventions. Communicate what nursing actions were implemented. ✚ Document care and patient responses to care. ✚ Give verbal reports as necessary.
Evaluating Measuring the degree to which goals/outcomes have been achieved and identifying factors that positively or negatively influence goal achievement	To determine whether to continue, modify or terminate the plan of care	Collaborate with patient and collect data related to desired outcomes. Judge whether goals/outcomes have been achieved. Relate nursing actions to patient outcomes. Make decisions about problem status. Review and modify the care plan as indicated or terminate nursing care. Document achievement of outcomes and modification of the care plan.

process, whereas the nursing process is directed toward a patient's responses to disease and illness.

✚ Decision making is involved in every phase of the nursing process. Nurses can be highly creative in determining when and how to use data to make decisions. They are not bound by standard responses and may apply their repertoire of skills and knowledge to assist patients. This facilitates the individualisation of the nurse's plan of care.

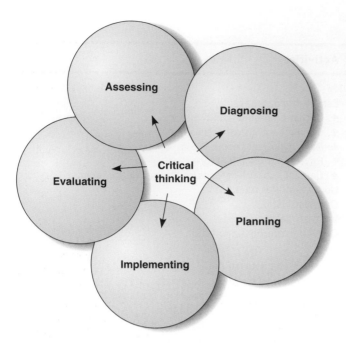

Figure 9-2 The five overlapping phases of the nursing process. Each phase depends on the accuracy of the preceding phase. Each phase involves critical thinking.

+ The nursing process is interpersonal and collaborative. It requires the nurse to communicate directly and consistently with patients and families to meet their needs. It also requires that nurses collaborate, as members of the health-care team, in a joint effort to provide quality patient care.
+ The universally applicable characteristic of the nursing process means that it is used as a framework for nursing care in all types of healthcare settings, with patients of all age groups.
+ Nurses must use a variety of critical-thinking skills to carry out the nursing process. Table 9-5 provides examples of critical thinking in the nursing process.

The Nursing Process in Action

Assessing

Assessing is the systematic and continuous collection, organisation, validation and documentation of **data** (information). In effect, assessing is a continuous process carried out during all phases of the nursing process. For example, in the evaluation phase, assessment is undertaken to determine the outcomes of the nursing strategies and to evaluate goal achievement. All phases of the nursing process depend on the accurate and complete collection of data.

There are four different types of assessments: initial assessment, problem-focused assessment, emergency assessment and time-lapsed reassessment (see Table 9-6 on page 146). Assessments vary according to their purpose, timing, time available and patient status.

Table 9-5 Examples of Critical Thinking in the Nursing Process

Nursing process phase	Critical-thinking activities
Assessing	Making reliable observations Distinguishing relevant from irrelevant data Distinguishing important from unimportant data Validating data Organising data Categorising data according to a framework Recognising assumptions
Diagnosing	Finding patterns and relationships among cues Identifying gaps in the data Making inferences Suspending judgement when lacking data Making interdisciplinary connections Stating the problem Examining assumptions Comparing patterns with norms Identifying factors contributing to the problem
Planning	Forming valid generalisations Transferring knowledge from one situation to another Developing evaluative criteria Hypothesising Making interdisciplinary connections Prioritising patient problems Generalising principles from other sciences
Implementing	Applying knowledge to perform interventions Testing hypotheses
Evaluating	Deciding whether hypotheses are correct Making criterion-based evaluations

Note: Adapted from Wilkinson, Judith M., *Nursing Process and Critical Thinking*, 3rd Edition, © 2001, pg 417. Reprinted by permission of Pearson Education Inc., Upper Saddle River, NJ.

Nursing assessments focus on a patient's responses to a health problem. A nursing assessment should include the patients perceived needs, health problems, related experience, health practices, values and lifestyles. To be most useful, the data collected should be relevant to a particular health problem. Therefore, nurses should think critically about what to assess. The assessment process involves four closely related activities: collecting data, organising data, validating data and documenting data (see Figure 9-3 on page 146).

Table 9-6 Types of Assessment

Type	Time performed	Purpose	Example
Initial assessment	Performed within specified time after admission to a healthcare agency	To establish a complete database for problem identification, reference and future comparison	Nursing admission assessment
Problem-focused assessment	Ongoing process integrated with nursing care	To determine the status of a specific problem identified in an earlier assessment. To identify new or overlooked problems	Hourly assessment of patients fluid intake and urinary output in a high-dependency area. Assessment of patient's ability to perform self-care while assisting with hygiene needs
Emergency assessment	During any physiological or psychological crisis of the patient	To identify life-threatening problems	Rapid assessment of a person's airway, breathing status and circulation during a cardiac arrest. Assessment of suicidal tendencies or potential for violence
Time-lapsed reassessment	Several months after initial assessment	To compare the patient's current status to baseline data previously obtained	Reassessment of a patient's functional health patterns in a home care or outpatient setting or, in a hospital, at shift change

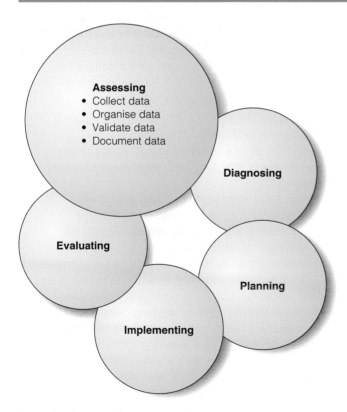

Figure 9-3 Assessing. The assessment process involves four closely related activities.

DATA

Collecting Data

Data collection is the process of gathering information about a patient's health status. It must be both systematic and con-tinuous to prevent the omission of significant data and reflect a patient's changing health status.

A **database** is all the information about a patient; it includes the nursing health history (see *Box 9-2*), physical assessment, the doctor's history notes and physical examination, results of laboratory and diagnostic tests, and material contributed by other health personnel. A nursing model or care pathway such as those described in Chapter 2 may also be used.

Patient data should include past history as well as current problems. For example, a history of an allergic reaction to penicillin is a vital piece of historical data. Past surgical procedures, complementary therapies and chronic diseases are also examples of historical data. Current data relate to present circumstances, such as pain, nausea, sleep patterns and religious practices. To collect data accurately, both the patient and nurse must actively participate.

Types of Data

Data can be subjective or objective. **Subjective data**, also referred to as **symptoms** or **covert data**, are apparent only to the person affected and can be described or verified only by that person. Itching, pain and feelings of worry are examples of subjective data. Subjective data include the patient's sensations, feelings, values, beliefs, attitudes and perception of personal health status and life situation.

Objective data, also referred to as **signs** or **overt data**, are detectable by an observer or can be measured or tested against an accepted standard. They can be seen, heard, felt or smelled, and they are obtained by observation or physical examination. For example, a discoloration of the skin or a blood pressure reading is objective data. During the physical examination, the nurse obtains objective data to validate subjective data and to

BOX 9-2 Components of a Nursing Health History

Biographic Data
Patient name, address, age, sex, marital status, occupation, religious preference, next of kin, family doctor/general practitioner.

Chief Complaint or Reason for Visit
The answer given to the question 'What is troubling you?' or 'What brought you to the hospital or clinic?' The chief complaint should be recorded in the patient's own words.

History of Present Illness
+ When the symptoms started
+ Whether the onset of symptoms was sudden or gradual
+ How often the problem occurs
+ Exact location of the distress/pain
+ Character of the complaint (e.g. intensity of pain or quality of sputum, sickness or discharge)
+ Activity in which the patient was involved when the problem occurred
+ Phenomena or symptoms associated with the chief complaint
+ Factors that aggravate or alleviate the problem

Past History
+ *Childhood illnesses*, such as chickenpox, mumps, measles, rubella (German measles), streptococcal infections, scarlet fever, rheumatic fever and other significant illnesses
+ *Childhood immunisations* and the date of the last tetanus immunisation
+ *Allergies* to drugs, animals, insects or other environmental agents, and the type of reaction that occurs
+ *Accidents and injuries*: how, when and where the incident occurred, type of injury, treatment received and any complications
+ *Hospitalisation for serious illnesses*: reasons for the hospitalisation, dates, surgery performed, course of recovery, and any complications
+ *Medications*: all currently used prescription and over-the-counter medications, such as aspirin, nasal spray, vitamins, herbal remedies or laxatives

Family History of Illness
To ascertain risk factors for certain diseases, the ages of siblings, parents and grandparents, and their current state of health or, if they are deceased, the cause of death are obtained. Particular attention should be given to disorders such as heart disease, cancer, diabetes, hypertension, hyperlipidaemia (high cholesterol), obesity, allergies, arthritis, tuberculosis, bleeding, alcoholism and any mental health disorders.

Lifestyle
+ *Personal habits*: the amount, frequency and duration of substance use (tobacco, alcohol, coffee, tea and illicit or recreational drugs)
+ *Diet*: description of a typical diet on a normal day or any special diet, number of meals and snacks per day, who cooks and shops for food, ethnically distinct food patterns and allergies
+ *Sleep/rest patterns*: usual daily sleep/wake times, difficulties sleeping and remedies used for difficulties
+ *Activities of daily living (ADLs)*: any difficulties experienced in the basic activities of eating, grooming, dressing, elimination and locomotion
+ *Instrumental activities of daily living*: any difficulties experienced in food preparation, shopping, transportation, housekeeping, laundry, and ability to use the telephone, handle finances and manage medications
+ *Recreation/hobbies*: exercise activity and tolerance, hobbies and other interests and vacations

Social Data
+ *Family relationships/friendships*: The patient's support system in times of stress (who helps in time of need?), what effect the patient's illness has on the family and whether any family problems are affecting the patient (see also Chapter 5).
+ *Ethnic affiliation*: Health customs and beliefs; cultural practices that may affect healthcare and recovery. See also detailed ethnic/cultural assessment guide in Chapter 5.
+ *Educational history*: Data about the patient's highest level of education attained and any past difficulties with learning.
+ *Occupational history*: Current employment status, the number of days missed from work because of illness, any history of accidents on the job, any occupational hazards with a potential for future disease or accident such as chemicals or industrial dust, the patient's need to change jobs because of past illness, the employment status of spouses or partners and the way childcare is handled, and the patient's overall satisfaction with the work.
+ *Economic status*: Information about how the patient is managing financially while in hospital and any consideration to effects to social benefits being received.

+ *Home and neighbourhood conditions*; Home safety measures and adjustments in physical facilities that may be required to help the patient manage a physical disability, activity intolerance and activities of daily living; the availability of social and community services to meet the patient's needs.

Psychologic Data

+ *Major stressors* experienced and the patient's perception of them
+ *Usual coping pattern* with a serious problem or a high level of stress
+ *Communication style*: ability to verbalise appropriate emotion; nonverbal communication –

such as eye movements, gestures, use of touch and posture; interactions with support persons; and the use of nonverbal behaviour and verbal expression

Patterns of Health Care

All healthcare resources the patient is currently using and has used in the past. These include the family doctor, specialists (e.g. ophthalmologist or gynaecologist), dentist, complementary practitioners (e.g. herbalist or reflexologist), health clinic or health centre; whether the patient considers the care being provided adequate; and whether access to healthcare is a problem.

Table 9-7 Examples of Subjective and Objective Data

Subjective	Objective
'I feel weak all over when I exert myself.'	Blood pressure 90/50 Apical pulse 104 Skin pale and clammy
Patient states he has a cramping pain in his abdomen. States, 'I feel sick to my stomach.'	Vomited 100 ml green-tinged fluid Abdomen firm and slightly distended Active bowel sounds auscultated in all four quadrants
'I'm short of breath.' Wife states: 'He doesn't seem so sad today.'	Lung sounds clear bilaterally; diminished in right lower lobe
'I would like to see the chaplain before surgery.'	Patient cried during interview Holding open Bible Has small silver cross on bedside table

complete the assessment phase of the nursing process. Information supplied by family members, significant others or other healthcare professionals is considered subjective if it is not based on fact. If the patient's relative states, 'Dad is very confused today,' that is subjective data. However, if she were to state, 'Dad couldn't remember his address or phone number today,' that is objective data.

A complete database of both subjective and objective data provides a baseline for comparing the patient's responses to nursing and medical interventions. Examples of subjective and objective data are shown in Table 9-7.

Sources of Data

Sources of data are primary or secondary. The patient is the primary source of data. Family members or other support persons, other health professionals, records and reports, laboratory and diagnostic tests, and relevant literature are secondary or indirect sources. In fact, all sources other than the patient are considered secondary sources.

The Patient

The best source of data is usually patients themselves, unless they are too ill, young or confused to communicate clearly. The patient can provide subjective data that no one else can offer.

Support People

Family members, friends and caregivers who know the patient well often can supplement or verify information provided by the patient. They might convey information about the patient's response to illness, the stresses the patient was experiencing before the illness, family attitudes on illness and health, and the patient's home environment.

Support people are an especially important source of data for a patient who is very young, unconscious or confused. In some cases – a patient who is physically or emotionally abused, for example – the person giving information may wish to remain anonymous. Before collecting data/information from support people, the nurse should ensure that the patient, if mentally able, accepts such input. The nurse should also indicate on the nursing history/notes that the data/information was obtained from a support person/significant other.

Patient Records/Notes

Patient records include information documented by various healthcare professionals. Patient records also contain data regarding their occupation, religion and marital status. By reviewing such records before interviewing the patient, the nurse can avoid asking questions for which answers have already been supplied. Repeated questioning can be stressful and annoying to patients and cause concern about the lack of communication among health professionals. Types of patient records include medical records, records of therapies, laboratory results, imaging such as x-ray and ultrasound. Increasingly the medium is moving from that of a 'hard' paper-based copy to the electronic health record. Higher proportions of hospitals and healthcare facilities now have most investigations such as laboratory and imaging available electronically within the healthcare setting. These systems tend to be closed systems unique to that hospital (group of hospitals) or healthcare setting to protect patient confidentiality and unauthorised illegal access.

Medical records (e.g. medical history, physical examination, operative report, progress notes and consultations recorded by doctors) are often a source of a patient's present and past health and illness patterns. These records can provide nurses with information about the patient's coping behaviours, health practices, previous illnesses and allergies.

Records of therapies provided by other health professionals, such as social workers, dietitians, occupational therapists or physiotherapists help the nurse obtain relevant data not expressed by the patient. For example, a social worker's/occupational therapist's report on a patient's home conditions or ability to cope at home alone can also be helpful to the nurse conducting an assessment.

Laboratory records/results also provide pertinent health information. For example, the determination of blood glucose level allows health professionals to monitor the administration of oral hypoglycaemic medications for the management of diabetes. Any laboratory data about a patient must be compared to the laboratory's norms for that particular test and for the patient's age, sex, and so on.

The nurse must always consider the information in patient records in light of the present situation. For example, if the most recent medical record is 10 years old, the patient health practices and coping behaviours are likely to have changed. Older adults may have numerous previous records. These are very useful and contribute to a full understanding of the health history, especially if the patient's memory is impaired, but may take some time to examine thoroughly.

Health Care Professionals

Because assessment is an ongoing process, verbal reports from other healthcare professionals serve as other potential sources of information about a patient's health. Nurses, social workers, physicians and physiotherapists, for example, may have information from either previous or current contact with the patient. Sharing of information among professionals is especially important to ensure continuity of care when patients are transferred to and from home and healthcare agencies. Therefore in some instances and healthcare settings a generic healthcare professional record is used in contrast to the traditional one profession one record system.

Data Collection Methods

The primary methods used to collect data are observing, interviewing and examining. Observation occurs whenever the nurse is in contact with the patient or significant others. Interviewing is used mainly while taking the nursing health history. Examining is the major method used in the physical health assessment.

In reality, the nurse uses all three methods simultaneously when assessing patients. For example, during the patient interview the nurse observes, listens, asks questions and mentally retains information to explore in the physiological examination.

Observing

To *observe* is to gather data by using the senses. Observation is a conscious, deliberate skill that is developed through effort and with an organised approach. Although nurses observe mainly through sight, most of the senses are engaged during careful observations. Examples of patient data observed through the senses are shown in Table 9-8.

Table 9-8 Using the Senses to Observe Patient Data

Sense	Example of patient data
Vision	Overall appearance (e.g. body size, general weight, posture, grooming); signs of distress or discomfort; facial and body gestures; skin colour and lesions; abnormalities of movement; nonverbal communication (e.g. signs of anger or anxiety); religious or cultural artefacts (e.g. books, icons, candles, beads)
Smell	Body or breath odours
Hearing	Ability to communicate; language spoken; ability to initiate conversation; ability to respond when spoken to; orientation to time, person and place; thoughts and feelings about self, others and health status
Touch	Skin temperature and moisture; muscle strength (e.g. hand grip); pulse rate, rhythm and volume; palpatory lesions (e.g. lumps, masses, nodules)

Observation has two aspects: (a) noticing the data and (b) selecting, organising and interpreting the data. A nurse who observes that a patient's face is flushed must relate that observation to, for example, body temperature, activity, environmental temperature and blood pressure. Errors can occur in selecting, organising and interpreting data. For example, a nurse might not notice certain signs, either because they are unexpected or because they do not conform to preconceptions about a patient's illness. Nurses often need to focus on specific data in order not to be overwhelmed by a multitude of data. Observing, therefore, involves discriminating among data, that is distinguishing data in a meaningful manner. For example, nurses caring for newborns learn to ignore the usual sounds of machines in the clinical area but respond quickly to an infant's cry or movement.

The experienced nurse is often able to attend to an intervention (e.g. give a bed bath or monitor an intravenous infusion) and at the same time make important observations (e.g. note a change in respiratory status or skin colour). The student nurse needs to learn to make observations and complete tasks simultaneously.

Nursing observations must be organised so that nothing significant is missed. Most nurses develop a particular sequence for observing events, usually focusing on the patient first. For example, a nurse walks into a patient's room and observes, in the following order:

1. Clinical signs of patient distress (e.g. pallor or flushing, laboured breathing, and behaviour indicating pain or emotional distress).
2. Threats to the patient's safety, real or anticipated (e.g. a lowered bed side/cot rail).
3. The presence and functioning of associated equipment (e.g. intravenous equipment and oxygen).
4. The immediate environment, including the people in it.

Interviewing

An **interview** is a planned communication or a conversation with a purpose, for example, to get or give information, identify problems of mutual concern, evaluate change, teach, provide support, or provide counselling or therapy. One example of the interview is the nursing health history, which is a part of the nursing admission assessment.

There are two approaches to interviewing: directive and nondirective. The **directive interview** is highly structured and elicits specific information. The nurse establishes the purpose of the interview and controls the interview, at least at the outset. The patient responds to questions but may have limited opportunity to ask questions or discuss concerns. Nurses frequently use directive interviews to gather and to give information when time is limited (e.g. in an emergency situation).

During a **nondirective interview**, or rapport-building interview, by contrast, the nurse allows the patient to control the purpose, subject matter and pacing. **Rapport** is an understanding between two or more people.

A combination of directive and nondirective approaches is usually appropriate during the information-gathering interview. The nurse begins by determining areas of concern for the patient. If, for example, a patient expresses worry about surgery, the nurse pauses to explore the patient's worry and to provide support. Simply noting the worry, without dealing with it, can leave the impression that the nurse does not care about the patient's concerns or dismisses them as unimportant.

Types of interview questions. Questions are often classified as closed or open ended, and neutral or leading. **Closed questions**, used in the directive interview, are restrictive and generally require only 'yes' or 'no' or short factual answers giving specific information. Closed questions often begin with 'when', 'where', 'who', 'what', 'do (did, does)' or 'is (are, was)'. Examples of closed questions are: 'What medication did you take?', 'Are you having pain now? Show me where it is', 'How old are you?', 'When did you fall?' The highly stressed person and the person who has difficulty communicating will find closed questions easier to answer than open-ended questions.

Open-ended questions, associated with the nondirective interview, invite patients to discover and explore, elaborate, clarify or illustrate their thoughts or feelings. An open-ended question specifies only the broad topic to be discussed, and invites answers longer than one or two words. Such questions give patients the freedom to divulge only the information that they are ready to disclose. The open-ended question is useful at the beginning of an interview or to change topics and to elicit attitudes.

Open-ended questions may begin with 'what' or 'how'. Examples of open-ended questions are: 'How have you been feeling lately?', 'What brought you to the hospital?', 'How did you feel in that situation?', 'Would you describe more about how you relate to your child?', 'What would you like to talk about today?'

The type of question a nurse chooses depends on the needs of the patient at the time. Nurses often find it necessary to use a combination of closed and open-ended questions throughout an interview to accomplish the goals of the interview and obtain needed information. See *Box 9-3* on page 150 for advantages and disadvantages of open-ended and closed questions.

A **neutral question** is a question the patient can answer without direction or pressure from the nurse, is open ended, and is used in nondirective interviews. Examples are: 'How do you feel about that?' and 'Why do you think you had the operation?' A **leading question**, by contrast, is usually closed, used in a directive interview, and thus directs the patient's answer. Examples are: 'You're stressed about surgery tomorrow, aren't you?' and 'You will take your medicine, won't you?' The leading question gives the patient less opportunity to decide whether the answer is true or not. Leading questions create problems if the patient, in an effort to please the nurse, gives inaccurate responses. This can result in inaccurate data.

> **BOX 9-3** Selected Advantages and Disadvantages of Open-Ended and Closed Questions
>
> ## Open-ended questions
>
> ### Advantages
>
> 1. They let the interviewee do the talking.
> 2. The interviewer is able to listen and observe.
> 3. They are easy to answer and non-threatening.
> 4. They reveal what the interviewee thinks is important.
> 5. They may reveal the interviewee's lack of information, misunderstanding of words, frame of reference, prejudices or stereotypes.
> 6. They can provide information the interviewer may not ask for.
> 7. They can reveal the interviewee's degree of feeling about an issue.
> 8. They can convey interest and trust because of the freedom they provide.
>
> ### Disadvantages
>
> 1. They take more time.
> 2. Only brief answers may be given.
> 3. Valuable information may be withheld.
> 4. They often elicit more information than necessary.
> 5. Responses are difficult to document and require skill in recording.
> 6. The interviewer requires skill in controlling an open-ended interview.
> 7. Responses require psychological insight and sensitivity from the interviewer.
>
> ## Closed questions
>
> ### Advantages
>
> 1. Questions and answers can be controlled more effectively
> 2. They require less effort from the interviewee.
> 3. They may be less threatening, since they do not require explanations or justifications.
> 4. They take less time.
> 5. Information can be asked for sooner than it would be volunteered.
> 6. Responses are easily documented.
> 7. Questions are easy to use and can be handled by unskilled interviewers.
>
> ### Disadvantages
>
> 1. They may provide too little information and require follow-up questions.
> 2. They may not reveal how the interviewee feels.
> 3. They do not allow the interviewee to volunteer possibly valuable information.
> 4. They may inhibit communication and convey lack of interest by the interviewer.
> 5. The interviewer may dominate the interview with questions.
>
> *Note*: From *Interviewing: Principles and Practices*, 10th edn (pp. 55–60), by C.J. Stewart and W.B. Cash, Jr, 2002, New York: McGraw-Hill. All rights reserved. Adapted with permission.

PLANNING THE INTERVIEW AND SETTING

Before beginning an interview, the nurse reviews available information, for example, the operative report, information about the current illness or literature about the patient's health problem. The nurse also reviews the healthcare setting data-collection form or set of nursing notes to identify what data must be collected and what data are within the nurse's discretion to collect based on the specific patient.

Each interview is influenced by time, place, seating arrangement or distance, and language.

Time

Nurses need to plan interviews with hospitalised patients when the patient is physically comfortable and free of pain, and when interruptions by friends, family and other health professionals are minimal. Nurses should schedule interviews with patients in their homes at a time selected by the patient wherever possible. The patient should be made to feel comfortable and unhurried.

Place

A well-lit, well-ventilated, moderate-sized room that is relatively free of noise, movements and interruptions encourages communication. In addition, a place where others cannot overhear or see the patient is desirable. (Remember curtains around a bed space in hospital are not sound proof.)

Seating Arrangement

A seating arrangement with the nurse behind a desk and the patient seated across creates a formal setting that suggests a business meeting between a superior and a subordinate. In contrast, a seating arrangement in which the parties sit on two chairs placed at right angles to a desk or table or a few feet apart, with no table between, creates a less formal atmosphere, and the nurse and patient tend to feel on equal terms. In groups, a horseshoe or circular chair arrangement can avoid a superior or head-of-the-table position. (This is especially important in mental health settings.)

By standing and looking down at a patient who is in bed or in a chair, the nurse risks intimidating the patient, who may perceive the nurse as having greater status. When a patient is in bed, the nurse can sit at a 45-degree angle to the bed. This position is less formal than sitting behind a table or standing at the foot of the bed. During an initial admission interview, a patient may feel less confronted if there is an overbed table between the patient and the nurse. Sitting on a patient's bed hems the patient in and makes staring difficult to avoid – it is also poor infection control practice.

Distance

The distance between the interviewer and interviewee should be neither too small nor too great, because people feel uncomfortable when talking to someone who is too close or too far away. Most people feel comfortable maintaining a distance of $1/2$ to 1 metre during an interview. Some patients require more or less personal space, depending on their cultural and personal needs (see *Box 9-4*).

BOX 9-4 Personal Space Variables

+ Accepted distance between individuals in conversation varies with ethnicity. It is about 8 to 12 inches (20–30 cm) in Arab countries, 18 inches (45 cm) in the USA, 24 inches (61 cm) in the UK and 36 inches (91 cm) in Japan.
+ Men of all cultures usually require more space than women.
+ Anxiety increases the need for space.
+ Direct eye contact increases the need for space. 'In East Asian and Scandinavian countries, direct eye contact is considered disrespectful' (O'Carroll, 2001: ¶7).
+ Physical contact is used only if it has a therapeutic purpose. Touch, even a simple hand on the shoulder, can be misinterpreted – especially between persons of opposite gender.

Note: From *'Getting Too Close (or Too Far) for Comfort,'* by E. O'Carroll, March 1, 2001. Retrieved 23 February 2003, from http://travel.boston.com/columns/sl/030502_close.html. Reprinted with permission from Smarter Living (www.smarterliving.com).

Language

Failure to communicate in language the patient can understand may be considered a form of discrimination. The nurse must convert complicated medical terminology into common English usage, and interpreters or translators are needed if the patient and the nurse do not speak the same language. Translating medical terminology is a specialised skill because not all persons fluent in the conversational form of the language are familiar with anatomical or other health terms. Interpreters, however, may make judgements about precise wording but also about subtle meanings that require additional explanation or clarification according to the specific language and ethnicity. They may edit the original source to make the meaning clearer or more culturally appropriate.

If giving written documents to patients, the nurse must determine that the patient can read in his or her native language. Live translation is preferred since the patient can then ask questions for clarification. Nurses must be cautious when asking family members, patient visitors or hospital nonprofessional staff to assist with translation. Services such as Language Line are available 24 hours a day in about 150 languages, for a fee paid by the healthcare setting. Many larger healthcare settings/hospitals are establishing their own on-call translator services for the languages commonly spoken in their geographical areas.

Even among patients who speak English, there may be differences in understanding terminology. Patients from different parts of the country may have strong accents; less well-educated and teen patients may ascribe different meanings to words. For example, 'cool' may imply something 'good' to one patient and something 'not warm' to another. The nurse must always confirm accurate understandings.

Stages of an Interview

An interview has three major stages: the opening or introduction, the body or development, and the closing.

The Opening

The opening can be the most important part of the interview because what is said and done at that time sets the tone for the remainder of the interview. The purposes of the opening are to establish rapport and orient the interviewee.

Establishing rapport is a process of creating goodwill and trust. It can begin with a greeting ('Good morning, Mr. Jones') or a self-introduction ('Good morning. I'm Becky James, a student nurse') accompanied by nonverbal gestures such as a smile, a handshake and a friendly manner. The nurse must be careful not to overdo this stage; too much superficial talk can arouse anxiety about what is to follow and may appear insincere.

In orientation, the nurse explains the purpose and nature of the interview, for example, what information is needed, how long it will take, and what is expected of the patient.

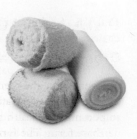

PRACTICE GUIDELINES

Communication during an Interview

+ Listen attentively, using all your senses, and speak slowly and clearly.
+ Use language the patient understands and clarify points that are not understood.
+ Plan questions to follow a logical sequence.
+ Ask only one question at a time. Double questions limit the patient to one choice and may confuse both the nurse and the patient.
+ Allow the patient the opportunity to look at things the way they appear to him or her and not the way they appear to the nurse or someone else.
+ Do not impose your own values on the patient.
+ Avoid using personal examples, such as saying, 'If I were you . . .'
+ Nonverbally convey respect, concern, interest and acceptance simply be self aware.
+ Use and accept silence to help the patient search for more thoughts or to organise them.
+ Use eye contact and be calm, unhurried and sympathetic.

The Body

In the body of the assessment interview, the patient communicates what they think, feel, know and perceive in response to questions from the nurse. Effective development of the interview demands that the nurse uses communication techniques that make both parties feel comfortable and serve the purpose of the interview.

The Closing

The nurse terminates the interview when the needed information has been obtained. In some cases, however, a patient terminates it, for example, when deciding not to give any more information or when unable to offer more information for some other reason – fatigue, for example. The closing is important for maintaining rapport and trust and for facilitating future interactions. The following techniques are commonly used to close an interview:

+ Offer to answer questions: 'Do you have any questions?' 'I would be glad to answer any questions you have.' Be sure to allow time for the patient to answer or the offer will be regarded as insincere.
+ Conclude by saying, 'Well, that's all I need to know for now' or 'Well, those are all the questions I have for now.' Preceding a remark with the word 'well' generally signals that the end of the interaction is near.
+ Thank the patient: 'Thank you for your time and help. The questions you have answered will be helpful in planning your nursing care.'
+ Express concern for the person's welfare and future: 'Take care of yourself' or 'I hope all goes well for you.'
+ Plan for the next meeting, if there is to be one, or state what will happen next. Include the day, time, place, topic and purpose: 'Let's get together again here on the 15th at 9:00 a.m. to see how you are managing then.' Or 'Mrs Smith, I will be responsible for visiting you three mornings a week to change your dressings. I will be in to see you each Monday, Wednesday and Friday between eight o'clock and noon. At those times, we can adjust your care if we need to.'
+ Provide a summary to verify accuracy and agreement. Summarising serves several purposes: it helps to terminate the interview, it reassures the patient that the nurse has listened, it checks the accuracy of the nurse's perceptions, it clears the way for new ideas and it helps the patient to note progress and forward direction. 'Let's review what we covered in this interview.' Summaries are particularly helpful for patients who are anxious or who have difficulty staying with the topic. 'Well, it seems to me that you are especially worried about your hospitalisation and chest pain because your father died of a heart attack five years ago. Is that correct? . . . I'll discuss this with you again tomorrow, and we'll decide what plans need to be made to help you.'

Examining

The physical assessment is a systematic data-collection method that uses observation (i.e. the senses of sight, hearing, smell and touch) to detect health problems. The physical assessment is carried out systematically. It may be organised according to the examiner's preference, in a head-to-toe approach or a body systems approach. Usually, the nurse first records a general impression about the patient's overall appearance and health status, for example, age, body size, mental and nutritional status, speech and behaviour. Then the nurse takes measurements such as vital signs (blood pressure, temperature, pulse and respirations), height, weight, visual acuity and skin inspection (see Chapter 15).

DATA MANAGEMENT

Organising Data

The nurse uses a written (or computerised) format that organises the assessment data systematically. This is often referred to as a nursing health history, nursing assessment or nursing database form. The format may be modified according to the patient's physical status such as one focused on musculoskeletal data for orthopaedic patients.

Nursing Conceptual Models

Most schools of nursing and healthcare settings have developed their own structured assessment format. Many of these are based on selected nursing theories (discussed earlier in Chapter 2). Four examples are Roper, Logan and Tierney's activities of living model, Gordon's functional health pattern framework, Orem's self-care model and Roy's adaptation model.

These structured models can be used as a means of assessing the patient and identifying self-care needs and deficits in a structured manner.

Body Systems Model

The body systems model focuses on abnormalities of the following anatomic systems:

+ integumentary (skin) system,
+ respiratory system,
+ cardiovascular system,
+ nervous system,
+ musculoskeletal system,
+ gastrointestinal system,
+ genitourinary system,
+ reproductive system,
+ immune system.

Maslow's Hierarchy of Needs

Maslow's hierarchy of needs (see Chapter 5) clusters data pertaining to the following:

+ physiological needs (survival needs),
+ safety and security needs,
+ love and belonging needs,
+ self-esteem needs,
+ self-actualisation needs.

Validating Data

The information gathered during the assessment phase must be complete, factual and accurate because the nursing diagnoses and interventions are based on this information. **Validation** is the act of 'double-checking' or verifying data to confirm that it is accurate and factual. Validating data helps the nurse complete these tasks:

+ Ensure that assessment information is complete.
+ Ensure that objective and related subjective data agree.
+ Obtain additional information that may have been overlooked.
+ Differentiate between cues and inferences. **Cues** are subjective or objective data that can be directly observed by the nurse; that is, what the patient says or what the nurse can see, hear, feel, smell or measure. **Inferences** are the nurse's interpretation or conclusions made based on the cues (e.g. a nurse observes the cues that an incision is red, hot and swollen; the nurse makes the inference that the incision is infected).
+ Avoid jumping to conclusions and focusing in the wrong direction to identify problems.

Not all data require validation. For example, data such as height, weight, birth date and most laboratory studies that can be measured with an accurate scale can be accepted as factual. As a rule, the nurse validates data when there are discrepancies between data obtained in the nursing interview (subjective data) and the physical assessment (objective data), or when the patient's statements differ at different times in the assessment. Guidelines for validating data are shown in Table 9-9 on page 154.

To collect data accurately, nurses need to be aware of their own biases, values and beliefs, and to separate fact from inference, interpretation and assumption. For example, a nurse seeing a man holding his arm to his chest might assume that he is experiencing chest pain, when in fact he has a painful hand.

To build an accurate database, nurses must validate assumptions regarding the patient's physical or emotional behaviour. In the previous example, the nurse should ask the patient why he is holding his arm to his chest. The patient's response may validate the nurse's assumptions or prompt further questioning.

Documenting Data

To complete the assessment phase, the nurse records patient data. Accurate documentation is essential and should include all data collected about the patient's health status. Data are recorded in a factual manner and not interpreted by the nurse. For example, the nurse records the patient's breakfast intake (objective data) as 'coffee 240 ml, juice 120 ml, 1 egg and 1 slice of toast,' rather than as 'appetite good' (a judgement). A judgement or conclusion such as 'appetite good' or 'normal appetite' may have different meanings for different people. To increase accuracy, the nurse records subjective data in the patient's own words. Restating in other words what someone says increases the chance of changing the original meaning.

DIAGNOSING

Diagnosing is the second phase of the nursing process. Although this is used extensively in the USA it is a system that is slowly developing within nursing in the UK. In this phase, nurses use critical-thinking skills to interpret assessment data

Table 9-9 Validating Assessment Data

Guidelines	Example
Compare subjective and objective data to verify the patient's statements with your observations.	Patient's perceptions of 'feeling hot' need to be compared with measurement of the body temperature.
Clarify any ambiguous or vague statements.	*Patient*: 'I've felt sick on and off for 6 weeks.' *Nurse*: 'Describe what your sickness is like. Tell me what you mean by "on and off".'
Be sure your data consist of cues and not inferences.	*Observation*: Dry skin and reduced tissue turgor. *Inference*: Dehydration. *Action*: Collect additional data that are needed to make the inference in the diagnosing phase. For example, determine the patient's fluid intake, amount and appearance of urine, and blood pressure.
Double-check data that are extremely abnormal.	*Observation*: A resting pulse of 30 beats per minute or a blood pressure of 210/95. *Action*: Repeat the measurement. Use another piece of equipment as needed to confirm abnormalities, or ask someone else to collect the same data.
Determine the presence of factors that may interfere with accurate measurement.	A crying infant will have an abnormal respiratory rate and will need quietening before accurate assessment can be made.
Use references (textbooks, journals, research reports) to explain phenomena.	A nurse considers tiny purple or bluish-black swollen areas under the tongue of an elderly patient to be abnormal until reading about physical changes of ageing. Such varicosities are common.

and identify patient strengths and problems. Diagnosing is a pivotal step in the nursing process. All activities preceding this phase are directed toward formulating the nursing diagnoses; all the care-planning activities following this phase are based on the nursing diagnoses (see Figure 9-4).

The identification and development of nursing diagnoses began formally in 1973. The first national conference to

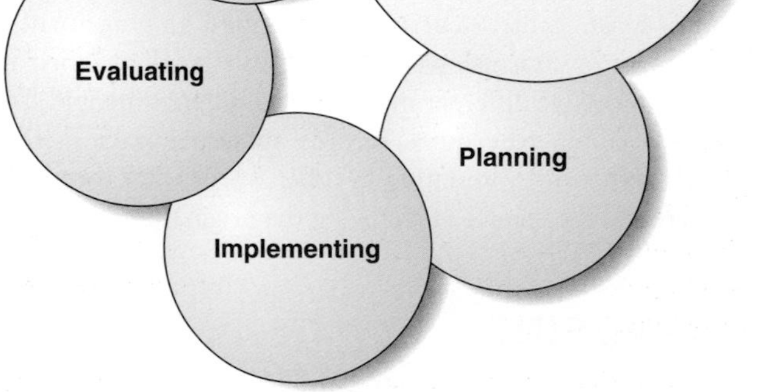

Figure 9-4 Diagnosing. The pivotal second phase of the nursing process, in which the nurse interprets assessment data, identifies patient strengths and health problems and formulates diagnostic statements.

identify nursing diagnoses was sponsored by the Saint Louis University School of Nursing and Allied Health Professions in 1973. Subsequent national conferences occurred in 1975, 1980 and every two years thereafter.

International recognition came with the First Canadian Conference in Toronto in 1977 and the International Nursing Conference in May 1987 in Calgary, Alberta, Canada. In 1982, the conference group accepted the name North American Nursing Diagnosis Association (NANDA), recognising the participation and contributions of nurses in the USA and Canada.

The purpose of NANDA is to define, refine and promote a taxonomy of nursing diagnostic terminology of general use to professional nurses. A **taxonomy** is a classification system or set of categories arranged on the basis of a single principle or set of principles. The members of NANDA include staff nurses, clinical specialists, faculty, directors of nursing, deans, theorists and researchers. The group has currently approved more than 150 nursing diagnosis labels for clinical use and testing. In 2000, Taxonomy I was revised and is now referred to as Taxonomy II.

Currently there is no UK equivalent of NANDA so where nursing diagnosis is applied in UK nursing practice the NANDA system is currently utilised.

NANDA Nursing Diagnoses

To use the concept of nursing diagnoses effectively in generating and completing a nursing care plan, the nurse must be familiar with the definitions of terms used, the types and the components of nursing diagnoses. Nursing diagnoses are not used in all healthcare settings within the UK and may not always form a full part of the nursing process explicitly.

Definitions

The term *diagnosing* refers to the reasoning process, whereas the term **diagnosis** is a statement or conclusion regarding the nature of a phenomenon. The standardised NANDA names for the diagnoses are called **diagnostic labels**; and the patient's problem statement, consisting of the diagnostic label plus **aetiology** (causal relationship between a problem and its related or risk factors), is called a **nursing diagnosis**.

In 1990, NANDA adopted an official working definition of nursing diagnosis: '. . . a clinical judgement about individual, family, or community responses to actual and potential health problems/life processes. Nursing diagnoses provide the basis for selection of nursing interventions to achieve outcomes for which the nurse is accountable' (as cited in NANDA International, 2003: 251). This definition implies the following:

+ Professional nurses (registered nurses) are responsible for making nursing diagnoses, even though other nursing personnel may contribute data to the process of diagnosing and may implement specified nursing care. The American Nurses Association *Standards of Clinical Nursing Practice* (1998) (the US equivalent of the NMC), states that nurses are accountable for this phase of the nursing process. The Joint Commission on Accreditation of Healthcare Organizations (JCAHO) – the equivalent of the UK Department of Health – requires evidence of nursing diagnoses in patients' medical records as well (JCAHO, 2001).
+ The domain of nursing diagnosis includes only those health states that nurses are educated and licensed to treat. For example, nurses are not educated to diagnose or treat diseases such as diabetes mellitus; this task is defined legally as within the practice of medicine. Yet nurses can diagnose and treat *deficient knowledge, ineffective coping* or *imbalanced nutrition*, all of which may accompany diabetes mellitus.
+ A nursing diagnosis is a judgement made only after thorough, systematic data collection.
+ Nursing diagnoses describe a continuum of health states: deviations from health, presence of risk factors and areas of enhanced personal growth.

Types of Nursing Diagnoses

The five types of nursing diagnoses are actual, risk, wellness, possible and syndrome.

1. An *actual diagnosis* is a patient problem that is present at the time of the nursing assessment. Examples are *ineffective breathing pattern* and *anxiety*. An actual nursing diagnosis is based on the presence of associated signs and symptoms.
2. A **risk nursing diagnosis** is a clinical judgement that a problem does not exist, but the presence of **risk factors** indicates that a problem is likely to develop unless nurses intervene. For example, all people admitted to a hospital have some possibility of acquiring an infection; however, a patient with diabetes or a compromised immune system is at higher risk than others. Therefore, the nurse would appropriately use the label *risk for infection* to describe the patient's health status.
3. A **wellness diagnosis** '[d]escribes human responses to levels of wellness in an individual, family or community that have a readiness for enhancement' (NANDA International, 2003: 263). Examples of wellness diagnosis would be *readiness for enhanced spiritual well-being* or *readiness for enhanced family coping*.
4. A **possible nursing diagnosis** is one in which evidence about a health problem is incomplete or unclear. A possible diagnosis requires more data either to support or to refute it. For example, an elderly widow who lives alone is admitted to the hospital. The nurse notices that she has no visitors and is pleased with attention and conversation from the nursing staff. Until more data are collected, the nurse may write a nursing diagnosis of **possible social isolation** related to unknown aetiology.
5. A **syndrome diagnosis** is a diagnosis that is associated with a cluster of other diagnoses (Alfaro-LeFevre, 1998). Currently six syndrome diagnoses are on the NANDA International list. *Risk for disuse syndrome*, for example, may be experienced by long-term bedridden patients. Clusters of diagnoses associated with this syndrome include *impaired physical mobility, risk for impaired tissue integrity, risk for activity intolerance, risk for constipation, risk for infection, risk for injury, risk for powerlessness, impaired gas exchange*, and so on.

Components of a NANDA Nursing Diagnosis

A nursing diagnosis has three components: (1) the problem and its definition, (2) the aetiology and (3) the defining characteristics. Each component serves a specific purpose.

Problem (Diagnostic Label) and Definition

The problem statement, or diagnostic label, describes the patient's health problem or response for which nursing therapy is given. It describes the patient's health status clearly and concisely in a few words. The purpose of the diagnostic label is to direct the formation of patient goals and desired outcomes. It may also suggest some nursing interventions.

To be clinically useful, diagnostic labels need to be specific; when the word *specify* follows a NANDA label, the nurse states the area in which the problem occurs, for example, *deficient knowledge (medications)* or *deficient knowledge (dietary adjustments)*.

Qualifiers are words that have been added to some NANDA labels to give additional meaning to the diagnostic statement; for example:

+ *deficient* (inadequate in amount, quality or degree; not sufficient; incomplete)
+ *impaired* (made worse, weakened, damaged, reduced, deteriorated)
+ *decreased* (lesser in size, amount or degree)

Table 9-10 Components of a Nursing Diagnosis Label

Diagnosis and definition	Aetiology/related factors	Defining characteristics
Activity intolerance: Insufficient physiological or psychological energy to endure or complete required or desired daily activities	Bedrest or immobility Generalised weakness Imbalance between oxygen supply/demand Sedentary lifestyle	Verbal report of fatigue or weakness Abnormal heart rate or blood pressure response to activity ECG changes reflecting arrhythmias or ischaemia Exertional discomfort or dyspnoea

Note: From *Nursing Diagnoses: Definitions and Classifications, 2007–2008*, by NANDA International, 2003, Philadelphia: Author. Reprinted with permission.

+ *ineffective* (not producing the desired effect)
+ *compromised* (to make vulnerable to threat).

Each diagnostic label approved by NANDA carries a definition that clarifies its meaning. For example, the definition of the diagnostic label *activity intolerance* is shown in Table 9-10.

Aetiology (Related Factors and Risk Factors)

The aetiology component of a nursing diagnosis identifies one or more probable causes of the health problem, gives direction to the required nursing therapy and enables the nurse to individualise the patient's care. As shown in Table 9-10, the probable causes of *activity intolerance* include sedentary lifestyle, generalised weakness, and so on. Differentiating among possible causes in the nursing diagnosis is essential because each may require different nursing interventions. Table 9-11 provides examples of problems that have different aetiologies and therefore require different interventions.

Defining Characteristics

Defining characteristics are the cluster of signs and symptoms that indicate the presence of a particular diagnostic label. For actual nursing diagnoses, the defining characteristics are the patient's signs and symptoms. For risk nursing diagnoses, no subjective and objective signs are present. Thus the factors that cause the patient to be more than 'normally' vulnerable to the problem form the aetiology of a risk nursing diagnosis.

The NANDA lists of defining characteristics are still being developed and refined. Characteristics are listed separately according to whether they are subjective or objective in nature.

Differentiating Nursing Diagnoses from Medical Diagnoses

A nursing diagnosis is a statement of nursing judgement and refers to a condition that nurses are permitted to treat. A medical diagnosis is made by a physician and refers to a condition that only a physician can treat. Medical diagnoses refer to disease processes – specific pathophysiological responses that are fairly uniform from one patient to another. In contrast, nursing diagnoses describe a patient's physical, sociocultural, psychological and spiritual responses to an illness or a health problem. See how these responses vary among individuals:

Seventy-year-old Joan Adams and 20-year-old Sarah Edwards both have rheumatoid arthritis. Their disease processes are much the same. X-ray studies show that in both patients, the extent of inflammation and the number of joints involved are similar, and both patients experience almost constant pain. Mrs Adams views her condition as part of the ageing process and is responding with acceptance. Ms Edwards, however, is responding with anger and hostility because she views her disease as a threat to her personal identity, role performance and self-esteem.

Table 9-11 Examples of Nursing Interventions to Address Different Aetiologies

Diagnostic label (problem)	Patient	Aetiology	Example of nursing interventions
Constipation	David Davies	Long-term laxative use	Work with Mr Davies to develop a plan for gradual withdrawal from the laxatives; teach components of a high-fibre diet.
	Aida Ede	Inactivity and insufficient fluid intake	Help Ms Ede develop an exercise regimen that she can follow at home; obtain information about her daily schedule and types of fluids she likes; help Ms Ede develop a plan for including sufficient amounts of fluids in her diet.
Ineffective breastfeeding	Zoe Ball	Breast engorgement	Teach Ms Ball to massage her breasts before feeding; use hot packs or hot shower before nursing infant.
	Binda Singh	Inexperience and lack of knowledge	Teach Ms Singh to feed infant on demand; show her how to be sure infant is sucking and swallowing; and demonstrate different holding positions for feedings.

A patient's medical diagnosis remains the same for as long as the disease process is present, but nursing diagnoses change as the patient's responses change. Ms Edwards response to her illness may change over time to become more similar to that of Mrs Adams.

Nurses have responsibilities related to both medical and nursing diagnoses. Nursing diagnoses relate to the nurse's **independent functions**, that is, the areas of healthcare that are unique to nursing and separate and distinct from medical management.

Nurses may not prescribe all the care for a nursing diagnosis, but if the problem is a nursing diagnosis, the nurse can prescribe most of the interventions needed for prevention or resolution. For example, most patients with a nursing diagnosis of *pain* have medical prescriptions for analgesics, but many independent nursing interventions can also alleviate pain (e.g. distraction techniques or teaching a patient to 'splint' an incision).

Differentiating Nursing Diagnoses from Collaborative Problems

A collaborative problem is a type of potential problem that nurses manage using both independent and physician-prescribed interventions. Independent nursing interventions for a collaborative problem focus mainly on monitoring the patient's condition and preventing development of the potential complication. Definitive treatment of the condition requires both medical and nursing interventions.

Collaborative problems tend to be present when a particular disease or treatment is present; that is, each disease or treatment has specific complications that are always associated with it. For example, a statement of collaborative problems is 'Potential complication of pneumonia: atelectasis, respiratory failure, pleural effusion, pericarditis and meningitis'.

Nursing diagnoses, by contrast, involve human responses, which vary greatly from one person to the next. Therefore, the same set of nursing diagnoses cannot be expected to occur with a particular disease or condition; moreover, a single nursing diagnosis may occur as a response to any number of diseases. For example, all postpartum/post birth maternity patients have similar collaborative problems, such as 'Potential complication of childbearing: postpartum haemorrhage', but not all new mothers have the same nursing diagnoses. Some might experience *impaired parenting* (delayed bonding), but most will not; some might have a *deficient knowledge* problem whereas others will not. Table 9-12 provides a comparison of nursing diagnoses, medical problems and collaborative problems.

Table 9-12 Comparison of Nursing Diagnoses, Medical Diagnoses and Collaborative Problems

Category	Nursing diagnoses	Medical diagnoses	Collaborative problems
Example	*Activity intolerance* related to decreased cardiac output	Myocardial infarction	Potential complication of myocardial infarction: congestive heart failure
Description	Describe human responses to disease process or health problem; consist of a one-, two- or three-part statement, usually including problem and aetiology	Describe disease and pathology; do not consider other human responses; usually consist of not more than three words	Involve human responses – mainly physiologic complications of disease, tests or treatments; consist of a two-part statement of situation/pathophysiology and the potential complication
Orientation and responsibility for diagnosing	Oriented to the individual; nurses responsible for diagnosing	Oriented to pathology; physician responsible for diagnosing; diagnosis not within the scope of nursing practice	Oriented to pathophysiology; nurses responsible for diagnosing
Treatment orders	Nurse orders most interventions to prevent and treat	Physician orders primary interventions to prevent and treat	Nurse collaborates with physician and other healthcare professionals to prevent and treat (require medical orders) for definitive treatment
Nursing focus	Treat and prevent	Implement medical orders for treatment and monitor status of condition	Prevent and monitor for onset or status of condition
Nursing actions	Independent	Dependent (primarily)	Some independent actions, but primarily for monitoring and preventing
Duration	Can change frequently	Remains the same while disease is present	Present when disease or situation is present
Classification system	Classification system is developed and being used but is not universally accepted	Well-developed classification system accepted by the medical profession	No universally accepted classification system

THE DIAGNOSTIC PROCESS

The diagnostic process uses the critical-thinking skills of analysis and synthesis. Critical thinking is a cognitive process during which a person reviews data and considers explanations before forming an opinion. Analysis is the separation into components, that is, the breaking down of the whole into its parts. Synthesis is the opposite, that is, the putting together of parts into the whole.

The diagnostic process is used continuously by most nurses. An experienced nurse may enter a patient's room and immediately observe significant data and draw conclusions about the patient. As a result of attaining knowledge, skill and expertise in the practice setting, the expert nurse may seem to perform these mental processes automatically. Novice nurses, however, need guidelines to understand and formulate nursing diagnoses. The diagnostic process has three steps:

1. analysing data,
2. identifying health problems, risks and strengths,
3. formulating diagnostic statements.

Analysing Data

In the diagnostic process, analysing involves the following steps:

1. Compare data against standards (identify significant cues).
2. Cluster cues (generate tentative hypotheses).
3. Identify gaps and inconsistencies.

For experienced nurses, these activities occur continuously rather than sequentially.

Comparing Data with Standards

Nurses draw on knowledge and experience to compare patient data to standards and norms and identify significant and relevant cues. A **standard** or **norm** is a generally accepted measure, rule, model or pattern. The nurse uses a wide range of standards, such as growth and development patterns, normal vital signs and laboratory values. A cue is considered significant if it does any of the following (Gordon, 2002):

+ Points to negative or positive change in a patient's health status or pattern. These may be positive or negative cues. For example, the patient states: 'I have recently experienced shortness of breath while climbing stairs' or 'I have not smoked for three months.'
+ Varies from norms of the patient population. The patient's pattern may fit within cultural norms but vary from norms of the general society. The patient may consider a pattern – for example, eating very small meals and having little appetite – to be normal. This pattern, however, may not be productive and may require further exploration.
+ Indicates a developmental delay. To identify significant cues, the nurse must be aware of the normal patterns and changes that occur as the person grows and develops. For example, by age nine months an infant is usually able to sit alone without support. The infant who has not accomplished this task needs further assessment for possible developmental delays.

Table 9-13 lists specific examples of patient cues and norms to which they may be compared.

Table 9-13 Comparing Cues to Standards and Norms

Type of cue	Patient cues	Standard/norm
Deviation from population norms	Height is 158 cm (5 ft 2 in). Woman with small frame. Weighs 109 kg.	Height and weight tables indicate that the 'ideal' weight for a woman 158 cm (5 ft 2 in) with a small frame is 49–53 kg.
Developmental delay	Child is 17 months old. Parents' state child has not yet attempted to speak. Child laughs aloud and makes cooing sounds.	Children usually speak their first word by 10 to 12 months of age.
Changes in patient's usual health status	States, 'I'm just not hungry these days.' Ate only 15% of food on breakfast tray. Has lost 13 kg in past three months.	Patient usually eats three balanced meals per day. Adults typically maintain stable weight.
Dysfunctional behaviour	Luke's mother reports that Luke has not left his room for two days. Luke is age 16. Luke has stopped attending school and has withdrawn from social contact.	Adolescents usually like to be with their peers; social group very important. Functional behaviour includes school attendance.
Changes in patient's usual behaviour	Mrs Mosford reports that lately her husband angers easily. 'Yesterday he even yelled at the dog.' 'He just seems so tense.'	Mr Mosford is usually relaxed and easygoing. He is friendly and kind to animals.

Clustering Cues

Data clustering or grouping cues is a process of determining the relatedness of facts and determining whether any patterns are present, whether the data represent isolated incidents, and whether the data are significant. This is the beginning of synthesis.

The nurse may cluster data inductively by combining data from different assessment areas to form a pattern. Or the nurse may begin with a framework, such as Gordon's functional health patterns, and cluster the subjective and objective data into the appropriate categories. The latter is a deductive approach to data clustering, or pattern formation.

Experienced nurses may cluster data as they collect and interpret it, as evidenced in remarks or thoughts such as 'I'm getting a picture of . . .' or 'This cue doesn't fit the picture.' The novice nurse does not have the knowledge base or the clinical experience that aids in recognising cues. Thus the novice must take careful assessment notes, search data for abnormal cues and use textbook resources for comparing the patient's cues with the defining characteristics and aetiologic factors of the accepted nursing diagnoses.

Data clustering involves making inferences about the data. The nurse interprets the possible meaning of the cues and labels the cue clusters with tentative diagnostic hypotheses.

Identifying Gaps and Inconsistencies in Data

Skilful assessment minimises gaps and inconsistencies in data. However, data analysis should include a final check to ensure that data are complete and correct.

Inconsistencies are conflicting data. Possible sources of conflicting data include measurement error, expectations and inconsistent or unreliable reports. For example, a nurse may learn from the nursing history that the patient reports not having seen a doctor in 15 years, yet during the physical health examination he states, 'My doctor takes my blood pressure every year.' All inconsistencies must be clarified before a valid pattern can be established.

Identifying Health Problems, Risks and Strengths

After data are analysed, the nurse and patient can together identify strengths and problems. This is primarily a decision-making process discussed earlier.

Determining Problems and Risks

After grouping and clustering the data, the nurse and patient together identify problems that support tentative actual, risk and possible diagnoses. In addition the nurse must determine whether the patient's problem is a nursing diagnosis, medical diagnosis or collaborative problem. See Figure 9-5.

Determining Strengths

At this stage, the nurse and patient also establish the patient's strengths, resources and abilities to cope. Most people have a clearer perception of their problems or weaknesses than of their strengths and assets, which they often take for granted. By

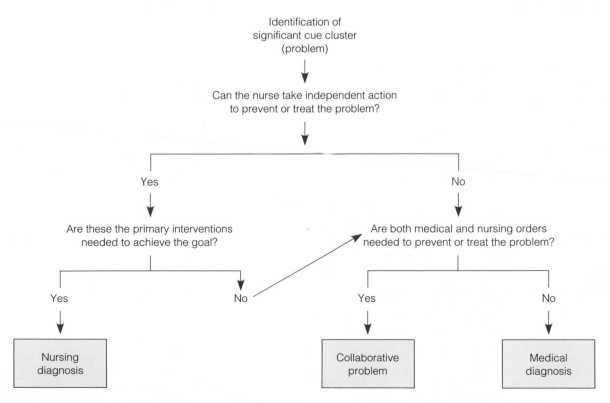

Figure 9-5 Decision tree for differentiating among nursing diagnoses, collaborative problems and medical diagnoses.

taking an inventory of strengths, the patient can develop a more well-rounded self-concept and self-image. Strengths can be an aid to mobilising health and regenerative processes.

A patient's strength might be weight that is within the normal range for age and height, thus enabling the patient to cope better with surgery. In another instance, a patient's strengths might be absence of allergies and being a nonsmoker.

A patient's strengths can be found in the nursing assessment record (health, home life, education, recreation, exercise, work, family and friends, religious beliefs and sense of humour, for example), the health examination and the patient's records.

Formulating Diagnostic Statements

Most nursing diagnoses are written as two-part or three-part statements, but there are variations of these.

Basic Two-Part Statements

The basic two-part statement includes the following:

1. *Problem (P)*: statement of the patient's response (NANDA label).
2. *Aetiology (E)*: factors contributing to or probable causes of the responses.

The two parts are joined by the words *related to* rather than *due to*. The phrase *due to* implies that one part causes or is responsible for the other part. By contrast, the phrase *related to* merely implies a relationship. Some examples of two-part nursing diagnoses are shown in *Box 9-5*.

Basic Three-Part Statements

The basic three-part nursing diagnosis statement is called the **PES format** and includes the following:

1. *Problem (P)*: statement of the patient's response (NANDA label).
2. *Aetiology (E)*: factors contributing to or probable causes of the response.
3. *Signs and symptoms (S)*: defining characteristics manifested by the patient.

Actual nursing diagnoses can be documented by using the three-part statement (see *Box 9-6*) because the signs and symptoms have been identified. This format cannot be used for risk diagnoses because the patient does not have signs and symptoms of the diagnosis.

BOX 9-5 Basic Two-Part Diagnostic Statement

Problem		Aetiology
Constipation	related to	prolonged laxative use
Ineffective Breastfeeding	related to	breast engorgement

The PES format is especially recommended for beginning diagnosticians because the signs and symptoms validate why the diagnosis was chosen and make the problem statement more descriptive.

The disadvantage of the PES format is that it can create very long problem statements, thereby making the problem and aetiology unclear. However, because the signs and symptoms can be helpful in planning nursing interventions, they should be easily accessible. To promote access without long problem statements, the nurse can record the signs and symptoms in the nursing notes instead of on the care plan. Another possibility, recommended for students, is to list the signs and symptoms on the care plan below the nursing diagnosis, grouping the subjective (S) and objective (O) data. The signs and symptoms are easily accessible, and the problem and aetiology stand out clearly. For example:

Noncompliance (diabetic diet) related to unresolved anger about diagnosis as manifested by:

S – 'I forget to take my medication.'
'I can't live without sugar in my food.'
O – Weight 98 kg [gain of 4.5 kg]
Blood pressure 190/100

One-Part Statements

Some diagnostic statements, such as wellness diagnoses and syndrome nursing diagnoses, consist of a NANDA label only. As the diagnostic labels are refined they tend to become more specific, so that nursing interventions can be derived from the label itself. Therefore, an aetiology may not be needed. For example, adding an aetiology to the label *rape-trauma syndrome* does not make the label any more descriptive or useful.

NANDA has specified that any new wellness diagnoses will be developed as one-part statements beginning with the words

BOX 9-6 Basic Three-Part Diagnostic Statement

Problem		Aetiology		Signs and symptoms
Situational low self-esteem	related to (r/t)	rejection by husband	as manifested by (a.m.b.)	hypersensitivity to criticism; states 'I don't know if I can manage by myself' and rejects positive feedback

readiness for enhanced followed by the desired higher level wellness (e.g. *readiness for enhanced parenting*).

Currently the NANDA list includes several wellness diagnoses. Some of these are *spiritual well-being, effective breastfeeding, health-seeking behaviours* and *anticipatory grieving*. These are usually accepted as one-part statements but may be made more explicit by adding a descriptor, for example, *health-seeking behaviours (low-fat diet)*.

Variations of Basic Formats

Variations of the basic one-, two- and three-part statements include the following:

+ Writing *unknown aetiology* when the defining characteristics are present but the nurse does not know the cause or contributing factors. One example is *noncompliance (medication regimen) related to unknown aetiology*.
+ Using the phrase *complex factors* when there are too many aetiologic factors or when they are too complex to state in a brief phrase. The actual causes of chronic low self-esteem, for instance, may be long term and complex, as in the following nursing diagnosis: *chronic low self-esteem related to complex factors*.
+ Using the word *possible* to describe either the problem or the aetiology. When the nurse believes more data are needed about the patient's problem or the aetiology, the word *possible* is inserted. Examples are *possible low self-esteem related to loss of job and rejection by family; altered thought processes possibly related to unfamiliar surroundings*.
+ Using *secondary to* to divide the aetiology into two parts, thereby making the statement more descriptive and useful. The part following *secondary to* is often a pathophysiological or disease process, as in *risk for impaired skin integrity related to decreased peripheral circulation secondary to diabetes*.
+ Adding a second part to the general response or NANDA label to make it more precise. For example, the diagnosis *impaired skin integrity* does not indicate the location of the problem. To make this label more specific, the nurse can add a descriptor as follows: *impaired skin integrity (left lateral ankle) related to decreased peripheral circulation*.

Collaborative Problems

Carpenito (1997) suggests that all collaborative (multidisciplinary) problems begin with the diagnostic label *potential complication* (PC). Nurses should include in the diagnostic statement both the possible complication they are monitoring and the disease or treatment that is present to produce it. For example, if the patient has a head injury and could develop increased intracranial pressure, the nurses should write the following:

Potential complication of head injury: Increased intracranial pressure

When monitoring for a group of complications associated with a disease or pathology, the nurse states the disease and follows it with a list of the complications:

Potential complication of pregnancy-induced hypertension: seizures, foetal distress, pulmonary oedema, hepatic/renal failure, premature labour, CNS haemorrhage

Evaluating the Quality of the Diagnostic Statement

In addition to using the correct format, nurses must consider the content of their diagnostic statements. The statements should, for example, be accurate, concise, descriptive and specific. The nurse must always validate the diagnostic statements with the patient and compare the patient's signs and symptoms to the NANDA defining characteristics. For risk problems, the nurse compares the patient's risk factors to NANDA risk factors.

Avoiding Errors in Diagnostic Reasoning

Some error is inherent in any human undertaking and diagnosis is no exception. However, it is important that nurses make nursing diagnoses with a high level of accuracy. Nurses can avoid some common errors of reasoning by recognising them and applying the appropriate critical-thinking skills. Error can occur at any point in the diagnostic process: data collection, data interpretation and data clustering. The following suggestions help to minimise diagnostic error:

+ *Verify*. Hypothesise possible explanations of the data, but realise that all diagnoses are only tentative until they are verified. Begin and end the diagnostic process by talking with the patient and family. When collecting data, ask them what their health problems are and what they believe the causes to be. At the end of the process, ask them to verify your diagnoses.
+ *Build a good knowledge base and acquire clinical experience*. Nurses must apply knowledge from many different areas to recognise significant cues and patterns and generate hypotheses about the data. To name only a few, principles from chemistry, anatomy and pharmacology each help the nurse understand patient data in a different way.
+ *Have a working knowledge of what is normal*. Nurses need to know the population norms for vital signs, laboratory tests, speech development, and so on. In addition, nurses must determine what is normal for a particular person, taking into account age, physical makeup, lifestyle, culture and the person's own perception of what is normal. For example, normal blood pressure for adults is in the range of 110/60 to 140/80. However, a nurse might obtain a reading of 90/50 that is perfectly normal for a particular patient. The nurse should compare findings to the patient's baseline when possible.
+ *Consult resources*. Both novices and experienced nurses should consult appropriate resources whenever in doubt about a diagnosis. Professional literature, nursing colleagues and other professionals are all appropriate resources.
+ *Base diagnoses on patterns – that is, on behaviour over time – rather than on an isolated incident*.

✦ *Improve critical-thinking skills.* These skills help the nurse to be aware of and avoid errors in thinking, such as overgeneralising, stereotyping, making unwarranted assumptions, and so on.

ONGOING DEVELOPMENT OF NURSING DIAGNOSES

In 1997, NANDA changed the name of its official journal from *Nursing Diagnosis* to *Nursing Diagnosis: The International Journal of Nursing Language and Classification.* The subtitle emphasises that nursing diagnosis is part of a larger, developing system of standardised nursing language worldwide. This system includes classifications of nursing interventions (NIC) and nursing outcomes (NOC) that are being developed by other research groups and linked to the NANDA diagnostic labels.

Research groups are examining what nurses do from different perspectives (diagnoses, interventions and outcomes) to clarify and communicate the role nurses play in the healthcare system. A standardised language will also enable nurses to implement a Nursing Minimum Data Set needed for computerised patient records.

LIFESPAN CONSIDERATIONS

Older Adults

Older adults tend to have multiple problems with complex physical and psychosocial needs when they are ill. If the nurse has done a thorough, accurate assessment, nursing diagnoses can be selected to cover all problems and, at the same time, prioritise the special needs. For example, if a patient is admitted with severe congestive heart failure, prompt attention will be focused on *decreased cardiac output* and *excess fluid volume*, with interventions selected to improve these areas quickly. As these conditions improve, then other nursing diagnoses, such as *activity intolerance* and *deficient knowledge* related to a new medication regime, might require more attention. They are all part of the same medical problem of congestive heart failure, but each nursing diagnosis has specific expected outcomes and nursing interventions. The patient's strengths should be an essential consideration in all phases of the nursing process.

PLANNING

Planning is a deliberative, individual, systematic phase of the nursing process that involves decision making and problem solving. In planning, the nurse refers to the patient's assessment data and diagnostic statements for direction in formulating care goals and designing the nursing interventions required to prevent, reduce or eliminate the patient's health problems (see Figure 9-6). A **nursing intervention** is 'any treatment, based upon clinical judgement and knowledge, that a nurse performs to enhance patient outcomes' (McCloskey and Bulechek, 2000: xix). The product of the planning phase is a patient care plan.

Although planning is basically the nurse's responsibility, input from the patient and support persons is essential if a plan is to be effective. Nurses should not plan for the patient, but encourage the patient to participate actively to the extent possible. In a home setting, the patient's support people and caregivers are the ones who implement the plan of care; thus, its effectiveness depends largely on them.

Types of Planning

Planning begins with the first patient contact and continues until the nurse–patient relationship ends, usually when the patient is discharged from the health setting or nurse's care in the community.

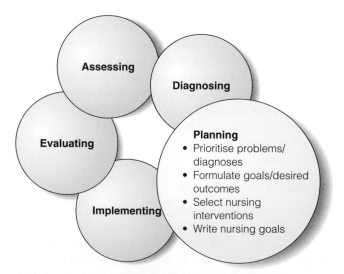

Figure 9-6 Planning. The third phase of the nursing process in which the nurse and patient develop goals/desired outcomes and nursing interventions to prevent, reduce or alleviate the patient's health problems.

Initial Planning

The nurse who performs the admission assessment usually develops the initial comprehensive plan of care. This nurse has the benefit of the patient's body language as well as some intuitive kinds of information that are not available solely from the written database. Planning should be initiated as soon as possible after the initial assessment, especially because of the trend toward shorter hospital stays.

Ongoing Planning

Ongoing planning is done by all nurses who work with the patient. As nurses obtain new information and evaluate the patient's responses to care, they can individualise the initial care plan further. Ongoing planning also occurs at the beginning of a shift as the nurse plans the care to be given that day. Using ongoing assessment data, the nurse carries out daily planning for the following purposes:

+ To determine whether the patient's health status has changed.
+ To set priorities for the patient's care during the shift.
+ To decide which problems to focus on during the shift.
+ To coordinate the nurse's activities so that more than one problem can be addressed at each patient contact.

Discharge Planning

Discharge planning, the process of anticipating and planning for needs after discharge, is a crucial part of comprehensive healthcare and should be addressed in each patient's care plan. Because the average stay of patients in acute care hospitals has become shorter, people are sometimes discharged still needing care. Although many patients are discharged to other agencies (e.g. long-term care facilities or nursing homes), such care is increasingly being delivered in the home. Effective discharge planning begins at first patient contact and involves comprehensive and ongoing assessment to obtain information about the patient's ongoing needs.

DEVELOPING NURSING CARE PLANS

The end product of the planning phase of the nursing process is a formal or informal plan of care. An **informal nursing care plan** is a strategy for action that exists in the nurse's mind. For example, the nurse may think, 'Mrs Lewis is very tired. I will need to reinforce her teaching after she is rested.' A **formal nursing care plan** is a written or computerised guide that organises information about the patient's care. The most obvious benefit of a formal written care plan is that it provides for continuity of care.

A **standardised care plan** is a formal plan that specifies the nursing care for groups of patients with common needs (e.g. all patients with myocardial infarction). An **individualised care plan** is tailored to meet the unique needs of a specific patient – needs that are not addressed by the standardised plan. It is important that all caregivers work toward the same outcomes and, if available, use approaches shown to be effective with a particular patient. Nurses also use the formal care plan for direction about what needs to be documented in patient progress notes and as a guide for delegating and assigning staff to care for patients. When nurses use the patient's nursing diagnoses to develop goals and nursing interventions, the result is a holistic, individualised plan of care that will meet the patient's unique needs.

Care plans include the actions nurses must take to address the patient's nursing diagnoses and produce the desired outcomes. The nurse begins the plan when the patient is admitted to the nursing care setting and constantly updates it throughout the patient's stay in response to changes in the patient's condition and evaluations of goal achievement. During the planning phase the nurse must (a) decide which of the patient's problems need individualised plans and which problems can be addressed by standardised plans and routine care, and (b) write individualised desired outcomes and nursing goals for patient problems that require nursing attention beyond pre-planned, routine care.

The complete plan of care for a patient is made up of several different documents that (a) describe the routine care needed to meet basic needs (e.g. hygiene, nutrition), (b) address the patient's nursing diagnoses and collaborative problems, and (c) specify nursing responsibilities in carrying out the medical plan of care (e.g. keeping the patient from eating or drinking before surgery; scheduling a laboratory test). A complete plan of care integrates dependent and independent nursing functions into a meaningful whole and provides a central source of patient information. Figure 9-7 on page 164 illustrates the various documents that may be included in a nursing care plan.

Standardised Approaches to Care Planning

Most health settings have devised a variety of pre-printed, standardised plans for providing essential nursing care to specified groups of patients who have certain needs in common (e.g. all patients with pneumonia). Standards of care, standardised care plans, protocols, policies and procedures are developed and accepted by the nursing staff in order to (a) ensure that minimally acceptable standards are met and (b) promote efficient use of nurses' time by removing the need to author common activities that are done over and over for many of the patients on a nursing unit/ward.

Standards of care describe nursing actions for patient with similar medical conditions rather than individuals, and they describe achievable rather than ideal nursing care. They define the interventions for which nurses are held accountable; they do not contain medical interventions.

Standardised care plans are pre-printed guides for the nursing care of a patient who has a need that arises frequently in the clinical area (e.g. a specific nursing diagnosis or all nursing diagnoses associated with a particular medical condition). They are written from the perspective of what care the patient

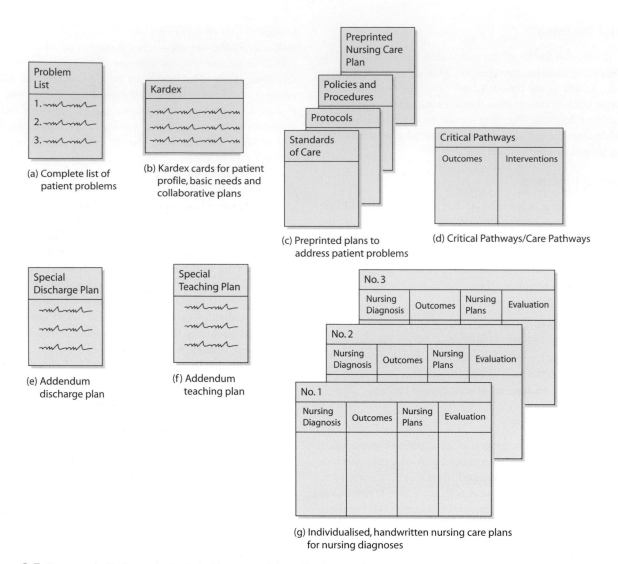

Figure 9-7 Documents that may be included in a complete patient care plan. (Note from Wilkinson, Judith M., *Nursing Process and Critical Thinking*, 3rd Edition, © 2001, pg 436. Reprinted by permission of Pearson Education, Inc, Upper Saddle River, NJ)

can expect. They should not be confused with standards of care. Although the two have some similarities, they have important differences. Figure 9-8, on page 166, shows a standardised care plan for *deficient fluid volume*. Standardised care plans:

+ Are kept with the patients individualised care plan on the ward. When the patient is discharged, they become part of the permanent medical record.
+ Provide detailed interventions and contain additions or deletions from the standards of care.
+ Typically are written in the nursing process format:

    Problem ⇒ Goals/Desired Outcomes ⇒ Nursing Interventions ⇒ Evaluation

+ Frequently include checklists, blank lines or empty spaces to allow the nurse to individualise goals and nursing interventions.

Like standards of care and standardised care plans, **protocols/ care pathways** are pre-printed to indicate the actions commonly required for a particular group of patients. For example, a clinical area may have a protocol for admitting a patient to the intensive care unit, for administering magnesium sulphate to a patient with pre-eclampsia or for caring for a patient receiving continuous epidural analgesia. Protocols may include both medical and nursing interventions.

Policies and **procedures** are developed to govern the handling of frequently occurring situations. For example, a hospital may have a policy specifying the number of visitors a patient may have. Some policies and procedures are similar to protocols and specify what is to be done, for example, in the case of cardiac arrest. If a policy covers a situation pertinent to patient care, it is usually noted on the care plan (e.g. 'Make social service referral according to policy manual'). Policies are institutional records and do not become a part of the care plan or permanent record.

Regardless of whether care plans are handwritten, computerised or standardised, nursing care must be individualised to fit the unique needs of each patient. In practice, a care plan

Aetiology	Desired Outcomes	Nursing Plan/Interventions (Identify Frequency)
✓Decreased oral intake ✓Nausea __Depression ✓Fatigue, weakness __Difficulty swallowing __Other:_____ ✓Excess fluid loss ✓Fever or increased metabolic rate ✓Diaphoresis ✓Vomiting __Diarrhoea __Burns __Other_____ **Defining Characteristics** ✓Insufficient intake ✓Negative balance of intake and output ✓Dry mucous membranes ✓Poor skin turgor __Concentrated urine __Hypernatraemia ✓Rapid, weak pulse __Falling B/P __Weight loss	✓Urinary output > 30 ml/hr ✓Urine specific gravity 1.005–1.025 ✓Serum Na⁺ normal ✓Mucous membranes moist ✓Skin turgor good ✓No weight loss ✓8-hour intake = _400 ml oral_ Other:	✓Monitor intake and output q_1_h ✓Weigh daily ✓Monitor serum electrolyte levels X 1 or until normal ✓Check skin turgor and mucous membranes q_8_h ✓Monitor temperature q_4_h ✓Administer prescribed IV therapy (Monitor according to protocol for Intravenous Therapy) 1000 ml D₅ LR at 100 ml/hr ✓Offer oral liquids q_1_h Type_clear, cold_ ✓Instruct client regarding amount, type and schedule of fluid intake ✓Assess understanding of type of fluid loss; teach accordingly ✓Mouth care prn with _mouthwash_ ✓Institute measures to reduce fever (e.g. lower room temperature, remove bed covers, offer cold liquids) Other Nursing Orders:_____ _Monitor urine specific gravity q shift_

Plan initiated by: _M. Medina RN_ Date _4-15-05_

Plan/outcomes evaluated_____ Date_____

Plan/outcomes evaluated_____ Date_____

Client: _Joe Bloggs_

Figure 9-8 A standardised care plan for the nursing diagnosis of Deficient Fluid Volume.

usually consists of both pre-printed and handwritten sections. The nurse uses standardised care plans for predictable, commonly occurring problems and handwrites an individual plan for unusual problems or problems needing special attention. For example, a standardised care plan for all 'patients with a medical diagnosis of pneumonia' would probably include a nursing diagnosis of *deficient fluid volume* and direct the nurse to assess the patient's hydration status.

Formats for Nursing Care Plans

Although formats differ from care setting to care setting, the care plan is often organised into four columns or categories: (a) nursing diagnoses, (b) goals/desired outcomes, (c) nursing interventions and (d) evaluation. Some agencies use a three-column plan in which evaluation is done in the goals column or in the nurses' notes; others have a five-column plan that adds a column for assessment data preceding the nursing diagnosis column.

Computerised Care Plans

Computers are increasingly being used to create and store nursing care plans. The computer can generate both standardised and individualised care plans. Nurses access the patients stored care plan from a centrally located terminal at the nurses' station or from terminals in patients' rooms. For an individualised plan the nurse chooses the appropriate diagnoses/problems from a menu suggested by the computer. The computer then lists possible goals and nursing interventions for those diagnoses/problems; the nurse chooses those appropriate for the patient and types in any additional goals and interventions or nursing actions not listed on the menu. The nurse can read the plan on the computer screen or print out an updated working copy.

Multidisciplinary (Collaborative) Care Plans

A **multidisciplinary care plan** is a standardised plan that outlines the care required for patients with common, predictable – usually medical – conditions. Such plans, also referred to as **collaborative care plans** and **critical or care pathways**, sequence the care that must be given on each day during the projected length of stay for the specific type of condition. Like the traditional nursing care plan, a multidisciplinary care plan can specify outcomes and nursing interventions to address patient problems (including nursing diagnoses/problems). However, it includes medical treatments to be performed by other healthcare providers as well.

The plan is usually organised with a column for each day, listing the interventions that should be carried out and the patient outcomes that should be achieved on that day. There are as many columns on the multidisciplinary care plan as the preset number of days allowed for the patients' diagnosis-related group (DRG). Multidisciplinary care plans do not include detailed nursing activities. They should be drawn from but do not replace standards of care and standardised care plans.

Guidelines for Writing Nursing Care Plans

The nurse should use the following guidelines when writing nursing care plans:

1. *Date and sign the plan.* The date the plan is written is essential for evaluation, review and future planning. The nurse's signature demonstrates accountability to the patient and to the nursing profession, since the effectiveness of nursing actions can be evaluated.

2. *Use category headings*: 'Nursing Problems', 'Goals/Desired Outcomes', 'Nursing Interventions' and 'Evaluation'. Include a date for the evaluation of each goal.

3. *Use standardised medical or English symbols and key words rather than complete sentences to communicate your ideas.* For example, write 'Turn and reposition 2h' rather than 'Turn and reposition the patient every two hours.' Or write 'Clean wound with H_2O_2 BD' rather than 'Clean the patient's wound with hydrogen peroxide twice a day, morning and evening.'

4. *Be specific.* Timing is very important when considering interventions so needs to be very clear.

5. *Refer to procedure books or other sources of information rather than including all the steps on a written plan.* For example, write 'See unit procedure book for tracheostomy care,' or attach a standard nursing plan about such procedures as cardiac pacemaker care and pre-operative or post-operative care.

6. *Tailor the plan to the unique characteristics of the patient by ensuring that the patient's choices, such as preferences about the times of care and the methods used, are included.* This reinforces the patient's individuality and sense of control. For example, the written nursing intervention 'Provide orange juice at breakfast rather than other juice' indicates that the patient was given a choice of beverages.

7. *Ensure that the nursing plan incorporates preventive and health maintenance aspects as well as restorative ones.* For example, carrying out the intervention 'Provide active-assistance ROM (range-of-motion) exercises to affected limbs 2h' prevents joint contractures and maintains muscle strength and joint mobility.

8. *Ensure that the plan contains interventions for ongoing assessment of the patient* (e.g. 'Inspect incision 8h').

9. *Include collaborative and coordination activities in the plan.* For example, the nurse may write interventions to ask a dietician or physiotherapist about specific aspects of the patient's care.

10. *Include plans for the patient's discharge and home care needs.* It is often necessary to consult and make arrangements with the community nursing team, social worker and specific agencies that supply patient information and needed equipment. Add teaching and discharge plans as addenda if they are lengthy and complex.

CLINICAL ANECDOTE

Craig, a first-year student: 'Planning the nursing care for a patient is the part that I find the hardest part of the nursing process. I have been told by some friends in their second and third years that the more experience you have the better. Writing goals is easy when you get the language right with the appropriate action verbs and understand some of the procedures better.'

THE PLANNING PROCESS

In the process of developing patient care plans, the nurse engages in the following activities:

+ setting priorities;
+ establishing patient goals/desired outcomes;
+ selecting nursing interventions;
+ writing nursing interventions.

Setting Priorities

Priority setting is the process of establishing a preferential sequence for addressing nursing interventions. The nurse and patient begin planning by deciding which nursing intervention requires attention first, which second, and so on. Instead of rank-ordering interventions, nurses can group them as having high, medium or low priority. Life-threatening problems, such as loss of respiratory or cardiac function, are designated as high priority. Health-threatening problems, such as acute illness and decreased coping ability, are assigned medium priority because they may result in delayed development or cause destructive physical or emotional changes. A low-priority problem is one that arises from normal developmental needs or that requires only minimal nursing support.

It is not necessary to resolve all high-priority intervention before addressing others. The nurse may partially address a high-priority intervention and then deal with an intervention of lesser priority. Furthermore, because patients usually have several problems, the nurse often deals with more than one intervention at a time.

Priorities change as the patient's responses, problems and therapies change. The nurse must consider a variety of factors when assigning priorities, including the following:

1. *Patient's health values and beliefs*: Values concerning health may be more important to the nurse than to the patient. For example, a patient may believe being home for the children to be more urgent than a health problem. When there is such a difference of opinion, the patient and nurse should discuss it openly to resolve any conflict. However, in a life-threatening situation the nurse usually must take the initiative.

2. *Patient's priorities*: Involving the patient in prioritising and care planning enhances cooperation. Sometimes, however, the patient's perception of what is important conflicts with the nurse's knowledge of potential problems or complications. For example, an elderly patient may not regard turning and repositioning in bed as important, preferring to be undisturbed. The nurse, however, aware of the potential complications of prolonged bed rest (e.g. muscle weakness and pressure sores), needs to inform the patient and carry out these necessary interventions.

3. *Resources available to the nurse and patient*: If money, equipment or personnel are scarce in a healthcare setting as is increasingly the case, then a problem may be given a lower priority than usual. Nurses in a home setting, for example, do not have the resources of a hospital. If the necessary resources are not available, the solution of that problem might need to be postponed, or the patient may need a referral. Patient resources, such as finances or coping ability, may also influence the setting of priorities. For example, a patient who is unemployed may defer dental treatment if not available via the NHS; a patient whose husband is terminally ill and dependent on her may feel unable to cope with nutritional guidance directed toward losing weight.

4. *Urgency of the health problem*: Regardless of the framework used, life-threatening situations require that the nurse assign them high priority. Situations that affect the integrity of the patient, that is, those that could have a negative or destructive effect on the patient, also have high priority. Such health problems as drug abuse and radical alteration of self-concept due to amputation can be destructive both to the individual and to the family.

5. *Medical treatment plan*: The priorities for treating health problems must be congruent with treatment by other health professionals. For example, a high priority for the patient might be to become mobile; however, if the medical treatment regimen calls for extended bed rest, then mobility must assume a lower priority in the nursing care plan. The nurse can provide or teach exercises to facilitate mobilisation later, provided the patient's health permits. The nursing intervention related to mobility is not ignored; it is merely deferred.

Establishing Patient Goals/Desired Outcomes

After establishing priorities, the nurse and patient set goals for each nursing problem. On a care plan the **goals/desired**

Table 9-14 Deriving Desired Outcomes from Nursing Diagnoses

Nursing diagnosis/identified problem	Opposite healthy responses (goals)	Desired outcomes
Impaired physical mobility: inability to bear weight on left leg, related to inflammation of knee joint	Improved mobility Ability to bear weight on left leg	Walk with crutches by end of week. Stand without assistance by end of the month.
Ineffective airway clearance related to poor cough effort, secondary to incision pain and fear of damaging sutures	Effective airway clearance	No skin pallor or cyanosis by 12 hours post-operation. Within 24 hours after surgery, will demonstrate good cough effort.

outcomes describe, in terms of observable patient responses, what the nurse hopes to achieve by implementing the nursing interventions.

Some nursing literature differentiates the terms by defining goals as broad statements about the patient's status and desired outcomes as the more specific, observable criteria used to evaluate whether the goals have been met. For example:

Goal (broad):   Improved nutritional status.
Desired outcome (specific):   Gain 5 kg by 25 April.

When goals are stated broadly, as in this example, the care plan must include both goals and desired outcomes. They are sometimes combined into one statement linked as follows:

Improved nutritional status as evidenced by weight gain of 5 kg by 25 April.

Writing the broad, general goal first may help students to think of the specific outcomes that are needed, but the broad goal is just a starting point for planning. It is the specific, observable outcomes that must be written on the care plan and used to evaluate patient progress. Table 9-14 shows both broad goals and specific outcomes.

Purpose of Desired Outcomes/Goals

Desired outcomes/goals serve the following purposes:

1. Provide direction for planning nursing interventions. Ideas for interventions come more easily if the desired outcomes state clearly and specifically what the nurse hopes to achieve.
2. Serve as criteria for evaluating patient progress. Although developed in the planning step of the nursing process, desired outcomes serve as the criteria for judging the effectiveness of nursing interventions and patient progress at the evaluation stage.
3. Enable the patient and nurse to determine when the problem has been resolved.
4. Help motivate the patient and nurse by providing a sense of achievement. As goals are achieved, both patient and nurse can see that their efforts have been worthwhile. This provides motivation to continue following the plan, especially when difficult lifestyle changes need to be made.

BOX 9-7 Examples of Action Verbs

Apply	Drink	Select
Assemble	Explain	Share
Breathe	Help	Sit
Choose	Identify	Sleep
Compare	Inject	State
Define	List	Talk
Demonstrate	Move	Transfer
Describe	Name	Turn
Differentiate	Prepare	Verbalise
Discuss	Report	

Long-Term and Short-Term Goals

Goals may be short term or long term. A short-term goal might be 'Patient will raise right arm to shoulder height by Friday 25 April.' In the same context, a long-term goal might be 'Patient will regain full use of right arm in six weeks.' Short-term goals are useful (a) for patients who require healthcare for a short time and (b) for those who are frustrated by long-term goals that seem difficult to attain and who need the satisfaction of achieving a short-term goal. In an acute care setting, much of the nurse's time is spent on the patient's immediate needs, so most goals are short term. However, patients in acute care settings also need long-term goals to guide planning for their discharge to long-term care settings or home, especially in a managed care environment. Long-term goals are often used for patients who live at home and have chronic health problems and for patients in nursing homes, extended care facilities and rehabilitation centres.

Components of Goal/Desired Outcome Statements

Goal/desired outcome statements should usually have the following four components:

1. *Subject.* The subject – a noun – is the patient, any part of the patient or some attribute of the patient, such as the patient's

pulse or urinary output. The subject is often omitted in goals; it is assumed that the subject is the patient unless indicated otherwise.

2. *Verb.* The verb specifies an action the patient is to perform, for example, what the patient is to do, learn or experience. Verbs that denote directly observable behaviours, such as *administer, show, walk*, must be used. See *Box 9-7*, on page 169, for some examples.

3. *Conditions or modifiers.* Conditions or modifiers may be added to the verb to explain the circumstances under which the behaviour is to be performed. They explain what, where, when or how. For example:
   - *Walks with the help of a stick* (how).
   - *After attending two support group diabetes meetings*, lists signs and symptoms of diabetes (when).
   - *When at home*, maintains weight at existing level (where).
   - Discusses *food pyramid and recommended daily servings* (what).

   Conditions need not be included if the criterion of performance clearly indicates what is expected.

4. *Criterion of desired performance.* The criterion indicates the standard by which a performance is evaluated or the level at which the patient will perform the specified behaviour. These criteria may specify time or speed, accuracy, distance and quality. To establish a time-achievement criterion, the nurse needs to ask 'How long?' To establish an accuracy criterion, the nurse asks 'How well?' Similarly, the nurse asks 'How far?' and 'What is the expected standard?' to establish distance and quality criteria, respectively. Examples are:
   - Weighs 75 kg *by 25 April* (time).
   - Lists *five out of six* signs of diabetes (accuracy).
   - Walks *one mile per day* (time and distance).
   - Administers insulin *using aseptic technique* (quality).

   Table 9-15 illustrates the format that should be used to write outcomes.

Guidelines for Writing Goals/Desired Outcomes

The following guidelines can help nurses write useful goals and desired outcomes:

1. Write goals and outcomes in terms of patient responses, not nurse activities. Beginning each goal statement with *the patient/name will* may help focus the goal on patient behaviours and responses. Avoid statements that start with *enable, facilitate, allow, let, permit* or similar verbs followed by the word *patient*. These verbs indicate what the nurse hopes to accomplish, not what the patient will do:
   - *Correct*: Patient will drink 100 ml of water per hour (patient behaviour)
   - *Incorrect*: Maintain patient hydration (nursing action).

2. Be sure that desired outcomes are realistic for the patient's capabilities, limitations and designated time span, if it is indicated. Limitations refers to finances, equipment, family support, social services, physical and mental condition and time. For example, the outcome 'Measures insulin accurately' may be unrealistic for a patient who has poor vision due to cataracts.

3. Ensure that the goals and desired outcomes are compatible with the therapies of other professionals. For example, the outcome 'Will increase the time spent out of bed by 15 minutes each day' is not compatible with a doctor's prescribed therapy of bed rest.

4. Make sure that each goal is derived from only one nursing problem. For example, the goal 'The patient will increase the amount of nutrients ingested and show progress in the ability to feed self' is derived from two nursing diagnoses: *feeding self-care deficit* and *impaired nutrition: less than body requirements*. Keeping the goal statement related to only one diagnosis/problem facilitates evaluation of care by ensuring that planned nursing interventions are clearly related to the diagnosis/problem identified.

5. Use observable, measurable terms for outcomes. Avoid words that are vague and require interpretation or judgement by the observer. For example, phrases such as *increase daily exercise* and *improve knowledge of nutrition* can mean different things to different people. If used in outcomes, these phrases can lead to disagreements about whether the outcome was met. These phrases may be suitable for a broad patient goal but are not sufficiently clear and specific to guide the nurse when evaluating patient responses.

Table 9-15 Components of Goals/Desired Outcomes

Subject	Verb	Conditions/modifiers	Criterion of desired performance
Patient	drinks	2,500 ml of fluid	daily (time)
Patient	administers	correct insulin dose	using aseptic technique (quality standard)
Patient	lists	three hazards of smoking (after reading literature)	(accuracy indicated by 'three hazards')
Patient	recalls	five symptoms of diabetes before discharge	(accuracy indicated by 'five symptoms')
Patient	walks	the length of the ward without a stick	by date of discharge (time)
Patient	measures	less than 10 inches in circumference	in 48 hours (time)
Patient	performs	leg ROM exercises as taught	every 8 hours (time)
Patient	identifies	foods high in salt from a prepared list	before discharge (time)
Patient	states	the purposes of his medications	before discharge (time)

6. Make sure the patient considers the goals/desired outcomes important and values them. Some outcomes, such as those for problems related to self-esteem, parenting and communication, involve choices that are best made by the patient or in collaboration with the patient.

Some patients may know what they wish to accomplish with regard to their health problem; others may not know all the outcome possibilities. The nurse must actively listen to the patient to determine personal values, goals and desired outcomes in relation to current health concerns. Patients are usually motivated and expend the necessary energy to reach goals they consider important.

Selecting Nursing Interventions and Activities

Nursing interventions and activities are the actions that a nurse performs to achieve patient goals. The specific interventions chosen should focus on eliminating or reducing the aetiology of the nursing diagnosis/problem identified, which is the second clause of the diagnostic statement.

Types of Nursing Interventions

Nursing interventions are identified and written during the planning step of the nursing process; however, they are actually performed during the implementing step. Nursing interventions include both direct and indirect care, as well as nurse-initiated, medical-initiated and other provider-initiated treatments. Direct care is an intervention performed through interaction with the patient. Indirect care is an intervention performed away from but on behalf of the patient such as interdisciplinary collaboration or management of the care environment.

Independent interventions are those activities that nurses perform on the basis of their knowledge and skills. They include physical care, ongoing assessment, emotional support and comfort, teaching, counselling, environmental management and making referrals to other healthcare professionals. McCloskey and Bulechek (2000) refer to these as *nurse-initiated treatments*. In performing an autonomous activity, the nurse determines that the patient requires certain nursing interventions; either carries these out or delegates them to other nursing personnel, and is accountable or answerable for the decision and the actions. An example of an independent action is planning and providing special mouth care for a patient after diagnosing/identifying *impaired oral mucous membranes.*

Dependent interventions are activities carried out according to specified routines. McCloskey and Bulechek (2000) call these *medical-initiated treatments*. Medical treatment commonly includes prescribed medications, intravenous therapy, diagnostic tests, treatments, diet and activity. The nurse is responsible for explaining, assessing the need for and administering the medical interventions. Nursing interventions may be written to individualise the medical treatment based on the patient's status.

Collaborative interventions are actions the nurse carries out in collaboration with other health team members, such as physiotherapists, social workers, dietitians and physicians. Collaborative nursing activities reflect the overlapping responsibilities of, and collegial relationships between, health personnel. For example, the doctor might recommend physiotherapy to teach the patient crutch-walking. The nurse would be responsible for informing the physiotherapy department and for coordinating the patient's care to include the physiotherapy sessions. When the patient returns to the ward, the nurse would assist with crutch-walking and collaborate with the physiotherapist to evaluate the patient's progress.

The amount of time the nurse spends in an independent versus a collaborative or dependent role varies according to the clinical area, type of institution and specific position of the nurse.

Considering the Consequences of Each Intervention

Usually several possible interventions can be identified for each nursing goal. The nurse's task is to choose those that are most likely to achieve the desired patient outcomes. The nurse begins by considering the risks and benefits of each intervention. An intervention may have more than one consequence. For example, 'Provide accurate information' could result in the following patient behaviours:

+ increased anxiety,
+ decreased anxiety,
+ wish to talk with the doctor,
+ desire to leave the hospital,
+ relaxation.

Determining the consequences of each intervention requires nursing knowledge and experience. For example, the nurse's experience may suggest that providing information the night before the patient's surgery may increase the patient's worry and tension, whereas maintaining the usual rituals before sleep is more effective. The nurse might then consider providing information several days before surgery.

Criteria for Choosing Nursing Interventions

After considering the consequences of the alternative nursing interventions, the nurse chooses one or more that are likely to be most effective. Although the nurse bases this decision on knowledge and experience, the patient's input is important.

The following criteria can help the nurse choose the best nursing interventions. The plan must be:

+ Safe and appropriate for the individual's age, health and condition.
+ Achievable with the resources available. For example, a community nurse might wish to include a nursing intervention for an elderly patient to 'Check blood glucose daily'; but in order for that to occur, either the patient must have intact sight, cognition and memory to carry this out independently, or daily visits from a community nurse must be available and achievable.

+ Congruent with the patient's values, beliefs and culture.
+ Congruent with other therapies (e.g. if the patient is not permitted food, the strategy of an evening snack must be deferred until health permits).
+ Based on nursing knowledge and experience or knowledge from relevant sciences (i.e. based on a rationale).
+ Within established standards of care as determined by law, and the policies of the institution. Many agencies have policies to guide the activities of health professionals and to safeguard patients. Rules for visiting hours and procedures to follow when a patient has a cardiac arrest are examples. If a policy does not benefit patients, nurses have a responsibility to bring this to the attention of the appropriate people.

Writing Nursing Interventions

After choosing the appropriate nursing interventions, the nurse writes them on the care plan. Nursing interventions are instructions for the specific individualised activities the nurse performs to help the patient meet established healthcare goals. The degree of detail included in the nursing intervention depends to some degree on the health personnel who will carry out the intervention.

Date

Nursing interventions are dated when they are written and reviewed regularly at intervals that depend on the individual's needs. In an intensive care unit, for example, the plan of care will be continually monitored and revised. In a community clinic, weekly or bi-weekly reviews may be indicated.

Action Verb

The action verb starts the intervention and must be precise. For example, 'Explain (to the patient) the actions of insulin' is a more precise statement than 'Teach (the patient) about insulin.' 'Measure and record ankle circumference daily at 0900 hrs' is more precise than 'Assess oedema of left ankle daily.' Sometimes a modifier for the verb can make the nursing intervention more precise. For example, 'Apply spiral bandage firmly to left lower leg' is more precise than 'Apply spiral bandage to left leg.'

Content

The content is the what and the where of the intervention. In the preceding order, 'spiral bandage' and 'left leg' state the what and where of the intervention. The content area in this example may also clarify whether the foot or toes are to be left exposed.

Time Element

The time element answers when, how long or how often the nursing action is to occur. Examples are 'Assist patient with bath at 0700 daily' and 'Administer analgesic 30 minutes prior to physiotherapy.'

Signature

The signature of the nurse planning the intervention shows the nurse's accountability and has legal significance.

LIFESPAN CONSIDERATIONS

Older Adults

When a patient is in an extended care facility or a long-term nursing home, interventions and medications often remain the same day after day. It is important to review the care plan on a regular basis, because changes in the condition of older adults may be subtle and go unnoticed. This applies to both changes of improvement or deterioration. Either one should receive attention so that appropriate revisions can be made in expected outcomes and interventions. Outcomes need to be realistic with consideration given to the patient's physical condition, emotional condition, support systems and mental status. Outcomes often have to be stated and expected to be completed in very small steps. For instance, a patient who has had a cerebrovascular accident may spend weeks learning to brush her own teeth or dress herself. When these small steps are successfully completed, it gives the patient a sense of accomplishment and motivation to continue working toward increasing self-care. This particular example also demonstrates the need to work collaboratively with other members of the multidisciplinary team, such as physiotherapists and occupational therapists, to develop the nursing care plan.

The nursing process is action oriented, patient centred and outcome directed. After developing a plan of care based on the assessing and diagnosing phases, the nurse implements the interventions and evaluates the desired outcomes. On the basis of this evaluation, the plan of care is either continued, modified or terminated. As in all phases of the nursing process, patients and support persons are encouraged to participate as much as possible.

IMPLEMENTING

In the nursing process, implementing is the phase in which the nurse implements the nursing interventions. **Implementing** consists of doing and documenting the **activities** that are the specific nursing actions needed to carry out the interventions. The nurse performs or delegates the nursing activities for the interventions that were developed in the planning step and then concludes the implementing step by recording nursing activities and the resulting patient responses.

Although the nurse may act on the patient's behalf (e.g. referring the patient to a community nurse for home care), professional standards support patient and family participation, as in all phases of the nursing process. The degree of participation depends on the patient's health status. For example, an unconscious man is unable to participate in his care and therefore needs to have care given to him. By contrast, a mobile patient may require very little care from the nurse and carry out healthcare activities independently.

Relationship of Implementing to Other Nursing Process Phases

The first three nursing process phases – assessing, diagnosing and planning – provide the basis for the nursing actions performed during the implementing step. In turn, the implementing phase provides the actual nursing activities and patient responses that are examined in the final phase, the evaluating phase. Using data acquired during assessment, the nurse can individualise the care given in the implementing phase, tailoring the interventions to fit a specific patient rather than applying them routinely to categories of patient (e.g. all patients with pneumonia).

While implementing nursing plans, the nurse continues to reassess the patient at every contact, gathering data about the patient's responses to the nursing activities and about any new problems that may develop. A nursing activity on the patient's care plan for *airway management* might read 'record oxygen saturation levels 4 hourly'. When performing this activity, the nurse is both carrying out the intervention (implementing) and performing an assessment.

Not every nursing action is directed by an intervention that follows from a nursing diagnosis/identified problem. Some routine nursing activities are, themselves, assessments. For example, all patients require hygiene, nutrition and elimination. When assisting the patient with these, nurses carry out actions that may involve assessment. For example, while bathing an elderly patient, the nurse observes a reddened area on the patient's sacrum. Or, when emptying a urinary catheter bag, the nurse measures 200 ml of strong-smelling, brown urine.

Implementing Skills

To implement the care plan successfully, nurses need cognitive, interpersonal and technical skills. These skills are distinct from one another; in practice, however, nurses use them in various combinations and with different emphasis, depending on the activity. For instance, when inserting a urinary catheter the nurse needs cognitive knowledge of the principles and steps of the procedure, interpersonal skills to inform and reassure the patient, and technical skill in draping the patient and manipulating the equipment.

The **cognitive skills** (intellectual skills) include problem solving, decision making, critical thinking and creativity. They are crucial to safe, intelligent nursing care. **Interpersonal skills** are all of the activities, verbal and nonverbal, people use when interacting directly with one another. The effectiveness of a nursing action often depends largely on the nurse's ability to communicate with others. The nurse uses therapeutic communication to understand the patient and in turn be understood. A nurse also needs to work effectively with others as a member of the healthcare team.

Interpersonal skills are necessary for all nursing activities: caring, comforting, advocating, referring, counselling and supporting are just a few. Interpersonal skills include conveying knowledge, attitudes, feelings, interest and appreciation of the patient's cultural values and lifestyle. Before nurses can be highly skilled in interpersonal relations, they must have self-awareness and sensitivity to others.

Technical skills are 'hands-on' skills such as manipulating equipment, giving injections and bandaging, moving, lifting and repositioning patients. These skills are also called tasks, procedures or psychomotor skills. The term *psychomotor* includes the interpersonal component, for example, the need to communicate with the patient.

Technical skills require knowledge and, frequently, manual dexterity. The number of technical skills expected of a nurse has greatly increased in recent years because of the increased use of technology, especially in acute care hospitals.

Process of Implementing

The process of implementing (see Figure 9-9, on page 174) normally includes:

+ reassessing the patient;
+ determining the nurse's need for assistance;
+ implementing the nursing interventions;
+ supervising the delegated care;
+ documenting nursing activities.

Reassessing the Patient

Just before implementing an intervention, the nurse must reassess the patient to make sure the intervention is still needed. Even though an intervention is written on the care plan, the patient's condition may have changed. For example, Gayle Tait has a nursing diagnosis of *disturbed sleep pattern* related to anxiety and unfamiliar surroundings. During night checks, the nurse discovers that Gayle is sleeping and therefore defers the back massage that had been planned as a relaxation strategy.

New data may indicate a need to change the priorities of care or the nursing activities. For example, a nurse begins to teach Ms Tuckett, who has diabetes, how to give herself insulin injections. Shortly after beginning the teaching, the nurse realises that Ms Tuckett is not concentrating on the lesson. Subsequent discussion reveals that she is worried about her eyesight and fears she is going blind. Realising that the patient's level of stress is interfering with her learning, the nurse ends the

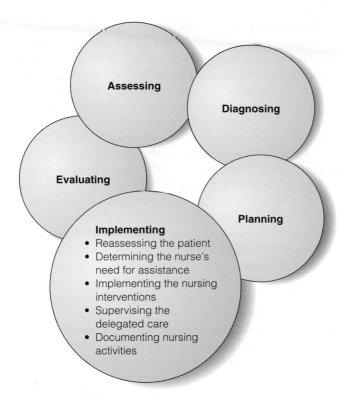

Figure 9-9 Implementing. The fourth phase of the nursing process, in which the nurse implements the nursing interventions and documents the care provided.

lesson and makes arrangements for a doctor to examine the patient's eyes. The nurse also provides supportive communication to help alleviate the patient's stress.

Determining the Nurse's Need for Assistance

When implementing some nursing interventions, the nurse may require assistance for one of the following reasons:

+ The nurse is unable to implement the nursing activity safely alone (e.g. mobilising an unsteady obese patient).
+ Assistance would reduce stress on the patient (e.g. turning a person who experiences acute pain when moved).
+ The nurse lacks the knowledge or skills to implement a particular nursing activity (e.g. a nurse who is not familiar with a particular model of traction equipment needs assistance the first time it is applied).

Implementing the Nursing Interventions

It is important to explain to the patient what interventions will be done, what sensations to expect, what the patient is expected to do and what the expected outcome is. For many nursing activities it is also important to ensure the patient's privacy, for example by closing doors, pulling curtains or covering the patient. The number and kind of direct nursing interventions is almost unlimited. Nurses also coordinate patient care. This activity involves scheduling patient contacts with other

departments (e.g. laboratory and radiographers, physiotherapists and occupational therapists) and serving as a liaison among the members of the healthcare team.

When implementing interventions, nurses should follow these guidelines:

+ Base nursing interventions on scientific knowledge, nursing research and professional standards of care (evidence-based practice) whenever possible. The nurse must be aware of the scientific rationale, as well as possible side effects or complications, of all interventions. For example, a patient prefers to take an oral medication after meals; however, this medication is not absorbed well in the presence of food. Therefore, the nurse will need to explain why this preference cannot be honoured.
+ Clearly understand the interventions to be implemented and question any that are not understood. The nurse is responsible for intelligent implementation of medical and nursing plans of care. This requires knowledge of each intervention, its purpose in the patient's plan of care, any contraindications (e.g. allergies) and changes in the patient's condition that may affect the intervention.
+ Adapt activities to the individual patient. A patient's beliefs, values, age, health status and environment are factors that can affect the success of a nursing action. For example, the nurse determines that a patient chokes when swallowing pills, so consults with the doctor and pharmacist to change the prescription to a liquid form of the medication.
+ Implement safe care. For example, when changing a sterile dressing, the nurse practises sterile technique to prevent infection; when giving a medication, the nurse administers the correct dosage by the ordered route.
+ Provide teaching, support and comfort. These independent nursing activities enhance the effectiveness of nursing care plans.
+ Be holistic. The nurse must always view the patient as a whole and consider the patient's responses in that context.
+ Respect the dignity of the patient and enhance the patient's self-esteem. Providing privacy and encouraging patients to make their own decisions are ways of respecting dignity and enhancing self-esteem.
+ Encourage patients to participate actively in implementing the nursing interventions. Active participation enhances the patient's sense of independence and control. However, patients vary in the degree of participation they desire. Some want total involvement in their care, whereas others prefer little involvement. The amount of desired involvement may be related to the severity of the illness; the patient's culture; or the patient's fear, understanding of the illness and understanding of the intervention.

Supervising Delegated Care

If care has been delegated to other healthcare personnel such as healthcare support workers or assistants, the nurse responsible for the patient's overall care must ensure that the activities have been implemented according to the care plan. Other caregivers may be required to communicate their activities to the nurse by documenting them on the patient record, reporting verbally or filling out a written form. The nurse validates and responds to any adverse findings or patient responses. This may involve modifying the nursing care plan.

Documenting Nursing Activities

After carrying out the nursing activities, the nurse completes the implementing phase by recording the interventions and patient responses in the nursing progress notes. These are a part of the permanent record for the patient. Nursing care must not be recorded in advance because the nurse may determine on reassessment of the patient that the intervention should not or cannot be implemented. For example, a nurse is authorised to inject 10 mg of morphine sulphate subcutaneously to a patient, but the nurse finds that the patient's respiratory rate is 4 breaths per minute. This finding contraindicates the administration of morphine (a respiratory depressant). The nurse withholds the morphine and reports the patient's respiratory rate to the nurse in charge and/or doctor.

The nurse may record routine or recurring activities (e.g. mouth care) in the patient record at the end of a shift. In the meantime, the nurse maintains a personal record of these interventions on a worksheet. In some instances, it is important to record a nursing intervention immediately after it is implemented. This is particularly true of the administration of medications and treatments because recorded data about a patient must be up to date, accurate and available to other nurses and healthcare professionals. Immediate recording helps safeguard the patient, for example, from receiving a duplicate dose of medication.

Nursing activities are communicated verbally as well as in writing. When a patient's health is changing rapidly, the charge nurse and/or the doctor may want to be kept up to date with verbal reports. Nurses also report patient status at a change of shift and on a patient's discharge to another ward or health agency in person, via a voice recording or in writing.

EVALUATING

To evaluate is to judge or to appraise. Evaluating is the fifth and last phase of the nursing process. In this context, **evaluating** is a planned, ongoing, purposeful activity in which patients and healthcare professionals determine (a) the patient's progress toward achievement of goals/outcomes and (b) the effectiveness of the nursing care plan. Evaluation is an important aspect of the nursing process because conclusions drawn from the evaluation determine whether the nursing interventions should be terminated, continued or changed.

Evaluation is continuous. Evaluation done while or immediately after implementing a nursing intervention enables the nurse to make on-the-spot modifications in an intervention. Evaluation performed at specified intervals (e.g. once a week for the patient at home) shows the extent of progress toward goal achievement and enables the nurse to correct any deficiencies and modify the care plan as needed. Evaluation continues until the patient achieves the health goals or is discharged from nursing care. Evaluation at discharge includes the status of goal achievement and the patient's self-care abilities with regard to follow-up care. Most agencies have a special discharge record for this evaluation.

Through evaluating, nurses demonstrate responsibility and accountability for their actions, indicate interest in the results of the nursing activities and demonstrate a desire not to perpetuate ineffective actions but to adopt more effective ones.

Relationship of Evaluating to Other Nursing Process Phases

Successful evaluation depends on the effectiveness of the steps that precede it. Assessment data must be accurate and complete so that the nurse can formulate appropriate nursing interventions and desired outcomes. The desired outcomes must be stated concretely in behavioural terms if they are to be useful for evaluating patient responses. And finally, without the implementing phase in which the plan is put into action, there would be nothing to evaluate.

The evaluating and assessing phases overlap. As previously stated, assessment (data collection) is ongoing and continuous at every patient contact. However, data are collected for different purposes at different points in the nursing process. During the assessment phase the nurse collects data for the purpose of making diagnoses. During the evaluation step the nurse collects data for the purpose of comparing it to pre-selected goals and judging the effectiveness of the nursing care. The act of assessing (data collection) is the same; the differences lie in (a) when the data are collected and (b) how the data are used.

CLINICAL ANECDOTE

Maria, a second-year student: '... evaluating the goals and care plan is easier now than my first year. I always used to feel nervous I would make the wrong evaluation. But I find now that I can do evaluation easier, now that I understand the procedures and interventions better, and how a person should respond to them. It is also easier toward the end of a clinical placement when I have got used to the standard procedures that happen there.'

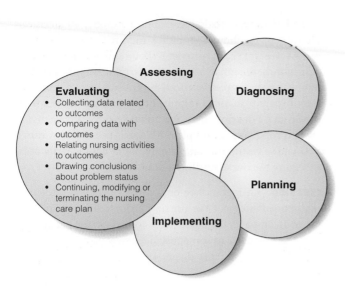

Figure 9-10 Evaluating. The final phase of the nursing process, in which the nurse determines the patient's progress toward goal achievement and the effectiveness of the nursing care plan. The plan may be continued, modified or terminated.

Process of Evaluating Patient Responses

Before evaluation, the nurse identifies the desired outcomes (indicators) that will be used to measure patient goal achievement. (This is done in the planning step.) Desired outcomes serve two purposes: they establish the kind of evaluative data that need to be collected and provide a standard against which the data are judged. For example, given the following expected outcomes, any nurse caring for the patient would know what data to collect:

+ Daily fluid intake will not be less than 2,500 ml.
+ Urinary output will balance with fluid intake.
+ Residual urine will be less than 100 ml.

The evaluation process has five components (see Figure 9-10):

1. Collecting data related to the desired outcomes.
2. Comparing the data with outcomes.
3. Relating nursing activities to outcomes.
4. Drawing conclusions about problem status.
5. Continuing, modifying or terminating the nursing care plan.

Collecting Data

Using the clearly stated, precise and measurable desired outcomes as a guide, the nurse collects data so that conclusions can be drawn about whether goals have been met. It is usually necessary to collect both objective and subjective data.

Some data may require interpretation. Examples of objective data requiring interpretation are the degree of tissue turgor of a dehydrated patient or the degree of restlessness of a patient with pain. When objective data need interpretation, the nurse may obtain the views of other nurses to substantiate whether change has occurred. Examples of subjective data needing

interpretation include complaints of nausea or pain by the patient. When interpreting subjective data, the nurse must rely upon either (a) the patient's statements (e.g. 'My pain is worse now than it was after breakfast') or (b) objective indicators of the subjective data, even though these indicators may require further interpretation (e.g. decreased restlessness, decreased pulse and respiratory rates, and relaxed facial muscles as indicators of pain relief). Data must be recorded concisely and accurately to facilitate the next part of the evaluating process.

Comparing the Data with Outcomes

If the first two parts of the evaluation process have been carried out effectively, it is relatively simple to determine whether a desired outcome has been met. Both the nurse and patient play an active role in comparing the patient's actual responses with the desired outcomes. Did the patient drink 3,000 ml of fluid in 24 hours? Did the patient walk unassisted the specified distance per day? When determining whether a goal has been achieved, the nurse can draw one of three possible conclusions:

+ The goal was met; that is, the patient response is the same as the desired outcome.
+ The goal was partially met; that is, either a short-term goal was achieved but the long-term goal was not, or the desired outcome was only partially attained.
+ The goal was not met.

After determining whether a goal has been met, the nurse writes an evaluative statement (either on the care plan or in the nurse's notes). An **evaluation statement** consists of two parts: a conclusion and supporting data. The conclusion is a statement that the goal/desired outcome was met, partially met or not met. The supporting data are the list of patient responses that support the conclusion, for example:

Goal met: Oral intake 300 ml more than output; skin turgor good; mucous membranes moist.

Relating Nursing Activities to Outcomes

The fourth aspect of the evaluating process is determining whether the nursing activities had any relation to the outcomes. It should never be assumed that a nursing activity was the cause of or the only factor in meeting, partially meeting or not meeting a goal.

For example, Mrs Joan Allen was obese and needed to lose 14 kg. When the nurse and patient drew up a care plan, one goal was 'Lose 1.4 kg by date X.' A nursing strategy in the care plan was 'Explain how to plan and prepare a 900-calorie diet.' On date X, the patient weighed herself and had lost 1.8 kg. The goal had been met – in fact, exceeded. It is easy to assume that the nursing strategy was highly effective. However, it is important to collect more data before drawing that conclusion. On questioning the patient, the nurse might find any of the following: (a) the patient planned a 900-calorie diet and prepared and ate the food; (b) the patient planned a 900-calorie diet but did not prepare the correct food; (c) the patient did not understand how to plan a 900-calorie diet, so she did not bother with it.

If the first possibility is found to be true, the nurse can safely judge that the nursing strategy 'Explain how to plan and prepare a 900-calorie diet' was effective in helping the patient lose weight. However, if the nurse learns that either the second or third possibility actually happened, then it must be assumed that the nursing strategy did not affect the outcome. The next step for the nurse is to collect data about what the patient actually did to lose weight. It is important to establish the relationship (or lack thereof) of the nursing actions to the patient responses.

Drawing Conclusions about Problem Status

The nurse uses the judgements about goal achievement to determine whether the care plan was effective in resolving, reducing or preventing patient problems. When goals have been met, the nurse can draw one of the following conclusions about the status of the patient's problem:

+ The actual problem stated in the nursing diagnosis/goal has been resolved; or the potential problem is being prevented and the risk factors no longer exist. In these instances, the nurse documents that the goals have been met and discontinues the care for the problem.
+ The potential problem stated in the nursing diagnosis/goal is being prevented, but the risk factors are still present. In this case, the nurse keeps the problem on the care plan.
+ The actual problem still exists even though some goals are being met. For example, a desired outcome on a patient's care plan is 'Will drink 3,000 ml of fluid daily.' Even though the data may show this outcome has been achieved, other data (dry oral mucous membranes) may indicate that there is *deficient fluid volume*. Therefore, the nursing interventions must be continued even though this one goal was met.

When goals have been partially met or when goals have not been met, two conclusions may be drawn:

1. The care plan may need to be revised, since the problem is only partially resolved. The revisions may need to occur during assessing, diagnosing or planning phases, as well as implementing.
   OR
2. The care plan does not need revision, because the patient merely needs more time to achieve the previously established goal(s). To make this decision, the nurse must assess why the goals are being only partially achieved, including whether the evaluation was conducted too soon.

Continuing, Modifying or Terminating the Nursing Care Plan

After drawing conclusions about the status of the patient's problems, the nurse modifies the care plan as indicated. Depending on the agency, modifications may be made by drawing a line through portions of the care plan, or marking portions using a highlighting pen, or writing 'Discontinued' and the date.

Whether or not goals were met, a number of decisions need to be made about continuing, modifying or terminating nursing care for each problem. Before making individual modifications, the nurse must first determine why the plan as a whole was not completely effective. This requires a review of the entire care plan and a critique of the nursing process steps involved in its development. See Table 9-16 for a checklist to use when reviewing a care plan. Although the checklist uses a closed-ended yes/no format, its only intent is to identify areas that require the nurse's further examination.

Assessing. An incomplete or incorrect database influences all subsequent steps of the nursing process and care plan. If data are incomplete, the nurse needs to reassess the patient and record the new data. In some instances, new data may indicate the need for new nursing diagnoses/interventions, new goals and new nursing plans.

Diagnosing. If the database is incomplete, new diagnostic statements/interventions may be required. If the database is complete, the nurse needs to analyse whether the problems were identified correctly and whether the nursing diagnoses are relevant to that database. After making judgements about problem status, the nurse revises or adds new diagnoses as needed to reflect the most recent patient data.

Planning: desired outcomes. If a nursing diagnosis is inaccurate, obviously the goal statement will need revision. If the nursing diagnosis is appropriate, the nurse then checks that the goals are realistic and attainable. Unrealistic goals require correction. The nurse should also determine whether priorities have changed and whether the patient still agrees with the priorities. Goals must also be written for any new nursing diagnoses.

Planning: nursing interventions. The nurse investigates whether the nursing interventions were related to goal achievement and whether the best nursing interventions were selected. Even when diagnoses and goals are appropriate, the nursing interventions selected may not have been the best ones to achieve the goal. New nursing interventions may reflect changes in the amount of nursing care the patient needs, scheduling changes, or rearrangement of nursing activities to group similar activities or to permit longer rest or activity periods for the patient. If new nursing diagnoses have been written, then new nursing interventions will also be necessary.

Implementing. Even if all sections of the care plan appear to be satisfactory, the manner in which the plan was implemented may have interfered with goal achievement. Before selecting new interventions, the nurse should check whether the nursing interventions were carried out. Other personnel may not have carried them out, either because the interventions were unclear or because they were unreasonable in terms of external constraints such as resources, staff and equipment.

After making the necessary modifications to the care plan, the nurse implements the modified plan and begins the nursing process cycle again.

Table 9-16 Evaluation Checklist

Assessing	Diagnosing	Planning	Implementing
____ Are data complete, accurate and validated? ____ Do new data require changes in the care plan?	____ Are nursing diagnoses relevant and accurate? ____ Are nursing diagnoses supported by the data? ____ Has problem status changed (i.e. potential, actual, risk)? ____ Are the diagnoses stated clearly and in correct format? ____ Have any nursing diagnoses been resolved?	**Desired outcomes** ____ Do new nursing diagnoses require new goals? ____ Are goals realistic? ____ Was enough time allowed for goal achievement? ____ Do the goals address all aspects of the problem? ____ Does the patient still concur with the goals? ____ Have patient priorities changed? **Nursing interventions** ____ Do nursing interventions need to be written for new nursing diagnoses or new goals? ____ Do the nursing interventions seem to be related to the stated goals? ____ Is there a rationale to justify each nursing order? ____ Are the nursing interventions clear, specific and detailed? ____ Are new resources available? ____ Do the nursing interventions address all aspects of the patient's goals? ____ Were the nursing orders actually carried out?	____ Was patient input obtained at each step of the nursing process? ____ Were goals and nursing interventions acceptable to the patient? ____ Did the caregivers have the knowledge and skill to perform the interventions correctly? ____ Were explanations given to the patient prior to implementing?

Evaluating the Quality of Nursing Care

In addition to evaluating goal achievement for individual patients, nurses are also involved in evaluating and modifying the overall quality of care given to groups of patients. This is an essential part of professional accountability.

Quality Assurance

A **quality-assurance (QA) programme** is an ongoing, systematic process designed to evaluate and promote excellence in the healthcare provided to patients. Quality assurance frequently refers to evaluation of the level of care provided in a health environment, but it may be limited to the evaluation of the performance of one nurse or more broadly involve the evaluation of the quality of the care in an environment or even in a region.

Quality assurance requires evaluation of three components of care: structure, process and outcome. Each type of evaluation requires different criteria and methods, and each has a different focus.

Structure evaluation focuses on the setting in which care is given. It answers this question: What effect does the setting have on the quality of care? Structural standards describe desirable environmental and organisational characteristics that influence care, such as equipment and staffing.

Process evaluation focuses on how the care was given. It answers questions such as these: Is the care relevant to the patient's needs? Is the care appropriate, complete and timely? Process standards focus on the manner in which the nurse uses the nursing process. Some examples of process criteria are 'Checks patient's identification band before giving medication' and 'Performs and records vital signs, once per shift.'

Outcome evaluation focuses on demonstrable changes in the patient's health status as a result of nursing care. Outcome criteria are written in terms of patient responses or health status, just as they are for evaluation within the nursing process. For example, 'How many patients undergoing hip repairs develop pneumonia?' or 'How many patients who have a colostomy experience an infection that delays discharge?'

Quality Improvement

Quality improvement (QI) is also known as continuous quality improvement (CQI), total quality management (TQM), performance improvement (PI) or persistent quality improvement (PQI). According to Schroeder (1994: 3), QI is

the commitment and approach used to continuously improve every process in every part of an organisation, with the intent of meeting and exceeding customer expectations and outcomes.

Unlike quality assurance, QI follows patient care rather than organisational structure, focuses on process rather than individuals, and uses a systematic approach with the intention of *improving* the quality of care rather than *ensuring* the quality of care. QI studies often focus on identifying and correcting a system's problems, such as duplication of services in a hospital or improving services.

Nursing Audit

An **audit** means the examination or review of records. A **retrospective audit** is the evaluation of a patient's record after discharge from a healthcare setting. *Retrospective* means 'relating to past events'. A **concurrent audit** is the evaluation of a patient's healthcare while the patient is still receiving care

within that environment. These evaluations use interviewing, direct observation of nursing care and review of clinical records to determine whether specific evaluative criteria have been met.

Another type of evaluation of care is the **peer review**. In nurse peer review, nurses functioning in the same capacity, that is, peers, appraise the quality of care or practice performed by other equally qualified nurses. The peer review is based on pre-established standards or criteria.

There are two types of peer reviews: individual and nursing audits. The individual peer review focuses on the performance of an individual nurse. The nursing audit focuses on evaluating nursing care through the review of records. The success of these audits depends on accurate documentation; auditors assume that if the data have not been recorded, the care has not been given.

RESEARCH NOTE

How Do We Know If Care Plans Are Patient Focused?

Kirrane (2001) undertook an audit in a neurology unit and acknowledged that there are very diverse views on the usefulness of nursing care plans, care pathways, interdisciplinary care maps and other related tools. She reported on literature supporting evidence of documentation that can speed nursing care and enhance accuracy of documentation. However, no evidence was available to indicate that care plans also were individualised based on patient-focused needs. The methodology chosen to evaluate the question in this institution was an audit tool. Five care plans on each of two neurology units were evaluated and, when possible, the patient or family was interviewed to determine their perspectives on the care plan. Although detailed results of the audit are not provided in the article, it is clear that the

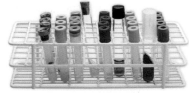

care plans had room for improvement relative to the study question.

Implications

In addition to forming qualitative judgements about the patient-focused nature of the care plans, the author used the results of the audit to provide staff development training in writing more objective and specific plans. Staff was strongly supported to author the plans in concert with the patient and family. A repeated audit 6 months later showed improvement in the use of appropriate documentation and individualisation. In addition, the second audit indicated that patients and families were more aware of the purpose and their role in care planning. The decision was made to have audits become a regular part of care evaluation and to continue to use the results for staff development.

Note: From 'An Audit of Care Planning on a Neurology Unit,' by C. Kirrane, 2001, *Nursing Standard*, 15(19), pp. 36–39.

LIFESPAN CONSIDERATIONS

Older Adults

Evaluation of goals, selected outcomes and interventions needs to be continuous, with ongoing assessment and reassessment of the situation. Priority needs can change quickly and must be reprioritised when problems occur. Older adults may have conditions that impair communication, such as aphasia from a cerebrovascular accident, dementia, multiple sclerosis or other neurological conditions. If this is the case, the nurse needs to

be even more astute in performing nonverbal assessments and detecting changes or problems. Relatives or carers could also be involved in the decision process. If evaluations are done often and thoroughly, changes can be made (even during the same shift) to improve care and intervene more effectively. Communication and interpersonal skills are as essential in the evaluation phase as they are in the initial assessment.

CRITICAL REFLECTION

Let us revisit the case study on page 136. Now that you have read this chapter you need to devise a plan of care for her using the nursing process. What questions would you ask yourself to check this assumption? How would you demonstrate that you are using the critical-thinking attitude of 'confidence in reasoning'? Critical thinkers look for subtle cues. Which cues in this situation require follow-up? What is the main problem you would write a care plan for?

CHAPTER HIGHLIGHTS

+ Critical thinking is an essential component of the decision-making aspect of the nursing process.
+ The nursing process comprises of assessment, diagnosing, planning, implementing and evaluating.
+ Nursing diagnosis is a relatively new concept in UK healthcare but has been developed and used extensively in the USA for many years.

+ When writing goals time frames are very important to measure if the goal has been achieved and assist evaluation.
+ The standard of language used for care planning needs to be concise and explicit to aid clarity in the care the patient receives.
+ Audit is a valuable tool in the healthcare setting to evaluate standards of care and further develop the healthcare delivery system.

REFERENCES

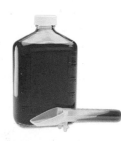

Alfaro-LeFevre, R. (1998) 'Applying the nursing process': A step-by-step guide (4th edn), Philadelphia/New York: Lippincott.

American Nurses Association (1998) Standards of clinical nursing practice (2nd edn), Kansas City, MO: Author.

Benner, P. (1984) From Novice to expert: Excellence and power in clinical nursing practice, Menlo Park, CA: Addison-Wesley.

Carpenito, L.J. (1997) Nursing diagnosis: Application to clinical practice (7th edn), Philadelphia: Lippincott-Raven.

Gordon, M. (2002) Manual of nursing diagnosis (10th edn), St. Louis, MO: Mosby.

Johnson, D.E. (1959) 'A philosophy of nursing', Nursing Outlook, 7, 198–200.

Joint Commission on Accreditation of Healthcare Organisations (2001) Accreditation manual for hospitals, Chicago, IL: Author.

Kirrane, C. (2001) 'An audit of care planning on a neurology unit', Nursing Standard, 15(19), 36–39.

McCloskey, J.C. and Bulechek, G.M. (Eds) (2000) Nursing interventions classification (NIC) (3rd edn), St. Louis, MO: Mosby.

NANDA International (2003) NANDA nursing diagnoses: Definitions and classification 2003–2004, Philadelphia: Author.

O'Carroll, E. (2001) Getting too close (or too far) for comfort. Available from http://www.travel.boston.com/columns/sl/030502_close.html. (Accessed on 23 February 2003.)

Orlando, I. (1961) The dynamic nurse–patient relationship, New York: Putnam.

Schroeder, P. (1994) Improving quality and performance: Concepts programs and techniques, St. Louis, MO: Mosby.

Stewart, C.J. and Cash, W.B., Jr (2002) Interviewing principles and practices (10th edn), New York: McGraw-Hill.

Wiedenbach, E. (1963) 'The helping art of nursing', American Journal of Nursing, 63(11), 54.

Wilkinson, J.M. (2001) Nursing process and critical thinking (3rd edn), Upper Saddle River, NJ: Prentice Hall.

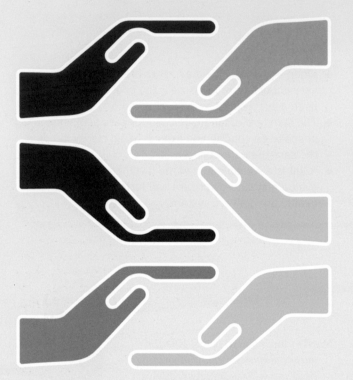

Chapter 10 Mental Health

Learning Outcomes

After completing this chapter, you will be able to:

+ Define the term mental health.

+ Discuss how alcohol and drug dependence can affect mental health.

+ Discuss mood disorders and memory problems, and their effects upon mental health.

+ Define the term schizophrenia.

+ Discuss post traumatic stress disorder.

CASE STUDY

During the early 1990s the traditional, large, Victorian type asylums/psychiatric hospitals that existed in counties throughout the UK were closed or reduced in size. This was to make way for more 'care in the community' for those with mental health problems, in keeping with the policy of the then UK government. During this move to care in the community in some counties it became apparent that some individuals in the 'asylums' had been there for the whole of their lives and were quite elderly.

These patients had either been born in the hospitals as illegitimate children of patients or had been placed in the hospitals because their childhood behaviour did not conform to the norms of society.

The majority of these few survivors of asylums of the late 19th and early 20th centuries had come to accept the institution as their permanent home and developed mental health problems as a result of their institutionalisation.

After reading this chapter you will be able to define mental health and discuss some of the mental health issues that are found in healthcare.

MENTAL HEALTH DEFINED

Mental health is a term used in a healthcare context to refer to an individual's psychological well-being or put simply the health of the mind. A **mental disorder** (any problem affecting mental health) may be defined as a mental illness, arrested or incomplete development of mind, psychopathic disorders and any other disorder or disability of the mind. It is important to differentiate at this stage that although a mental disorder is defined in this manner a learning disability is a separate concept and will be discussed later.

Mental illness is not legally clearly defined in the Mental Health Act 1983 (see Chapter 3) and the courts have considered a definition unnecessary. The legal system therefore suggests that the test should be what the ordinary sensible person would decide on a case-by-case basis. Most admissions under the Mental Health Act 1983 requiring the category of mental disorder to be specified are admissions of individuals with a diagnosis of a mental illness. The conditions that are generally accepted as falling under the category of 'mental illness' include schizophrenia and mood disorders.

The Mental Health Act 1983 defines three other forms of mental disorder:

1. Severe mental impairment: 'a state of arrested or incomplete development of mind which includes severe impairment of intelligence and social functioning and is associated with abnormally aggressive or seriously irresponsible conduct on the part of the person concerned.'
2. Mental impairment: 'a state of arrested or incomplete development of mind (not amounting to a severe mental impairment) which includes significant impairment of intelligence and social functioning and is associated with abnormally aggressive or seriously irresponsible conduct on the part of the person concerned.'
3. Psychopathic disorder: 'a persistent disorder or disability of mind (whether or not including significant impairment of intelligence) which results in abnormally aggressive or seriously irresponsible conduct on the part of the person concerned.'

Historically, within the UK, especially in the late 19th and early 20th centuries a person could be institutionalised in an asylum (the then current term for a mental health hospital), if they had a baby outside of marriage or were classed as sexually deviant (homosexual or bi-sexual). Also, following both the First and Second World Wars soldiers returning from the battle fields who suffered what we would now term post traumatic stress disorder (PTSD) were frequently placed in asylums. Even those who would be regularly drunk in some counties within the UK could be placed into an asylum for 'treatment'. This institutionalisation was society's way of dealing with the problem – out of sight out of mind.

Fortunately society has advanced over the past century in its understanding of mental health issues and how this group of patients is treated. The Mental Health Act 1983 states that a person cannot be treated as mentally disordered solely on the grounds of 'promiscuity or other immoral conduct, sexual deviancy or dependence on alcohol or drugs'.

Terms used within the Mental Health Act are legal, and not medical, categories. While recognising these terms have no legal meaning in the context of the Mental Health Act, many people, in particular people who use mental health services, prefer terms such as 'mental health problems' and 'mental distress' when describing their experience.

Patients with mental health problems frequently feel there is a stigma attached to their illness and they are viewed by society as 'mad'. It is imperative when dealing with those patients who have mental health problems to consider their needs in a sensitive manner regardless of illness type, age, gender, ethnicity, sexual orientation or religious belief system.

SUBSTANCE ABUSE/MISUSE

Alcohol and drug dependence tend to be the two commonest forms of substance misuse encountered within healthcare. Frequently the use of alcohol and drugs may begin as a recreational activity for various reasons such as social, peer pressure or escapism from reality; it may then become a problem of dependence.

In the UK 90% of people drink alcohol as part of normal social culture, an aspect we feel comfortable with as a society. Moderate drinking does not cause many problems; however over the past three decades society has become wealthier and alcohol has become cheaper. Frequently alcohol is used by many to relax after a busy day at work or while engaging in social recreational activities. Many individuals are starting to drink at a younger age and are drinking ever-increasing volumes of alcohol. More than one in four men and about one in seven women are drinking more than is medically safe for them. According to the Department of Health, around one in eight men are physically addicted to alcohol.

Alcohol affects the brain in several ways. First, the body develops a tolerance. Alcohol is like many other drugs that act on the brain, such as tranquillisers. Regular intake reduces the effects that the substance has upon the body. This then results in the need to drink increasing volumes to get the desired affect. Tolerance is a powerful part of becoming addicted to alcohol and directly relates to the dependency effects. Excessive alcohol can also lead to a variety of psychological and physiological conditions. Alcohol dementia or memory loss may develop with prolonged use, rather like Alzheimer's dementia. Unlike Alzheimer's this dementia does not have an age dependent onset and can occur at any age with excessive alcohol use.

Psychosis is also quite common in long-term drinkers who start to hear voices as a result of progressive damage caused by excessive alcohol intake. Dependence is a significant problem – if a heavy drinker stops drinking suddenly, they may develop withdrawal symptoms such as shaking, nervousness and hallucinations.

Suicide and alcohol dependence are closely associated, 40% of men who try to kill themselves have had a long-standing alcohol problem. Of these, 70% who succeed in killing themselves have drunk alcohol before doing so.

The connection between alcohol, depression, suicide and self-harm is one which has been studied for some time. Rates of self-harm and suicide are higher in individuals who suffer with alcohol dependency. An explanation for this is that alcohol acts as an agent that causes depression and tiredness by changing the chemical balance of the brain. Hangovers create a cycle of waking up feeling ill, anxious, jittery and guilty. Regular drinking can make life depressing – family arguments, poor work, unreliable memory and sexual problems.

The dependent person will drink alcohol to relieve anxiety or depression, resulting in further depression. Alcohol may help with forgetting problems for a while, make one relax and overcome any shyness, or can make talking easier and more fun regardless of setting. However if an individual is depressed and lacking in energy, it can be tempting to use alcohol to help them cope with life and keep going. The problem is that it is easy to slip into drinking regularly, using it like a medication. The benefits soon wear off, the drinking becomes part of a routine, and the individual has to keep drinking ever-increasing volumes to get the same effect.

Recommended Limits

An acceptable recommended volume of alcohol consumption has been established by the Department of Health and is measured in units (see Table 10-1). One unit is the equivalent of 10 grams of alcohol – the amount in a standard pub measure of spirits, a half pint of normal strength beer or lager, or a small glass of wine. If a man and woman of the same weight drink the same amount of alcohol, the woman will have a much higher alcohol concentration in her bodily organs than the man due to difference in metabolism. For this reason the safe recommended limit is lower for women (14 units per week) than for men (21 units per week). Although this safe recommended limit has been established, individuals may socially only drink once or twice a week and then 'binge' drink. So how much alcohol is consumed at any one time is also important. These recommended safe limits assume that alcohol consumption is spread out through the week. In any one day, it is recommended for a man to drink no more than four units and for a woman to drink no more than three units. Drinking over eight units in a day for men, or six units for women is classed as 'binge' drinking.

Even drinking above the safe limit on one night, but still remaining within the recommended limit for the week, can be a health issue. There is some evidence that even a couple of days of binge drinking may start to kill off brain cells. This was previously considered only to occur in people who drank continuously for long periods of time. Binge drinking also seems to be connected with an increased risk of early death in middle-aged men and associated health problems.

These guidelines are approximate and may vary depending on the brand chosen and the size of measure. All alcohol sold in the UK above 1.2% ABV (Alcohol By Volume) should state how strong it is in percentages (%). The higher the percentage the greater the alcohol concentration. Pub measures are generally considerably smaller than the amount we pour ourselves at home.

Table 10-1 A guide to the amount of alcohol found in standard measures of different drinks

Beer, cider and alcopops	Strength ABV	Half pint	Pint	Bottle/can (330 ml)	Bottle/can (500 ml)	Bottle (1 l)
Ordinary strength beer, lager or cider (e.g. draught beer, Woodpecker)	3-4%	1	2	1.5	1.9	-
'Export' strength beer, lager or cider (e.g. Stella, Budweiser, Heineken, Kronenbourg, Strongbow)	5%	1.25	2.5	2	2.5	-
Extra strong beer, lager or cider (e.g. Special Brew, Diamond White, Tennants Extra)	8-9%	2.5	4.5	3	4.5	9
Alcopops (e.g. Bacardi Breezer, Smirnoff Ice, Reef, Archers, Hooch)	5%	-	-	1.7	-	-

Wines and spirits	Strength ABV	Small glass/pub measure	Wine glass	Bottle (750 ml)
Table wine	10-12%	-	1.5	9
Fortified wine (sherry, martini, port)	15-20%	0.8	2-3	14
Spirits (whisky, vodka, gin)	40%	1	-	30

Managing and Controlling Consumption

When assessing alcohol consumption most individuals will underestimate the amount they drink. In order to accurately assess consumption a diary of how much alcohol consumed over the course of a week may be kept. This can give a clearer indication of whether an individual is drinking to excess. It may also help to highlight any risky situations – regular times, places and with certain people when we seem to drink more (see Table 10-2).

The earliest warning signs of alcohol dependency may be summarised as:

+ Regular use of alcohol as a way of coping with feelings of anger, frustration, anxiety or depression.
+ Regular use of alcohol to feel confident.
+ The individual gets hangovers regularly.
+ Drinking affects the individual's relationships with other people.
+ Drinking makes the individual feel disgusted, angry or suicidal.
+ Other people notice that when the individual drinks they become gloomy, embittered or aggressive.
+ The individual needs to drink more and more to feel good.
+ The individual disengages and stops doing other things to spend more time drinking.
+ The individual starts to feel shaky and anxious the morning after a previous night's drinking.
+ To control anxieties and shaking the individual drinks to stop these feelings.
+ The individual starts drinking earlier in the day.

For individuals who consume too much alcohol, as part of their management plan, targets have to be set in order to reduce the amount that is consumed. Situations in which there is a high risk of consuming alcohol should be avoided and these can be identified by the individual from the diary of alcohol consumption kept previously. The individual must also have a high level of motivation to wish to stop consuming excessive alcohol quantities. Distraction strategies may be effective in reducing consumption such as undertaking some form of physical activity/exercise instead of consuming alcohol. Strategies such as this tend to be more effective when they are undertaken with a friend or relative present as a support mechanism and social contact. Friends or relatives can also be used to assist with monitoring the effectiveness of interventions as they tend to be more objective than the individual.

When excessive alcohol use is suddenly stopped very few individuals have no problems, whereas the majority develop some form of withdrawal symptom. Withdrawal symptoms can include craving for alcohol, shaking/tremors, restlessness and in the extreme fits. These symptoms are frequently managed with medications prescribed to manage the specific problem the patient is experiencing.

Depression is a frequent common symptom as many heavy drinkers feel depressed when they are drinking; most will feel better within a few weeks of stopping. The most effective strategy is to manage the excessive alcohol consumption first and then consider interventions to manage the depression if it has not improved after a few weeks. Strategies that may be affective in managing the associated depression may include counselling, psychotherapy or the use of medications such as anti-depressants.

As part of the overall management plan for the patient it is important to consider aspects of teaching the patient regarding appropriate alcohol consumption (see *Box 10-1*).

Drug Dependence

Drug dependence like alcohol misuse can be due to a variety of reasons. The dependence may be for the effects the drug has, such as a feeling of escapism and well-being, or due to over reliance upon a particular prescribed medication and its habit-

Table 10-2 Diary

Day	How much?	When?	Where?	Who with?	Units	Total
Monday						
Tuesday						
Wednesday						
Thursday						
Friday						
Saturday						
Sunday						
Total for week						

BOX 10-1 Dos and Don'ts of Drinking Safely

Explain to the patient that the following strategies for consuming alcohol can be effective in preventing excess consumption.

+ Do sip your drink slowly - don't gulp it down.
+ Do space your drinks with a nonalcoholic drink in between.
+ Don't drink on an empty stomach. Have something to eat first.
+ Don't drink every day. Have two or three alcohol-free days in the week.
+ Do provide nonalcoholic drinks as well as alcohol on social occasions.
+ Do ask your doctor or pharmacist if it is safe to drink with any medicine that you have been prescribed.
+ Do keep to the target (amount of alcohol per week) you have set yourself.
+ Do check your drinking every few weeks with your drinking diary.

---

forming side effects. Drugs of dependence and misuse may either be prescription medications or of the drugs considered illicit or recreational. Prescription drugs that are dependence forming and frequently misused may include benzodiazepines such as diazepam or temazepam. Frequently opiate or opiate derivative analgesics are also misused including morphine, pethidine and codeine.

More frequently illicit or recreational drugs are used mainly by the teenage to late thirties age group. Drugs in this category may include hallucinogenics such as LSD, cannabis and ecstasy; stimulants such as amphetamines or cocaine; or anabolic steroids for body building of muscle bulk. All of the drugs used for recreational purposes can be habit forming and have serious consequences for the health of the individual. Alarmingly these drugs can be purchased quite easily in many places such as pubs and clubs; this may be one of the reasons for their increase in recent years.

Cannabis

Cannabis is probably the drug most frequently used recreationally and will be discussed as an example of a habit-forming drug of misuse. There has been much debate in recent years about the legalisation of cannabis for its potential health benefits to certain groups of patient such as those with progressive neurological disorders. However, legally it remains a habit-forming drug of misuse.

It is estimated that up to two million people in the UK smoke cannabis on a recreational basis. Half of all 16–29 year-olds have tried it at least once. Despite government warnings about health risks, many people have the misconception that it is a harmless substance that helps you to relax and 'chill' – a drug that, unlike alcohol and cigarettes, might even be good for your physical and mental health. On the other hand, recent research has suggested that it can be a major cause of psychotic illnesses in those who are genetically vulnerable.

Cannabis sativa and *cannabis indica* are members of the nettle family that have grown wild throughout the world for centuries. Both plants have been used for a variety of purposes including hemp to make rope and textiles, as a medical herb and as the popular recreational drug.

The plant is used as either the resin – a brown/black lump, known as bhang, ganja, hashish, resin, etc.; or the dried leaves – known as grass, marijuana, spliff, weed, etc. *Skunk* is one of the stronger types of cannabis which is grown specifically for its higher concentration of psychoactive ingredients. It is named after the pungent smell it gives off during growing. It can be grown either under grow lights or in a greenhouse, often using hydroponics (growing in nutrient rich liquids rather than soil) techniques. There are hundreds of other varieties of cannabis with exotic names such as AK-47 or Destroyer.

Street cannabis can come in a wide variety of strengths, so it is often not possible to judge exactly what is being used in any one particular session. It is used most commonly in the form of resin or the dried leaves being mixed with tobacco and smoked as a 'spliff' or 'joint'. The smoke is inhaled strongly and held in the lungs for a number of seconds. It can also be smoked in a pipe, a water pipe or smoke is collected in a container before inhaling it. Some individuals used it as a brewed tea or cooked in cakes.

More than half of its psychologically active chemical ingredient are absorbed into the blood when smoked. These compounds tend to build up in fatty tissues throughout the body, so it takes a long time to be excreted in the urine. This is why cannabis can be detected in urine up to 56 days after it has last been used.

The Legal Situation

Legally, before January 2004, cannabis was classified as a Class B drug, alongside amphetamines and barbiturates. This dates from 1928, when Egyptian and South African doctors stated that heavy use could cause mental disturbances. Currently it is a Class C drug, in the same group as anabolic steroids and tranquillisers such as valium and temazepam. It is still illegal to have it and the maximum penalty for possession is two years. The decision to reclassify cannabis was recently reconsidered by the Government's Advisory Council on the Misuse of Drugs (ACMD) because of worries about possible connections with mental health problems and the increased strength of the cannabis that is now widely used. The decision was taken in January 2006 to keep cannabis as a Class C drug under the Misuse of Drugs Act 1971 (see Chapter 3). This means that the maximum penalties are:

+ for possession: a two-year prison sentence or an unlimited fine, or both;
+ for dealing/supplying: a 14-year prison sentence or an unlimited fine, or both.

Despite its legal status the use of cannabis continues as a recreational drug in high proportions.

Research

How cannabis affects the mind and body has been subject to much research because of its potential future health benefits. Research by Adams and Martin (1996) discovered that there are about 60 compounds and 400 chemicals in an average cannabis plant. The four main compounds are called delta-9-tetrahydrocannabinol (delta-9-THC), cannabidiol, delta-8-tetrahydrocannabinol and cannabinol. Apart from cannabidiol (CBD), these compounds are psychoactive, the strongest one being delta-9-tetrahydrocannabinol. The stronger varieties of the plant contain little cannabidiol, while the delta-9-THC content is a lot higher.

When cannabis is smoked, its compounds rapidly enter the bloodstream and are transported directly to the brain and other parts of the body. The feeling of being 'stoned' or 'high' is caused mainly by the delta-9-THC binding to cannabinoid receptors in the brain. The brain receptors are the sites on brain cells where certain substances can stick or bind for a while. If this happens, it has an effect on the cell and the nerve impulses it produces. There are also cannabis-like substances produced naturally by the brain itself – these are called endocannabinoids. Most of the brain receptors are found in the parts of the brain that influence pleasure, memory, thought, concentration, sensory and time perception. Cannabis compounds can also affect the eyes, the ears, the skin and the stomach.

The effects that are experienced with cannabis use as with all drugs of misuse can either be pleasant or unpleasant. During a pleasant experience a 'high' or sense of relaxation, happiness, sleepiness, colours appearing more intense and music sounding better may be experienced. However around one in 10 cannabis users have unpleasant experiences, including confusion, hallucinations, anxiety and paranoia. The same person may have either pleasant or unpleasant effects depending on their mood and circumstances with each use. These feelings are usually only temporary but as the drug can stay in the system for some weeks, the effect can be more long-lasting than users realise. Long-term use can have a depressant effect, reducing motivation, similar to the effects experienced with alcohol misuse.

Fergusson et al. (2003) in their research also indicated that cannabis may interfere with a person's capacity to concentrate and organise and use information. This effect seems to last several weeks after use, which can cause particular problems for students who alarmingly account for a fairly high proportion of users. This is supported by a large study in New Zealand by McGee et al. (2000) that followed up 1,265 children for 25 years. It found that cannabis use in adolescence was linked to poor school performance, but that there was no direct connection between the two. It looked as though it was simply because cannabis use encouraged a way of life that did not help with schoolwork!

Cannabis seems to have a similar effect on people at work. There is no evidence that cannabis causes specific health hazards in the workplace. But users are more likely to leave work without permission, spend work time on personal matters or simply daydream which is a particular danger when working with machinery. Cannabis users themselves report that drug use has interfered with their work and social life. A review of the research (Janowsky et al. (1976a); Janowsky et al. (1976b); Yesavage et al. (1985); Leirer et al. (1989); Leirer and Yesavage (1991)) on the effect of cannabis on pilots (in flying simulators), revealed that those who had used cannabis made far more mistakes, both major and minor, than when they had not smoked cannabis. The worst effects were in the first four hours, although they persisted for at least 24 hours, even when the pilot had no sense at all of being 'high'.

Accidents and Depression

Like any drug of misuse driving a motorised vehicle after using a substance can have an increased risk of associated accidents. In New Zealand, Blows et al. (2005) noted that those who smoked regularly, and had smoked before driving, were more likely to be injured in a car crash. A study in France by Laumon et al. (2005) looked at over 10,000 drivers who were involved in fatal car crashes. Even when the influence of alcohol was taken into account, cannabis users were twice as likely to be the cause of a fatal crash than to be one of the victims.

There is growing evidence to suggest that people with serious mental illness, including depression and psychosis, are more likely to use cannabis or have used it for long periods of time in the past. Regular use of the drug appears to have doubled the risk of developing a psychotic episode or long-term schizophrenia. Some research by Henquet et al. (2005) has strongly suggested that there is a clear link between early cannabis use and later mental health problems in those with a genetic vulnerability – and that there is a particular issue with the use of cannabis by adolescents.

A study by Rey et al. (2002) following 1,600 Australian school-children, aged 14–15 for seven years, found that while children who use cannabis regularly have a significantly higher risk of depression, the opposite was not the case – children who already suffered from depression were not more likely than anyone else to use cannabis. However, adolescents who used cannabis daily were five times more likely to develop depression and anxiety in later life.

Another associated risk with cannabis use is schizophrenia. Three studies (Arendt et al. (2005); Fergusson et al. (2003); Patton et al. (2002)) followed large numbers of people over several years, and showed that those people who use cannabis have a higher than average risk of developing schizophrenia. If you start smoking cannabis before the age of 15, you are four times more likely to develop a psychotic disorder by the time you are 26. The studies found no evidence of self-medication. It seemed that, the more cannabis someone used, the more likely they were to develop symptoms. Recent research in Europe by Arseneault et al. (2002) has suggested that people who have a family background of mental illness, so probably have a genetic vulnerability anyway, are more likely to develop schizophrenia if they use cannabis as well.

Research in Denmark by Van Os *et al.* (2002) suggests that individuals may experience a cannabis psychosis with prolonged use. This is a short-lived psychotic disorder that seems to be brought on by cannabis use but which subsides fairly quickly once the individual has stopped using it. It is quite rare though as in the whole of Denmark only around 100 new cases per year were noted. The research did however note that three quarters of those studied had a different psychotic disorder diagnosed within the next year; and nearly half still had a psychotic disorder three years later.

It is therefore probable that nearly half of those diagnosed as having cannabis psychosis were actually showing the first signs of a more long-lasting psychotic disorder, such as schizophrenia.

Like many of the drugs misused cannabis can be addictive and all seem to have similar mechanisms. The addiction develops via a mechanism similar to that of alcohol dependence. First a tolerance develops, whereby the individual needs to take more and more to get the same effect. Eventually withdrawal symptoms occur and include; craving, decreased appetite, sleep difficulty, weight loss, aggression anger, irritability, restlessness and strange dreams.

A pattern develops in personality with individuals who become dependent upon drugs of misuse. The user feels they have to have the substance and spends much of their life seeking, buying and using it. They cannot stop even when other important parts of their life (family, school, work) suffer. Self-esteem decreases and eventually the individual will become socially disengaged.

Assessment and Overcoming Dependence

Assessment of any individual with a substance misuse problem is essential to determine the extent of their dependence. *Box 10-2* shows some assessment questions that may be used when assessing a patient.

Individuals who have a dependence upon substances may need a combination of counselling, psychotherapy and medication to overcome their dependence. This is best achieved by mental health professionals specialised in the particular substance that is being abused in order to overcome the associated symptoms and problems. A strategy that may be used to assist the individual could include the nurse helping to:

+ draw up a list of reasons for wanting to change;
+ planning how the patient will change;
+ thinking about coping with withdrawal symptoms;
+ having a back-up plan;
+ considering what support mechanism and supportive friends or relatives the patient can use to facilitate the process.

MENTAL HEALTH DISORDERS

Schizophrenia

Schizophrenia is a relatively common mental health disorder that affects one in every 100 people. It affects men and women equally and seems to be more common in city areas and in some minority ethnic groups. It is rare before the age of 15, but can start at any time after this, most often between the ages of 15 and 35.

Hallucinations

These are among some of the most common symptoms associated with schizophrenia but can also be associated with other mental health disorders. A **hallucination** can affect any of the senses but usually occurs when the individual hears, smells, feels or sees something, when there is nothing (or nobody) actually there to account for it. In schizophrenia, the commonest hallucination is that of hearing voices. They sound completely real

---

BOX 10-2 Assessment Questions for Drug and ALcohol Misuse

If the patient answers yes to any of the questions they may have a dependence problem.

1. Has taking drugs/alcohol stopped being fun?
2. Do you ever get high/drunk alone?
3. Is it hard for you to imagine a life without drugs/alcohol?
4. Do you find that your friends are determined by your drugs/alcohol use?
5. Do you take drugs/alcohol to avoid dealing with your problems?
6. Do you take drugs/alcohol to cope with your feelings?
7. Does your drug/alcohol use let you live in a privately defined world?

8. Have you ever failed to keep promises you made about cutting down or controlling your drugs/alcohol?
9. Have drugs/alcohol caused problems with memory, concentration or motivation?
10. When your drugs/alcohol supply is nearly finished, do you feel anxious or worried about how to get more?
11. Do you plan your life around your drugs/alcohol use?
12. Have friends or relatives ever complained that your drugs/alcohol use is damaging your relationship with them?

to the individual and can be described as coming from outside the person, although other people cannot hear them. The individual may hear them in different places or may hear them coming from a particular object, such as a television. The voices may talk to the individual directly or they may talk to each other about the individual. It can often be described as if the individual is over-hearing a conversation; voices can be pleasant but are often rude, critical, abusive or just plain irritating.

Frequently an individual may feel that they have to do what the voices say; even if they are telling the individual to harm themselves or to do something which the individual knows is wrong. Much of the time individuals tend to ignore the voices but often they can cause depression and frustration. The voices are not imaginary, but are actually created by the mind. Brain scans have shown that the part of the brain that is active when someone experiences auditory hallucinations is the part that is active when the individual is talking or forming words in their mind. It is as though the brain mistakes the individual's own thoughts for real voices.

Auditory hallucinations can also be associated with other mental health disorders including depression. In depression the voices are critical and repeat the same word or phrase over and over again, lowering the self-esteem of the individual.

Delusions

A **delusion** is a belief that the individual holds with complete conviction, although it seems to be based on a misinterpretation or misunderstanding of situations or events. While the individual has no doubts, other people consider the belief as mistaken, strange or unrealistic. The individual may feel that they cannot really discuss the belief or cannot explain it – they 'just know'. Delusions associated with schizophrenia tend to develop over a period of time and may or may not be proceeded by hallucinations. Initially the individual may consider something strange is going on over a period of weeks or months but cannot explain it. Delusions may also be of a paranoid nature where the individual believes they are being persecuted by a family, friends or an imaginary threat.

Causes of Schizophrenia

The cause of schizophrenia is not fully understood but is considered to be a combination of several different factors which will be different for different people. Genetically one in 10 people with schizophrenia have a parent with the illness. Studies of twins have demonstrated how much is due to genes and how much to upbringing. Identical twins have exactly the same genetic make-up as each other, down to the last molecule of DNA. If one identical twin has schizophrenia, their twin has about a 50:50 chance of having it too. Nonidentical twins do not have the same genetic make-up as each other. If one of them has schizophrenia, the risk to the other twin is just slightly more than for any other brother or sister.

These findings hold true even if twins are adopted and brought up in different families. This suggests that the difference is due to genes rather than upbringing (see Table 10-3).

Table 10-3 Chances of Developing Schizophrenia

Relatives with schizophrenia	Chance of developing schizophrenia
None	1 in 100
1 parent	1 in 10
1 identical twin (same genetic make up)	1 in 2
1 nonidentical twin (different genetic make up)	1 in 80

Research by Fanous *et al.* (2001) suggests that genes account for about half of the risk of developing schizophrenia. Currently the combination of genes responsible for this illness have not been identified. Brain damage is another potential explanation for the illness. Brain scans show that, compared with people who do not suffer from the illness, there are differences in the brains of some people with schizophrenia. For some people with schizophrenia, parts of their brain may not have developed normally because of problems during birth that affect the supply of oxygen to the brain, or viral infections during the early months of pregnancy.

As discussed earlier, alcohol and drug abuse can increase the risk of developing schizophrenia. Stress is another closely associated factor: personal difficulties often seem to happen shortly before symptoms worsen. An example could be a sudden event like a car accident, bereavement or moving home. It could also be an everyday problem, such as difficulty with work or studies. Long-term stress, such as family tensions, can worsen symptoms.

Statistically, individuals with schizophrenia rarely require hospital treatment and are able to settle down, work and have lasting relationships. In the long term, for every five people who develop schizophrenia:

+ One in five will get better within five years of their first episode of schizophrenia.
+ Three in five will get better, but will still have some symptoms. They will have times when their symptoms get worse.
+ One in five will continue to have troublesome symptoms.

PSYCHOLOGICAL TREATMENTS

Cognitive Behavioural Therapy (CBT)

CBT may be undertaken by clinical psychologists, psychiatrists or nurse therapists. The therapist helps the individual to:

+ Identify problems that are most troublesome for them. These could be thoughts, experiences or ways of behaving.
+ Look at the individual's self-perception – their 'thinking habits'.
+ Look at the individual's self-reaction – their 'behaving habits'.
+ Look at how the individual's thoughts affect their behaviour.

+ Work out if any of these thinking or behaving habits are unrealistic or unhelpful.
+ Work out if there are other ways of thinking about these things or reacting to them that would be more helpful.
+ Try out new ways of thinking and behaving.
+ See if these work. If they do help the individual encourage their use regularly. If they do not, find others which do work.

This kind of therapy can help the individual to feel better about their personality and to learn new ways of solving problems. Cognitive therapy can also help an individual to cope with troublesome hallucinations or delusional ideas. Most people have between eight and 20 sessions lasting about one hour. For CBT to be effective at least ten meetings over a period of about six months need to be implemented.

Medication

Medication is frequently used in combination with psychological treatments as part of a treatment plan. The aim of the medication treatment is to reduce the effect of the symptoms upon the individual's life. Medication is usually prescribed to weaken delusions and hallucinations gradually, over a period of a few weeks; improve clarity of thought; and increase individual motivation and ability to self-care.

The medication may either be prescribed to be taken regularly via the oral route or via a 'depot injection' which is given at weekly intervals or every two, three or four weeks. Most of the depot injections are older, typical antipsychotics, but one of the atypicals, Risperidone, is now available in this form.

The effectiveness of medication is quite significant: approximately four in five people get help from them. Medication tends to control the disorder but does not cure it and it needs to be taken continuously to prevent the redevelopment of symptoms.

Typical Antipsychotics

In the mid-1950s, several medications appeared that could reduce the symptoms of schizophrenia. They became known as **antipsychotic medications**. These older drugs are called typical or first-generation antipsychotics (see Table 10-4). They work by reducing the action of a dopamine in the brain, which is a chemical messenger.

These drugs frequently have a number of side-effects including:

+ Stiffness and shakiness like Parkinson's disease, along with feeling sluggish and slow in thinking. In most cases, this will mean too much of the medication is being taken. It should be reduced to a level at which these symptoms disappear. If higher doses are needed, these side-effects can be controlled with anti-Parkinsonian medication.
+ Uncomfortable restlessness (akathisia).
+ Problems with sexual life.
+ A long-term side-effect is tardive dyskinesia (TD) – persistent movements, usually of the mouth and tongue. This affects about one in 20 people every year who are taking these medications.

Atypical Antipsychotics

Over the past 10 years, several newer medications have been developed and licensed for use. They work on a different range of chemical messengers in the brain (such as serotonin) and are called atypical or second-generation anti-psychotics (see Table 10-5). They are less likely to cause Parkinsonian side-effects, although they may cause weight gain and problems with sexual function. They may also help the negative symptoms on which the older drugs have very little effect. They also appear much less likely to produce tardive dyskinesia. Many people who use these newer medications have found the side-effects less troublesome than those of the older medications. Side-effects include:

Table 10-4 Some Typical Antipsychotics

Tablets	Trade name	Normal daily dose (mg)	Max. daily dose (mg)
Chlorpromazine	Largactil	75-300	1,000
Haloperidol	Haldol	3-15	30
Pimozide	Orap	4-20	20
Trifluoperazine	Stelazine	5-20	
Sulpiride	Dolmatil	200-800	2,400
Depot injections (may be given every 2-4 weeks)	Trade name	Normal 2-weekly dose	Max. 2-weekly dose
Haloperidol	Haldol	50	
Flupenthixol decanoate	Depixol	40	
Fluphenazine decanoate	Modecate	12.5-100	
Pipothiazine palmitate	Piportil	50	
Zuclopenthixol decanoate	Clopixol	200	

Table 10-5 Some Atypical Antipsychotics

Tablets	Trade name	Normal daily dose (mg)	Max. daily dose (mg)
Amisulpiride	Solian	50-800	1,200
Aripiprazole	Abilify	10-30	
Clozapine	Clozaril	200-450	900
Olanzapine	Zyprexa	10-20	20
Quetiapine	Seroquel	300-450	750
Risperidone	Risperdal	4-6	16
Sertindole	Serdolect	12-20	24
Zotepine	Zoleptil	75-200	300
Depot injections	**Trade name**	**Normal 2-weekly dose**	**Max. 2-weekly dose**
Risperidone	Risperdal Consta	25	50

+ sleepiness and slowness,
+ weight increase,
+ interference with sex life,
+ increased chance of developing diabetes,
+ in high doses, some atypicals may produce the same Parkinsonian side-effects as the typicals.

Clozapine

This atypical antipsychotic medication is worth special consideration as it is the only medication that has been proven to be more effective for individuals who do not respond to other sorts of antipsychotics. It also appears to reduce suicide in people with schizophrenia. Clozapine has many of the same side-effects as other atypical antipsychotics, but may also increase salivation. A significant side-effect is the suppressant effect it has upon bone marrow development. This leads to a shortage of white cells which causes vulnerability to infection. If this occurs, the medication is discontinued as quickly as possible to allow the bone marrow to recover. Weekly blood tests are undertaken for the first six months of taking Clozapine, then every two weeks and eventually four-weekly.

DEPRESSION AND ITS EFFECTS

Bipolar Disorder

Bipolar disorder used to be called manic depression. As the name suggests, it is characterised by mood swings or episodes that are far beyond what most people experience in their normal life. The extremes are: low – feelings of intense depression and despair; 'depressive'; and high – feelings of elation, 'manic'. Mixed feelings may also be experienced – for example, depressed mood with the restlessness and the over-activity of a manic episode. Typically, an individual will usually experience both depressive and manic episodes, but some will have only manic ones.

Bipolar disorder affects about one in every 100 adults at some point in their life. It can start at any time during or after the teenage years, although it is unusual for it to start after the age of 40. Men and women are affected equally. Bipolar disorder is divided into four main types.

1. **Bipolar I** – The individual has experienced at least one high or manic episode (see below), which has lasted for longer than one week. Some individuals will have only manic episodes, although most will also have depressive episodes, while others will have more depressive episodes than manic episodes. Untreated manic episodes generally last three to six months, depressive episodes rather longer – six to 12 months without treatment.
2. **Bipolar II** – There has been more than one episode of major depression, but only mild manic episodes (referred to as 'hypomania').
3. **Rapid cycling** – There are more than four mood swings in a 12-month period. This affects around one in 10 people with bipolar disorder and can happen with both types I and II.
4. **Cyclothymia** – The mood swings are not as severe as those in full bipolar disorder, but may continue for longer. This can, sometimes, develop into full bipolar disorder.

The causes of bipolar disorder are not fully understood but research suggests that it is hereditary; a chemical imbalance may be present in the brain and this is why the symptoms of bipolar disorder can often be controlled with medication. Frequently, acute episodes may be brought on by stressful experiences or physical illness.

Symptoms of Depression

The feeling of depression is something we all experience from time to time. It can even help us to recognise and deal with problems in our lives. For individuals with clinical depression or bipolar disorder, their depressive feelings will be worse, go on for longer and make it harder to tackle the daily tasks and problems of living. Someone with this sort of depression is more likely to have the physical symptoms discussed later. If an individual develops a depressive episode, they may have many of these symptoms:

Emotions

+ Feelings of unhappiness that do not go away;
+ losing interest in things;
+ being unable to enjoy things;
+ feeling restless and agitated;
+ losing self-confidence;
+ feeling useless, inadequate and hopeless;
+ feeling more irritable than usual;
+ thinking of suicide.

Thinking

+ Finding it hard to make even simple decisions;
+ difficulty in concentrating.

Physical

+ Losing appetite and weight;
+ difficulty in getting to sleep;
+ waking earlier than usual;
+ feeling utterly tired;
+ constipation;
+ loss of sexual drive.

Behaviour

+ Difficulty in starting or completing tasks;
+ crying a lot – or feeling like you want to cry, but not being able to;
+ avoiding contact with other people.

When depressed it is virtually impossible to function in employment or indeed complete any of the activities of daily living. Those individuals that are depressed find it virtually impossible to see a future and may feel continually emotional.

Mania

Mania is an exaggeration of feelings that we all experience from time to time. It is the opposite of depression – a feeling of well-being, energy and optimism. These feelings can be so intense that the individual can lose contact with reality. When this happens, they may believe strange things about their personality, making bad judgements and behave in embarrassing, harmful and sometimes even dangerous ways. Like depression, it can make it difficult or impossible to deal with life in an effective way. A period of mania can, if untreated, destroy relationships and work. When it is not so extreme, the word 'hypomania' is used to describe it. In an episode of mania, the following changes may be noted:

Emotional

+ Very happy and excited;
+ irritated with other people who don't share the same optimistic outlook;
+ feeling more important than usual.

Thinking

+ Full of new and exciting ideas;
+ moving quickly from one idea to another;
+ hearing voices that other people can't hear.

Physical

+ Full of energy;
+ unable or unwilling to sleep;
+ increased interest in sex.

Behaviour

+ Making plans that are grandiose and unrealistic;
+ very active and moving very quickly;
+ behaving in a bizarre way;
+ speaking very quickly – if mood is very high, it can be difficult for other people to understand what is being talked about;
+ making odd decisions on the spur of the moment, sometimes with disastrous consequences;
+ recklessly spending your money;
+ becoming over-familiar or recklessly critical with other people;
+ less inhibited in general behaviour.

In the middle of a first manic episode, an individual may not realise that there is anything wrong, it will often be friends, family or colleagues that note a change. Frequently an individual will feel quite insulted if someone tries to point this out as they may well feel better than they ever have done before. The problem with feeling like this is that it increasingly detaches the individual from day-to-day reality. And when they have recovered from one of these episodes, they will often regret the things that they said and did while they were high.

Psychotic Symptoms

If an episode of mania or depression becomes very severe, experiences may become so intense that the individual in effect loses contact with reality. During a manic episode, there will be a tendency for the individual to hold grandiose beliefs, for example that they are on an important mission or that they have special powers. If they are depressed, they feel uniquely guilty, that they are worse than anybody else or even that they do not exist. As well as these unusual beliefs, they may experience hallucinations.

It used to be thought that, between episodes of depression and mania, people with bipolar disorder revert back to normal behaviour patterns. While this may be true for some, it is now known that this is not the case for many people with bipolar disorder. They continue to experience low levels of depressive symptoms and mild problems in thinking even when they appear, to other people, to be 'back to normal'.

MEDICATION - MOOD STABILISERS

Mood stabilisers tend to be the main form of treatment for this bipolar disorder. There are several mood stabilisers, most of which are also effective in treating epilepsy. However, lithium (a naturally occurring salt) was the first medication that was found to be helpful in stabilising moods.

Lithium

Lithium has been used as a mood stabiliser for 50 years but its action mechanism is still unclear. It can be used to treat both manic and depressive episodes. The main consideration is getting the level of lithium in the body right; too low and it will not work, too high and it will become toxic. Treatment with lithium is usually started by a psychiatrist. Regular blood tests have to be performed to ensure the appropriate dose has been prescribed. Once the dose is stabilised, the prescribing and monitoring of lithium treatment can be taken over by the individual's GP.

The amount of lithium in blood is very sensitive to how much, or how little, water there is in the body. If an individual becomes dehydrated, the level of lithium in the blood will rise and they will be more likely to get side-effects or even toxic effects. So, it is essential to advise a patient on lithium to drink plenty of water; more in hot weather or if they are more active; and to use coffee and tea in moderation because of their diuretic effects. It usually takes up to three months for lithium to reach a concentration in the body that is effective for a treatment level.

Side-effects can occur in the first few weeks after starting lithium treatment. They can be irritating and unpleasant, but often disappear or get better with time. Most common side-effects include:

+ feeling thirsty;
+ passing more urine than usual;
+ weight gain.

Less common side-effects (these can usually be improved by lowering the dose) are:

+ blurred vision;
+ slight muscle weakness;
+ occasional diarrhoea;
+ fine trembling of the hands;
+ a feeling of being mildly ill.

If the level of lithium in blood is too high, the individual may experience:

+ vomiting;
+ staggering;
+ slurred speech.

Initially blood tests are required every few weeks to make sure that the right level of lithium has been prescribed. Lithium levels have to be monitored for the duration of the therapy but less often after the first few months. In some cases, long-term use of lithium can affect the kidneys or the thyroid gland.

Other Mood Stabilisers Which May Be Prescribed

While lithium is probably the most effective mood stabiliser, reducing the incidence of relapse by 30–40%, sodium valproate, an anti-convulsant, could be just as effective, but there is not yet enough evidence to be sure. The latter should not be prescribed to women of child-bearing age. Carbamazepine is slightly less effective. It is not generally recommended but, if it has worked previously, there is no reason to change it. Finally, there is also evidence that atypical antipsychotic medications (such as Olanzapine) can act as mood stabilisers.

Depressive Episodes

Antidepressant medication will usually need to be added to any mood stabiliser medication. The most commonly used antidepressants are the 'SSRI' medications. These affect the action of serotonin, and seem to be less likely than other kinds of antidepressant to push someone into a manic episode. The older tricyclic antidepressants should be avoided for this reason.

If a recent manic episode or a rapid-cycling disorder has occurred, an antidepressant is more likely to push the individual into a manic swing. It is frequently safer to increase the dose of the mood stabiliser without an antidepressant. Antidepressants usually take between two and six weeks to work properly, but sleep and appetite often improve first. Antidepressants should be continued for at least eight weeks after there has been a major improvement in the depression, and then should be reduced slowly.

There is evidence that, if repeated depressive episodes occur but have never switched to mania, while the individual is on antidepressants, they can continue on a combined mood stabiliser and antidepressant treatment to prevent further episodes. If the individual has had manic episodes, then it is not advisable to continue antidepressants long term.

Mania and Mixed Depressive Episodes

If an antidepressant is being taken, it should be stopped. The first line of treatment may be a mood stabiliser or antipsychotic medication, either alone or in combination. Antipsychotic medications are generally used in schizophrenia, but also help to reduce the overactivity, grandiosity, sleeplessness and agitation of a manic episode.

The older antipsychotics (e.g. Chlorpromazine, Haloperidol) have some unpleasant side-effects such as stiffness, shakiness, dizziness and dry mouth. However, some of the newer drugs (Risperidone, Olanzapine) can improve manic symptoms without many of the unpleasant side-effects of the older drugs.

Once the treatment has started the symptoms could improve within a few days, but may take several weeks for a full recovery.

Psychological Treatments

Inbetween episodes of mania or depression, psychological treatment can be helpful. This should be around 16 one-hour sessions over a period of six to nine months. Psychological treatment usually includes:

+ psychoeducation – to find out more about bipolar disorder;
+ mood monitoring – to help identify when mood swings are extreme;
+ mood strategies – to help prevent mood swings developing into a full-blown manic or depressive episode;
+ help to develop general coping skills.
+ cognitive behavioural therapy (CBT) for depression.

Box 10-3 gives some pointers that patients can use to prevent or lessen the effects of mood swings.

MEMORY PROBLEMS

The human mind is remarkably fast, faster than the most advanced computers, but yet we still forget things. We usually forget those things we do not really need to remember. What were you doing at exactly this time last year? or last month? or last week? Unless those were very special days, like Christmas or anniversaries, you probably will not remember. If you go back as far as your childhood, you can certainly remember some things, but only a few. You may remember your first day at primary school and your seventh birthday, but not every day at school or all the other birthdays. We often do not bother to remember things when the information is usually to hand. For example, what is the date today? Most people look at their newspaper or watch. We even forget some of the things we really need to remember. Most of us have spent frustrating minutes searching for our keys, documents or a vital tool. It is normal to forget, especially in modern life when we have so much to consider and do in such a short period of time.

Most of the time we can live comfortably with our limitations, including the fact that we forget. But as we grow older, the time comes when we start to forget more than we used to. This can not only be frustrating but also a concern for some older adults. Frequently, as memory recall becomes poorer, concern may be expressed that dementia is developing and loss of independence can occur.

BOX 10-3 Stopping the Mood Swings and Helping Yourself

Self-Monitoring
Learn how to recognise the signs that your mood is swinging out of control, so you can get help early. By doing this, it may be possible to avoid both full blown episodes and hospital admissions. By keeping a mood diary, you may be better able to identify the things in your life that are helpful - and those that are not.

Knowledge
Find out as much as you can about your illness and how you can be helped.

Stress
If possible, avoid particularly stressful situations - these can trigger off a manic or depressive episode. It is impossible to avoid all stresses, so it can be helpful to learn ways of handling stress better. You can do relaxation training yourself with audio cassette tapes, join a relaxation group or seek advice from a clinical psychologist.

Relationships
Episodes of depression or mania can cause great strain on friends and family - you may find that you have to rebuild some relationships after an episode. It is helpful if you have at least one person that you can rely on and confide in. When you are well, try explaining the illness to people who are important to you. They need to understand what happens to you, and what to do.

Activities
It is vital to balance your life between work, leisure and relationships with your family and friends. You can bring on a manic episode if you get too busy when you feel well.

Make sure that you have enough time to relax and unwind. If you are unemployed, think about taking courses or doing some volunteer work that has nothing to do with mental illness.

Exercise
Reasonably intense exercise for 20 minutes or so, three times a week, seems to have a positive effect on mood.

Fun
Make sure you regularly do things that you enjoy and that give your life meaning.

Continue with Medication
It may be tempting to stop taking your medication before your doctor recommends - unfortunately this will often lead to an early relapse. One way of feeling better about continuing with the treatment is to discuss this with your doctor and your family when you are well.

There are numerous explanations for memory problems other than dementia. Depression can affect memory recall. When we are depressed, we tend to see only the bad things about ourselves and the world. We may condemn ourselves unfairly for relatively unimportant human failings. We tend to withdraw into ourselves and may not notice what is going on around us. So, we may not remember things because we did not notice them in the first place.

People who are depressed may also become **agitated** and this will make it hard to concentrate. If the depression is particularly bad, our thinking may actually slow down (**retardation**). Both agitation and retardation make it difficult for depressed people to remember as well as they normally would. Sometimes the memory problems caused by depression will show up on tests. They can be so bad that other people may actually think that the sufferer has dementia and this is known as **pseudo-dementia**.

In spite of this, depressed people are usually no more than normally forgetful. However, older depressed people often think they are 'going senile'. In fact, older people who complain to their doctors of bad memory are much more likely to be suffering from depression than dementia.

If we are very anxious or worried, we may not be able to concentrate. We may panic when we really need to remember something. This often happens in exams or interviews. **Anxiety** can affect memory at any age.

Most of our powers weaken as we get older, and memory is no exception. This makes it harder to learn new skills in later life, although not impossible. Many people over 65 do not let this put them off, and are able to finish university courses. However, many older people do gradually find it harder to remember. This is called **age associated memory impairment (AAMI)**.

The main problem seems to be that, the older we are, the longer it takes us to get the information from our memory when we need it. This may be partly because we have more memories than we did when we were young. It may be like looking for a book in a library. It is easier to find a book on a single shelf than if it is hidden somewhere in the middle of hundreds of others in a large bookcase. Another common problem is difficulty in putting a name to a face. This affects most people, to some degree, from around the age of 50. Another problem can crop up when we remember that something happened, but do not know when it did. Ordinary memory tests may not demonstrate AAMI, but it may be uncovered by tests that measure the time taken to give a correct answer.

Other psychological factors that can affect memory include boredom, tiredness or sleepiness. This may become a particular problem for a patient in a healthcare setting where there is continuous noise over a 24-hour period that affects the ability of the individual to rest.

Memory may be affected by poor hearing and sight, alcohol and tranquillisers, chronic pain and head injuries. It may also be affected by a number of medical conditions. Before a diagnosis of dementia or a mental health problem is made investigations should be undertaken to rule out physical illness such as:

+ An under-active thyroid gland – this slows the whole body, including the brain.
+ Severe heart or lung disease – these starve the brain of oxygen.
+ Diabetes – both high and low levels of sugar interfere with the way the brain works.
+ Infections – of the body (like pneumonia in an old person or a child) or the brain (like meningitis and encephalitis) can also cause memory problems.

Dementia

This is the most serious cause of memory problems. It affects very few people under the age of 65. However, the recent scare about the new variant Creutzfeld-Jakob disease (nvCJD) arising from bovine spongiform encephalitis (BSE) has made the general public aware that although rare, it does happen.

Dementia mainly affects older people. After the age of 65, the risk of developing it doubles every five years. Over the age of 80, about one in five people suffer from some degree of dementia. It is important to remember though that four out of five people over the age of 80 are not suffering from dementia. There are several causes, but the commonest is **Alzheimer's disease**.

As well as the forgetfulness, several other problems may occur:

+ Difficulty in finding the right words. At its worse, the sufferer's speech will become completely incomprehensible. It works both ways – they will no longer be able to understand other people's writing or speech.
+ Difficulty with skills learnt early in life, like dressing and using a knife and fork.
+ Failure of intelligence, judgement and logic (e.g. giving one's mother's age as the same as one's own, saying it is summer when it is snowing).
+ Personality change: becoming irritable, withdrawn, rude, scruffy, idle, uninterested.
+ Suspiciousness.
+ Anxiety and depression (arising from the sense of 'losing one's mind').
+ Refusing to accept that something is wrong, even though it is so obvious to others. This may mean that the sufferer refuses the help they clearly need.
+ Uncharacteristic behaviour, including reluctance to wash or to change clothes, wandering, becoming incontinent and aggressive.
+ Becoming unable to look after oneself.

Eventually the forgetfulness of dementia becomes a serious problem. If a person with dementia is taken away from familiar surroundings, on holiday for example, they may start to get lost. It is common to forget what time, day, date, month or year it is, or where they live or where they are now. Those affected may lose things or leave them behind, and may start to believe that someone is stealing their possessions. They may forget to pass on messages, or may repeat them in a rather scrambled way. They may say the same things again and again, because they cannot remember what they have just said. As the condition worsens, someone with dementia may get lost in familiar surroundings – even in their own homes. Most distressingly, they may fail to recognise their nearest and dearest.

Dementia nearly always gets steadily worse. It may take a few months (as in the case of classical CJD) or a few years (as in Alzheimer's starting in a person over 65). It may happen quickly, but more often it is gradual. Sometimes a series of small strokes, one after another, may cause dementia. They produce sudden, small worsenings of the dementia. There may be a period of a year or so between them when there is little change. This type of dementia may be hereditary.

Some people, while they have insight, realise their limitations and adapt to them. They are able to accept that they have to depend more on others, and so can have a say in the arrangements that relatives have to make for them. Others, however, vigorously refuse to admit that there is anything wrong with them – they can be particularly hard to help.

Causes of Dementia

The exact causes of most dementias are unknown, but there are some clues. It may run in families, as Alzheimer's sometimes does. It is very common in sufferers of Down's syndrome. A severe head injury at some stage in life may increase the risk.

High blood pressure and cholesterol, diabetes, smoking, drinking, and being over-weight all increase the risk of dementia (and associated physiological illnesses), because they all cause problems with the blood supply to the brain. One particular type of dementia occurs in people with Parkinson's disease. **Korsakoff's syndrome** is a type of dementia that can occur in younger people. It mainly affects the memory for recent events. This is caused by lack of vitamin B_1 (thiamine) and, in the UK, is most often due to drinking too much alcohol. Lastly, there are infections such as Creutzfeldt-Jakob syndrome and AIDS.

Management Strategies

Strategies that may be useful for an individual with memory problems include:

+ Take notice – and notes.
+ Get organised.
+ Use a diary.
+ Keep fit.
+ Don't miss regular health checks.
+ Use your mind, don't lose it.
+ Memory aids.
+ External aids.
+ Remember – nobody's perfect!

See also *Box 10-4*.

BOX 10-4 Patients with Memory Problems: Coping Strategies and Advice

Take notice
You can't remember what you never heard or saw in the first place. So you need to keep yourself alert and make yourself notice the things that you need to. For instance, you may find it helpful to repeat the name of a person you have just met. If you don't want to lose something, tell yourself aloud where you are putting it.

Taking notes can be useful
Writing down messages will help you to remember. It also gives you something on paper with which to remind yourself.

Get organised
You are more likely to remember things if you are organised. For instance, if you are tidy, you are more likely to know where you have put things. If you have a regular routine you are more likely to remember what you are supposed to be doing. This doesn't mean that you have to be obsessed with tidiness and routine, but it does mean that you may have to take a bit more time over it to organise yourself.

Use a diary
If you keep a diary of what you've been doing, you can look up what happened yesterday or last week. If you are busy, you really need to keep an appointments diary – but you do have to remember to look at it! It's particularly embarrassing to have missed something when it was in your diary all the time.

Keep fit
It's easier to have a healthy mind if you have a healthy body. This means getting regular exercise, eating and drinking moderately, and not smoking. If your eyesight is poor or you are a bit deaf, make sure you have the proper spectacles or hearing aids. This will help you to be aware of what is happening and will help you to hear what other people are saying. It will certainly help you to keep up to date. Try not to use sleeping tablets and tranquillisers – you'll be more alert.

Regular health checks
Many doctors do regular health checks of their elderly patients every year. These can help you to sort out any problems with your physical health, but can also help to diagnose Alzheimer's early. There are some new treatments which may hold back the disease for a year or so, and they're most likely to be effective if they are used early. If you are depressed, your doctor will be able to start you on antidepressants. Your memory will often improve as your depression lifts.

Use your mind

If you don't use your body, it weakens. If you stay in bed for weeks, your leg muscles shrink and you are likely to find it difficult to walk. It may be that if you don't use your mind, a similar thing may happen. We know that intelligent, well-educated people seem to experience fewer memory problems as they get older. This may be because they have a better memory in the first place and so take longer to develop problems. It may also be that, being in the habit of using their minds to study, learn and solve problems, they don't 'switch off' after retirement. So hobbies such as quizzes, crosswords, reading, learning passages or poems, and card games, may help to offset the effects of ageing. Endless snoozing, putting your feet up too much, and being a 'couch-potato' may make them worse.

Reality orientation

This is a means of helping people with dementia remember where they are, the day, date and time and what is happening. This is done by constantly telling them these things and getting them to repeat what they have been told. It is a bit tedious but, up to a point, it works.

Mnemonics

These are tricks to help us memorise particular things. A useful one is '30 days hath September' - for the lengths of the months.

External aids

Most of us check what day it is by looking at a calendar or the day's newspaper. We regularly use alarms to wake us, but can also use them to remind you of things to do. Leave things you will need to take out by the front door or where you are unlikely to miss them. Put your pills by your toothbrush, this can remind you to take them when you clean your teeth. Pills are now often packaged so that you can check whether you've taken today's or not.

Nobody's perfect

Most people who think their memory is going have a normal memory that isn't perfect. Younger people will explain their memory lapses saying that they are hung over, in love, too busy or 'scatty' - they won't think they have Alzheimer's disease. If this happens to older people, they tend to think they have dementia, even when they haven't.

POST-TRAUMATIC STRESS DISORDER

In our everyday lives, any of us can have an experience that is overwhelming, frightening and beyond our control. We could find ourselves in a car crash, the victim of an assault or see an accident. Emergency services workers are more likely to have such experiences – they often have to deal with horrifying scenes. Likewise soldiers may be shot or blown up, and see friends killed or injured. Most people, in time, get over experiences like this without needing help. In some people, though, traumatic experiences set off a reaction that can last for many months or years. This is termed **post-traumatic stress disorder** (PTSD).

PTSD can start after any traumatic event. A traumatic event is one where the individual can see that they are in danger, their life is threatened, or where significant injury or distress of others is observed. Some typical traumatic events could be:

+ serious road accidents,
+ military combat,
+ violent personal assault (sexual assault, physical attack, abuse, robbery, mugging),
+ being taken hostage,
+ terrorist attack,
+ being a prisoner-of-war,
+ natural or man-made disasters,
+ being diagnosed with a life-threatening illness.

Even hearing about an unexpected injury or the violent death of a family member or close friend can start PTSD.

Common Symptoms of PTSD

The symptoms of PTSD can start after a delay of weeks or even months but usually appear within six months of a traumatic event occurring. Many people feel grief-stricken, depressed, anxious, guilty and angry after a traumatic experience. As well as these understandable emotional reactions, there are three main types of symptoms produced by such an experience:

1. **Flashbacks and nightmares**: The individual relives the event, again and again. This can happen both as a 'flashback' in the day and as nightmares when during sleep. These can be so realistic that it feels as though the individual is living through the experience all over again. They see it in their mind, but may also feel the emotions and physical sensations of what happened – fear, sweating, smells, sounds, pain. Ordinary things can trigger off flashbacks. For instance, if you had a car crash in the rain, a rainy day might start a flashback.

2. **Avoidance and numbing**: It can be just too upsetting to relive the experience over and over again. So individuals distract themselves. They keep their minds busy by losing themselves in a hobby, working very hard, or spending their time absorbed in crossword or jigsaw puzzles. They avoid places and people that remind them of the trauma, and try not to talk about it. They may deal with the pain of their feelings by trying to feel nothing at all – by becoming emotionally numb. They communicate less with other people, who then find it hard to live or work with them.

3. **Being 'on guard'**: An individual may stay alert all the time, as if they are looking out for danger. They cannot relax. This is termed hyper-vigilance. They feel anxious and find it hard to sleep. It may also be noted that the individual is jumpy and irritable.

Other Symptoms

Emotional reactions to stress are often accompanied by:

+ muscle aches and pains,
+ diarrhoea,
+ irregular heartbeats,
+ headaches,
+ feelings of panic and fear,
+ depression,
+ drinking too much alcohol,
+ using drugs (including painkillers).

The majority of individuals exposed to a significant stressful event will develop a form of PTSD. This is an 'acute stress reaction'. Over a few weeks, most people slowly come to terms with what has happened, and their stress symptoms start to disappear.

About one in three people will find that their symptoms just carry on and that they cannot come to terms with what has happened. It is as though the process has got stuck. The symptoms of post-traumatic stress, although normal in themselves, become a problem – or PTSD – when they go on for too long.

The more disturbing the experience, the more likely the individual to develop PTSD, and mechanisms including psychological and physiological may influence the individual's probability of experiencing PTSD.

Psychological

When we are frightened, we remember things very clearly. Although it can be distressing to remember these things, it can help us to understand what happened and, in the long run, help us to survive.

+ The flashbacks, or replays, force us to think about what has happened. We can decide what to do if it happens again. After a while, we learn to think about it without becoming upset.
+ It is tiring and distressing to remember a trauma. Avoidance and numbing keep the number of replays down to a manageable level.
+ Being 'on guard' means that we can react quickly if another crisis happens. We sometimes see this happening with survivors of an earthquake, when there may be second or third shocks. It can also give us the energy for the work that is needed after an accident or crisis.

But we do not want to spend the rest of our life going over it. We only want to think about it when we have to – if we find ourselves in a similar situation.

Physical

Adrenaline is a hormone our bodies produce when we are under stress. It pumps up the body to prepare it for action. When the stress disappears, the level of adrenaline should go back to normal. In PTSD, it may be that the vivid memories of the trauma keep the levels of adrenaline high. This will make a person tense, irritable and unable to relax or sleep well.

The hippocampus is the part of the brain that processes memories. High levels of stress hormones, like adrenaline, can stop it from working properly – like blowing a fuse. This means that flashbacks and nightmares continue because the memories of the trauma cannot be processed. If the stress goes away and the adrenaline levels get back to normal, the brain is able to repair the damage itself, like other natural healing processes in the body. The disturbing memories can then be processed and the flashbacks and nightmares will slowly disappear.

Children and PTSD

PTSD can develop at any age. Younger children may have upsetting dreams of the actual trauma, which then change into nightmares of monsters. They often relive the trauma in their play. For example, a child involved in a serious road traffic accident might re-enact the crash with toy cars, over and over again. They may lose interest in things they used to enjoy. They may find it hard to believe that they will live long enough to grow up. They often complain of stomach-aches and headaches.

Treatment

Just as there are both physical and psychological aspects to PTSD, so there are both physical and psychological treatments for it.

Psychotherapy

All the effective psychotherapies for PTSD focus on the traumatic experiences that have produced the symptoms rather than the individual's past life. The individual cannot change or forget what has happened, but they can learn to think differently about it, about the world and about their life.

The individual needs to be able to remember what happened, as fully as possible, without being overwhelmed by fear and distress. These therapies help to put words to the traumatic experiences. By remembering the event, going over it and making sense of it, the mind can do its normal job of storing the memories away and moving on to other things. When the individual starts to feel safe again and in control of their feelings, they will not need to avoid the memories as much. They can gain more control over their memories so that they only think about them when they want to, rather than having them erupt into their mind spontaneously.

All these treatments should be given by specialists in the treatment of PTSD. The sessions should be at least weekly, every week, with the same therapist, and should usually continue for

8-12 weeks. Although sessions will usually last around an hour, they may sometimes last up to 90 minutes.

Group therapy may also be effective and involves meeting with a group of other people who have been through the same or a similar traumatic event. The fact that other people in the group do have some idea of what the individual has experienced can make it much easier to talk about what has happened.

Medication

SSRI antidepressant tablets will both reduce the strength of PTSD symptoms and relieve any depression that is also present. Treatment with SSRI drugs usually continues for up to 12 months. Soon after starting an antidepressant, some people may find that they feel more anxious, restless or suicidal. These feelings usually pass in a few days. Occasionally, if someone is so distressed that they cannot sleep or think clearly, anxiety-reducing medication may be necessary such as benzo-diazepines. These tablets should usually not be prescribed for more than 10 days or so.

Body-focused Therapies

These can help to control the distress of PTSD. They can also reduce hyperarousal, or the feeling of being 'on guard' all the time. These therapies include physiotherapy and osteopathy, but also complementary therapies such as massage, acupuncture, reflexology, yoga, meditation and tai chi. They all help to develop ways of relaxing and managing stress.

The National Institute for Health and Clinical Excellence (NICE) guidelines suggest that trauma-focused psychological therapies (CBT) should be offered before medication, wherever possible.

CRITICAL REFLECTION

Let us revisit the case study on page 180. Now that you have read the chapter, name three mental health illnesses. Under what sections of the Mental Health Act can a person be admitted to hospital against their will? What treatments are used for mental health illness other than medication?

CHAPTER HIGHLIGHTS

+ Mental health is a term used in a healthcare context to refer to an individual's psychological well-being, or put simply the health of the mind.
+ A mental disorder is any problem affecting mental health.
+ Mental illness is not clearly legally defined in the Mental Health Act 1983.
+ Alcohol and drug dependence tend to be the two commonest forms of substance misuse encountered within healthcare.
+ More than one in four men and about one in seven women are drinking more than is medically safe for them.
+ Suicide and alcohol dependence are closely associated: 40% of men who try to kill themselves have had a long-standing alcohol problem.
+ Drugs of dependence and misuse may either be prescription medications or of the drugs considered as illicit or recreational drugs.
+ Cannabis is probably the drug most frequently used recreationally in the UK.
+ Assessment of any individual with a substance misuse problem is essential to determine the extent of their dependence.
+ Schizophrenia is a relatively common mental health disorder that affects one in every 100 people.
+ Both medication and psychological techniques can be used in the treatment of schizophrenia.
+ Bipolar disorder affects about one in every 100 adults at some point in their life.
+ Bipolar disorder is divided into four main types.
+ Memory problems can occur as a result of physiological illness, psychological problems or dementia.
+ PTSD can be experienced by an individual following a particularly stressful event.
+ Strategies to manage PTSD may include counselling, psychotherapy or developing new coping strategies.

GUIDANCE AND FURTHER INFORMATION

For the full text of Acts and Regulations mentioned in this chapter see www.legislation.hmso.gov.uk.

UK Trauma Group has links to a selection of materials with helpful information for the general public and for health professionals about post-traumatic stress reactions, see www.uktrauma.org.uk.

Information on PTSD is available from the National Center for PTSD (USA), see www.ncptsd.org/disaster.html.

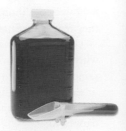

REFERENCES

Adams, I.B. and Martin, B.R. (1996) 'Cannabis: pharmacology and toxicology in animals and humans', *Addiction*, 91(11), 1585–1614.

Arendt, M., Rosenberg, R., Foldager, L. and Perto, G. (2005) 'Cannabis-induced psychosis and subsequent schizophrenia-spectrum disorders: follow-up study of 535 incident cases', *British Journal of Psychiatry*, 187, 510–515.

Arseneault, L., Cannon, M., Poulton, R., Murray, R., Caspi, A. and Moffit, T.E. (2002) 'Cannabis use in adolescence and risk for adult psychosis: longitudinal prospective study', *British Medical Journal*, 325: 1212–1213.

Blows, S., Ivers, R.Q., Connor. J., Ameratunga, S., Woodward, M. and Norton, R. (2005) 'Marijuana use and car crash injury', *Addiction*, 100(5), 605–611.

Fanous, A., Gardner, C., Walsh, D. and Kendler, K.S. (2001) 'Relationship between positive and negative symptoms of schizophrenia and schizotypal symptoms in nonpsychotic relatives', *Archives of General Psychiatry*, 58, 669–673.

Fergusson, D.M., Horwood, L.J. and Beautrais, A.L. (2003) 'Cannabis and educational achievement', *Addiction*, 98(12), 1681–1692.

Fergusson, D.M., Horwood, L.J. and Ridder, E.M. (2005) 'Test of causal linkages between cannabis use and psychotic symptoms, *Addition*, 100(3), 354–366.

Henquet, C., Krabbendam, L., Spauwen, J., Kaplan, C.D., Lieb, R., Wittchen, H.U. and Van Os, J. (2005) 'Prospective cohort study of cannabis use, predisposition for psychosis, and psychotic symptoms in young people', *British Medical Journal*, 330(7481), 11–14.

Janowsky, D.S., Meacham, M.P., Blaine, J.D., Schoor, M. and Bozzetti, L.P. (1976a) 'Marjuana effects on simulated flying ability', *American Journal of Psychiatry*, 133(4), 384–388.

Janowsky, D.S., Meacham, M.P., Blaine, J.D., Schoor, M. and Bozzetti, L.P. (1976b) 'Simulated flying performance after marijuana intoxication', *Aviation Space Environment Medicine*, 47(2), 124–128.

Laumon, B., Gadegbeku, B., Martin, J.L., Biecheler, M.B. and the SAM Group (2005) 'Cannabis intoxication and fatal road crashes in France: population based case-control study', *British Medical Journal*, 331, 1371–1377.

Leirer, V.O. and Yesavage, J.A. (1991) 'Marijuana carry-over effects on aircraft pilot performance', *Aviation, Space, and Environmental Medicine*, 62, 221–227.

Leirer, V.O., Yesavage, J.A. and Morrow, D.G. (1989) 'Marijuana, aging, and task difficulty effects on pilot performance', *Aviation, Space, and Environmental Medicine*, 60, 1145–1152.

McGee, R., Williams, S., Poulton, R. and Moffitt, T. (2000) 'A longitudinal study of cannabis use and mental health from adolescence to early adulthood', *Addiction*, 95, 491–503.

Patton, G.C., Coffey, C., Carlin, J.B., Degenhardt, L., Lynskey, M. and Hall, W. (2002) 'Cannabis use and mental health in young people: cohort study', *British Medical Journal*, 325, 1195–1198.

Rey, J.M., Sawyer, M.G., Raphael, B., Paton, G.C. and Lynskey, M. (2002) 'Mental health of teenagers who use cannabis: Results of an Australian survey', *British Journal of Psychiatry*, March, 180, 216–221.

Van Os, J., Bak, M., Hanssen, M., Bijl, R.V., de Graaf, R. and Verdoux, H. (2002) 'Cannabis use and psychosis: A longitudinal population-based study', *American Journal of Epidemiology*, 156, 319–327.

Yesavage, J.A., Leirer, V.O., Denari, M. and Hollister, L.E. (1985) 'Carry-over effects of marijuana intoxication on aircraft pilot performance; a preliminary report', *American Journal of Psychiatry*, 142, 1325–1329.

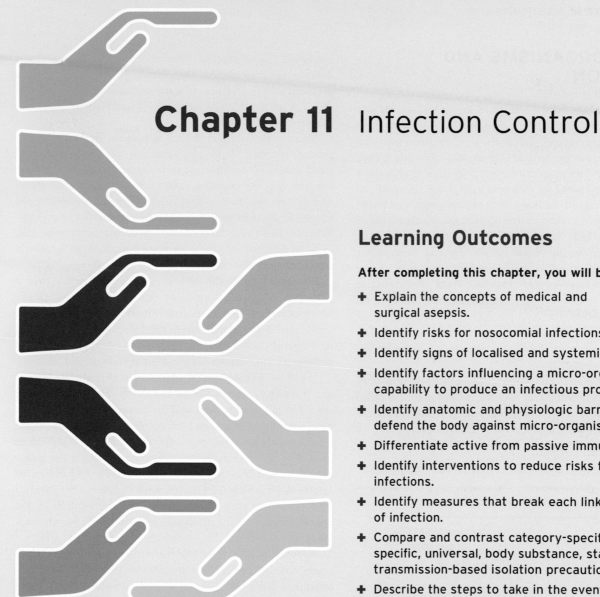

Chapter 11 Infection Control

Learning Outcomes

After completing this chapter, you will be able to:

+ Explain the concepts of medical and surgical asepsis.

+ Identify risks for nosocomial infections.

+ Identify signs of localised and systemic infections.

+ Identify factors influencing a micro-organism's capability to produce an infectious process.

+ Identify anatomic and physiologic barriers that defend the body against micro-organisms.

+ Differentiate active from passive immunity.

+ Identify interventions to reduce risks for infections.

+ Identify measures that break each link in the chain of infection.

+ Compare and contrast category-specific, disease-specific, universal, body substance, standard and transmission-based isolation precaution systems.

+ Describe the steps to take in the event of a blood-borne pathogen exposure.

+ Correctly implement aseptic practices, including handwashing, donning and removing a facemask, gowning, donning and removing disposable gloves, bagging articles and managing equipment used for isolation situations.

CASE STUDY

The *Daily Express* newspaper had, on 31 March 2007, yet another headline, 'New Superbug Kills 17 - Danger threatening our hospitals'. A member of your family is extremely concerned about your safety working in the healthcare environment after yet another report in the media of patients being infected with hospital acquired 'super bugs'. You explain to them about infection control and how the chain of infection works, and how it is possible to prevent the spread of infection by good hand hygiene practices. You also explain why you do not wear your uniform to and from clinical practice and why it is washed separately at a higher temperature to other clothes.

The family member is reassured following your explanation and asks you to teach them the hand hygiene techniques used in clinical practice in preparation for when they go to visit family and friends in hospital. You teach them these techniques and again emphasise the importance of good hand hygiene and infection control to prevent the spread of infection.

MICRO-ORGANISMS AND INFECTION

Nurses are directly involved in providing a biologically safe environment. Micro-organisms exist everywhere: in water, in soil and on body surfaces such as the skin, intestinal tract and other areas open to the outside (e.g. mouth, upper respiratory tract, vagina and lower urinary tract). Most micro-organisms are harmless, and some are even beneficial in that they perform essential functions in the body. Some micro-organisms found in the intestines (e.g. enterobacteria) produce substances called **bacteriocins**, which are lethal to related strains of bacteria. Others produce antibiotic-like substances and toxic metabolites that repress the growth of other micro-organisms. Some micro-organisms are normal **resident flora** (the collective vegetation in a given area) in one part of the body, yet produce infection in another. For example, *Escherichia coli* is a normal inhabitant of the large intestine but a common cause of infection of the urinary tract. Table 11-1 provides a list of common resident micro-organisms.

An **infection** is an invasion of body tissue by micro-organisms and their proliferation there. Such a micro-organism is called an *infectious agent*. If the micro-organism produces no clinical evidence of disease, the infection is called *asymptomatic* or

Table 11-1 Examples of Common Resident Micro-Organisms

Body area	Micro-organisms
Skin	*Staphylococcus epidermidis* *Propionibacterium acnes* *Staphylococcus aureus* *Corynebacterium xerosis* *Pityrosporum oxale* (yeast)
Nasal passages	*Staphylococcus aureus* *Staphylococcus epidermidis*
Oropharynx	*Streptococcus pneumoniae*
Mouth	*Streptococcus mutans* *Lactobacillus* *Bacteroides* *Actinomyces*
Intestine	*Bacteroides* *Fusobacterium* *Eubacterium* *Lactobacillus* *Streptococcus* Enterobacteriaceae *Shigella* *Escherichia coli*
Urethral orifice	*Staphylococcus epidermidis*
Urethra (lower)	*Proteus*
Vagina	*Lactobacillus* *Bacteroides* *Clostridium* *Candida albicans*

subclinical. Some subclinical infections can cause significant damage, for example, cytomegalovirus (CMV) infection in a pregnant woman can lead to significant disease in the unborn child. A detectable alteration in normal tissue function, however, is called **disease**.

Micro-organisms vary in their **virulence** (i.e. their ability to produce disease). Micro-organisms also vary in the severity of the diseases they produce and their degree of communicability. For example, the common cold virus is more readily transmitted than the bacillus that causes leprosy (*Mycobacterium leprae*). If the infectious agent can be transmitted to an individual by direct or indirect contact, through a vector or vehicle, or as an airborne infection, the resulting condition is called a **communicable disease**.

Pathogenicity is the ability to produce disease; thus a pathogen is a micro-organism that causes disease. Many micro-organisms that are normally harmless can cause disease under certain circumstances. A 'true' pathogen causes disease or infection in a healthy individual. An **opportunistic pathogen** causes disease only in a susceptible individual.

Infectious diseases are the major cause of death worldwide, and a leading cause of illness and death. The control of the spread of micro-organisms and the protection of people from communicable diseases and infections are carried out on the international, national, regional, community and individual level. The World Health Organization (WHO) is the major regulatory agency at the international level. The Department of Health is the principal UK public health agency at the national level concerned with disease prevention and control. At the regional level, health authorities and local health boards track epidemics and illnesses as reports are made in a local area.

Asepsis is the freedom from disease-causing micro-organisms. To decrease the possibility of transferring micro-organisms from one place to another, asepsis is used. There are two basic types of asepsis: medical and surgical. **Medical asepsis** includes all practices intended to confine a specific micro-organism to a specific area, limiting the number, growth and transmission of micro-organisms. In medical asepsis, objects are referred to as **clean**, which means the absence of almost all micro-organisms, or **dirty** (soiled, contaminated), which means likely to have micro-organisms, some of which may be capable of causing infection.

Surgical asepsis, or **sterile technique**, refers to those practices that keep an area or object free of all micro-organisms; it includes practices that destroy all micro-organisms and spores. Surgical asepsis is used for all procedures involving the sterile areas of the body.

Sepsis is the state of infection and can take many forms, including septic shock.

(Aseptic technique is discussed in more detail in Chapter 14.)

Types of Micro-organisms Causing Infections

Four major categories of micro-organisms cause infection in humans: bacteria, viruses, fungi and parasites. **Bacteria** are by far the most common infection-causing micro-organisms. Several hundred species can cause disease in humans and can live and be transported through air, water, food, soil, body tissues and fluids and inanimate objects. Most of the micro-organisms in Table 11-1 are bacteria. **Viruses** consist primarily of nucleic acid and therefore must enter living cells in order to reproduce. Common virus families include the rhinovirus (causes the common cold), hepatitis, herpes and human immunodeficiency virus. **Fungi** include yeasts and moulds. *Candida albicans* is a yeast considered to be normal flora in the human vagina. **Parasites** live on other living organisms. They include protozoa such as the one that causes malaria, helminths (worms) and arthropods (mites, fleas, ticks).

TYPES OF INFECTIONS

Colonisation is the process by which strains of micro-organisms become resident flora. In this state, the micro-organisms may grow and multiply but do not cause disease. Infection occurs when newly introduced or resident micro-organisms succeed in invading a part of the body where the host's defence mechanisms are ineffective and the pathogen causes tissue damage. The infection becomes a disease when the signs and symptoms of the infection are unique and can be differentiated from other conditions.

Infections can be local or systemic. A **local infection** is limited to the specific part of the body where the micro-organisms remain. If the micro-organisms spread and damage different parts of the body, it is a **systemic infection**. When a culture of the person's blood reveals micro-organisms, the condition is called **bacteraemia**. When bacteraemia results in systemic infection, it is referred to as **septicaemia**.

There are also **acute** or **chronic infections**. Acute infections generally appear suddenly or last a short time. A chronic infection may occur slowly, over a very long period, and may last months or years.

Nosocomial Infections

Nosocomial infections are classified as infections that are associated with the delivery of healthcare services in a healthcare environment. Nosocomial infections can either develop during a patient's stay in a clinical area or manifest after discharge. Nosocomial micro-organisms (e.g. MRSA (Methicillin Resistant Staphylococcus Aureus); Clostridium difficile tuberculosis and HIV) may also be acquired by health personnel working in the facility and can cause significant illness and time lost from work.

Nosocomial infections have received increasing attention in recent years and affect significant patient numbers every year. The most common settings where nosocomial infections develop are hospital surgical or medical intensive care units. The most common sites for nosocomial infections are the urinary tract, the respiratory tract, bloodstream and wounds. The micro-organisms that cause nosocomial infections can originate from the patient themselves (an **endogenous** source) or from the hospital environment and hospital personnel (**exogenous** sources). Most nosocomial infections appear to have endogenous sources. *Escherichia coli, Staphylococcus aureus* and enterococci are the most common infecting micro-organisms.

A number of factors contribute to nosocomial infections. **Iatrogenic infections** are the direct result of diagnostic or therapeutic procedures. One example of an iatrogenic infection is bacteraemia that results from an intravascular line. Not all nosocomial infections are iatrogenic, nor are all nosocomial infections preventable.

Another factor contributing to the development of nosocomial infections is the compromised host, that is, a patient whose normal defences have been lowered by surgery or illness.

The hands of personnel are a common vehicle for the spread of micro-organisms. Insufficient handwashing is thus an important factor contributing to the spread of nosocomial micro-organisms.

> **CLINICAL ALERT**
>
> *A person does not need to have an identified infection in order to pass potentially infective micro-organisms to another person. Even normal micro-organisms for one person can infect another person.*

The cost of nosocomial infections to the patient, the clinical area, and funding sources is great. Nosocomial infections extend hospitalisation time, increase patients' time away from work, cause disability and discomfort, and even result in loss of life (see Table 11-2 on page 202).

CHAIN OF INFECTION

Six links make up the chain of infection (Figure 11-1 on page 202): the aetiological agent, or micro-organism; the place where the organism naturally resides (reservoir); a portal of exit from the reservoir; a method (mode) of transmission; a portal of entry into a host; and the susceptibility of the host.

Aetiological Agent

The extent to which any micro-organism is capable of producing an infectious process depends on the number of micro-organisms present, the virulence and potency of the micro-organisms (pathogenicity), the ability of the micro-organisms to enter the body, the susceptibility of the host, and the ability of the micro-organisms to live in the host's body.

Some micro-organisms, such as the smallpox virus (now eradicated worldwide), have the ability to infect almost all susceptible people after exposure. By contrast, micro-organisms such as the tuberculosis bacillus infect a relatively small number of the population who are susceptible and exposed, usually people who are poorly nourished, who are living in crowded

Table 11-2 Nosocomial Infections

Most common micro-organisms	Causes
Urinary tract	
Escherichia coli	Improper catheterisation technique
Enterococcus species	Contamination of closed drainage system
Pseudomonas aeruginosa	Inadequate handwashing
Surgical sites	
Staphylococcus aureus (may be resistant to treatment)	Inadequate handwashing
Enterococcus species	Improper dressing change technique
Pseudomonas aeruginosa	
Bloodstream	
Coagulase-negative staphylococci	Inadequate handwashing
Staphylococcus aureus	Improper intravenous fluid, tubing and site care technique
Enterococcus species	
Pneumonia	
Staphylococcus aureus	Inadequate handwashing
Pseudomonas aeruginosa	Improper suctioning technique
Enterobacter species	

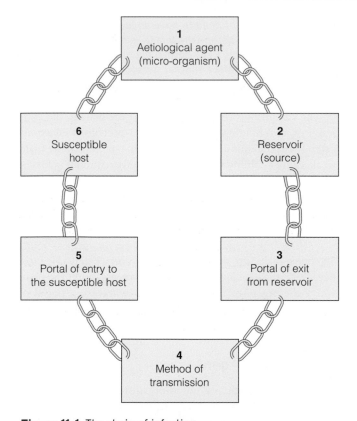

Figure 11-1 The chain of infection.

conditions, or whose immune systems are less competent (such as older adults or those with HIV or cancer).

Reservoir

There are many **reservoirs** or sources of micro-organisms. Common sources are other humans, the patient's own micro-organisms, plants, animals or the general environment. People are the most common source of infection for others and for themselves (see Table 11-3). For example, the person with an influenza virus frequently spreads it to others. A **carrier** is a person or animal reservoir of a specific infectious agent that usually does not manifest any clinical signs of disease. The *Anopheles* mosquito reservoir carries the malaria parasite but is unaffected by it. The carrier state may also exist in individuals with a clinically recognisable disease such as the dog with rabies. Under either circumstance, the carrier state may be of short duration (temporary or transient carrier) or long duration (chronic carrier). Food, water and faeces also can be reservoirs.

Portal of Exit from Reservoir

Before an infection can establish itself in a host, the micro-organisms must leave the reservoir. Common human reservoirs and their associated portals of exit are summarised in Table 11-3.

Method of Transmission

After a micro-organism leaves its source or reservoir, it requires a means of transmission to reach another person or host through a receptive portal of entry. There are three mechanisms:

1. *Direct transmission.* Direct transmission involves immediate and direct transfer of micro-organisms from person to person through touching, biting kissing or sexual intercourse. Droplet spread is also a form of direct transmission but can occur only if the source and the host are within a few metres of each other. Sneezing, coughing, spitting, singing or talking can project droplet spray into the conjunctiva or onto the mucous membranes of the eye, nose or mouth of another person.

2. *Indirect transmission.* Indirect transmission may be either vehicle-borne or vector-borne.
   - **Vehicle-borne transmission**. A *vehicle* is any substance that serves as an intermediate means to transport and

Table 11-3 Human Body Area Reservoirs, Common Infectious Micro-Organisms and Portals of Exit

Body area	Common infectious organisms	Portals of exit
Respiratory tract	Parainfluenza virus	Nose or mouth through sneezing, coughing, breathing or talking
	Mycobacterium tuberculosis *Staphylococcus aureus*	
Gastrointestinal tract	Hepatitis A virus	Mouth: saliva, vomitus; anus: faeces; ostomies
	Salmonella species	
Urinary tract	*Escherichia coli* enterococci *Pseudomonas aeruginosa*	Urethral meatus and urinary diversion
Reproductive tract	*Neisseria gonorrhoeae*	Vagina: vaginal discharge; Urinary meatus: semen, urine
	Treponema pallidum Herpes simplex virus type 2 Hepatitis B virus (HBV)	
Blood	Hepatitis B virus	Open wound, needle puncture site, any disruption of intact skin or mucous membrane surfaces
	Human immunodeficiency virus (HIV) *Staphylococcus aureus* *Staphylococcus epidermidis*	
Tissue	*Staphylococcus aureus* *Escherichia coli* *Proteus* species *Streptococcus* beta-haemolytic A or B	Drainage from cut or wound

introduce an infectious agent into a susceptible host through a suitable portal of entry. Fomites (inanimate materials or objects), such as handkerchiefs, toys, soiled clothes, cooking or eating utensils, and surgical instruments or dressings, can act as vehicles. Water, food, blood, serum and plasma are other vehicles. For example, food or water may become contaminated by a food handler who carries the hepatitis A virus. The food is then ingested by a susceptible host.

- **Vector-borne transmission.** A *vector* is an animal or flying or crawling insect that serves as an intermediate means of transporting the infectious agent. Transmission may occur by injecting salivary fluid during biting or by depositing faeces or other materials on the skin through the bite wound or a traumatised skin area.

3. *Airborne transmission.* **Airborne transmission** may involve droplets or dust. **Droplet nuclei**, the residue of evaporated droplets emitted by an infected host such as someone with tuberculosis, can remain in the air for long periods. Dust particles containing the infectious agent (e.g. *Clostridium difficile* spores from the soil) can also become airborne. The material is transmitted by air currents to a suitable portal of entry, usually the respiratory tract, of another person.

Portal of Entry to the Susceptible Host

Before a person can become infected, micro-organisms must enter the body. The skin is a barrier to infectious agents; however, any break in the skin can readily serve as a portal of entry. Often, micro-organisms enter the body of the host by the same route they used to leave the source.

Susceptible Host

A susceptible host is any person who is at risk for infection. A **compromised host** is a person 'at increased risk', an individual who for one or more reasons is more likely than others to acquire an infection. Impairment of the body's natural defences and a number of other factors can affect susceptibility to infection. Examples include age (the very young or the very old); patients receiving immune suppression treatment for cancer, chronic illness or following a successful organ transplant; and those with immune deficiency conditions.

BODY DEFENCES AGAINST INFECTION

Individuals normally have defences that protect the body from infection. These defences can be categorised as nonspecific and specific. **Nonspecific defences** protect the person against all micro-organisms, regardless of prior exposure. **Specific (immune) defences**, by contrast, are directed against identifiable bacteria, viruses, fungi or other infectious agents.

Nonspecific Defences

Nonspecific body defences include anatomical and physiological barriers, and the inflammatory response.

Anatomical and Physiological Barriers

Intact skin and mucous membranes are the body's first line of defence against micro-organisms. Unless the skin and mucosa become cracked and broken, they are an effective barrier against bacteria. Fungi can live on the skin, but they cannot penetrate it. The dryness of the skin also is a deterrent to bacteria. Bacteria are most plentiful in moist areas of the body, such as the perineum and axillae. Resident bacteria of the skin also prevent other bacteria from multiplying. They use up the available nourishment, and the end products of their metabolism inhibit other bacterial growth. Normal secretions make the skin slightly acidic; acidity also inhibits bacterial growth.

The nasal passages have a defensive function. As entering air follows the tortuous route of the passage, it comes in contact with moist mucous membranes and cilia. These trap micro-organisms, dust and foreign materials. The lungs have alveolar **macrophages** (large phagocytes). **Phagocytes** are cells that ingest micro-organisms, other cells and foreign particles.

Each body orifice also has protective mechanisms. The oral cavity regularly sheds mucosal epithelium to rid the mouth of colonisers. The flow of saliva and its partially buffering action help prevent infections. Saliva contains microbial inhibitors, such as lactoferrin, lysozyme and secretory IgA.

The eye is protected from infection by tears, which continually wash micro-organisms away and contain inhibiting lysozyme. The gastrointestinal tract also has defences against infection. The high acidity of the stomach normally prevents microbial growth. The resident flora of the large intestine help prevent the establishment of disease-producing micro-organisms. Peristalsis also tends to move microbes out of the body.

The vagina also has natural defences against infection. When a girl reaches puberty, lactobacilli ferment sugars in the vaginal secretions, creating a vaginal pH of 3.5 to 4.5. This low pH inhibits the growth of many disease-producing micro-organisms. The entrance to the urethra normally harbours many micro-organisms. These include *Staphylococcus epidermidis coagulase* (from the skin) and *Escherichia coli* (from faeces). It is believed that the urine flow has a flushing and bacteriostatic action that keeps the bacteria from ascending the urethra. An intact mucosal surface also acts as a barrier.

Inflammatory Response

Inflammation is a local and nonspecific defensive response of the tissues to an injurious or infectious agent. It is an adaptive mechanism that destroys or dilutes the injurious agent, prevents further spread of the injury, and promotes the repair of damaged tissue. It is characterised by five signs: (a) pain, (b) swelling, (c) redness, (d) heat and (e) impaired function of the part, if the injury is severe. Commonly, words with the suffix *-itis* describe an inflammatory process. For example, *appendicitis* means inflammation of the appendix; *gastritis* means inflammation of the stomach.

CLINICAL ALERT

An easy way to remember the signs of inflammation are the rhyming Latin words: rubor *(redness),* tumor *(swelling),* colour/calor *(heat), and* dolor *(pain).*

Injurious agents can be categorised as physical agents, chemical agents and micro-organisms. *Physical agents* include mechanical objects causing trauma to tissues, excessive heat or cold, and radiation. *Chemical agents* include external irritants (e.g. strong acids, alkalis, poisons and irritating gases) and internal irritants (substances manufactured within the body such as excessive hydrochloric acid in the stomach). *Micro-organisms* include the broad groups of bacteria, viruses, fungi and parasites.

A series of dynamic events is commonly referred to as the three stages of the inflammatory response:

+ *First stage*: vascular and cellular responses;
+ *Second stage*: exudate production;
+ *Third stage*: reparative phase.

These three phases are discussed in depth in Chapter 14.

Specific Defences

Specific defences of the body involve the immune system. An **antigen** is a substance that induces a state of sensitivity or immune responsiveness (**immunity**). If the proteins originate in a person's own body, the antigen is called an **autoantigen**.

The immune response has two components: antibody-mediated defences and cell-mediated defences. These two systems provide distinct but overlapping protection.

Antibody-mediated Defences

Another name for the *antibody-mediated defences* is **humoral immunity** (or **circulating immunity**) because these defences reside ultimately in the B lymphocytes and are mediated by antibodies produced by B cells. **Antibodies**, also called **immunoglobulins**, are part of the body's plasma proteins. The antibody-mediated responses defend primarily against the extracellular phases of bacterial and viral infections.

There are two major types of immunity: active and passive (see Table 11-4). In **active immunity**, the host produces antibodies in response to natural antigens (e.g. infectious micro-organisms) or artificial antigens (e.g. vaccines). B cells are activated when they recognise the antigen. They then differentiate into plasma cells, which secrete the antibodies, and serum proteins that bind specifically to the foreign substance and initiate a variety of elimination responses. The B cell may produce antibody molecules of five classes of immunoglobulins designated by letters and usually written as IgM, IgG, IgA, IgD and IgE. The presence of IgM in a laboratory analysis shows current infection. Before the antibody response can become effective, the phagocytic cells of the blood bind and ingest foreign substances. The rate of binding and phagocytosis increases if IgG antibodies (which indicate past infection and

Table 11-4 Types of Immunity

Type	Antigen or antibody source	Duration
1 Active	Antibodies are produced by the body in response to an antigen.	Long
a. Natural	Antibodies are formed in the presence of active infection in the body.	Lifelong
b. Artificial	Antigens (vaccines or toxoids) are administered to stimulate antibody production.	Many years; the immunity must be reinforced by booster
2. Passive	Antibodies are produced by another source, animal or human.	Short
a. Natural	Antibodies are transferred naturally from an immune mother to her baby through the placenta or in colostrum.	6 months to 1 year
b. Artificial	Immune serum (antibody) from an animal or another human is injected.	2 to 3 weeks

subsequent immunity) are present. With **passive immunity** (or **acquired immunity**), the host receives natural (e.g. from a nursing mother) or artificial (e.g. from an injection of immune serum) antibodies produced by another source.

Cell-Mediated Defences

The **cell-mediated defences**, or **cellular immunity**, occur through the T-cell system. On exposure to an antigen, the lymphoid tissues release large numbers of activated T cells into the lymph system. These T cells pass into the general circulation. There are three main groups of T cells: (a) helper T cells, which help in the functions of the immune system; (b) cytotoxic T cells, which attack and kill micro-organisms and sometimes the body's own cells; and (c) suppressor T cells, which can suppress the functions of the helper T cells and the cytotoxic T cells. When cell-mediated immunity is lost, as occurs with human immunodeficiency virus (HIV) infection, an individual is 'defenceless' against most viral, bacterial and fungal infections.

FACTORS INCREASING SUSCEPTIBILITY TO INFECTION

Whether a micro-organism causes an infection depends on a number of factors already mentioned. One of the most

important factors is host susceptibility, which is affected by age, heredity, level of stress, nutritional status, current medical therapy and pre-existing disease processes.

Age influences the risk of infection. Newborns and older adults have reduced defences against infection. Infections are a major cause of death of newborns, who have immature immune systems and are protected only for the first two or three months by immunoglobulins passively received from the mother. Between one and three months of age, infants begin to synthesise their own immunoglobulins. Immunisations against diphtheria, tetanus and pertussis are usually started at two months, when the infant's immune system can respond. Guidelines change frequently regarding childhood immunisations, up-to-date guidelines can be accessed from the Department of Health website.

With advancing age, the immune responses again become weak. Although there is still much to learn about ageing, it is known that immunity to infection decreases with advancing age. Because of the prevalence of influenza and its potential for causing death, the Department of Health recommends annual immunisation against influenza for older adults and for persons with chronic cardiac, respiratory, metabolic and renal disease. Pneumococcal vaccine is recommended for older adults last vaccinated more than ten years previously.

LIFESPAN CONSIDERATIONS

Older Adults
Normal ageing may predispose older adults to increased risk of infection and delayed healing. Organs and biochemical agents that are protective when a person is younger often change in structure and function with increasing age and then provide a decrease in their protective ability. Changes take place in the skin, respiratory tract,

gastrointestinal system, kidneys and immune system. If unchallenged, these systems work well to maintain homoeostasis for the individual, but if compromised by stress, illness, infections, treatments or surgeries, they find it difficult to keep up and therefore are not able to provide adequate protection. Special considerations for older adults are:

+ Nutrition is often poor in older adults and certain components, especially adequate protein, are necessary to build up and maintain the immune system.
+ Diabetes mellitus, which occurs more frequently in the elderly, increases the risk of infection and delayed healing by causing an alteration in nutrition and impaired peripheral circulation, which decrease the oxygen transport to the tissues.
+ The immune system reacts slowly to the introduction of antigens, allowing the antigen to reproduce itself several times before it is recognised by the immune system. T-cell effectiveness is often decreased due to immaturity.
+ The normal inflammatory response is delayed. This often causes atypical responses to infections with unusual presentations. Instead of displaying redness, swelling, and fever usually associated with infections, atypical symptoms such as confusion and disorientation, agitation, incontinence, falls, lethargy and general fatigue are often seen first.

Recognising these changes in older adults is important in early detection and treatment of related potential for infections and delayed healing. Nursing interventions to promote prevention are:

+ Provide and teach ways to improve nutritional status.
+ Use strict aseptic technique to decrease chance of infections (especially nosocomial infections in healthcare environments).
+ Encourage older adults to have regular immunisations for flu and pneumonia.
+ Be alert to subtle atypical signs of infection and act quickly to diagnose and treat.

Heredity influences the development of infection in that some people have a genetic susceptibility to certain infections. For example, some may be deficient in serum immunoglobulins, which play a significant role in the internal defence mechanism of the body.

The nature, number and duration of physical and emotional stressors can influence susceptibility to infection. Stressors elevate blood cortisone. Prolonged elevation of blood cortisone decreases anti-inflammatory responses, depletes energy stores, leads to a state of exhaustion and decreases resistance to infection. For example, a person recovering from a major operation or injury is more likely to develop an infection than a healthy person.

Resistance to infection depends on adequate nutritional status. Because antibodies are proteins, the ability to synthesise antibodies may be impaired by inadequate nutrition, especially when protein reserves are depleted (e.g. as a result of injury, surgery or debilitating diseases such as cancer).

Some medical therapies predispose a person to infection. For example, radiation treatments for cancer destroy not only cancerous cells but also some normal cells, thereby rendering them more vulnerable to infection. Some diagnostic procedures may also predispose the patient to an infection, especially when the skin is broken or sterile body cavities are penetrated during the procedure.

Certain medications also increase susceptibility to infection. Antineoplastic (anticancer) medications may depress bone marrow function, resulting in inadequate production of white blood cells necessary to combat infections. Anti-inflammatory medications, such as adrenal corticosteroids, inhibit the inflammatory response, an essential defence against infection. Even some antibiotics used to treat infections can have adverse effects. Antibiotics may kill resident flora, allowing the proliferation of strains that would not grow and multiply in the body under normal conditions. Certain antibiotics can also induce resistance in some strains of organisms.

Any disease that lessens the body's defences against infection places the patient at risk. Examples are chronic pulmonary disease, which impairs ciliary action and weakens the mucous barrier; peripheral vascular disease, which restricts blood flow; burns, which impair skin integrity; chronic or debilitating diseases, which deplete protein reserves; and such immune system diseases as leukaemia and aplastic anaemia, which alter the production of white blood cells. Diabetes mellitus is a major underlying disease predisposing patients to infection because compromised peripheral vascular status and increased serum glucose levels increase susceptibility.

NURSING MANAGEMENT

ASSESSING

During the assessing phase of the nursing process, the nurse obtains the patient's history, conducts the physical assessment, and gathers laboratory data.

Patient History

During the patient history, the nurse assesses (a) the degree to which a patient is at risk of developing an infection and (b) any patient complaints suggesting

 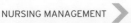

the presence of an infection. The nurse needs to collect data regarding the factors influencing the development of infection; especially existing disease process, history of recurrent infections, current medications and therapeutic measures, current emotional stressors, nutritional status and history of immunisations (see the *Assessment interview* on page 211).

Physiological Assessment

Signs and symptoms of an infection vary according to the body area involved. For example, sneezing, watery or mucoid discharge from the nose and nasal stuffiness commonly occur with an infection of the nose and sinuses; urinary frequency and possible cloudy or discoloured urine often occur with a urinary infection. Commonly the skin and mucous membranes are involved in a local infectious process, resulting in

+ localised swelling;
+ localised redness;
+ pain or tenderness with palpation or movement;
+ palpable heat at the infected area;
+ loss of function of the body part affected, depending on the site and extent of involvement.

In addition, open wounds may exude drainage of various colours.

Signs of *systemic infection* include:

+ fever;
+ increased pulse and respiratory rate, if the fever is high;
+ malaise and loss of energy;
+ anorexia and, in some situations, nausea and vomiting;
+ enlargement and tenderness of lymph nodes that drain the area of infection.

Laboratory Data

Laboratory data that indicate the presence of an infection include the following:

+ elevated leukocyte (white blood cell or WBC) count;
+ increases in specific types of leukocytes as revealed in the differential WBC count – specific types of white blood cells are increased or decreased in certain infections;
+ elevated *erythrocyte sedimentation rate (ESR)* – red blood cells normally settle slowly, but the rate increases in the presence of an inflammatory process;
+ urine, blood, sputum or other drainage **cultures** (laboratory cultivations of micro-organisms in a special growth medium) that indicate the presence of pathogenic micro-organisms.

PLANNING

The major goals for patients susceptible to infection are to:

+ maintain or restore defences;
+ avoid the spread of infectious organisms;
+ reduce or alleviate problems associated with the infection.

Desired outcomes depend on the individual patient's condition. Nursing strategies to meet the three broad goals stated above generally include using meticulous handwashing, medical and surgical aseptic techniques to prevent the spread of potentially infectious micro-organisms, implementing measures to support the defences of a susceptible host, and teaching patients about protective measures to prevent infections and the spread of infectious agents when an infection is present.

Planning for Community Care

Patients being discharged following hospital care for an infection often require continued care to completely eliminate the infection or to adapt to a chronic state. In addition, such patients may be at increased risk for reinfection or development of an opportunistic infection following therapy for existing pathogens.

In preparation for discharge, the nurse needs to know the patient's and family's risks, needs, strengths and resources. The *Teaching: Community care* box on page 212 describes the specific assessment data required before establishing a discharge plan. Using the data gathered about the home situation, the nurse tailors the teaching plan for the patient and family (see the *Teaching: Wellness care* box on page 212).

IMPLEMENTING

Whenever possible, the nurse implements strategies to prevent infection. If infection cannot be prevented, the nurse's goal is to prevent the spread of the infection within and between persons, and to treat the existing infection. In the sections that follow, specific nursing activities are described that interfere in the chain of infection to prevent and control transmission of infectious organisms, and that promote care of the infected patient. These activities are summarised in Table 11-5.

Preventing Nosocomial Infections

Meticulous use of medical and surgical asepsis is necessary to prevent transport of potentially infectious micro-organisms. As discussed previously in this chapter, nosocomial infections are those acquired in relation to healthcare services. Many nosocomial infections can be prevented using proper handwashing techniques, environmental controls, sterile technique when warranted, and identification and management of patients at risk for infections.

Handwashing

Handwashing is important in every setting, including hospitals. It is considered one of the most effective infection control measures. Any patient may harbour micro-organisms that are currently harmless to the patient yet potentially harmful to another person or to the same patient if they find a portal of

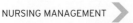

NURSING MANAGEMENT

Table 11-5 Nursing Interventions that Break the Chain of Infection

Link	Interventions	Rationale
Aetiologic agent or (micro-organism)	Ensure that articles are correctly cleaned and disinfected or sterilised before use eliminate micro-organisms.	Correct cleaning, disinfecting and sterilising reduce/eradicate micro-organisms
	Educate patients and support persons about appropriate methods to clean, disinfect and sterilise articles.	Knowledge of ways to reduce or eliminate micro-organisms reduces the numbers of micro-organisms present and the likelihood of transmission.
Reservoir (source)	Change dressings and bandages when they are soiled or wet.	Moist dressings are ideal environments for micro-organisms to grow and multiply.
	Assist patients to carry out appropriate skin and oral hygiene.	Hygienic measures reduce the numbers of resident and transient micro-organisms and the likelihood of infection.
	Dispose of damp, soiled linens appropriately.	Damp, soiled linens harbour more micro-organisms than dry linens.
	Dispose of faeces and urine in appropriate receptacles.	Urine and faeces in particular contain many micro-organisms.
	Ensure that all fluid containers, such as bedside water jugs and suction and drainage bottles, are covered or capped.	Prolonged exposure increases the risk of contamination and promotes microbial growth.
	Empty suction and drainage bottles at the end of each shift or before they become full, or according to agency policy.	Drainage harbours micro-organisms that, if left for long periods, proliferate and can be transmitted to others.
Portal of exit from the reservoir	Avoid talking, coughing or sneezing over open wounds or sterile fields, and cover the mouth and nose when coughing and sneezing.	These measures limit the number of micro-organisms that escape from the respiratory tract.
Method of transmission	Wash hands between patient contacts, after touching body substances, and before performing invasive procedures or touching open wounds.	Handwashing is an important means of controlling and preventing the transmission of micro-organisms.
	Instruct patients and support persons to wash hands before handling food or eating, after eliminating and after touching infectious material.	
	Wear gloves when handling secretions and excretions.	Gloves and gowns prevent soiling of the hands and clothing.
	Wear gowns/disposable plastic aprons if there is danger of soiling clothing with body substances.	
	Place discarded soiled materials in moisture-proof clinical waste bags.	Moisture-proof bags prevent the spread of micro-organisms to others.
	Hold used bedpans steadily to prevent spillage, and dispose of urine and faeces in appropriate receptacles.	Faeces in particular contain many micro-organisms.
	Initiate and implement aseptic precautions for all patients.	All patients may harbour potentially infectious micro-organisms that can be transmitted to others.
	Wear masks and eye protection when in close contact with patients who have infections transmitted by droplets from the respiratory tract.	Masks and eyewear reduce the spread of droplet-transmitted micro-organisms.
	Wear masks and eye protection when sprays of body fluid are possible (e.g. during irrigation procedures).	Masks and eye protection provide protection from micro-organisms in patients' body substances.
Portal of entry to the susceptible host	Use sterile technique for invasive procedures (e.g. injections, catheterisations).	Invasive procedures penetrate the body's natural protective barriers to micro-organisms.
	Use sterile technique when exposing open wounds or handling dressings.	Open wounds are vulnerable to microbial infection.
	Place used disposable needles and syringes in puncture-resistant containers sharps containers for disposal.	Injuries from needles contaminated by blood or body fluids from an infected patient or carrier are a primary cause of HBV and HIV transmission to healthcare workers.
	Provide all patients with their own personal care items.	People have less resistance to another person's micro-organisms than to their own.
Susceptible host	Maintain the integrity of the patient's skin and mucous membranes.	Intact skin and mucous membranes protect against invasion by micro-organisms.
	Ensure that the patient receives a balanced diet.	A balanced diet supplies proteins and vitamins necessary to build or maintain body tissues.
	Educate the public about the importance of immunisations.	Immunisations protect people against virulent infectious diseases.

entry. It is important that both the nurses' and the patients' hands be washed at the following times to prevent the spread of micro-organisms: before eating, after using the bedpan or toilet, and after the hands have come in contact with any body substances, such as sputum or drainage from a wound. In addition, healthcare workers should wash their hands before and after giving care of any kind to every patient.

For routine patient care, antimicrobial foam, hand gel or vigorous handwashing under a stream of water for at least 10 seconds using liquid soap or antimicrobial liquid soap should be performed. Antimicrobial soaps are usually provided in high-risk areas, such as the intensive care units, and are frequently supplied in dispensers at the sink. Studies have shown that the convenience of antimicrobial foams and gels, which do not require soap and water, may increase healthcare worker's adherence to hand cleansing (Bischoff *et al.*, 2000).

It is important to recognise that handwashing with either plain soap or antimicrobial soap can damage the skin through the drying effect of the detergents or chemicals. If the nurse develops dermatitis, the patient may be at higher risk because handwashing does not decrease bacterial counts on skin with dermatitis. The nurse is also at higher risk because the normal skin barrier has been broken. Although lotions, moisturisers and emollients have been tried, no research has yet confirmed their effectiveness in decreasing the problem.

Procedure 11-1 describes proper handwashing techniques.

PROCEDURE 11-1 Handwashing

Purposes

+ To reduce the number of micro-organisms on the hands
+ To reduce the risk of transmission of micro-organisms to patients
+ To reduce the risk of cross-contamination among patients
+ To reduce the risk of transmission of infectious organisms to oneself

Assessment

+ Presence of factors increasing susceptibility to infection
+ Use of immunosuppressive medications
+ Recent diagnostic procedures or treatments that penetrated the skin or a body cavity
+ Current nutritional status
+ Signs and symptoms indicating the presence of an infection:
  • Localised signs, such as swelling, redness, pain or tenderness with palpation or movement, palpable heat at site, loss of function of affected body part, presence of exudate
  • Systemic indications, such as fever, increased pulse and respiratory rates, lack of energy, anorexia, enlarged lymph nodes

Planning

Determine the location of running water and soap or soap substitutes.

Equipment

+ Soap
+ Warm running water
+ Disposable towels
+ Alcohol hand gel

Implementation

Preparation

+ Assess the hands.
+ Nails should be kept short. *Short, natural nails are less likely to harbour micro-organisms, scratch a patient or puncture gloves.*
+ Remove all jewellery. *Micro-organisms can lodge in the settings of jewellery and under rings.*

Removal facilitates proper cleaning of the hands and arms.
+ Check hands for breaks in the skin, such as hangnails or cuts. *A nurse who has open sores may require a clinical placement with decreased risk for transmission of infectious organisms.*

Performance

1. If you are washing your hands where the patient can observe you, explain to the patient what you are going to do and why it is necessary.
2. Turn on the water, and adjust the flow.
   - There are several common types of tap controls: hand-operated handles; elbow controls (move these with the elbows instead of the hands); infrared controls (motion in front of the sensor causes water to start and stop flowing automatically).
   - Adjust the flow so that the water is warm. *Warm water removes less of the protective oil of the skin than hot water.*
3. Wet the hands thoroughly by holding them under the running water, and apply soap to the hands.
   - Hold the hands lower than the elbows so that the water flows from the arms to the fingertips. *The water should flow from the least contaminated to the most contaminated area; the hands are generally considered more contaminated than the lower arms.*
   - If the soap is liquid, apply 2 to 4 ml.
4. Thoroughly wash and rinse the hands.
   - Use firm, rubbing and circular movements to wash the palm, back and wrist of each hand. Interlace the fingers and thumbs, and move the hands back and forth (Figure 11-2). Continue this motion for 10 seconds. *The circular action helps remove micro-organisms mechanically. Interlacing the fingers and thumbs cleans the interdigital spaces.*
   - Rub the fingertips against the palm of the opposite hand. *The nails and fingertips are commonly missed during handwashing.*
   - Rinse the hands.

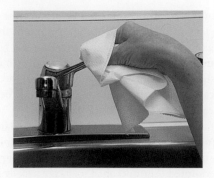

Figure 11-3 Using a paper towel to grasp the handle of a hand-operated tap.

5. Thoroughly dry the hands and arms.
   - Dry hands and arms thoroughly with a paper towel. *Moist skin becomes chapped readily; chapping produces lesions.*
   - Discard the paper towel in the appropriate container.
6. Turn off the water.
   - Use a new paper towel to grasp a hand-operated control (Figure 11-3). *This prevents the nurse from picking up micro-organisms from the tap handles.*

Variation: Handwashing Before Sterile Techniques

+ Apply the soap and wash as described in step 4 above, but hold the hands higher than the elbows during this handwash. Wet the hands and forearms under the running water, letting it run from the fingertips to the elbows so that the hands become cleaner than the elbows (see Figure 11-4). *In this way, the water runs from the area that now has the fewest micro-organisms to areas with a relatively greater number.*

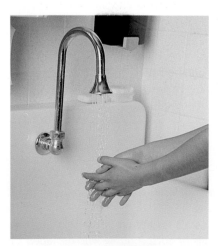

Figure 11-2 Interlacing the fingers during handwashing.

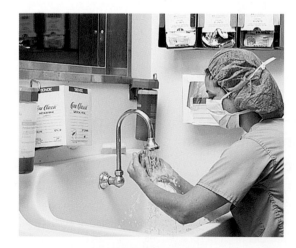

Figure 11-4 The hands are held higher than the elbows during a handwash before sterile technique.

+ Apply the soap and wash as described in step 6 above, maintaining the hands uppermost.
+ After washing and rinsing, use a towel to dry one hand thoroughly in a rotating motion from the

fingers to the elbow. Use a new towel to dry the other hand and arm. *A clean towel prevents the transfer of micro-organisms from one elbow (least clean area) to the other hand (cleanest area).*

Evaluation

There is no traditional evaluation of the effectiveness of the individual nurse's handwashing. Institutional infection control departments monitor the occurrence of patient infections and investigate those situations in which healthcare providers are implicated in the transmission of infectious organisms. Research has repeatedly shown the positive impact of careful handwashing on patient health associated with prevention of infection. Checks may be performed periodically on staff

handwashing with the use of an ultraviolet glow box. The nurse washes their hands thoroughly drying them to remove any contamination. A small amount of UV 'glow gel' is applied and rubbed thoroughly into hands as though the hands are being washed. The hands are then placed under a UV light source to see any areas missed during handwashing.

Common areas missed include the backs of the hands, web spaces between fingers and finger nails.

ASSESSMENT INTERVIEW

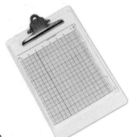

Patients at Risk of Infections

+ When were you last immunised for diphtheria, tetanus, poliomyelitis, rubella, measles, influenza, hepatitis and pneumococcal pneumonia?
+ When did you last have a tuberculin/heaf skin test?
+ What infections have you had in the past and how were these treated?
+ Have any of these infections recurred?
+ Are you taking any antibiotics, anti-inflammatory medications such as aspirin or ibuprofen, or medications for cancer?

+ Have you had any recent diagnostic procedure or therapy that penetrated through your skin or a body cavity?
+ What past surgeries have you had?
+ How would you describe your eating habits? Do you eat a variety of different types of foods?
+ Do you take vitamins?
+ On a scale of 1 to 10, how would you rate the stress you have experienced in the past six months?
+ Have you experienced any loss of energy, loss of appetite, nausea, headache or other signs associated with specific body systems (e.g. difficulty urinating, urinary frequency or a sore throat)?

Note: As with all history taking, the nurse must individualise the specific terms used, examples given to the patient, and teaching techniques used to validate agreement on the meaning of words according to the patient's culture, language spoken and education or intellectual abilities.

TEACHING: COMMUNITY CARE

Environmental Management

+ Discuss injury-proofing the home to prevent the possibility of further tissue injury (e.g. use of padding, handrails, removal of hazards).
+ Explore ways to control the environmental temperature and airflow (especially if patient has an airborne pathogen).
+ Determine the advisability of visitors and family members in proximity to the patient.
+ Describe ways to manipulate the bed, the room and other household facilities.

Infection Control

+ Teach proper handwashing and related hygienic measures to all family members.
+ Discuss antimicrobial soaps and effective disinfectants.
+ Ensure access to and proper use of gloves and other barriers as indicated by the type of infection or risk.
+ Discuss the relationship between hygiene, rest, activity and nutrition in the chain of infection.

+ Instruct about proper administration of medication.
+ Instruct about cleaning reusable equipment and supplies.

Infection Protection

+ Teach the patient and family members the signs and symptoms of infection, and when to contact a healthcare provider.
+ Teach the patient and family members how to avoid infections.
+ Suggest techniques for safe food preservation and preparation.
+ Emphasise the need for proper immunisations of all family members.

Wound Care

+ Teach the patient and family the signs of wound healing and of wound infection.
+ Explain the proper technique for changing the dressing and disposing of the soiled one.
+ Delineate the factors that promote wound healing.

TEACHING: WELLNESS CARE

Preventing Infections in the Home

+ Wash your hands before handling foods, before eating, after toileting, before and after any required home care treatment, and after touching any body substances (e.g. wound drainage).
+ Keep your fingernails short, clean and well manicured to eliminate rough edges or hangnails, which can harbour micro-organisms.
+ Do not share personal care items: toothbrush, washcloths and towels.
+ Wash raw fruits and vegetables before eating them.
+ Refrigerate all opened and unpackaged foods.
+ Clean used equipment with soap and water, and disinfect it with a chlorine bleach solution.

+ Place contaminated dressings and other disposable items containing body fluids in moisture-proof clinical waste bags.
+ Put used needles in a puncture-resistant sharps container.
+ Clean obviously soiled linen separately from other laundry. Rinse in cold water, wash in hot water if possible and add a cup of bleach to the wash.
+ Avoid coughing, sneezing or breathing directly on others. Cover the mouth and nose to prevent the transmission of airborne micro-organisms.
+ Be aware of any signs or symptoms of an infection, and report these immediately to your healthcare contact person.
+ Maintain a sufficient fluid intake to promote urine production and output. This helps flush the bladder and urethra of micro-organisms.

CLINICAL ANECDOTE

When I started as a student nurse I would be really afraid of catching an infection from a patient and wear gloves all the time when I did things. Now I am not so afraid and only wear gloves when I need to but wash my hands frequently and use alcohol hand gel between every patient.

Debbie, third-year student nurse

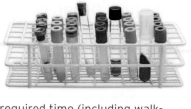

RESEARCH NOTE

Will a Soap-and-Water Alternative Increase Compliance with Handwashing?

Alcohol-based hand gels are available to the general public and to healthcare institutions as a substitute for soap-and-water handwashing of physically clean hands. However, limited research has been conducted on the effectiveness of these gels from the perspectives of their ability to kill micro-organisms, affect handwashing frequency, or impact skin condition. In this study by Earl *et al.* (2001), researchers designed three phases to specifically address the question of frequency of handwashing by nurses, physicians and ancillary personnel (technicians and therapists) in two intensive care units.

In phase I, prior to any intervention, the number of opportunities to wash hands was compared to actual compliance with handwashing over four weeks. In phase II, alcohol gel dispensers were installed inside and outside of patient rooms and both opportunities and occurrences for handwashing with either soap-and-water or gel were counted for four weeks. Phase III examined opportunities and occurrences for handwashing between 10 and 14 weeks after installation of the dispensers.

The results were as follows: phase I, 39.6% compliance; phase II, 52.6%; phase III, 57%. The highest rates of compliance were by ancillary personnel, followed by nursing staff and then physicians. The alcohol gel was used instead of soap about 50% to 60% of the time.

Although total amount of required time (including walking to the sinks) was not determined, less actual time was spent in hand antisepsis with gel in phase III (7.5 seconds) than with soap-and-water in phase I (9.4 seconds).

Implications

Although the gel dispensers succeeded in increasing the percentage of compliance with hand degerming, the researchers expressed concern that the final rate was still only about 60% of the incidences requiring antisepsis. However, the gel did take less time and was most likely more effective than the inadequate nine-second soap use. The authors recognised weaknesses in the study, including the common Hawthorne effect. This effect states that the participants' behaviour may change purely by knowing that a study is being conducted. In this case, the healthcare providers may have paid more attention to hand antisepsis than they would have had the study not been performed. In addition, it is not possible to extrapolate these results to other institutions and types of care units.

However, this study is an important example of the need to assess, intervene and reassess effectiveness of procedures designed to increase the safety and health of both providers and patients. The study could easily be replicated in other settings and the results expanded to include other variables such as cost and true time savings.

Note: From 'Improved Rates of Compliance with Hand Antisepsis Guidelines: A Three-Phase Observational Study,' by M.L. Earl, M.M. Jackson and L.S. Rickman, 2001, *American Journal of Nursing*, 101(3), pp. 26–33.

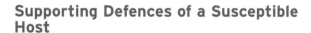

Supporting Defences of a Susceptible Host

People are constantly in contact with micro-organisms in the environment. Normally a person's natural defences ward off the development of an infection. **Susceptibility** is the degree to which an individual can be affected, that is, the likelihood of an organism causing an infection in that person. The following measures can reduce a person's susceptibility:

+ *Hygiene.* Intact skin and mucous membranes are one barrier against micro-organisms entering the body. In addition, good oral care reduces the likelihood of an oral infection. Regular and thorough bathing and shampooing remove micro-organisms and dirt that can result in an infection.
+ *Nutrition.* A balanced diet enhances the health of all body tissues, helps keep the skin intact and promotes the skin's ability to repel micro-organisms. Adequate nutrition enables tissues to maintain and rebuild themselves and helps keep the immune system functioning well.

+ *Fluid.* Fluid intake permits fluid output that flushes out the bladder and urethra, removing micro-organisms that could cause an infection.
+ *Rest and sleep.* Adequate rest and sleep are essential to health and to renewing energy (see Chapter 21).
+ *Stress.* Excessive stress predisposes people to infections. Nurses can assist patients to learn stress-reducing techniques.
+ *Immunisations.* The use of immunisations has dramatically decreased the incidence of infectious diseases. It is recommended that immunisations begin shortly after birth and be completed in early childhood except for boosters. Immunisations may be given by injection, inhalation, oral solutions or nasal sprays. They are frequently given in combination to minimise multiple injections. Because there are frequent changes to immunisation schedules, it is advisable to update immunisation schedules yearly.

There are immunisation programmes for high-risk groups such as healthcare personnel, older adults who are chronically ill and people travelling to foreign countries. For example, hepatitis B vaccine is recommended for all healthcare workers.

Cleaning, Disinfecting and Sterilising

The first links in the chain of infection, the aetiologic agent and the reservoir, are interrupted by the use of **antiseptics** (agents that inhibit the growth of some micro-organisms) and **disinfectants** (agents that destroy pathogens other than spores), and by sterilisation.

Cleaning

Cleanliness inhibits the growth of micro-organisms. When cleaning visibly soiled objects such as beds contaminated with faeces, nurses must always wear gloves to avoid direct contact with infectious micro-organisms. Most objects used in the care of patients, whether forceps or drawsheets, can be cleaned by rinsing them in cold water to remove any organic material, washing them with hot soapy water, then rinsing them again to remove the soap. The following steps should be followed when cleaning objects in a hospital.

1. Rinse the article with cold water to remove organic material. *Hot water coagulates the protein of organic material and tends to make it adhere.* Examples of organic material are blood and pus.
2. Wash the article in hot water and soap. *The emulsifying action of soap reduces surface tension and facilitates the removal of substances. Washing dislodges the emulsified substances.*
3. Use an abrasive, such as a stiff-bristled brush, to clean equipment with grooves and corners. *Friction helps dislodge foreign material.*
4. Rinse the article well with warm to hot water.
5. Dry the article; it is now considered clean.
6. Clean the brush and sink. These are considered soiled until they are cleaned appropriately, usually with a disinfectant.

Disinfecting

A disinfectant is a chemical preparation, such as hypochlorite (bleach), used on inanimate objects. Disinfectants are frequently caustic and toxic to tissues. An antiseptic is a chemical preparation used on skin or tissue. Disinfectants and antiseptics often have similar chemical components, but the disinfectant is a more concentrated solution.

Both antiseptics and disinfectants are said to have bactericidal or bacteriostatic properties. A *bactericidal* preparation destroys bacteria, whereas a *bacteriostatic* preparation prevents the growth and reproduction of some bacteria. Although some agents are active against a broad array of bacteria, if a specific micro-organism is identified, an agent known to be effective against it should be selected. Spore-forming bacteria such as *Clostridium difficile* (commonly referred to as *C. difficile*), which is a frequent cause of nosocomial diarrhoea, and *Bacillus anthracis* (anthrax) may be inhibited by only a few of the agents normally effective against other forms of bacteria. Table 11-6 lists commonly used antiseptics and disinfectants.

When disinfecting articles, nurses need to follow local policy and consider the following:

✛ The type and number of infectious organisms. Some micro-organisms are readily destroyed, whereas others require longer contact with the disinfectant.
✛ The recommended concentration of the disinfectant and the duration of contact.
✛ The temperature of the environment. Most disinfectants are intended for use at room temperature.
✛ The presence of soap. Some disinfectants are ineffective in the presence of soap or detergent.
✛ The presence of organic materials. The presence of saliva, blood, pus or excretions can readily inactivate many disinfectants.
✛ The surface areas to be treated. The disinfecting agent must come into contact with all surfaces and areas.

Sterilising

Sterilisation is a process that destroys all micro-organisms, including spores and viruses. Four commonly used methods of sterilisation are moist heat, gas, boiling water and radiation.

Moist heat. For sterilising, moist heat (steam) can be employed in two ways: as steam under pressure or as free steam. Steam under pressure attains temperatures higher than the boiling point. Autoclaves sterilisers supply steam under pressures of 15 to 17 lb and temperatures of 121°C to 123°C.

Table 11-6 Commonly Used Antiseptics and Disinfectants, Effectiveness and Use

| Agent | Effective against | | | | | |
	Bacteria	Tuberculosis	Spores	Fungi	Viruses	Use on
Isopropyl and ethyl alcohol	X	X		X	X	Hands, vial stoppers
Chlorine/hypochlorite (bleach)	X	X	X	X	X	Blood spills
Hydrogen peroxide	X	X	X	X	X	Surfaces
Iodophors	X	X	X	X	X	Equipment; intact skin and tissues if diluted
Phenol	X	X		X	X	Surfaces
Chlorhexidine gluconate (Hibiclens)	X				X	Hands
Triclosan (Bacti-Stat)	X					Hands, intact skin

Gas. Ethylene oxide gas destroys micro-organisms by interfering with their metabolic processes. It is also effective against spores. Its advantages are good penetration and effectiveness for heat-sensitive items. Its major disadvantage is its toxicity to humans.

Boiling water. This is the most practical and inexpensive method for sterilising in the home. The main disadvantage is that spores and some viruses are not killed by this method. The water temperature rises no higher than 100°C. Boiling a minimum of 15 minutes is advised for disinfection of articles in the home.

Radiation. Both ionising and non ionising radiation can be used for disinfection and sterilisation. Ultraviolet light, a type of non ionising radiation, can be used for disinfection. Its main drawback is that the ultraviolet rays do not penetrate deeply. Ionising radiation is used effectively in industry to sterilise foods, drugs and other items that are sensitive to heat. Its main advantage is that it is effective for items difficult to sterilise; its chief disadvantage is that the equipment is very expensive.

Nurses should be familiar with the cleaning, disinfecting and sterilising protocols of the clinical area in which they practise and should be prepared to teach patients and family members appropriate techniques for home care.

ISOLATION PRECAUTIONS

Isolation refers to measures designed to prevent the spread of infections or potentially infectious micro-organisms to health personnel, patients and visitors. Various infection control measures are used to decrease the risk of transmission of micro-organisms in hospitals.

Universal precautions (UP), techniques should be used with all patients to decrease the risk of transmitting unidentified pathogens. Universal precautions interfere with the spread of **blood borne pathogens**, those micro-organisms carried in blood and body fluids that are capable of infecting other persons with serious and difficult to treat viral infections, namely, hepatitis B virus, hepatitis C virus and HIV.

The **body substance isolation (BSI)** system employs generic infection control precautions for all patients except those with the few diseases transmitted through the air. The BSI system (Jackson, 1993), is based on three premises:

1. All people have an increased risk for infection from micro-organisms placed on their mucous membranes and nonintact skin.
2. All people are likely to have potentially infectious micro-organisms in all of their moist body sites and substances.
3. An unknown portion of patients and healthcare workers will always be colonised or infected with potentially infectious micro-organisms in their blood and other moist body sites and substances.

The term *body substance* includes blood, some body fluids, and urine, faeces, wound drainage, oral secretions and any other body product or tissue.

Figure 11-5 Biohazard alert.

In addition to other actions and precautions discussed in this chapter, significant emphasis is placed on avoiding injury due to sharp instruments, measures to be taken in case of exposure to bloodborne pathogens and communication about biohazards to employees. Legislation requires that warning labels be affixed to containers of regulated waste and to refrigerators and freezers containing blood or other potentially infectious materials. The labels required are fluorescent orange or orange-red and feature the biohazard legend shown in Figure 11-5.

Compromised Patients

Compromised patients (those highly susceptible to infection) are often infected by their own micro-organisms, by micro-organisms on the inadequately washed hands of healthcare personnel, and by nonsterile items (food, water, air and patient-care equipment). Patients who are severely compromised include those who:

+ have diseases, such as leukaemia, that depress the patient's resistance to infectious organisms;
+ have extensive skin impairments, such as severe dermatitis or major burns, which cannot be effectively covered with dressings.

ISOLATION PRACTICES

Initiation of practices to prevent the transmission of micro-organisms is generally a nursing responsibility and is based on a comprehensive assessment of the patient. This assessment takes into account the status of the patient's normal defence mechanisms, the patient's ability to implement necessary precautions and the source and mode of transmission of the infectious agent. The nurse then decides whether to wear gloves, gowns, masks and protective eyewear. In all patient situations, *nurses must wash their hands before and after giving care.*

In addition to the precautions cited within this chapter, the nurse implements aseptic precautions when performing many specific therapies. The following are some examples:

+ Use strict aseptic technique when performing any invasive procedure (e.g. suctioning an airway or inserting a urinary catheter) and when changing surgical dressings.
+ Handle needles and syringes carefully to avoid needle-stick injuries.
+ Change intravenous tubing and solution containers according to local policy (e.g. every 48 to 72 hours).
+ Check all sterile supplies for expiration date and intact packaging.
+ Prevent urinary infections by maintaining a closed urinary drainage system with a downhill flow of urine. Provide regular catheter care, and clean the perineal area with soap and water. Keep the drainage bag and spout off the floor.
+ Implement measures to prevent impaired skin integrity and to prevent accumulation of secretions in the lungs (e.g. encourage the patient to move, cough and breathe deeply at least every two hours).

Personal Protective Equipment

All healthcare providers must apply clean or sterile gloves, gowns, masks and protective eyewear according to the risk of exposure to potentially infective materials.

Gloves

Gloves are worn for three reasons:

1. They protect the hands when the nurse is likely to handle any body substances, for example, blood, urine, faeces, sputum, mucous membranes and non intact skin.
2. Gloves reduce the likelihood of nurses transmitting their own endogenous micro-organisms to individuals receiving care. Nurses who have open sores or cuts on the hands must wear gloves for protection.
3. Gloves reduce the chance that the nurse's hands will transmit micro-organisms from one patient to another.

In all situations, gloves are changed between patient contacts. The hands are washed each time gloves are removed for two primary reasons: (a) the gloves may have imperfections or be damaged during wearing so that they could allow micro-organism entry and (b) the hands may become contaminated during glove removal.

Many of the gloves used in infection control are made of latex rubber, as are various other items used in healthcare (catheters, blood pressure cuffs, rubber sheets, intravenous tubing, stockings and adhesive bandages). Because of the frequent use of gloves, patients with chronic illnesses and healthcare workers have increasingly reported allergic reactions to latex. Latex gloves lubricated by powder or cornstarch are particularly allergenic because the latex allergen adheres to the powder, which is aerosolised during glove use and inhaled by the user. Latex gloves that are labelled 'hypoallergenic' still contain measurable latex and should not be used by or on persons with known latex sensitivity. Recent studies show some level of latex allergy in 6% to 17% of healthcare personnel (Corbin, 2002). The people at greatest risk for developing latex allergies are those with other allergic conditions and those who have had frequent or long-term exposure to latex.

Latex allergies can be either local or systemic and may take the form of dermatitis, urticaria (hives), asthma or anaphylaxis. Patients and healthcare workers should be assessed for possible allergies through a thorough history taking and screening. Ask patients if they have had any adverse reactions to items such as balloons, condoms or dishwashing or utility gloves. Strategies to avoid sensitisation or exposure to latex include use of nonlatex products, nonlatex barriers between latex products and the skin, and gloves that are unpowdered or washed before use. People with significant allergies should have no contact with latex products.

Procedure 11-2 describes application and removal of gloves.

Gowns

Clean or disposable impervious (water-resistant) gowns or plastic aprons are worn during procedures when the nurse's uniform is likely to become soiled. *Single-use gown technique* (using a gown only once before it is discarded or laundered) is the usual practice in hospitals. After the gown is worn, the nurse discards it (if it is paper) or places it in a laundry hamper (see *Procedure 11-2*). Before leaving the patient's room, the nurse must wash their hands.

Sterile gowns may be indicated when the nurse changes the dressings of a patient with extensive wounds (e.g. burns).

Face Masks

Masks are worn to reduce the risk for transmission of organisms by the droplet contact and airborne routes, and by splatters of body substances. Masks may be under the following conditions:

+ By those close to the patient if the infection (e.g. measles, mumps or acute respiratory diseases in children) is transmitted by large-particle aerosols (droplets). Large-particle aerosols are transmitted by close contact and generally travel short distances (about 1 m).
+ By all persons entering the room if the infection (e.g. pulmonary tuberculosis and SARS) is transmitted by small-particle aerosols (droplet nuclei). Small-particle aerosols remain suspended in the air and thus travel greater distances by air. Special masks that provide a tighter face seal and better filtration may be used for these infections.

Various types of masks differ in their filtration effectiveness and fit. Single-use disposable surgical masks are effective for use while the nurse provides care to most patients but should be changed if they become wet or soiled. These masks are discarded in the waste container after use. Disposable particulate respirators of different types may be effective for droplet transmission, splatters and airborne micro-organisms. Some respirators now available are effective in preventing inhalation of tuberculin organisms.

During certain techniques requiring surgical asepsis (sterile technique), masks are worn (a) to prevent droplet contact transmission of exhaled micro-organisms to the sterile field or to a patient's open wound and (b) to protect the nurse from splashes of body substances from the patient.

Because the effectiveness of disposable masks and respirators against airborne micro-organisms is questionable, clinical areas should usually not assign susceptible caregivers to patients with the specific airborne disease in question. However, caregivers who are immune to specific diseases (e.g. chickenpox, tuberculosis, measles, mumps and rubella) can provide care to patients with these diseases. Guidelines for donning and removing face masks are shown in *Procedure 11-2*.

Eyewear

Protective eyewear (goggles, glasses or face shields) and masks may be indicated in situations where body substances may splatter the face (see *Procedure 11-2*). If the nurse wears prescription eyeglasses, goggles may be worn over the glasses. The protective eyewear must extend around the sides of the glasses.

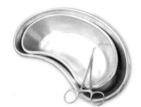

PROCEDURE 11-2 Donning and Removing Personal Protective Equipment (Gloves, Gown, Mask, Eyewear)

Purposes

+ To protect healthcare workers and patients from transmission of potentially infective materials

Assessment

Consider which activities will be required while the nurse is in the patient's room at this time. *This will determine which personal protective equipment is required.*

Planning

+ Application and removal of personal protective equipment can be time consuming. Arrange for the care of your other patients if indicated.
+ Determine which supplies are present within the patient's room and which must be brought with you.
+ Consider if special handling is indicated for removal of any specimens or other materials from the room.

Equipment

As indicated according to which activities will be performed. Ensure that extra supplies are easily available.

+ Gown
+ Mask
+ Eyewear
+ Clean gloves

Implementation

Preparation

See *Procedure 11-1* for preparation for handwashing. Remove or secure all loose items such as nametags or jewellery.

Performance

1. Explain to the patient what you are going to do, why it is necessary, and how they can cooperate.
2. Wash your hands.

3. Don a clean gown.
   - Pick up a clean gown, and allow it to unfold in front of you without allowing it to touch any area soiled with body substances.
   - Slide the arms and the hands through the sleeves.
   - Fasten the ties at the neck to keep the gown in place.
   - Overlap the gown at the back as much as possible, and fasten the waist ties or belt (see Figure 11-6 on page 218). *Overlapping securely*

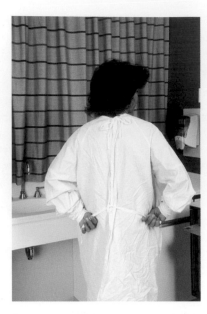

Figure 11-6 Overlapping the gown at the back to cover the nurse's uniform.

covers the uniform at the back. Waist ties keep the gown from falling away from the body and prevent inadvertent soiling of the uniform.

4. Don the face mask.
   - Locate the top edge of the mask. The mask usually has a narrow metal strip along the edge.
   - Hold the mask by the top two strings or loops.
   - Place the upper edge of the mask over the bridge of the nose, and tie the upper ties at the back of the head or secure the loops around the ears. If glasses are worn, fit the upper edge of the mask under the glasses. *With the edge of the mask under the glasses, clouding of the glasses is less likely to occur.*
   - Secure the lower edge of the mask under the chin, and tie the lower ties at the nape of the neck (see Figure 11-7). *To be effective, a mask must cover both the nose and the mouth, because air moves in and out of both.*
   - If the mask has a metal strip, adjust this firmly over the bridge of the nose. *A secure fit prevents both the escape and the inhalation of micro-organisms around the edges of the mask and the fogging of eyeglasses.*
   - Wear the mask only once, and do not wear any mask longer than the manufacturer recommends or once it becomes wet. *A mask should be used only once because it becomes ineffective when moist.*
   - Do not leave a used face mask hanging around the neck.

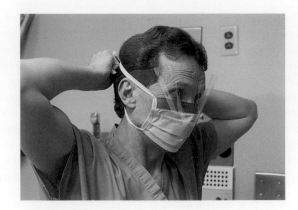

Figure 11-7 A facemask and eye protection covering the nose, mouth and eyes.

5. Don protective eyewear if it is not combined with the face mask.
6. Don clean disposable gloves.
   - No special technique is required.
   - If you are wearing a gown, pull the gloves up to cover the cuffs of the gown. If you are not wearing a gown, pull the gloves up to cover the wrists.
7. To remove soiled personal protective equipment, remove the gloves first since they are the most soiled.
   - If wearing a gown that is tied at the waist in front, undo the ties before removing gloves.
   - Remove the first glove by grasping it on its palmar surface just below the cuff, taking care to touch only glove to glove (see Figure 11-8). *This keeps the soiled parts of the used gloves from touching the skin of the wrist or hand.*

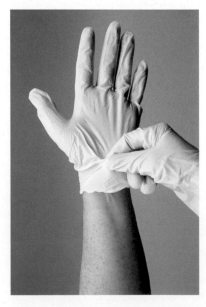

Figure 11-8 Plucking the palmar surface below the cuff of a contaminated glove.

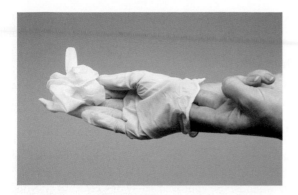

Figure 11-9 Inserting fingers to remove the second contaminated glove.

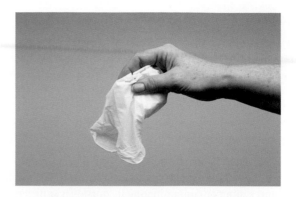

Figure 11-10 Holding contaminated gloves, which are inside out.

- Pull the first glove completely off by inverting or rolling the glove inside out.
- Continue to hold the inverted removed glove by the fingers of the remaining gloved hand. Place the first two fingers of the bare hand inside the cuff of the second glove (see Figure 11-9). *Touching the outside of the second soiled glove with the bare hand is avoided.*
- Pull the second glove off to the fingers by turning it inside out. This pulls the first glove inside the second glove. *The soiled part of the glove is folded to the inside to reduce the chance of transferring any micro-organisms by direct contact.*
- Using the bare hand, continue to remove the gloves, which are now inside out, and dispose of them in the refuse container (Figure 11-10).

8. Wash your hands.
9. Remove the mask.
   - If using a mask with strings, first untie the *lower* strings of the mask. *This prevents the top part of the mask from falling onto the chest.*
   - Untie the top strings and, while holding the ties securely, remove the mask from the face.

This prevents hand contact with the moistened, contaminated portion of the mask.
Or
If side loops are present, lift the side loops up and away from the ears and face.
   - Discard a disposable mask in the waste container.
   - Wash the hands again if they have become contaminated by accidentally touching the soiled part of the mask.

10. Remove the gown when preparing to leave the room. Unless a gown is grossly soiled with body substances, no special precautions are needed to remove it. If a gown is grossly soiled:
    - Avoid touching soiled parts on the outside of the gown, if possible. *The top part of the gown may be soiled, for example, if you have been holding an infant with a respiratory infection.*
    - Grasp the gown along the inside of the neck and pull down over the shoulders.
    - Roll up the gown with the soiled part inside, and discard it in the appropriate container.

11. Remove protective eyewear and dispose of properly or place in the appropriate receptacle for cleaning.

Evaluation

Conduct any follow-up indicated during your care of the patient. If there has been any failure of the equipment and exposure to potentially infective materials is suspected, follow the steps in the *Practice guidelines* on page 223.

Ensure that an adequate supply of equipment is available for the next healthcare provider.

Disposal of Soiled Equipment and Supplies

Many pieces of equipment are supplied for single use only and are disposed of after use. Some items, however, are reusable. Clinical areas have specific policies and procedures for handling soiled equipment (e.g. disposal, cleaning, disinfecting and sterilising); the nurse needs to become familiar with these practices in the employing area. Appropriate handling of soiled equipment and supplies is essential for two main reasons:

1. to prevent inadvertent exposure of healthcare workers to articles contaminated with body substances;
2. to prevent contamination of the environment.

Bagging

Most articles do not need to be placed in bags unless they are contaminated, or likely to have been contaminated, with infective material such as pus, blood, body fluids, faeces or respiratory secretions. Contaminated articles need to be enclosed in a sturdy bag impervious to micro-organisms before they are removed from the room of any patient. Clinical waste bags are always colour coded yellow with a biohazard warning mark.

+ A single bag, if it is sturdy and impervious to micro-organisms, and if the contaminated articles can be placed in the bag without soiling or contaminating its outside is sufficient.
+ Double-bagging if the above conditions are not met.
+ Place *nondisposable* or *reusable* equipment that is visibly soiled in a labelled bag before removing it from the patient's room or cubicle, and send it to a central processing area for decontamination. Some areas may require that glass bottles or jars and metal items be placed in separate bags from rubber and plastic items. Glass and metal can be sterilised in an autoclave, but rubber and plastic are damaged by this process and must be cleaned by other methods, such as gas sterilisation.
+ Disassemble special procedure trays into component parts. Some components are disposable; others need to be sent to the laundry or central services for cleaning and decontaminating.
+ Bag soiled clothing before sending it home or to the hospital laundry.

Linens

Handle soiled linen as little as possible and with the least agitation possible before placing it in the laundry hamper. This prevents gross microbial contamination of the air and persons handling the linen. Close the bag before sending it to the laundry in accordance with agency practice.

Laboratory Specimens

Laboratory specimens, if placed in a leakproof container with a secure lid with a biohazard label, need no special precautions. Use care when collecting specimens to avoid contaminating the outside of the container. Containers that are visibly contaminated on the outside should be placed inside a sealable plastic bag before sending them to the laboratory. This prevents personnel from having hand contact with potentially infective material.

Dishes

Dishes require no special precautions. Soiling of dishes can largely be prevented by encouraging patients to wash their hands before eating. Some agencies use paper dishes for convenience, which are disposed of in the refuse container.

Blood Pressure Equipment

Blood pressure equipment needs no special precautions unless it becomes contaminated with infective material. If it does become contaminated, follow local policy. Cleaning procedures vary according to whether it is a wall or portable unit.

Thermometers

Nondisposable used thermometers are generally disinfected after use. Check local policy.

Disposable Needles, Syringes and Sharps

Place needles, syringes and 'sharps' (e.g. lancets, scalpels and broken glass) into a sharps disposal container. To avoid puncture wounds, use approved safety or needleless systems where possible and do not detach needles from the syringe or recap the needle before disposal.

Transporting Patients with Infections

Transporting patients with infections outside their own rooms is avoided unless absolutely necessary. If a patient must be moved, the nurse implements appropriate precautions and measures to prevent soilage of the environment. For example, the nurse ensures that any draining wound is securely covered or places a surgical mask on the patient who has an airborne infection. In addition, the nurse notifies personnel at the receiving area of any infection risk so that they can maintain necessary precautions. Follow local protocol.

Psychosocial Needs of Isolation Patients

Patients requiring isolation precautions can develop several problems as a result of the separation from others and of the special precautions taken in their care. Two of the most common are sensory deprivation and decreased self-esteem related to feelings of inferiority. *Sensory deprivation* occurs when the environment lacks normal stimuli for the patient, for example, communication with others. Nurses should therefore be alert to common clinical signs of sensory deprivation: boredom, inactivity, slowness of thought, daydreaming, increased sleeping, thought disorganisation, anxiety, hallucinations and panic.

A patient's *feeling of inferiority* can be due to the perception of the infection itself or to the required precautions. In Western culture, many people place a high value on cleanliness, and the idea of being 'soiled', 'contaminated' or 'dirty' can give patients the feeling that they are at fault and substandard. Although this is obviously not true, the infected persons may feel 'not as good' as others and blame themselves.

Nurses need to provide care that prevents these two problems or deals with them positively. Nursing interventions include the following:

+ Assess the individual's need for stimulation.
+ Initiate measures to help meet the need, including regular communication with the patient and diversionary activities, such as toys for a child and books, television or radio for an adult; provide a variety of foods to stimulate the patient's sense of taste; stimulate the patient's visual sense by providing a view or an activity to watch.

- Explain the infection and the associated procedures to help patients and their support people understand and accept the situation.
- Demonstrate warm, accepting behaviour. Avoid conveying to the patient any sense of annoyance about the precautions or any feelings of revulsion about the infection.
- Do not use stricter precautions than are indicated by the diagnosis or the patient's condition.

Sterile Gloves

Sterile gloves may be donned by the open method or the closed method. The open method is most frequently used outside the operating department because the closed method requires that the nurse wear a sterile gown. Gloves are worn during many procedures to maintain the sterility of equipment and to protect a patient's wound.

Sterile gloves are packaged with a cuff of about 5 cm and with the palms facing upward when the package is opened. The package usually indicates the size of the glove (e.g. size 6 or 7½).

Latex, nitrile and vinyl sterile gloves are available to protect the nurse from contact with blood and body fluids. Latex and nitrile are more flexible than vinyl, mould to the wearer's hands, allow freedom of movement, and have the added feature of resealing tiny punctures automatically. Therefore, wear latex or nitrile gloves when performing tasks (a) that demand flexibility, (b) that place stress on the material (e.g. turning stopcocks, handling sharp instruments or tape) and (c) that involve a high risk of exposure to pathogens. Vinyl gloves should be chosen for tasks unlikely to stress the glove material, requiring minimal precision, and with minimal risk of exposure to pathogens.

Procedure 11-3 describes how to don and remove sterile gloves by the open method.

PROCEDURE 11-3 Donning and Removing Sterile Gloves (Open Method)

Purposes

- To enable the nurse to handle or touch sterile objects freely without contaminating them
- To prevent transmission of potentially infective organisms from the nurse's hands to patients at high risk for infection

Assessment

Review the patient's record and orders to determine exactly what procedure will be performed that requires sterile gloves. Check the patient record and ask about latex allergies.

Planning

Think through the procedure, planning which steps need to be completed before the gloves can be applied. Determine what additional supplies are needed to perform the procedure for this patient. Always have an extra pair of sterile gloves available.

Equipment

- Packages of sterile gloves

Implementation

Preparation

Ensure the sterility of the package of gloves.

Performance

1. Explain to the patient what you are going to do, why it is necessary and how they can cooperate, and gain informed consent. Discuss how the results will be used in planning further care or treatments.
2. Observe other appropriate infection control procedures (see Procedures 11-1 and 11-2).
3. Provide for patient privacy.

4. Open the package of sterile gloves.
   - Place the package of gloves on a clean, dry surface. *Any moisture on the surface could contaminate the gloves.*
   - Some gloves are packed in an inner as well as an outer package. Open the outer package without contaminating the gloves or the inner package.
   - Remove the inner package from the outer package.

- Open the inner package according to the manufacturer's directions. Some manufacturers provide a numbered sequence for opening the flaps and folded tabs to grasp for opening the flaps. If no tabs are provided, pluck the flap so that the fingers do not touch the inner surfaces. *The inner surfaces, which are next to the sterile gloves, will remain sterile.*

5. Put the first glove on the dominant hand.
   - If the gloves are packaged so that they lie side by side, grasp the glove for the dominant hand by its folded cuff edge (on the palmar side) with the thumb and first finger of the nondominant hand. Touch only the inside of the cuff (see Figure 11-11). *The hands are not sterile. By touching only the inside of the glove, the nurse avoids contaminating the outside.*
   Or
   - If the gloves are packaged one on top of the other, grasp the cuff of the top glove as above, using the opposite hand.
   - Insert the dominant hand into the glove and pull the glove on. Keep the thumb of the inserted hand against the palm of the hand during insertion (see Figure 11-12). *If the thumb is kept*

against the palm, it is less likely to contaminate the outside of the glove.
   - Leave the cuff turned down.
6. Put the second glove on the nondominant hand.
   - Pick up the other glove with the sterile gloved hand, inserting the gloved fingers under the cuff and holding the gloved thumb close to the gloved palm (see Figure 11-13). *This helps prevent accidental contamination of the glove by the bare hand.*
   - Pull on the second glove carefully. Hold the thumb of the gloved first hand as far as possible from the palm (see Figure 11-14). *In this position, the thumb is less likely to touch the arm and become contaminated.*
   - Adjust each glove so that it fits smoothly, and carefully pull the cuffs up by sliding the fingers under the cuffs.
7. Remove and dispose of used gloves.
   - There is no special technique for removing sterile gloves. If they are soiled with secretions, remove them by turning them inside out. See removal of disposable gloves in Procedure 11-2.
8. Document that sterile technique was used in the performance of the procedure.

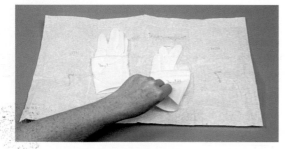

Figure 11-11 Picking up the first sterile glove.

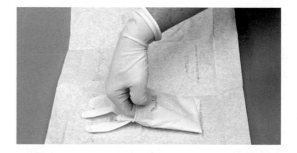

Figure 11-13 Picking up the second sterile glove.

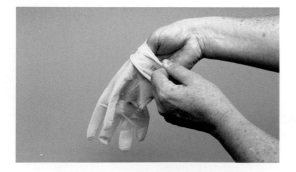

Figure 11-12 Putting on the first sterile glove.

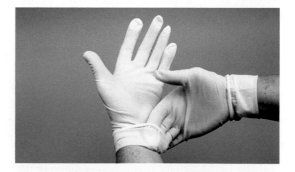

Figure 11-14 Putting on the second sterile glove.

Evaluation

Conduct any follow-up indicated during your care of the patient. Ensure that adequate numbers and types of sterile supplies are available for the next healthcare provider.

INFECTION CONTROL FOR HEALTHCARE WORKERS

There are three major modes of transmission of infectious materials in the clinical setting:

1. Puncture wounds from contaminated needles or other sharps
2. Skin contact, which allows infectious fluids to enter through wounds and broken or damaged skin
3. Mucous membrane contact, which allows infectious fluids to enter through mucous membranes of the eyes, mouth and nose.

Using proper precautions with general medical asepsis, appropriately using personal protective equipment (gloves, masks, gowns, goggles, shoe covers, special resuscitative equipment), and avoiding carelessness in the clinical area will place the caregiver at significantly less risk for injury. The chance of a healthcare worker becoming infected following exposure to pathogens varies widely – estimates range from 30% for hepatitis B (nonimmune workers), to 1.8% for hepatitis C, to 0.3% for HIV (CDC, 1997). Measures to be taken in case of possible exposure to these viruses are outlined in the Practice guidelines box (see below). Hepatitis C, a worldwide epidemic greater than HIV, has become a significant concern to all healthcare workers since there is currently no vaccine against the virus nor post-exposure prophylaxis. Prevention remains the primary goal.

The Department of Health requires that healthcare employers make the hepatitis B vaccine and vaccination series available to all employees. Other vaccinations may also be made available (e.g. nurses working in an obstetric area should be vaccinated against rubella to protect pregnant mothers and their foetuses).

CLINICAL ALERT

Nurses should consider in advance whether or not they would want prophylaxis for HIV exposure since this must be started within one hour of exposure.

PRACTICE GUIDELINES

Steps to Follow after Exposure to Blood-borne Pathogens

+ Report the incident immediately to appropriate personnel within the clinical area.
+ Complete an injury report.
+ Seek appropriate evaluation and follow-up. This includes:
  • identification and documentation of the source individual when feasible
  • testing of the source for hepatitis B, hepatitis C and HIV when feasible and consent is given
  • making results of the test available to the source individual's healthcare provider
  • testing of blood of exposed nurse (with consent) for hepatitis B, hepatitis C and HIV antibodies
  • post-exposure prophylaxis if medically indicated
  • medical and psychological counselling regarding personal risk of infection or risk of infecting others.
+ For a puncture/laceration:
  • encourage bleeding
  • wash/clean the area with soap and water
  • initiate first-aid and seek treatment if indicated.
+ For a mucous membrane exposure (eyes, nose, mouth), saline or water flush for five to 10 minutes.

Post-exposure Protocol (PEP)

HIV:
+ For 'high-risk' exposure (high blood volume *and* source with a high HIV titre): three-drug treatment is recommended. Must be started within one hour.
+ For 'increased risk' exposure (high blood volume *or* source with a high HIV titre): three-drug treatment is recommended. Must be started within one hour.
+ For 'low-risk' exposure (neither high blood volume nor source with a high HIV titre): two-drug treatment is considered. Must be started within one hour.
+ Drug prophylaxis continues for four weeks.
+ Drug regimens vary.
+ HIV antibody tests done shortly after exposure (baseline) and six weeks, three months and six months afterward.

Hepatitis B
+ Anti-HBs testing one to two months after last vaccine dose.

Hepatitis C
+ Anti-HCV and ALT at baseline and four to six months after exposure.

ROLE OF THE INFECTION CONTROL NURSE

All healthcare organisations must have multidisciplinary infection control committees. Representatives from the clinical laboratory, cleaning maintenance, catering and patient care areas should be included. An important member of this committee is the infection control nurse. This nurse is specially trained to be knowledgeable about the latest research and practices in preventing, detecting and treating infections. All infections are reported to the nurse in a manner that allows for recording and analysing statistics that can assist in improving infection control practices. In addition, the infection control nurse may be involved in employee education and implementation of the blood-borne pathogen exposure control plan.

Evaluating Outcomes

Using data collected during care – vital signs, lung sounds, skin status, characteristics of urine or other drainage, laboratory blood values, and so on – the nurse judges whether patient outcomes have been achieved.

If outcomes are not achieved, the nurse may need to consider questions such as the following:

+ Were appropriate measures implemented to prevent skin breakdown and lung infection?
+ Was strict aseptic technique implemented for invasive procedures?
+ Are prescribed medications affecting the immune system?
+ Is patient placement appropriate to reduce the risk of transmission of micro-organisms?
+ Did the patient and family misunderstand or fail to comply with necessary instructions?

CRITICAL REFLECTION

Mrs Lewis is a 76-year-old woman who is independent, lives alone and prefers not to rely on others unless absolutely necessary. She was active and healthy until about six months ago, at which time she developed a persistent upper respiratory infection. Because she was unable to obtain or prepare foods, she lost weight and became very weak. She finally sought medical attention, but she has not yet fully recovered. Her GP has admitted Mrs Lewis to the acute medical ward for shortness of breath, productive cough, dehydration and nutritional deficiency.

Now that you have read this chapter what data support Mrs Lewis's increased risk of pneumonia? What other information or assessment data would be helpful to you when planning care for Mrs Lewis? You recognise that standard precautions are instituted for all hospitalised patients. Explain why the use of such precautions may not prevent the spread of Mrs Lewis's respiratory infection to other susceptible patients. What can you do to prevent the spread of Mrs Lewis's infection to other hospitalised patients and at the same time prevent Mrs Lewis from getting infections from other patients?

CHAPTER HIGHLIGHTS

+ Micro-organisms are everywhere. Most are harmless and some are beneficial; however, many can cause infection in susceptible persons.
+ Effective control of infectious disease is an international, national, community and individual responsibility.
+ Asepsis is the freedom from infection or infectious material.
+ Medical aseptic practices limit the number, growth and transmission of micro-organisms.
+ Surgical aseptic practices keep an area or objects free of all micro-organisms.
+ The incidence of nosocomial infections is significant. Major sites for these infections are the respiratory and urinary tracts, the bloodstream and wounds.
+ Factors that contribute to nosocomial infection risks are invasive procedures, medical therapies, the existence of a large number of susceptible persons, inappropriate use of antibiotics, and insufficient handwashing after patient contact and after contact with body substances.
+ An infection can develop if the links in the chain of infection – infectious agent, reservoir, portal of exit, mode of transmission, portal of entry and susceptible host – are not interrupted.
+ Intact skin and mucous membranes are the body's first line of defence against micro-organisms.
+ Some normal body flora release bacteriocins and antibiotic-like substances that inhibit microbial growth and destroy foreign bacteria.
+ Some body secretions (e.g. saliva and tears) contain enzymes that act as antibacterial agents.

+ The inflammatory response limits physical, chemical and microbial injury and promotes repair of injured tissue.
+ Immunity is the specific resistance of the body to infectious agents.
+ Acquired immunity is active or passive and in either case may be naturally or artificially induced.
+ Especially at risk of acquiring an infection are the very young or old; those with poor nutritional status, a deficiency of serum immunoglobulins, multiple stressors, insufficient immunisations or an existing disease process; and those receiving certain medical therapies.
+ Preventing infections in healthy or ill persons and preventing the transmission of micro-organisms from infected patients to others are major nursing functions.
+ The nurse must be knowledgeable about sources and modes of transmission of micro-organisms.
+ Micro-organisms are invisible, and nurses have an ethical obligation to ensure that appropriate aseptic measures are taken to protect patients, support people and health personnel, including themselves.
+ All healthcare providers must apply clean or sterile gloves, gowns, masks and protective eyewear according to the risk of exposure to potentially infective materials.
+ Should a healthcare worker be exposed to substances with high risk of transmitting blood-borne pathogens, postexposure practices and consideration of prophylactic treatment must be followed immediately.

REFERENCES

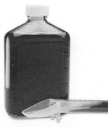

Bischoff, W.E., Reynolds, T.M., Sessler, C.N., Edmond, M.B. and Wenzel, R.P. (2000) 'Handwashing compliance by healthcare workers: The impact of introducing an accessible, alcohol-based hand antiseptic', *Archives of Internal Medicine*, 160, 1017–1021.

Centers for Disease Control (CDC) (1997) '1997 USPHS/IDSA guidelines for the prevention of opportunistic infections in persons infected with human immunodeficiency virus', *Morbidity and Mortality Weekly Report*, 46(RR12), 1–46.

Corbin, D.E. (2002) 'Latex allergy and dermatitis', *Occupational Health and Safety*, 71(36–38), 89.

Earl, M.E., Jackson, M.M. and Rickman, L.S. (2001) 'Improved rates of compliance with hand antisepsis guidelines: A three-phase observational study', *American Journal of Nursing*, 101(3), 26–33.

Jackson, M.M. (1993) 'Infection precautions: what works and what does not', *CRNA: The Clinical Forum for Nurse Anesthetists*, 4(2), 77–82.

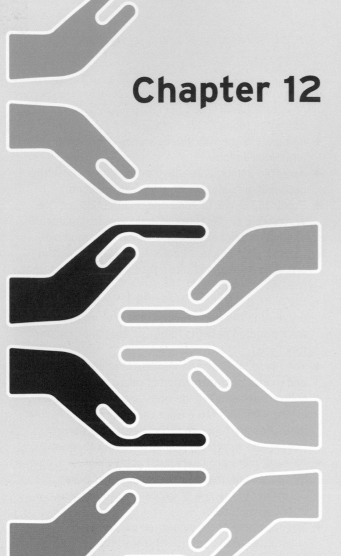

Chapter 12

Moving and Handling:
Promoting the Safety of the Patient and the Nurse

Learning Outcomes

After completing this chapter, you will be able to:

+ Discuss the implications of manual handling in practice.

+ Discuss the regulations that controls manual handling.

+ Discuss the professional responsibilities when handling a patient.

+ Identify the four emergency situations when a person can be manually lifted.

+ Identify the components of the spine.

+ Discuss the principles of safer handling.

+ Perform a risk assessment when handling a patient or object.

+ Describe how to lift an inanimate object.

+ Describe a range of handling manoeuvres.

CASE STUDY

Two sisters aged 26 and 22 years, with profound physical and learning disabilities, are being cared for at home by their parents and social service home carers as they are unable to do anything for themselves. Some of the care needed involves manually lifting and moving the sisters as they do not like being lifted in a hoist. However the council has decided that in response to health and safety requirements it is introducing a no lifting ban. As a result, the council is refusing to employ carers to look after the sisters in their own home and have decided to place the sisters in a care home. The council has even refused the sisters' parents' offer to pay for the home carers, resulting in the parents having to care for their daughters. The family therefore decide to take the council to the high court.

This is an actual manual handling case, *A & B, X & Y v East Sussex County Council* (2003). By the end of this chapter you will be able to understand the reasons why this case was problematic for the council.

INTRODUCTION

Back injuries currently cost the National Health Service (NHS) £400 million each year with one in four nurses having to take time off work as a result of a back injury (Department of Health, 2004). Such statistics have prompted the NHS and social services to prioritise moving and handling.

However, it is not just the healthcare professional that is at risk of injury. Chell (2003), writing on the implications of poor manual handling practices, states that patients too are at risk of injury from inappropriate handling techniques. Indeed, the National Back Pain Association (1998), an independent national charity aimed at helping people to manage and prevent back pain, states that poor manual handling techniques can lead to patients suffering from shoulder dislocation, damaged nerves and soft tissue injuries. Despite these facts, it has been reported that many nurses continue to use poor manual handling techniques, blaming staff shortages, poor supervision and inadequate provision of handling equipment.

CLINICAL ANECDOTE

I was a healthcare support worker before coming to do my nurse training and I know now that my manual handling practice was awful even though I had manual handling training provided by the Trust. Now, since beginning my training, I can see the error of my ways and understand the potential damage that I could have done to my back. At the end of the day God only gave me one back so I have to look after it if I want to continue nursing.

Anonymous student nurse

LEGAL AND PROFESSIONAL RESPONSIBILITIES

The law within the UK with regard to the moving and handling of patients has two clear goals; first to prevent injury and second to compensate the handler when an injury occurs. The no manual lifting policy implemented by East Sussex County Council was imposed to protect their employees from injury and to avoid having to pay compensation if injuries occurred. However, the law must also consider the patient's needs and their human rights (discussed later in the chapter). This has and continues to be a 'balancing act' within law.

Accident Prevention

The **Health and Safety at Work Act 1974** (abbreviated to HSWA 74) clearly states that an employer must ensure the

BOX 12-1 HSWA 74 Employer Duties

The employer must:

+ Provide and maintain any work equipment required, e.g. hoists, trolleys, etc.
+ Ensure that there are no health risks to employee when using, handling, storing or transporting articles and/or substances, e.g. the storage of chemicals.
+ Provide information, instruction, training and supervision necessary to ensure health and safety, e.g. fire training.
+ Maintain any place of work, ensuring there is adequate and safe access to, and that there is a safe and accessible exit from, the place of work, e.g. providing ramps for disabled employees.
+ Provide and maintain the work environment, ensuring that there are adequate facilities for welfare at work, e.g. adequate facilities for employees to eat, such as a canteen.

health, safety and welfare at work of its employees, as far as it is reasonably practicable. This means that the employer has a duty to provide safe equipment, information, training and instruction of health and safety issues, for example, fire training, and also provide the employee with a healthy working environment, for example, no smoking environments (see *Box 12-1*). However it is important to note that the employee also has a duty to take reasonable care of their own health and safety (see *Box 12-2*).

BOX 12-2 HSWA 74 Employee Duties

The employee owes a duty to the employer to:

+ Obey reasonable and lawful instructions.
+ Act with reasonable care and skill.
+ Take reasonable care for their own health and safety and for those who may be affected by their acts or omissions.
+ Use all work equipment and safety devices provided by the employer in accordance with the training and instruction provided.
+ Use equipment and any other safe systems of work provided for the employee by the employer in order to minimise the risk of injury to the employee to the lowest level reasonably practicable.

The term 'reasonably practicable' means that the employer's duty is not absolute. If the benefit is minimal and the cost is considerable the employer may not have to comply with the duty. However, if the employer fails to meet the duty when it is reasonably practical to do so, it may face either criminal prosecution from the Health and Safety Executive (HSE) or a civil suit from its employee.

The judgment made in the case of *A & B, X & Y v East Sussex County Council* (2003) EWHC 167 (Admin) held that although it is important to protect the rights of the employees, the local authority should also have considered the two sisters' rights. This would involve very careful and balanced decision making but would not mean that the rights of the two sisters should override the rights of the carers or that the rights of the carers should override the rights of the sisters. However, the court conceded that it may mean that the carers might have to work with higher, but not unacceptable, levels of risk.

In addition to HSWA 74 other regulations help to regulate the issue of manual handling in the workplace. The **Manual Handling Operations Regulations 1992**, as amended by the **Health and Safety Miscellaneous Amendments Regulations 2002 (MHOR 92)** sets very specific duties for the employer in relation to manual handling in the workplace (see *Box 12-3*), while the **Provision and Use of Work Equipment Regulations 1992 (PUWER)** aims to prevent or control the risk to an individual's health and safety from work equipment such as photocopiers, hoists, etc. and sets out a number of requirements that the employer must adhere to (see *Box 12-4*). The **Lifting Operations and Lifting Equipment Regulations 1998 (LOLER)** (see *Box 12-5*), on the other hand, regulates lifting equipment used in the workplace and like PUWER it sets out requirements that the employer must adhere to. Any breach by the employer under any or all of these regulations can result in criminal prosecution.

It is the LOLER regulations that East Sussex County Council were trying to uphold. In addition to accident prevention, the

---

BOX 12-4 The Provision and Use of Work Equipment Regulations 1992 (PUWER)

Regulates work equipment such as hoists which must be:

+ Suitable for their intended use.
+ Safe for use, maintained in a safe condition and inspected to ensure they are safe for use.
+ Used only by people who have had adequate information, instruction and training.
+ Accompanied by suitable safety measures such as instructions, warnings and markings.

BOX 12-5 The Lifting Operations and Lifting Equipment Regulations 1998 (LOLER)

These regulations require that lifting equipment is:

+ Strong and stable enough for its use and is marked with safe working loads, i.e. the weight that can safely be lifted with the equipment.
+ Positioned and installed to minimise any risks.
+ Used safely by competent personnel who have planned its use and have organised the lifting task.
+ Inspected regularly by competent persons.

Source: Health and Safety Executive (1998) *Simple Guide to the Lifting Operations and Lifting Equipment Regulations 1998*, Caerphilly, Wales: HSE.

BOX 12-3 Manual Handling Operations Regulations 1992 (MHOR 92)

The basic duties of the employer include:

+ Hazardous manual handling should be avoided if reasonably practicable.
+ Make a suitable and sufficient assessment of any hazardous manual handling which cannot be avoided.
+ Reduce the risk of injury so far as is reasonably practicable.
+ Provide information about the load and centre of weight.
+ Any assessment must be reviewed if there are significant changes.

---

council was trying to avoid paying compensation to any injured employees caring for the sisters.

Compensation for the Injured Handler

HSWA 74 clearly sets out the employer's duties (see Box 12-1 earlier), but a breach of these duties does not automatically entitle the injured handler to compensation. Nevertheless, common law, a uniform set of laws derived from custom and practice of judges, places duties on the employer to take reasonable care regarding the safety of its employees and to ensure that they are not placed under any unnecessary risk. In addition to this, the employer is also responsible for the negligence of the employees even when the employer is not at fault. This is known as **vicarious liability**.

Despite HSWA 74 stating that a breach of duties does not entitle the injured handler to compensation, the introduction of new regulations – the Management of Health and Safety at Work and Fire Precautions (Workplace) (Amendment) Regulations 2003 does entitle the injured handler to claim compensation if the employer has failed to comply with the Management of Health and Safety at Work Regulations 1999 (MHSWR).

In order to claim compensation for an alleged failure to comply with MHSWR 99, the injured handler must also prove that the injury sustained was due to the failure. This requires that the injured handler has expert medical evidence that unequivocally proves that the injury was due to the failure.

Employee Duties

It is not only the employer who has duties to the employee; the employee has duties that they must comply with (see Box 12-2 earlier). If injured, failure to comply with these duties could result in a reduction in the amount of compensation awarded, if successful.

These duties sometimes provide healthcare professionals with manual handling dilemmas. Where the employer has not complied with the obligations under MHOR 92 and the employee is put in the position of coping with inappropriate equipment, inadequate training and poor staffing levels, then when presented with a situation where a patient has to be moved does the healthcare professional have the right to refuse? It could be argued that a request to move or handle a patient in circumstances that could cause injury and where it is reasonably practical to avoid that risk is an unlawful order. However, healthcare professionals have a duty of care to meet the needs of patients. According to Griffith and Stevens (2003), lecturers with a background in law and manual handling, this may mean that the healthcare professional may be required to manually handle a patient even if there is a risk of injury to the handler. But does this breach their professional responsibilities?

Professional Responsibilities

Nurses and midwives are accountable to the Nursing and Midwifery Council (NMC), which aims to protect the public by setting and maintaining professional standards. As a result, all nurses and midwives are subject to the NMC's 'Code of Professional Conduct' (2004), a set of standards aimed at informing the professions and the public of the standard of professional conduct expected from a nurse or midwife (see *Box 12-6*).

These standards state that all nurses and midwives must adhere to the laws of the country in which they are practising. This is important when considering manual handling as the law clearly states that employers have a duty to ensure the health and safety of their employees as far as is reasonably practicable and that employees have a reciprocating duty. This means that nurses have a duty to take reasonable care of their own health and safety. However, in the past, nurses have been brought before the NMC and UK Central Council (UKCC), the predecessor of the NMC, to face allegations of professional misconduct for refusing to lift patients.

BOX 12-6 The Nursing and Midwifery Council's Code of Professional Conduct

When caring for patients the nurse/midwife must:

+ Respect the patient as an individual.
+ Obtain consent before any treatment or care is given.
+ Protect confidential information.
+ Cooperate with others in the team.
+ Maintain professional knowledge and competence.
+ Be trustworthy.
+ Act to identify and minimise risk to patients.

Source: NMC (2004) *Code of Professional Conduct: Standards for Conduct, Performance and Ethics*, London: NMC.

One such case found a nurse facing the UKCC for refusing to perform an unsafe lift and accused of conduct unbefitting a registered nurse (*U.K.C.C. v Lalis Lillian Grant* (as reported in the *Nursing Standard*, 18 February 1989). In this case, the nurse was found not guilty of professional misconduct. The guidance of the UKCC was that any refusal to manually handle a patient should be fully documented, clearly stating the reasons for the decision made (Smith, 2005).

HUMAN RIGHTS

Everyone, including patients and health and social care workers, is protected by the Human Rights Act 1998. Human rights are the rights all individuals have just because they are human beings. These rights not only affect matters of life and death, like freedom from torture and killing, but also affect the individual's rights in everyday life: what they can say and do, their beliefs, their right to a fair trial along with other similar fundamental rights (see *Box 12-7* on page 230).

The case of *A & B, X & Y v East Sussex County Council* centred on the human rights of the two sisters. The specific issues highlighted in this case are shown in *Box 12-8* on page 230. Specifically it was argued that using mechanical lifts to move the sisters in all situations breached their human rights. This argument was supported by the Disability Rights Commission, who stated that East Sussex County Council's policy regarding manual lifting should not restrict the sisters' rights to autonomy, privacy or dignity.

However, it is important to state that it is not only the sisters who had rights, the carers too had rights that needed to be upheld. A balance needed to be struck between the rights of the sisters to treatment respecting personal dignity and not to be deprived of valuable activities, and the rights of the carer not to

BOX 12-7 The Human Rights Act 1998

The main provisions set out by the Human Rights Act are:

Right	Issues arising from the right
Right to life	Abortion; availability of life-saving treatments; euthanasia.
Prohibition of torture	Respecting the dignity of vulnerable people
Prohibition of slavery	Slavery was effectively abolished in 1774
Right to liberty and security	Detention of the mentally ill
Right to a fair trial	Right to legal representation; right to silence
No punishment without law	Criminal law must be certain and an offence at the time it was committed
Right to respect for private and family life	Care orders; fertility treatment
Freedom of thought, conscience and religion	Certain employment practices
Freedom of expression	Restrictions on the media with regard to privacy
Freedom of assembly and association	Right to belong to a trade union
Right to marry	Arranged marriages; same-sex marriages.
Prohibition of discrimination	Prohibits discrimination on the grounds of race, colour, sex, language, religion, political opinion, national or social origin or any other status.
Protection of property	Planning; access to environmental information
Right to education	School exclusions; special educational needs
Right to free elections	Right to vote
Abolition of the death penalty	No person should be put to death for a crime committed

BOX 12-8 Specific Issues Highlighted in the *East Sussex County Council* Case

+ Moving in a hoist appeared to cause the sisters distress.
+ When bathing, the sisters slipped down in the bath and went under the water.
+ Swimming was difficult as the sisters needed to be lifted into the water.
+ The sisters could not be taken shopping as they would have to be lifted to be toileted.

BOX 12-9 Situations Where It Is Deemed Appropriate to Manually Lift People.

+ If a person is threatened by bomb or bullet.
+ If a person is threatened by fire.
+ If a person is threatened with drowning.
+ If a person is in a collapsing building.

be exposed to undue risk of physical harm. However, the RCN guidance had advised that 'manual lifting of patients is to be eliminated in all but exceptional or life-threatening situations'. These situations are outlined in *Box 12-9*.

The Human Rights Act 1998 also prohibits torture, inhuman or degrading treatment, but what constitutes this is 'a matter of fact and degree in each case' (Griffith and Stevens, 2003). Thus, to refuse to manual handle or lift a patient who is at risk of developing pressures sores, if the patient refused to be moved in any other way (e.g. by using a hoist) would breach the human rights of the patient and thereby may be seen as unlawful.

In the *East Sussex County Council* case the judge made a number of important observations, including:

+ manual lifting is an inherent feature of caring for the disabled;
+ a blanket ban on manual lifting is likely to be unlawful;
+ all lifts required to maintain a person's dignity and quality of life must be performed somehow;
+ a significant amount of manual handling may be required to facilitate a disabled person's right to participate in community life.

The judgment made in this case is rather complex and has been interpreted differently by opposing parties. The Disability Rights Commission, an independent body established to end discrimination and promote equality for disabled people, who supported the sisters, felt the judgment heralded a victory for them and disabled people as it meant that the sisters could be manually lifted in certain circumstances. However, the actual judgment was that the carers would be expected to lift the sisters once each day. This means that they could be manually lifted into the bath, for example, but could not be lifted out of the bath and therefore would need to be hoisted or moved by some other means.

Since the judgment did state that in certain circumstances the carers would be expected to lift the sisters it is important to consider some of the principles of safe handling of people.

THE SPINE

The spine or vertebral column extends from the base of the skull to the pelvis and is made up of 33 individual bones or

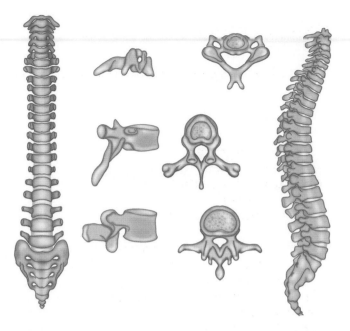

Figure 12-2 Facet joints of spine.

vertebrae. These individual bones give the spine strength and flexibility. The 33 vertebrae are divided into regions:

+ seven cervical (neck) vertebrae,
+ 12 thoracic (chest) vertebrae,
+ five lumbar (lower back) vertebrae,
+ five sacrum and four coccyx, which are fused together (see Figure 12-1).

Each of the vertebrae is linked together by facet joints. These joints allow the vertebrae to move against one another and give the spine its flexibility. The facets are the bony prominences that meet between each vertebra. There are two facet joints between each pair of vertebrae (see Figure 12-2) that extend and flex over one another.

One quarter of the spine's length is made up by the intervertebral discs, which are fibrocartilaginous cushions and act as shock absorbers for the spine protecting the brain, vertebrae and nerves. Intervertebral discs are nonvascular and therefore depend on the end plates of each of the vertebra for nutrients. The discs allow for movement within the spine. It is damage to these discs that cause most back pain. This condition is commonly referred to as 'a slipped disc' or prolapsed disc. This is where the disc slips out of position (see Figure 12-3 on page 232).

Each disc is made up of an annulus fibrosus and a nucleus pulposus (see Figure 12-4 on page 232). The annulus fibrosus is made up of concentric circles of collagen that connects to the vertebral end plates, and can be likened to a car tyre and encapsulates the nucleus pulposus. The nucleus pulposus contains a gel like substance that resists compression.

Although the vertebral column is strong and flexible, it still requires support from a number of muscles and ligaments. In fact there are over 30 muscles that support the spine giving it stability and allowing for mobility (see Table 12-1 on page 232).

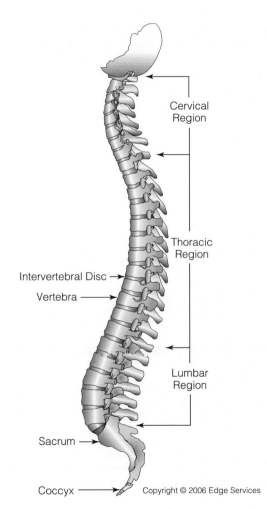

Figure 12-1 The spine.

Manual handling illustrations © EDGE Services (2006) reproduced by kind permission of EDGE Services – The Manual Handling Training Co. Ltd (01904 677853) sourced from People Handling & Risk Assessment Key Trainer's Certificate course materials.

The views expressed in this text book, generally and with specific reference to manual handling, do not necessarily reflect the views, approach, company policies or course content of training programmes of EDGE Services – The Manual Handling Training Co. Ltd.

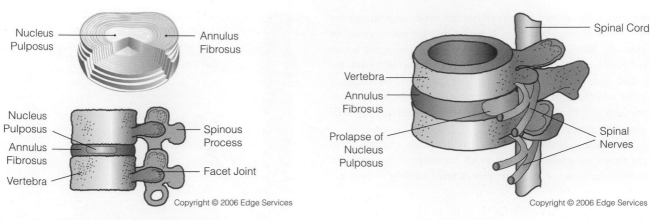

Copyright © 2006 Edge Services   Copyright © 2006 Edge Services

Figure 12-3 Prolapsed intervertebral disc.   **Figure 12-4** Intervertebral disc.

Manual handling illustrations © EDGE Services (2006) reproduced by kind permission of EDGE Services – The Manual Handling Training Co. Ltd (01904 677853) sourced from People Handling & Risk Assessment Key Trainer's Certificate course materials.

The views expressed in this text book, generally and with specific reference to manual handling, do not necessarily reflect the views, approach, company policies or course content of training programmes of EDGE Services – The Manual Handling Training Co. Ltd.

Table 12-1 Spinal Muscles

Cervical muscles	Function
Sternocleidomastoid	Extends and rotates head, flexes vertebral column
Scalenus	Flexes and rotates neck
Spinalis Cervicis	Extends and rotates head
Spinalis Capitus	Extends and rotates head
Semispinalis Cervicis	Extends and rotates vertebral column
Semispinalis Capitus	Rotates head and pulls backward
Splenius Cervicis	Extends vertebral column
Longus Colli Cervicis	Flexes cervical vertebrae
Longus Capitus	Flexes head
Rectus Capitus Anterior	Flexes head
Rectus Capitus Lateralis	Bends head laterally
Iliocostalis Cervicis	Extends cervical vertebrae
Longissimus Cervicis	Extends cervical vertebrae
Longissimus Capitus	Rotates head and pulls backward
Rectus Capitus Posterior Major	Extends and rotates head
Rectus Capitus Posterior Minor	Extends head
Obliquus Capitus Inferior	Rotates atlas
Obliquus Capitus Superior	Extends and bends head laterally

Thoracic muscles	Function
Longissimus Thoracis	Extension, lateral flexion of vertebral column, rib rotation
Iliocostalis Thoracis	Extension, lateral flexion of vertebral column, rib rotation
Spinalis Thoracis	Extends vertebral column
Semispinalis Thoracis	Extends and rotates vertebral column
Rotatores Thoracis	Extends and rotates vertebral column

Lumbar muscles	Function
Psoas Major	Flexes thigh at hip joint and vertebral column
Intertransversarii Lateralis	Lateral flexion of vertebral column
Quadratus Lumborum	Lateral flexion of vertebral column
Interspinales	Extends vertebral column
Intertransversarii Mediales	Lateral flexion of vertebral column
Multifidus	Extends and rotates vertebral column
Longissimus Lumborum	Extends and rotates vertebral column
Iliocostalis Lumborum	Extension, lateral flexion of vertebral column, rib rotation

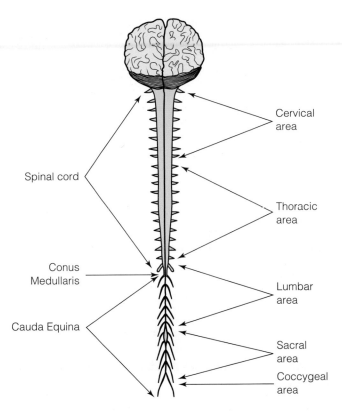

Figure 12-5 The spinal cord.

The purpose of the vertebral column is two-fold; it gives us mobility, flexibility and allows us to stand up but also acts as a protective casing for the spinal cord, which passes down through the middle of the vertebral column in the spinal canal (see Figure 12-5). The spinal nerves branch off at each level of the vertebral column and carry nerve impulses to and from various parts of the body.

Although the spine is relatively robust, back pain is the most common cause of absence from work in the UK. In 1998 a survey performed by the Department of Health (1999) found that 40% (2,200 out of 5,500) of the UK population surveyed had suffered back pain during that year. Many believe that back pain is caused by one specific incident but this is rarely the case. Indeed most back pain is cause by an accumulation of damage over many years as a result of six possible factors:

1. poor posture – how we stand and sit;
2. poor body mechanics – how we use our body to pull, lift or push objects;
3. the way we live and work – repetitive motions (e.g. shopping, lifting a child, sitting for too long and not being able to relax);
4. loss of flexibility – stiffening up, unable to have a full range of movement;
5. poor physical condition – loss of stamina and strength;
6. age – weakens the spine.

Usually damage to the spine has already occurred before pain is felt. However a painful episode can be triggered by something as simple as a sneeze or twisting to put shopping into a trolley

or bending down to put a patient's slippers on. But what do you do if you suffer with back pain? A recent Welsh strategy for tackling absence from work due to back pain suggests:

+ *Staying active – back muscles weaken if they are not used.*
+ *Take control – do not allow the pain to control your life, continue as if normal and take regular analgesia if needed.*
+ *Stay in control – by keeping active as usually the pain will subside.*

(Welshbacks, 2006)

In order to prevent back injury there are a number of principles that should be adhered to – these are termed the principles of biomechanics.

PRINCIPLES OF BIOMECHANICS

Biomechanics is the study of the mechanics of living organisms and ranges from the inner workings of the cell to the development of bones and muscles. An understanding of the basic principles of biomechanics is important as they can help prevent damage to the spine.

There are three main principles of biomechanics that are important when considering moving patients or objects. They are:

1. centre of gravity,
2. stable base,
3. keeping external levers short.

Principle 1 – Using the Centre of Gravity

Everything has a centre of gravity. The centre of gravity is where the total mass or weight of the object is concentrated. For uniform objects such as a brick, the centre of gravity will always be in the middle of the object (see Figure 12-6).

The human body also has a centre of gravity but unlike the brick whose dimensions remain constant, the human body changes its dimensions at will from sitting to standing, from

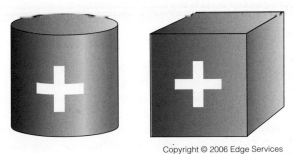

Copyright © 2006 Edge Services

Figure 12-6 Uniform objects centre of gravity.

Manual handling illustrations © EDGE Services (2006) reproduced by kind permission of EDGE Services - The Manual Handling Training Co. Ltd (01904 677853) sourced from People Handling & Risk Assessment Key Trainer's Certificate course materials.

The views expressed in this text book, generally and with specific reference to manual handling, do not necessarily reflect the views, approach, company policies or course content of training programmes of EDGE Services - The Manual Handling Training Co. Ltd.

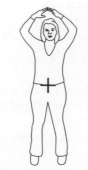

Figure 12-7 Centre of gravity of a human.

Manual handling illustrations © EDGE Services (2006) reproduced by kind permission of EDGE Services - The Manual Handling Training Co. Ltd (01904 677853) sourced from People Handling & Risk Assessment Key Trainer's Certificate course materials.

The views expressed in this text book, generally and with specific reference to manual handling, do not necessarily reflect the views, approach, company policies or course content of training programmes of EDGE Services - The Manual Handling Training Co. Ltd.

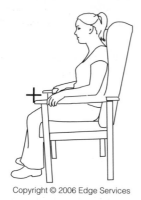

Figure 12-8 Centre of gravity outside the body making it difficult to stand.

Manual handling illustrations © EDGE Services (2006) reproduced by kind permission of EDGE Services - The Manual Handling Training Co. Ltd (01904 677853) sourced from People Handling & Risk Assessment Key Trainer's Certificate course materials.

The views expressed in this text book, generally and with specific reference to manual handling, do not necessarily reflect the views, approach, company policies or course content of training programmes of EDGE Services - The Manual Handling Training Co. Ltd.

crouching to lying. When standing upright the centre of gravity is usually situated around the navel (belly button) (see Figure 12-7).

The lower the centre of gravity is to the floor the more stable the body is, such as when we are on all fours. The higher the centre of gravity the less stable the body becomes, such as when the arms are raised above the head.

If the centre of gravity is within the body, stability is increased and it is easier to move. However if the centre of gravity is outside the body, the body is less stable and more difficult to move. For instance when sitting all the way back in a chair the centre of gravity is outside the body, standing from this position is difficult (see Figure 12-8). However if we sit forward in the chair the centre of gravity comes closer to the body making it easier to stand (see Figure 12-9).

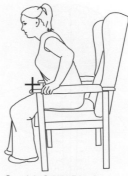

Figure 12-9 Leaning forward brings the centre of gravity closer to the body.

Manual handling illustrations © EDGE Services (2006) reproduced by kind permission of EDGE Services - The Manual Handling Training Co. Ltd (01904 677853) sourced from People Handling & Risk Assessment Key Trainer's Certificate course materials.

The views expressed in this text book, generally and with specific reference to manual handling, do not necessarily reflect the views, approach, company policies or course content of training programmes of EDGE Services - The Manual Handling Training Co. Ltd.

Principle 2 - Using a Stable Base

When standing, the feet and the area between them acts as the base of support for the body (see Figure 12.10). In order to remain stable the line of gravity should be within the base of support. Humans tend to be more stable when their feet are placed shoulder width apart and knees slightly bent (which brings the centre of gravity closer to the floor) (see Figure 12-11, on page 235).

Principle 3 - Keeping the External Levers Short

The term 'external levers' in manual handling refers to the arms. These need to be kept as short as possible: therefore keeping the

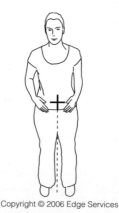

Figure 12-10 Knees slightly bent and feet shoulder width apart provides stability.

Manual handling illustrations © EDGE Services (2006) reproduced by kind permission of EDGE Services - The Manual Handling Training Co. Ltd (01904 677853) sourced from People Handling & Risk Assessment Key Trainer's Certificate course materials.

The views expressed in this text book, generally and with specific reference to manual handling, do not necessarily reflect the views, approach, company policies or course content of training programmes of EDGE Services - The Manual Handling Training Co. Ltd.

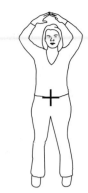

Figure 12-7 Centre of gravity of a human.

Manual handling illustrations © EDGE Services (2006) reproduced by kind permission of EDGE Services - The Manual Handling Training Co. Ltd (01904 677853) sourced from People Handling & Risk Assessment Key Trainer's Certificate course materials.

 The views expressed in this text book, generally and with specific reference to manual handling, do not necessarily reflect the views, approach, company policies or course content of training programmes of EDGE Services - The Manual Handling Training Co. Ltd.

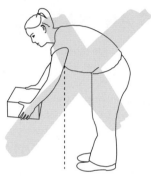

Figure 12-12 Bending forward causes instability and increased tension in the muscles of the back.

Manual handling illustrations © EDGE Services (2006) reproduced by kind permission of EDGE Services - The Manual Handling Training Co. Ltd (01904 677853) sourced from People Handling & Risk Assessment Key Trainer's Certificate course materials.

 The views expressed in this text book, generally and with specific reference to manual handling, do not necessarily reflect the views, approach, company policies or course content of training programmes of EDGE Services - The Manual Handling Training Co. Ltd.

load (weight) closer to the body ultimately brings the centre of gravity closer to the body, resulting in added stability.

 If we consider a person leaning forward to lift an object as in Figure 12-12, a common position that many of us adopt, then the centre of gravity moves outside of the body, which causes instability. In order to keep the body as stable as possible the muscles and ligaments of the back are put under a great deal of stress. If the person were to stay in this position for long the muscles would become fatigued. If the person then lifts the object they will find it extremely difficult as only minor muscles are available for the manoeuvre. Basically in this position the person is at increased risk of injury.

 Therefore to prevent injury, keep the arms short and close to the body, and bend the knees with the feet slightly apart (see Figure 12-13). This keeps the centre of gravity within the body resulting in stability.

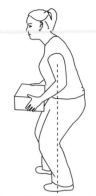

Figure 12-13 Keeping the arms short, knees bent and feet a shoulder width apart reduces the tension on the muscles of the back.

Manual handling illustrations © EDGE Services (2006) reproduced by kind permission of EDGE Services - The Manual Handling Training Co. Ltd (01904 677853) sourced from People Handling & Risk Assessment Key Trainer's Certificate course materials.

 The views expressed in this text book, generally and with specific reference to manual handling, do not necessarily reflect the views, approach, company policies or course content of training programmes of EDGE Services - The Manual Handling Training Co. Ltd.

These three principles to safer handling can then be applied to moving and handling any object including patients. However before contemplating moving an object or person there is one more point to consider, risk assessment.

RISK ASSESSMENT

The Manual Handling Operations Regulations 1992, as discussed earlier, set out some clear guidelines for the manual handling of an object or person (see Figure 12-14 on page 236). As part of these guidelines, MHOR 92 clearly states that manual handling should be avoided but if it cannot then the hazards and risks associated with the handling should be fully assessed.

 A hazard is the potential to cause harm, for example, lifting a person on your own has the potential to cause you harm (i.e. back injury) while a risk is the likelihood and severity of that harm occurring. So, for the previous example, it is highly likely that you would injure your back if you were to lift a person on your own and that injury could actually cause you to have persistent long-term back pain.

 In order to risk assess a manual handling procedure we need to consider the following:

Task	What you are doing. Does it involve stooping, bending, twisting, reaching upwards, carrying long distances, etc.
Individual	Are you capable of moving the object? Are you pregnant? Do you have an injury that could prevent you from performing the task? Are you overweight? Do you have the necessary knowledge? Have you had appropriate training?

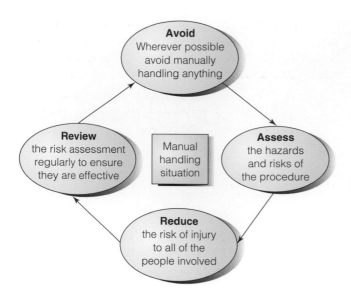

Figure 12-14 Manual Handling Operations Regulations 1992 requirements.

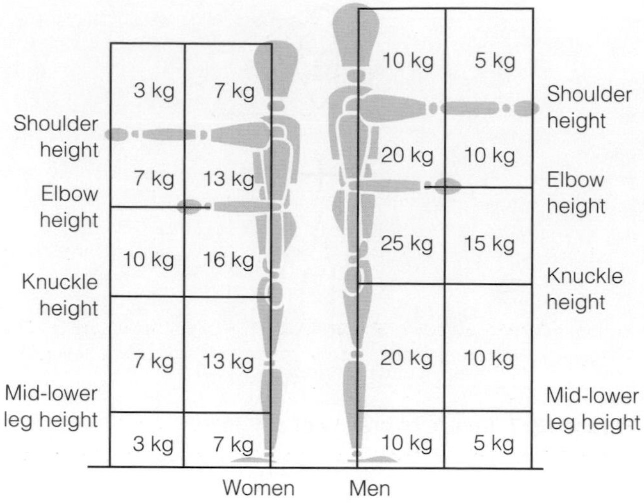

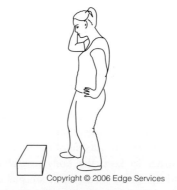

Figure 12-15 The Health and Safety Executive's Guidelines for Handling Loads.

Load	Is it heavy, bulky, unwieldy? Do you know its weight? Is it hot, cold or sharp? (see Figure 12-15)
Environment	Are there slippery floors, variations in levels? Are there leads, equipment in the way? Are the conditions hot, cold or humid?

The acronym TILE, can be quickly and easily used informally to risk assess a manual handling procedure and can also be used for more formal documented risk assessments as undertaken in many hospital and home environments by nurses.

HANDLING AN INANIMATE LOAD

It is probably a misconception that the only handling a nurse does is that of patient handling, but it is far more likely that a nurse will handle inanimate objects such as intravenous fluid boxes, beds, lockers and chairs. Nurses also have personal lives where they lift shopping from a trolley into the boot of a car or unload a washing machine and carry the heavy basket to the tumble dryer. Therefore it is important that the nurse applies the principles of safe manual handling to all aspects of their life. *Box 12-10* considers the safe lifting of a box from the floor to a shelf.

BOX 12-10 Lifting a Box from the Floor to a Shelf

First risk assess the manoeuvre using TILE.

T – Do I need to lift this box?

Where do you want to move the item? Does moving the box require bending or stooping?

Does the manoeuvre involve long carrying distances? What could I do to reduce the risk of injury, e.g. can I move the box by some other means for example using a hoist or trolley.

I – Am I capable of lifting this box. Am I in good health at the moment?

L – How do I know I can lift this weight? What does the box contain? Can the contents be moved individually?

E – Are the floors slippery? Are there any potential hazards such as other people, furniture, leads and cables? (See Figure 12-16.)

If you feel that it is safe to proceed after doing the risk assessment, you need to consider your approach to the lift, in particular the positioning of your feet. Place your feet apart ensuring that you are in a

Copyright © 2006 Edge Services

Figure 12-16 Risk assess the manoeuvre before starting.

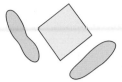

Figure 12-17 Put your leading foot forward.

stable position. Put your leading foot forward. (See Figure 12-17.)

Your knees should be bent but you sould not be kneeling on the floor. Your arms should be between the legs, and shoulders should be in line with your hips. Hands should maintain a secure grip on the box. Remember to keep the natural curves of the spine. (See Figure 12-18.)

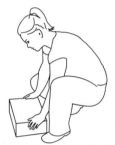

Copyright © 2006 Edge Services

Figure 12-18 Bend the knees, keep your arm between your legs and securely grip the box.

Manual handling illustrations © EDGE Services (2006) reproduced by kind permission of EDGE Services - The Manual Handling Training Co. Ltd (01904 677853) sourced from People Handling & Risk Assessment Key Trainer's Certificate course materials.

   The views expressed in this text book, generally and with specific reference to manual handling, do not necessarily reflect the views, approach, company policies or course content of training programmes of EDGE Services - The Manual Handling Training Co. Ltd.

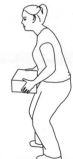

Copyright © 2006 Edge Services

Figure 12-19 Lead with your head and raise the box smoothly.

Manual handling illustrations © EDGE Services (2006) reproduced by kind permission of EDGE Services - The Manual Handling Training Co. Ltd (01904 677853) sourced from People Handling & Risk Assessment Key Trainer's Certificate course materials.

   The views expressed in this text book, generally and with specific reference to manual handling, do not necessarily reflect the views, approach, company policies or course content of training programmes of EDGE Services - The Manual Handling Training Co. Ltd.

When you are ready to lift, lead with your head, that is keep your head up, looking where you are going. Then raise your body lifting the box smoothly without any jarring. (See Figure 12-19.)

Keep the load as close to the body as possible. Remember not to twist or turn your body. If you need to change direction use your feet. (See Figure 12-20.)

When you reach the shelf, place the box down as close to your body as possible, you can then move the box to the desired position once it is on the shelf. (See Figure 12-21.)

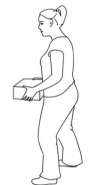

Copyright © 2006 Edge Services

Figure 12-20 Keep the load close to the body.

Manual handling illustrations © EDGE Services (2006) reproduced by kind permission of EDGE Services - The Manual Handling Training Co. Ltd (01904 677853) sourced from People Handling & Risk Assessment Key Trainer's Certificate course materials.

   The views expressed in this text book, generally and with specific reference to manual handling, do not necessarily reflect the views, approach, company policies or course content of training programmes of EDGE Services - The Manual Handling Training Co. Ltd.

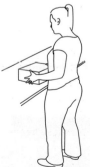

Copyright © 2006 Edge Services

Figure 12-21 Place the box on the shelf and readjust its position if needed.

Manual handling illustrations © EDGE Services (2006) reproduced by kind permission of EDGE Services - The Manual Handling Training Co. Ltd (01904 677853) sourced from People Handling & Risk Assessment Key Trainer's Certificate course materials.

   The views expressed in this text book, generally and with specific reference to manual handling, do not necessarily reflect the views, approach, company policies or course content of training programmes of EDGE Services - The Manual Handling Training Co. Ltd.

PATIENT HANDLING

Handling patients is a key component of the nurse's role. The nurse needs to be aware of the legal and professional responsibilities surrounding handling patients in order to have a clear understanding of the implications of such a task.

The principles of safer handling and biomechanics – risk assessment, using the centre of gravity, stable base, keeping external levers short – apply to both inanimate objects and people. According to the RCN (2002), when nursing small children and babies it would be impossible to eradicate lifting but in these circumstances the nurse should apply common-sense and prevent injury to themselves by taking measures such as choosing the correct cot for the weight of the child.

The following procedures (*Procedures 12-1* to *12-12*) demonstrate how to perform particular handling tasks using the principles of safer handling. Many handling tasks involve more than one nurse or nursing assistant and in these cases it is important that one of the nurses acts as team leader in order that the task be undertaken smoothly.

PROCEDURE 12-1 Moving a Person from Sitting to Standing

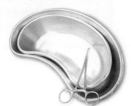

Purpose

+ To promote a sense of well-being
+ To check and/or relieve pressure areas and maintain skin integrity
+ To aid the recovery of the patient
+ To stimulate circulation

Assessment

Assess:

+ Risk assess the procedure using TILE
+ The patient's ability to stand by assessing mobility, strength and ability to understand (see *Box 12-11*)
+ Fatigue
+ Presence of pain and need for adjunctive measures (e.g. an analgesic) before standing the patient

---

Planning

+ Plan the procedure with any assistants including the patient (*promotes concordance*)
+ Encourage the patient to do as much as possible for themselves (*increasing mobility aids recovery and rehabilitation*)
+ Gather any equipment that may be needed
+ Ensure patient is properly dressed (*ensures the patient's dignity is maintained*)
+ Ensure the patient is wearing appropriate footwear or is barefooted (*ill fitting shoes, slippers or feet in stockings can lead to falls*)

Equipment

+ Tubular slide sheets (see Figure 12-22)
+ Flexi disc (see Figure 12-23)
+ Handling belt (see Figure 12-24)

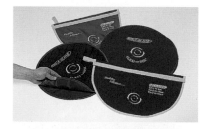

Figure 12-23 Flexi disc. © Phil-e-slide patient handling system.

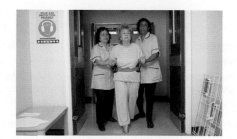

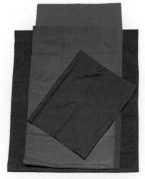

Figure 12-22 Tubular slide sheets.

Figure 12-24 Handling belt.

Implementation

Performance

1. Explain to the patient what you are going to do, why it is necessary and how they can cooperate (*promotes concordance*).
2. If needed, observe appropriate infection control procedures.
3. Prepare the patient and the environment.
4. If the patient is being returned to bed ensure that the bed is prepared and at the correct height for the patient with the head of the bed tilted up.
5. The patient needs to lean forward with their head over their knees, usually placing the hand on the arms of the chair will help stabilise the patient (see Figure 12-25).
6. Encourage the patient to move forward in the chair by walking on the cheeks of their bottom.
7. If the patient is unable to do this then you may consider using tubular slide sheets, which should be placed underneath the patient. If you do use slide sheets then you must adhere to the safety guidelines for their use (see *Box 12-12*).
8. Once the patient is toward the front of the chair the feet need to be positioned slightly apart or in a walk stance position and positioned posterior to the knees.
9. When ready to stand, the patient should gain momentum by leaning back, then forward in a rocking motion while pushing down on the arms of

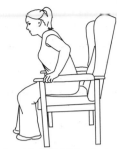

Copyright © 2006 Edge Services

Figure 12-25 Leaning forward and putting their hands on the arms of the chair or on their knees stabilises the patient.

Manual handling illustrations © EDGE Services (2006) reproduced by kind permission of EDGE Services – The Manual Handling Training Co. Ltd (01904 677853) sourced from People Handling & Risk Assessment Key Trainer's Certificate course materials.

The views expressed in this text book, generally and with specific reference to manual handling, do not necessarily reflect the views, approach, company policies or course content of training programmes of EDGE Services – The Manual Handling Training Co. Ltd.

the chair. The nurse can say 'Ready, steady, stand' to help the coordination of the movement.

10. For reassurance, the nurse can place their hands on the patient's shoulder or can use a handling belt, ensuring that they do not lift the patient or bend or stoop during the procedure.
11. Once standing the patient can then turn if needed to the bed or if they are unable to do this the nurse can use the Flexi Disc on the floor to turn the patient toward the bed or chair.

Evaluation

+ Note the patient's tolerance of the procedure (e.g. respiratory rate and effort, pulse rate, behaviour, cooperation).

+ Document procedure and findings in the nursing notes.

BOX 12-11 Assessing a Patient's Mobility, Strength and Understanding

Before performing the following, the nurse must gain consent from the patient:

+ Ask the patient when they moved last and how they felt.
+ Ask the patient if they can feel their hands, arms, feet and legs. *This checks understanding and sensation.*
+ Apply pressure to the patient's knee by placing your hand on their knee then ask the patient to lift their knee; repeat for other knee. *The patient should be able to lift both knees with equal strength.*
+ Place your hand on top of the patient's foot and ask the patient to lift their foot off the floor or bed. *The patient should be able to lift both feet with equal strength.*

+ Ask the patient to place their hands on the arms of the chair and lift themselves off the chair slightly. *The patient should be able to lift themselves slightly off the chair.*
+ Ask the patient to squeeze your hand tightly with their left hand, repeat with right hand. *The patient should be able to squeeze equally with both hands. This checks understanding, sensation and strength.*
+ Explain to the patient what the manoeuvre involves and ask the patient to repeat the requirements. *This checks understanding.*

If in any doubt at any stage do not move the patient.

BOX 12-12 Slide Sheets

+ Slide sheets are made from specialised flexible fabric that has been designed to reduce friction during handling procedures.
+ There are different types of slide sheets made by a number of different companies.
+ The main types are tubular slide sheets and flat slide sheets.
+ Tubular slide sheets are tubes of fabric that have a low friction inner surface (usually shiny surface) which slides over itself and can be used for the seated patient or a patient who is lying down.
+ Flat sheets are sheets of fabric that have a low friction surface. These must be used in pairs unless advised by the manufacturer. When using in pairs, the low friction surfaces must be next to one another (shiny surface to shiny surface).

Safety While Using Slide Sheets

+ Because of the slippery nature of the slide sheets they may not be suitable for all handling procedures with all patients. Assess the individual situation and patient before using.
+ If the low friction surfaces are not together, this can cause added stress on the nurse's back and potentially cause injury.
+ You must receive training before using slide sheets as with all manual handling equipment.
+ Once used, do not put the slide sheet on the floor as it is a slipping hazard.
+ Slide sheets should be for single patient use.
+ Most slide sheets can be washed when soiled and between patients.
+ Disposable slide sheets are for single patient use and then should be disposed of.

Removing Tubular Slide Sheets

+ Place your hand between the layers of the tubular sheet.
+ Grasp the opposite corner and pull the tube inside out in the direction you have just moved the patient: so if you have moved the patient up the bed you should pull to the top of the bed (see Figure 12-26).

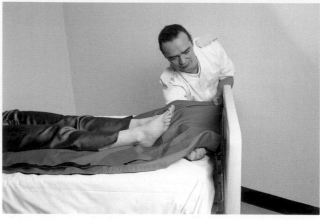

A

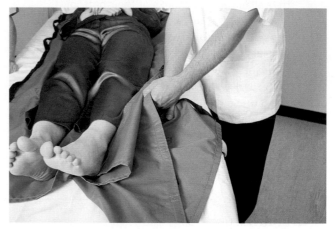

B

Figure 12-26 Removing tubular and flat sheets.

Removing Flat Slide Sheets

+ Place your hand between the two layers of the sheets.
+ Grasp the opposite corner bottom sheet and pull it over the top of itself (shiny surface to shiny surface) in the direction you have just moved the patient (see Figure 12-26).
+ Grasp the opposite corner of the top sheet and pull it under itself (shiny surface to shiny surface) in the direction you have just moved the patient.

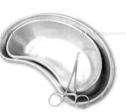

PROCEDURE 12-2 Moving a Person from a Lying Position to Standing

Purpose

+ To promote a sense of well-being
+ To check and/or relieve pressure areas and maintain skin integrity
+ To aid the recovery of the patient
+ To stimulate circulation

Assessment

Assess:

+ Risk assess the procedure using TILE
+ The patient's ability to stand by assessing mobility, strength and ability to understand (see Box 12-11)
+ Fatigue
+ Presence of pain and need for adjunctive measures (e.g. an analgesic) before standing the patient

Planning

+ Plan the procedure with any assistants including the patient (*promotes concordance*)
+ Encourage the patient to do as much as possible for themselves (*increasing mobility aids recovery and rehabilitation*)
+ Gather any equipment that may be needed
+ Ensure patient is properly dressed (*ensures the patient's dignity is maintained*)
+ Ensure the patient is wearing appropriate footwear or is barefooted (*ill fitting shoes, slippers or feet in stockings can lead to falls*)

Equipment

+ Tubular slide sheets (see Figure 12-22 on page 238)
+ Flexi disc (see Figure 12-23 on page 238)
+ Handling belt (see Figure 12-24 on page 238)

Implementation

Performance

1. Explain to the patient what you are going to do, why it is necessary and how they can cooperate (*this promotes concordance*)
2. If needed, observe appropriate infection control procedures.
3. Prepare the patient and the environment.
4. If the patient is to sit in a chair ensure this is correctly positioned.
5. The patient needs to roll themselves onto their side or be assisted on to their side by the nurse and their assistants (see Procedure 12-5 on page 246).
6. The patient should then be encouraged to push the uppermost part of the arm onto the bed so they are able to lift their head and trunk (see Figure 12-27).
7. The opposite arm can then be used to take their weight and raise the trunk.
8. If the patient then swings their legs over the edge of the bed the pelvis will become vertical and help the patient into a sitting position.
9. If the patient is unable to swing their legs over the edge of the bed then you may consider using tubular slide sheets, which should be placed underneath the patient's legs. If you do use slide

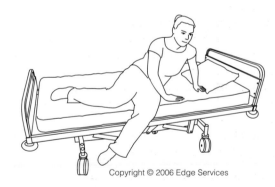

Copyright © 2006 Edge Services

Figure 12-27 Encourage the patient to push up from the bed using their arms.

Manual handling illustrations © EDGE Services (2006) reproduced by kind permission of EDGE Services – The Manual Handling Training Co. Ltd (01904 677853) sourced from People Handling & Risk Assessment Key Trainer's Certificate course materials.

The views expressed in this text book, generally and with specific reference to manual handling, do not necessarily reflect the views, approach, company policies or course content of training programmes of EDGE Services – The Manual Handling Training Co. Ltd.

sheets then you must adhere to the safety guidelines for their use (see Box 12-12).

10. Once the patient is on the edge of the bed they should be encouraged to stabilise themselves by positioning their arms on either side of their hips (see Figure 12-28 on page 242).

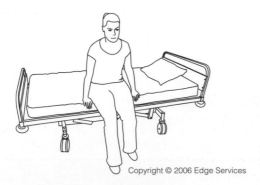

Copyright © 2006 Edge Services

Figure 12-28 Encourage the patient to place their hands on the bed to stabilise themselves.

Manual handling illustrations © EDGE Services (2006) reproduced by kind permission of EDGE Services – The Manual Handling Training Co. Ltd (01904 677853) sourced from People Handling & Risk Assessment Key Trainer's Certificate course materials.

The views expressed in this text book, generally and with specific reference to manual handling, do not necessarily reflect the views, approach, company policies or course content of training programmes of EDGE Services – The Manual Handling Training Co. Ltd.

11. To stand, the patient's feet need to be positioned slightly apart or in a walk stance position and positioned posterior to the knees.
12. When ready to stand, the patient should gain momentum by leaning back, then forward in a rocking motion while pushing down on the bed. The nurse can say 'Ready, steady, stand' to help the coordination of the movement.
13. For reassurance, the nurse can place their hands on the patient's shoulder or can use a handling belt, ensuring that they do not lift the patient or bend or stoop during the procedure.
14. Once standing the patient can then turn if needed to the chair or if they are unable to do this the nurse can use the Flexi Disc on the floor to turn the patient toward the bed or chair.

Evaluation

+ Note the patient's tolerance of the procedure (e.g. respiratory rate and effort, pulse rate, behaviour, cooperation).

+ Document procedure and findings in the nursing notes.

PROCEDURE 12-3 Moving a Person from the Floor to Sitting or Standing

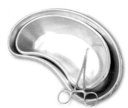

Purpose

+ To raise the fallen patient

+ To aid the recovery of the patient

Assessment

Assess:

+ Risk assess the procedure using TILE
+ The patient's ability to stand by assessing mobility, strength and ability to understand (see *Box 12-11* on page 239)
+ Fatigue

+ Presence of pain and need for adjunctive measures (e.g. an analgesic) before standing the patient
+ Any medical injuries as a result of the fall

Planning

+ Plan the procedure with any assistants including the patient (*promotes concordance*)
+ Encourage the patient to do as much as possible for themselves (*increasing mobility aids recovery and rehabilitation*)
+ Gather any equipment that may be needed
+ Ensure patient is properly dressed (*ensures the patient's dignity is maintained*)

+ Ensure the patient is wearing appropriate footwear or is barefooted (*ill fitting shoes, slippers or feet in stockings can lead to falls*)

Equipment

+ Two chairs

Implementation

Performance

1. Explain to the patient what you are going to do, why it is necessary and how they can cooperate. *This promotes concordance.*
2. If needed, observe appropriate infection control procedures.
3. Prepare the patient and the environment.
4. If the patient is being returned to bed ensure that the bed is prepared and at the correct height for the patient with the head of the bed tilted up.
5. Ask the patient to roll onto their side or assist them onto their side.

6. Once on their side ask them to place both their hands on the floor and push their head and trunk off the floor (see Figure 12-29).
7. The patient then can position themselves on 'all fours'. If needed they can rest in this position (see Figure 12-30).
8. Place a chair in front of the patient and ask the patient to pull themselves up onto it (see Figure 12-31).
9. Once standing another chair can be positioned behind them in order for them to sit down (see Figure 12-32).

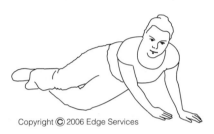

Copyright © 2006 Edge Services

Figure 12-29 Encourage the patient to push up from the floor using their arms.

Manual handling illustrations © EDGE Services (2006) reproduced by kind permission of EDGE Services - The Manual Handling Training Co. Ltd (01904 677853) sourced from People Handling & Risk Assessment Key Trainer's Certificate course materials.

The views expressed in this text book, generally and with specific reference to manual handling, do not necessarily reflect the views, approach, company policies or course content of training programmes of EDGE Services - The Manual Handling Training Co. Ltd.

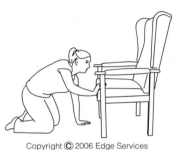

Copyright © 2006 Edge Services

Figure 12-31 Place a chair in front of the patient so they can pull themselves up.

Manual handling illustrations © EDGE Services (2006) reproduced by kind permission of EDGE Services - The Manual Handling Training Co. Ltd (01904 677853) sourced from People Handling & Risk Assessment Key Trainer's Certificate course materials.

The views expressed in this text book, generally and with specific reference to manual handling, do not necessarily reflect the views, approach, company policies or course content of training programmes of EDGE Services - The Manual Handling Training Co. Ltd.

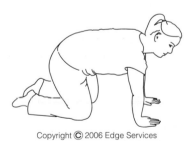

Copyright © 2006 Edge Services

Figure 12-30 The patient can rest on all fours.

Manual handling illustrations © EDGE Services (2006) reproduced by kind permission of EDGE Services - The Manual Handling Training Co. Ltd (01904 677853) sourced from People Handling & Risk Assessment Key Trainer's Certificate course materials.

The views expressed in this text book, generally and with specific reference to manual handling, do not necessarily reflect the views, approach, company policies or course content of training programmes of EDGE Services - The Manual Handling Training Co. Ltd.

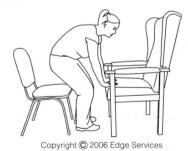

Copyright © 2006 Edge Services

Figure 12-32 Place another chair behind so they can sit down.

Manual handling illustrations © EDGE Services (2006) reproduced by kind permission of EDGE Services - The Manual Handling Training Co. Ltd (01904 677853) sourced from People Handling & Risk Assessment Key Trainer's Certificate course materials.

The views expressed in this text book, generally and with specific reference to manual handling, do not necessarily reflect the views, approach, company policies or course content of training programmes of EDGE Services - The Manual Handling Training Co. Ltd.

Evaluation

+ Note the patient's tolerance of the procedure (e.g. respiratory rate and effort, pulse rate, behaviour, cooperation).
+ Note any injuries.
+ Document procedure and findings in the nursing notes.

PROCEDURE 12-4 Assisting a Patient to Walk

Purpose

+ To promote a sense of well-being
+ To aid the recovery of the patient
+ To stimulate circulation

Assessment

Assess:

+ Risk assess the procedure using TILE
+ The patient's ability to walk by assessing mobility, strength and ability to understand (see *Box 12-11* on page 239)
+ Fatigue
+ Presence of pain and need for adjunctive measures (e.g. an analgesic) before walking the patient

Planning

+ Plan the procedure with any assistants including the patient (*promotes concordance*)
+ Ensure patient is properly dressed (*ensures the patient's dignity is maintained*)
+ Ensure the patient is wearing appropriate footwear or is barefooted (*ill fitting shoes, slippers or feet in stockings can lead to falls*)

Equipment

No equipment needed

Implementation

Performance

1. Explain to the patient what you are going to do, why it is necessary and how they can cooperate (*promotes concordance*).
2. If needed, observe appropriate infection control procedures.
3. Prepare the patient and the environment.
4. Stand to the side of the patient, half a step behind them.
5. Ask the patient to place their hand in your furthest hand using a palm to palm grip (see Figure 12-33).
6. The nurse's closest hand can be placed on the patient's back for reassurance.
7. The nurse can then walk with the patient at the patient's pace.

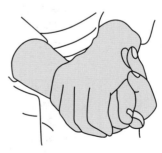

Figure 12-33 Palm to palm grip avoiding thumb hold.

8. If needed another nurse or nursing assistant can push a wheelchair behind the patient in case they need to rest.

Evaluation

+ Note the patient's tolerance of the procedure (e.g. respiratory rate and effort, pulse rate, behaviour, cooperation).
+ Document procedure and findings in the nursing notes.

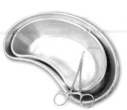

PROCEDURE 12-5 Turning a Patient in Bed and Positioning in a 30° Tilt

Purpose

+ To promote a sense of well-being
+ To check and/or relieve pressure areas and maintain skin integrity
+ To reposition the patient
+ To aid the recovery of the patient
+ To stimulate circulation

Assessment

Assess:

+ Risk assess the procedure using TILE
+ The patient's haemodynamic stability
+ Fatigue
+ Presence of pain and need for adjunctive measures (e.g. an analgesic) before turning the patient

Planning

+ Plan the procedure with any assistants including the patient (*promotes concordance*)
+ Encourage the patient to do as much as possible for themselves (*increasing mobility aids recovery and rehabilitation*)
+ Gather any equipment that may be needed
+ Ensure dignity is maintained by drawing curtains, and closing windows and doors

Equipment

Two or three pillows

Implementation

Performance

1. Explain to the patient what you are going to do, why it is necessary and how they can cooperate (*promotes concordance*).
2. If needed, observe appropriate infection control procedures.
3. Prepare the patient and the environment.
4. Usually one or two nurses or nursing assistants are required to turn a patient in bed.
5. The nurses should position themselves at the heaviest parts of the patient, which is usually the trunk and upper legs.
6. The bed should be positioned so that all involved in moving the patient are comfortable.
7. Position the patient to aid moving (see Figure 12-34).
8. The nurse closest to the patient's head should place one hand on the patient's shoulder and one on their hip. While the other nurse should place one hand on the patient's hip and the other should be used to guide the legs over. No pressure should be applied to the knee joint as this can cause injury to the patient.
9. When ready to move the patient the team leader should say 'Ready, steady, roll'. The nurses will then roll the patient.

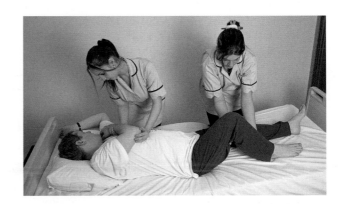

Figure 12-34 Position the patient in bed ready to roll. Head turned to the direction of the roll, opposite arm across chest and opposite leg bent.

10. Once over on their side, pillows can be placed behind the patient and between the patient's knees.
11. The patient should then be rested back onto the pillows.
12. The same process can be used for changing sheets and checking pressure areas.

Evaluation

+ Note the patient's tolerance of the procedure (e.g. respiratory rate and effort, pulse rate, behaviour, cooperation).

+ Document procedure and findings in the nursing notes.

PROCEDURE 12-6 Moving a Supine Patient Up and Down the Bed

Purpose

+ To promote a sense of well-being
+ To reposition the patient
+ To aid the recovery of the patient
+ To stimulate circulation and respiratory function

Assessment

Assess:

+ Risk assess the procedure using TILE
+ The patient's haemodynamic stability
+ Fatigue
+ Presence of pain and need for adjunctive measures (e.g. an analgesic) before moving the patient

Planning

+ Plan the procedure with any assistants including the patient (*promotes concordance*)
+ Encourage the patient to do as much as possible for themselves (*increasing mobility aids recovery and rehabilitation*)
+ Gather any equipment that may be needed
+ Ensure dignity is maintained by drawing curtains, and closing windows and doors

Equipment

Flat slide sheets

Implementation

Performance

1. Explain to the patient what you are going to do, why it is necessary and how they can cooperate (*promotes concordance*).
2. If needed, observe appropriate infection control procedures.
3. Prepare the patient and the environment.
4. Ask the patient to turn onto their side or assist the patient to roll (see Procedure 12-5).
5. Position the flat sheets under the patient, ensuring they are positioned correctly
   (see Box 12-12 on page 240 for the principles of flat slide sheets).
6. Roll the patient back onto their back and ensure that the slide sheets are pulled through.
7. Tilt the bed in the direction you wish the patient to move.
8. Push or pull the patient up or down the bed.
9. Reposition the bed and removing the flat slide sheets (see *Box 12-12* on page 240).

Evaluation

+ Note the patient's tolerance of the procedure (e.g. respiratory rate and effort, pulse rate, behaviour, cooperation).

+ Document procedure and findings in the nursing notes.

PROCEDURE 12-7 Transferring a Patient from Bed to Bed/Trolley with the Patient in a Lying Position

Purpose

+ To move the patient to a more suitable bed or mattress
+ To transfer the patient to or from theatre

Assessment

Assess:

+ Risk assess the procedure using TILE
+ The patient's haemodynamic stability
+ Fatigue

+ Presence of pain and need for adjunctive measures (e.g. an analgesic) before standing the patient

Planning

+ Plan the procedure with any assistants including the patient (*promotes concordance*)
+ Encourage the patient to do as much as possible for themselves (*increasing mobility aids recovery and rehabilitation*)
+ Gather any equipment that may be needed
+ Ensure dignity is maintained by drawing curtains, and closing windows and doors

Equipment

+ Lateral transfer aid (see Figure 12-35)

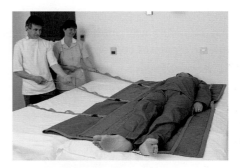

Figure 12-35 Lateral transfer aid. © Phil-e-slide patient handling system.

Implementation

Performance

1. Explain to the patient what you are going to do, why it is necessary and how they can cooperate (*promotes concordance*).
2. If needed, observe appropriate infection control procedures.
3. Prepare the patient and the environment.
4. A minimum of two healthcare staff are required for this move depending on the size of the patient and haemodynamic stability.
5. The nurse should ask the patient to roll away from the other bed/trolley or should be assisted to roll (see *Procedure 12-5* on page 245).
6. Once the patient is over on their side the nurse can position the lateral transfer aid under the patient.

7. The patient can then be rolled back on to the bed and the other bed or trolley can then be positioned next to and slightly lower than the bed the patient is on. Ensure the brakes are on each of the beds.
8. Ask the patient to place their hands across their chest or down by their sides.
9. Once ready to transfer the team leader can say 'Ready, steady, slide', the nurses will then hand over hand pull the patient across from one bed to the other (see Figure 12-35).
10. Once the patient is on the other bed or trolley the lateral transfer aid can be removed.
11. The patient can then be made comfortable on the bed or trolley.

Evaluation

+ Note the patient's tolerance of the procedure (e.g. respiratory rate and effort, pulse rate, behaviour, cooperation).

+ Document procedure and findings in the nursing notes.

PROCEDURE 12-8 Transferring a Patient from Bed to Chair in a Seated Position

Purpose

+ To promote a sense of well-being
+ To reposition the patient
+ To aid the recovery of the patient
+ To stimulate circulation

Assessment

Assess:

+ Risk assess the procedure using TILE
+ The patient's ability by assessing mobility, strength and ability to understand (see *Box 12-11* on page 240)
+ Fatigue
+ Presence of pain and need for adjunctive measures (e.g. an analgesic) before moving the patient

Planning

+ Plan the procedure with any assistants including the patient (*promotes concordance*)

+ Encourage the patient to do as much as possible for themselves (*increasing mobility aids recovery and rehabilitation*)
+ Gather any equipment that may be needed
+ Ensure dignity is maintained by drawing curtains, and closing windows and doors

Equipment

+ Curved or straight seated transfer aid (see Figure 12-36)
+ Bed ladder if needed (see Figure 12-37)

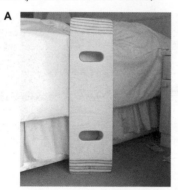

A

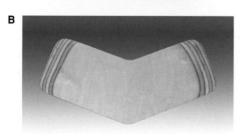

B

Figure 12-36 Straight and curved seated lateral transfer aids.

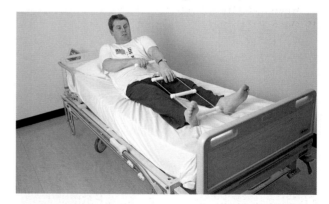

Figure 12-37 Bed ladder.

Implementation

Performance

1. Explain to the patient what you are going to do, why it is necessary and how they can cooperate (*promotes concordance*).
2. If needed, observe appropriate infection control procedures.
3. Prepare the patient and the environment.

4. Ask the patient to get into a seated position or assist them into a seated position using the bed or a bed ladder.
5. If the chair has arms that can be lowered a straight seated transfer board is needed with the chair positioned directly next to the bed (see Figure 12-38).

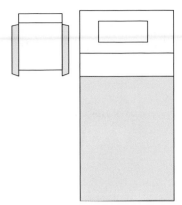 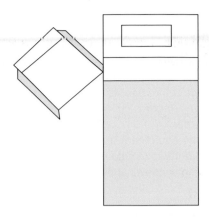

Figure 12-38 Place the chair next to the bed.

Figure 12-39 If the chair does not have arms that lower then place the chair at a 45-degree angle to the bed.

6. Place the transfer aid under the patient's buttock ensuring that the board bridges the gap between the bed and chair.
7. Instruct the patient *not* to put their hands under the end of the board as this can cause injury. Instead tell the patient to use the handles provided or place their hand flat on the transfer aid.
8. The patient may then begin to slide themselves across between the bed and chair.
9. If using a normal arm chair, it will need to be positioned at an angle for transferring using a curved seated transfer aid (see Figure 12-39).
10. The patient may need to bring themselves to the edge of the bed in order to slide across when using the curved transfer aid.
11. Once across onto the chair ensure the patient is comfortable.

12. If the patient has a tendency to slide forward or slump in the chair they may need to use a one-way slide sheet (see Figure 12-40) which allows them to slide back in the chair but does not allow them to slide forward in the chair.

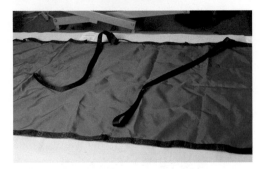

Figure 12-40 One-way slide sheet.

Evaluation

+ Note the patient's tolerance of the procedure (e.g. respiratory rate and effort, pulse rate, behaviour, cooperation).
+ Document procedure and findings in the nursing notes.

PROCEDURE 12-9 Hoisting a Patient from Bed to Chair

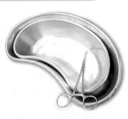

Purpose

+ To promote a sense of well-being
+ To reposition the patient
+ To aid the recovery of the patient
+ To stimulate circulation

Assessment

Assess:

+ Risk assess the procedure using TILE
+ The patient's ability by assessing mobility, strength and ability to understand (see *Box 12-11* on page 240)
+ Fatigue
+ Presence of pain and need for adjunctive measures (e.g. an analgesic) before hoisting the patient

Planning

+ Plan the procedure with any assistants including the patient (*promotes concordance*).
+ Encourage the patient to do as much as possible for themselves (*increasing mobility aids recovery and rehabilitation*).
+ Gather any equipment that may be needed.
+ Ensure dignity is maintained by drawing curtains, and closing windows and doors.

Equipment

+ Suitable hoist (see Figure 12-41)
+ Suitable sling for the hoist and patient (see Figure 12-42)

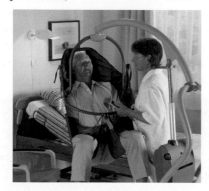

Figure 12-41 Hoist that lifts the whole body.

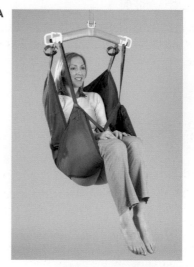

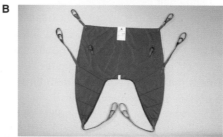

Figure 12-42 Universal sling.

Implementation

Performance

1. Explain to the patient what you are going to do, why it is necessary and how they can cooperate (*promotes concordance*).
2. If needed, observe appropriate infection control procedures.
3. Prepare the patient and the environment.
4. Ask the patient to roll onto their side or assist them to roll (see *Procedure 12-5* on page 245).
5. Place the appropriate sling (see *Box 12-13* on how to choose the appropriate sling) under the patient and ask the patient to roll back onto their back.
6. Position the hoist over the patient (make sure the brakes are off on the hoist), lower and attach the sling to the hoist (see *Box 12-14* on the safe use of hoists).

7. If the patient is competent and the hoist has a remote control, then the patient can control the lift.
8. Raise the patient slightly off the bed and check that the hoist is comfortable for the patient.
9. The patient can then be raised further but only enough so that they are able to clear the bed.
10. The hoist can then be moved so that the patient is over the chair.
11. Again if competent the patient can lower themselves into the chair.
12. Ensure the patient is right in the back of the chair. Sometimes tilting the chair can help to position the patient correctly in the chair.
13. Once in the chair the sling can be removed.
14. Ensure that the patient is comfortable before leaving the patient.

Evaluation

+ Note the patient's tolerance of the procedure (e.g. respiratory rate and effort, pulse rate, behaviour, cooperation).

+ Document procedure and findings in the nursing notes.

CLINICAL ALERT

With hoists that lift the whole person, the hoist has to find its centre of gravity. If the brakes are put on the hoist when lifting, it is liable to fall over as it cannot find its centre of gravity.

BOX 12-13 Choosing an Appropriate Sling

Slings are the most important component of a hoist system as a sling is the interface between the patient and the hoist. So when choosing the type and size of sling to use consider the following:

+ Different makes of hoist have different sling.
+ Also there are different slings for different handling procedures such as for bathing and toileting.
+ Check the label of the sling to ensure that it is appropriate sling for the type of hoist you are using.
+ Check the safe working load of sling (maximum weight that the sling will lift) usually found on the label.
+ Check that the safe working load of the sling is less than the safe working load of the hoist, the maximum weight that can be lifted would be the weight denoted on the sling.
+ The sling should not be soiled and if so slings usually can be washed.
+ All attachments of the sling should be checked to ensure that they are in good working order.

+ If there are signs of fraying or damage to the sling do not use it.

Sizing Slings
+ Slings are usually colour coded for sizing. However it is important to note that different companies use different colours for different sizes: for example, yellow may denote small size with one company but with another may denote medium size.
+ The sling should fit comfortably around the patient: too big and the patient may feel that they are going to fall out; too small and the patient may find it uncomfortable.
+ Specific sizing will depend on the type of sling used but generally you need to measure the sling against the patient's back to ensure that there is enough length from shoulder to buttocks and from arm to arm across the back.

You must receive training on the use of hoists and their slings.

BOX 12-14 Safe Use of A Hoist

Hoist Checks
+ Check that the hoist is the type needed for the handling procedure: for example, for standing a patient a stand aid hoist is needed.
+ Check the safe working load of the hoist.
+ Check when it was serviced last (usually a sticker on the frame of the hoist).
+ Check that it looks in good working order.
+ If it is dirty is can be cleaned with soap and water or alcohol wipes.
+ Check that the battery is charged, if not change or charge it.
+ Check that the mechanism works.
+ Check that all attachments are in working order and attached properly.

+ Check the brakes are in good working order.
+ Check the wheels of the hoist run smoothly.

Using the Hoist
+ When using a hoist act confidently, as this will reduce the patient's fear.
+ When lowering the jig or cross bar of the hoist to attach the sling ensure that it does not hit the patient.
+ Raise the hoist smoothly; do not stop and start the lift as this can frighten the patient.
+ The maximum distance that a hoist should be pushed is 10 metres, less if it is over carpeted flooring.

Training must be received before using a hoist.

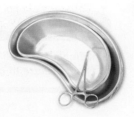

PROCEDURE 12-10 Using a Stand Aid Hoist to Move a Patient

Purpose

+ To promote a sense of well-being
+ To reposition the patient
+ To aid the recovery of the patient
+ To stimulate circulation

Assessment

Assess:

+ Risk assess the procedure using TILE
+ The patient's ability to stand by assessing mobility, strength and ability to understand (see *Box 12-11*)
+ Fatigue
+ Presence of pain and need for adjunctive measures (e.g. an analgesic) before standing the patient

Planning

+ Plan the procedure including the patient (*promotes concordance*)
+ Encourage the patient to do as much as possible for themselves (*increasing mobility aids recovery and rehabilitation*)
+ Gather any equipment that may be needed
+ Ensure dignity is maintained by drawing curtains, and closing windows and doors

Equipment

+ Suitable stand aid hoist (see Figure 12-43)
+ Suitable sling for the hoist and patient

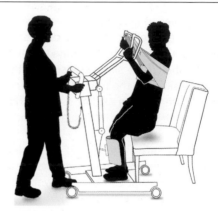

Figure 12-43 Stand aid hoist.

Implementation

Performance

1. Explain to the patient what you are going to do, why it is necessary and how they can cooperate (*promotes concordance*).
2. If needed, observe appropriate infection control procedures.
3. Prepare the patient and the environment.
4. Place the appropriate sling (see Box 12-13 on how to choose the appropriate sling) under the patient.
5. Position the hoist over the patient (make sure the brakes are on), lower and attach the sling to the hoist (see *Box 12-14*).
6. Ask the patient to place their feet on the platform of the hoist and push their knees into the knee braces of the hoist.

7. If the patient is competent and the hoist has a remote control, then the patient can control the lift.
8. Raise the patient slightly off the chair and check that the sling is comfortable for the patient.
9. The patient can then be raised further so they are standing in the hoist.
10. The hoist's brakes can then be removed and the patient moved to the desired location.
11. Once at the desired location, the patient can be lowered and the sling and hoist removed.
12. Ensure that the patient is comfortable before leaving the patient.

Evaluation

+ Note the patient's tolerance of the procedure (e.g. respiratory rate and effort, pulse rate, behaviour, cooperation).
+ Document procedure and findings in the nursing notes.

CLINICAL ALERT

For stand aid hoists the brakes must be left on when lifting the patient because the centre of gravity for the hoist will be the person's legs.

CRITICAL REFLECTION

Let us revisit the case study on page 226. Now that you have read this chapter, reflect on why you think a 'no lifting policy' was problematic for East Sussex County Council? What legal and professional responsibilities would prevent a 'no lifting policy' being implemented?

CHAPTER HIGHLIGHTS

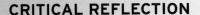

+ Back injuries currently cost the NHS £400 million each year with one in four nurses having to take time off work as a result of a back injury.
+ The law within the UK with regard to the moving and handling of patients has two clear goals: first to prevent injury and second to compensate the handler when an injury occurs.
+ The Health and Safety at Work Act 1974 clearly states that an employer must ensure the health, safety and welfare at work of its employees, as far as it is reasonably practicable.
+ However, it is important to note that the employee also has a duty to take reasonable care of their own health and safety.
+ The Manual Handling Operations Regulations 1992 (MHOR 92), as amended by the Health and Safety Miscellaneous Amendments Regulations 2002 sets very specific duties for the employer in relation to manual handling in the workplace.
+ The Provision and Use of Work Equipment Regulations 1992 (PUWER) aims to prevent or control the risk to an individual's health and safety from work equipment such as photocopiers, hoists, etc. and sets out a number of requirements that the employer must adhere to.

+ The Lifting Operations and Lifting Equipment Regulations 1998 (LOLER), on the other hand, regulates lifting equipment used in the workplace and like PUWER it sets out requirements that the employer must adhere to.
+ Any breach by the employer under any or all of these regulations can result in criminal prosecution.
+ Everyone, including patients and health and social care workers, is protected by the Human Rights Act 1998.
+ The spine or vertebral column extends from the base of the skull to the pelvis and is made up of 33 individual bones or vertebrae.
+ An understanding of basic principles of biomechanics is important as this can help prevent damage to the spine.
+ A hazard is the potential to cause harm, for example, lifting a person on your own has the potential to cause you harm that is back injury.
+ A risk is the likelihood and severity of that harm occurring. The acronym TILE can be quickly and easily used to informally risk assess a manual handling procedure and can also be used for more formal documented risk assessments as used in many hospital and home environments by nurses.

GUIDANCE

For the full text of Acts and Regulations mentioned in this chapter see www.legislation.hmso.gov.uk.

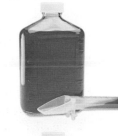

REFERENCES

Chell, P. (2003) 'Moving and handling: implications of bad practice', *Nursing and Residential Care*, 5(6), 276–279.

Department of Health (1999) *The prevalence of back pain in Great Britain in 1998*, London: Crown Copyright.

Department of Health (2004) *The manager's guide: Back in work campaign*, London: Crown Copyright.

Griffith, R. and Stevens, M. (2003) 'Manual handling and the lawfulness of no-lift policies', *Nursing Standard*, 18(21), 39–43.

Health and Safety Executive (1998) *Simple guide to the lifting operations and lifting equipment regulations 1998*, Caerphilly: HSE.

National Back Pain Association (1998) *The guide to the handling of patients* (4th edn), London: RCN.

NMC (2004) *Code of professional conduct: Standards for conduct, performance and ethics*, London: NMC.

RCN (2002) *Code of practice for patient handling*, London: RCN.

Smith, J. (Ed.) (2005) *The guide to the handling of people*, Middlesex: Backcare.

Welshbacks (2006) *Don't take back pain lying down*, Cardiff: NHS Wales. Available from http://www.welshbacks.com. (Accessed on 7 December 2006.)

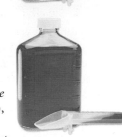

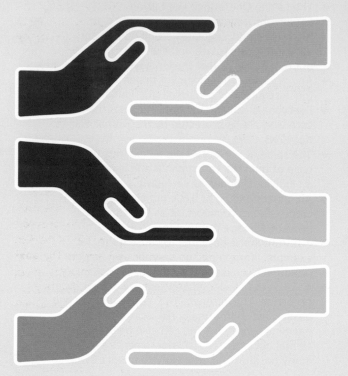

Chapter 13 Hygiene

Learning Outcomes

After completing this chapter, you will be able to:

+ Describe hygienic care that nurses provide to patients.

+ Identify factors influencing personal hygiene.

+ Identify normal and abnormal assessment findings while providing hygiene care.

+ Apply the nursing process to common problems related to hygienic care of the skin, feet, nails, mouth, hair, eyes, ears and nose.

+ Identify the purposes of bathing.

+ Explain specific ways in which nurses help hospitalised patients with hygiene.

+ Describe steps for identified hygienic-care procedures.

+ Identify steps in removing contact lenses and inserting and removing artificial eyes.

+ Describe steps for removing, cleaning and inserting hearing aids.

+ Identify safety and comfort measures underlying bed-making procedures.

CASE STUDY

Joan is 45 years old and has suffered an injury affecting her nervous system. This injury also affects her ability to perform unaided activities of daily living including attending to her own personal hygiene needs. As a relatively young person Joan is expressing feelings of distress when receiving assistance from members of the nursing team which in turn is making her mood low and causing depression.

Joan's husband shows you a picture of a very smartly dressed lady with immaculate make up and perfect hair style. Her husband comments that she would spend hours ensuring she was 'perfect' to go anywhere. As you reflect upon this image and look at the lady in front of you it is easy to appreciate why Joan is so upset and distressed.

In consultation with Joan a plan of care is designed that assists her to be as independent as possible to attend to her own needs with minimal assistance. The plan also incorporates aspects of her lifestyle considerations prior to her admission to your care.

After reading this chapter you will be able to discuss the importance of maintaining personal hygiene.

INTRODUCTION

Hygiene is the science of health and its maintenance. Personal **hygiene** is the self-care by which people attend to such functions as bathing, toileting, general body hygiene and grooming. Hygiene is a highly personal matter determined by individual values and practices. It involves care of the skin, hair, nails, teeth, oral and nasal cavities, eyes, ears and perineal-genital areas.

It is important for nurses to know exactly how much assistance a patient needs for hygienic care. Patients may require help after urinating or defecating, after vomiting, and whenever they become soiled, for example, from wound drainage or from profuse perspiration. Table 13-1 lists factors that influence hygiene practices.

HYGIENIC CARE

Morning care is provided to patients as they awaken in the morning or after breakfast. A patient who requires assistance would have their elimination needs provided for, an assisted wash, bath or shower, perineal care, skin pressure areas checked, oral, nail and hair care. Making the patient's bed is part of morning care.

Prior to the patient settling for the night elimination needs should be provided for, hands and face washed as necessary, and oral care performed. Individuals frequently need additional care during the day or night as necessary including assistance with elimination. Additionally a patient who is diaphoretic (sweating profusely) may need more frequent bathing and a change of clothes and linen.

SKIN

The skin is the largest organ of the body. It serves five major functions:

1. It protects underlying tissues from injury by preventing the passage of micro-organisms. The skin and mucous membranes are considered the body's first line of defence.
2. It regulates the body temperature. Cooling of the body occurs through the heat loss processes of evaporation of perspiration, and by radiation and conduction of heat from the body when the blood vessels of the skin are vasodilated. Body heat is conserved through lack of perspiration and vasoconstriction of the blood vessels.
3. It secretes **sebum**, an oily substance that (a) softens and lubricates the hair and skin, (b) prevents the hair from becoming brittle, and (c) decreases water loss from the skin when the external humidity is low. Because fat is a poor conductor of heat, sebum (d) lessens the amount of heat lost from the skin. Sebum also (e) has a **bactericidal** (bacteria-killing) action.
4. It transmits sensations through nerve receptors, which are sensitive to pain, temperature, touch and pressure.
5. It produces and absorbs vitamin D in conjunction with ultraviolet rays from the sun, which activate a vitamin D precursor present in the skin.

The normal skin of a healthy person has transient and resident micro-organisms that are not usually harmful.

Sudoriferous (sweat) glands are on all body surfaces except the lips and parts of the genitals. The body has from two to five million, which are all present at birth. They are most numerous on the palms of the hands and the soles of the feet. Sweat glands are classified as apocrine and eccrine. The **apocrine glands**, located largely in the axillae and anogenital areas, begin to function at puberty under the influence of androgens. Although they produce sweat almost constantly, apocrine glands are of little use in thermoregulation. The secretion of these glands is odourless, but when decomposed or acted on by bacteria on the skin, it takes on a musky, unpleasant odour. The **eccrine glands** are important physiologically. They are more numerous than the apocrine glands and are found chiefly on the palms of the hands, the soles of the feet and forehead. The sweat they produce cools the body through evaporation. Sweat is made up of water, sodium, potassium, chloride, glucose, urea and lactate.

Table 13-1 Factors Influencing Individual Hygienic Practices

Factor	Variables
Culture	Society places a high value on cleanliness. Many people bathe or shower once or twice a day, whereas people from some cultures will bathe once a week only. Some cultures consider privacy essential for bathing, whereas others practise communal bathing. Body odour is offensive in some cultures and accepted as normal in others.
Religion	Ceremonial washings are practised by some religions.
Environment	Finances may affect the availability of facilities for bathing. For example, homeless people may not have warm water available; soap, shampoo, shaving equipment and deodorants may be too expensive for people who have limited resources.
Developmental level	Children learn hygiene in the home. Practices vary according to the individual's age; for example, pre-schoolers can carry out most tasks independently with encouragement.
Health and energy	Ill people may not have the motivation or energy to attend to hygiene. Some patients who have neuromuscular impairments/illness may be unable to perform hygienic care.
Personal preferences	Some people prefer a shower to a bath.

NURSING MANAGEMENT

ASSESSING

Assessment of the patient's skin and hygienic practices is included within the majority of nursing care models. The assessment should usually include (a) a nursing health history to determine the patient's skin care practices, self-care abilities and past or current skin problems; (b) physical assessment of the skin; and (c) identification of patients at risk for developing skin impairments.

Patient History

Data about the patient's skin care practices enable the nurse to incorporate the patient's needs and preferences as much as possible in the plan of care. Andrews and Boyle (2003) suggest that people in most Western cultures try to disguise natural body odours by bathing frequently and using deodorant, cologne or perfumes. Immigrants from other countries where water is scarce may bathe less often than people from countries where water is more accessible.

Assessment of the patient's self-care abilities determines the amount of nursing assistance and the type of bath (e.g. bed, immersion bath or shower) best suited for the patient.

Important considerations include the patient's balance (for bath and shower), ability to sit unsupported (in the bath or bed), activity tolerance, coordination, adequate muscle strength, appropriate joint range of motion, vision, and the patient's preferences. Cognition and motivation are also essential. Patients whose cognitive function is impaired or whose illness alters energy levels and motivation will usually need more assistance. It is important for the nurse to determine the patient's functional level and to maintain and promote as much independence as possible. This also enables the nurse to identify the individual's potential for growth and rehabilitation. There are several models of functional levels of self-care.

The presence of past or current skin problems alerts the nurse to specific nursing interventions or referrals the patient may require. Many skin care conditions have implications for hygienic care. The patient may provide descriptions of these problems during the nursing assessment, or the nurse may observe some during the physical examination that follows. Common skin problems and implications for nursing interventions are shown in Table 13-2. Questions to elicit information about the patient's skin care practices, self-care abilities and skin problems are shown in the *Assessment questions*.

Table 13-2 Common Skin Problems

Problem and appearance	Nursing implications
Abrasion Superficial layers of the skin are scraped or rubbed away. Area is reddened and may have localised bleeding or serous weeping.	1. Prone to infection; therefore, wound should be kept clean and dry. 2. Do not wear rings or jewellery when providing care to avoid causing abrasions to patients. 3. Use appropriate moving and handling techniques.
Excessive dryness Skin can appear flaky and rough.	1. Prone to infection if the skin cracks; therefore, provide alcohol-free lotions to moisturise the skin and prevent cracking. 2. Use no soap, or use nonirritating soap and limit its use. Rinse skin thoroughly because soap can be irritating and drying. 3. Encourage increased fluid intake if health permits to prevent dehydration.
Ammonia dermatitis (nappy rash) Caused by skin bacteria reacting with urea in the urine. The skin becomes reddened and is sore.	1. Keep skin dry and clean by applying protective ointments containing zinc oxide to areas at risk (e.g. buttocks and perineum). 2. If reusable nappy in use boil the infant's nappy or wash them with an antibacterial detergent to prevent infection. Rinse nappy well because detergent is irritating to an infant's skin.
Acne Inflammatory condition with papules and pustules.	1. Keep the skin clean to prevent secondary infection. 2. Treatment varies widely.
Erythema Redness associated with a variety of conditions, such as rashes, exposure to sun, elevated body temperature.	1. Wash area carefully to remove excess micro-organisms. 2. Apply antiseptic spray or lotion to prevent itching, promote healing and prevent skin breakdown.
Hirsutism Excessive hair on a person's body and face, particularly in women.	1. Remove unwanted hair by using depilatories, shaving, electrolysis or tweezing. 2. Enhance patient's self-concept.

ASSESSMENT QUESTIONS THAT MAY BE USED

Skin Hygiene

Skin Care Practices
+ What are your usual showering or bathing times?
+ What hygienic products do you routinely use (e.g. bath oils, powder, facial cleansing creams, body lotions or creams, deodorants, antiperspirants)?
+ What facial cosmetic products do you use?
+ How and when do you clean makeup applicators? (Applicators should be kept clean, and products used around the eyes in particular should be discarded after four months to prevent bacterial and fungal infections.)
+ What hygienic or cosmetic products do you not use because of the skin problems they create (e.g. skin dryness or allergic reactions)?

Self-care Abilities
+ Do you have any problems managing your hygienic practices (e.g. baths and facial care)? If so, what are these?

+ How can the nurses best assist you?

Skin Problems
+ Do you have any tendency toward skin dryness, itchiness, rashes, bruising, excessive perspiration or lack of perspiration? Have you had skin or scalp lesions in the past?
+ Do you have any allergic tendencies? If so, what?

Positive responses to any of these require further exploration in terms of duration (When did it start?); frequency (How often have you had this?); description of lesion or rash; any associated signs, such as fever or nausea; aggravating factors (e.g. season of the year, stress, occupation, medication, recent travel, housing, personal contact); alleviating factors (e.g. medications, lotions, home remedies); and any family history of the problem.

BOX 13-1 Aetiologies of Self-care Deficits

+ Decreased or lack of motivation
+ Weakness or tiredness
+ Pain or discomfort
+ Perceptual or cognitive impairment
+ Inability to perceive body part or spatial relationship
+ Neuromuscular or musculoskeletal impairment
+ Medically imposed restriction
+ Therapeutic procedure restraining mobility (e.g. intravenous infusion, cast)
+ Severe anxiety
+ Environmental barriers

Physical Assessment

When assisting with bathing and other hygienic care, the nurse often has the opportunity to collect information about skin discoloration, uniformity of colour, texture, turgor, temperature, intactness and lesions.

Difficulties encountered by the patient in performing bathing activities include the inability to wash the body or body parts, to obtain or get to a water source, and to regulate water temperature or flow. Difficulties in dressing and grooming include inability to obtain, put on, take off, fasten or replace articles of clothing; and to maintain appearance at a satisfactory level. Toileting problems may involve difficulties getting to the toilet or commode or sitting on and rising from it. In addition, the patient may experience problems manipulating clothing for toileting, carrying out proper toilet hygiene, or flushing the toilet or emptying the commode. The reasons (aetiologies or related factors) for these problems are varied (see Box 13-1).

+ Deficient knowledge related to:
  • lack of experience with skin condition (acne) and need to prevent secondary infection;
  • new therapeutic regimen to manage skin problems;
  • lack of experience in providing hygiene care to dependent person;
  • unfamiliarity with devices available to facilitate sitting on or rising from toilet.
+ Situational low self-esteem related to:
  • visible skin problem (e.g. acne or alopecia);
  • body odour.

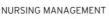

PLANNING

In planning care, the nurse and, if appropriate, the patient and/or family set outcomes for each problem identified. The nurse then performs nursing interventions and activities to achieve the patient outcomes.

The specific, detailed nursing activities taken by the nurse may include assisting dependent patient with bathing, skin care and perineal care; instructing patients/families about appropriate hygienic practices and alternative methods for dressing; and demonstrating use of assistive equipment and adaptive activities in conjunction with other members of the multidisciplinary team.

Planning to assist a patient with personal hygiene includes consideration of the patient's personal preferences, health and limitations; the best time to give the care; and the equipment, facilities and personnel available. A patient's personal preferences – about when and how to bathe, for example – should be followed as long as they are compatible with the their health and the equipment available. Nurses should provide whatever assistance the patient requires, either directly or by delegating this task to other nursing support personnel.

Planning for Home Care

To provide for continuity of care, it is important that the nurse assess the patient's and family's abilities for care and the need for referrals and home health services. In addition, the nurse needs to determine the patient's learning needs.

A home care assessment of the patient's normal home environment is usually performed by the Occupational Therapist.

IMPLEMENTING

The nurse applies the general guidelines for skin care while providing one of the various types of baths available to patients. *Procedure 13-1* on page 262 describes how to bathe an adult or paediatric patient.

General Guidelines for Skin Care

1. *An intact, healthy skin is the body's first line of defence.* Nurses need to ensure that all skin care measures prevent injury and irritation. Scratching the skin with jewellery or long, sharp fingernails must be avoided. Harsh rubbing or use of rough towels and washcloths can cause tissue damage, particularly when the skin is irritated or when circulation or sensation is diminished. Bottom bed sheets are kept taut and free from wrinkles to reduce friction and abrasion to the skin. Top bed linens are arranged to prevent undue pressure on the toes. When necessary, bed cradles on footboards are used to keep bedclothes off the feet.

2. *The degree to which the skin protects the underlying tissues from injury depends on the general health of the cells, the amount of subcutaneous tissue and the dryness of the skin.* Skin that is poorly nourished and dry is less easily protected and more vulnerable to injury. When the skin is dry, lotions or

---

COMMUNITY CARE CONSIDERATIONS

Hygiene

Patient and Environment

+ *Self-care abilities for hygiene:* Assess the patient's ability to bathe, to regulate water flow with taps, to dress and undress, to groom and to use the toilet.
+ *Self-care aids required:* Determine if there is a need for a bath/shower seat (see Figure 13-1, see overleaf), a hand shower, a nonskid surface or mat in the bath or shower, hand bars on the sides of the bath (see Figure 13-2, see overleaf), or a raised toilet seat.
+ *Facilities:* Check for the presence of laundry facilities and running water.
+ *Mechanical barriers:* Note furniture obstructing access to the bathroom and toilet, or a doorway too narrow for a wheelchair.

Family

+ *Caregiver availability, skills and responses:* Determine whether individuals are available and able to assist with bathing, dressing, toileting, nail care, hair shampoo, shopping for hygienic or grooming aids, and so on.

+ *Education needs:* Assess whether the caregiver needs instruction in how to assist the patient in and out of the bath, on and off the toilet, and so on.
+ *Family role changes and coping:* Assess effects of patient's illness on financial status, parenting, spousal roles, sexuality and social roles.

Community

+ Explore resources that will provide assistance with bathing, laundry and foot care (e.g. home healthcare, podiatrist).
+ Consult a social worker as needed to coordinate placement of a patient unable to remain in the home or to identify community resources that will help the patient stay in the home.
+ Consider assistance from the physiotherapist to assess, develop and improve the patient's motor function; (b) a community nurse to provide follow-up for care, teaching and support; and (c) an occupational therapist to assess and develop abilities to perform activities of daily living.

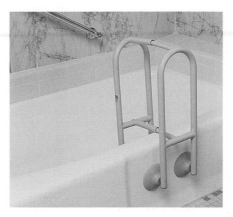

Figure 13-1 Shower seat in the home.

Figure 13-2 Hand bars on the sides of the bath.

creams with moisturising agents can be applied, and bathing is limited to once or twice a week because frequent bathing removes the natural oils of the skin and causes dryness.

3. *Moisture in contact with the skin for more than a short time can result in increased bacterial growth and irritation.* After a bath, the patient's skin is dried carefully. Particular attention is paid to areas such as the axillae, the groin, beneath the breasts and between the toes, where the potential for irritation is greatest. A non-irritating dusting powder, such as baby talcum, tends to reduce moisture and can be applied to these areas after they are dried. Patients who are incontinent of urine or faeces or who perspire excessively are provided with immediate skin care to prevent skin irritation.

4. *Body odours are caused by resident skin bacteria acting on body secretions.* Cleanliness is the best deodorant. Commercial deodorants and antiperspirants can be applied only after the skin is cleaned. Deodorants diminish odours, whereas antiperspirants reduce the amount of perspiration. Neither should be applied immediately after shaving, because of the possibility of skin irritation, nor are they used on skin that is already irritated.

5. *Skin sensitivity to irritation and injury varies among individuals and in accordance with their health.* Generally speaking, skin sensitivity is greater in infants, very young children and older people. A person's nutritional status also affects sensitivity. Emaciated or obese persons tend to experience more skin irritation and injury. The same tendency is seen in individuals with poor dietary habits and insufficient fluid intake. Even in healthy persons, skin sensitivity is highly variable. Some people's skin is sensitive to chemicals in skin care agents and cosmetics. Hypoallergenic cosmetics and soaps or soap substitutes are now available for these people. The nurse needs to ascertain whether the patient has any sensitivities and what agents are appropriate to use.

6. *Agents used for skin care have selective actions and purposes.* Commonly used agents are described in Table 13-3.

Table 13-3 Agents Commonly Used on the Skin

Agent	Action
Soap	Lowers surface tension and thus helps in cleaning. Some soaps contain antibacterial agents, which can change the natural flora of the skin.
Detergent	Used instead of soap for cleaning. Some people who are allergic to soaps may not be allergic to detergents, and vice versa.
Bath oil	Used in bathwater; provides an oily film on the skin that softens and prevents chapping. Oils can make the bath surface slippery, and patients should be instructed about safety measures (e.g. using nonskid bath surface or mat).
Skin cream, lotion	Provides a film on the skin that prevents evaporation and therefore chapping.
Powder	Can be used to absorb water and prevent friction. For example, powder under the breasts can prevent skin irritation. Some powders are antibacterial.
Deodorant	Masks or diminishes body odours.
Antiperspirant	Reduces the amount of perspiration.

NURSING MANAGEMENT

Bathing

Bathing removes accumulated oil, perspiration, dead skin cells and some bacteria. The nurse can appreciate the quantity of oil and dead skin cells produced when observing a person after the removal of a cast that has been on for six weeks. The skin is crusty, flaky and dry underneath the cast. Applications of oil over several days are usually necessary to remove the debris.

Excessive bathing, however, can interfere with the intended lubricating effect of the sebum, causing dryness of the skin. This is an important consideration, especially for older adults, who produce less sebum.

In addition to cleaning the skin, bathing also stimulates circulation. A warm or hot bath dilates superficial arterioles, bringing more blood and nourishment to the skin. Vigorous rubbing has the same effect. Rubbing with long smooth strokes from the distal to proximal parts of extremities (from the point farthest from the body to the point closest) is particularly effective in facilitating venous blood flow unless there is some underlying condition (e.g. blood clot) that would preclude this.

Bathing also produces a sense of well-being. It is refreshing and relaxing and frequently improves morale, appearance and self-respect. Some people take a morning shower for its refreshing, stimulating effect. Others prefer an evening bath because it is relaxing. These effects are more evident when a person is ill. For example, it is not uncommon for patients who have had a restless or sleepless night to feel relaxed, comfortable and sleepy after a morning bath.

Bathing offers an excellent opportunity for the nurse to assess all patients. The nurse can observe the condition of the patient's skin and physical conditions such as sacral oedema or rashes. While assisting a patient with a bath, the nurse can also assess the patient's psychosocial needs, such as orientation to time and ability to cope with the illness. Learning needs, such as a diabetic patient's need to learn foot care, can also be assessed.

Categories

Two categories of baths are given to patients: cleaning and therapeutic. **Cleaning baths** are given chiefly for hygiene purposes and include these types:

+ *Complete bed bath.* The nurse washes the entire body of a dependent patient in bed.
+ *Self-help bed bath.* Patients confined to bed are able to bathe themselves with help from the nurse for washing the back and perhaps the feet.
+ *Partial bath (abbreviated bath).* Only the parts of the patient's body that might cause discomfort or odour, if neglected, are washed: the face, hands, axillae, perineal area and back. Omitted are the arms, chest, abdomen, legs and feet. The nurse provides this care for dependent patients and assists self-sufficient patients confined to bed by washing their backs. Some ambulatory patients prefer to take a partial bath at the sink. The nurse can assist them by washing their backs.

+ *Immersion bath.* Immersion baths are often preferred to bed baths because it is easier to wash and rinse in a bath. Baths are also used for therapeutic interventions. The amount of assistance the nurse offers depends on the abilities of the patient. There are specially designed baths for dependent patients. These baths greatly reduce the work of the nurse in moving and handling patients in and out of the bath and offer greater benefits than a sponge bath in bed.

Sponge baths are suggested for the newborn because daily immersion baths are not considered necessary. After the bath, the infant should be immediately dried and wrapped to prevent heat loss. Parents need to be advised that the infant's ability to regulate body temperature has not yet fully developed. Infants perspire minimally, and shivering starts at a lower temperature than it does in adults; therefore, infants lose more heat before shivering begins. In addition, because the infant's body surface area is very large in relation to body mass, the body loses heat readily.

+ *Shower.* Many ambulatory patients are able to use shower facilities and require only minimal assistance from the

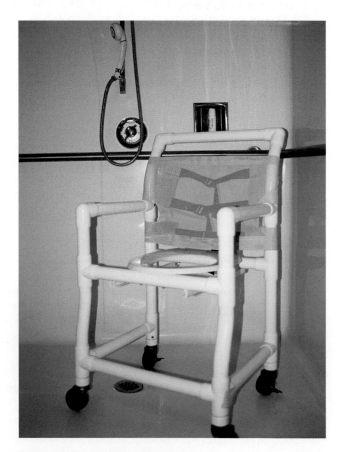

Figure 13-3 A shower chair.

nurse. Patients in long-term care settings are often given showers with the aid of a shower chair. The wheels on the shower chair allow patients to be transported from their room to the shower. The shower chair also has a commode seat to facilitate cleansing of the patient's perineal area during the shower process (see Figure 13-3).

The water for a bath should feel comfortably warm to the patient. People vary in their sensitivity to heat; generally, the temperature should be 32°C to 42°C. Most patients will verify a suitable temperature. Patients with decreased circulation or cognitive problems will not be able to verify the temperature. Therefore, the nurse must check the water

temperature to avoid patient injury with water that is too hot. The water for a bed bath should be changed when it becomes dirty or cold.

Therapeutic baths are given for physical effects, such as to soothe irritated skin or to treat an area (e.g. the perineum). Medications may be placed in the water. A therapeutic bath is generally taken in a bath one-third or one-half full. The patient remains in the bath for a designated time, often 20 to 30 minutes. If the patient's back, chest and arms are to be treated, these areas need to be immersed in the solution. The bath temperature is generally included as part of the prescription. *Procedure 13-1* provides guidelines for bathing patients.

CLINICAL ANECDOTE

Children are especially prone to accidental injury with hot water in baths so the nurse should always be alert. Sarah, a third-year student, describes seeing an injured child on a paediatric ward. 'David, an 18-month-old, had been admitted to the ward after he was put into a bath by his mother that was too hot. I will never forget seeing the burns on his legs and buttocks. His mother was so upset that she had hurt her precious baby. I will always

check the temperature of water even more so now before putting anyone into a bath. I always feel that if the water is too hot for my hand then it is too hot for the patient. I never want to see anyone accidentally injured, I cannot imagine how the mother felt.'

Sarah, a third-year student

PROCEDURE 13-1 Bathing an Adult or Paediatric Patient

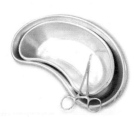

Purposes

+ To remove transient micro-organisms, body secretions and excretions, and dead skin cells
+ To stimulate circulation to the skin
+ To produce a sense of well-being
+ To promote relaxation and comfort
+ To prevent or eliminate unpleasant body odours

Assessment

Assess:

+ Condition of the skin (colour, texture and turgor, presence of pigmented spots, temperature, lesions, excoriations and abrasions)
+ Fatigue
+ Presence of pain and need for adjunctive measures (e.g. an analgesic) before the bath
+ Range of motion of the joints
+ Any other aspect of health that may affect the patient's bathing process (e.g. mobility, strength, cognition)
+ Need for use of clean gloves during the bath

Planning

Equipment

+ Basin or sink with warm water (check water temperature comfortable for patient requirements)
+ Soap and soap dish
+ Towels, washcloth, clean gown or pyjamas or clothes as needed, additional bed linen, if required
+ Gloves, if appropriate (e.g. presence of body fluids or open lesions)
+ Personal hygiene articles (e.g. deodorant, powder, lotions)
+ Shaving equipment for male patients
+ Table for bathing equipment
+ Laundry bag as required

Implementation

Preparation

Before bathing a patient, determine (a) the purpose and type of bath the patient needs; (b) self-care ability of the patient; (c) any movement or positioning precautions specific to the patient; (d) other care the patient may be receiving, such as physiotherapy or x-rays, in order to coordinate all aspects of healthcare and prevent unnecessary fatigue; (e) patient's comfort level with being bathed by someone else; and (f) necessary bath equipment and towels.

Caution is needed when bathing patients who are receiving intravenous therapy or have multiple connections to equipment. Easy-to-remove gowns that have Velcro or snap fasteners along the sleeves may be used. If a special gown is not available, the nurse needs to pay special attention when changing the patient's gown after the bath (or whenever the gown becomes soiled). General guidelines are provided in *Box 13-2* on page 267. These guidelines do not apply if the patient has an Intravenous infusion pump or controller. In this situation, either use a special gown or do not put the sleeve of a gown over the patient's involved arm.

Performance

1. Explain to the patient what you are going to do, why it is necessary and how he or she can cooperate. Discuss with the patient the plan for bathing and explain any unfamiliar procedures to the patient.
2. Wash hands and observe other appropriate infection control procedures.
3. Provide for patient privacy by drawing the curtains around the bed or closing the door to the room.
4. Prepare the patient and the environment.
   - Invite a family member or significant other to participate if desired.
   - Close windows and doors to ensure the room is a comfortable temperature. *Air currents increase loss of heat from the body by convection.*
   - Offer the patient a bedpan or urinal or ask whether the patient wishes to use the toilet or commode. *Warm water and activity can stimulate*

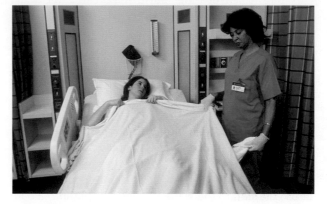

Figure 13-4 Remove top sheet from under the bath towel.

the need to void. The patient will be more comfortable after voiding, and voiding before cleaning the perineum is advisable.

   - Encourage the patient to perform as much personal self-care as possible. *This promotes independence, exercise and self-esteem.*
   - During the bath, assess each area of the skin carefully.

For a bed bath

5. Prepare the bed and position the patient appropriately.
   - Position the bed at a comfortable working height. Lower the side rail on the side close to you. Keep the other side rail up *(if in use)*. Assist the patient to move near you. *This avoids undue reaching and straining and promotes good body mechanics.*
   - Place a towel over the top sheet. Remove the top sheet from under the towel by starting at patient's shoulders and moving linen down toward the patient's feet (Figure 13-4). Ask the patient to grasp and hold the top of the bath towel while pulling linen to the foot of the bed. *The towel provides comfort, warmth and privacy.* *Note*: If the bed linen is to be reused, place it over the bedside chair. If it is to be changed, place it in the linen skip.
   - Remove patient's gown/clothing while keeping the patient covered with the towel.

6. Make a bath mitt with the washcloth. *A bath mitt retains water and heat better than a cloth loosely held and prevents ends of washcloth from dragging across the skin.* See Figure 13-5 for the triangular method and Figure 13-6 for the rectangular method.

7. Wash the face. *Begin the bath at the cleanest area and work downward toward the feet.*
   • Place towel under patient's head.
   • Wash the patient's eyes with water only and dry them well. Use a separate corner of the washcloth for each eye. *Using separate corners prevents transmitting micro-organisms from one eye to the other. Wipe from the inner to the outer canthus (Figure 13-7). This prevents secretions from entering the nasolacrimal ducts.*
   • Ask whether the patient wants soap used on the face. *Soap has a drying effect, and the face, which is exposed to the air more than other body parts, tends to be drier.*
   • Wash, rinse and dry the patient's face, ears and neck.
   • Remove the towel from under the patient's head.

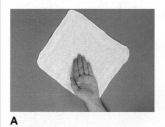 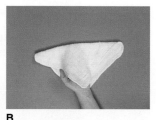 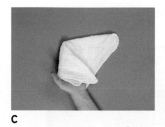 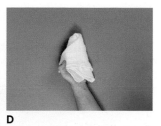

A   B   C   D

Figure 13-5 Making a bath mitt, triangular method. (A) Lay your hand on the washcloth; (B) fold the top corner over your hand; (C) fold the side corners over your hand; (D) tuck the second corner under the cloth on the palm side to secure the mitt.

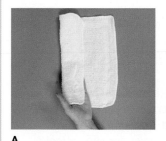 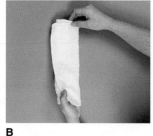 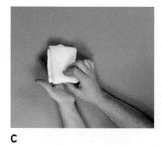

A   B   C

Figure 13-6 Making a bath mitt, rectangular method. (A) Lay your hand on the washcloth and fold one side over your hand; (B) fold the second side over your hand; (C) fold the top of the cloth down and tuck it under the folded side against your palm to secure the mitt.

8. Wash the arms and hands. (Omit the arms for a partial bath.)
   • Place a towel lengthwise under the arm away from you. *It protects the bed from becoming wet.*
   • Wash, rinse and dry the arm by elevating the patient's arm and supporting the patient's wrist and elbow (Figure 13-8). Use long, firm strokes from wrist to shoulder, including the axillary area. *Firm strokes from distal to proximal areas promote circulation by increasing venous blood return.*
   • Apply deodorant or powder if desired.
   • (Optional) Place a towel on the bed and put a washbasin on it. Place the patient's hands in the basin. *Many patients enjoy immersing their hands in the basin and washing themselves. Soaking loosens dirt under the nails.* Assist the patient as needed to wash, rinse and dry the hands, paying particular attention to the spaces between the fingers.
   • Repeat for hand and arm nearest you. Exercise caution if an intravenous infusion is present, and check its flow after moving the arm.

9. Wash the chest and abdomen. (Omit the chest and abdomen for a partial bath. However, the areas under a woman's breast may require bathing if this area is irritated or if the patient has significant perspiration under the breast.)

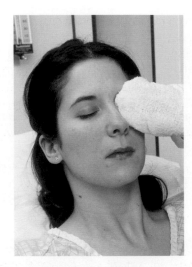

Figure 13-7 Using a separate corner of the washcloth for each eye, wipe from the inner to the outer canthus.

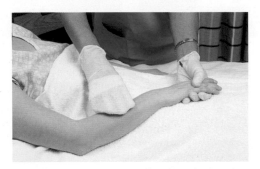

Figure 13-8 Washing the far arm using long, firm strokes from wrist to shoulder area.

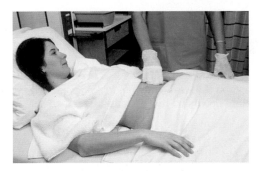

Figure 13-9 Washing the chest and abdomen.

- Place bath towel lengthwise over chest. Fold bath blanket down to the patient's pubic area. *Keeps the patient warm while preventing unnecessary exposure of the chest.*
- Lift the bath towel off the chest, and bathe the chest and abdomen with your mitted hand using long, firm strokes (Figure 13-9). Give special attention to the skin under the breasts and any other skin folds particularly if the patient is overweight. Rinse and dry well.
- Replace the towel when the areas have been dried.

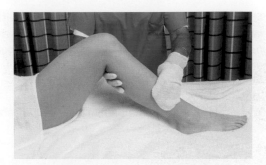

Figure 13-10 Washing far leg.

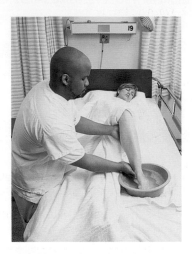

Figure 13-11 Soaking a foot in a basin.

10. Wash the legs and feet. (Omit legs and feet for a partial bath.)
    - Expose the leg farthest from you by folding the towel toward the other leg being careful to keep the perineum covered. *Covering the perineum promotes privacy and maintains the patient's dignity.*
    - Lift leg and place the bath towel lengthwise under the leg. Wash, rinse and dry the leg using long, smooth, firm strokes from the ankle to the knee to the thigh (Figure 13-10). *Washing from the distal to proximal areas promotes circulation by stimulating venous blood flow.*
    - Reverse the coverings and repeat for the other leg.
    - Wash the feet by placing them in the basin of water (Figure 13-11).
    - Dry each foot. Pay particular attention to the spaces between the toes. If you prefer, wash one foot after that leg before washing the other leg.
    - Obtain fresh, warm bathwater now or when necessary. *Water may become dirty or cold. Because surface skin cells are removed with washing, the bathwater from dark-skinned patients may be dark, however, this does not*

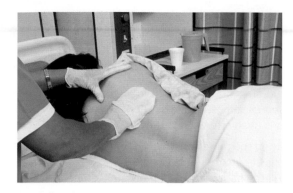

Figure 13-12 Washing the back.

mean the patient is dirty. Raise side rails when refilling basin. *This ensures the safety of the patient.*

11. Wash the back and then the perineum.
    - Assist the patient into a prone or side-lying position facing away from you. Place the bath towel lengthwise alongside the back and buttocks while keeping the patient covered with the towel as much as possible. *This provides warmth and undue exposure.*
    - Wash and dry the patient's back, moving from the shoulders to the buttocks, and upper thighs, paying attention to the gluteal folds (Figure 13-12).
    - Assist the patient to the supine position and determine whether the patient can wash the perineal area independently. If the patient cannot do so, cover the patient as shown in *Procedure 13-2* on page 269 and wash the area.

12. Assist the patient with grooming aids such as powder, lotion or deodorant.
    - Use powder sparingly. Release as little as possible into the atmosphere. *This will avoid irritation of the respiratory tract by powder inhalation. Excessive powder can cause caking, which leads to skin irritation.*
    - Help the patient put on fresh clothing.
    - Assist the patient to care for hair, mouth and nails. Some people prefer or need mouth care prior to their bath.

For an immersion bath or shower

13. Prepare the patient and the bath.
    - Fill the bath about one-third to one-half full of water, put cold water in before hot. *Sufficient water is needed to cover the perineal area.*
    - Cover all intravenous catheters or wound dressings with plastic coverings, and instruct the patient to prevent wetting these areas if possible.
    - Put a rubber bath mat or towel on the floor of the tub if safety strips are not on the tub floor. *These prevent slippage of the patient during the bath or shower.*

14. Assist the patient into the shower or tub.
    - Assist the patient taking a standing shower with the initial adjustment of the water temperature and water flow pressure, as needed. Some patients need a chair to sit on in the shower because of weakness. Hot water can cause elderly people to feel faint.
    - If the patient requires considerable assistance with an immersion bath, a hydraulic chair may be required (see Variation below).
    - Explain how the patient can signal for help, leave the patient for 2–5 minutes. For safety reasons, do not leave a patient with decreased cognition or patients who may be at risk (e.g. history of seizures, syncope).

15. Assist the patient with washing and getting out of the bath.
    - Wash the patient's back, lower legs and feet, if necessary.
    - Assist the patient out of the bath. If the patient is unsteady, place a bath towel over the patient's shoulders and drain the water before the patient attempts to get out of it. *Draining the water first lessens the likelihood of a fall. The towel prevents chilling.*

16. Dry the patient, and assist with follow-up care.
    - Follow step 12.
    - Assist the patient back to his or her room.
    - Clean the bath or shower in accordance with local policy, discard the used linen in the laundry skip.

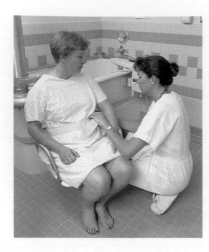

Figure 13-13 Secure the seat belt before moving the patient in a hydraulic bath chair.

17. Document:
  - Type of bath given (i.e. complete, partial, or self-help).
  - Skin assessment, such as excoriation, erythema, exudates, rashes, drainage or skin breakdown.
  - Nursing interventions related to skin integrity.
  - Ability of the patient to assist or cooperate with bathing.
  - Patient response to bathing.

- Educational needs regarding hygiene.
- Information or teaching shared with the patient or their family.

Variation: bathing using a hydraulic bath chair

A hydraulic lift, often used in long-term care or rehabilitation settings, can facilitate the transfer of a patient who is unable to walk to the bath.

✚ Bring the patient to the bathroom in a wheelchair or shower chair.
✚ Fill the bath and check the water temperature with a bath thermometer *to avoid thermal injury to the patient.*
✚ Lower the hydraulic chair lift to its lowest point, outside the bath.
✚ Transfer the patient to the chair lift and secure the seat belt (Figure 13-13).
✚ Raise the chair lift above the bath.
✚ Support the patient's legs as the chair is moved over the bath *to avoid injury to the legs.*
✚ Position the patient's legs down into the water and slowly lower the chair lift into the bath.
✚ Assist in bathing the patient, if appropriate.
✚ Reverse the procedure when taking the patient out of the bath.
✚ Dry the patient and transport them back to their room.

Evaluation

✚ Note the patient's tolerance of the procedure (e.g. respiratory rate and effort, pulse rate, behaviours, statements regarding comfort).
✚ Conduct appropriate follow up, such as:
  - Condition and integrity of skin (dryness, turgor, redness, lesions, and so on);

  - Patient strength;
  - Percentage of bath done without assistance.
✚ Relate to prior assessment data, if available.

BOX 13-2 Changing a Hospital Gown for a Patient with an intravenous Infusion

✚ Slip the gown completely off the arm without the infusion and onto the tubing connected to the arm with the infusion.
✚ Holding the container above the patient's arm, slide the sleeve up over the container to remove the used gown.
✚ Place the clean gown sleeve for the arm with the infusion over the container as if it were an extension of the patient's arm, from the inside of the gown to the sleeve cuff.

✚ Rehang the container. Slide the gown carefully over the tubing toward the patient's hand.
✚ Guide the patient's arm and tubing into the sleeve, taking care not to pull on the tubing.
✚ Assist the patient to put the other arm into the second sleeve of the gown and fasten as usual.
✚ Check the rate of flow of the infusion to make sure it is correct before leaving the bedside.

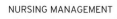

LIFESPAN CONSIDERATIONS

Bathing

Infants

+ Sponge baths are suggested for the newborn because daily immersion baths are not considered necessary. After the bath, the infant should be immediately dried and wrapped. Parents need to be advised that the infant's ability to regulate body temperature has not yet fully developed and newborns' bodies lose heat readily.

Children

+ Encourage a child's participation appropriate for developmental level.
+ Closely supervise children in the bath. Do not leave them unattended.

Adolescents

+ Assist adolescents if they need help to choose deodorants and antiperspirants. Secretions from newly active sweat glands react with bacteria on the skin, causing a pungent odour.

Older Adults

+ Changes of ageing can decrease the protective function of the skin in older adults. These changes include fragile skin, less oil and moisture and a decrease in elasticity.
+ To minimise skin dryness in older adults, avoid excessive use of soap. The ideal time to moisturise the skin is immediately after bathing.
+ Avoid powder because it causes moisture loss and is a hazardous inhalant.
+ Protect older adults and children from injury related to hot water burns.

COMMUNITY CARE CONSIDERATIONS

Hygiene

Suggest that the patient or family do the following:

+ Consider purchasing a bath seat that fits in the bath or shower.
+ Install a hand shower for use with a bath seat and shampooing.
+ Use a nonskid surface on the bath or shower.

+ Install hand bars on both sides of the bath or shower to facilitate transfers in and out of the bath or shower.
+ Carefully monitor the temperature of the bathwater.
+ Apply lotion and oil *after* a bath, not during, because these solutions can make a bath surface slippery.

Long-Term Care Setting

From a historical perspective, the bath has always been a part of nursing care and considered a component of the 'art' of nursing. In today's nursing world, however, the bath is seen as 'basic' and often delegated to nonprofessionals (Hektor and Touhy, 1997).

In spite of the previously listed therapeutic values associated with bathing, the choice of bathing procedure often depends on the amount of time available to the nurse or support worker and the patient's self-care ability. Nursing authors (Brawley, 2002; Hektor and Touhy, 1997; Rader, Lavelle *et al.*, 1996; Skewes, 1997) challenge nurses to switch from a task-centred approach to an individualised and aesthetic approach to bathing, especially for the older person in a long-term care setting.

The bath routine (e.g. day, time and number/week) for patients in healthcare settings is often determined by local policy, such that the bath becomes routine and depersonalised versus therapeutic, satisfying and person focused. An individualised approach focusing on therapeutic and comforting outcomes of bathing is especially important for patients with dementia.

Providing personal hygiene to a patient with dementia is often an ongoing challenge. Being sensitive to the rhythm of their behaviour and looking for cues can often offset problems related to this. Patients with dementia, whether they are at home or in a healthcare facility, often have certain times of the day when they are more agitated – these are times to avoid doing things that will increase their fear and agitation. It is sometimes helpful to wait awhile (e.g. half an hour or so) and then try giving the bath because they may forget that they were protesting and be willing to participate.

NURSING MANAGEMENT

Perineal-Genital Care

Perineal-genital care is also referred to as *perineal care* or *peri-care*. Perineal care as part of the bed bath is embarrassing for many patients. Nurses also may find it embarrassing initially, particularly with patients of the opposite sex. Most patients who require a bed bath from the nurse are able to clean their own genital areas with minimal assistance. The nurse may need to hand a moistened washcloth and soap to the patient, rinse the washcloth and provide a towel.

Because some patients are unfamiliar with terminology for the genitals and perineum, it may be difficult for nurses to explain what is expected. Most patients, however, understand what is meant if the nurse simply says, 'I'll give you a washcloth to finish your bath.' Older patients may be familiar with the term *private parts*. Whatever expression the nurse uses, it needs to be one that the patient understands and one that the nurse finds comfortable to use.

The nurse needs to provide perineal care efficiently and matter-of-factly. Nurses should wear gloves while providing this care for the comfort of the patient and to protect themselves from infection. *Procedure 13-2* explains how to provide perineal-genital care.

> ### CLINICAL ALERT
>
> *Always wash or wipe from 'clean to dirty'. For a female, cleanse perineal area from front to back. For a male, cleanse the urinary meatus by moving in a circular motion from centre of urethral opening around the glans.*

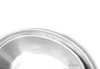
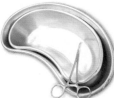

PROCEDURE 13-2 Providing Perineal-Genital Care

Purposes

+ To remove normal perineal secretions and odours
+ To promote patient comfort

Assessment

Assess for the presence of:

+ Irritation, excoriation, inflammation, swelling
+ Excessive discharge
+ Odour; pain or discomfort
+ Urinary or faecal incontinence

+ Recent rectal or perineal surgery
+ Indwelling catheter

Determine:

+ Perineal-genital hygiene practices
+ Self-care abilities

Planning

Equipment

Perineal-genital care provided in conjunction with the bed bath:

+ Bath towel
+ Clean gloves
+ Wash bowl with warm water
+ Soap
+ Washcloth

Special perineal-genital care:

+ Bath towel
+ Clean gloves
+ Gauze swabs
+ Solution bottle, or container filled with warm water or a prescribed solution
+ Bedpan to receive rinse water
+ Moisture-resistant bag or receptacle for used swabs
+ Perineal/incontinence pad

Implementation

Preparation

+ Determine whether the patient is experiencing any discomfort in the perineal-genital area.

+ Obtain and prepare the necessary equipment and supplies.

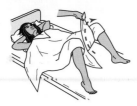

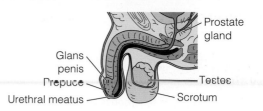

Figure 13-14 Draping the patient for perineal-genital care.

Figure 13-16 Male genitals.

Performance

1. Explain to the patient what you are going to do, why it is necessary and how they can cooperate, being particularly sensitive to any embarrassment felt by the patient.
2. Wash hands and observe other appropriate infection control procedures (e.g. clean gloves).
3. Provide for patient privacy by drawing the curtains around the bed or closing the door to the room.
4. Prepare the patient:
   - Fold the top bed linen to the foot of the bed and fold the gown up to expose the genital area.
   - Place a towel under the patient's hips. *The towel prevents the bed from becoming soiled.*
5. Position and drape the patient and clean the upper inner thighs.

   ### For females
   - Position the female in a back-lying position with the knees flexed and spread well apart.
   - Cover her body and legs with the towel. Drape the legs by tucking the bottom corners of the towel under the inner sides of the legs (Figure 13-14). *Minimum exposure lessens embarrassment and helps to provide warmth.* Bring the middle portion of the base of the blanket up over the pubic area.
   - Put on gloves, wash and dry the upper inner thighs.

   ### For males
   - Position the male patient in a supine position with knees slightly flexed and hips slightly externally rotated.
   - Put on gloves, wash and dry the upper inner thighs.
6. Inspect the perineal area.
   - Note particular areas of inflammation, excoriation or swelling, especially between the labia in females and the scrotal folds in males.
   - Also note excessive discharge or secretions from the orifices and the presence of odours.
   - Wash and dry the perineal-genital area.

   ### For females
   - Clean the labia majora. Then spread the labia to wash the folds between the labia majora and the labia minora (Figure 13-15). *Secretions that tend*

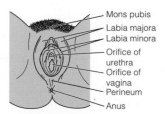

Figure 13-15 Female genitals.

to collect around the labia minora facilitate bacterial growth.
- Use separate quarters of the washcloth for each stroke, and wipe from the pubis to the rectum. For menstruating women and patients with indwelling catheters, use clean wipes, or gauze. Take a clean wipe/gauze for each stroke. *Using separate quarters of the washcloth or new gauzes prevents the transmission of micro-organisms from one area to the other. Wipe from the area of least contamination (the pubis) to that of greatest (the rectum).*
- Rinse the area well. Dry the perineum thoroughly, paying particular attention to the folds between the labia. *Moisture supports the growth of many micro-organisms.*

For males
- Wash and dry the penis, using firm strokes. *Handling the penis firmly may prevent an erection.*
- If the patient is uncircumcised, retract the prepuce (foreskin) to expose the glans penis (the tip of the penis) for cleaning. Replace the foreskin after cleaning the glans penis (Figure 13-16). *Retracting the foreskin is necessary to remove the smegma that collects under the foreskin and facilitates bacterial growth. Replacing the foreskin prevents constriction of the penis, which may cause oedema.*
- Wash and dry the scrotum. The posterior folds of the scrotum may need to be cleaned when the buttocks are cleaned (see step 9). *The scrotum tends to be more soiled than the penis because of its proximity to the rectum; thus it is usually cleaned after the penis.*

8. Inspect perineal orifices for intactness.
   - Inspect particularly around the urethra in patients with indwelling catheters. *A catheter may cause excoriation around the urethra.*
9. Clean between the buttocks.
   - Assist the patient to turn onto the side facing away from you.
   - Pay particular attention to the anal area and posterior folds of the scrotum in males. Clean the anus with toilet tissue before washing it, if necessary.
   - Dry the area well.
   - For post child delivery or menstruating females, apply a perineal pad as needed from front to back. *This prevents contamination of the vagina and urethra from the anal area.*
10. Document any unusual findings such as redness, excoriation, skin breakdown, discharge or drainage and any localised areas of tenderness.

Evaluation

+ Relate current assessments to previous assessments.
+ Conduct appropriate follow-up such as prescribed ointment for excoriation.

Patient teaching: Patients often need information about dry skin, skin rashes and acne.

EVALUATING

Using data collected during care, the nurse judges whether desired outcomes have been achieved. If the outcomes are not achieved, the nurse explores reasons why. For example:

+ Did the nurse overestimate the patient's functional abilities (physical, mental, emotional) for self-care?
+ Were provided instructions not clear to the patient?

+ Were appropriate assistive devices or supplies not available to the patient?
+ Did the patient's condition change?
+ Were required analgesics provided before hygienic care?
+ What currently prescribed medications and therapies could affect the patient's abilities or tissue integrity?
+ Is the patient's fluid and food intake adequate or appropriate to maintain skin and mucous membrane moisture and integrity?

TEACHING: PATIENT CARE

Skin Problems and Care

Dry Skin

+ Use cleansing creams to clean the skin rather than soap or detergent, which cause drying and, in some cases, allergic reactions.
+ Use bath oils, but take precautions to prevent falls caused by slippery bath surfaces.
+ Thoroughly rinse soap or detergent, if used, from the skin.
+ Bathe less frequently when environmental temperature and humidity are low.
+ Increase fluid intake.
+ Humidify the air with a humidifier or by keeping a tub or sink full of water.
+ Use moisturising or emollient creams that contain lanolin, petroleum jelly or cocoa butter to retain skin moisture.

Skin Rashes

+ Keep the area clean by washing it with a mild soap. Rinse the skin well, and pat it dry.
+ To relieve itching, try a tepid bath or soak. Some over-the-counter preparations, may help but should be used with full knowledge of the product.
+ Avoid scratching the rash to prevent inflammation, infection and further skin lesions.
+ Choose clothing carefully. Too much can cause perspiration and aggravate a rash.

Acne

+ Wash the face frequently with soap or detergent and hot water to remove oil and dirt.
+ Avoid using oily creams, which aggravate the condition.
+ Avoid using cosmetics that block the ducts of the sebaceous glands and the hair follicles.
+ Never squeeze or pick at the lesions. This increases the potential for infection and scarring.

FEET

The feet are essential for ambulation and merit attention even when people are confined to bed. Each foot contains 26 bones, 107 ligaments and 19 muscles. These structures function together for both standing and walking.

Developmental Variations

At birth, a baby's foot is relatively unformed. The arches are supported by fatty pads and do not take their full shape until five to six years of age. During childhood, the bones and small muscles of the feet are easily damaged by tight, binding stockings and ill-fitting shoes. For normal development, it is impor-

tant that the arches be supported and that the bony structure and the feet grow with no external restrictions. Feet are not fully grown until about age 20. Healthy feet remain relatively unchanged during life. However, the elderly often require special attention for their feet. For example, reduced blood supply and accompanying arteriosclerosis can make a foot prone to ulcers and infection following trauma.

> ### CLINICAL ALERT
>
> *Patients with diabetes are at high risk for lower extremity amputations (LEA). Routine foot assessment and patient education in proper foot care can significantly reduce the risk for LEA.*

NURSING MANAGEMENT

ASSESSING

Assessment of the patient's feet includes identifying patients at risk for foot problems.

Nursing Health History

The nurse determines the patient's history of (a) normal nail and foot care practices, (b) type of footwear worn, (c) self-care abilities, (d) presence of risk factors for foot problems, (e) any foot discomfort and (f) any perceived problems with foot mobility. To elicit such data, the nurse may ask the patient the questions provided in the *Assessment interview*.

Physical Assessment

Each foot and toe is inspected for shape, size and presence of lesions and is palpated to assess areas of tenderness, oedema and circulatory status. Normally, the toes are straight and flat. Table 13-4 lists physical assessment methods for the feet. Common foot problems include calluses, corns, unpleasant odours, plantar warts, fissures between the toes and fungal infections such as athlete's foot.

A **callus** is a thickened portion of epidermis, a mass of keratotic material. Most calluses are painless and flat and are found on the bottom or side of the foot over a bony prominence. Calluses are usually caused by pressure from shoes. They

ASSESSMENT INTERVIEW

Foot Hygiene

Foot Care Practices
+ How often do you wash your feet and cut your toenails?
+ What hygiene products do you usually use on your feet (e.g. soap, foot powder or deodorant, lotion or cream)?
+ What type of shoes and socks do you wear?
+ How often do you change your socks or put on clean socks?
+ Do you ever go barefoot? If so, when, where and how often?

Self-care Abilities
+ Do you have any problems managing your foot care? If so, what are these?
+ How can the nurses best help you?

Foot Problems and Risk Factors
+ Do you have any problems with foot odour?
+ Do you have any foot discomfort? If so, where? When does this occur? What do you do to relieve the discomfort? Does this discomfort affect how you walk?
+ Have you noticed any problems with foot mobility (e.g. joint stiffness)?
+ Do you have diabetes, any circulatory problems with feet (e.g. swelling, changes in skin colour, arthritis) or any instances of prolonged exposure to chemicals or water?

Table 13-4 Assessment of the Feet

Method	Normal findings	Deviations from normal
Inspect all skin surfaces, particularly between the toes, for cleanliness, odour, dryness, inflammation, swelling, abrasions or other lesions.	Intact skin Absence of swelling or inflammation	Excessive dryness Areas of inflammation or swelling (e.g. corns, calluses) Fissures Scaling and cracking of skin (e.g. athlete's foot) Plantar warts
Palpate anterior and posterior surfaces of ankles and feet for oedema.	No swelling	Swelling or pitting oedema
Palpate dorsalis pedis pulse on dorsal surface of foot.	Strong, regular pulses in both feet	Weak or absent pulses
Compare skin temperature of both feet.	Warm skin temperature	Cool skin temperature in one or both feet

can be softened by soaking the foot in warm water with Epsom salts, and abraded with pumice stones or similar abrasives. Creams will help to keep the skin soft and prevent the formation of calluses.

A **corn** is a keratosis caused by friction and pressure from a shoe. It commonly occurs on the fourth or fifth toe, usually on a bony prominence such as a joint. Corns are usually conical (circular and raised). The base is the surface of the corn and the apex is in deeper tissues, sometimes even attached to bone. Corns are generally removed surgically. They are prevented from reforming by relieving the pressure on the area (i.e. wearing comfortable shoes), and massaging the tissue to promote circulation. The use of oval corn pads should be avoided because they increase pressure and decrease circulation.

Unpleasant odours occur as a result of perspiration and its interaction with micro-organisms. Regular and frequent washing of the feet and wearing clean hosiery help to minimise odour. Foot powders and deodorants also help to prevent this problem.

Plantar warts appear on the sole of the foot. These warts are caused by the virus papovavirus hominis. They are moderately contagious. The warts are frequently painful and often make walking difficult. Curettage of the warts may be performed, freeze them with solid carbon dioxide several times, or apply salicylic acid.

Fissures, or deep grooves, frequently occur between the toes as a result of dryness and cracking of the skin. The treatment of choice is good foot hygiene and application of an antiseptic to prevent infection. Often a small piece of gauze is inserted between the toes in applying the antiseptic and left in place to assist healing by allowing air to reach the area.

> **CLINICAL ALERT**
>
> *Patients with diabetes often have extremely dry skin. Tell them to use a nonperfumed lotion and to avoid putting lotion between the toes. Advise them not to soak their feet in water because it is drying to the skin.*

Athlete's foot, or **tinea pedis** (ringworm of the foot), is caused by a fungus. The symptoms are scaling and cracking of the skin, particularly between the toes. Sometimes small blisters form, containing a thin fluid. In severe cases, the lesions may also appear on other parts of the body, particularly the hands. Treatments usually involve the application of commercial antifungal ointments or powders. Prevention is important. Common preventive measures are keeping the feet well ventilated, drying the feet well after bathing, wearing clean socks or stockings, and not going barefoot in public showers.

An **ingrown toe nail**, the growing inward of the nail into the soft tissues around it, most often results from improper nail trimming. Pressure applied to the area causes localised pain. Treatment involves frequent, hot antiseptic soaks and surgical removal of the portion of nail embedded in the skin. Preventing recurrence involves appropriate instruction and adherence to proper nail-trimming techniques.

Identifying Patients at Risk

Because of reduced peripheral circulation to the feet, patients with diabetes or peripheral vascular disease are particularly prone to infection if skin breakage occurs. Many foot problems can be prevented by teaching the patient simple foot care guidelines (see *Teaching: patient care*).

PLANNING

Planning involves (a) identifying nursing interventions that will help the patient maintain or restore healthy foot care practices and (b) establishing desired outcomes for each patient. Interventions may include teaching the patient about correct nail and foot care, proper footwear, wearing the correct size and ways to prevent potential foot problems (e.g. infection, injury and decreased circulation). For patients with self-care difficulties, the nurse plans a schedule for soaking the patient's feet and assisting with regular cleaning and trimming of nails (if not contraindicated). Foot and nail care is often provided during the patient's bath but may be provided at any time in the day to accommodate the patient's preference or schedule. The frequency of foot care is determined by the nurse and patient and is based on objective assessment data and the patient's specific problems. For some patients feet may need to be bathed daily; for those whose feet perspire excessively, bathing more than once a day may be necessary.

IMPLEMENTING

Procedure 13-3 describes how to provide foot care. See also the discussion of nails. During these procedures, the nurse has the opportunity to teach the patient appropriate methods for foot care, that is, methods designed to prevent tissue injury and infection (see *Teaching: patient care*).

EVALUATING

Examples of desired outcomes for foot hygiene include the patient being able to:

+ Participate in self-care (foot hygiene) to optimal level of capacity (specify)
+ Describe hygienic and other interventions (e.g. proper footwear) to maintain skin integrity, prevent infection and maintain peripheral tissue perfusion
+ Demonstrate optimal foot hygiene, as evidenced by
  (a) Intact, smooth, soft, hydrated and warm skin
  (b) Intact cuticles and skin surrounding nails
  (c) Correct foot care and nail care practices.

TEACHING: PATIENT CARE

Foot Care

+ Wash the feet daily, and dry them well, especially between the toes.
+ When washing, inspect the skin of the feet for breaks or red or swollen areas. Use a mirror if needed to visualise all areas.
+ To prevent burns, check the water temperature before immersing the feet.
+ Use creams or lotions to moisten the skin, or soak the feet in warm water with Epsom salts to avoid excessive drying of the skin of the feet. Lotion will also soften calluses. A lotion that reduces dryness effectively is a mixture of lanolin and mineral oil.
+ To prevent or control an unpleasant odour due to excessive foot perspiration, wash the feet frequently and change socks and shoes at least daily. Special deodorant sprays or absorbent foot powders are also helpful.
+ File the toenails rather than cutting them to avoid skin injury. File the nails straight across the ends of the toes. If the nails are too thick or misshapen to file, consult a podiatrist.
+ Wear clean stockings or socks daily. Avoid socks with holes or darns that can cause pressure areas.
+ Wear correctly fitting shoes that neither restrict the foot nor rub on any area; rubbing can cause corns and calluses. Check worn shoes for rough spots in the lining. Break in new shoes gradually by increasing the wearing time 30 to 60 minutes each day.
+ Avoid walking barefoot, because injury and infection may result. Wear slippers in public showers and in change areas to avoid contracting athlete's foot or other infections.
+ Several times each day exercise the feet to promote circulation. Point the feet upward, point them downward and move them in circles.
+ Avoid wearing constricting garments such as knee-high elastic stockings and avoid sitting with the legs crossed at the knees, which may decrease circulation.
+ When the feet are cold, use extra blankets and wear warm socks rather than using heating pads or hot water bottles, which may cause burns. Test bathwater before stepping into it.
+ Wash any cut on the foot thoroughly and apply a mild antiseptic.
+ Avoid self-treatment for corns or calluses. Pumice stones and some callus and corn applications are injurious to the skin. Consult a podiatrist first.
+ Notify the physician if you notice abnormal sores or drainage, pain or changes in temperature, colour and sensation of the foot.

PROCEDURE 13-3 Providing Foot Care

Purposes

+ To maintain the skin integrity of the feet
+ To prevent foot infections
+ To prevent foot odours
+ To assess or monitor foot problems

Assessment

Determine

+ History of any problems with foot odour, foot discomfort, foot mobility, circulatory problems (e.g. swelling, changes in skin colour and/or temperature, and pain), structural problems (e.g. bunion, hammer toe or overlapping digits)
+ Usual foot care practices (e.g. frequency of washing feet and cutting nails, foot hygiene products used, how often socks are changed, whether the patient ever goes barefoot, whether the patient sees a podiatrist)

Assess

+ Skin surfaces for cleanliness, odour, dryness and intactness
+ Each foot and toe for shape, size, presence of lesions (e.g. corn, callus, wart or rash), and areas of tenderness, ankle oedema
+ Skin temperatures of the two feet to assess circulatory status and the dorsalis pedis pulses
+ Self-care abilities (e.g. any problems managing foot care)

Planning

Equipment

+ Washbowl containing warm water
+ Pillow
+ Moisture-resistant disposable pad
+ Towels
+ Soap
+ Washcloth
+ Toenail cleaning and trimming equipment
+ Lotion or foot powder

Implementation

Performance

1. Explain to the patient what you are going to do, why it is necessary and how they can cooperate.
2. Wash hands and observe other appropriate infection control procedures.
3. Provide for patient privacy by drawing the curtains around the bed or closing the door to the room.
4. Prepare the equipment and the patient.
   - Fill the washbowl with warm water. *Warm water promotes circulation, comforts and refreshes.*
   - Assist the ambulatory patient to a sitting position in a chair, or the bed patient to a supine or semi-Fowler's position.
   - Place a pillow under the bed patient's knees. *This provides support and prevents muscle fatigue.*
   - Place the washbowl on the moisture-resistant pad at the foot of the bed for a bed patient or on the floor in front of the chair for an ambulatory patient.
   - For a bed patient, pad the rim of the washbowl with a towel. *The towel prevents undue pressure on the skin.*
5. Wash the foot and soak it.
   - Place one of the patient's feet in the bowl and wash it with soap, paying particular attention to the interdigital areas. Prolonged soaking is generally not recommended for diabetic patients or individuals with peripheral vascular disease. *Prolonged soaking may remove natural skin oils, thus drying the skin and making it more susceptible to cracking and injury.*
   - Rinse the foot well to remove soap. *Soap irritates the skin if not properly removed.*
   - Rub callused areas of the foot with the washcloth. *This helps remove dead skin layers.*
   - If the nails are brittle or thick and require trimming, replace the water and allow the foot to soak for 10-20 minutes. *Soaking softens the nails and loosens debris under them.*
   - Clean the nails as required. *This removes excess debris that harbours micro-organisms.*
   - Remove the foot from the basin and place it on the towel.
6. Dry the foot thoroughly and apply lotion or foot powder.
   - Blot the foot gently with the towel to dry it thoroughly, particularly between the toes. *Harsh rubbing can damage the skin. Thorough drying reduces the risk of infection.*
   - Apply lotion or cream. *This lubricates dry skin.* or
   - Apply a foot powder containing a non-irritating deodorant if the feet tend to perspire excessively. *Foot powders have greater absorbent properties than regular bath powders; some also contain menthol, which makes the feet feel cool.*
7. If local policy permits, trim the nails of the first foot while the second foot is soaking.
   - See the discussion on nails for the appropriate method to trim nails. Note that in many healthcare settings toenail trimming requires a chiropodist or is contraindicated for patients with diabetes mellitus, toe infections and peripheral vascular disease, unless performed by a podiatrist.
8. Document any foot problems observed.
   - Foot care is not generally recorded unless problems are noted.
   - Record any signs of inflammation, infection, breaks in the skin, corns, troublesome calluses, bunions and pressure areas. This is of particular importance for patients with peripheral vascular disease and diabetes.

Evaluation

+ Inspect nails and skin after the soak.
+ Compare to prior assessment data.

NAILS

Nails are normally present at birth. They continue to grow throughout life and change very little until people are elderly. At that time, the nails tend to be tougher, more brittle and in some cases thicker. The nails of an older person normally grow less quickly than those of a younger person and may be ridged and grooved.

NURSING MANAGEMENT

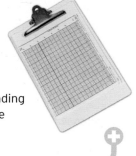

ASSESSING

During the nursing assessment, the nurse explores the patient's usual nail care practices, self-care abilities and any problems associated with them (see the *Assessment interview* box below). Physical assessment involves inspection of the nails (e.g. nail shape and texture, nail bed colour and tissues surrounding the nails).

PLANNING

The nurse identifies measures that will assist the patient to develop or maintain healthy nail care practices. A schedule of nail care needs to be established.

IMPLEMENTING

To provide nail care, the nurse needs a nail cutter or sharp scissors, a nail file, hand lotion or mineral oil to lubricate any dry tissue around the nails, and a bowl of water to soak the nails if they are particularly thick or hard.

One hand or foot is soaked, if needed, and dried; then the nail is cut or filed straight across beyond the end of the finger or toe. Avoid trimming or digging into nails at the lateral corners. This predisposes the patient to ingrown toenails. Patients who have diabetes or circulatory problems should have their nails filed rather than cut; inadvertent injury to tissues can occur if scissors are used. After the initial cut or filing, the nail is filed to round the corners, and the nurse cleans under the nail. The nurse then gently pushes back the cuticle, taking care not to injure it. The next finger or toe is cared for in the same manner. Any abnormalities, such as an infected cuticle or inflammation of the tissue around the nail, are recorded and reported.

EVALUATING

Examples of desired outcomes for nail hygiene include the patient being able to:

+ Demonstrate healthy nail care practices, as shown by:
  (a) Clean, short nails with smooth edges
  (b) Intact cuticles and hydrated surrounding skin
+ Describe factors contributing to the nail problem.
+ Describe preventive interventions for the specific nail problem.
+ Demonstrate nail care as instructed.

In addition, the patient should have pink nail beds and quick return of nail bed colour after capillary refill test.

ASSESSMENT INTERVIEW

Nail Hygiene

+ What are your usual nail care practices?
+ Do you have any problems managing your nail care? If so, what are these?
+ Have you had any problems associated with your nails (e.g. inflammation of the tissue surrounding the nail, injury, prolonged exposure to water or chemicals, circulatory problems)?

MOUTH

Each tooth has three parts: the crown, the root and the pulp cavity (see Figure 13-17). The crown is the exposed part of the tooth, which is outside the gum. It is covered with a hard substance called enamel. The ivory-coloured internal part of the crown below the enamel is the dentin. The root of a tooth is embedded in the jaw and covered by a bony tissue called cementum. The pulp cavity in the centre of the tooth contains the blood vessels and nerves.

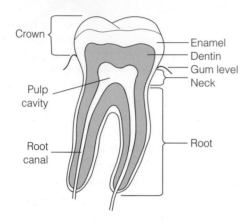

Figure 13-17 The anatomic parts of a tooth.

Developmental Variations

Teeth usually appear five to eight months after birth. Baby-bottle syndrome may result in decay of all of the upper teeth and the lower posterior teeth (Pillitteri, 2003: 824). This syndrome occurs when an infant is put to bed with a bottle of sugar water, formula, milk or fruit juice. The carbohydrates in the solutions causes demineralisation of the tooth enamel, which leads to tooth decay.

By the time children are two years old, they usually have all 20 of their temporary deciduous teeth (see Figure 13-18). At about age six or seven, children start losing their deciduous teeth, and these are gradually replaced by the 32 permanent teeth (see Figure 13-19). By age 25, most people have all of their permanent teeth.

The incidence of periodontal disease increases during pregnancy because the rise in female hormones affects gingival tissue and increases its reaction to bacterial plaque. Many pregnant women experience more bleeding from the gingival sulcus during brushing and increased redness and swelling of the **gingiva** (the gum).

Some older adults may have few permanent teeth left, and some have dentures. Loss of teeth occurs mainly because of **periodontal disease** (gum disease) rather than **dental caries** (cavities); however, caries are also common in middle-aged adults.

Some receding of the gums and a brownish pigmentation of the gums occur with age. Because saliva production decreases with age, dryness of the oral mucosa is a common finding in older people.

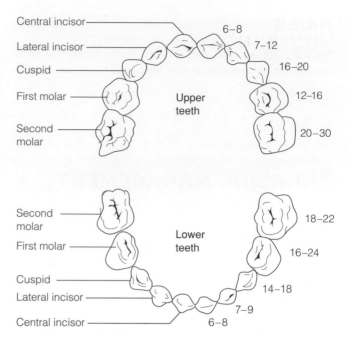

Figure 13-18 Temporary teeth and their times of eruption (stated in months).

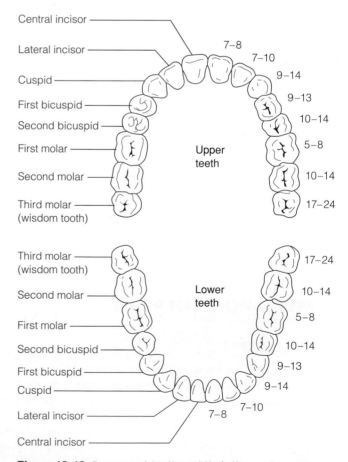

Figure 13-19 Permanent teeth and their times of eruption (stated in years).

NURSING MANAGEMENT

ASSESSING

Assessment of the patient's mouth and hygiene practices includes (a) a nursing health history, (b) physical assessment of the mouth and (c) identification of patients at risk for developing oral problems.

Nursing Health History

During the nursing health history, the nurse obtains data about the patient's oral hygiene practices, including dental visits, self-care abilities and past or current mouth problems. Data about the patient's oral hygiene help the nurse determine learning needs and incorporate the patient's needs and preferences in the plan of care. Assessment of the patient's self-care abilities determines the amount and type of nursing assistance to provide. Patients whose hand coordination is impaired, whose cognitive function is impaired, whose illness alters energy levels and motivation, or whose therapy imposes restrictions on activities will need assistance from the nurse. Information about past or current problems alerts the nurse to specific interventions required or referrals that may be necessary. Questions to elicit this information are shown in the *Assessment interview* on page 278.

Physical Assessment

Dental caries (cavities) and periodontal disease are the two problems that most frequently affect the teeth. Both problems are commonly associated with plaque and tartar deposits. **Plaque** is an *invisible* soft film that adheres to the enamel surface of teeth; it consists of bacteria, molecules of saliva and remnants of epithelial cells and leukocytes. When plaque is unchecked, tartar (dental calculus) is formed. **Tartar** is a visible, hard deposit of plaque and dead bacteria that forms at the gum lines. Tartar buildup can alter the fibres that attach the teeth to the gum and eventually disrupt bone tissue. Periodontal disease is characterised by **gingivitis** (red, swollen gingiva), bleeding, receding gum lines and the formation of pockets between the teeth and gums. In advanced periodontal disease (**pyorrhea**), the teeth are loose and pus is evident when the gums are pressed. Table 13-5 lists additional problems of the mouth.

Identifying Patients at Risk

Certain patients are prone to oral problems because of lack of knowledge or the inability to maintain oral hygiene. Among these are seriously ill, confused, comatose, depressed and dehydrated patients. In addition, people with nasogastric tubes or receiving oxygen are likely to develop dry oral mucous membranes, especially if they breathe through their mouths. Patients who have had oral or jaw surgery must have meticulous oral hygiene care to prevent the development of infections.

Healthy-appearing individuals, too, may be at risk. High-risk variables such as inadequate nutrition, lack of money for dental care, excessive intake of refined sugars and family

Table 13-5 Common Problems of the Mouth

Problem	Description	Nursing implications
Halitosis	Bad breath	Teach or provide regular oral hygiene.
Glossitis	Inflammation of the tongue	As above
Gingivitis	Inflammation of the gums	As above
Periodontal disease	Gums appear spongy and bleeding	As above
Reddened or excoriated mucosa		Check for ill-fitting dentures.
Excessive dryness of the buccal mucosa		Increase fluid intake as health permits.
Cheilosis	Cracking of lips	Lubricate lips, use antimicrobial ointment to prevent infection as prescribed.
Dental caries	Teeth have darkened areas, may be painful	Advise patient to see a dentist.
Sordes	Accumulation of foul matter (food, micro-organisms and epithelial elements) in the mouth	Teach or provide regular cleaning.
Stomatitis	Inflammation of the oral mucosa	Teach or provide regular cleaning.
Parotitis	Inflammation of the parotid salivary glands	Teach or provide regular oral hygiene.

ASSESSMENT INTERVIEW

Oral Hygiene

Oral Hygiene Practices

+ What are your usual mouth care and/or denture care practices?
+ What oral hygiene products do you routinely use (e.g. mouthwash, type of toothpaste, dental floss, denture cleaner)?
+ When was your last dental examination, and how often do you see your dentist?

Self-care Abilities

+ Do you have any problems managing your mouth care?

Past or Current Mouth Problems

+ Have you had or do you have any problems such as bleeding, swollen or reddened gums, ulcerations, lumps or tooth pain?

---

history of periodontal disease also need to be identified. Some older people may also be at risk, for example, those who choose salty and enamel-eroding sugary foods because of a decline in their number of taste buds. The decreased saliva production in older adults, which produces a dry mouth and thinning of the oral mucosa, is another factor.

A dry mouth can be aggravated by poor fluid intake, heavy smoking, alcohol use, high salt intake, anxiety and many medications. Medications that can cause dryness of the mouth include diuretics; laxatives, if used excessively; and tranquillisers, such as chlorpromazine and diazepam. Some chemotherapeutic agents used to treat cancer also cause oral dryness and lesions. A common side-effect of the anticonvulsant drug phenytoin is gingival hyperplasia. Optimal oral hygiene (e.g. brushing with a soft toothbrush and flossing) is needed.

Patients who are receiving or have received radiation treatments to the head and neck may have permanent damage to salivary glands. This results in a very dry mouth and can often be treated by providing a thick liquid called *artificial saliva*. Some patients prefer to just sip on liquids to moisten their mouth. Radiation can also cause damage to teeth and jaw structure, with actual damage occurring years after the radiation.

PLANNING

In planning care, the nurse and, if appropriate, the patients and/or family set outcomes for identified problem or self-care deficit. The nurse then performs nursing interventions and activities to achieve the patient outcomes.

During the planning phase, the nurse also identifies interventions that will help the patient achieve these goals. Specific, detailed nursing activities taken by the nurse may include the following:

+ Monitor regularly for dryness of the oral mucosa.
+ Monitor for signs and symptoms of glossitis (inflammation of the tongue) and stomatitis (inflammation of the mouth).

+ Assist dependent patients with oral care.
+ Provide special oral hygiene for patients who are debilitated, unconscious or have lesions of the mucous membranes or other oral tissues.
+ Teach patients about good oral hygiene practices and other measures to prevent tooth decay.
+ Reinforce oral hygiene regimen as part of discharge teaching.

IMPLEMENTING

Good oral hygiene includes daily stimulation of the gums, mechanical brushing and flossing of the teeth, and flushing of the mouth. The nurse is often in a position to help people maintain oral hygiene by helping or teaching them to clean the teeth and oral cavity, by inspecting whether patients (especially children) have done so, or by actually providing mouth care to patients who are ill or incapacitated. The nurse can also be instrumental in identifying problems that require the intervention of a dentist or oral surgeon and arranging a referral.

Promoting Oral Health Through the Life Span

A major role of the nurse in promoting oral health is to teach patients about specific oral hygienic measures.

Infants and Toddlers

Most dentists recommend that dental hygiene should begin when the first tooth erupts and be practised after each feeding. Cleaning can be accomplished by using a wet washcloth or small gauze moistened with water.

Dental caries occur frequently during the toddler period, often as a result of the excessive intake of sweets or a prolonged use of the bottle during naps and at bedtime. The nurse should give parents the following instructions to promote and maintain dental health:

+ Beginning at about 18 months of age, brush the child's teeth with a soft toothbrush. Use only a toothbrush moistened with water at first and introduce toothpaste later. Use one that contains fluoride.

+ Schedule an initial dental visit for the child at about two or three years of age, as soon as all 20 primary teeth have erupted.

+ Some dentists recommend an inspection type of visit when the child is about 18 months old to provide an early pleasant introduction to the dental examination.

+ Seek professional dental attention for any problems such as discolouring of the teeth, chipping, or signs of infection such as redness and swelling.

Pre-school and School-age Children

Because deciduous teeth guide the entrance of permanent teeth, dental care is essential to keep these teeth in good repair. Abnormally placed or lost deciduous teeth can cause misalignment of permanent teeth. Fluoride remains important at this stage to prevent dental caries. Pre-schoolers need to be taught to brush their teeth after eating and to limit their intake of refined sugars. Parental supervision may be needed to ensure the completion of these self-care activities. Regular dental checkups are required during these years when permanent teeth appear.

Adolescents and Adults

Proper diet and tooth and mouth care should be evaluated and reinforced to adolescents and adults. Specific measures to prevent tooth decay and periodontal disease are listed in *Procedure 13-4* on page 280.

Brushing and Flossing the Teeth

Thorough brushing of the teeth is important in preventing tooth decay. The mechanical action of brushing removes food particles that can harbour and incubate bacteria. It also stimulates circulation in the gums, thus maintaining their healthy firmness. One of the techniques recommended for brushing teeth is called the sulcular technique, which removes plaque and cleans under the gingival margins. Many toothpastes are marketed. Fluoride toothpaste is often recommended because of its antibacterial protection.

Caring for Artificial Dentures

Some people have artificial teeth in the form of a plate – a complete set of teeth for one jaw. A person may have a lower plate or an upper plate or both. When only a few artificial teeth are needed, the individual may have a bridge rather than a plate. A bridge may be fixed or removable. Artificial teeth are fitted to the individual and usually will not fit another person. People who wear dentures or other types of oral prostheses should

be encouraged to use them. Those who do not wear their prostheses are prone to shrinkage of the gums, which results in further tooth loss.

Like natural teeth, artificial dentures collect micro-organisms and food. They need to be cleaned regularly, at least once a day. They can be removed from the mouth, scrubbed with a toothbrush, rinsed and reinserted. Some people use commercial cleaning compounds for plates.

Assisting Patients with Oral Care

When providing mouth care for partially or totally dependent patients, the nurse should wear gloves to guard against infections. Other required equipment includes a curved kidney basin that fits snugly under the patient's chin to receive the rinse water and a towel to protect the patient and the bedclothes (see *Procedure 13-4* on page 280).

Foam swabs are often used in clinical areas to clean the mouths of dependent patients (see Figure 13-20). These swabs are convenient and effective in removing excess debris from the teeth and mouth but should be used infrequently and for short periods (i.e. less than three days) because they do not remove plaque that is at the base of the teeth. Increasingly clinical policies are being changed to remove these swabs from clinical areas and recommend the use of a toothbrush instead.

Most people prefer privacy when they take their artificial teeth out to clean them. Many do not like to be seen without their teeth; one of the first requests of many post-operative patients is 'May I have my teeth in, please?' The Variation section in *Procedure 13-4* on page 280 describes how to clean artificial dentures.

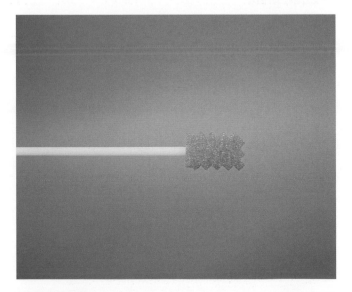

Figure 13-20 Example of foam swab used to clean mouth of a dependent patient.

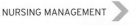
NURSING MANAGEMENT

Patients with Special Oral Hygiene Needs

For the patient who is debilitated or unconscious or who has excessive dryness, sores or irritations of the mouth, it may be necessary to clean the oral mucosa and tongue in addition to the teeth. Depending on the health of the patient's mouth, special care may be needed every two to eight hours.

Mouth care for unconscious or debilitated people is important because their mouths tend to become dry and consequently predisposed to infections. Saliva has antiviral, antibacterial and antifungal effects (Walton *et al.*, 2001: 40). Dryness occurs because the patient cannot take fluids by mouth, is often breathing through the mouth, or may be receiving oxygen that tends to dry the mucous membranes.

CLINICAL ALERT

Long-term use of lemon-glycerine swabs can lead to further dryness of the mucosa and changes in tooth enamel. Mineral oil is contraindicated because aspiration of it can initiate an infection (lipid pneumonia).

Procedure 13-5 on page 283) focuses on oral care for the unconscious person but may be adapted for conscious persons who are seriously ill or have mouth problems.

PROCEDURE 13-4 Brushing and Flossing the Teeth

Purposes

+ To remove food particles from around and between the teeth
+ To remove dental plaque

+ To enhance the patient's feelings of well-being
+ To prevent sores and infection of the oral tissues

Assessment

+ Determine the extent of the patient's self-care abilities
+ Assess the patient's usual mouth care practices
+ Inspect lips, gums, oral mucosa and tongue for deviations from normal

+ Identify presence of oral problems such as tooth caries, halitosis, gingivitis and loose or broken teeth
+ Check if the patient has bridgework or wears dentures. If the patient has dentures, ask if any tenderness or soreness is present and, if so, the location of the area(s) for ongoing assessment

Planning

Equipment

Brushing and flossing

+ Towel
+ Disposable gloves
+ Curved basin (kidney basin)
+ Toothbrush
+ Cup of tepid water
+ Toothpaste
+ Mouthwash if required

For cleaning artificial dentures

+ Disposable gloves
+ Tissue or piece of gauze
+ Denture container
+ Clean washcloth
+ Toothbrush or stiff-bristled brush
+ Toothpaste or denture cleaner
+ Tepid water
+ Container of mouthwash if required
+ Curved basin (kidney basin)
+ Towel

Implementation

Preparation

Assemble all the necessary equipment.

Performance

1. Explain to the patient what you are going to do, why it is necessary and how they can cooperate.

2. Wash hands and observe other appropriate infection control procedures (e.g. disposable gloves). *Wearing gloves while providing mouth care prevents the nurse from acquiring infections. Gloves also prevent transmission of micro-organisms to the patient.*

3. Provide for patient privacy by drawing the curtains around the bed or closing the door to the room.

4. Prepare the patient.
   - Assist the patient to a sitting position in bed, if health permits. If not, assist the patient to a side-lying position with the head turned *so liquid may be prevented from draining down the patient's throat.*

5. Prepare the equipment.
   - Place the towel under the patient's chin.
   - Put on disposable gloves.
   - Moisten the bristles of the toothbrush with tepid water and apply the toothpaste to the toothbrush.
   - Use a soft toothbrush (a small one for a child) and the patient's choice of toothpaste.
   - For the patient who must remain in bed, place or hold the curved basin under the patient's chin, fitting the small curve around the chin or neck.
   - Inspect the mouth and teeth.

6. Brush the teeth.
   - Hand the toothbrush to the patient, or brush the patient's teeth as follows:

   (a) Hold the brush against the teeth with the bristles at a 45-degree angle. The tips of the outer bristles should rest against and penetrate under the gingival sulcus (see Figure 13-21). The brush will clean under the sulcus of two or three teeth at one time. *This sulcular technique removes plaque and cleans under the gingival margins.*

   (b) Move the bristles up and down using a vibrating or jiggling motion from the sulcus to the crowns of the teeth (see Figure 13-22).

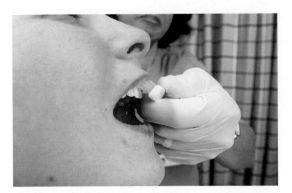

Figure 13-21 The sulcular technique: place the bristles at a 45-degree angle with the tips of the outer bristles under the gingival margins.

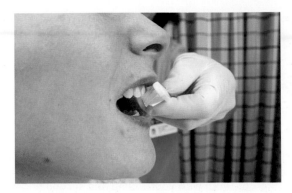

Figure 13-22 Brushing from the sulcus to the crown of the teeth.

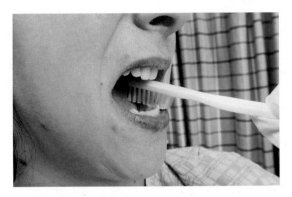

Figure 13-23 Brushing the biting surfaces.

(c) Repeat until all outer and inner surfaces of the teeth and sulci of the gums are cleaned.

(d) Clean the biting surfaces by moving the brush back and forth over them in short strokes (see Figure 13-23).

(e) If the tongue is coated, brush it gently with the toothbrush. *Brushing removes accumulated materials and coatings. A coated tongue may be caused by poor oral hygiene and low fluid intake. Brushing gently and carefully helps prevent gagging or vomiting.*

   - Hand the patient the water cup or mouthwash to rinse the mouth vigorously. Then ask the patient to spit the water and excess toothpaste into the basin. *Vigorous rinsing loosens food particles and washes out already loosened particles.*
   - Repeat the preceding steps until the mouth is free of toothpaste and food particles.
   - Remove the curved basin and help the patient wipe the mouth.

7. Remove and dispose of equipment appropriately.
   - Remove and clean the curved basin.
   - Remove and discard the gloves.

8. Document assessment of the teeth, tongue, gums and oral mucosa. Include any problems such as sores or inflammation, bleeding and swelling of the gums.

Variation: artificial dentures

1. Remove the dentures.
   - Put on gloves. *Wearing gloves protects the nurse and patient from infection.*
   - If the patient cannot remove the dentures, take the tissue or gauze, grasp the upper plate at the front teeth with your thumb and second finger, and move the denture up and down slightly (see Figure 13-24). *The slight movement breaks the suction that holds the plate on the roof of the mouth.*
   - Lower the upper plate, move it out of the mouth, and place it in the denture container.
   - Lift the lower plate, turning it so that the left side, for example, is slightly lower than the right, to remove the plate from the mouth without stretching the lips. Place the lower plate in the denture container.
   - Remove a partial denture by exerting equal pressure on the border of each side of the denture, not on the clasps, which can bend or break.

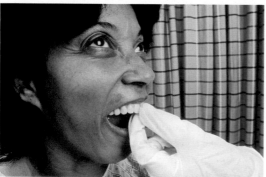

Figure 13-24 Removing the top dentures by first breaking the suction.

2. Clean the dentures.
   - Take the denture container to a sink. Take care not to drop the dentures *as they may break*. Place a washcloth in the bowl of the sink *to prevent damage if the dentures are dropped.*
   - Using a toothbrush or special stiff-bristled brush, scrub the dentures with the cleaning agent and tepid water. Hot water is not used *because heat will change the shape of some dentures*.

- Rinse the dentures with tepid running water. *Rinsing removes the cleaning agent and food particles.*
   - (a) If the dentures are stained, soak them in a commercial cleaner. Be sure to follow the manufacturer's directions. To prevent corrosion, dentures with metal parts should not be soaked overnight.

3. Inspect the dentures and the mouth.
   - Observe the dentures for any rough, sharp or worn areas that could irritate the tongue or mucous membranes of the mouth, lips and gums.
   - Inspect the mouth for any redness, irritated areas or indications of infection.
   - Assess the fit of the dentures. People who have them should see a dentist at least once a year to check the fit and the presence of any irritation to the soft tissues of the mouth.

4. Return the dentures to the mouth.
   - Offer some mouthwash and a curved basin to rinse the mouth. If the patient cannot insert the dentures independently, insert the plates one at a time. Hold each plate at a slight angle while inserting it, to avoid injuring the lips (see Figure 13-25).

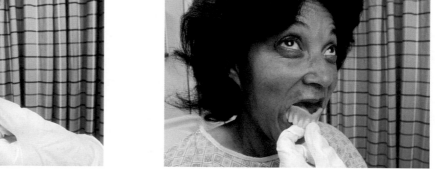

Figure 13-25 Inserting the dentures at a slight angle.

5. Assist the patient as needed.
   - Wipe the patient's hands and mouth with the towel.
   - If the patient does not want to or cannot wear the dentures, store them in a denture container with water. Label the container with the patient's name and identification number.
6. Remove and discard gloves.
7. Document all assessments and include any problems such as an irritated area on the mucous membrane.

PROCEDURE 13-5 Providing Special Oral Care

Purposes

+ To maintain the intactness and health of the lips, tongue and mucous membranes of the mouth
+ To prevent oral infections
+ To clean and moisten the membranes of the mouth and lips

Assessment

+ Inspect lips, gums, oral mucosa and tongue for deviations from normal
+ Identify presence of oral problems such as tooth caries, halitosis, gingivitis and loose or broken teeth
+ Assess for gag reflex, when appropriate

Planning

Equipment

+ Towel
+ Curved basin (kidney basin)
+ Disposable clean gloves
+ Toothbrush
+ Cup of tepid water
+ Toothpaste or denture cleaner
+ Tissue or piece of gauze to remove dentures (optional)
+ Denture container as needed
+ Mouthwash
+ Suction catheter with suction apparatus (optional)
+ Foam swabs and cleaning solution for cleaning the mucous membranes

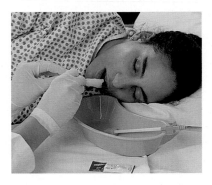

Figure 13-26 Position of patient and placement of curved basin when providing special mouth care.

Performance

1. Explain to the patient and the family what you are going to do and why it is necessary.
2. Wash hands and observe other appropriate infection control procedures (e.g. disposable gloves).
3. Provide for patient privacy by drawing the curtains around the bed or closing the door to the room.
4. Prepare the patient.
   - Position the unconscious patient in a side-lying position, with the head of the bed lowered. *In this position, the saliva automatically runs out by gravity rather than being aspirated into the lungs.* This position is the one of choice for the unconscious patient receiving mouth care. If the patient's head cannot be lowered, turn it to one side. *The fluid will readily run out of the mouth or pool in the side of the mouth, where it can be suctioned.*
   - Place the towel under the patient's chin.
   - Place the curved basin against the patient's chin and lower cheek to receive the fluid from the mouth (see Figure 13-26).
   - Put on gloves.

5. Clean the teeth and rinse the mouth.
   - If the person has natural teeth, brush the teeth as described in Procedure 13-4 on page 280. Brush gently and carefully to avoid injuring the gums. If the patient has artificial teeth, clean them as described in the Variation component of Procedure 13-4 on page 280.
   - Rinse the patient's mouth by drawing about 10 ml of water or alcohol-free mouthwash into a syringe and injecting it gently into each side of the mouth. *If the solution is injected with force, some of it may flow down the patient's throat and be aspirated into the lungs.*
   - Watch carefully to make sure that all the rinsing solution has run out of the mouth into the basin. If not, suction the fluid from the mouth. *Fluid remaining in the mouth may be aspirated into the lungs.*
   - Repeat rinsing until the mouth is free of toothpaste, if used.
6. Inspect and clean the oral tissues.
   - If the tissues appear dry or unclean, clean them with the foam swabs, toothbrush or gauze and cleaning solution following local policy.

- Picking up a moistened foam swab, wipe the mucous membrane of one cheek. If no foam swabs are available, wrap a small gauze square around a tongue depressor and moisten it. Discard the swab or tongue depressor in a clinical waste container; use a fresh one to clean the next area. *Using separate applicators for each area of the mouth prevents the transfer of micro-organisms from one area to another.*
- Clean all mouth tissues in an orderly progression, using separate applicators: the cheeks, roof of the mouth, base of the mouth and tongue.

- Observe the tissues closely for inflammation and dryness.
- Rinse the patient's mouth as described in step 5.
- Remove and discard gloves.

7. Ensure patient comfort.
   - Remove the basin, and dry around the patient's mouth with the towel. Replace artificial dentures, if indicated.
8. Document assessment of the teeth, tongue, gums and oral mucosa. Include any problems such as sores or inflammation and swelling of the gums.

Evaluation

✚ Consider the patient's medical diagnosis and treatment (e.g. chemotherapy, oxygen) and the necessary nursing interventions related to oral hygiene.

✚ Conduct an ongoing assessment, if appropriate, of the oral mucosa, gums, tongue and lips.
✚ Conduct appropriate follow-up such as a referral to a dentist for dental caries.

LIFESPAN CONSIDERATIONS

Oral Hygiene

Infants

✚ Most dentists recommend that dental hygiene should begin when the first tooth erupts and be practised after each feeding. Cleaning can be accomplished by using a wet washcloth or small gauze moistened with water.

Children

✚ Beginning at about 18 months of age, brush the child's teeth with a soft toothbrush. Use only a toothbrush moistened with water. Introduce toothpaste later and use one that contains fluoride.

Older Adults

✚ Oral care is often difficult for certain older adults to perform due to problems with dexterity or cognitive problems with dementia.
✚ Most long-term healthcare facilities have dentists that come on a regular basis to see patients with special needs.
✚ Dryness of the oral mucosa is a common finding in older adults because saliva production decreases with age.
✚ Promoting good oral hygiene can have a positive effect on the individual's ability to eat.

EVALUATING

Using data collected during care – status of oral mucosa, lips, tongue, teeth, and so on – the nurse judges whether desired outcomes have been achieved.

If outcomes are not achieved, the nurse and patient need to explore the reasons before modifying the care plan. Examples of questions to consider are as follows:

✚ Did the nurse overestimate the patient's functional abilities?
✚ Is the patient's hand coordination or cognitive function impaired?
✚ Did the patient's condition change?
✚ Has there been a change in the patient's energy level and/or motivation?

HAIR

The appearance of the hair often reflects a person's feelings of self-concept and socio-cultural well-being. Becoming familiar with hair care needs and practices that may be different than our own is an important aspect of providing competent nursing care to all patients. People who feel ill may not groom their hair as before. A dirty scalp and hair are itchy, uncomfortable and can have an odour. The hair may also reflect state of health (e.g. excessive coarseness and dryness may be associated with endocrine disorders such as hypothyroidism).

Each person has particular ways of caring for hair. Many dark-skinned people need to oil their hair daily because it tends to be dry. Oil prevents the hair from breaking and the scalp from drying. A wide-toothed comb is usually used because finer combs pull and break the hair. Some people brush their hair vigorously before retiring; others comb their hair frequently.

Developmental Variations

Newborns may have **lanugo** (the fine hair on the body of the foetus, also referred to as *down* or *woolly hair*) over their shoulders, back and sacrum. This generally disappears, and the hair distribution on the eyebrows, head and eyelashes of young children subsequently becomes noticeable. Some newborns have hair on their scalps; others are free of hair at birth but grow hair over the scalp during the first year of life.

Pubic hair usually appears in early puberty followed in about six months by the growth of axillary hair. Boys develop facial hair in later puberty.

In adolescence, the sebaceous glands increase in activity as a result of increased hormone levels. As a result, hair follicle openings enlarge to accommodate the increased amount of sebum, which can make the adolescent's hair more oily.

In older adults, the hair is generally thinner, grows more slowly and loses its colour as a result of ageing tissues and diminishing circulation. Men often lose their scalp hair and may become completely bald. This phenomenon may occur even when a man is relatively young. The older person's hair also tends to be drier than normal. With age, axillary and pubic hair becomes finer and scanter, in contrast to the eyebrows, which become bristly and coarse. Many women develop hair on their faces, which may be a concern to them. All these changes can affect the patient's body image.

NURSING MANAGEMENT

ASSESSING

Assessment of the patient's hair, hair care practices and potential problems includes a nursing health history and physical assessment.

NURSING HEALTH HISTORY

During the patient history/assessment the nurse elicits data about usual hair care, self-care abilities, history of hair or scalp problems, and conditions known to affect the hair.

Chemotherapeutic agents and radiation of the head may cause **alopecia** (hair loss). Hypothyroidism may cause the hair to be thin, dry and/or brittle. Use of some hair dyes and curling or straightening preparations can cause the hair to become dry and brittle. Questions to elicit these data are shown in the *Assessment interview*.

Physical Assessment

Problems identified may include dandruff, hair loss, pediculosis, scabies and hirsutism.

ASSESSMENT INTERVIEW

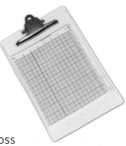

Hair Care

Hair Care Practices
+ What are your usual hair care practices?
+ What hair care products do you routinely use (e.g. hair spray, lubricant, shampoo, conditioners, hair dye, curling or straightening preparations)?

Self-care Abilities
+ Do you have any problems managing your hair?

Past or Current Hair Problems
+ Have you had any of the following conditions or therapies: recent chemotherapy, hypothyroidism, radiation of the head, unexplained loss of hair, growth of excessive body hair?

Dandruff

Often accompanied by itching, **dandruff** appears as a diffuse scaling of the scalp. In severe cases it involves the auditory canals and the eyebrows. Dandruff can usually be treated effectively with a commercial shampoo. In severe or persistent cases, the patient may need specialist prescribed shampoo.

Hair Loss

Hair loss and growth are continual processes. Some permanent thinning of hair normally occurs with ageing. Baldness, common in men, is thought to be a hereditary problem for which there is no known remedy other than the wearing of a hairpiece or a costly surgical hair transplant, in which hair is taken from the back or the sides of the scalp and surgically moved to the hairless area. Although some medications are being developed, their long-term outcomes are unknown.

Pediculosis (Lice)

Lice are parasitic insects that infest mammals. Infestation with lice is called **pediculosis**. Hundreds of varieties of lice infest humans. Three common kinds are *Pediculus capitis* (the head louse), *Pediculus corporis* (the body louse) and *Pediculus pubis* (the crab louse).

Pediculus capitis is found on the scalp and tends to stay hidden in the hairs; similarly, *Pediculus pubis* stays in pubic hair. *Pediculus corporis* tends to cling to clothing, so that when a patient undresses, the lice may not be in evidence on the body; these lice suck blood from the person and lay their eggs on the clothing. The nurse can suspect their presence in the clothing if (a) the person habitually scratches, (b) there are scratches on the skin and (c) there are haemorrhagic spots on the skin where the lice have sucked blood.

Head and pubic lice lay their eggs on the hairs; the eggs look like oval particles, similar to dandruff, clinging to the hair. Bites and pustular eruptions may also be noticed at the hair lines and behind the ears.

Lice are very small, greyish white and difficult to see. The crab louse in the pubic area has red legs. Lice may be contracted from infested clothes and direct contact with an infested person.

The treatment often includes topical pediculicides. Another treatment, occlusive agents, is used by some. The idea is that an oily substance, such as olive oil, smothers the lice and they die.

Removal of nits (eggs) after applying the treatment is not necessary to prevent spread but most people remove them for aesthetic reasons (Frankowski and Weiner, 2002). Fine-toothed 'nit' combs are available. Transmission is from head-to-head contact and it is suggested that the hair care items and bedding of the person who has the lice infestation be washed with hot water.

Scabies

Scabies is a contagious skin infestation by the itch mite. The characteristic lesion is the burrow produced by the female mite as it penetrates into the upper layers of the skin. Burrows are short, wavy, brown or black, threadlike lesions most commonly observed between the webs of the fingers and the folds of the wrists and elbows. The mites cause intense itching that is more pronounced at night because the increased warmth of the skin has a stimulating effect on the parasites. Secondary lesions caused by scratching include vesicles, papules, pustules, excoriations and crusts. Treatment involves thorough cleansing of the body with soap and water to remove scales and debris from crusts, and then an application of a scabicide lotion. All bed linens and clothing should be washed in very hot or boiling water.

Hirsutism

The growth of excessive body hair is called **hirsutism**. The acceptance of body hair in the axillae and on the legs is largely dictated by culture. In Western culture, the well-groomed woman, as depicted in magazines, has no hair on her legs or under her axillae. Excessive facial hair on a woman is thought unattractive in most Western and Asian cultures. For example, some Japanese brides follow the custom of shaving their faces the day before the wedding.

The cause of excessive body hair is not always known. Older women may have some on their faces, and women in menopause may also experience the growth of facial hair. Excessive body hair may be due to the action of the endocrine system. Heredity is also thought to influence the pattern of hair distribution.

PLANNING

In planning care, the nurse and, if appropriate, the patient and/or family set outcomes for each identified nursing problem. The nurse then performs nursing interventions and activities to achieve the patient outcomes.

The specific, detailed nursing activities taken by the nurse to assist the patient should take into account the patient's personal preferences, health and energy resources as well as the time, equipment and personnel available. Often, patients like to receive hair care after a bath, before receiving visitors, and before retiring.

IMPLEMENTING

Hair needs to be brushed or combed daily and washed, as needed, to keep it clean. Nurses may need to provide hair care for patients who cannot meet their own self-care needs.

Brushing and Combing Hair

To be healthy, hair needs to be brushed daily. Brushing has three major functions: It stimulates the circulation of blood in the scalp, it distributes the oil along the hair shaft, and it helps to arrange the hair.

Long hair may present a problem for patients confined to bed because it may become matted. It should be combed and brushed at least once a day to prevent this. A brush with stiff bristles provides the best stimulation to blood circulation in the scalp. The bristles should not be so sharp that they injure the patient's scalp, however. A comb with dull, even teeth is advisable. A comb with sharp teeth might injure the scalp; combs that are too fine can pull and break the hair. Some patients are pleased to have their hair tied neatly in the dark-skinned people often have thicker, drier, curlier hair than light-skinned people. Very curly hair may stand out from the scalp. Although the shafts of curly or kinky hair look strong and wiry, they have less strength than straight hair shafts and can break easily.

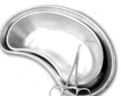

PROCEDURE 13-6 Providing Hair Care for Patients

Purposes

+ To increase the patient's sense of well-being

+ To assess or monitor hair or scalp problems (e.g. matted hair or dandruff)

Assessment

Determine

+ History of the following conditions or therapies: recent chemotherapy, hypothyroidism, radiation of the head, unexplained hair loss and growth of excessive body hair
+ Usual hair care practices and routinely used hair care products (e.g. hair spray, shampoo, conditioners, hair oil preparation, hair dye, curling or straightening preparations)
+ Whether wetting the hair will make it difficult to comb. Kinky hair is easier to comb when wet, however, it is very difficult to comb when it dries (Jackson, 1998: 102).

Assess

+ Condition of the hair and scalp. Is the hair straight, curly, kinky? Is the hair matted or tangled? Is the scalp dry?
+ Evenness of hair growth over the scalp, in particular, any patchy loss of hair; hair texture, oiliness, thickness or thinness; presence of lesions, infections or infestations on the scalp; presence of hirsutism
+ Self-care abilities (e.g. any problems managing hair care)

Planning

Equipment

+ Clean brush and comb
+ A wide-toothed comb is usually used for many black-skinned people because finer combs pull the hair into knots and may also break the hair

+ Towel
+ Hair oil preparation, if appropriate

Implementation

Performance

1. Explain to the patient what you are going to do, why it is necessary and how they can cooperate and gain informed consent.
2. Wash hands and observe other appropriate infection control procedures.
3. Provide for patient privacy by drawing the curtains around the bed or closing the door to the room.

4. Position and prepare the patient appropriately.
   • Assist the patient who can sit to move to a chair. *Hair is more easily brushed and combed when the individual is in a sitting position.* If health permits, assist a patient confined to a bed to a sitting position by raising the head of the bed. Otherwise, assist the patient to alternate side-lying positions, and do one side of the head at a time.

- If the patient remains in bed, place a clean towel over the pillow and the patient's shoulders. Place it over the sitting patient's shoulders. *The towel collects any removed hair, dirt and scaly material.*
- Remove any pins or ribbons in the hair.

5. Remove any mats or tangles gradually.
   - Mats can usually be pulled apart with fingers or worked out with repeated brushings.
   - If the hair is very tangled, rub alcohol or an oil, such as mineral oil, on the strands to help loosen the tangles.
   - Comb out tangles in a small section of hair toward the ends. Stablilise the hair with one hand and comb toward the ends of the hair with the other hand. *This avoids scalp trauma.*

6. Brush and comb the hair.
   - For short hair, brush and comb one side at a time. Divide long hair into two sections by parting it down the middle from the front to the back. If the hair is very thick, divide each section into front and back subsections or into several layers.

7. Arrange the hair as neatly and attractively as possible, according to the individual's desires.
   - Braiding long hair helps prevent tangles.

8. Document assessments and special nursing interventions. Daily combing and brushing of the hair are not normally recorded.

CLINICAL ALERT

Excessively matted or tangled hair may be infested with lice.

EVALUATION

+ Conduct ongoing assessments for problems such as dandruff, alopecia, pediculosis, scalp lesions or excessive dryness or matting.
+ Evaluate effectiveness of medication (e.g. for treating pediculosis), if appropriate.

Shampooing the Hair

Hair should be washed as often as needed to keep it clean. There are several ways to shampoo patients' hair, depending on their health, strength and age. The patient who is well enough to take a shower can shampoo while in the shower. The patient who is unable to shower may be given a shampoo while sitting on a chair in front of a sink. The back-lying patient who can move to a stretcher can be given a shampoo on a stretcher wheeled to a sink. The patient who must remain in bed can be given a shampoo with water brought to the bedside.

Shampoo basins to catch the water and direct it to the washbasin or other receptacle are usually made of plastic or metal. A bowl or large jug can be used as a receptacle for the shampoo water. If possible, the receptacle should be large enough to hold all shampoo water so that it does not have to be emptied during the shampoo.

Water used for the shampoo should be warm enough for an adult or child and be comfortable and not injure the scalp. Dry shampoos are also available. They will remove some of the dirt, odour and oil. Their main disadvantage is that they dry the hair and scalp.

How often a person needs a shampoo is highly individual, depending largely on the person's activities and the amount of sebum secreted by the scalp. Oily hair tends to look stringy and dirty, and it feels unclean to the person. *Procedure 13-7* explains how to provide a shampoo for a patient confined to bed.

PROCEDURE 13-7 Shampooing the Hair of a Patient Confined to Bed

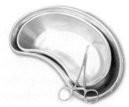

Purposes

+ To clean the hair and increase the patient's sense of well-being

---

Assessment

+ Determine routinely used shampoo products
+ Assess:

+ Any scalp problems
+ Activity tolerance of the patient

Planning

Equipment

- Comb and brush
- Plastic sheet or pad
- Two bath towels
- Shampoo basin
- Washcloth or pad

- Receptacle for the shampoo water
- Cotton balls (optional)
- Jug of water
- Liquid or cream shampoo
- Hair dryer if required

Implementation

Preparation

- Determine the type of shampoo to be used (e.g. medicated shampoo).
- Determine the best time of day for the shampoo. Discuss this with the patient. A person who must remain in bed may find the shampoo tiring. Choose a time when the patient is rested and can rest after the procedure.

Performance

1. Explain to the patient what you are going to do, why it is necessary if appropriate and how they can cooperate.
2. Wash hands and observe other appropriate infection control procedures as needed.
3. Provide for patient privacy by drawing the curtains around the bed or closing the door to the room.
4. Position and prepare the patient appropriately.
   - Assist the patient to the side of the bed from which you will work.
5. Arrange the equipment.
   - Put the plastic sheet or pad on the bed under the head. *The plastic keeps the bedding dry.*
   - Remove the pillow from under the individual's head, and place it under the shoulders unless there is some underlying condition (e.g. neck surgery, arthritis of the neck). *This hyperextends the neck.*
   - Tuck a bath towel around the patient's shoulders. *This keeps the shoulders dry.*
   - Place the shampoo basin under the head (see Figure 13-27), putting a folded washcloth or pad where the patient's neck rests on the edge of the basin. If the patient is on a stretcher, the neck can rest on the edge of the sink with the washcloth as padding. *Padding supports the muscles of the neck and prevents undue strain and discomfort.*
   - Fanfold the top bedding down to the waist, and cover the upper part of the patient with a towel. *The folded bedding will stay dry, and the bath*

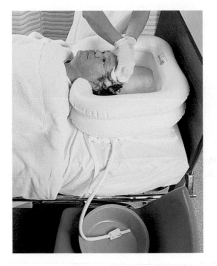

Figure 13-27 Shampooing the hair of a patient confined to bed. Note the shampoo basin and the receptacle below.

towel, which can be discarded after the shampoo, will keep the patient warm.
   - Place the receiving receptacle on a table or chair at the bedside. Put the spout of the shampoo basin over the receptacle.
6. Protect the patient's eyes and ears.
   - Place a damp washcloth over the patient's eyes. *The washcloth protects the eyes from soapy water. A damp washcloth will not slip.*
   - Place cotton balls in the patient's ears if indicated. *These keep water from collecting in the ear canals.*
7. Shampoo the hair.
   - Wet the hair thoroughly with the water.
   - Apply shampoo to the scalp. Make a good lather with the shampoo while massaging the scalp with the pads of your fingertips. Massage all areas of the scalp systematically, for example, starting at the front and working toward the back of the head. *Massaging stimulates the blood circulation in the scalp. The pads of the fingers are used so that the fingernails will not scratch the scalp.*

- Rinse the hair briefly, and apply shampoo again.
- Make a good lather and massage the scalp as before.
- Rinse the hair thoroughly this time to remove all shampoo. *Shampoo remaining in the hair may dry and irritate the hair and scalp.*
- Squeeze as much water as possible out of the hair with your hands.

8. Dry the hair thoroughly.
- Rub the patient's hair with a heavy towel.

- Dry the hair with the dryer. Set the temperature at 'warm'.
- Continually move the dryer to prevent burning the patient's scalp.

9. Ensure patient comfort.
- Assist the person confined to bed to a comfortable position.
- Arrange the hair using a clean brush and comb.

10. Document the shampoo and any assessments.

Evaluation

+ Conduct ongoing assessments such as any scalp problems or intolerance to the procedure.

Report any problems noted to the nurse in charge.

LIFESPAN CONSIDERATIONS

Hair Care

Infants

+ Shampoo an infant's hair daily to prevent seborrhea.

Children

+ Monitor **school-age children for nits (pediculosis)**.

Older Adults

+ Ensure adequate warmth for elders when shampooing their hair, because they are susceptible to chilling.

Beard and Moustache Care

Beards and moustaches also require daily care. The most important aspect of the care is to keep them clean. Food particles tend to collect in beards and moustaches, and they need washing and combing periodically. Patients may also wish a beard or moustache trim to maintain a well-groomed appearance.

Male patients patients often shave or are shaved after a bath/shower. See *Box 13-3* for the steps involved in shaving facial hair with a safety razor.

BOX 13-3 Using a Safety Razor to Shave Facial Hair

+ Wear gloves in case facial nicks occur and you come in contact with blood.
+ Apply shaving cream or soap and water to soften the bristles and make the skin more pliable.
+ Hold the skin taut, particularly around creases, to prevent cutting the skin.
+ Hold the razor so that the blade is at a 45-degree angle to the skin, and shave in short, firm strokes in the direction of hair growth (see Figure 13-28).
+ After shaving the entire area, wipe the patient's face with a wet washcloth to remove any remaining shaving cream and hair.
+ Dry the face well, then apply aftershave lotion or powder as the patient prefers.
+ To prevent irritating the skin, pat on the lotion with the fingers and avoid rubbing the face.

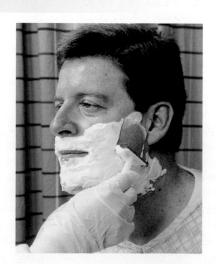

Figure 13-28 Shaving in the direction of hair growth.

EVALUATING

Using data collected during care, the nurse judges whether desired outcomes have been achieved. Examples of patient outcomes that are measurable or observable include the patient being able to:

+ Perform hair grooming with assistance (specify)
+ Exhibit clean, well-groomed, resilient hair with a healthy sheen
+ Reduce or get rid of scalp lesions or infestations
+ Describe factors, interventions and preventive measures for specific hair problem (e.g. dandruff).

EYES

Normally eyes require no special hygiene, because lacrimal fluid continually washes the eyes, and the eyelids and lashes prevent the entrance of foreign particles. Special interventions are needed, however, for unconscious patients and for patients recovering from eye surgery or having eye injuries, irritations or infections. In unconscious patients, the blink reflex may be absent, and excessive drainage may accumulate along eyelid margins. In patients with eye trauma or eye infections, excessive discharge or drainage is common. Excessive secretions on the lashes need to be removed before they dry on the lashes as crusts. Individuals who wear eyeglasses, contact lenses or an artificial eye also may require instruction from and care by the nurse.

NURSING MANAGEMENT

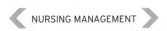

ASSESSING

Assessment of the patient's eyes includes a nursing health assessment and physical assessment.

Nursing Health History

During the patient history, the nurse obtains data about the patient's eyeglasses or contact lenses, recent examination by an ophthalmologist, and any history of eye problems and related treatments. Questions to elicit these data are shown in the *Assessment interview* on page 292.

Physical Assessment

In physical assessment, all external eye structures are inspected for signs of inflammation, excessive drainage, encrustations or other obvious abnormalities.

PLANNING

In planning care, the nurse identifies nursing activities that will assist the individual to maintain the integrity of the eye structures or a prosthesis and to prevent eye injury and infection.

IMPLEMENTING

Nursing activities may include teaching individuals about how to insert, clean and remove contact lenses or a prosthesis, and ways to protect the eyes from injury and strain.

Eye Care

Dried secretions that have accumulated on the lashes need to be softened and wiped away. Soften dried secretions by placing a sterile gauze moistened with sterile water or normal saline over the lid margins. Wipe the loosened secretions from the inner canthus of the eye to the outer canthus to prevent the particles and fluid from draining into the lacrimal sac and nasolacrimal duct.

If the patient is unconscious and lacks a blink reflex or cannot close the eyelids completely, drying and irritation of the cornea must be prevented. Lubricating eye drops may be prescribed. *Box 13-4* on page 292 gives suggestions for providing eye care for the comatose patient.

Eyeglass Care

It is essential that the nurse exercise caution when cleaning eyeglasses to prevent breaking or scratching the lenses. Glass

ASSESSMENT INTERVIEW

Eyes

For Patients Who Wear Eyeglasses
+ When do you use your glasses?
+ What is your vision like with and without the glasses?

For Patients Who Wear Contact Lenses
+ How often do you wear lenses? Daily? On special occasions?
+ How long do you wear your lenses in a given day, including sleep time?
+ Do you have any problems with the lenses (e.g. cleaning, insertion, removal, damage)?
+ Do you carry an emergency identification label to alert others to remove the lenses and ensure appropriate care in an emergency? (If not, advise the patient to acquire one.)
+ What are your insertion and removal procedures?
+ What are your cleaning and storage procedures?

+ Have you had any problems with either or both eyes or eyelids, such as excessive tearing, burning, redness, sensitivity to light, swelling or feelings of dryness? Describe them.
+ Are you using any eyedrops or ointments? (These medications can combine chemically with soft lenses and cause lens damage and eye irritation.)

For All Patients
+ When did you last have your eyesight tested?
+ Are you currently taking any eye medication? If so, provide name, dosage and frequency.
+ Do you have any of the following eye problems: difficulty reading or seeing objects, blurring of vision, tearing, spots or floaters, photophobia (sensitivity to light), burning, itching, pain, double vision, flashing lights or halos around lights?

BOX 13-4 Eye Care for the Comatose Patient

When a comatose patient's corneal reflex is impaired, eye care is essential to keep moist the areas of the cornea that are exposed to air.

+ Administer moist compresses to cover the eyes every two to four hours.
+ Clean the eyes with saline solution and gauze swabs. Wipe from the inner to outer canthus. This prevents debris from being washed into the nasolacrimal duct.

+ Use a new gauze for each wipe. This prevents extending infection in one eye to the other eye.
+ Instill ophthalmic ointment or artificial tears into the lower lids as ordered. This keeps the eyes moist.
+ If the patient's corneal reflex is absent, keep the eyes moist with artificial tears and protect the eye with a protective shield.
+ Monitor the eyes for redness, exudate or ulceration.

---

lenses can be cleaned with warm water and dried with a soft tissue that will not scratch the lenses. Plastic lenses are easily scratched and may require special cleaning solutions and drying tissues. When not being worn, all glasses should be placed in an appropriately labelled case and stored at the patient's bedside.

Contact Lens Care

Contact lenses, thin curved discs of hard or soft plastic, fit on the cornea of the eye directly over the pupil. They float on the tear layer of the eye. For some people, contact lenses offer several advantages over eyeglasses: (a) they cannot be seen and

thus have cosmetic value; (b) they are highly effective in correcting some astigmatisms; (c) they are safer than glasses for some physical activities; (d) they do not fog, as eyeglasses do; and (e) they provide better vision in many cases.

Contact lenses may be either hard or soft or a compromise between the two types – gas-permeable lenses. *Hard contact lenses* are made of a rigid, unwettable, airtight plastic that does not absorb water or saline solutions. They usually cannot be worn for more than 12–14 hours and are rarely recommended for first-time wearers.

Soft contact lenses cover the entire cornea. Being more pliable and soft, they mould to the eye for a firmer fit. The duration of extended wear varies by brand from 1–30 days or

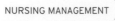

NURSING MANAGEMENT

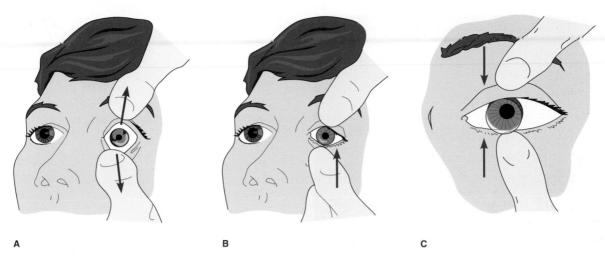

A   **B**   **C**

Figure 13-29 Removing hard contact lenses.

more. Eye specialists recommend that long-wear brands be removed and cleaned at least once a week. These lenses require scrupulous care and handling.

Gas-permeable lenses are rigid enough to provide clear vision but are more flexible than the traditional hard lens. They permit oxygen to reach the cornea, thus providing greater comfort, and will not cause serious damage to the eye if left in place for several days.

Most patients normally care for their own contact lenses. In general, each lens manufacturer provides detailed cleaning instructions. Depending on the type of lens and cleaning method used, warm tap water, normal saline, or special rinsing or soaking solutions may be used.

All users should have a special container for their lenses. Some contain a solution so that the lenses are stored wet; in others, the lenses are dry. Each lens container has a slot or cup with a label indicating whether it is for the right or left lens. It is essential that the correct lens be stored in the appropriate slot so that it will be placed in the correct eye.

Removing Contact Lenses

Hard contact lenses must be positioned directly over the cornea for proper removal. If the lens is displaced, the nurse asks the patient to look straight ahead, and gently exerts pressure on the upper and lower lids to move the lens back onto the cornea. Figure 13-29 shows the steps needed to remove a hard lens. To avoid lens mixups, the nurse places the first lens in its designated cup in the storage base before removing the second lens (see Figure 13-30).

Removal of soft lenses varies in two ways. First, have the patient look forward. Retract the lower lid with one hand. Using the pad of the index finger of the other hand, move the lens down to the inferior part of the sclera. This reduces the risk of damage to the cornea. Second, remove the lens by gently pinching the lens between the pads of the thumb and index finger. Pinching causes the lens to double up, so that air enters

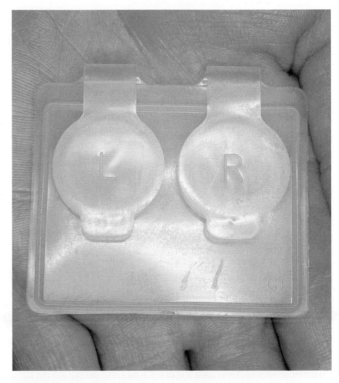

Figure 13-30 Storing lenses. Place the first lens in its designated cup in the storage case before removing the second lens. This avoids mixing up two potentially different lenses. (David Parker/Science Photo Library/Photo Researchers, Inc.)

underneath the lens, overcoming the suction and allowing removal. Use the pads of the fingers to prevent scratching the eye or the lens with the fingernails. Figure 13-31 on page 294 shows an individual removing her own contact lens using the method described. Please note that a nurse should wear gloves.

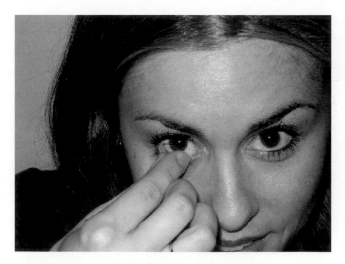

Figure 13-31 Removing a soft lens by pinching it between the pads of the thumb and index finger. (Lester Lefkowitz/Corbis.)

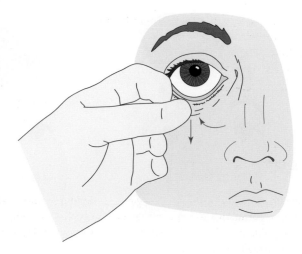

Figure 13-32 Removing an artificial eye by retracting the lower eyelid and exerting slight pressure below the eyelid.

Inserting Contact Lenses

Seriously ill patients whose contact lenses have been removed will not need them reinserted until they become more active in their care and require the lenses to see properly. Contact lenses need to be lubricated in a sterile, nonirritating wetting solution (usually a saline solution) before they are inserted. The wetting solution helps the lens glide over the cornea, thus reducing the risk of injury. Most patients, when well, will reinsert the lenses independently.

Artificial Eyes

Artificial eyes are usually made of glass or plastic. Some are permanently implanted; others are removed regularly for cleaning. Most individuals who wear a removable artificial eye follow their own care regimen. Even for an unconscious patient, daily removal and cleaning are not necessary.

To remove an artificial eye, the nurse puts on clean gloves and retracts the patient's lower eyelid down over the infra-orbital bone while exerting slight pressure below the eyelid to overcome the suction (see Figure 13-32). An alternate method is to compress a small rubber bulb and apply the tip directly to the eye. As the nurse gradually releases the finger pressure on the bulb, the suction of the bulb counteracts the suction holding the eye in the socket and draws the eye out of the socket.

The eye is cleaned with warm normal saline and placed in a container filled with water or saline solution. The socket and tissues around the eye are usually cleaned with cotton wipes and normal saline. To reinsert the eye, the nurse uses the thumb and index finger of one hand to retract the eyelids, exerting pressure on the supraorbital and infraorbital bones. Holding the eye between the thumb and index finger of the other hand, the nurse slips the eye gently into the socket (see Figure 13-33).

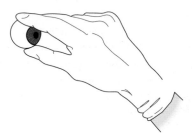

Figure 13-33 Holding an artificial eye between the thumb and index finger for insertion.

General Eye Care

Many individuals may need to learn specific information about care of the eyes. Some examples follow.

+ Avoid home remedies for eye problems. Eye irritations or injuries at any age should be treated medically and immediately.
+ If dirt or dust gets into the eyes, clean them copiously with clean, tepid water as an emergency treatment.
+ Take measures to guard against eyestrain and to protect vision, such as maintaining adequate lighting for reading and obtaining shatterproof lenses for glasses.
+ Schedule regular eye examinations, particularly after age 40, to detect problems such as cataracts and glaucoma.

EVALUATING

Using data collected during care, the nurse judges whether desired outcomes have been achieved. Examples of desired outcomes to evaluate the effectiveness of nursing interventions follow.

+ Conjunctive and sclera free of inflammation
+ Eyelids free of secretions
+ No tearing
+ No eye discomfort

+ Demonstrates appropriate methods of caring for contact lenses
+ Describes interventions to prevent eye injury and infection.

EARS

Normal ears require minimal hygiene. Individuals who have excessive **cerumen** (earwax) and dependent patients who have hearing aids may require assistance from the nurse. Hearing aids are usually removed before surgery.

Cleaning the Ears

The auricles of the ear are cleaned during the bed bath. The nurse or patient must remove excessive cerumen that is visible or that causes discomfort or hearing difficulty. Visible cerumen may be loosened and removed by retracting the auricle up and back. If this measure is ineffective, irrigation is necessary. Patients need to be advised never to use keys, toothpicks or cotton-tipped applicators to remove cerumen. Keys and toothpicks can injure the ear canal and rupture the tympanic membrane; cotton-tipped applicators can cause wax to become impacted within the canal.

Care of Hearing Aids

A hearing aid is a battery-powered, sound-amplifying device used by persons with hearing impairments. It consists of a microphone that picks up sound and converts it to electric energy, an amplifier that magnifies the electric energy electronically, a receiver that converts the amplified energy back to sound energy, and an earmould that directs the sound into the ear. There are several types of hearing aids:

+ *Behind-the-ear (BTE, or postaural) aid.* This is the most widely used type because it fits snugly behind the ear. The hearing aid case, which holds the microphone, amplifier and receiver, is attached to the earmould by a plastic tube (see Figure 13-34).
+ *In-the-ear aid (ITE, or intra-aural).* This one-piece aid has all its components housed in the earmould (see Figure 13-35).
+ *In-the-canal (ITC) aid.* This is the most compact and least visible aid, fitting completely inside the ear canal. In addition to having cosmetic appeal, the ITC does not interfere with telephone use or the wearing of eyeglasses. However, it is not suitable for individuals with progressive hearing loss; it requires adequate ear canal diameter and length for a good fit; and it tends to plug with cerumen more than other aids.
+ *Eyeglasses aid.* This is similar to the behind-the-ear aid, but the components are housed in the temple of the

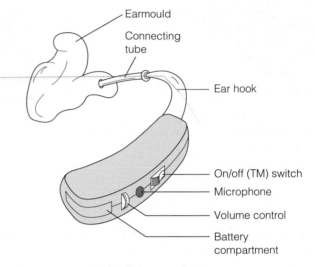

Figure 13-34 A behind-the-ear hearing aid.

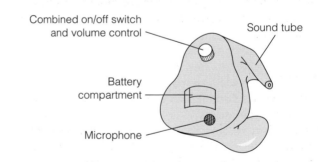

Figure 13-35 An in-the-ear hearing aid.

eyeglasses. A hearing aid can be in one or both temples of the glasses.
+ *Body hearing aid.* This pocket-sized aid, used for more severe hearing losses, clips onto an undergarment, shirt pocket or harness carrier supplied by the manufacturer. The case, containing the microphone and amplifier, is connected by a cord to the receiver, which snaps into the earpiece.

For correct functioning, hearing aids require appropriate handling during insertion and removal, regular cleaning of the earmould, and replacement of dead batteries. With proper care, hearing aids generally last 5–10 years. Earmoulds generally need readjustment every 2–3 years. *Procedure 13-8* on page 296 describes how to remove, clean and insert a hearing aid.

PROCEDURE 13-8 Removing, Cleaning and Inserting a Hearing Aid

Purpose

+ To maintain proper hearing aid function

Assessment

Determine if the individual has experienced any problems with the hearing aid and hearing aid practices.

Assess for the presence of inflammation, excessive wax, drainage or discomfort in the external ear.

Planning

Equipment

+ Individual's hearing aid
+ Soap, water and towels or a damp cloth

+ New battery (if needed)

Implementation

Performance

1. Explain to the patient what you are going to do, why it is necessary and how they can cooperate.
2. Wash hands and observe other appropriate infection control procedures.
3. Provide for patient privacy by drawing the curtains around the bed or closing the door to the room.
4. Remove the hearing aid.
   - Turn the hearing aid off and lower the volume. The on/off switch may be labelled 'O' (off), 'M' (microphone), 'T' (telephone) or 'TM' (telephone/microphone). *The batteries continue to run if the hearing aid is not turned off.*
   - Remove the earmould by rotating it slightly forward and pulling it outward.
   - If the hearing aid is not to be used for several days, remove the battery. *Removal prevents corrosion of the hearing aid from battery leakage.*
   - Store the hearing aid in a safe place and label with individual's name. Avoid exposure to heat and moisture. *Proper storage prevents loss or damage.*
5. Clean the earmould.
   - Detach the earmould if possible. Disconnect the earmould from the receiver of a body hearing aid or from the hearing aid case of behind-the-ear and eyeglass hearing aids where the tubing meets the hook of the case. Do not remove the earmould if it is glued or secured by a small metal ring. *Removal facilitates cleaning and prevents inadvertent damage to the other parts.*
   - If the earmould is detachable, soak it in a mild soapy solution. Rinse and dry it well. Do not

   use isopropyl alcohol. *Alcohol can damage the hearing aid.*
   - If the earmould is not detachable or is for an in-the-ear aid, wipe the earmould with a damp cloth.
   - Check that the earmould opening is patent. Blow any excess moisture through the opening or remove debris (e.g. earwax) with a pipe cleaner or toothpick.
   - Reattach the earmould if it was detached from the rest of the hearing aid.
6. Insert the hearing aid.
   - Determine from the patient if the earmould is for the left or the right ear.
   - Check that the battery is inserted in the hearing aid. Turn off the hearing aid, and make sure the volume is turned all the way down. *A volume that is too loud is distressing.*
   - Inspect the earmould to identify the ear canal portion. Some earmoulds are fitted for only the ear canal and concha; others are fitted for all the contours of the ear. The canal portion, common to all, can be used as a guide for correct insertion.
   - Line up the parts of the earmould with the corresponding parts of the patient's ear.
   - Rotate the earmould slightly forward, and insert the ear canal portion.
   - Gently press the earmould into the ear while rotating it backward.
   - Check that the earmould fits snugly by asking the patient if it feels secure and comfortable.

- Adjust the other components of a behind-the-ear or body hearing aid.
- Turn the hearing aid on and adjust the volume according to the individual's needs.

7. Correct problems associated with improper functioning.
   - If the sound is weak or there is no sound:
   (a) Ensure that the volume is turned high enough.
   (b) Ensure that the earmould opening is not clogged.
   (c) Check the battery by turning the hearing aid on, turning up the volume, cupping your hand over the earmould, and listening. A constant whistling sound indicates the battery is functioning. If necessary, replace the battery. Be sure that the negative (−) and positive (+) signs on the battery match those where indicated on the hearing aid.
   (d) Ensure that the ear canal is not blocked with wax, which can obstruct sound waves.
   - If the individual reports a whistling sound or squeal after insertion:
   (a) Turn the volume down.
   (b) Ensure that the earmould is properly attached to the receiver.
   (c) Reinsert the earmould.

8. Document pertinent data.
   - The removal and the insertion of a hearing aid are not normally recorded.
   - Report and record any problems the patient has with the hearing aid.

Evaluation

✚ Speak to the patient in a normal conversational tone and observe patient behaviours.

✚ Compare the patient's hearing ability to previous assessments.

NOSE

Nurses usually need not provide special care for the nose, because patients can ordinarily clear nasal secretions by blowing gently into a soft tissue. When the external nares are encrusted with dried secretions, they should be cleaned with a cotton-tipped applicator or moistened with saline or water. The applicator should not be inserted beyond the length of the cotton tip; inserting it further may cause injury to the mucosa.

SUPPORTING A HYGIENIC ENVIRONMENT

Because people are usually confined to bed when ill, often for long periods, the bed becomes an important element in the patient's life. A place that is clean, safe and comfortable contributes to the individual's ability to rest and sleep and to a sense of well-being. Basic furniture in a healthcare environment includes the bed, bedside table, overbed table, one or more chairs and a storage space for clothing. Most bed units also have a call light, light fixtures, electric outlets and hygienic equipment in the bedside table. Two types of equipment often installed in an acute care facility are a suction outlet for several kinds of suction and an oxygen outlet for most oxygen equipment.

Hospital Beds

The frame of a hospital bed is divided into three sections. This permits the head and the foot to be elevated separately. Most hospital beds have electric motors to operate the movable joints. The motor is activated by pressing a button or moving a small lever, located either at the side of the bed or on a small panel separate from the bed but attached to it by a cable, which the patient can readily use. Common bed positions are shown in Table 13-6 on page 298.

Mattresses

Mattresses are usually covered with a water-repellent material that resists soiling and can be cleaned easily. Most mattresses have handles on the sides called lugs by which the mattress can be moved.

Many special mattresses are also used in hospitals to relieve pressure on the body's bony prominences, such as the heels. They are particularly helpful for individuals confined to bed for a long time.

Side Rails/Cot Sides

Side rails, or safety sides, are used on both hospital beds and trolleys. They are of various shapes and sizes and are usually made of metal. A bed can have two full-length side rails or four

Table 13-6 Commonly Used Bed Positions

Flat Head of bed Foot of bed	Mattress is completely horizontal.	Patient sleeping in a variety of bed positions, such as back-lying, side-lying and prone (face down) To maintain spinal alignment for clients with spinal injuries To assist patients to move and turn in bed Bed-making by nurse
Fowler's position	Semi-sitting position in which head of bed is raised to angle of at least 45°. Knees may be flexed or horizontal.	Convenient for eating, reading, visiting, watching TV Relief from lying positions To promote lung expansion for client with respiratory problem To assist a patient to a sitting position on the edge of the bed
Semi-Fowler's position	Head of bed is raised only to 30° angle.	Relief from lying position To promote lung expansion
Trendelenburg's position	Head of bed is lowered and the foot raised in a straight incline.	To promote venous circulation in certain clients To provide postural drainage of basal lung lobes
Reverse Trendelenburg's position	Head of bed raised and the foot lowered. Straight tilt in direction opposite to Trendelenburg's position.	To promote stomach emptying and prevent oesophageal reflex in client with hiatus hernia

half- or quarter-length side rails (also called split rails). Devices to raise and lower side rails differ. Often one or two knobs are pulled to release the side and permit it to be moved. When side rails are being used, it is important that the nurse never leaves the bedside while the rail is lowered. Some side rails have two positions: up and down. Others have three: high, intermediate and low.

For decades, the use of side rails has been routine practice with the rationale that the side rails serve as a safe and effective means of preventing patients from falling out of bed. Research, however, has not validated this assumption. In fact, several studies have shown that raised side rails do not deter older patients from getting out of bed unassisted and have led to more serious falls, injuries and even death (Talerico and Capazuti, 2001). Alternatives to side rails do exist and can include low-height bed, mats placed at the side of the bed, motion sensors and bed alarms.

Bed Cradles

A bed cradle is a device designed to keep the top bedclothes off the feet, legs and even abdomen of a patient. The bedclothes

are arranged over the device and may be pinned in place. There are several types of bed cradles. One of the most common is a curved metal rod that fits over the bed. Part of the cradle fits under the mattress, and small metal brackets press down on each side of the mattress to keep the cradle in place. The frame of some cradles extends over half of the width of the bed, above one leg.

Intravenous Stands

Intravenous stands usually made of metal, support intravenous (IV) infusion containers while fluid is being administered to a patient. These rods were traditionally freestanding on the floor beside the bed. Now, intravenous stands are often attached to the hospital beds.

MAKING BEDS

Nurses need to be able to prepare hospital beds in different ways for specific purposes. In most instances, beds are made after the patient receives certain care and when beds are

PRACTICE GUIDELINES

Bed-Making

+ Always work with a colleague, never alone. Wash hands thoroughly after handling a patient's bed linen. Linens and equipment that have been soiled with secretions and excretions harbour micro-organisms that can be transmitted to others directly or by the nurse's hands or uniform.
+ Hold soiled linen away from uniform.
+ Linen for one patient is never (even momentarily) placed on another patient's bed.
+ Place soiled linen directly in a portable linen skip or tucked into a pillow case at the end of the bed before it is gathered up for disposal.
+ Do not shake soiled linen in the air because shaking can disseminate secretions and excretions and the micro-organisms they contain.
+ When stripping and making a bed, conserve time and energy by stripping and making up one side as much as possible before working on the other side.
+ To avoid unnecessary trips to the linen supply area, gather all linen before starting to strip a bed.

unoccupied. At times, however, nurses need to make an occupied bed or prepare a bed for a patient who is having surgery (an anaesthetic, post-operative or surgical bed). Regardless of what type of bed equipment is available, whether the bed is occupied or unoccupied, or the purpose for which the bed is being prepared, certain practice guidelines pertain to all bed-making.

Unoccupied Bed

An unoccupied bed can be either closed or open. Generally the top covers of an open bed are folded back (thus the term *open*

bed) to make it easier for a patient to get in. Open and closed beds are made the same way, except that the top sheet, blanket and bedspread of a *closed bed* are drawn up to the top of the bed and under the pillows.

Beds are often changed after bed baths. The linen can be collected before the bath. The linen is not usually changed unless it is soiled. Unfitted sheets, blankets and bedspreads are mitred at the corners of the bed. The purpose of mitring is to secure the bedclothes while the bed is occupied. Figure 13-36 shows how to mitre the corner of a bed. *Procedure 13-9* on page 300 explains how to change an unoccupied bed.

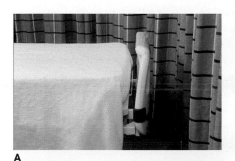
A

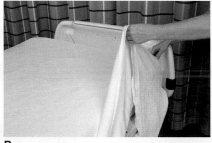
B

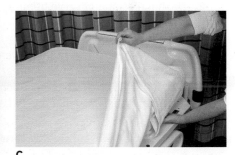
C

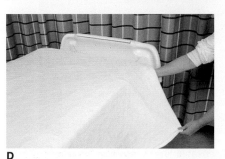
D

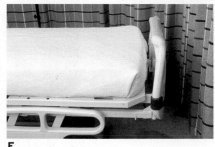
E

Figure 13-36 Mitring the corner of a bed.

PROCEDURE 13-9 Changing an Unoccupied Bed

Purposes

+ To promote the individual's comfort
+ To provide a clean neat environment for the patient
+ To provide a smooth, wrinkle-free bed foundation, thus minimising sources of skin irritation

Assessment

+ Assess the patient's health status to determine that the person can safely get out of bed
+ Note all the tubes and equipment connected to the patient *because this may influence the need for additional linens or waterproof pads*

Planning

Equipment

+ Two flat sheets
+ Cloth drawsheet (optional)
+ One blanket
+ One bedspread
+ Waterproof drawsheet or waterproof pads (optional)
+ Pillowcase(s) for the head pillow(s)
+ Plastic laundry bag or portable linen hamper/skip, if available

Implementation

Preparation

Determine what linens the patient may already have in the room *to avoid stockpiling of unnecessary extra linens.*

Performance

1. Explain to the patient what you are going to do, why it is necessary and how they can cooperate.
2. Wash hands and observe other appropriate infection control procedures.
3. Provide for patient privacy.
4. Place the fresh linen on the patient's chair or overbed table; do not use another patient's bed. *This prevents cross-contamination (the movement of micro-organisms from one patient to another) via soiled linen.*
5. Assess and assist the patient out of bed.
   - Make sure that this is an appropriate and convenient time for the patient to be out of bed.
   - Assist the patient to a comfortable chair.
6. Raise the bed to a comfortable working height.
7. Strip the bed.
   - Check bed linens for any items belonging to the patient and detach the call bell or any drainage tubes from the bed linen.
   - Loosen all bedding systematically, starting at the head of the bed on the far side and moving around the bed up to the head of the bed on the near side. *Moving around the bed systematically prevents stretching and reaching and possible muscle strain.*
   - Remove the pillowcases, if soiled, and place the pillows on the bedside chair near the foot of the bed.
   - Fold reusable linens, such as the bedspread and top sheet on the bed, into fourths. First, fold the linen in half by bringing the top edge even with the bottom edge, and then grasp it at the centre of the middle fold and bottom edges (see Figure 13-37). *Folding linens saves time and energy when reapplying the linens on the bed.*
   - Remove the waterproof pad and discard it if soiled.

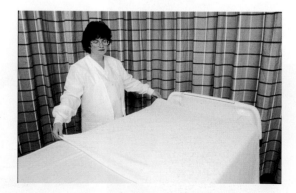

Figure 13-37 Fold reusable linens into fourths when removing them from the bed.

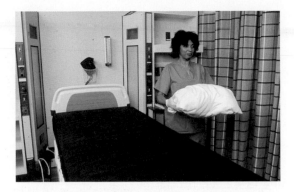

Figure 13-38 Roll soiled linen inside bottom sheet and hold away from body.

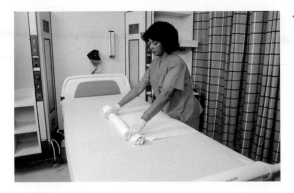

Figure 13-40 Placing drawsheet on bed.

- Roll all soiled linen inside the bottom sheet, hold it away from your uniform, and place it directly in the linen hamper (see Figure 13-38). *These actions are essential to prevent the transmission of micro-organisms to the nurse and others.*
- Grasp the mattress securely, using the lugs if present, and move the mattress up to the head of the bed.

7. Apply the bottom sheet and drawsheet.
- Place the folded bottom sheet with its centre fold on the centre of the bed. Make sure the sheet is hem side down for a smooth foundation. Spread the sheet out over the mattress, and allow a sufficient amount of sheet at the top to tuck under the mattress (see Figure 13-39). *The top of the sheet needs to be well tucked under to remain securely in place, especially when the head of the bed is elevated.* Place the sheet along the edge of the mattress at the foot of the bed and do not tuck it in (unless it is a contour or fitted sheet).
- Mitre the sheet at the top corner on the near side (Figure 13-36, earlier) and tuck the sheet under the mattress, working from the head of the bed to the foot.

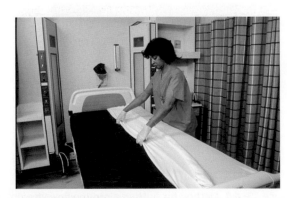

Figure 13-39 Placing bottom sheet on bed.

- If a waterproof drawsheet is used, place it over the bottom sheet so that the centrefold is at the centreline of the bed and the top and bottom edges extend from the middle of the patient's back to the area of the midthigh or knee. Fanfold the uppermost half of the folded drawsheet at the centre or far edge of the bed and tuck in the near edge (see Figure 13-40).
- Lay the cloth drawsheet over the waterproof sheet in the same manner.
- *Optional:* Before moving to the other side of the bed, place the top linens on the bed hemside up, unfold them, tuck them in and mitre the bottom corners. *Completing one entire side of the bed at a time saves time and energy.*

8. Move to the other side and secure the bottom linens.
- Tuck in the bottom sheet under the head of the mattress, pull the sheet firmly and mitre the corner of the sheet.
- Pull the remainder of the sheet firmly so that there are no wrinkles. *Wrinkles can cause discomfort for the patient. Tuck the sheet in at the side.*
- Complete this same process for the drawsheet(s).

9. Apply or complete the top sheet, blanket and spread.
- Place the top sheet, hemside up, on the bed so that its centrefold is at the centre of the bed and the top edge is even with the top edge of the mattress.
- Unfold the sheet over the bed.
- *Optional:* Make a vertical or a horizontal toe pleat in the sheet to provide additional room for the patient's feet.
  (a) *Vertical toe pleat:* Make a fold in the sheet 5–10 cm perpendicular to the foot of the bed (see Figure 13-41 on page 302).

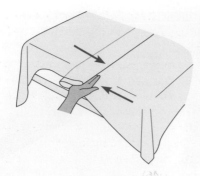

Figure 13-41 A vertical toe pleat.

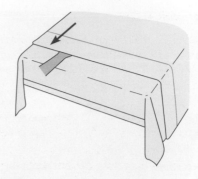

Figure 13-42 A horizontal toe pleat.

(b) Horizontal toe pleat: Make a fold in the sheet 5–10 cm across the bed near the foot (see Figure 13-42).

Loosening the top covers around the feet after the patient is in bed is another way to provide additional space.

- Follow the same procedure for the blanket and the spread, but place the top edges about 15 cm from the head of the bed to allow a cuff of sheet to be folded over them.
- Tuck in the sheet, blanket and spread at the foot of the bed, and mitre the corner, using all three layers of linen. Leave the sides of the top sheet, blanket and spread hanging freely unless toe pleats were provided.
- Fold the top of the top sheet down over the spread, providing a cuff (see Figure 13-43). *The cuff of sheet makes it easier for the patient to pull the covers up.*
- Move to the other side of the bed and secure the top bedding in the same manner.
10. Put clean pillowcases on the pillows as required.
    - Grasp the closed end of the pillowcase at the centre with one hand.
    - Gather up the sides of the pillowcase and place them over the hand grasping the case.

Then grasp the centre of one short side of the pillow through the pillowcase (see Figure 13-44).
- With the free hand, pull the pillowcase over the pillow.
- Adjust the pillowcase so that the pillow fits into the corners of the case and the seams are straight. *A smoothly fitting pillowcase is more comfortable than a wrinkled one.*
- Place the pillows appropriately at the head of the bed.
11. Provide for patient comfort and safety.
    - Attach the signal cord so that the patient can conveniently use it. Some cords have clamps that attach to the sheet or pillowcase.
    - If the bed is currently being used by a patient, either fold back the top covers at one side or fanfold them down to the centre of the bed. *This makes it easier for the patient to get into the bed.*
    - Place the bedside table and the overbed table so that they are available to the patient.
    - Leave the bed in the high position if the patient is returning by trolley or place in the low position if the patient is returning to bed after being out of bed.

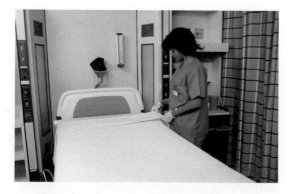

Figure 13-43 Making a cuff of the top linens.

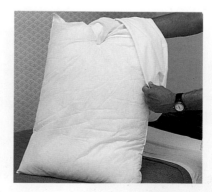

Figure 13-44 Method for putting a clean pillowcase on a pillow.

Variation: surgical bed

While the patient is in the operating theatre, the patient's bed is prepared for the post-operative phase. In some clinical areas, the patient is brought back to the ward on a trolley and transferred to the bed in the room. In others, the patient's bed is brought to the operating department and the patient is transferred there. In the latter situation, the bed needs to be made with clean linens as soon as the patient goes to theatre so that it can be taken to the operating department when needed.

+ Strip the bed.
+ Place and leave the pillows on the bedside chair. *Pillows are left on a chair to facilitate transferring the patient into the bed.*
+ Apply the bottom linens as for an unoccupied bed.
+ Place the top covers (sheet, blanket and bedspread) on the bed as you would for an unoccupied bed. Do not tuck them in, mitre the corners or make a toe pleat.

+ Make a cuff at the top of the bed as you would for an unoccupied bed. Fold the top linens up from the bottom.
+ On the side of the bed where the patient will be transferred, fold up the two outer corners of the top linens so they meet in the middle of the bed forming a triangle (see Figure 13-45).
+ Pick up the apex of the triangle and fanfold the top linens lengthwise to the other side of the bed *to facilitate the patient's transfer into the bed* (see Figure 13-46).
+ Leave the bed in high position with the side rails down. *The high position facilitates the transfer of the patient.*
+ Lock the wheels of the bed if the bed is not to be moved. *Locking the wheels keeps the bed from rolling when the patient is transferred from the trolley to the bed.*

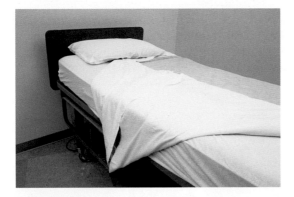

Figure 13-45 Fold up the two outer corners of the top linens forming a triangle.

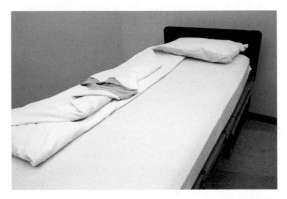

Figure 13-46 Surgical bed. The linens are horizontally fanfolded to the other side of the bed to facilitate transfer of the patient into the bed.

Evaluation

+ Make sure the call light is accessible to the patient.
+ Relate patient parameters of activity (e.g. pulse and respirations) to previous assessment data

particularly if the patient has been on bedrest for an extended period of time or it is the first time that the patient is getting out of bed after surgery.

Changing an Occupied Bed

Some patients may be too weak to get out of bed. Either the nature of their illness may contraindicate their sitting out of bed, or they may be restricted in bed by the presence of traction or other therapies. When changing an occupied bed (see *Procedure 13-10* on page 304), the nurse works quickly and disturbs the patient as little as possible to conserve the patient's energy, using the following guidelines:

+ Maintain the patient in good body alignment. Never move or position a patient in a manner that is contraindicated by the patient's health. Obtain help to ensure safety.
+ Move the patient gently and smoothly. Rough handling can cause the patient discomfort and abrade the skin.
+ Explain what you plan to do throughout the procedure before you do it. Use terms that the patient can understand.
+ Use the bed-making time, like the bed bath time, to assess and meet the patient's needs.

PROCEDURE 13-10 Changing an Occupied Bed

Purposes

+ To conserve the patient's energy and maintain current healthy status
+ To promote patient comfort
+ To provide a clean, neat environment for the patient
+ To provide a smooth, wrinkle-free bed foundation, thus minimising sources of skin irritation

Assessment

+ Note specific precautions for moving and positioning the patient
+ Determine presence of incontinence or excessive drainage from other sources indicating the need for protective waterproof pads
+ Assess skin condition and need for special mattress, footboard or heel protectors

Planning

Equipment

+ Two flat sheets
+ Cloth drawsheet (optional)
+ One blanket
+ One bedspread
+ Waterproof drawsheet or waterproof pads (optional)
+ Pillowcase(s) for the head pillow(s)
+ Plastic laundry bag or portable linen hamper, if available

Implementation

Performance

1. Explain to the patient what you are going to do, why it is necessary and how they can cooperate.
2. Wash hands and observe other appropriate infection control procedures. Put on disposable gloves if linen is soiled with body fluids.
3. Provide for patient privacy.
4. Remove the top bedding.
   • Remove any equipment attached to the bed linen, such as a signal light.
   • Loosen all the top linen at the foot of the bed and remove the spread and the blanket.
   • Leave the top sheet over the patient (the top sheet can remain over the patient if it is being changed and if it will provide sufficient warmth).
5. Change the bottom sheet and drawsheet.
   • Assist the patient to turn on the side facing away from the side where the clean linen is.
   • Raise the side rail nearest the patient. *This protects the patient from falling.* If there is no side rail, have another nurse support the patient at the edge of the bed.
   • Loosen the foundation of the linen on the side of the bed near the linen supply.

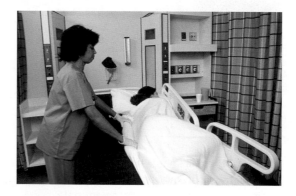

Figure 13-47 Moving soiled linen as close to the patient as possible.

   • Fanfold the drawsheet and the bottom sheet at the centre of the bed (see Figure 13-47), as close to the patient as possible. *Doing this leaves the near half of the bed free to be changed.*
   • Place the new bottom sheet on the bed, and vertically fanfold the half to be used on the far side of the bed as close to the patient as possible (see Figure 13-48). Tuck the sheet under the near half of the bed and mitre the corner if a contour sheet is not being used.

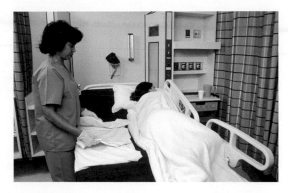

Figure 13-48 Placing new bottom sheet on half of the bed.

- Place the clean drawsheet on the bed with the centre fold at the centre of the bed. Fanfold the uppermost half vertically at the centre of the bed and tuck the near side edge under the side of the mattress (Figure 13-49).
- Assist the patient to roll over toward you onto the clean side of the bed. The patient rolls over the fanfolded linen at the centre of the bed.

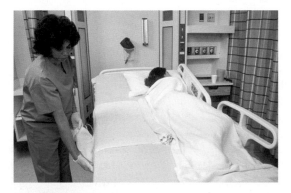

Figure 13-49 Placing clean drawsheet on the bed.

- Move the pillows to the clean side for the patient's use. Raise the side rail before leaving the side of the bed.
- Move to the other side of the bed and lower the side rail.
- Remove the used linen and place it in the portable hamper.
- Unfold the fanfolded bottom sheet from the centre of the bed.
- Facing the side of the bed, use both hands to pull the bottom sheet so that it is smooth and tuck the excess under the side of the mattress.
- Unfold the drawsheet fanfolded at the centre of the bed and pull it tightly with both hands. Pull the sheet in three sections: (a) face the side of the bed to pull the middle section, (b) face the far top corner to pull the bottom section and (c) face the far bottom corner to pull the top section.
- Tuck the excess drawsheet under the side of the mattress.

6. Reposition the patient in the centre of the bed.
   - Reposition the pillows at the centre of the bed.
   - Assist the patient to the centre of the bed. Determine what position the patient requires or prefers and assist the patient to that position.

7. Apply or complete the top bedding.
   - Spread the top sheet over the patient and either ask the patient to hold the top edge of the sheet or tuck it under the shoulders.
   - Complete the top of the bed.

8. Ensure continued safety of the patient.
   - Raise the side rails. Place the bed in the low position before leaving the bedside.
   - Attach the signal cord to the bed linen within the patient's reach.
   - Put items used by the patient within easy reach.

Evaluation

+ Conduct appropriate follow-up, such as determining patient's comfort and safety, patency of all drainage tubes and patient's access to call light to summon help when needed.

CRITICAL REFLECTION

Let us revisit the case study on page 254. Now that you have read this chapter what approaches might you use if you feel that the patient does need her hair shampooed and needs to have her personal care attended to? What advantages do bathing patients and attending to their personal hygiene have for the nurse?

CHAPTER HIGHLIGHTS

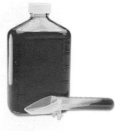

+ Patients' hygienic practices are influenced by numerous factors including culture, religion, environment, developmental level, health and energy and personal preferences.
+ The major functions of the skin are to: protect underlying tissues; help regulate body temperature; secrete sebum; transmit sensations through nerve receptors for sensory perception; and produce and absorb vitamin D in conjunction with ultraviolet rays from the sun.
+ When planning hygiene care, the nurse must take the patient's preferences into consideration.
+ Nurses provide perineal-genital care for patients who are unable to do so for themselves.
+ Nurses can often teach patients how to prevent foot problems.

+ Oral hygiene should include daily dental flossing and mechanical brushing of the teeth.
+ Regular dental checkups and fluoride supplements are recommended to maintain healthy teeth.
+ Nurses provide special oral care to patients who are unconscious or debilitated.
+ Hair care includes daily combing and brushing and regular shampooing.
+ Nurses may need to assist dependent patients with their artificial eyes, eyeglasses and contact lenses.
+ Patients with a hearing aid may require nursing assistance with the device.
+ Changing bed linens is a part of maintaining hygiene.
+ It is important to keep beds clean and comfortable for patients.

REFERENCES

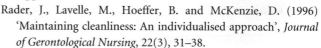

Andrews, M.M. and Boyle, J.S. (2003) *Transcultural concepts in nursing care* (4th edn), Philadelphia: Lippincott Williams and Wilkins.

Brawley, E.C. (2002) 'Bathing environments: How to improve the bathing experience', *Alzheimer's Care Quarterly*, 3(1), 38–41.

Frankowski, B.L. and Weiner, L.B. (2002) 'Head lice', *Pediatrics*, 110(3), 638–643.

Hektor, L.M. and Touhy, T.A. (1997) The history of the bath: From art to task? *Journal of Gerontological Nursing*, 23(5), 7–15.

Jackson, F. (1998) 'The ABC's of black hair and skin care', *The ABNF Journal*, 9(5), 100–104.

Pillitteri, A. (2003) *Maternal and child health nursing: Care of the child bearing and child-rearing family* (4th edn), Philadelphia: Lippincott Williams and Wilkins.

Rader, J., Lavelle, M., Hoeffer, B. and McKenzie, D. (1996) 'Maintaining cleanliness: An individualised approach', *Journal of Gerontological Nursing*, 22(3), 31–38.

Skewes, S. (1997) 'Bathing: It's a tough job!', *Journal of Gerontological Nursing*, 23(5), 45–49.

Talerico, K.A. and Capezuti, E. (2001) 'Myths and facts about side rails', *American Journal of Nursing*, 101(7), 43–48.

Walton, J.C., Miller, J. and Tordecilla, L. (2001) 'Elder oral assessment and care', *MEDSURG Nursing*, 10(1), 37–44.

Chapter 14

Skin Integrity and Wound Care

Learning Outcomes

After completing this chapter, you will be able to:

+ Describe factors affecting skin integrity.

+ Identify patients at risk for pressure ulcer formation and describe the four stages of pressure ulcer development.

+ Differentiate primary and secondary wound healing.

+ Describe the three phases of wound healing.

+ Identify the main complications of and factors that affect wound healing.

+ Discuss assessment information required when assessing a patient with a wound.

+ Identify essential aspects of planning care to maintain skin integrity and promote wound healing.

+ Discuss measures to prevent pressure ulcer formation.

+ Describe nursing strategies to treat pressure ulcers, promote wound healing and prevent complications of wound healing.

+ Identify purposes of commonly used wound dressing materials and binders.

CASE STUDY

Maggot or larval therapy has been around for hundreds of years. Ambroise Pare (1509-1590), chief surgeon to King Charles IX and Henry III, first noted wounds infested with maggots during the Battle of St Quentin (in 1557). Then in the 19th century Napoleon's Surgeon in Chief, Baron Dominic Larrey, reported that the presence of maggots in battle wounds prevented infection and accelerated healing. However there is no evidence that either of these surgeons deliberately introduced maggots into wounds.

The real founder of maggot therapy though is William Baer (1872-1931) who was the Clinical Professor of Orthopaedic Surgery in Maryland, USA. Baer documented how he treated two First World War soldiers, one of which had a compound fracture (where the broken bone breaks through the skin) of the femur (thigh) bone and the other had large wounds to his abdomen and scrotum. Both men had been overlooked on the battlefield for seven days, but did not show any signs of fever or septicaemia. When their clothes were removed Baer found that the wounds were filled with thousands of maggots. When the maggots were removed, to Baer's amazement, the wounds were clean and there was even granulating tissue in them.

Baer went on to treat four children with osteomyelitis (bone infection) with unsterilised maggots with great success. However some of his subsequent patients he treated with unsterilised maggots were not so lucky – they developed tetanus. Baer concluded that he would have to use sterile maggots for future patients. Eventually Baer developed a way of ensuring that the maggots were sterile by exposing them to a concoction of mercuric chloride, alcohol and hydrochloric acid.

Today larval therapy is a common treatment for many necrotic wounds. Maggots both debride (remove the dead tissue) and remove bacteria from the wound. They are available loose or within dressings and are becoming an acceptable treatment with healthcare professionals and patients alike.

This chapter will consider skin integrity and the importance of assessment. It will also consider some treatments available for patients with wounds.

INTRODUCTION

The skin is the largest organ in the body and serves a variety of important functions in maintaining health and protecting the individual from injury. Important nursing functions are maintaining skin integrity and promoting wound healing. Impaired skin integrity is not a frequent problem for most healthy people but is a threat to older people; to patients with restricted mobility, chronic illnesses or trauma; and to those undergoing invasive procedures. To protect the skin and manage wounds effectively, the nurse must understand the factors affecting skin integrity, the physiology of wound healing and specific measures that promote optimal skin conditions.

SKIN INTEGRITY

Intact skin refers to the presence of normal skin and skin layers uninterrupted by wounds. The appearance of the skin and skin integrity are influenced by intrinsic factors such as genetics, age and the underlying health of the individual as well as extrinsic factors such as activity, nutrition and smoking.

Genetics and heredity determine many aspects of a person's skin, including skin colour, sensitivity to sunlight and allergies.

Age influences skin integrity in that the skin of both the very young and the very old is more fragile and susceptible to injury than that of most adults. Wounds tend to heal more rapidly in infants and children, however.

Many chronic illnesses and their treatments affect skin integrity. People with impaired peripheral arterial circulation may have skin on the legs that appears shiny, has lost its hair distribution and damages easily. Some medications, corticosteroids for example, cause thinning of the skin and allow it to be much more readily harmed (Charman et al., 2000). Many medications increase sensitivity to sunlight and can predispose one to severe sunburns. Some of the most common ones that cause this damage are certain antibiotics, chemotherapy drugs for cancer (Bellnier et al., 2006), and some psychotherapeutic drugs. Poor nutrition alone can interfere with the appearance and function of normal skin.

TYPES OF WOUNDS

Wounds may be described according to how they are acquired (see Table 14-1) and may be intentional or unintentional.

Wounds are also classified by depth, that is, the tissue layers involved in the wound (see Box 14-1).

Table 14-1 Types of Wounds

Type	Cause	Description and characteristics
Incision	Sharp instrument (e.g. knife or scalpel)	Open wound; deep or shallow
Contusion	Blow from a blunt instrument	Closed wound, skin appears ecchymotic (bruised) because of damaged blood vessels
Abrasion	Surface scrape, either unintentional (e.g. scraped knee from a fall) or intentional (e.g. dermal abrasion to remove pockmarks)	Open wound involving the skin
Puncture	Penetration of the skin and often the underlying tissues by a sharp instrument, either intentional or unintentional	Open wound
Laceration	Tissues torn apart, often from accidents (e.g. with machinery)	Open wound; edges are often jagged
Penetrating wound	Penetration of the skin and the underlying tissues, usually unintentional (e.g. from a bullet or metal fragments)	Open wound

BOX 14-1 Classifying Wounds by Depth

Partial thickness: Confined to the skin, that is, the dermis and epidermis; heal by regeneration.

Full thickness: Involving the dermis, epidermis, subcutaneous tissue and possibly muscle and bone; require connective tissue repair.

PRESSURE ULCERS

Pressure ulcers were previously called **decubitus ulcers**, *pressure sores* or *bedsores*. A pressure ulcer is an area of localised tissue damage believed to be caused by a combination of pressure, shear and friction (European Pressure Ulcer Advisory Panel (EPUAP), 1999).

Pressure ulcers are a problem in both primary and acute care settings. According to Bennett *et al.* (2004) 412,000 individuals will develop a new pressure ulcer each year, putting an immense strain on the finances of the NHS. Bennett *et al.* (2004) goes on to say that pressure ulcers costs the health and social care system approximately £1.77 billion each year.

Aetiology of Pressure Ulcers

Pressure ulcers are due to localised **ischaemia**, a deficiency in the blood supply to the tissue. The tissue is caught between two hard surfaces, usually the surface of the bed and the bony skeleton. When blood cannot reach the tissue, the cells are deprived of oxygen and nutrients, the waste products of metabolism accumulate in the cells and the tissue consequently dies. Prolonged, unrelieved pressure also damages the small blood vessels.

After the skin has been compressed, it appears pale, as if the blood had been squeezed out of it. When pressure is relieved, the skin takes on a bright red flush, called **reactive hyperaemia**, which is the body's mechanism for preventing pressure ulcers. The flush is due to **vasodilation**, a process in which extra blood floods to the area to compensate for the preceding period of impeded blood flow.

Two other factors frequently act in conjunction with pressure to produce pressure ulcers: friction and shearing force. **Friction** is force acting parallel to the skin surface. For example, sheets rubbing against skin create friction. Friction can abrade the skin, that is, remove the superficial layers, making it more prone to breakdown.

Shearing force is a parallel force that twists and stretches tissues in opposite directions and causes tissue ischaemia by moving vessels laterally and impeding the flow of blood. This can be best illustrated by observing a patient sitting up in bed. The body will tend to slide downwards towards the foot of the bed. This downward movement is transmitted to the sacral bone and the deep tissues. At the same time, the skin over the sacrum tends not to move because of the adherence between the skin and the bed sheets. The skin and superficial tissues are thus relatively unmoving in relation to the bed surface, whereas the deeper tissues are firmly attached to the skeleton and move downward. This causes a shearing force in the area where the deeper tissues and the superficial tissues meet.

Risk Factors

Several factors contribute to the formation of pressure ulcers: immobility and inactivity, inadequate nutrition, faecal and urinary incontinence, decreased mental capacity, diminished sensation, excessive body heat, ageing and the presence of certain chronic conditions.

Immobility

Immobility refers to a reduction in the amount and control of movement a person has. Normally people move when they experience discomfort due to pressure on an area of the body. Healthy people rarely exceed their tolerance to pressure. However, paralysis, extreme weakness, pain or any cause of decreased activity can hinder a person's ability to change positions independently and relieve the pressure, even if the person can perceive the pressure. According to Margolis *et al.* (2003) immobility is consistently a determining factor in the development of pressure ulcers.

Inadequate Nutrition

According to Russell (2000) adequate nutrition is needed to maintain skin integrity. Prolonged inadequate nutrition causes weight loss, muscle atrophy and the loss of subcutaneous tissue. These three reduce the amount of padding between the skin and the bones, thus increasing the risk of pressure ulcer development. More specifically, inadequate intake of protein, carbohydrates, fluids and vitamin C contribute to pressure ulcer formation.

CLINICAL ANECDOTE

The worst wound I ever saw was a pressure ulcer. The lady came into hospital from a nursing home with the wound. The pressure ulcer was on her sacrum and you could see the bone. It was disgusting. Funnily enough the patient didn't seem to have much pain with it. I guess it was so deep that the nerves had been damaged.

Nicola Davies, staff nurse

Hypoproteinemia (abnormally low protein content in the blood), due either to inadequate intake or abnormal loss, predisposes the patient to dependent oedema. Oedema (the presence of excess fluid in the tissues) makes skin more prone to injury by decreasing its elasticity, resilience and vitality. Oedema increases the distance between the capillaries and the cells, thereby slowing the diffusion of oxygen to the tissue cells and of metabolites away from the cells.

Faecal and Urinary Incontinence

Moisture from incontinence promotes skin **maceration** (tissue softened by prolonged wetting or soaking) and makes the epidermis more easily eroded and susceptible to injury. Digestive enzymes in faeces also contribute to skin **excoriation** (area of loss of the superficial layers of the skin). Any accumulation of secretions or excretions is irritating to the skin, harbours micro-organisms, and makes an individual prone to skin breakdown and infection. Cooper and Gray (2001) recognise that incontinence is a major causative factor in pressure ulcer development and state that maintaining skin integrity for a patient with incontinence is challenging for healthcare professionals.

Decreased Mental Capacity

Individuals with a reduced level of awareness, for example, those who are unconscious or heavily sedated, are at risk for pressure ulcers because they are less able to recognise and respond to pain associated with prolonged pressure (Bours *et al.*, 2001).

Diminished Sensation

Paralysis, stroke or other neurological disease may cause loss of sensation in a body area. Loss of sensation reduces a person's ability to respond to injurious heat and cold and to feel the tingling ('pins and needles') that signals loss of circulation. Keller *et al.* (2002) suggest that this is a particular problem with intensive care patients as they have reduced sensation due to analgesics and sedation and are unable to feel the painful stimuli of pressure so do not feel the need to or cannot change position to relieve the pressure.

Excessive Body Heat

Body heat is another factor in the development of pressure ulcers. An elevated body temperature increases the metabolic rate, thus increasing the cells' need for oxygen. This increased need is particularly severe in the cells of an area under pressure, which are already oxygen deficient. Severe infections with accompanying elevated body temperatures may affect the body's ability to deal with the effects of tissue compression.

Advanced Age

The ageing process brings about several changes in the skin and its supporting structures, making the older person more prone to impaired skin integrity. These changes include the following:

+ loss of lean body mass;
+ generalised thinning of the epidermis;
+ decreased strength and elasticity of the skin due to changes in the collagen fibres of the dermis;
+ increased dryness due to a decrease in the amount of oil produced by the sebaceous glands;
+ diminished pain perception due to a reduction in the number of cutaneous end organs responsible for the sensation of pressure and light touch.

Ayello and Braden (2002) suggest that people aged over 80 are at increased risk of pressure ulcers and therefore should be taken into account when measuring a patient's risk of developing pressure ulcers.

Chronic Medical Conditions

Certain chronic conditions such as diabetes and cardiovascular disease are risk factors for skin breakdown and delayed healing. These conditions compromise oxygen delivery to tissues by poor perfusion and thus cause poor and delayed healing and increase risk of pressure sores. Margolis *et al.* (2003) suggest that the presence of a medical condition such as diabetes increases the patient's likelihood of developing pressure ulcers and states identification of these medical conditions should override identification of other risk factors such as incontinence and immobility.

Other Factors

Other factors contributing to the formation of pressure ulcers are poor lifting techniques (RCN, 2001), incorrect positioning, repeated injections in the same area, hard support surfaces, and incorrect application of pressure-relieving devices.

Stages of Pressure Ulcer Formation

The four recognised stages of pressure ulcer formation related to observable tissue damage are shown in Figure 14-1.

WOUND HEALING

For living organisms, the ability to repair tissue that has been damaged is imperative to survival. Regardless of the severity of the injury, there are two mechanisms for the repair of tissue: regeneration (renewal of tissues) or connective tissue repair (replacement of the damaged tissue with a scar). Humans have limited ability to regenerate new tissue, but tend to heal by connective tissue repair.

Healing can be considered in terms of *types of healing* and *phases of healing*.

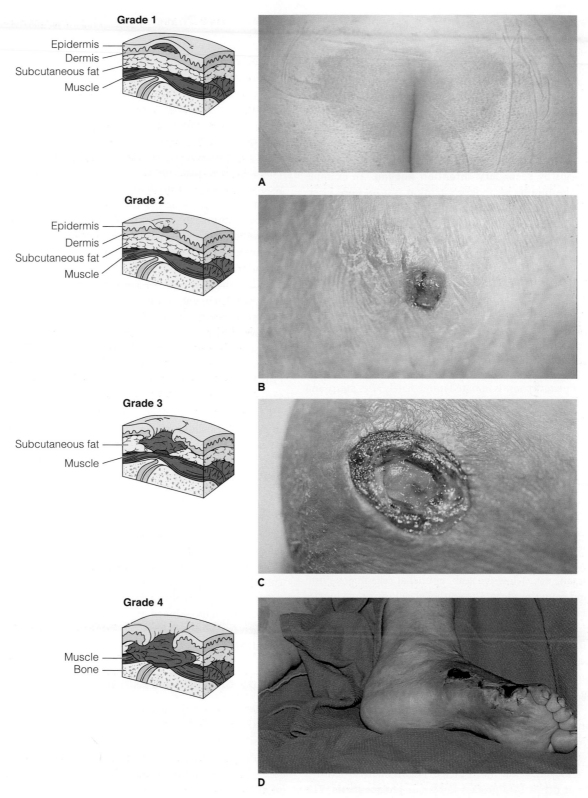

Figure 14-1 Four grades of pressure ulcers. *A*, grade 1: nonblanchable erythema signalling potential ulceration; *B*, grade 2: partial-thickness skin loss (abrasion, blister or shallow crater) involving the epidermis and possibly the dermis; *C*, grade 3: full-thickness skin loss involving damage or necrosis of subcutaneous tissue that may extend down to, but not through, underlying fascia. The ulcer presents clinically as a deep crater with or without undermining of adjacent tissue. *D*, grade 4: full-thickness skin loss with tissue necrosis or damage to muscle, bone or supporting structures, such as a tendon or joint capsule. Undermining and sinus tracts may also be present. (Line Art From 'Clinical Practice Guideline, Pressure Ulcers in Adults: Prediction and Prevention,' by U.S. Department of Health and Human Services, PPPPUA, Pub. no. 92-0047, 1992, Rockville, MD: Public Health Service. Reprinted with permission.) EPUAP (2003) Classification system.

Types of Wound Healing

There are two types of healing, influenced by the amount of tissue loss. **Primary intention healing** occurs where the tissue surfaces have been **approximated** (closed) and there is minimal or no tissue loss; it is characterised by the formation of minimal granulation tissue and scarring. An example of wound healing by primary intention is a closed surgical incision.

A wound that is extensive and involves considerable tissue loss, and in which the edges cannot or should not be approximated, heals by **secondary intention healing**. An example of wound healing by secondary intention is a pressure ulcer. Secondary intention healing differs from primary intention healing in three ways: (a) the repair time is longer, (b) the scarring is greater and (c) the susceptibility to infection is greater.

Stages of Wound Healing

Wound healing can be broken down into three stages: inflammatory, proliferative and maturation or remodelling.

Inflammatory Phase

The *inflammatory phase* is initiated immediately after injury and lasts three to six days. Two major processes occur during this phase: haemostasis and phagocytosis.

Haemostasis (the cessation of bleeding) results from vasoconstriction of the larger blood vessels in the affected area, retraction (drawing back) of injured blood vessels, the deposition of **fibrin** (connective tissue) and the formation of blood clots in the area. The blood clots, formed from blood platelets, provide a matrix of fibrin that becomes the framework for cell repair. A scab also forms on the surface of the wound. Consisting of clots and dead and dying tissue, this scab serves to aid haemostasis and inhibit contamination of the wound by micro-organisms. Below the scab, epithelial cells migrate into the wound from the edges. The epithelial cells serve as a barrier between the body and the environment, preventing the entry of micro-organisms.

The inflammatory phase also involves vascular and cellular responses intended to remove any foreign substances and dead and dying tissues. The blood supply to the wound increases, bringing with it oxygen and nutrients needed in the healing process. The area appears reddened and oedematous as a result.

During cell migration, leukocytes (specifically, neutrophils) move into the interstitial space. These are replaced about 24 hours after injury by macrophages, which arise from the blood monocytes. These macrophages engulf micro-organisms and cellular debris by a process known as **phagocytosis**. The macrophages also secrete an angiogenesis factor (AGF), which stimulates the formation of epithelial buds at the end of injured blood vessels. The microcirculatory network that results sustains the healing process and the wound during its life. This inflammatory response is essential to healing, and measures that impair inflammation, such as steroid medications, can place the healing process at risk.

Proliferative Phase

The *proliferative phase*, the second phase in healing, extends from day three or four to about day 21 post-injury. Fibroblasts (connective tissue cells), which migrate into the wound starting about 24 hours after injury, begin to synthesise collagen. **Collagen** is a whitish protein substance that adds tensile strength to the wound. As the amount of collagen increases, so does the strength of the wound, thus the chance that the wound will open progressively decreases. If the wound is sutured, a raised 'healing ridge' appears under the intact suture line. In a wound that is not sutured, the new collagen is often visible.

Capillaries grow across the wound, increasing the blood supply. Fibroblasts move from the bloodstream into the wound, depositing fibrin. As the capillary network develops, the tissue becomes a translucent red colour. This tissue, called **granulation tissue**, is fragile and bleeds easily.

When the skin edges of a wound are not sutured, the area must be filled in with granulation tissue. When the granulation tissue matures, marginal epithelial cells migrate to it, proliferating over this connective tissue base to fill the wound. If the wound does not close by epithelialisation, the area becomes covered with dried plasma proteins and dead cells. This is called **eschar**. Initially, wounds healing by secondary intention seep blood-tinged (serosanguineous) drainage. Later, if they are not covered by epithelial cells, they become covered with thick, grey, fibrinous tissue that is eventually converted into dense scar tissue.

Maturation Phase

The *maturation phase* begins about day 21 and can extend one or two years after the injury. Fibroblasts continue to synthesise collagen. The collagen fibres themselves, which were initially laid in a haphazard fashion, reorganise into a more orderly structure. During maturation, the wound is remodelled and contracted. The scar becomes stronger but the repaired area is never as strong as the original tissue. In some individuals, particularly dark-skinned persons, an abnormal amount of collagen is laid down. This can result in a hypertrophic scar, or **keloid**.

Kinds of Wound Drainage

Exudate is material, such as fluid and cells, which has escaped from blood vessels during the inflammatory process and is deposited in tissue or on tissue surfaces. The nature and amount of exudate vary according to the tissue involved, the intensity and duration of the inflammation, and the presence of micro-organisms.

There are three major types of exudate: serous, purulent and sanguineous (haemorrhagic). A **serous exudate** consists chiefly of serum (the clear portion of the blood) derived from blood and the serous membranes of the body. It looks watery and has few cells. An example is the fluid in a blister from a burn.

A **purulent exudate** is thicker than serous exudate because of the presence of **pus**, which consists of leukocytes, liquefied dead tissue debris and dead and living bacteria. Purulent exudates vary in colour, some acquiring tinges of blue, green or yellow. The colour may depend on the causative organism.

Haemorrhagic exudate consists of large amounts of red blood cells, indicating damage to capillaries that is severe enough to allow the escape of red blood cells from plasma. This type of exudate is frequently seen in open wounds.

> **CLINICAL ALERT**
>
> *A bright haemorrhagic exudate indicates fresh bleeding, whereas dark sanguineous exudate denotes older bleeding.*

Mixed types of exudates are often observed. A *haemoserous* (consisting of clear and blood-tinged drainage) exudate is commonly seen in surgical incisions.

Complications of Wound Healing

Several untoward events can occur to interfere with the healing of a wound. These include excessive bleeding, infection and dehiscence.

Haemorrhage

Some escape of blood from a wound is normal. **Haemorrhage** (massive bleeding), however, is abnormal. It may be caused by a dislodged clot, a slipped stitch or erosion of a blood vessel, for example.

Internal haemorrhage may be detected by swelling or distention in the area of the wound and, possibly, by the presence of blood in a surgical drain. Some patients will have a **haematoma**, a localised collection of blood underneath the skin that may appear as a reddish blue swelling (bruise). A large haematoma may be dangerous in that it places pressure on blood vessels and can thus obstruct blood flow.

The risk of haemorrhage is greatest during the first 48 hours after surgery. Haemorrhage is an emergency; the nurse should apply pressure dressings to the area and monitor the patient's vital signs. Medical advice should be sought immediately as the patient may need to be taken to theatre for surgical intervention.

Infection

Colonisation is the presence of micro-organisms without illness or reaction. Most if not all wounds are contaminated as the skin is surrounded by micro-organisms. These micro-organisms compete with the new cells in the wound for oxygen and nutrition and as a result can delay wound healing. If these micro-organisms multiply excessively or invade tissues, infection can result. If a wound and surrounding tissues become infected there are generally a few tell-tale signs including:

+ pain,
+ change in the colour of the wound bed,
+ malodorous (offensive smelling) exudate,
+ heat,
+ swelling.

If infection is suspected the nurse should swab the wound and send it for culture and sensitivity. This test will identify the micro-organism and suggest a drug that the micro-organism is sensitive to. Severe infection causes fever and elevated white blood cell count. Patients who are immunosuppressed are especially susceptible to wound infections.

A wound can be infected with micro-organisms at the time of injury, during surgery or postoperatively. Wounds that occur as a result of injury (e.g. bullet and knife wounds) are most likely to be contaminated at the time of injury. Surgery involving the intestines can also result in infection from the micro-organisms inside the intestine.

Dehiscence

Dehiscence is the partial or total rupturing of a sutured wound. Dehiscence usually involves an abdominal wound in which the layers below the skin also separate. A number of factors, including obesity, poor nutrition, multiple trauma, failure of suturing, excessive coughing, vomiting and dehydration, heighten a patient's risk of wound dehiscence. Wound infection can be the cause of the wound dehiscing (Tobon *et al.*, 2003).

Dehiscence may be preceded by sudden straining, such as coughing or sneezing. It is not unusual for a patient to feel that 'something has given away'. When dehiscence occurs, the wound should be quickly supported by large sterile dressings, the patient should be placed in a bed in a position that puts as little pressure on the wound as possible. The surgeon must be notified because immediate surgical repair of the area may be necessary.

Factors Affecting Wound Healing

Characteristics of the individual such as age, nutritional status, lifestyle and medications influence the speed of wound healing.

Developmental Considerations

Healthy children and adults often heal more quickly than older people, who are more likely to have chronic diseases that hinder healing. For example, reduced liver function can impair the synthesis of blood clotting factors. Box 14-2 on page 314 lists factors inhibiting wound healing in older adults.

Nutrition

Wound healing places additional demands on the body. Patients with wounds require a diet rich in protein, carbohydrates, lipids, vitamins A and C and minerals, such as iron, zinc and copper (Anderson, 2005). Malnourished patients may require time to improve their nutritional status before surgery, if this is possible.

BOX 14-2 Factors Inhibiting Wound Healing in Older Adults

+ Vascular changes associated with ageing, such as atherosclerosis and atrophy of capillaries in the skin, can impair blood flow to the wound.
+ Collagen tissue is less flexible, which increases the risk of damage from pressure, friction and shearing.
+ Scar tissue is less elastic.
+ Changes in the immune system may reduce the formation of the antibodies and monocytes necessary for wound healing.

+ Nutritional deficiencies may reduce the numbers of red blood cells and leukocytes, thus impeding the delivery of oxygen and the inflammatory response essential for wound healing. Oxygen is needed for the synthesis of collagen and the formation of new epithelial cells.
+ Having diabetes or cardiovascular disease increases the risk of delayed healing due to impaired oxygen delivery to these tissues.
+ Cell renewal is slower, leading to delayed healing.

Lifestyle

People who exercise regularly tend to have good circulation and because blood brings oxygen and nourishment to the wound, they are more likely to heal quickly. Smoking reduces the amount of functional haemoglobin in the blood, thus limiting the oxygen-carrying capacity of the blood, and constricts arterioles (Whiteford, 2003).

Medications

Anti-inflammatory drugs (e.g. steroids and aspirin) interfere with healing as they prevent the necessary inflammation of the wound (Dahners and Mullis, 2004). Prolonged use of antibiotics may make a person susceptible to wound infection by resistant organisms.

NURSING MANAGEMENT

ASSESSING

Assessment of Skin Integrity

The nurse conducts an examination of the skin as part of the initial and ongoing assessment of the patient.

Assessment

During the initial assessment of the patient, the nurse elicits information regarding the integrity of the patient's skin. In particular, the nurse obtains information regarding skin diseases, previous bruising, general skin condition, skin lesions and usual healing of wounds. By examining and feeling the skin the nurse can gain information on the patient's skin colour, skin turgor (elasticity), presence of oedema (swelling) and the characteristics of any wounds that may be present. Particular attention should be paid to skin condition in areas most likely to break down: in skin folds such as under the breasts, in areas that are frequently moist such as the perineum, and in areas that receive extensive pressure such as the coccyx and trochanters (hips) (see Figure 14-2).

Risk Assessment Tools

Patients may be at risk of pressure ulcers therefore the nurse should assess the patient's likelihood of developing pressure ulcers. Several risk assessment tools are available that provide the nurse with systematic means of identifying patients at high risk for pressure ulcer development.

The most common pressure ulcer risk assessment tool used in the UK is the Waterlow risk assessment scale which was developed in 1984 by Judy Waterlow a British State Registered Nurse. The tool is a simplistic scoring system when used with the nurses clinical judgement can indicate the patient's risk of developing pressure ulcers (Waterlow, 1997). The score provides objective data for the prevention and management of patients at risk of developing pressure ulcers (see Figure 14-3).

Another tool available within the UK is the Braden Scale for Predicting Pressure Sore Risk which was published in 1987 by Bergstrom, Braden, Laguzza and Holman. Their scale consists of six subscales: sensory perception, moisture, activity, mobility, nutrition, and friction and shear (see Figure 14-4 on page 316).

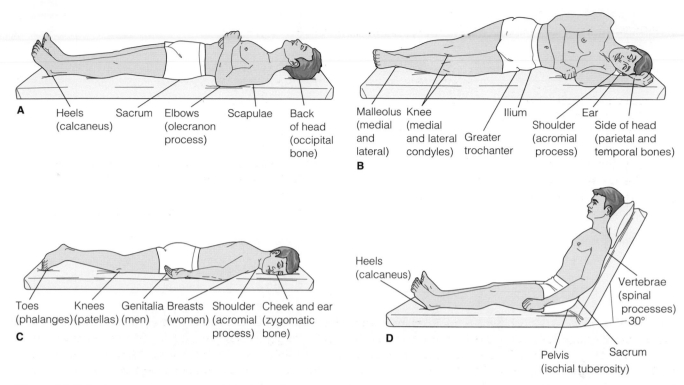

Figure 14-2 Body pressure areas: in *A*, supine position; *B*, lateral position; *C*, prone position; *D*, Fowler's position.

WATERLOW PRESSURE ULCER PREVENTION/TREATMENT POLICY
RING SCORES IN TABLE, ADD TOTAL. MORE THAN 1 SCORE/CATEGORY CAN BE USED

BUILD/WEIGHT FOR HEIGHT	◆	SKIN TYPE VISUAL RISK AREAS	◆	SEX AGE	◆	MALNUTRITION SCREENING TOOL (MST) Nutrition Vol.15, No.6 1999 – Australia		
AVERAGE BMI = 20–24.9	0	HEALTHY	0	MALE	1	A – HAS PATIENT LOST WEIGHT RECENTLY	B – WEIGHT LOSS SCORE	
		TISSUE PAPER	1	FEMALE	2	YES – GO TO B	0.5 – 5kg = 1	
ABOVE AVERAGE BMI = 25–29.9	1	DRY	1	14–49	1	NO – GO TO C	5 – 10kg = 2	
		OEDEMATOUS	1	50–64	2	UNSURE – GO TO C AND	10 – 15kg = 3	
OBESE BMI > 30	2	CLAMMY. PYREXIA	1	65–74	3	SCORE 2	> 15kg = 4	
		DISCOLOURED	1				unsure = 2	
BELOW AVERAGE BMI < 20	3	GRADE 1	2	75–80	4	C – PATIENT EATING POORLY OR LACK OF APPETITE 'NO' = 0; 'YES' SCORE = 1	NUTRITION SCORE If > 2 refer for nutrition assessment/Intervention	
BMI=Wt(Kg)/Ht (m)²		BROKEN/SPOTS GRADE 2–4	3	81+	5			

CONTINENCE	◆	MOBILITY	◆	SPECIAL RISK				
COMPLETE/ CATHETERISED	0	FULLY	0	TISSUE MALNUTRITION	◆	NEUROLOGICAL DEFICIT		◆
		RESTLESS/FIDGETY	1					
URINE INCONT.	1	APATHETIC	2	TERMINAL CACHEXIA	8	DIABETES, MS, CVA		4–6
FAECAL INCONT.	2	RESTRICTED	3	MULTIPLE ORGAN FAILURE	8	MOTOR/SENSORY		4–6
URINARY + FAECAL INCONTINENCE	3	BEDBOUND e.g. TRACTION	4	SINGLE ORGAN FAILURE (RESP, RENAL, CARDIAC.)	5	PARAPLEGIA (MAX OF 6)		4–6
		CHAIRBOUND e.g. WHEELCHAIR	5	PERIPHERAL VASCULAR DISEASE	5	MAJOR SURGERY or TRAUMA		
SCORE						ORTHOPAEDIC/SPINAL		5
10+ AT RISK				ANAEMIA (Hb < 8)	2	ON TABLE > 2 HR#		5
15+ HIGH RISK				SMOKING	1	ON TABLE > 6 HR#		8
20+ VERY HIGH RISK				MEDICATION – CYTOTOXICS, LONG TERM/HIGH DOSE STEROIDS, ANTI-INFLAMMATORY MAX OF 4				

Scores can be discounted after 48 hours provided patient is recovering normally

Figure 14-3 Waterlow Pressure Ulcer Prevention Risk Assessment Tool.

BRADEN SCALE FOR PREDICTING PRESSURE SORE RISK

Patient's Name _____   Evaluator's Name _____   Date of Assessment

SENSORY PERCEPTION Ability to respond meaningfully to pressure-related discomfort	**1. Completely Limited:** Unresponsive (does not moan, flinch or grasp) to painful stimuli, due to diminished level of consciousness or sedation, OR limited ability to feel pain over most of body surface.	**2. Very Limited:** Responds only to painful stimuli. Cannot communicate discomfort except by moaning or restlessness, OR has a sensory impairment which limits the ability to feel pain or discomfort over 1/2 of body.	**3. Slightly Limited:** Responds to verbal commands but cannot always communicate discomfort or need to be turned, OR has some sensory impairment which limits ability to feel pain or discomfort in 1 or 2 extremities.	**4. No Impairment:** Responds to verbal commands. Has no sensory deficit which would limit ability to feel or voice pain or discomfort.
MOISTURE Degree to which skin is exposed to moisture	**1. Constantly Moist:** Skin is kept moist almost constantly by perspiration, urine, etc. Dampness is detected every time patient is moved or turned.	**2. Moist:** Skin is often but not always moist. Linen must be changed at least once a shift.	**3. Occasionally Moist:** Skin is occasionally moist, requiring an extra linen change approximately once a day.	**4. Rarely Moist:** Skin is usually dry; linen requires changing only at routine intervals.
ACTIVITY Degree of physical activity	**1. Bedfast:** Confined to bed.	**2. Chairfast:** Ability to walk severely limited or nonexistent. Cannot bear own weight and/or must be assisted into chair or wheelchair.	**3. Walks Occasionally:** Walks occasionally during day but for very short distances, with or without assistance. Spends majority of each shift in bed or chair.	**4. Walks Frequently:** Walks outside the room at least twice a day and inside room at least once every 2 hours during waking hours.
MOBILITY Ability to change and control body position	**1. Completely Immobile:** Does not make even slight changes in body or extremity position without assistance.	**2. Very Limited:** Makes occasional slight changes in body or extremity position but unable to make frequent or significant changes independently.	**3. Slightly Limited:** Makes frequent though slight changes in body or extremity position independently.	**4. No Limitations:** Makes major and frequent changes in position without assistance.
NUTRITION Usual food intake pattern	**1. Very Poor:** Never eats a complete meal. Rarely eats more than 1/3 of any food offered. Eats 2 servings or less of protein (meat or dairy products) per day. Takes fluids poorly. Does not take a liquid dietary supplement, OR is NPO and/or maintained on clear liquids or IVs for more than 5 days.	**2. Probably Inadequate:** Rarely eats a complete meal and generally eats only about 1/2 of any food offered. Protein intake includes only 3 servings of meat or dairy products per day. Occasionally will take a dietary supplement, OR receives less than optimum amount of liquid diet or tube feeding.	**3. Adequate:** Eats over half of most meals. Eats a total of 4 servings of protein (meat, dairy products) each day. Occasionally will refuse a meal, but will usually take a supplement if offered, OR is on a tube feeding or TPN regimen, which probably meets most of nutritional needs.	**4. Excellent:** Eats most of every meal. Never refuses a meal. Usually eats a total of 4 or more servings of meat and dairy products. Occasionally eats between meals. Does not require supplementation.
FRICTION AND SHEAR	**1. Problem:** Requires moderate to maximum assistance in moving. Complete lifting without sliding against sheets is impossible. Frequently slides down in bed or chair, requiring frequent repositioning with maximum assistance. Spasticity, contractures or agitation leads to almost constant friction.	**2. Potential Problem:** Moves feebly or requires minimum assistance. During a move skin probably slides to some extent against sheets, chair, restraints or other devices. Maintains relatively good position in chair or bed most of the time but occasionally slides down.	**3. No Apparent Problem:** Moves in bed and in chair independently and has sufficient muscle strength to lift up completely during move. Maintains good position in bed or chair at all times.	

Total Score _____

Figure 14-4 Braden Scale for Predicting Pressure Sore Risk. (From 'Clinical Practice Guideline, Pressure Ulcers in Adults: Prediction and Prevention,' by U.S. Department of Health and Human Services, PPPPUA Pub no. 92-0047, pp. 16-17, 1992, Rockville, MD: Public Health Service. Copyright © Barbara Braden and Nancy Bergstrom, 1988. Reprinted with permission.)

NURSING MANAGEMENT

Table 14-2 Norton's Pressure Area Risk Assessment Form (Scoring System)

A. General physical condition		B. Mental state		C. Activity		D. Mobility		E. Incontinence	
Good	4	Alert	4	Ambulatory	4	Full	4	Absent	4
Fair	3	Apathetic	3	Walks with help	3	Slightly limited	3	Occasional	3
Poor	2	Confused	2	Chairbound	2	Very limited	2	Usually urinary	2
Very bad	1	Stuporous	1	Bedfast	1	Immobile	1	Double	1

Note: From *An Investigation of Geriatric Nursing Problems in Hospitals*, by D. Norton, R. McLaren, and A.N. Exton-Smith, 1975, Edinburgh, UK: Churchill Livingstone. Reprinted with permission.

A total of 23 points is possible. An adult who scores 15 to 18 points is considered at risk, scores of 13 to 14 indicate moderate risk, 10 to 12 high risk, and 9 or less very high risk (Ayello and Braden, 2001). For best results, nurses should be trained in proper use of the scale (Bergstrom *et al.*, 1994).

Norton's Pressure Area Risk Assessment Form Scale (Table 14-2) includes the categories of general physical condition, mental state, activity, mobility and incontinence. A category of medications was added in 1987, resulting in a possible score of 24. Scores of 15 or 16 should be viewed as indicators, not predictors, of risk (Anthony, 1987). The Braden and Norton tools should be used when the patient is initially assessed and at regular intervals thereafter, particularly if the patient's condition changes. This increases awareness of specific risk factors and serves as assessment data from which care delivery can be planned and implemented.

Assessment of Wounds

Nurses play a vital role in the management of wounds. In order to manage a wound effectively, the patient should be fully assessed. Wound assessment should be done in conjunction with a holistic assessment of the patient. Wound assessment is shown in the *Practice guidelines* on page 320.

As part of the assessment process, photographs can be taken weekly as a visual record of the progress of chronic wounds, although it is important to note that nurses may have to seek consent from the patient before taking the photographs.

When caring for patients with full thickness (see Box 14-1 on page 311) wounds it is important to establish if there is evidence of undermining or sinus tract formation. To fully assess the size of the wound, the nurse gently explores the undermined area with a thin, flexible probe. Do not use a cotton-tipped swab since it can leave fibres behind in the wound. Once the end of the tract is reached, gently raise the probe so that the bulge created by the end can be seen and its length measured on the skin surface. However the nurse should bear in mind that probing a wound can be painful and can cause bleeding. If excessive bleeding occurs apply pressure and seek medical advice.

Sinus tracts are often caused by infection and have significant drainage. They may be treated using antibiotics,

PRACTICE GUIDELINES

Assessing Common Pressure Sites

+ Be sure the lighting is good, preferably natural or fluorescent, because incandescent lights can create a transilluminating effect.
+ Regulate the environment before beginning the assessment so that the room is neither too hot nor too cold. Heat can cause the skin to flush; cold can cause the skin to blanch or become cyanotic.
+ Inspect pressure areas (see Figure 14-2) for any whitish or reddened spots; discoloration can be caused by impaired blood circulation to the area. It should disappear in a few minutes when rubbing restores circulation.
+ Inspect pressure areas for abrasions and excoriations. An abrasion can occur when skin rubs against a sheet (e.g. when the patient is pulled). Excoriations can occur when the skin has prolonged contact with body secretions or excretions or with dampness in skin folds.
+ Palpate the surface temperature of the skin over the pressure areas (warm your hands first). Normally, the temperature is the same as that of the surrounding skin. Increased temperature is abnormal and may be due to inflammation or blood trapped in the area.
+ Palpate over bony prominences and dependent body areas for the presence of oedema, which feels spongy.

NURSING MANAGEMENT

irrigation, surgical incision to open and drain the tract, or vacuum therapy for large tracts (Butcher, 2002).

Laboratory Tests

Laboratory tests can often support the nurse's clinical assessment of the wound's progress in healing. A decreased white cell (leucocyte) count can delay healing and increase the possibility of infection. A haemoglobin level below normal range indicates poor oxygen delivery to the tissues. Blood coagulation studies are also significant. Prolonged coagulation times can result in excessive blood loss and prolonged clot absorption. Hypercoagulability can lead to intravascular clotting. Intra-arterial clotting can result in a deficient blood supply to the wound area. Serum protein analysis provides an indication of the body's nutritional reserves for rebuilding cells. Wound cultures can either confirm or rule out the presence of infection. Sensitivity studies are helpful in the selection of appropriate antibiotic therapy. The nurse obtains a wound culture whenever an infection is suspected.

Procedure 14-1 provides guidelines to obtain a specimen of wound drainage.

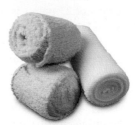

PRACTICE GUIDELINES

The Assessment of Wounds

Should include:

+ location of the wound
+ dimensions and depth of the wound
+ extent of tissue loss
+ characteristics of wound base
+ exudates (type, colour, odour)
+ condition of surrounding skin
+ signs of infection
+ the presence of any foreign material
+ presence of pain associated with the wound.

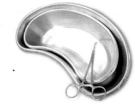

PROCEDURE 14-1 Collecting a Wound Swab for Culture and Sensitivity

Purposes

+ To identify the micro-organisms potentially causing an infection and the antibiotics to which they are sensitive

Assessment

Assess

+ For signs of infection in the wound, e.g. pain, inflammation (remember this can be a normal part of the healing process), exudates (type, volume, colour, odour)
+ For systemic signs of infection such as fever, chills or elevated white blood cell count (WBC).

Wound swabs should only be taken if clinically indicated. The nurse should use their clinical judgement when assessing for infection before doing a wound swab. This is important as almost all wounds are colonised with micro-organisms, therefore a wound swab will almost always show micro-organisms. However colonisation with micro-organisms poses very little risk to the patient, whereas infection causes localised problems such as malodorous exudate and pain and systemic problems such as fever. Colonisation with micro-organisms requires no treatment whereas infection requires the use of antibiotics. Over prescribing antibiotics leads to resistant bacteria such as Multi-Resistant Staphylococcus Aureus (MRSA).

Planning

Before collecting the specimen, ensure collection of equipment and that an appropriate microbiology form is completed. Remember when collecting wound specimens the wound should not be cleansed prior to collection.

Equipment

+ Clean gloves
+ Sterile gloves
+ Sterile dressing set
+ Normal saline (for cleansing after collection of the specimen)
+ Culture tube with swab
+ Appropriate sterile wound dressing
+ Completed microbiology form

Implementation

Preparation

If appropriate, administer analgesia 30 minutes before the procedure if the patient is complaining of pain at the wound site.

Performance

1. Explain to the patient what you are going to do, why it is necessary and how they can cooperate. Discuss how the results will be used in planning further care or treatments.
2. Wash hands and observe other appropriate infection control procedures (e.g. gloves and apron).
3. Provide for patient privacy.
4. Remove any dressings that cover the wound.
   - Put on clean gloves.
   - Remove the dressing, and observe any drainage on the dressing.
   - Determine the amount of the drainage, for example, 'one 2 × 2 gauze saturated with pale yellow drainage'.
   - Discard the dressing in the clinical waste disposal unit.
   - Remove your gloves and dispose of them properly.
5. Wash hands again and open the sterile dressing set using aseptic technique.
6. Assess the wound.
   - Put on sterile gloves.
   - Assess the appearance of the tissues in and around the wound and the drainage. Infection can cause reddened tissues with a thick discharge, which may be foul smelling, whitish or coloured.
7. Obtain the specimen by rotating the swab back and forth over the wound. Then return the swab to the culture tube, taking care not to touch the top or the outside of the tube.
8. Cleanse the wound if appropriate.
9. Dress the wound with an appropriate dressing.
10. Arrange for the specimen to be transported to the laboratory immediately. Be sure to include the completed requisition.
11. Document all relevant information.
   - Record on the patient's chart the taking of the specimen and source.
   - Include the date and time, the appearance of the wound, the colour, consistency, amount and odour of any drainage, the type of culture collected and any discomfort experienced by the patient.

Evaluation

+ Compare findings of wound assessment and drainage to previous assessments to determine any changes.
+ Report the culture results to the doctor or nurse practitioner.
+ Conduct appropriate follow-up such as administering medications as ordered.

IMPLEMENTING

Nursing interventions for maintaining skin integrity and wound care involve supporting wound healing, preventing pressure ulcers, treating pressure ulcers, dressing and cleaning wounds, applying heat and cold, and supporting and immobilising wounds.

Supporting Wound Healing

There are three major areas in which nurses can help patients develop optimal conditions for wound healing: obtaining sufficient nutrition and fluids, preventing wound infections and proper positioning.

Nutrition and Fluids

Patients should be assisted to take in at least 2,500 ml of fluids a day unless conditions contraindicate this amount. Although there is no evidence that excessive doses of vitamins or minerals enhance wound healing, adequate amounts are extremely important. The nurse should ensure that patients receive sufficient protein, vitamins C, A, B_1 and B_5 and zinc (Anderson, 2005).

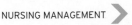
NURSING MANAGEMENT

BOX 14-3 Guidelines for Preventing Infection and the Transmission of Blood-borne Pathogens

Universal precautions

+ Wear gloves and apron when touching blood and body fluids, mucous membranes or nonintact skin of all patients, and when handling items or surfaces soiled with blood or body fluids.
+ Wash hands thoroughly and/or apply alcohol gel after removing gloves, and if contaminated with blood or body fluids.

Wound care

+ Wash hands and/or apply alcohol gel before and after caring for wounds.
+ Wear gloves, apron, surgical masks and protective eyewear as appropriate if procedures commonly cause droplets or splashing of blood or body fluids (e.g. wound irrigation).
+ Touch an open or fresh surgical wound only when wearing sterile gloves or using a sterile instrument.
+ Remove or change dressings over closed wounds when they become wet.

Preventing Infection

There are two main aspects to controlling wound infection: preventing micro-organisms from entering the wound and preventing the transmission of blood borne pathogens to or from the patient to others (see Box 14-3).

Positioning

To promote wound healing, patients must be positioned to keep pressure off the wound. Changes of position and transfers can be accomplished without shear or friction damage. In addition to proper positioning, the patient should be assisted to be as mobile as possible because activity enhances circulation. If the patient cannot move independently, range-of-motion exercises and regular repositioning should be implemented.

Preventing Pressure Ulcers

To reduce the likelihood of pressure ulcer development in all patients, the nurse employs a variety of preventive measures (i.e. skin hygiene) to maintain the skin integrity and educates the patient and family about how to prevent pressure ulcers.

Providing Nutrition

Because an inadequate intake of calories, protein, vitamins and iron is believed to be a risk factor for pressure ulcer development, nutritional supplements should be considered for nutritionally compromised patients. The diet should be similar to that which supports wound healing, as discussed earlier. Monitor weight regularly to help assess nutritional status. Pertinent lab work should also be monitored including lymphocyte count, protein (especially albumin) and haemoglobin.

Maintaining Skin Hygiene

When bathing the patient, the nurse should minimise the force and friction applied to the skin, using mild cleansing agents that minimise irritation and dryness and that do not disrupt the skin's 'natural barriers'. Also, avoid using hot water, which increases skin dryness and irritation. The patient's skin should be kept clean and dry and free of irritation and maceration by urine, faeces, sweat, incomplete drying after a bath, soap or alcohol. Apply skin protection if indicated. Moisture or skin barriers are very effective in preventing moisture or drainage from collecting on the skin.

Avoiding Skin Trauma

Providing the patient with a smooth, firm and wrinkle-free foundation on which to sit or lie helps prevent skin trauma. To prevent injury due to friction and shearing forces, patients must be positioned, transferred and turned correctly.

Frequent shifts in position, even if only slight, effectively change pressure points. The patient should shift weight every 15–30 minutes and, whenever possible, exercise or ambulate to stimulate blood circulation.

Providing Pressure Relieving Equipment

In order for circulation to remain uncompromised, pressure on the bony prominences should remain below capillary pressure for as much time as possible through a combination of turning, positioning and use of pressure-relieving surfaces. Mean capillary pressure can be estimated at 20 mm Hg although this varies (de Graaff *et al.*, 2002).

There are a number of devices available to relieve pressure. Decisions regarding which device to use should be based on a holistic assessment of the individual and should include the level of risk, comfort and general health state. According to the Royal College of Nursing (RCN, 2001) patients who are considered to be at risk of pressure ulcers should not be nursed on foam mattresses but should be placed on alternating pressure mattresses or high tech pressure redistributing systems. Also the RCN (2001) strongly advise that sheepskins, whether genuine or synthetic, should not be used as pressure relieving aids. Table 14-3 lists selected mechanical devices for reducing pressure on body parts.

Table 14-3 Mechanical Devices for Reducing Pressure on Body Parts

Device	Description/comments
Gel or viscoelastic filled pads	Polyvinyl, silicone or Silastic pads filled with a gelatinous substance similar to fat.
Pillows and wedges (foam, gel, air, fluid)	Can raise a body part (e.g. heels) off the bed or surface.
Foam mattress	Foam moulds to the body.
Alternating pressure mattress	Composed of a number of cells in which the pressure alternately increases and decreases; uses a pump (see Figure 14-5).
Air fluidised bed (high-air-loss bed)	Forced temperature-controlled air is circulated around millions of tiny silicone-coated beads, producing a fluid-like movement. Provides uniform support to body contours. Decreases skin maceration by its drying effect. Moisture from the patient penetrates the bed sheet and soaks the beads. Air flow forces the beads away from the patient and rapidly dries the sheet. (see Figure 14-6).
Static low-air-loss (LAL) bed	Consists of many air-filled cushions divided into four or five sections. Separate controls permit each section to be inflated to a different level of firmness; thus pressure can be reduced on bony prominences but increased under other body areas for support (see Figure 14-7).
Active or second-generation LAL bed	Like the static LAL bed, but in addition greatly pulsates or rotates from side to side, thus stimulating capillary blood flow and facilitating movement of pulmonary secretions.

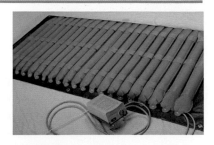

Figure 14-5 Alternating pressure mattress (Ease). (Courtesy of EASE.)

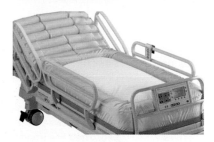

Figure 14-6 Air-fluidised bed (Clinitron). (Courtesy of Hill-Rom Services, Inc. Reprinted with permission. All rights reserved.)

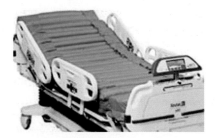

Figure 14-7 Low-air-loss bed. (Therapulse®) II. Courtesy of KCI Licensing, Inc. 9/2007.

Treating Pressure Ulcers

Pressure ulcers are a challenge for nurses because of the number of variables involved (e.g. risk factors, types of ulcers and degrees of impairment) and the numerous treatment/dressings available. Existing and potential infections are the most serious complications of pressure ulcers. In treating pressure ulcers, nurses should follow the local trust's policies and national guidelines. Prompt treatment can prevent further tissue damage and pain and facilitate wound healing. See Table 14-4 on page 324 regarding dressings for pressure ulcers.

Pressure ulcer treatment usually combines effective wound care with pressure reducing techniques and holistic management of the patient such as maintaining adequate nutritional intake.

Pressure ulcer wounds should be cleansed with sterile saline in hospitals, however in the patient's home tap water can be used as research suggests there is no clinical advantage for using sterile saline for chronic wounds (Fernandez *et al.*, 2002) and it is acceptable for some individuals to cleanse the area by means of showering particularly for large or awkward areas. Minimal mechanical force should be used when cleansing the wound as this will delay healing. The wound should only be cleansed with antiseptics if clinically indicated.

Tissue that is non-viable should be removed in order to reduce the risk of infection, facilitate healing and aid assessment of the wound. The removal of non-viable tissue can be achieved by a number of techniques including surgery, autolysis (breakdown of the dead tissue by self produced enzymes),

Table 14-4 Dressings for Pressure Ulcers

Dressing	Mechanism of action	Grade			
		1	2	3	4
Transparent barrier	Retains wound moisture, allows gas exchange, does not stick to wound surface.	✓	✓		
Hydrocolloid	Occlusive, repels moisture and dirt, maintains moist wound environment.	✓		✓	
Hydrogel	Maintains moist wound environment.		✓	✓	✓
Alginate	Maintains moist wound environment, absorbs exudate.			✓	✓

Note: Some dressings may be used on other pressure ulcer grades. See Figure 14-1 on page 311 for European Pressure Ulcer Advisory Panel Pressure Ulcer Grading and Classification.

Table 14-5 Selected Types of Wound Dressings

Dressing	Description	Purpose	Examples
Transparent adhesive films/wound barriers	Adhesive plastic, semi permeable, nonabsorbent dressings allow exchange of oxygen between the atmosphere and wound bed. They are impermeable to bacteria and water.	To provide protection against contamination and friction; to maintain a clean moist surface that facilitates cellular migration; to provide insulation by preventing fluid evaporation; and to facilitate wound assessment. For procedure for applying this dressing see *Procedure 14-2*	Op-Site, Tegaderm, Bioclusive
Impregnated nonadherent dressings	Woven or nonwoven cotton or synthetic materials are impregnated with petrolatum, saline, zinc-saline, antimicrobials or other agents. Require secondary dressings to secure them in place, retain moisture and provide wound protection.	To cover, soothe and protect partial- and full-thickness wounds without exudate	Adaptic, Carrasyn, Xeroform
Hydrocolloids	Waterproof adhesive wafers, pastes or powders. Wafers, designed to be worn for up to seven days, consist of two layers. The inner adhesive layer has particles that absorb exudate and form a hydrated gel over the wound; the outer film provides a seal.	To absorb exudate; to produce a moist environment that facilitates healing but does not cause maceration of surrounding skin; to protect the wound from bacterial contamination, foreign debris and urine or faeces; and to prevent shearing. For procedure for applying this dressing see *Procedure 14-3* on page 325	DuoDerm, Comfeel, Tegasorb, Granuflex
Hydrogels	Glycerin or water-based non-adhesive jellylike sheets, granules or gels are oxygen permeable, unless covered by a plastic film. May require secondary occlusive dressing.	To liquefy necrotic tissue or slough, rehydrate the wound bed and fill in dead space	Aquasorb, Elasto-Gel, Vigilon
Polyurethane foams	Nonadherent hydrocolloid dressings; these need to have their edges taped down or sealed. Require secondary dressings to obtain an occlusive environment. Surrounding skin must be protected to prevent maceration.	To absorb light to moderate amounts of exudate; to debride wounds	Lyofoam, Allevyn
Exudate absorbers (alginates)	Nonadherent dressings of powder, beads or granules, ropes, sheets or paste conform to the wound surface and absorb up to 20 times their weight in exudate; require a secondary dressing.	To provide a moist wound surface by interacting with exudate to form a gelatinous mass; to absorb exudate; to eliminate dead space or pack wounds; and to support debridement	Sorbsan, Kaltostat

enzymatic (use of topical ointments to promote debridement (removal of dead tissue)) and larval (maggot) therapy.

Surgical removal of non-viable tissue can range from the use of scissors or scalpel at the bedside to full surgery. The use of hydrocolloids and hydrogels dressings aid the autolysis of non-viable tissue by providing a moist environment.

Dressing Wounds

Dressings are applied for the following purposes:

+ To protect the wound from mechanical injury
+ To protect the wound from microbial contamination
+ To provide or maintain a moist environment
+ To provide thermal insulation
+ To absorb drainage or debride a wound or both
+ To prevent haemorrhage (when applied as a pressure dressing or with elastic bandages)
+ To splint or immobilise the wound site and thereby facilitate healing and prevent injury.

Types of Dressing

Various dressing materials are available to cover wounds. The type of dressing used depends on (a) the location, size and type of the wound; (b) the amount of exudate; (c) whether the wound requires debridement or is infected; and (d) such considerations as frequency of dressing change, ease or difficulty of dressing application and cost. Table 14-5 describes these materials.

PROCEDURE 14-2 Applying a Transparent Wound Barrier

Purposes

+ To provide a moist wound environment and promote wound healing
+ To protect the wound from trauma and infectious agents
+ To facilitate assessment of wound healing

Assessment

Assess

+ Appearance and size of the wound or at-risk skin area
+ Amount and character of exudate
+ For complaints of discomfort
+ For signs of infection such as fever, chills or elevated WBC count

Planning

Equipment

+ Clean gloves
+ Sterile gloves (optional)
+ Hair scissors or clippers
+ Alcohol or acetone to remove adhesive from old dressing
+ Clinical waste bag
+ Saline and gauze or syringe for wound irrigation
+ Wound barrier dressing
+ Scissors

Implementation

Preparation

Review patient's notes regarding frequency and type of dressing change. Ensure where possible that the dressing is done at a time that is convenient for the patient (e.g. not at visiting time).

Performance

1. Explain to the patient what you are going to do, why it is necessary and how they can cooperate. Discuss how the results will be used in planning further care or treatments.

2. Wash hands and observe appropriate infection control procedures.

3. Provide for patient privacy. Assist the patient to a comfortable position in which the wound can be readily exposed. Expose only the wound area, using a sheet or towel to cover the patient, if necessary. *Undue exposure is physically and psychologically distressing to most people.*

4. Apply clean gloves and remove the existing dressing, discarding it in the clinical waste bag. If after the dressing is removed, adhesive remains on the skin this can be cleaned using alcohol or acetone. However you must be careful that the wound is not touched with this fluid as it can be extremely painful for the patient.

5. Clean the wound if indicated.
   - Put on clean or sterile gloves in accordance with local policy.
   - Clean the wound using tap water, saline or antiseptic as indicated.
   - Dry the surrounding skin with dry gauze.

6. Assess the wound.

7. Apply the wound barrier.
   - Remove part of the paper backing on the dressing (see Figure 14-8).
   - Apply the dressing at one edge of the wound site, allowing at least 2.5 cm (1 inch) coverage of the skin surrounding the wound.
   - Gently lay or press the barrier over the wound. Keep it free of wrinkles, but avoid stretching it

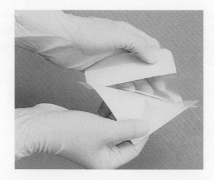

Figure 14-8 A transparent wound dressing.

too tightly. *A stretched dressing restricts mobility.*
   - Remove and dispose of gloves appropriately.

8. Assess the wound at least daily.
   - Determine the extent of serous fluid accumulation under the dressing, wound healing and the need to repair the dressing.
   - If excessive serum has accumulated, consider replacing the transparent wound barrier with a more absorbent type of dressing, such as hydrocolloid.
   - If the dressing is leaking, remove it and apply another dressing.

9. Document the dressing change, wound status and the patient's response in the patient notes. Many clinical areas have use wound assessment charts in order to accurately document information regarding the patient and their wound (see Figure 14-9).

Description of Pressure Ulcers and Classification

Stage I: Characterised by erythema that does not resolve within minutes of pressure relief. Skin remains intact.

Stage II: Partial thickness loss of skin involving the epidermis or dermis – may involve both. The ulcer is superficial and may present as a blister, abrasion or shallow crater. Free of eschar.

Stage III: Full thickness loss which goes through the dermis to the subcutaneous tissue but does not extend through the underlying fascia. Appears as a crater and may include undermining.

Stage IV: Full thickness skin loss with extensive damage through the subcutaneous tissue to the fascia and may involve muscle layers, joint and/or bone.

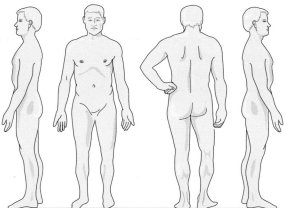

- IDENTIFY LOCATION OF ALL PRESSURE ULCERS ABOVE BY NUMBERING (1, 2, 3): IF MORE THAN 3, USE ADDITIONAL SHEET.

- COMPLETE CHART BELOW FOR SITE #1, USE REVERSE SIDE FOR SITES 2 & 3.

Patient Admitted On: _____

Date Sheet Initiated: _____

Pressure relief methods in use:

❑ Low Airloss Bed

❑ Low Airloss Mattress Overlay

❑ Turning Q2h when pt. supine and Q1h if HOB↑

❑ Pressure Reducing Mattress Overlay

❑ Other _____

Date MD notified of ulcer:

_____

Figure 14-9 Wound/skin documentation sheet.

DOCUMENT WEEKLY AND P.R.N. SIGNIFICANT CHANGE IN ULCER'S APPEARANCE

SITE #1: LOCATION	DESCRIBE TREATMENT:				FREQUENCY:
DATE / TIME					
DIMENSIONS: LENGTH (in. cm.)					
WIDTH					
DEPTH					
ODOUR (None or Foul)					
DESCRIBE DRAINAGE (Purulent, Serous, Serosanguinous) and AMOUNT (Scant, Moderate, Copious)					
STAGE (See Above)					
COMMENTARY: i.e.: Describe tissue surrounding ulcer: is there undermining? % necrotic vs % granular, etc.					
NURSE					

WOUND/SKIN DOCUMENTATION SHEET

Figure 14-9 *(continued)*

Evaluation

+ Perform follow-up based on findings that deviate from expected or normal for the patient. Relate findings to previous assessment information if available.

+ Report significant deviations from normal to the doctor.

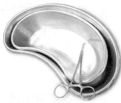

PROCEDURE 14-3 Applying a Hydrocolloid Dressing

Purposes

+ To maintain a moist wound surface and promote healing
+ To prevent the entrance of micro-organisms into the wound

+ To minimise wound discomfort
+ To promote autolysis of necrotic material by white blood cells
+ To decrease the frequency of dressing changes

Assessment

Assess

+ Appearance and size of the wound or at-risk skin area
+ Amount and character of exudate
+ For complaints of discomfort
+ For signs of infection such as fever, chills or elevated WBC count

Planning

If possible, review the patient notes to note details regarding previous hydrocolloid dressing changes.

Equipment

+ Clean gloves
+ Sterile gloves (optional)
+ Dressing set including scissors
+ Clinical waste bag
+ Sterile gauze and saline (if required)
+ Hydrocolloid dressing at least 3-4 cm (1.5 inch) larger than wound on all four sides.

Implementation

Preparation

+ Review the care plan for information regarding frequency and type of dressing change.
+ Change the dressing if it leaks, is dislodged or develops an odour. Otherwise, it may remain in place up to one week.
+ If possible, schedule the dressing change at a time convenient for the patient. Some dressing changes require only a few minutes and others can take much longer.

Performance

1. Explain to the patient what you are going to do, why it is necessary and how they can cooperate. Discuss how the results will be used in planning further care or treatments.
2. Wash hands and observe appropriate infection control procedures.
3. Provide for patient privacy. Assist the patient to a comfortable position in which the wound can be readily exposed. Expose only the wound area, using a bath blanket to cover the patient, if necessary. *Undue exposure is physically and psychologically distressing to most people.*
4. Apply clean gloves and remove the existing dressing, discarding it into the clinical waste bag.
5. Thoroughly clean the skin area around the wound.
   - Put on clean gloves.
   - Clean the skin well but gently with normal saline or a mild cleansing agent. Always rinse

the adjacent skin well before applying a dressing.
   - Clip the hair about 5 cm (2 inch) around the wound area if indicated.
   - Leave the residue that is difficult to remove on the skin. It will wear off in time. Attempts to remove residue can irritate the surrounding skin.
   - Remove gloves and dispose of them in the clinical waste bag.
6. Clean the wound if indicated.
   - Put on clean or sterile gloves in accordance with local policy.
   - Clean the wound, preferably using irrigation technique
   - Dry the surrounding skin with dry gauze.
7. Assess the wound.
8. Apply the dressing.
   - Follow the manufacturer's instructions. Hold the dressing in place for about one minute with your hand. *The warmth helps the dressing conform and adhere.*
   - Remove and dispose of the gloves.
9. Assess and change the dressing as indicated.
   - Inspect the dressing at least daily for leakage, dislodgement, odour and wrinkling.
   - Change the dressing if any of these signs are present.
10. Document the dressing change and the patient's response in the patient record.

Evaluation

+ Relate findings from dressing change to previous assessment information.
+ Report any significant changes to doctor or nurse specialist.

Cleaning Wounds

Wound cleaning involves the removal of debris (i.e. foreign materials, excess slough, necrotic tissue and excess exudate). It is important to point out that exudates should only be removed if it is excessive as it is believed to contain growth factors and nutrients vital to wound healing (Bell, 2004). In order to make a decision about whether to cleanse a wound, the nurse must fully assess the wound.

The choices of cleaning agent and method depend largely on local policy, however antiseptics and disinfectants are not recommended as they have been found to be inactivated by body fluid, can damage healing tissue and can lead to systemic toxicity (Farstvedt *et al.*, 2004). Although many local policies advocate the use of 0.9% saline to cleanse wounds (Davies, 1999), some studies have shown that the risk of infection does not increase if tap water is used to cleanse the wound (Fernandez *et al.*, 2002).

Nurses are guided by evidence-based practice and local policy when deciding whether to cleanse a wound and what cleanser to use. Recommended guidelines for cleaning wounds are shown in the *Practice guidelines* below.

Cleansing Technique

The most common ways of cleansing a wound is by swabbing and irrigation, however showering and bathing are acceptable options for some individual patients (Selim *et al.*, 2001). Cleansing a wound with cotton wool or gauze is not recommended as they can leave fibres behind which can lead to infection (Dowsett *et al.*, 2004). It is also believed that the pressure exerted on the wound during swabbing can be detrimental to the wound (Oliver, 1997).

The technique of choice for cleansing a wound is irrigation (Horrocks, 2006), however there are problems associated with this technique. Too much irrigation pressure and new tissue is damaged while too little pressure does not remove debris (Davies *et al.*, 2005).

PRACTICE GUIDELINES

Cleaning Wounds

+ Use solutions such as isotonic saline or tap water to clean or irrigate wounds (Fernandez *et al.*, 2002).
+ When possible, warm the solution to body temperature before use. *This prevents lowering the wound temperature, which slows the healing process.*
+ If a wound is grossly contaminated by foreign material, bacteria, slough or necrotic tissue, clean the wound at every dressing change. *Foreign bodies and devitalised tissue act as a focus for infection and can delay healing.*
+ If a wound is clean, has little exudate, and reveals healthy granulation tissue, avoid cleaning. *Unnecessary cleaning can delay wound healing by traumatising newly produced, delicate tissues, reducing the surface temperature of the wound, and removing exudate which itself may have bactericidal properties.*

+ Use gauze squares. Avoid using cotton balls and other products that shed fibres onto the wound surface. *The fibres become embedded in granulation tissue and can act as foci for infection. They may also stimulate 'foreign body' reactions, prolonging the inflammatory phase of healing and delaying the healing process.*
+ Clean superficial noninfected wounds by irrigating them with normal saline. *The hydraulic pressure of an irrigating stream of fluid dislodges contaminating debris and reduces bacterial colonisation.*
+ *To retain wound moisture,* avoid drying a wound after cleaning it.
+ Clean from the wound in an outward direction to avoid transferring organisms from the surrounding skin into the wound.

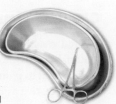

PROCEDURE 14-4 Irrigating a Wound

Purposes

+ To clean the area

+ To apply heat and hasten the healing process

Assessment

Assess

+ The patient's care plan and notes to determine previous appearance and size of the wound
+ The character of the exudate

+ Presence of pain and the time of the last pain medication
+ Clinical signs of systemic infection
+ Allergies to the wound irrigation agent or tape

Planning

+ Before irrigating a wound, determine (a) the type of irrigating solution to be used, (b) the frequency of irrigations and (c) the temperature of the solution.
+ If possible, schedule the irrigation at a time convenient for the patient. Some irrigations require only a few minutes and others can take much longer.

Equipment

+ Sterile dressing equipment and dressing materials
+ Sterile syringes (e.g. a 30 to 60 ml syringe)
+ Sterile gallipot for the irrigating solution
+ Clinical waste bag
+ Receiver for the irrigation returns
+ Irrigating solution warmed to body temperature
+ Clean gloves
+ Sterile gloves
+ Moisture-proof sterile drape

Implementation

Preparation

Check that the irrigating fluid is at the proper temperature.

Performance

1. Explain to the patient what you are going to do, why it is necessary and how they can cooperate. Discuss how the results will be used in planning further care or treatments.
2. Wash hands and observe appropriate infection control procedures.
3. Provide for patient privacy.
4. Prepare the patient.
   - Assist the patient to a position in which the irrigating solution will flow by gravity from the upper end of the wound to the lower end and then into the basin.
   - Place the waterproof drape over the patient and the bed.
   - Put on clean gloves and remove and discard the old dressing.
   - Assess the wound and drainage.

   - Remove and discard clean gloves and wash hands.
5. Prepare the equipment.
   - Open the sterile dressing pack and supplies.
   - Pour the cleansing solution into the gallipot.
   - Position the receiver below the wound to receive the irrigating fluid.
6. Irrigate the wound.
   - Instil a steady stream of irrigating solution into the wound. Make sure all areas of the wound are irrigated.
   - Use either a syringe with a catheter tip to flush the wound (Figure 14-10).
   - Continue irrigating until the solution becomes clear (no exudate is present). *The irrigation washes away tissue debris and drainage so that later returns are clearer.*
   - Dry the area around the wound. *Moisture left on the skin promotes the growth of micro-organisms and can cause skin irritation and breakdown.*

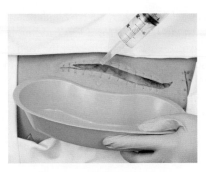

Figure 14-10 Irrigating a wound.

7. Assess and dress the wound.
   - Assess the appearance of the wound again, noting in particular the type and amount of exudate still present and the presence and extent of granulation tissue.
   - Using aseptic technique, apply a dressing to the wound based on the amount of drainage expected (see Table 14-5 on page 322).
8. Document the irrigation and the patient's response in the patient notes.

Evaluation

+ Relate findings from dressing change to previous assessment information.
+ Report any significant changes to doctor or nurse specialist.

Many of the techniques described here for dressing wounds may be combined depending on the specific type of wound. In addition, therapies are constantly being designed and evaluated. One example is *vacuum-assisted closure* (VAC), which refers to the use of suction equipment to apply negative pressure to a variety of large or nonhealing wounds. This therapy has been shown to speed tissue generation, reduce swelling around the wound and enhance wound healing by providing a moist and protected environment (Mendez-Eastman, 2002).

Supporting and Immobilising Wounds

Bandages and binders serve various purposes:

+ supporting a wound (e.g. a fractured bone);
+ immobilising a wound (e.g. a strained shoulder);
+ applying pressure (e.g. elastic bandages on the lower extremities to improve venous blood flow);
+ securing a dressing (e.g. for an extensive abdominal surgical wound).

There are several types of bandages and binders and several ways in which they are applied. When correctly applied, they promote healing, provide comfort and can prevent injury (see the *Practice guidelines* below).

Bandages

A **bandage** is a strip of cloth used to wrap some part of the body. Bandages are available in various widths, most commonly 1.5 to 7.5 cm and are usually supplied in rolls for easy application to a body part.

PRACTICE GUIDELINES

Bandaging

+ Whenever possible, bandage the part in its normal position, with the joint slightly flexed *to avoid putting strain on the ligaments and the muscles of the joint.*
+ Pad between skin surfaces and over bony prominences *to prevent friction from the bandage and consequent abrasion of the skin.*
+ Always bandage body parts by working from the distal to the proximal end *to aid the return flow of venous blood.*
+ Bandage with even pressure *to prevent interference with blood circulation.*

+ Whenever possible, leave the end of the body part (e.g. the toe) exposed *so that you will be able to determine the adequacy of the blood circulation to the extremity.*
+ Cover dressings with bandages at least 5 cm beyond the edges of the dressing *to prevent the dressing and wound from becoming contaminated.*
+ Face the patient when applying a bandage *to maintain uniform tension and the appropriate direction of the bandage.*

Many types of materials are used for bandages. Gauze is one of the most commonly used, because it is light and porous and readily moulds to the body. It is also relatively inexpensive, so it is generally discarded when soiled. Gauze is used to retain dressings on wounds and to bandage the fingers, hands, toes and feet. It supports dressings and at the same time permits air to circulate, while elastic conforming bandages are applied to provide pressure to an area.

The width of the bandage used depends on the size of the body part to be bandaged. For example, a 2.5 cm (1 inch) bandage is used for a finger, a 5 cm bandage for an arm, and a 7.5 or 10 cm bandage for a leg. Padding (e.g. abdominal pads and gauze squares) is frequently used to cover bony prominences (e.g. the elbow) or to separate skin surfaces (e.g. the fingers).

Before applying a bandage, the nurse needs to know its purpose and to assess the area requiring support (see the *Practice guidelines* below). When bandages are used to secure dressings, the nurse wears gloves to prevent contact with body fluids.

PRACTICE GUIDELINES

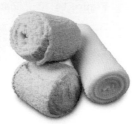

Assessing before Applying Bandages or Binders

+ Inspect and palpate the area for swelling.
+ Inspect for the presence of and status of wounds (open wounds will require a dressing before a bandage or binder is applied).
+ Note the presence of drainage (amount, colour, odour, viscosity).
+ Inspect and palpate for adequacy of circulation (skin temperature, colour and sensation). Pale or cyanotic skin, cool temperature, tingling and numbness can indicate impaired circulation.
+ Ask the patient about any pain experienced (location, intensity, onset, quality).
+ Assess the ability of the patient to reapply the bandage or binder when needed.
+ Assess the capabilities of the patient regarding activities of daily living (e.g. to eat, dress, comb hair, bathe) and assess the assistance required during the convalescence period.

Basic Turns for Roller Bandages

Applying bandages to various parts of the body involves one or more of five basic bandaging turns.

1. *Circular* turns are used to anchor bandages and to terminate them. Circular turns usually are not applied directly over a wound because of the discomfort the bandage would cause.
2. *Spiral* turns are used to bandage parts of the body that are fairly uniform in circumference, for example, the upper arm or upper leg.
3. *Spiral reverse* turns are used to bandage cylindrical parts of the body that are not uniform in circumference, for example, the lower leg or forearm.
4. *Recurrent* turns are used to cover distal parts of the body, for example, the end of a finger, the skull or the stump of an amputation.
5. *Figure-eight* turns are used to bandage an elbow, knee or ankle, because they permit some movement after application.

Circular Turns

+ Hold the bandage in your dominant hand, keeping the roll uppermost, and unroll the bandage about 8 cm. This length of unrolled bandage allows good control for placement and tension.
+ Apply the end of the bandage to the part of the body to be bandaged. Hold the end down with the thumb of the other hand (see Figure 14-11).

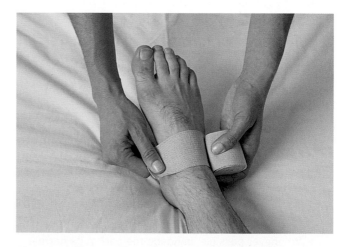

Figure 14-11 Starting a bandage with two circular turns.

+ Encircle the body part a few times or as often as needed, making sure that each layer overlaps one-half to two-thirds of the previous layer. This provides even support to the area.
+ The bandage should be firm, but not too tight. Ask the patient if the bandage feels comfortable. A tight bandage can interfere with blood circulation, whereas a loose bandage does not provide adequate protection.
+ Secure the end of the bandage with tape or a safety pin over an uninjured area. Pins can cause discomfort when situated over an injured area.

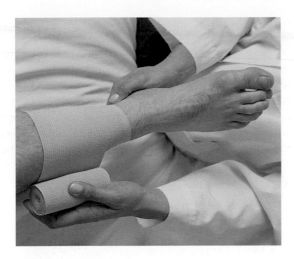

Figure 14-12 Applying spiral turns.

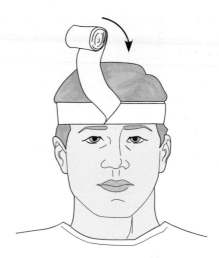

Figure 14-14 Starting a recurrent bandage.

Spiral Turns

✦ Make two circular turns. Two circular turns anchor the bandage.

✦ Continue spiral turns at about a 30-degree angle, each turn overlapping the preceding one by two-thirds the width of the bandage (see Figure 14-12).

✦ Terminate the bandage with two circular turns and secure the end as described for circular turns.

Spiral Reverse Turns

✦ Anchor the bandage with two circular turns, and bring the bandage upward at about a 30-degree angle.

✦ Place the thumb of your free hand on the upper edge of the bandage (see Figure 14-13, part A). The thumb will hold the bandage while it is folded on itself.

✦ Unroll the bandage about 15 cm, and then turn your hand so that the bandage falls over itself (see Figure 14-13, part B).

✦ Continue the bandage around the limb, overlapping each previous turn by two-thirds the width of the bandage. Make

each bandage turn at the same position on the limb so that the turns of the bandage will be aligned (see Figure 14-13, part C).

✦ Terminate the bandage with two circular turns, and secure the end as described for circular turns.

Recurrent Turns

✦ Anchor the bandage with two circular turns.

✦ Fold the bandage back on itself, and bring it centrally over the distal end to be bandaged (see Figure 14-14).

✦ Holding it with the other hand, bring the bandage back over the end to the right of the centre bandage but overlapping it by two-thirds the width of the bandage.

✦ Bring the bandage back on the left side, also overlapping the first turn by two-thirds the width of the bandage.

✦ Continue this pattern of alternating right and left until the area is covered. Overlap the preceding turn by two-thirds the bandage width each time.

✦ Terminate the bandage with two circular turns (see Figure 14-15 on page 332). Secure the end appropriately.

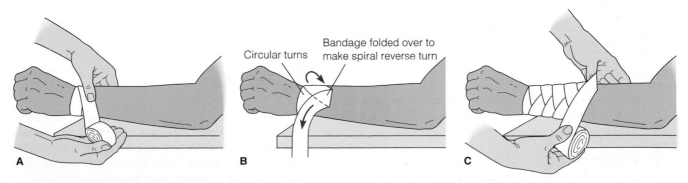

Circular turns   Bandage folded over to make spiral reverse turn

A   B   C

Figure 14-13 Applying spiral reverse turns.

NURSING MANAGEMENT ▶

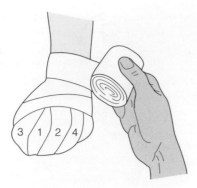

Figure 14-15 Completing a recurrent bandage.

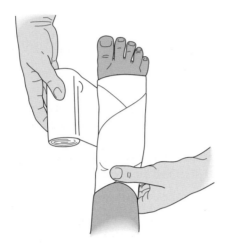

Figure 14-16 Applying a figure-eight bandage.

Figure-Eight Turns

+ Anchor the bandage with two circular turns.
+ Carry the bandage above the joint, around it and then below it, making a figure-eight (see Figure 14-16).
+ Continue above and below the joint, overlapping the previous turn by two-thirds the width of the bandage.
+ Terminate the bandage above the joint with two circular turns and then secure the end appropriately.

Tubular Support and Retention Bandages

Tubular retention bandages are made out of a gauze material and are used to retain dressings. They are particularly useful when dressing awkward areas such as the trunk of the body. Tubular support bandages are elasticated and when applied in a double layer can support strains and sprains of limbs.

Binders A **binder** is a type of bandage designed for a specific body part, for example, the triangular binder (sling) fits the arm. Binders are used to support large areas of the body, such as the abdomen, arm or chest.

Triangular Arm Sling

+ Ask the patient to flex the elbow to an 80-degree angle or less, depending on the purpose. The thumb should be facing

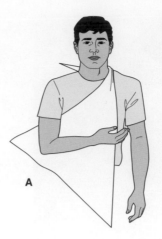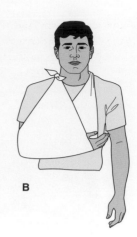

Figure 14-17 Large arm sling.

upward or inward toward the body. *An 80-degree angle is sufficient to support the forearm, to prevent swelling of the hand, and to relieve pressure on the shoulder joint (e.g. to support the paralysed arm of a stroke patient whose shoulder might otherwise become dislocated). A more acute angle is preferred if there is swelling of the hand (see how to apply a sling for maximum hand elevation, below).*
+ Place one end of the unfolded triangular binder over the shoulder of the uninjured side so that the binder falls down the front of the chest of the patient with the point of the triangle (apex) under the elbow of the injured side.
+ Take the upper corner and carry it around the neck until it hangs over the shoulder on the injured side.
+ Bring the lower corner of the binder up over the arm to the shoulder of the injured side. Using a square knot, secure this corner to the upper corner at the side of the neck on the injured side (see Figure 14-17, part A). *A square knot will not slip. Tying the knot at the side of the neck prevents pressure on the bony prominences of the vertebral column at the back of the neck.*
+ Make sure the wrist is supported, to maintain alignment.
+ Fold the sling neatly at the elbow and secure it with safety pins or tape. It may be folded and fastened at the front (see Figure 14-17, part B).
+ Remove the sling periodically to inspect the skin for indications of irritation, especially around the site of the knot.

It is important to note that once the dressing or bandage is applied, circulation beyond that dressing bandage should be checked. The nurse must note the colour of the skin, temperature, any sensation of 'pins and needles' or numbness.

EVALUATING

Evaluation of the care provided as measured against the desired outcomes should be undertaken as usual. Ongoing assessment judges whether patient outcomes have been achieved, in particular the nurse assesses skin integrity (particularly over bony prominences), nutritional and fluid intake, and signs of healing. If outcomes are not achieved, the nurse should explore the reasons why and consider other interventions to achieve the desired outcomes.

Wound management is one of the most challenging and varied roles within nursing. Effective wound management requires knowledge of wound healing, assessment and dressings. Generally wound management is not a role that can be delegated to nursing assistants as it requires a level of expertise to make rational decisions and evaluate previous treatment.

Key to wound management is accurate documentation. Assessment of the whole person is vital in understanding the underlying factors that could affect wound healing. This along with assessment of the wound should provide the nurse with the information to establish effective treatment. It is important to note that no dressing will ever heal a wound – the wound is healed from the inside out – and for some patients their wounds will never heal as their underlying condition is not conducive with healing.

CRITICAL REFLECTION

Let us revisit the case study on page 307. Now that you have read this chapter, how can you aid patient concordance with this type of treatment? How would you begin to assess a patient with a necrotic pressure ulcer? What intrinsic and extrinsic factors could affect wound healing?

CHAPTER HIGHLIGHTS

+ Maintaining skin integrity is an important function of the nurse.
+ Wounds are described as clean, clean-contaminated, contaminated or dirty (infected). Wounds are also classified by depth as partial thickness or full thickness. In addition, wounds are classified according to how they are acquired, as incisions, contusions, abrasions, punctures, lacerations and penetrating wounds.
+ A pressure ulcer is any lesion caused by unrelieved pressure that results in damage to underlying tissues. Pressure ulcers usually occur over bony prominences.
+ Two other factors that act in conjunction with pressure to produce a pressure ulcer are friction and shearing forces.
+ Several factors increase the risk for the development of pressure ulcers: immobility and inactivity, inadequate nutrition, faecal and urinary incontinence, decreased mental status, diminished sensation, excessive body heat and advanced age.
+ There are four grades of pressure ulcer development, which vary according to the degree of tissue damage.
+ There are two types of wound healing, which are distinguished by the amount of tissue loss: primary intention healing and secondary intention healing.
+ The wound-healing process has three phases: inflammatory, proliferative and maturation.

+ Major types of wound exudate are serous, purulent and haemorrhagic. Exudate can be a combination of two or three of these types.
+ The main complications of wound healing are haemorrhage, infection and dehiscence, each of which is identifiable by specific clinical signs and symptoms.
+ Factors affecting wound healing include developmental stage, nutritional status, lifestyle, medications and the presence of infection.
+ Several risk assessment tools are available to identify patients at risk for pressure ulcer development. They include scoring systems to evaluate a person's degree of risk.
+ Meticulous skin examination of common pressure ulcer sites by the nurse is an important ongoing assessment activity for patients at risk.
+ When a pressure ulcer is present, the nurse describes the ulcer in terms of location, size, depth, stage, colour, status of wound margins and surrounding skin, and specific signs of infection, if present.
+ Wound assessment is an ongoing process to evaluate healing. The nurse assesses wounds by visual inspection, palpation and the sense of smell. Essential information acquired from the assessment of wounds include wound appearance, size, drainage, swelling and pain.

+ Laboratory tests that may be used to assess the progress of wound healing include leukocyte count, haemoglobin, blood coagulation studies, serum protein analysis and wound cultures. Nurses are usually responsible for obtaining specimens of wound drainage for culture.

+ Major goals for patients at risk for developing pressure ulcers are to maintain skin integrity and to avoid potential associated risks.

+ Nursing interventions to prevent the formation of pressure ulcers include conducting ongoing assessment of risk factors and skin status, providing skin care to maintain skin integrity, ensuring adequate nutrition, implementing measures to avoid skin trauma, providing supportive devices and patient education.

+ Treatment for pressure ulcers varies according to the stage of the ulcer and local policy.

+ Major nursing responsibilities related to wound care include assisting the patient in obtaining sufficient nutrition and fluids, preventing wound infections and proper positioning.

+ Wound care may involve cleaning wounds, changing dressings, irrigating and applying bandages and binders.

+ Various dressing materials are available to protect wounds, absorb exudate and keep the wound bed moist, thus facilitating healing.

+ Synthetic dressings have been developed for use with specific types of wounds. These include transparent adhesive films, hydrocolloids, hydrogels, polyurethane foams and exudate absorbers. The nurse must be aware of the specific purposes of each and their indications for use.

+ The type of dressing used depends on (a) location, size and type of the wound; (b) amount of exudate; (c) whether or not the wound requires debridement, is infected or has sinus tracts; and (d) such considerations as frequency of dressing change, ease or difficulty of dressing applications and cost.

REFERENCES

Anderson, B. (2005) 'Nutrition and wound healing: the necessity of assessment', *British Journal of Nursing*, 14(19 Suppl.), S30, S32, S34, S36, S38.

Anthony, D. (1987) 'Norton revises risk scores', *Nursing Times*, 83, 6.

Ayello, E.A. and Braden, B. (2002) 'How and why to do pressure ulcer risk assessment', *Advances in Skin and Wound Care*, 15(3), 125–133.

Ayello, E.A. and Braden, B. (2001) 'Why is pressure ulcer risk assessment so important?', *Nursing*, 31(11), 74–79.

Bell, E.S. (2004) 'Managing a breast sinus wound in the community: a care study', *British Journal of Nursing*, 13(21), 1276–1279.

Bellnier, D.A., Greco, W.R., Nava, H., Loewen, G.M., Oseroff, A.R. Dougherty, T.J. (2006) 'Mild skin photosensitivity in cancer patients following injection of Photochlor (2-[1-hexyloxyethyl]-2-devinyl pyropheophorbide-a; HPPH) for photodynamic therapy', *Cancer Chemotherapy Pharmacology*, 57, 40–45.

Bennett, G. Dealey, C. and Posnet, J. (2004) 'The cost of pressure ulcers in the UK', *Age and Ageing*, 33, 230–235.

Bergstrom, N., Allman, R.M., Alvarez, A.M., Bennett, M.A., Carlson, C.E., Frantz, R.A., *et al.* (1994) *Pressure ulcer treatment: clinical practice guideline number 15. Quick reference guide for clinicians* (Publication No. 95-0653), Rockville, MD: Agency for Health Care Policy and Research, Public Health Service, US Department of Health and Human Services.

Bours, G.J.J.W., De Laat, E., Halfens, R.J.G. and Lubbers, M. (2001) 'Prevalence, risk factors and prevention of pressure ulcers in Dutch intensive care units – results of a cross-sectional survey', *Intensive Care Medicine*, 27, 1599–1605.

Butcher, M. (2002) 'Wound care: Managing wound sinuses', *Nursing Times*, 98(2), 63–65.

Charman, C.R., Morris, A.D. and Williams, H.C. (2000) 'Topical corticosteroid phobia in patients with atopic eczema', *British Journal of Dermatology*, 142, 931–936.

Cooper, P. and Gray, D. (2001) 'Comparison of two skin care regimes for incontinence', *British Journal of Nursing*, 10(6 Suppl.), S6–S20.

Dahners, L.E. and Mullis, B.H. (2004) 'Effect of non-steroidal anti-inflammatory drugs on bone formation and soft tissue healing', *Journal of American Academic Orthopaedic Surgery*, 12(3), 130–143.

Davies, C.E., Turton, G., Woolfrey, G., Elley, R. and Taylor, M. (2005) 'Exploring debridement options for chronic venous leg ulcers', *British Journal of Nursing*, 14(7), 393–397.

Davies, C. (1999) 'Cleansing rites and wrongs', *Nursing Times*, 95(43), 71–73.

de Graaff, J.C., Ubbink, D., Lagarde, S.M. and Jacobs, M.J. (2002) 'The feasibility and reliability of capillary blood pressure measurements in the fingernail fold', *Microvascular Research*, 63, 270–278.

Dowsett, C., Edwards-Jones, V. and Davies, S. (2004) 'Infection control for wound bed preparation', *British Journal of Community Nursing*, 9(9 Time supp), 12–17.

European Pressure Ulcer Advisory Panel (EPUAP) (2003) *Classification System*, www.epuap.org.uk. (Accessed 4 July 2005.)

European Pressure Ulcer Advisory Panel (EPUAP) (1999) 'Guidelines on treatment of pressure ulcers', *EPUAP Review*, 1, 31–33.

Farstvedt, E., Stashak, T.S. and Othic, A. (2004) 'Update on topical wound medication', *Clinical Techniques in Equine Practice*, 3(2), 164–172.

Fernandez, R., Griffiths, R. and Ussia, C. (2002) 'Water for wound cleansing', *Cochrane Database Systematic Review*, 4.

Horrocks, A. (2006) 'Prontosan wound irrigation and gel: management of chronic wounds', *British Journal of Nursing*, 15(22), 1222–1228.

Keller, B.P.J.A., Wille, J., van Ramshorst, B. and van der Werken, C. (2002) 'Pressure ulcers in intensive care patients: a review of risks and prevention', *Intensive Care Medicine*, 28, 1379–1388.

Margolis, D.J., Knauss, J., Bilker, W. and Baumgarten, M. (2003) 'Medical conditions as risk factors for pressure ulcers in an outpatient setting', *Age and Ageing*, 32, 259–264.

Mendez-Eastman, S. (2002) 'Negative-pressure wound therapy', *Nursing*, 32(5), 58–63.

Norton, D., McLaren, R. and Exton-Smith, A.N. (1975). *An investigation of geriatric nursing problems in hospital*, Edinburgh: Churchill Livingstone.

Oliver, L. (1997) 'Wound cleansing', *Nursing Standard*, 11(20), 47–56.

Royal College of Nursing (2001) *Clinical practice guidelines: pressure ulcer risk assessment and prevention*, London: RCN.

Russell, L. (2000) 'Malnutrition and pressure ulcers: nutritional assessment tools', *British Journal of Nursing*, 9(4), 194–204.

Selim, P., Bashford, C. and Grossman, C. (2001) 'Evidence-based practice: tap water cleansing of leg ulcers in the community', *Journal of Clinical Nursing*, 10, 372–379.

Tobon, A., Arango, M., Fernandez, D. and Restrepo, A. (2003) 'Mucormycosis (zygomycosis) in a heart-kidney transplant recipient. Recovery after Posaconazole Therapy', *Clinical Infectious Diseases*, 36, 1488–1491.

US Department of Health and Human Services (1992) *Clinical practice guidelines, pressure ulcers in adults: Prediction and prevention*, Rockville, MD: Public Health Service.

Waterlow, J. (1997) 'Practical use of the Waterlow tool in the community', *British Journal of Community Nursing*, 2(2), 83–86.

Whiteford, L. (2003) 'Nicotine, CO and HCN: the detrimental effects of smoking on wound healing', *British Journal of Community Nursing*, 8(12 supp): S22–S26.

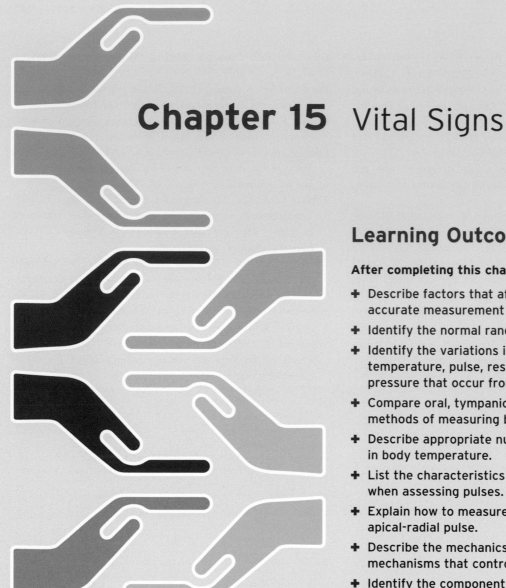

Chapter 15 Vital Signs

Learning Outcomes

After completing this chapter, you will be able to:

+ Describe factors that affect the vital signs and accurate measurement of them.

+ Identify the normal ranges for each vital sign.

+ Identify the variations in normal body temperature, pulse, respirations and blood pressure that occur from infancy to old age.

+ Compare oral, tympanic, rectal and axillary methods of measuring body temperature.

+ Describe appropriate nursing care for alterations in body temperature.

+ List the characteristics that should be included when assessing pulses.

+ Explain how to measure the apical pulse and the apical-radial pulse.

+ Describe the mechanics of breathing and the mechanisms that control respirations.

+ Identify the components of a respiratory assessment.

+ Differentiate systolic from diastolic blood pressure.

+ Describe five phases of Korotkoff's sounds.

+ Describe various methods and sites used to measure blood pressure.

+ Discuss measurement of blood oxygenation using pulse oximetry.

CASE STUDY

Rosa Granville is a 72-year-old lady who lives with her daughter Francine at their family business in a rural community. Her daughter has noticed Rosa has not been well for the past few months complaining of dizziness, loss of balance and falls. Francine contacts her family doctor who agrees to visit Rosa at home.

After a home visit by the doctor and some initial investigations including the recording of base line vital signs, it is decided that the community nurse will visit Rosa three times a week to monitor her vital signs. When the community nurse assesses Rosa utilising the nursing process and a model of care, a care plan is devised which is family centred. The agreed care plan suggests Rosa and Francine record patterns of symptoms In a diary and the community nurse will visit Rosa at varying times during the day three times a week. The care plan includes the recording of blood pressure (both lying and standing), pulse and respirations at each of the planned visits.

After visiting Rosa for two weeks a pattern emerges that her blood pressure is lower in the mornings and a significant difference is noted when this is recorded from a lying to standing position. Symptoms are also worse at this time. The results are discussed and the care plan amended with the consideration the falls Rosa has been experiencing could be due to 'postural hypotension' in the mornings.

After reading this chapter you will be able to discuss vital signs and their role in assessing a patient's stability.

INTRODUCTION

Vital signs are the physiological measures nurses record in clinical situations to assess the clinical status of patients in their care and to monitor for changes. The vital signs include body temperature, pulse, respirations and blood pressure. Pulse oximetry is also commonly measured at the same time as the traditional vital signs – this is a measurement of blood oxygen saturation. These signs, which should be looked at in total, are checked to monitor the functions of the body. The signs reflect changes in function that otherwise might not be observed. Monitoring a patient's vital signs should not be an automatic or routine procedure; it should be a thoughtful, scientific assessment. Vital signs, which should be evaluated with reference to the patient's present and prior health status, are compared to the patient's usual 'base line' (if known) and accepted normal standards (see Table 15-1).

When and how often to assess a specific patient's vital signs are chiefly nursing judgements, depending on the patient's health status. A patient's vital signs may be recorded on a routine basis as part of an identified care plan, however if there is a change in the patient's condition then the vital signs may need to recorded more frequently. Examples of times to assess vital signs are listed in *Box 15-1*.

Often, someone other than the registered nurse, such as a care assistant or healthcare support worker, may record a patient's routine vital signs in a clinical area. Even when the recording of vital signs is not performed by a registered nurse the registered nurse remains ultimately accountable for the interpretation of the recorded values. When this clinical intervention is delegated the support staff should report all findings to the registered nurse immediately when completed.

BOX 15-1 Times to Assess Vital Signs

+ On admission to a clinical area to obtain baseline data
+ When a patient has a change in health status or reports symptoms such as chest pain or feeling hot, dizzy or faint
+ Before and after surgical intervention or an invasive procedure
+ Before and/or after the administration of a medication that could affect the respiratory or cardiovascular systems, for example, before giving a digitalis preparation (Digoxin)
+ Before and after any nursing intervention that could affect the vital signs (e.g. mobilising a patient who has been on bed rest)

BODY TEMPERATURE

Body temperature reflects the balance between the heat produced and the heat lost from the body, measured in heat units called *degrees*. There are two kinds of body temperature: core temperature and surface temperature. **Core temperature** is the temperature of the deep tissues of the body, such as the abdominal cavity and pelvic cavity. It remains relatively constant. The normal core body temperature is a range of temperatures (see Figure 15-1 on page 338). The **surface temperature** is the temperature of the skin, the subcutaneous tissue and fat. It, by contrast, rises and falls in response to the environment.

Table 15-1 Variations in Normal Vital Signs by Age

Age	Oral temperature in degrees celsius	Pulse (average and ranges)	Respirations (average and ranges)	Blood pressure (mm Hg)
Newborns	36.8 (axillary)	130 (80-180)	35 (30-80)	73/55
1 year	36.8 (axillary)	120 (80-140)	30 (20-40)	90/55
5-8 years	37	100 (75-120)	20 (15-25)	95/57
10 years	37	70 (50-90)	19 (15-25)	102/62
Teen	37	75 (50-90)	18 (15-20)	120/80
Adult	37	80 (60-100)	16 (12-20)	120/80
Older adult (>70 years)	37	70 (60-100)	16 (15-20)	Possible increased diastolic

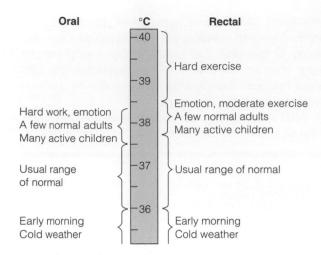

Figure 15-1 Estimated ranges of body temperatures in normal persons. (*Note:* Adapted from *Fever and the Regulation of Body Temperature*, by E.F. DuBois, 1948, Springfield, IL: Charles C. Thomas. Reprinted with permission.)

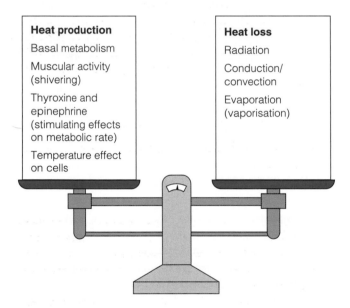

Figure 15-2 As long as heat production and heat loss are properly balanced, body temperature remains constant. Factors contributing to heat production (and temperature rise) are shown on the left side of the scale; those contributing to heat loss (and temperature fall) are shown on the right side of the scale. (*Note:* From *Human Anatomy and Physiology*, 4th edn (p. 953), by E.N. Marieb, 1998, Menlo Park, CA: Benjamin/Cummings. Adapted with permission.)

The body continually produces heat as a by-product of metabolism. When the amount of heat produced by the body equals the amount of heat lost, the person is in **heat balance** (see Figure 15-2).

A number of factors affect the body's heat production. The most important are these five:

1. *Basal metabolic rate.* The **basal metabolic rate (BMR)** is the rate of energy utilisation in the body required to maintain essential activities such as breathing. Metabolic rates decrease with age. In general, the younger the person, the higher the BMR (Marieb, 1998: 952).

2. *Muscle activity.* Muscle activity, including shivering, increases the metabolic rate.

3. *Thyroxine output.* Increased thyroxine output increases the rate of cellular metabolism throughout the body. This effect is called **chemical thermogenesis**, the stimulation of heat production in the body through increased cellular metabolism.

4. *Epinephrine (adrenaline), norepinephrine (noradrenaline) and sympathetic stimulation.* These hormones immediately increase the rate of cellular metabolism in many body tissues. Epinephrine and norepinephrine directly affect liver and muscle cells, thereby increasing cellular metabolism.

5. *Fever.* Fever increases the cellular metabolic rate and thus increases the body's temperature further.

Heat is lost from the body through radiation, conduction, convection and vaporisation. **Radiation** is the transfer of heat from the surface of one object to the surface of another without contact between the two objects, mostly in the form of infrared rays. For example, radiation accounts for 60% of the heat lost by a nude person standing in a room at normal room temperature (Guyton, 1996: 912).

Conduction is the transfer of heat from one molecule to a molecule of lower temperature. Conductive transfer cannot take place without contact between the molecules and normally accounts for minimal heat loss except, for example, when a body is immersed in cold water. The amount of heat transferred depends on the temperature difference and the amount and duration of the contact.

Convection is the dispersion of heat by air currents. The body usually has a small amount of warm air adjacent to it. This warm air rises and is replaced by cooler air, and so people always lose a small amount of heat through convection.

Vaporisation is continuous evaporation of moisture from the respiratory tract and from the mucosa of the mouth and from the skin. This continuous and unnoticed water loss is called **insensible water loss**, and the accompanying heat loss is called **insensible heat loss**. Insensible heat loss accounts for about 10% of basal heat loss. When the body temperature increases, vaporisation accounts for greater heat loss.

Regulation of Body Temperature

The system that regulates body temperature has three main parts: sensors in the peripheral body shell and in the body core, an integrator in the hypothalamus, and an effector system that adjusts the production and loss of heat. Most sensors or sensory receptors are in the skin. The skin has more receptors for cold than warmth. Therefore, skin sensors detect cold more efficiently than warmth.

When the skin becomes chilled over the entire body, three physiologic processes to increase the body temperature take place:

1. Shivering increases heat production.
2. Sweating is inhibited to decrease heat loss.
3. Vasoconstriction decreases heat loss.

The **hypothalamic integrator**, the centre that controls the core temperature, is located in the preoptic area of the hypothalamus. When the sensors in the hypothalamus detect heat, they send out signals intended to reduce the temperature, that is, to decrease heat production and increase heat loss. When the cold sensors are stimulated, signals are sent out to increase heat production and decrease heat loss.

The signals from the cold-sensitive receptors of the hypothalamus initiate effectors, such as vasoconstriction, shivering and the release of epinephrine, which increases cellular metabolism and hence heat production. When the warmth-sensitive receptors in the hypothalamus are stimulated, the effector system sends out signals that initiate sweating and peripheral vasodilatation. Also, when this system is stimulated, the person consciously makes appropriate adjustments, such as putting on additional clothing in response to cold or turning on a fan in response to heat.

Factors Affecting Body Temperature

Nurses should be aware of the factors that can affect a patient's body temperature so that they can recognise normal temperature variations and understand the significance of body temperature measurements that deviate from normal. Among the factors that affect body temperature are the following:

1. *Age.* The infant is greatly influenced by the temperature of the environment and must be protected from extreme changes. Children's temperatures continue to be more variable than those of adults until puberty. Many older people, particularly those over 75 years old, are at risk of hypothermia (temperatures below 36°C) for a variety of reasons, such as inadequate diet, loss of subcutaneous fat, lack of activity and reduced thermoregulatory efficiency. Older people are also particularly sensitive to extremes in the environmental temperature due to decreased thermoregulatory controls.
2. *Diurnal variations (circadian rhythms).* Body temperatures normally change throughout the day, varying as much as 1.0°C between the early morning and the late afternoon. The point of highest body temperature is usually reached between 20.00 and 24.00 hours (8:00 p.m. and midnight), and the lowest point is reached during sleep between 04.00 and 06.00 hours (4:00 and 6:00 a.m.) (see Figure 15-3).
3. *Exercise.* Hard work or strenuous exercise can increase body temperature to as high as 38.3 to 40°C measured rectally.
4. *Hormones.* Women usually experience more hormone fluctuations than men. In women, progesterone secretion at the time of ovulation raises body temperature by about 0.3 to 0.6°C above basal temperature (Ladewig *et al.*, 1998).
5. *Stress.* Stimulation of the sympathetic nervous system can increase the production of epinephrine and norepinephrine, thereby increasing metabolic activity and heat

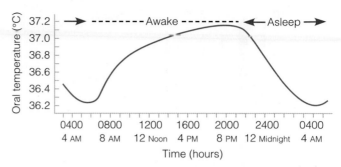

Figure 15-3 Range of oral temperatures during 24 hours for a healthy young adult.

production. Nurses may anticipate that a highly stressed or anxious patient could have an elevated body temperature for that reason.
6. *Environment.* Extremes in environmental temperatures can affect a person's temperature regulatory systems. If the temperature is assessed in a very warm room and the body temperature cannot be modified by convection, conduction or radiation, the temperature will be elevated. Similarly, if the patient has been outside in extremely cold weather without suitable clothing, the body temperature may be low.

Alterations in Body Temperature

There are two primary alterations in body temperature: pyrexia and hypothermia.

Pyrexia

A body temperature above the usual range is called **pyrexia, hyperthermia** or (in lay terms) **fever**. A very high temperature, such as 41°C, is called **hyperpyrexia** (see Figure 15-4 on page 340). The patient who has a raised temperature is referred to as **febrile**; the one who has not is **afebrile**.

Four common types of pyrexia are intermittent, remittent, relapsing and constant. During an **intermittent pyrexia**, the body temperature alternates at regular intervals between periods of raised and periods of normal or subnormal temperatures. During a **remittent pyrexia**, a wide range of temperature fluctuations (more than 2°C) occurs over the 24-hour period, all of which are above normal. In a **relapsing pyrexia**, short febrile periods of a few days are interspersed with periods of one or two days of normal temperature. During a **constant pyrexia**, the body temperature fluctuates minimally but always remains above normal. A temperature that rises to pyrexia level rapidly following a normal temperature and then returns to normal within a few hours is called a **pyrexia spike**.

The clinical signs of fever vary with the onset, course and abatement stages of the fever (see *Box 15-2* on page 340). These signs occur as a result of changes in the set point of the temperature control mechanism regulated by the hypothalamus. Under normal conditions, whenever the core temperature rises

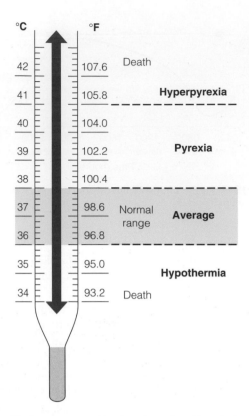

Figure 15-4 Terms used to describe alterations in body temperature (oral measurements) and ranges in Celsius (centigrade). (National Heart, Lung and Blood Institute, part of the National Institutes of Health and the US Department of Health and Human Services.)

BOX 15-2 Clinical Signs of Raised Temperature

Onset (Cold or Chill Stage)
+ Increased heart rate
+ Increased respiratory rate and depth
+ Shivering
+ Pallid, cold skin
+ Complaints of feeling cold
+ Cyanotic nail beds
+ 'Goose pimples' appearance of the skin
+ Cessation of sweating

Course
+ Absence of chills
+ Skin that feels warm
+ Photosensitivity
+ Glassy-eyed appearance
+ Increased pulse and respiratory rates
+ Increased thirst
+ Mild to severe dehydration
+ Drowsiness, restlessness, delirium or convulsions
+ Herpetic lesions of the mouth
+ Loss of appetite (if the fever is prolonged)
+ Malaise, weakness and aching muscles

Defervescence (temperature abatement)
+ Skin that appears flushed and feels warm
+ Sweating
+ Decreased shivering
+ Possible dehydration

above 37°C, the rate of heat *loss* is increased, resulting in a fall in temperature toward the set-point level. Conversely, when the core temperature falls below 37°C, the rate of heat *production* is increased, resulting in a rise in temperature toward the set point.

During a raised temperature the set point of the hypothalamic thermostat changes suddenly from the normal level to a higher than normal value (e.g. 39.5°C) as a result of the effects of tissue destruction, pyrogenic substances or dehydration on the hypothalamus. Although the set point changes rapidly, the core body temperature (i.e. the blood temperature) reaches this new set point only after several hours. During this interval, the usual heat production responses that cause elevation of the body temperature occur: chills, feeling of coldness, cold skin due to vasoconstriction, and shivering.

When the core temperature reaches the new set point, the person feels neither cold nor hot and no longer experiences chills. Depending on the degree of temperature elevation, other signs may occur during the course of the pyrexia. Very high temperatures, such as 41 to 42°C, damage the cells throughout the body, particularly in the brain where destruction of neuronal cells is irreversible. Damage to the liver, kidneys and other body organs can also be great enough to disrupt functioning and eventually cause death.

When the cause of the high temperature is suddenly removed, the set point of the hypothalamic thermostat is suddenly reduced to a lower value, perhaps even back to the original normal level. In this instance, the hypothalamus now attempts to lower the temperature to 37°C, and the usual heat loss responses causing a reduction of the body temperature occur: excessive sweating and a hot, flushed skin due to sudden vasodilatation. This sudden change of events is known as the *crisis*, the *flush* or the *defervescent (abatement) stage* of a pyrexic condition.

Nursing interventions for a patient who has a pyrexia are designed to support the body's normal physiological processes, provide comfort and prevent complications. During the course of pyrexias, the nurse needs to monitor the patient's vital signs closely.

Nursing measures during the chill phase are designed to help the patient decrease heat loss. At this time, the body's physiological processes are attempting to raise the core temperature to the new set-point temperature. During the flush or crisis phase, the body processes are attempting to lower the core temperature to the reduced or normal set-point temperature. At this time, the nurse takes measures to increase heat loss and decrease heat production. Nursing interventions for a patient with a pyrexia are shown in *Box 15-3*.

BOX 15-3 Nursing Interventions for Pyrexial Patients

+ Monitor vital signs.
+ Assess skin colour and temperature.
+ Monitor white blood cell count, and relevant laboratory reports for indications of infection or dehydration.
+ Remove excess blankets when the patient feels warm, but provide extra warmth when the patient feels chilled.
+ Provide adequate nutrition and fluids (e.g. 2,500–3,000 ml per day) to meet the increased metabolic demands and prevent dehydration.
+ Measure intake and output accurately.
+ Reduce physical activity to limit heat production, especially during the flush stage.
+ Administer antipyretics (drugs that reduce the level of temperature such as Paracetamol) as prescribed.
+ Provide oral hygiene to keep the mucous membranes moist.
+ Provide a tepid sponge bath to increase heat loss through conduction.
+ Provide dry clothing and bed linen.

Hypothermia

Hypothermia is a core body temperature below the lower limit of normal. The three physiological mechanisms of hypothermia are (a) excessive heat loss, (b) inadequate heat production to counteract heat loss and (c) impaired hypothalamic thermoregulation. The clinical signs of hypothermia are listed in *Box 15-4*.

Hypothermia may be accidental or induced. Accidental hypothermia can occur as a result of (a) exposure to a cold environment, (b) immersion in cold water and (c) lack of

BOX 15-4 Clinical Signs of Hypothermia

+ Decreased body temperature, pulse and respirations
+ Severe shivering (initially)
+ Feelings of cold and chills
+ Pale, cool, waxy skin
+ Hypotension
+ Decreased urinary output
+ Lack of muscle coordination
+ Disorientation
+ Drowsiness progressing to coma

BOX 15-5 Nursing Interventions for Patients with Hypothermia

+ Provide a warm environment.
+ Provide dry clothing.
+ Apply warm blankets.
+ Keep limbs close to body.
+ Cover the patient's scalp with a cap or turban.
+ Supply warm oral or intravenous fluids.
+ Apply warming pads.

adequate clothing, shelter or heat. In older people the problem can be compounded by a decreased metabolic rate and the use of sedatives.

Managing hypothermia involves removing the patient from the cold and rewarming the patient's body. For the patient with mild hypothermia, the body is rewarmed by applying blankets; for the patient with severe hypothermia, a rewarming blanket (an electronically controlled blanket that provides a specified temperature either via direct heat or warm air) is applied and warm intravenous fluids may be given. Wet clothing, which increases heat loss because of the high conductivity of water, should be replaced with dry clothing. See *Box 15-5* for nursing interventions for patents who have hypothermia.

Induced hypothermia is the deliberate lowering of the body temperature to decrease the need for oxygen by the body tissues. Induced hypothermia can involve the whole body or a body part. It is sometimes indicated prior to surgical intervention (e.g. cardiac and brain surgery).

Assessing Body Temperature

The four most common sites for measuring body temperature are oral, rectal, axillary and the tympanic membrane. Each of the sites has advantages and disadvantages (see Table 15-2 on page 342).

The body temperature is frequently measured *orally*. This method reflects changing body temperature more quickly than the rectal method. If a patient has been taking cold or hot food or fluids or smoking, the nurse should wait 30 minutes before taking the temperature orally to ensure that the temperature of the mouth is not affected by the temperature of the food, fluid or warm smoke.

Rectal temperature readings are considered to be very accurate, although very rarely recorded in clinical practice. In some clinical areas, taking temperatures rectally is not advised for patients with myocardial infarction. It is believed that inserting a rectal thermometer can produce vagal stimulation, which in turn can cause myocardial damage. However, not all authorities share this belief. Rectal temperatures are contraindicated for patients who are undergoing rectal surgery, have diarrhoea or diseases of the rectum, are immuno-suppressed, have a clotting disorder or have significant haemorrhoids.

Table 15-2 Advantages and Disadvantages of Four Sites for Body Temperature Measurement

Site	Advantages	Disadvantages
Oral	Accessible and convenient	Glass thermometers can break if bitten.
		Inaccurate if patient has just ingested hot or cold food or fluid or smoked.
		Could injure the mouth following oral surgery.
Rectal	Reliable measurement	Inconvenient and more unpleasant for patients; difficult for patient who cannot turn to the side.
		Could injure the rectum following rectal surgery.
		A rectal glass thermometer does not respond to changes in arterial temperatures as quickly as an oral thermometer, a fact that may be potentially dangerous for febrile patients because misleading information may be acquired.
		Presence of stool may interfere with thermometer placement. If the stool is soft, the thermometer may be embedded in stool rather than against the wall of the rectum.
		(No longer used routinely for reasons of safety)
Axillary (in the arm pit)	Safe and noninvasive	The thermometer must be left in place a long time to obtain an accurate measurement.
Tympanic membrane	Readily accessible; reflects the core temperature. Very fast.	Can be uncomfortable and involves risk of injuring the membrane if the probe is inserted too far.
		Repeated measurements may vary. Right and left measurements can differ.
		Presence of cerumen/ear wax can affect the reading.

The axilla is the preferred site for measuring temperature in newborns because it is accessible and offers no possibility of rectal perforation. However, some research indicates that the axillary method is inaccurate when assessing a pyrexia (Bindler and Ball, 2003). Nurses should check local policy and protocol when taking the temperature of newborns, infants, toddlers and children. Adult patients for whom the axillary method of temperature assessment is appropriate include those with oral inflammation or wired jaws, patients recovering from oral surgery, patients who cannot breathe through their noses, irrational or confused patients, and patients for whom other temperature sites are contraindicated.

The *tympanic membrane*, or nearby tissue in the ear canal, is another site for core body temperature. Like the sublingual oral site, the tympanic membrane has an abundant arterial blood supply, primarily from branches of the external carotid artery. Because temperature sensors applied directly to the tympanic membrane can be uncomfortable and involve risk of membrane injury or perforation, noninvasive infrared thermometers are now used. Electronic tympanic thermometers are found extensively in both inpatient hospital and primary care settings.

In addition to the four common sites for measuring temperature, the forehead may also be used using a chemical thermometer. Forehead temperature measurements are most useful for infants and children where a more invasive measurement is not necessary. If the forehead indicates a temperature elevation, a glass or electronic thermometer should be used to obtain a more accurate measurement.

Types of Thermometers

Traditionally, body temperatures were measured using *mercury-in-glass thermometers*. Glass thermometers can be hazardous, however, due to exposure to mercury, which is toxic to humans, and broken glass should the thermometer crack or break. Some clinical areas no longer use mercury-in-glass thermometers. In some cases, plastics have replaced glass and safer chemicals have replaced mercury in modern versions of the thermometer. Thus, the nurse may still encounter this type of thermometer and must be well versed in its safe use.

Although the amount of mercury in a thermometer (or in a flourescent light bulb) is minimal, should it break, cleanup involves several 'dos and don'ts'. Unsealed mercury slowly vaporises into the air and these mercury vapors are toxic. Keep children and animals away from the area. Wearing rubber gloves, wipe mercury beads off clothing, skin or other disposable items with a paper towel placed immediately into a plastic bag. Discard the item. If the spill is on a porous material that cannot be discarded (e.g. carpet), a specialist mercury spill kit may be required. If the mercury is on a hard surface, use folded stiff cardboard to slowly gather the beads and pour them into a wide-mouthed container. Use a torch to search for the beads since the light will reflect off the mercury. Dispose of all items used in the cleanup in a plastic bag that is well sealed. Wash thoroughly after any contact with spilt mercury. Keep the area well ventilated for several days. Do not use any type of vacuum cleaner or broom since these will disperse the mercury and will

CENTIGRADE

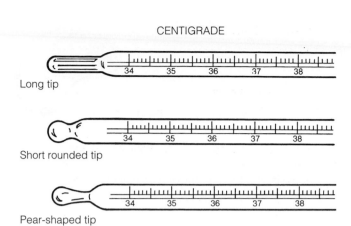

Long tip

Short rounded tip

Pear-shaped tip

Three types of thermometer tips (Centigrade scale)

Figure 15-5 Three types of thermometer tips (centigrade scale).

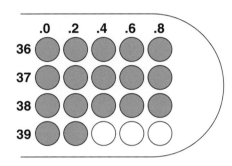

Figure 15-6 A chemical thermometer showing a reading of 39.2°C.

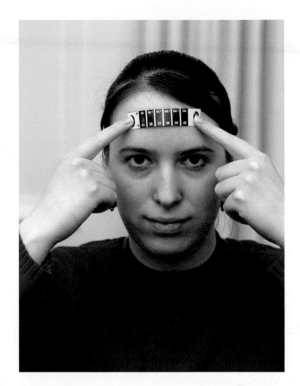

Figure 15-7 A temperature-sensitive skin tape.

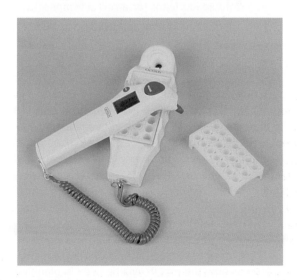

Figure 15-8 An infrared (tympanic) thermometer used to measure the tympanic membrane temperature.

be contaminated. Do not pour the mercury down a toilet or drain and do not wash or reuse contaminated materials.

Oral thermometers may have long, short, slender or rounded tips (see Figure 15-5). A rounded thermometer can be used at the rectal as well as other sites. In some clinical areas, thermometer ends may be colour coded; for example, blue thermometers may be used for rectal temperatures and red/silver/clear ones for oral and axillary temperatures.

Chemical disposable thermometers are also used to measure body temperatures. Chemical thermometers using liquid crystal dots or bars or heat-sensitive tape or patches applied to the forehead change colour to indicate temperature. Some of these are single use and others may be reused several times. One type that has small chemical dots at one end is shown in Figure 15-6. To read the temperature, the nurse notes the highest reading among the dots that have changed colour.

Temperature-sensitive tape may also be used to obtain a general indication of body surface temperature. It does not indicate the core temperature. The tape contains liquid crystals that change colour according to temperature. When applied to the skin, usually of the forehead or abdomen, the temperature digits on the tape respond by changing colour (see Figure 15-7).

The skin area should be dry. After the length of time specified by the manufacturer (e.g. 15 seconds), a colour appears on the tape. This method is particularly useful at home and for infants whose temperatures are to be monitored.

Infrared thermometers sense body heat in the form of infrared energy given off by a heat source, which in the ear canal is primarily the tympanic membrane (see Figure 15-8). The infrared thermometer makes no contact with the tympanic membrane.

Procedure 15-1 on page 344 shows the steps in assessing body temperature.

PROCEDURE 15-1 Assessing Body Temperature

Purposes

+ To establish baseline data for subsequent evaluation
+ To identify whether the core temperature is within normal range
+ To determine changes in the core temperature in response to specific therapies (e.g. antipyretic medication, immunosuppressive therapy, invasive procedure)
+ To monitor patients at risk for imbalanced body temperature (e.g. patients at risk for infection or diagnosis of infection; those who have been exposed to temperature extremes)

Assessment

Assess

+ Clinical signs of pyrexia
+ Clinical signs of hypothermia
+ Site most appropriate for measurement
+ Factors that may alter core body temperature

Planning

Equipment

+ Thermometer
+ Thermometer sheath or cover
+ Water-soluble lubricant for a rectal temperature
+ Disposable gloves
+ Towel for axillary temperature
+ Tissues/alcohol wipes

Implementation

Preparation

Check that all equipment is functioning normally. If necessary, shake a glass thermometer down to below 35°C. *The indicator fluid will not fall below the starting level if the patient's temperature is less than that. Beginning with the thermometer on a very low temperature allows the nurse to note that the indicator fluid has risen to the patient's actual temperature.*

Performance

1. Explain to the patient what you are going to do, why it is necessary and how they can cooperate. Discuss how the results will be used in planning further care or treatments.
2. Wash hands and observe appropriate infection control procedures. Apply gloves if performing a rectal temperature.
3. Consider patient privacy.
4. Place the patient in the appropriate position (e.g. lateral position for inserting a rectal thermometer).
5. Place the thermometer (see *Box 15-6* on page 346):
   • Apply a protective sheath or probe cover if appropriate.
   • Lubricate a rectal thermometer.
6. Wait the appropriate amount of time: 2–3 minutes for an oral or rectal temperature using a glass thermometer, 6–9 minutes for an axillary temperature with a glass thermometer. Electronic and tympanic thermometers will indicate that the reading is complete through a light or tone. Check package instructions for length of time to wait prior to reading chemical dot or tape thermometers.
7. Remove the thermometer and discard the cover or wipe with a tissue if necessary.
8. Read the temperature, if the temperature is obviously too high, too low or inconsistent with the patient's condition, recheck it with a thermometer known to be functioning properly.
9. Clean the thermometer in accordance with local infection control policy.
10. Document the temperature on the patient's observation chart (see Figure 15-9). A rectal temperature may be recorded with an 'R' next to the value or with the mark on a graphic sheet circled. An axillary temperature may be recorded with PA or marked on a graphic sheet with an X.

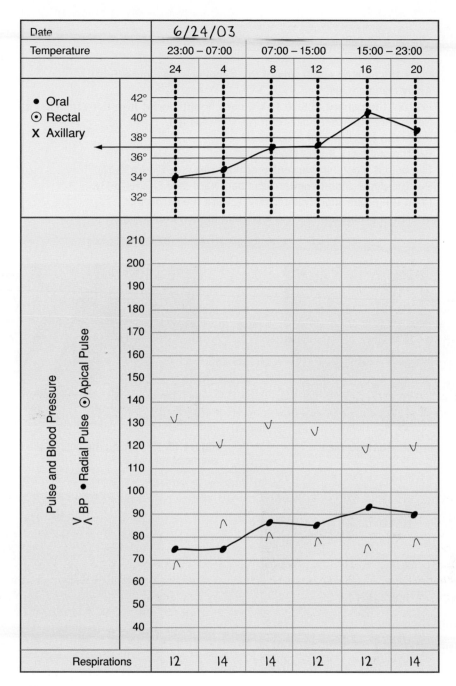

Date	6/24/03					
Temperature	23:00 – 07:00		07:00 – 15:00		15:00 – 23:00	
	24	4	8	12	16	20

Figure 15-9 Vital signs graphic record.

Evaluation

+ Compare the temperature measurement to baseline data, normal range for age of patient, and patient's previous temperatures. Analyse considering time of day and any additional influencing factors and other vital signs.

+ Conduct appropriate follow-up such as notifying the medical staff, administering a medication or adjusting the patient's environment. This includes teaching the patient how to lower an elevated temperature through actions such as increasing fluid intake, coughing and deep breathing, or removing heavy coverings.

BOX 15-6 Thermometer Placement

Oral	Place the bulb on either side of the frenulum (see Figure 15-10).
Rectal	Apply clean gloves.
	Instruct the patient to take a slow deep breath during insertion (see Figure 15-11).
	Never force the thermometer if resistance is felt.
	Insert 3.5 cm (1½ inch) in adults.
Axillary	Pat the axilla dry if very moist.
	The bulb is placed in the centre of the axilla (see Figure 15-12).
Tympanic	Pull the pinna slightly upward and backward (see Figure 15-13).
	Point the probe slightly anteriorly, toward the eardrum.
	Insert the probe slowly using a circular motion until snug.

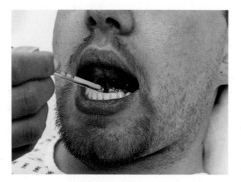

Figure 15-10 Oral thermometer placement.

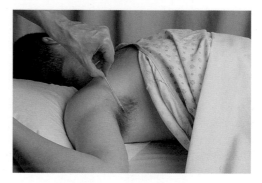

Figure 15-12 Placing the bulb of the thermometer in the centre of the axilla.

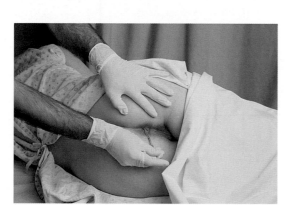

Figure 15-11 Inserting a rectal thermometer.

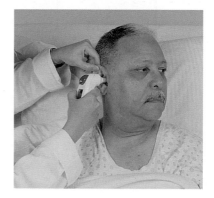

Figure 15-13 Pull the pinna of the ear up and back while inserting the tympanic thermometer.

PULSE

The **pulse** is a wave of blood created by contraction of the left ventricle of the heart. Generally the pulse wave represents the stroke volume output and the amount of blood that enters the arteries with each ventricular contraction. **Compliance** of the arteries is their ability to contract and expand. When a person's arteries lose their elasticity, as can happen in old age, greater pressure is required to pump the blood into the arteries.

Cardiac output is the volume of blood pumped into the arteries by the heart and equals the result of the stroke volume (SV) times the heart rate (HR) per minute. For example, 65 ml × 70 beats per minute = 4.55 l per minute. When an adult is resting, the heart pumps about 5 litres of blood each minute.

In a healthy person, the pulse reflects the heartbeat; that is, the pulse rate is the same as the rate of the ventricular contractions of the heart. However, in some types of cardiovascular disease, the heartbeat and pulse rates can differ. For example, a patient's heart may produce very weak or small pulse waves that are not detectable in a peripheral pulse far from the heart. In these instances, the nurse should assess the heartbeat and the peripheral pulse. A **peripheral pulse** is a pulse located away from the heart, for example, in the foot, wrist or neck. The **apical pulse**, in contrast, is a central pulse; that is, it is located at the apex of the heart.

Factors Affecting the Pulse

The rate of the pulse is expressed in beats per minute (BPM). A pulse rate varies according to a number of factors. The nurse should consider each of the following factors when assessing a patient's pulse:

+ *Age.* As age increases, the pulse rate gradually decreases. See Table 15-1 on page 337 for specific variations in pulse rates from birth to adulthood.
+ *Gender.* After puberty, the average male's pulse rate is slightly lower than the female's.
+ *Exercise.* The pulse rate normally increases with activity. The rate of increase in the professional athlete is often less than in the average person because of greater cardiac size, strength and efficiency.
+ *Pyrexia.* The pulse rate increases (a) in response to the lowered blood pressure that results from peripheral vasodilatation associated with elevated body temperature and (b) because of the increased metabolic rate.
+ *Medications.* Some medications decrease the pulse rate, and others increase it. For example, cardiotonics (e.g. digitalis preparations – Digoxin) decrease the heart rate, whereas epinephrine/adrenaline increases it.
+ *Hypovolaemia.* Loss of blood from the vascular system normally increases pulse rate. In adults the loss of circulating volume results in an adjustment of the heart rate to increase blood pressure as the body compensates for the lost blood volume. Adults can usually lose up to 10% of their normal circulating volume without adverse effects.
+ *Stress.* In response to stress, sympathetic nervous stimulation increases the overall activity of the heart. Stress increases the rate as well as the force of the heartbeat. Fear and anxiety as well as the perception of severe pain stimulate the sympathetic system.
+ *Position changes.* When a person is sitting or standing, blood usually pools in dependent vessels of the venous system. Pooling results in a transient decrease in the venous blood return to the heart and a subsequent reduction in blood pressure and increase in heart rate.
+ *Pathology.* Certain diseases such as some heart conditions or those that impair oxygenation can alter the resting pulse rate.

LIFESPAN CONSIDERATIONS

Temperature

Infants
+ Using the axillary site, you may need to hold the infant's arm against the chest (see Figure 15-14).
+ Axillary route may not be as accurate as other routes for detecting a pyrexia in children (Bindler and Ball, 2003).
+ The tympanic route is fast and convenient. Place infant supine and stabilise the head. Pull the pinna straight back and slightly downward. Direct the probe tip anteriorly and insert far enough to seal the canal.
+ Avoid the tympanic route in a child with active ear infections or tympanic membrane drainage tubes.
+ The rectal route is least desirable in infants.

Children
+ Tympanic or axillary sites are commonly preferred.
+ For the tympanic route, have the child held on an adult's lap with the child's head held gently against the adult for support. Pull the pinna straight back and upward for children over age three (see Figure 15-15 on page 348).
+ Avoid the tympanic route in a child with active ear infections or tympanic membrane drainage tubes.
+ The oral route may be used for children over age three but non-breakable, electronic thermometers are recommended.
+ For a rectal temperature place the child prone across your lap or in a side-lying position with the knees flexed. Insert the thermometer 1 inch into the rectum. (Very few clinical areas advocate this route.)

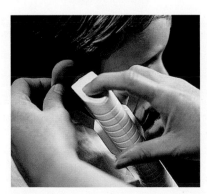

Figure 15-14 Tympanic temperature.

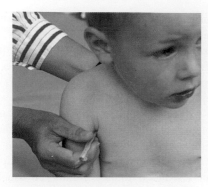

Figure 15-15 Axillary thermometer placement.

Older Adults

+ Older adults' temperatures tend to be lower than those of middle-age adults.
+ Older adults' temperatures are strongly influenced by both environmental and internal temperature

changes. Their thermoregulation control processes are not as efficient as when they are younger and they are at higher risk for both hypothermia and hyperthermia.

+ Older adults can develop significant build up of ear cerumen/wax that may interfere with tympanic thermometer readings.
+ Older adults are more likely to have haemorrhoids. Inspect the anus before taking a rectal temperature.
+ Older adults temperatures may not be a valid indication of the seriousness of the pathology of a disease. They may have pneumonia or a urinary tract infection and have only a slight temperature elevation. Other symptoms, such as confusion and restlessness, may be displayed and need follow-up to determine if there is an underlying process.

Pulse Sites

A pulse may be measured in nine sites (see Figure 15-16).

1. Temporal, where the temporal artery passes over the temporal bone of the head. The site is superior (above) and lateral to (away from the midline of) the eye.
2. Carotid, at the side of the neck where the carotid artery runs between the trachea and the sternocleidomastoid muscle.

> **CLINICAL ALERT**
>
> *Never press both carotids at the same time because this can cause a reflex drop in blood pressure or pulse rate.*

3. Apical, at the apex of the heart. In an adult this is located on the left side of the chest, about 8 cm to the left of the sternum (breastbone) and at the fourth fifth or sixth intercostal space (area between the ribs). For a child seven to nine years of age, the apical pulse is located at the fourth or fifth intercostal spaces. Before four years of age it is left of the midclavicular line (MCL); between four and six years, it is at the MCL (see Figure 15-17).
4. Brachial, at the inner aspect of the biceps muscle of the arm or medially in the antecubital space.
5. Radial, where the radial artery runs along the radial bone, on the thumb side of the inner aspect of the wrist.
6. Femoral, where the femoral artery passes alongside the inguinal ligament.
7. Popliteal, where the popliteal artery passes behind the knee.
8. Posterior tibial, on the medial surface of the ankle where the posterior tibial artery passes behind the medial malleolus.

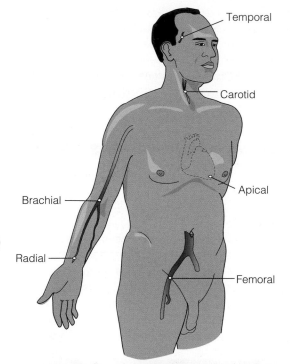

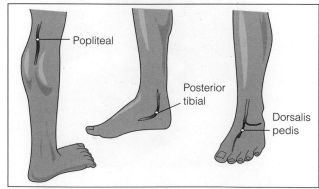

Figure 15-16 Nine sites for assessing pulse.

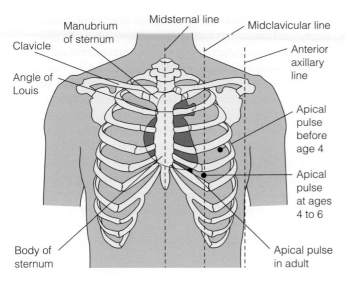

Figure 15-17 Location of the apical pulse for a child under four years, a child four to six years, and an adult.

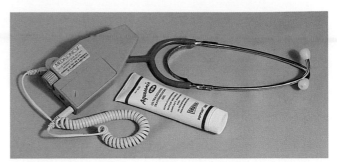

Figure 15-18 A Doppler ultrasound stethoscope (DUS).

Table 15-3 Reasons for Using Specific Pulse Site

Pulse site	Reasons for use
Radial	Readily accessible
Temporal	Used when radial pulse is not accessible
Carotid	Used in cases of cardiac arrest Used to determine circulation to the brain
Apical	Routinely used for infants and children up to three years of age Used to determine discrepancies with radial pulse Used in conjunction with some medications
Brachial	Used to measure blood pressure Used during cardiac arrest for infants
Femoral	Used in cases of cardiac arrest Used for infants and children Used to determine circulation to a leg
Popliteal	Used to determine circulation to the lower leg
Posterior tibial	Used to determine circulation to the foot
Pedal	Used to determine circulation to the foot

9. Pedal (dorsalis pedis), where the dorsalis pedis artery passes over the bones of the foot, on an imaginary line drawn from the middle of the ankle to the space between the big and second toes. The radial site is most commonly used in adults. It is easily found in most people and readily accessible. Some reasons for use of each site are given in Table 15-3.

Assessing the Pulse

A pulse is commonly assessed by palpation (feeling) or auscultation (hearing). The middle three fingertips are used for palpating all pulse sites except the apex of the heart. A stethoscope is used for assessing apical pulses and foetal heart tones. A Doppler ultrasound stethoscope (DUS; see Figure 15-18) is used for pulses that are difficult to assess. The DUS headset has earpieces similar to standard stethoscope earpieces, but it has a long cord attached to a volume-controlled audio unit and an ultrasound transducer. The DUS detects movement of red blood cells through a blood vessel. In contrast to the conventional stethoscope, it excludes environmental sounds.

A pulse is normally palpated by applying moderate pressure with the three middle fingers of the hand. The pads on the most distal aspects of the finger are the most sensitive areas for detecting a pulse. With excessive pressure one can obliterate a pulse, whereas with too little pressure one may not be able to detect it. Before the nurse assesses the resting pulse, the patient should assume a comfortable position. The nurse should also be aware of the following:

+ Any medication that could affect the heart rate.
+ Whether the patient has been physically active. If so, wait 10–15 minutes until the patient has rested and the pulse has slowed to its usual rate.
+ Any baseline data about the normal heart rate for the patient. For example, a physically fit athlete may have a heart rate below 60 BPM.
+ Whether the patient should assume a particular position (e.g. sitting). In some patients, the rate changes with the position because of changes in blood flow volume and autonomic nervous system activity.

When assessing the pulse, the nurse collects the following data: the rate, rhythm, volume, arterial wall elasticity and presence or absence of bilateral equality. An excessively fast heart rate (e.g. over 100 BPM in an adult) is referred to as **tachycardia**. A heart rate in an adult of 60 BPM or less is called **bradycardia**. If a patient has either tachycardia or bradycardia, the apical pulse should be assessed.

The **pulse rhythm** is the pattern of the beats and the intervals between the beats. Equal time elapses between beats of a normal pulse. A pulse with an irregular rhythm is referred to as a **dysrhythmia** or **arrhythmia**. It may consist of random, irregular beats or a predictable pattern of irregular beats. When a dysrhythmia is detected, the apical pulse should be assessed. An electrocardiogram (ECG) is necessary to define the dysrhythmia further.

Pulse volume, also called the pulse strength or amplitude, refers to the force of blood with each beat. Usually, the pulse volume is the same with each beat. It can range from absent to bounding. A normal pulse can be felt with moderate pressure of the fingers and can be obliterated with greater pressure. A forceful or full blood volume that is obliterated only with difficulty is called a full or bounding pulse. A pulse that is readily obliterated with pressure from the fingers is referred to as weak, feeble or thready.

The **elasticity of the arterial wall** reflects its expansibility or its deformities. A healthy, normal artery feels straight, smooth, soft and pliable. Older people often have inelastic arteries that feel twisted (tortuous) and irregular upon palpation.

When assessing a peripheral pulse to determine the adequacy of blood flow to a particular area of the body, the nurse should also assess the corresponding pulse on the other side of the body. The second assessment gives the nurse data with which to compare the pulses. For example, when assessing the blood flow to the right foot, the nurse assesses the right dorsalis pedis pulse and then the left dorsalis pedis pulse. If the patient's right and left pulses are the same, the patient's dorsalis pedis pulses are bilaterally equal.

Procedure 15-2 provides guidelines for assessing a peripheral pulse, *Procedure 15-3* on page 352 for an apical pulse and *Procedure 15-4* on page 354 for an apical-radial pulse.

PROCEDURE 15-2 Assessing a Peripheral Pulse

Purposes

+ To establish baseline data for subsequent evaluation
+ To identify whether the pulse rate is within normal range
+ To determine whether the pulse rhythm is regular and the pulse volume is appropriate
+ To compare the equality of corresponding peripheral pulses on each side of the body
+ To monitor and assess changes in the patient's health status
+ To monitor patients at risk for pulse alterations (e.g. those with a history of heart disease or experiencing cardiac arrhythmias, haemorrhage, acute pain, infusion of large volumes of fluids, pyrexia)

Assessment

Assess

+ Clinical signs of cardiovascular alterations, other than pulse rate, rhythm or volume (e.g. dyspnoea [difficult respirations], fatigue, pallor, cyanosis [bluish discoloration of skin and mucous membranes], palpitations, syncope [fainting], impaired peripheral tissue perfusion as evidenced by skin discoloration and cool temperature)
+ Factors that may alter pulse rate (e.g. emotional status and activity level)
+ Site most appropriate for assessment

Planning

Equipment

+ Watch with a second hand or indicator
+ If using a digital ultrasound stethoscope (DUS), the transducer probe, the stethoscope headset, transmission gel and tissues/wipes

Implementation

Preparation

If using a DUS check that the equipment is functioning normally.

Performance

1. Explain to the patient what you are going to do, why it is necessary and how they can cooperate. Discuss how the results will be used in planning further care or treatments.
2. Wash hands and observe appropriate infection control procedures.
3. Provide for patient privacy.

4. Select the pulse point. Normally, the radial pulse is taken, unless it cannot be exposed or circulation to another body area is to be assessed.

5. Assist the patient to a comfortable resting position. When the radial pulse is assessed, with the palm facing downward, the patient's arm can rest alongside the body or the forearm can rest at a 90-degree angle across the chest. For the patient who can sit, the forearm can rest across the thigh, with the palm of the hand facing downward or inward.

6. Palpate and count the pulse. Place two or three middle fingertips lightly and squarely over the pulse point (see Figure 15-19). *Using the thumb is contraindicated because the thumb has a pulse that the nurse could mistake for the patient's pulse.*
   - Count for one minute. An irregular pulse also requires taking the apical pulse.

7. Assess the pulse rhythm and volume.
   - Assess the pulse rhythm by noting the pattern of the intervals between the beats. A normal pulse has equal time periods between beats.
   - Assess the pulse volume. A normal pulse can be felt with moderate pressure, and the pressure is equal with each beat. A forceful pulse volume is full; an easily obliterated pulse is weak.

8. Document the pulse rate, rhythm and volume and your actions in patient observations chart. Also record pertinent related data such as variation in pulse rate compared to normal for the patient and abnormal skin colour and skin temperature in the nurse's notes.

Variation: using a DUS

✦ If used, plug the stethoscope headset into one of the two output jacks located next to the volume control. DUS units may have two jacks so that a second person can listen to the signals.

✦ Apply transmission gel either to the probe at the narrow end of the plastic case housing the transducer, or to the patient's skin. *Ultrasound beams do not travel well through air. The gel makes an airtight seal, which then promotes optimal ultrasound wave transmission.*

✦ Press the 'on' button.

✦ Hold the probe against the skin over the pulse site. Use a light pressure, and keep the probe in contact with the skin (see Figure 15-20 on page 352). *Too much pressure can stop the blood flow and obliterate the signal.*

✦ Adjust the volume if necessary. Distinguish artery sounds from vein sounds. The artery sound (signal) is distinctively pulsating and has a pumping quality. The venous sound is

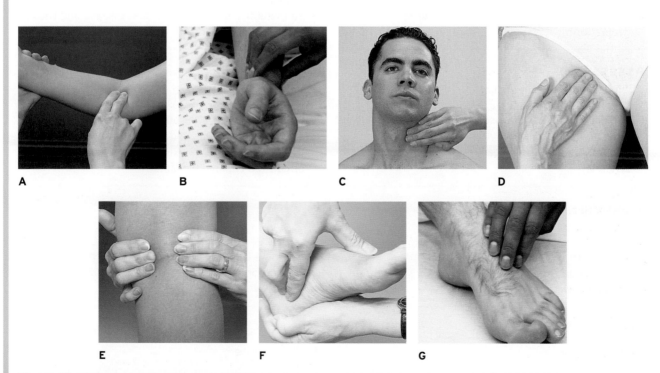

A   B   C   D

E   F   G

Figure 15-19 Assessing the pulses: *A*, brachial; *B*, radial; *C*, carotid; *D*, femoral; *E*, popliteal; *F*, posterior tibial; and *G*, pedal (dorsalis pedis).

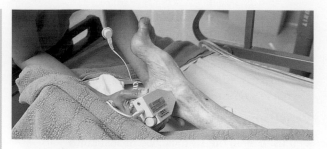

Figure 15-20 Using a (Doppler) ultrasound stethoscope to assess the posterior tibial pulse.

intermittent and varies with respirations. Both artery and vein sounds are heard simultaneously through the DUS because major arteries and veins are situated close together throughout the body. If arterial sounds cannot be easily heard, then reposition the probe.

✛ After assessing the pulse, remove all gel from the probe to prevent damage to its surface. Clean the transducer with aqueous solutions. *Alcohol or other disinfectants may damage the face of the transducer. Remove all gel from the patient.*

Evaluation

✛ Compare the pulse rate to baseline data or normal range for age of patient.

✛ Relate pulse rate and volume to other vital signs; pulse rhythm and volume to baseline data and health status.

✛ If assessing peripheral pulses, evaluate equality, rate and volume in corresponding extremities.

✛ Conduct appropriate follow-up such as notifying the medical staff or administering medication.

PROCEDURE 15-3 Assessing an Apical Pulse

Purposes

✛ To obtain the heart rate of newborns, infants and children 2-3 years old or of an adult with an irregular peripheral pulse

✛ To establish baseline data for subsequent evaluation

✛ To determine whether the cardiac rate is within normal range and the rhythm is regular

✛ To monitor patients with cardiac disease and those receiving medications to improve heart action

Assessment

Assess

✛ Clinical signs of cardiovascular alterations, other than pulse rate, rhythm or volume (e.g. dyspnoea, fatigue, pallor, cyanosis, syncope)

✛ Factors that may alter pulse rate (e.g. emotional status, activity level, and medications that affect heart rate such as digoxin, beta blockers or calcium channel blockers)

Planning

Equipment

✛ Watch with a second hand or indicator
✛ Stethoscope
✛ Antiseptic wipes

✛ If using a DUS, the transducer probe, the stethoscope headset, transmission gel and tissues/wipes

Implementation

Preparation

If using a DUS, check that the equipment is functioning normally.

Performance

1. Explain to the patient what you are going to do, why it is necessary and how they can cooperate.

Discuss how the results will be used in planning further care or treatments.

2. Observe appropriate local infection control procedures.

3. Provide for patient privacy.

4. Position the patient appropriately in a comfortable supine position or in a sitting position. Expose the area of the chest over the apex of the heart.

5. Locate the apical impulse. This is the point over the apex of the heart where the apical pulse can be most clearly heard. It is also referred to as the **point of maximal impulse (PMI)**.

   - Palpate the angle of Louis (the angle between the manubrium, the top of the sternum and the body of the sternum). It is palpated just below the suprasternal notch and is felt as a prominence (see Figure 15-17 on page 349).
   - Slide your index finger just to the left of the patient's sternum and palpate the second intercostal space.
   - Place your middle or next finger in the third intercostal space, and continue palpating downward until you locate the fifth intercostal space.
   - Move your index finger laterally along the fifth intercostal space toward the MCL. Normally, the apical impulse is palpable at or just medial to the MCL (see Figure 15-17 on page 349).

6. Auscultate and count heartbeats.

   - Use antiseptic wipes to clean the earpieces and diaphragm of the stethoscope after use. *The diaphragm needs to be cleaned and disinfected if soiled with body substances and before and after each use.*
   - Warm the diaphragm of the stethoscope by holding it in the palm of the hand for a moment. *The metal of the diaphragm is usually cold and can startle the patient when placed immediately on the chest.*
   - Insert the earpieces of the stethoscope into your ears in the direction of the ear canals, or slightly forward, *to facilitate hearing*.
   - Tap your finger lightly on the diaphragm *to be sure it is the active side of the head*. If necessary, rotate the head to select the diaphragm side (see Figure 15-21).
   - Place the diaphragm of the stethoscope over the apical impulse and listen for the normal S1 and S2 heart sounds, which are heard as 'lub-dub' (see Figure 15-22). *The heartbeat is normally loudest over the apex of the heart.* Each lub-dub is counted as one heartbeat. *The two heart sounds are produced by closure of the valves of the heart. The S1 heart sound (lub) occurs when the*

A

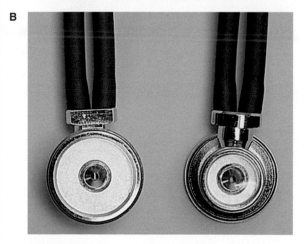

B

Figure 15-21 *A*, stethoscope with both a bell-shaped and flat-disc amplifier. *B*, Close-up of a flat-disc amplifier (left) and a bell amplifier (right).

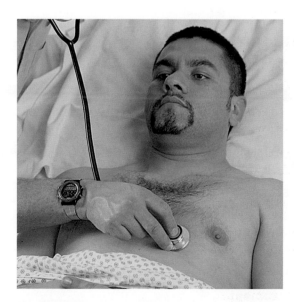

Figure 15-22 Taking an apical pulse using the flat disc of the stethoscope. Note how the amplifier is held against the chest.

atrioventricular valves close after the ventricles have been sufficiently filled. The S2 heart sound (dub) occurs when the semilunar valves close after the ventricles empty.

- If the rhythm is regular or irregular, count the heartbeats for one minute.
- Assess the rhythm of the heartbeat by noting the pattern of intervals between the beats. A normal pulse has equal time periods between beats.

- Assess the strengths (volume) of the heartbeat. Normally, the heartbeats are equal in strength and can be described as strong or weak.
7. Document the pulse site, rate, rhythm and volume and your actions in the patient observation chart. Also record pertinent related data such as variation in pulse rate compared to normal for the patient and abnormal skin colour and skin temperature.

Evaluation

+ Relate pulse rate to other vital signs; pulse rhythm to baseline data and health status.
+ Report to the medical staff any abnormal findings such as irregular rhythm, and reduced ability to hear the heartbeat, pallor, cyanosis, dyspnoea, tachycardia or bradycardia.
+ Conduct appropriate follow-up such as administering medication prescribed based on apical heart rate.

Apical Pulse Assessment

Assessment of the apical pulse is indicated for patients whose peripheral pulse is irregular or unavailable as well as for patients with known cardiovascular, pulmonary and renal diseases. It is commonly assessed prior to administering medications that affect heart rate. The apical site is also used to assess the pulse for new-borns, infants and children up to 2–3 years old. *Procedure 15-3* on page 352 presents guidelines for assessing the apical pulse.

Apical-Radial Pulse Assessment

An **apical-radial pulse** may need to be assessed for patients with certain cardiovascular disorders. Normally, the apical and radial rates are identical. An apical pulse rate greater than a radial pulse rate can indicate that the thrust of the blood from the heart is too feeble for the wave to be felt at the peripheral pulse site, or it can indicate that vascular disease is preventing impulses from being transmitted. Any discrepancy between the two pulse rates is called a **pulse deficit** and needs to be reported promptly. In no instance is the radial pulse greater than the apical pulse.

An apical-radial pulse can be taken by two nurses or one nurse, although the two-nurse technique may be more accurate. *Procedure 15-4* outlines the steps for assessing an apical-radial pulse.

PROCEDURE 15-4 Assessing an Apical-Radial Pulse

Purpose

+ To determine adequacy of peripheral circulation or presence of pulse deficit

Assessment

Assess

+ Clinical signs of hypovolaemic shock (hypotension, pallor, cyanosis and cold, clammy skin)

Planning

Equipment

+ Watch with a second hand or indicator
+ Stethoscope
+ Antiseptic wipes

Implementation

Preparation

If using the two-nurse technique, ensure that the other nurse is available at this time.

Performance

1. Explain to the patient what you are going to do, why it is necessary and how they can cooperate. Discuss how the results will be used in planning further care or treatments.
2. Observe appropriate local infection control procedures.
3. Provide for patient privacy.
4. Position the patient appropriately. Assist the patient to assume the position described for taking the apical pulse. Position the patient appropriately in a comfortable supine position or to a sitting position. Expose the area of the chest over the apex of the heart. If previous measurements were taken, determine what position the patient assumed, and use the same position. *This ensures an accurate comparative measurement*.
5. Locate the apical and radial pulse sites. In the two-nurse technique, one nurse locates the apical impulse by palpation or with the stethoscope while the other nurse palpates the radial pulse site (see *Procedures 15-2* and *15-3*).
6. Count the apical and radial pulse rates.

Two-nurse Technique

+ Place the watch where both nurses can see it. The nurse who is taking the radial pulse may hold the watch.
+ Decide on a time to begin counting. A time when the second hand is on 12, 3, 6 or 9 or an even number on digital clocks is usually selected. The nurse taking the radial pulse says 'Start' at the same time. *This ensures that simultaneous counts are taken.*
+ Each nurse counts the pulse rate for 60 seconds. Both nurses end the count when the nurse taking the radial pulse says 'Stop'. *A full 60-second count is necessary for accurate assessment of any discrepancies between the two pulse sites.*
+ The nurse who assesses the apical rate also assesses the apical pulse rhythm and volume (i.e. whether the heartbeat is strong or weak). If the pulse is irregular, note whether the irregular beats come at random or at predictable times.
+ The nurse assessing the radial pulse rate also assesses the radial pulse rhythm and volume.

One-nurse Technique

+ Assess the apical pulse for 60 seconds.
+ Assess the radial pulse for 60 seconds.

7. Document the apical and radial (AR) pulse rates, rhythm, volume and any pulse deficit on the patient observation chart. Also record related data such as variation in pulse rate compared to normal for the patient and other pertinent observations, such as pallor, cyanosis or dyspnoea.

Evaluation

+ Relate pulse rate and rhythm to other vital signs, to baseline data and to general health status.
+ Report to the medical staff any changes from previous measurements or any discrepancy between the two pulses.
+ Conduct appropriate follow-up such as administering medication or other actions to be taken for a discrepancy in the AR pulse rates.

LIFESPAN CONSIDERATIONS

Pulse

Infants

+ Use the apical pulse for the heart rate of newborns, infants and children 2–3 years old to establish baseline data for subsequent evaluation, to determine whether the cardiac rate is within normal range, and to determine if the rhythm is regular.
+ Place a baby in a supine position. Crying and physical activity will increase the pulse rate. For this reason, take the apical pulse rate of infants and small children before assessing body temperatures.
+ Locate the apical pulse in the fourth intercostal space, lateral to the midclavicular line during infancy.
+ Brachial, popliteal and femoral pulses may be palpated. Due to a normally low blood pressure and rapid heart rate, infants' other distal pulses may be hard to feel.

Children

+ To take a peripheral pulse, position the child comfortably in the adult's arms or have the adult remain close by. This may decrease anxiety and yield more accurate results.
+ To assess the apical pulse, assist a young child to a comfortable supine or sitting position.
+ Demonstrate the procedure to the child using a stuffed animal or doll, and allow the child to handle the stethoscope before beginning the procedure. This will decrease anxiety and promote cooperation.
+ The apex of the heart is normally located in the fourth intercostal space in young children; fifth intercostal space in children seven years of age and over.

+ Locate the apical impulse along the fourth intercostal space, between the MCL and the anterior axillary line (see Figure 15-17 earlier).

Older Adults

+ If the patient has severe hand or arm tremors, the radial pulse may be difficult to count.
+ Cardiac changes in older adults, such as decrease in cardiac output, sclerotic changes to heart valves and dysarhythmias often indicate that obtaining an apical pulse will be more accurate.
+ Older adults often have decreased peripheral circulation so that pedal pulses should also be checked for regularity, volume and symmetry.

RESPIRATIONS

Respiration is the act of breathing. **External respiration** refers to the interchange of oxygen and carbon dioxide between the alveoli of the lungs and the pulmonary blood. **Internal respiration**, by contrast, takes place throughout the body; it is the interchange of these same gases between the circulating blood and the cells of the body tissues.

Inhalation or **inspiration** refers to the intake of air into the lungs. **Exhalation** or **expiration** refers to breathing out or the movement of gases from the lungs to the atmosphere. **Ventilation** is also used to refer to the movement of air in and out of the lungs.

There are basically two types of breathing: **costal (thoracic) breathing** and **diaphragmatic (abdominal) breathing**. Costal breathing involves the external intercostal muscles and other accessory muscles, such as the sternocleidomastoid muscles. It can be observed by the movement of the chest upward and outward. By contrast, diaphragmatic breathing involves the contraction and relaxation of the diaphragm, and it is observed by the movement of the abdomen, which occurs as a result of the diaphragm's contraction and downward movement.

Mechanics and Regulation of Breathing

During *inhalation*, the following processes normally occur (see Figure 15-23): The diaphragm contracts (flattens), the ribs move upward and outward, and the sternum moves outward, thus enlarging the thorax and permitting the lungs to expand. During *exhalation* (see Figure 15-24), the diaphragm relaxes, the ribs move downward and inward, and the sternum moves inward, thus decreasing the size of the thorax as the lungs are compressed. Normally breathing is carried out automatically and effortlessly. A normal adult inspiration lasts 1–1.5 seconds, and an expiration lasts 2–3 seconds.

Respiration is controlled by (a) respiratory centres in the medulla oblongata and the pons of the brain and (b) by chemoreceptors located centrally in the medulla and peripherally in

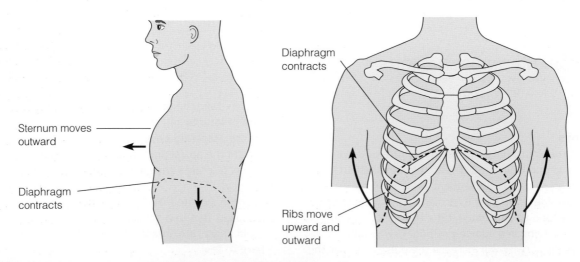

Figure 15-23 Respiratory inhalation, *Left*: lateral view; *Right*: anterior view.

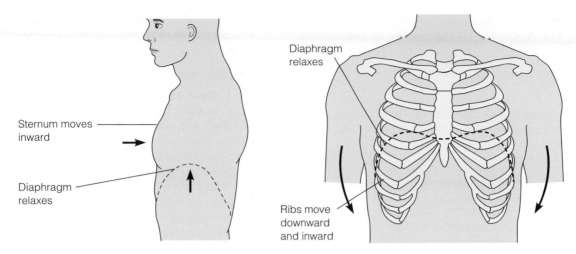

Sternum moves inward

Diaphragm relaxes

Diaphragm relaxes

Ribs move downward and inward

Figure 15-24 Respiratory exhalation. *Left:* lateral view; *Right:* anterior view.

the carotid and aortic bodies. These centres and receptors respond to changes in the concentrations of oxygen (O_2), carbon dioxide (CO_2) and hydrogen (H^+) in the arterial blood.

Assessing Respirations

Resting respirations should be assessed when the patient is relaxed because exercise affects respirations, increasing their rate and depth. Anxiety is likely to affect respiratory rate and depth as well. Respirations may also need to be assessed after exercise to identify the patient's tolerance to activity. Before assessing a patient's respirations, a nurse should be aware of the following:

+ the patient's normal breathing pattern;
+ the influence of the patient's health problems on respirations;
+ any medications or therapies that might affect respirations;
+ the relationship of the patient's respirations to cardiovascular function.

The rate, depth, rhythm and quality and effectiveness of respirations should be assessed.

The *respiratory rate* is normally described in breaths per minute. Breathing that is normal in rate and depth iscalled **eupnoea**. Abnormally slow respirations are referred to as **bradypnoea**, and abnormally fast respirations are called **tachypnoea** or **polypnoea**. **Apnoea** is the absence of breathing. For the respiratory rates for different age groups, see Table 15-1 on page 337.

Factors Affecting Respirations

Several factors influence respiratory rate. Those that increase the rate include exercise (increases metabolism), stress (readies the body for 'fight or flight'), increased environmental temperature and lowered oxygen concentration at increased altitudes. Factors that may decrease the respiratory rate include decreased environmental temperature, certain medications (e.g. narcotics) and increased intracranial pressure.

The *depth* of a person's respirations can be established by watching the movement of the chest. Respiratory depth is generally described as normal, deep or shallow. *Deep respirations* are those in which a large volume of air is inhaled and exhaled, inflating most of the lungs. *Shallow respirations* involve the exchange of a small volume of air and often the minimal use of lung tissue. During a normal inspiration and expiration, an adult takes in about 500 ml of air. This volume is called the **tidal volume**.

Body position also affects the amount of air that can be inhaled. People in a supine position experience two physiological processes that suppress respiration: an increase in the volume of blood inside the thoracic cavity and compression of the chest. Consequently, patients lying on their back have poorer lung aeration, which predisposes them to the stasis of fluids and subsequent infection. Certain medications also affect the respiratory depth. For example, narcotics such as morphine and large doses of barbiturates depress the respiratory centres in the brain, thereby depressing the respiratory rate and depth. **Hyperventilation** refers to very deep, rapid respirations; **hypoventilation** refers to very shallow respirations.

Respiratory rhythm refers to the regularity of the expirations and the inspirations. Normally, respirations are evenly spaced. Respiratory rhythm can be described as *regular* or *irregular*.

Respiratory quality or **character** refers to those aspects of breathing that are different from normal, effortless breathing. Two of these are the amount of effort a patient must exert to breathe and the sound of breathing. Usually, breathing does not require noticeable effort; some patients, however, breathe only with decided effort, referred to as *laboured breathing*.

The *sound* of breathing is also significant. Normal breathing is silent, but a number of abnormal sounds such as a wheeze are obvious to the nurse's ear. Many sounds occur as a result of the presence of fluid in the lungs and are most clearly heard with a stethoscope. For details about altered breathing patterns and terms used to describe various patterns and sounds, see *Box 15-7* on page 358.

The steps for assessing respirations are shown in *Procedure 15-5* on page 358.

BOX 15-7 Altered Breathing Patterns and Sounds

Breathing Patterns

Rate
+ *Tachypnoea* – quick, shallow breaths
+ *Bradypnoea* – abnormally slow breathing
+ *Apnoea* – cessation of breathing

Volume
+ *Hyperventilation* – overexpansion of the lungs characterised by rapid and deep breaths
+ *Hypoventilation* – underexpansion of the lungs, characterised by shallow respirations

Rhythm
+ *Cheyne-Stokes breathing* – rhythmic waxing and waning of respirations, from very deep to very shallow breathing and temporary apnoea

Ease or Effort
+ *Dyspnoea* – difficult and laboured breathing during which the individual has a persistent, unsatisfied need for air and feels distressed
+ *Orthopnoea* – ability to breathe only in upright sitting or standing positions

Breath Sounds

Audible without Amplification
+ *Stridor* – a shrill, harsh sound heard during inspiration with laryngeal obstruction
+ *Stertor* – snoring or sonorous respiration, usually due to a partial obstruction of the upper airway
+ *Wheeze* – continuous, high-pitched musical squeak or whistling sound occurring on expiration and sometimes on inspiration when air moves through a narrowed or partially obstructed airway
+ *Bubbling* – gurgling sounds heard as air passes through moist secretions in the respiratory tract

Chest Movements
+ *Intercostal retraction* – indrawing between the ribs
+ *Substernal retraction* – indrawing beneath the breastbone
+ *Suprasternal retraction* – indrawing above the clavicles

Secretions and Coughing
+ *Haemoptysis* – the presence of blood in the sputum
+ *Productive cough* – a cough accompanied by expectorated secretions
+ *Nonproductive cough* – a dry, harsh cough without secretions

PROCEDURE 15-5 Assessing Respirations

Purposes
+ To acquire baseline data against which future measurements can be compared
+ To monitor abnormal respirations and respiratory patterns and identify changes
+ To assess respirations before the administration of a medication such as morphine (an abnormally slow respiratory rate may warrant withholding the medication)
+ To monitor respirations following the administration of a general anaesthetic or any medication that influences respirations
+ To monitor patients at risk for respiratory alterations (e.g. those with pyrexia, pain, acute anxiety, chronic obstructive pulmonary disease, respiratory infection, pulmonary oedema or emboli, chest trauma or constriction, brain stem injury)

Assessment

Assess
+ Skin and mucous membrane colour (e.g. cyanosis or pallor)
+ Position assumed for breathing (e.g. use of orthopnoeic position)
+ Signs of cerebral anoxia (e.g. irritability, restlessness, drowsiness or loss of consciousness)
+ Chest movements (e.g. retractions between the ribs or above or below the sternum)
+ Activity tolerance
+ Chest pain
+ Dyspnoea
+ Medications affecting respiratory rate

Planning

Equipment
+ Watch with a second hand or indicator

Implementation

Preparation

For a routine assessment of respirations, choose a suitable time to monitor the respirations. A patient who has been exercising will need to rest for a few minutes to permit the accelerated respiratory rate to return to normal.

Performance

1. Explain to the patient what you are going to do, why it is necessary and how they can cooperate. Discuss how the results will be used in planning further care or treatments.
2. Observe appropriate local infection control procedures.
3. Provide for patient privacy.
4. Observe or palpate and count the respiratory rate.
   - The patient's awareness that you are counting the respiratory rate could cause the patient voluntarily to alter the respiratory pattern. If you anticipate this, place a hand against the patient's chest to feel the chest movements with breathing, or place the patient's arm across the chest and observe the chest movements while supposedly taking the radial pulse.
   - Count the respiratory rate for 60 seconds. An inhalation and an exhalation count as one respiration.
5. Observe the depth, rhythm and character of respirations.
   - Observe the respirations for depth by watching the movement of the chest and ensure the patient is unaware you are counting their respirations otherwise they will change the breathing pattern. *During deep respirations a large volume of air is exchanged; during shallow respirations a small volume is exchanged.*
   - Observe the respirations for regular or irregular rhythm. *Normally, respirations are evenly spaced.*
   - Observe the character of respirations – the sound they produce and the effort they require. *Normally, respirations are silent and effortless.*
6. Document the respiratory rate, depth, rhythm and character on the appropriate record.

Evaluation

- Relate respiratory rate to other vital signs, in particular pulse rate, respiratory rhythm and depth to baseline data and health status.
- Report to the medical staff respiratory rate significantly above or below the normal range and any notable change in respirations from previous assessments; irregular respiratory rhythm; inadequate respiratory depth; abnormal character of breathing - orthopnoea, wheezing, stridor or bubbling; and any complaints of dyspnoea.
- Conduct appropriate follow-up such as administering appropriate medications or treatments, positioning the patient to ease breathing, and requesting involvement of other members of the healthcare team such as the physiotherapist.

LIFESPAN CONSIDERATIONS

Respirations

Infants

- An infant or child who is crying will have an abnormal respiratory rate and will need quietening before respirations can be accurately assessed.
- If necessary, place your hand gently on the infant's abdomen to feel the rapid rise and fall during respirations.

Children

- Because young children are diaphragmatic breathers, observe the rise and fall of the abdomen.

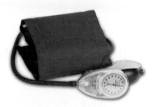

If necessary, place your hand gently on the abdomen to feel the rapid rise and fall during respirations.

Older Adults

- Ask the patient to remain quiet or count respirations after taking the pulse.
- Older adults experience anatomical and physiological changes that cause the respiratory system to be less efficient. Any changes in rate or type of breathing should be reported immediately.

The effectiveness of respirations is measured in part by the uptake of oxygen from the air into the blood and the release of carbon dioxide from the blood into expired air. The amount of haemoglobin in arterial blood that is saturated with oxygen can be measured indirectly through pulse oximetry. Using a pulse oximeter monitor applied to the patient's finger, toe or other site provides a digital readout of both the patient's pulse rate and the oxygen saturation (see *Procedure 15-7* on page 370).

CLINICAL ANECDOTE

'I frequently find it hard to count a patient's respiratory rate as they always try to talk to you as you are counting. So I often pretend I'm counting their pulse by placing the patient's hand on their chest with me holding the wrist. I then make the excuse that if they talk I lose count so it is then easier to count their pulse rate more accurately in one minute.'

Kate, second-year student nurse

BLOOD PRESSURE

Arterial blood pressure is a measure of the pressure exerted by the blood as it flows through the arteries. Because the blood moves in waves, there are two blood pressure measures: the **systolic pressure**, which is the pressure of the blood as a result of contraction of the ventricles, that is, the pressure of the height of the blood wave; and the **diastolic pressure**, which is the pressure when the ventricles are at rest. Diastolic pressure, then, is the lower pressure, present at all times within the arteries. The difference between the diastolic and the systolic pressures is called the **pulse pressure**.

Blood pressure is measured in millimetres of mercury (mm Hg) and recorded as a fraction. The systolic pressure is written over the diastolic pressure. The average blood pressure of a healthy adult is 120/80 mm Hg. A number of conditions are reflected by changes in blood pressure. Because blood pressure can vary considerably among individuals, it is important for the nurse to know a specific patient's baseline blood pressure. For example, if a patient's usual blood pressure is 180/100 mm Hg, and it is assessed following surgery to be 120/80 mm Hg, this significant drop in pressure must be reported to the medical staff.

Determinants of Blood Pressure

Arterial blood pressure is the result of several factors: the pumping action of the heart, the peripheral vascular resistance (the resistance supplied by the blood vessels through which the blood flows), and the blood volume and viscosity.

Pumping Action of the Heart

When the pumping action of the heart is weak, less blood is pumped into arteries (lower cardiac output), and the blood pressure decreases. When the heart's pumping action is strong and the volume of blood pumped into the circulation increases (higher cardiac output), the blood pressure increases.

Peripheral Vascular Resistance

Peripheral resistance can increase blood pressure. The diastolic pressure especially is affected. Some factors that create resistance in the arterial system are the capacity of the arterioles and capillaries, the compliance of the arteries and the viscosity of the blood.

The internal diameter or capacity of the arterioles and the capillaries determines in great part the peripheral resistance to the blood in the body. The smaller the space within a vessel, the greater the resistance. Normally, the arterioles are in a state of partial constriction. Increased vasoconstriction raises the blood pressure, whereas decreased vasoconstriction lowers the blood pressure.

If the elastic and muscular tissues of the arteries are replaced with fibrous tissue, the arteries lose much of their ability to constrict and dilate. This condition, most common in middle-aged and elderly adults, is known as **arteriosclerosis**.

Blood Volume

When the blood volume decreases (e.g. as a result of a haemorrhage or dehydration), the blood pressure decreases because of decreased fluid in the arteries. Conversely, when the volume increases (e.g. as a result of a rapid intravenous infusion), the blood pressure increases because of the greater fluid volume within the circulatory system.

Blood Viscosity

Blood pressure is higher when the blood is highly **viscous** (thick), that is, when the proportion of red blood cells to the blood plasma is high. This proportion is referred to as the **haematocrit**. The viscosity increases markedly when the haematocrit is more than 60% to 65%.

Factors Affecting Blood Pressure

Among the factors influencing blood pressure are age, exercise, stress, race, obesity, sex, medications, diurnal variations and disease processes.

+ *Age.* Newborns have a mean systolic pressure of about 75 mm Hg. The pressure rises with age, reaching a peak at the onset of puberty and then tends to decline somewhat. In older people, elasticity of the arteries is decreased – the arteries are more rigid and less yielding to the pressure of the blood. This produces an elevated systolic pressure. Because the walls no longer retract as flexibly with decreased pressure, the diastolic pressure is also high (see Table 15-1 earlier).

+ *Exercise.* Physical activity increases the cardiac output and hence the blood pressure; thus 20–30 minutes of rest following exercise is indicated before the resting blood pressure can be reliably assessed.

+ *Stress.* Stimulation of the sympathetic nervous system increases cardiac output and vasoconstriction of the arterioles, thus increasing the blood pressure reading; however, severe pain can decrease blood pressure greatly by inhibiting the vasomotor centre and producing vasodilatation.

+ *Gender.* After puberty, females usually have lower blood pressures than males of the same age; this difference is thought to be due to hormonal variations. After menopause, women generally have higher blood pressures than before.

+ *Medications.* Many medications may increase or decrease the blood pressure.

+ *Obesity.* Both childhood and adult obesity predispose to hypertension.

+ *Diurnal variations.* Pressure is usually lowest early in the morning, when the metabolic rate is lowest, then rises throughout the day and peaks in the late afternoon or early evening.

+ *Disease process.* Any condition affecting the cardiac output, blood volume, blood viscosity and/or compliance of the arteries has a direct effect on the blood pressure.

Hypertension

A blood pressure that is persistently above normal is called **hypertension**. It is usually asymptomatic and is often a contributing factor to myocardial infarctions (heart attacks). An elevated blood pressure of unknown cause is called *primary hypertension.* An elevated blood pressure of known cause is called *secondary hypertension.* Hypertension is a widespread health problem. A systolic blood pressure greater than 130 or diastolic greater than 85 requires follow-up (see Table 15-4). The diagnosis of hypertension is made when the average of two or more diastolic readings on two visits subsequent to the initial assessment is 90 mm Hg or higher or when the average of multiple systolic blood pressure readings is higher than 140 mm Hg. Factors associated with hypertension include thickening of the arterial walls, which reduces the size of the arterial lumen, and inelasticity of the arteries as well as such lifestyle factors as cigarette smoking, obesity, heavy alcohol consumption, lack of physical exercise, high blood cholesterol levels and continued exposure to stress. Follow-up care should include lifestyle changes conducive to lowering the blood pressure as well as monitoring the pressure itself.

Hypotension

Hypotension is a blood pressure that is below normal, that is, a systolic reading consistently between 85 and 110 mm Hg in an adult whose normal pressure is higher than this. **Orthostatic hypotension** is a blood pressure that falls when the patient sits or stands. It is usually the result of peripheral vasodilatation in which blood leaves the central body organs, especially the brain, and moves to the periphery, often causing the person to feel faint. Hypotension can also be caused by analgesics such as morphine sulphate, bleeding, severe burns and dehydration. It is important to monitor hypotensive patients carefully to prevent falls. When assessing for orthostatic hypotension:

+ Place the patient in a supine position for 2–3 minutes.
+ Record the patient's pulse and blood pressure.

Table 15-4 Recommendations for Follow-up Based on Initial Blood Pressure Measurements for Adults Without Acute End Organ Damage

Initial blood pressure (MMHG)*	SBP MMHG	DBP MMHG	Follow-up recommended
Normal	<120	and <80	Recheck in 2 years
Prehypertension	120-139	or 80-89	Recheck in 1 year**
Stage 1 hypertension	140-159	or 90-99	Confirm within 2 months***
Stage 2 hypertension	≥160	or ≥100	Evaluate or refer to source of care within 1 month. For those with higher pressures (e.g. >180/110 mmHg), evaluate and treat immediately or within 1 week, depending on clinical situation and complications

SBP = systolic blood pressure; DBP = diastolic blood pressure.

* If systolic and diastolic categories are different, follow recommendations for shorter time follow-up (e.g. 160/86 mmHg should be evaluated or referred to source of care within 1 month).

** Modify the scheduling of follow-up according to reliable information about past BP measurements, other cardiovascular risk factors, or target organ disease.

*** Provide advice about lifestyle modifications.

Source: Tables 3 and 4 (pp. 12 and 18), *The Seventh Report of the Joint National Committee on Prevention, Detection, Evaluation, and Treatment of High Blood Pressure*. London: The National Heart, Lung and Blood Institute.

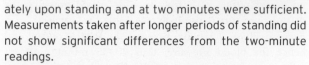

RESEARCH NOTE

How Long Should a Patient Lie and Stand When Taking Orthostatic Blood Pressures?

Lack of agreement within the research literature and in their own institution regarding the technique for measuring orthostatic blood pressures led these authors (Lance et al., 2000) to conduct this study. Thirty-five normal participants exercised, had their pulse and blood pressure measured when rested, then had pulse, blood pressure and dizziness measured when standing. The variables were the length of time required for resting to produce baseline values and the minimum time standing to return indications of blood pressure drop or dizziness.

The results of the study showed that 10 minutes of resting were needed for baseline values. This was longer than the five-minute departmental standard and shorter than the 15-minute nursing unit practice. Pulse, blood pressure and dizziness readings taken immediately upon standing and at two minutes were sufficient. Measurements taken after longer periods of standing did not show significant differences from the two-minute readings.

Implications

The authors acknowledged that their results could not be easily extrapolated to the broader population since their participants were healthy, young (under 25 years old) adults. However, they felt secure enough with their results to implement the standard in their institution while recommending further study on patients with higher risk of orthostatic variations. The article is clear and well written and would easily permit replication of the research. Nurses should pursue the investigation of similar clinical practices that are unstudied or have conflicting results in the published literature.

Note: From 'Comparison of Different Methods of Obtaining Orthostatic Vital Signs,' by R. Lance *et al.*, 2000, *Clinical Nursing Research*, 9, pp. 479-491.

+ Assist the patient to slowly sit or stand. Support the patient in case of faintness.
+ After one minute in the upright position, recheck the pulse and blood pressure in the same sites as previously.
+ Record the results. A rise in pulse of 40 beats per minute or a drop in blood pressure of 30 mm Hg indicates abnormal orthostatic vital signs.

Assessing Blood Pressure

Blood pressure is measured with a *blood pressure cuff*, a *sphygmomanometer* and a *stethoscope*. The blood pressure cuff consists of a rubber bag that can be inflated with air. It is called the *bladder* (see Figure 15-25). It is covered with cloth and has two tubes attached to it. One tube connects to a rubber bulb that inflates the bladder. When turned counterclockwise, a small valve on the side of this bulb releases the air in the bladder. When the valve is tightened (turned clockwise), air pumped into the bladder remains there.

The other tube is attached to a sphygmomanometer. The sphygmomanometer indicates the pressure of the air within the bladder. There are two types of sphygmomanometers: *aneroid* and *mercury* (see Figure 15-26). The aneroid sphygmomanometer is a calibrated dial with a needle that points to the calibrations.

The mercury sphygmomanometer is a calibrated cylinder filled with mercury. The pressure is indicated at the point to

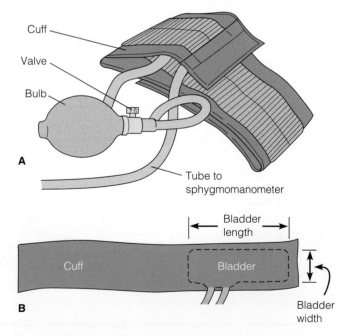

Figure 15-25 *A*, A blood pressure cuff and bulb; *B*, the bladder inside the cuff.

which the rounded curve of the **meniscus** (the crescent-shaped dome) rises (see Figure 15-27). The blood pressure reading should be made with the eye at the level of the rounded curve in order to be accurate.

A

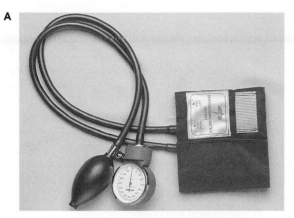

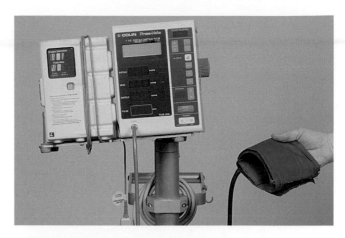

Figure 15-28 Automatic blood pressure monitors register systolic, diastolic and mean blood pressures.

B

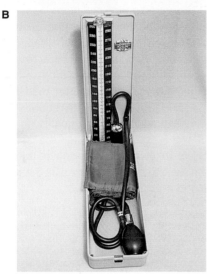

Figure 15-26 Blood pressure equipment: *A*, an aneroid manometer and cuff; *B*, a mercury manometer and cuff.

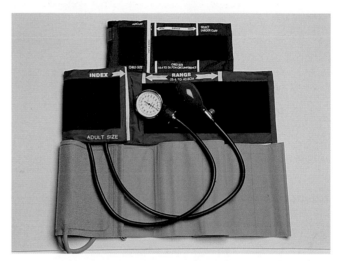

Figure 15-29 Three standard cuff sizes: a small cuff for an infant, small child or frail adult; a normal adult-size cuff; and a large cuff for measuring the blood pressure on the leg or on the arm of an obese adult.

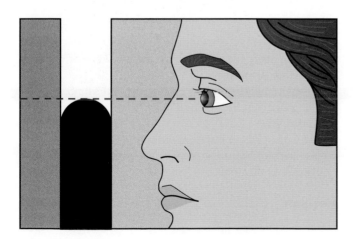

Figure 15-27 To obtain an accurate reading from a mercury manometer, position the meniscus at eye level.

Some clinical areas use *electronic sphygmomanometers* (see Figure 15-28), which eliminate the need to listen to the sounds of the patient's systolic and diastolic blood pressures through a stethoscope. Electronic blood pressure devices should be

calibrated periodically to check accuracy in accordance with manufacturer guidelines and local policy.

Blood pressure cuffs come in various sizes because the bladder must be the correct width and length for the patient's arm (see Figure 15-29). If the bladder is too narrow, the blood pressure reading will be erroneously elevated; if it is too wide, the reading will be erroneously low. The width should be 40% of the circumference, or 20% wider than the diameter of the midpoint of the limb on which it is used. The arm circumference, not the age of the patient, should always be used to determine bladder size. The nurse can also determine whether the width of a blood pressure cuff is appropriate: Lay the cuff lengthwise at the midpoint of the upper arm, and hold the outermost side of the bladder edge laterally on the arm. With the other hand, wrap the width of the cuff around the arm, and ensure that the width is 40% of the arm circumference (see Figure 15-30 on page 364).

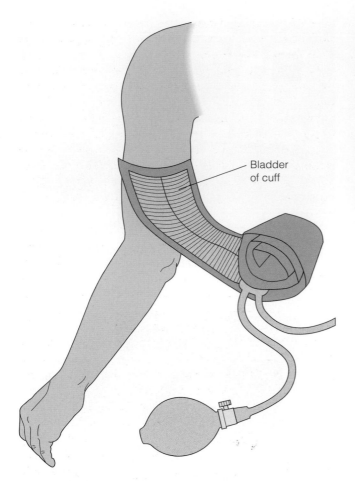

Figure 15-30 Determining that the bladder of a blood pressure cuff is 40% of the arm circumference or 20% wider than the diameter of the mid-point of the limb.

The length of the bladder also affects the accuracy of measurement. The bladder should be sufficiently long to cover at least two-thirds of the limb's circumference.

Blood pressure cuffs are made of nondistensible material so that an even pressure is exerted around the limb. Most cuffs are held in place by Velcro. Others have a cloth bandage that is long enough to encircle the limb several times; this type is closed by tucking the end of the bandage into one of the bandage folds.

Blood Pressure Sites

The blood pressure is usually assessed in the patient's arm using the brachial artery and a standard stethoscope. Assessing the blood pressure on a patient's thigh is usually indicated in these situations:

+ The blood pressure cannot be measured on either arm (e.g. because of burns or other trauma).
+ The blood pressure in one thigh is to be compared with the blood pressure in the other thigh.

Blood pressure is not measured on a patient's arm or thigh in the following situations:

BOX 15-8 Korotkoff's Sounds

These are the sounds listened for when recording blood pressure manually with a stethoscope and sphygmomanometer.

Phase 1 The pressure level at which the first faint, clear tapping or thumping sounds are heard. These sounds gradually become more intense. To ensure that they are not extraneous sounds, the nurse should identify at least two consecutive tapping sounds. The first tapping sound heard during deflation of the cuff is the systolic blood pressure.

Phase 2 The period during deflation when the sounds have a muffled, whooshing or swishing quality.

Phase 3 The period during which the blood flows freely through an increasingly open artery and the sounds become crisper and more intense and again assume a thumping quality but softer than in phase 1.

Phase 4 The time when the sounds become muffled and have a soft, blowing quality.

Phase 5 The pressure level when the last sound is heard. This is followed by a period of silence. The pressure at which the last sound is heard is the diastolic blood pressure in adults.*

*In clinical areas where the fourth phase is considered the diastolic pressure, three measures are recommended (systolic pressure, diastolic pressure and phase 5). These may be referred to as systolic, first diastolic and second diastolic pressures. The phase 5 (second diastolic pressure) reading may be zero; that is, the muffled sounds are heard even when there is no air pressure in the blood pressure cuff. In some instances, muffled sounds are never heard, in which case a dash is inserted where the reading would normally be recorded (e.g. 190/-/110).

+ The shoulder, arm or hand (or the hip, knee or ankle) is injured or diseased.
+ A cast or bulky bandage is on any part of the limb.
+ The patient has had removal of axilla (or hip) lymph nodes on that side.
+ The patient has an intravenous infusion in that limb.
+ The patient has an arteriovenous fistula (e.g. for renal dialysis) in that limb.

Methods

Blood pressure can be assessed directly or indirectly. *Direct (invasive monitoring) measurement* involves the insertion of a catheter into the brachial, radial or femoral artery. Arterial pressure is represented as wavelike forms displayed on an oscilloscope. With correct placement, this pressure reading is highly accurate.

Two *noninvasive indirect methods* of measuring blood pressure are the *auscultatory* and *palpatory* methods. The *auscultatory method* is most commonly used in hospitals, clinics and

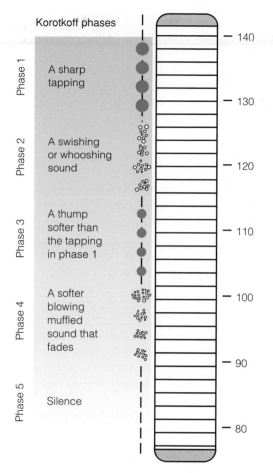

Figure 15-31 Korotkoff's sounds can be differentiated into five phases. In the illustration the blood pressure is 138/90 or 138/102/90.

homes. Required equipment is a sphygmomanometer, a cuff and a stethoscope. When carried out correctly, the auscultatory method is relatively accurate.

When taking a blood pressure using a stethoscope, the nurse identifies five phases in the series of sounds called **Korotkoff's sounds** (see Figure 15-31). First the nurse pumps the cuff up to about 30 mm Hg above the point where the pulse is no longer felt; that is the point when the blood flow in the artery is stopped. Then the pressure is released slowly (2–3 mm Hg per sound) while the nurse observes the readings on the manometer and relates them to the sounds heard through the stethoscope. Five phases occur but may not always be audible (see *Box 15-8*).

The *palpatory method* is sometimes used when Korotkoff's sounds cannot be heard and electronic equipment to amplify the sounds is not available, or to prevent misdirection from the presence of an auscultatory gap occurs. An **auscultatory gap**, which occurs particularly in hypertensive patients, is the temporary disappearance of sounds normally heard over the brachial artery when the cuff pressure is high followed by the reappearance of the sounds at a lower level. This temporary disappearance of sounds occurs in the latter part of phase 1 and phase 2 and may cover a range of 40 mm Hg. If a palpated estimation of the systolic pressure is not made prior to auscultation, the nurse may begin listening in the middle of this range and underestimate the systolic pressure. In the palpatory method of blood pressure determination, instead of listening for the blood flow sounds, using light to moderate pressure the nurse palpates the pulsations of the artery as the pressure in the cuff is released. The pressure is read from the sphygmomanometer when the first pulsation is felt.

Procedure 15-6 shows the steps in assessing blood pressure.

PROCEDURE 15-6 Assessing Blood Pressure

Purposes

+ To obtain a baseline measure of arterial blood pressure for subsequent evaluation
+ To determine the patient's haemodynamic status (e.g. stroke volume of the heart and blood vessel resistance)
+ To identify and monitor changes in blood pressure resulting from a disease process and medical therapy (e.g. presence or history of cardiovascular disease, renal disease, circulatory shock or acute pain; rapid infusion of fluids or blood products)

Assessment

Assess

+ Signs and symptoms of hypertension (e.g. headache, ringing in the ears, flushing of face, nosebleeds, fatigue)
+ Signs and symptoms of hypotension (e.g. tachycardia, dizziness, mental confusion, restlessness, cool and clammy skin, pale or cyanotic skin)
+ Factors affecting blood pressure (e.g. activity, emotional stress, pain and time the patient last smoked or ingested caffeine)

Planning

Equipment

+ Stethoscope
+ Blood pressure cuff of the appropriate size

+ Sphygmomanometer

Implementation

Preparation

1. Ensure that the equipment is intact and functioning properly. Check for leaks in the rubber tubing of the sphygmomanometer.
2. Make sure that the patient has not smoked or ingested caffeine within 30 minutes prior to measurement.

Performance

1. Explain to the patient what you are going to do, why it is necessary and how they can cooperate. Discuss how the results will be used in planning further care or treatments.
2. Observe appropriate local infection control procedures.
3. Provide for patient privacy.
4. Position the patient appropriately.
   • The adult patient should be sitting unless otherwise specified. Both feet should be flat on the floor *since legs crossed at the knee result in elevated systolic and diastolic blood pressures* (Foster-Fitzpatrick *et al.*, 1999).
   • The elbow should be slightly flexed with the palm of the hand facing up and the forearm supported at heart level. Readings in any other position should be specified. The blood pressure is normally similar in sitting, standing and lying positions, but it can vary significantly by position in certain persons. *The blood pressure increases when the arm is below heart level and decreases when the arm is above heart level.*
   • Expose the upper arm.
5. Wrap the deflated cuff evenly around the upper arm. Locate the brachial artery (see Figure 15-19 earlier). Apply the centre of the bladder directly over the artery. *The bladder inside the cuff must be directly over the artery to be compressed if the reading is to be accurate.*
   • For an adult, place the lower border of the cuff approximately 2.5 cm (1 inch) above the antecubital space.
6. If this is the patient's initial examination, perform a preliminary palpatory determination of systolic pressure. *The initial estimate tells the nurse the maximal pressure to which the manometer needs to be elevated in subsequent determinations. It also prevents underestimation of the systolic pressure or overestimation of the diastolic pressure should an auscultatory gap occur.*
   • Palpate the brachial artery with the fingertips.
   • Close the valve on the pump by turning the knob clockwise.
   • Pump up the cuff until you no longer feel the brachial pulse. At that pressure the blood cannot flow through the artery. Note the pressure on the sphygmomanometer at which pulse is no longer felt. *This gives an estimate of the maximum pressure required to measure the systolic pressure.*
   • Release the pressure completely in the cuff, and wait 1–2 minutes before making further measurements. *A waiting period gives the blood trapped in the veins time to be released. Otherwise, false high systolic readings will occur.*
7. Position the stethoscope appropriately.
   • Cleanse the earpieces with alcohol or recommended disinfectant.
   • Insert the ear attachments of the stethoscope in your ears so that they tilt slightly forward. *Sounds are heard more clearly when the ear attachments follow the direction of the ear canal.*
   • Ensure that the stethoscope hangs freely from the ears to the diaphragm. *Rubbing the stethoscope against an object can obliterate the sounds of the blood within an artery.*
   • Place the bell side of the amplifier of the stethoscope over the brachial pulse. *Because the blood pressure is a low-frequency sound, it is best heard with the bell-shaped diaphragm.* Hold the diaphragm with the thumb and index finger.
8. Auscultate the patient's blood pressure.
   • Pump up the cuff until the sphygmomanometer reads 30 mm Hg above the point where the brachial pulse disappeared by palpation as in point 6.
   • Release the valve on the cuff carefully so that the pressure decreases at the rate of 2–3 mm Hg per second. *If the rate is faster or slower an error in measurement may occur.*

- As the pressure falls, identify the manometer reading at each of the five phases, if possible.
- Deflate the cuff rapidly and completely.
- Wait 1-2 minutes before making further determinations. *This permits blood trapped in the veins to be released.*
- Repeat the above steps once or twice as necessary to confirm the accuracy of the reading.

9. If this is the patient's initial examination, repeat the procedure on the patient's other arm. There should be a difference of no more than 10 mm Hg between the arms. The arm found to have the higher pressure should be used for subsequent examinations.

Variation: obtaining a blood pressure by the palpation method

If it is not possible to use a stethoscope to obtain the blood pressure or if the Korotkoff sounds cannot be heard, palpate the radial or brachial pulse site as the cuff pressure is released. The manometer reading at the point where the pulse reappears represents a blood pressure between what would be auscultated systolic and diastolic values.

Variation: taking a thigh blood pressure

+ Help the patient to assume a prone position. If the patient cannot assume this position, measure the blood pressure while the patient is in a supine position with the knee slightly flexed. Slight flexing of the knee will facilitate placing the stethoscope on the popliteal space (see Figure 15-32).
+ Expose the thigh, taking care not to expose the patient unduly.

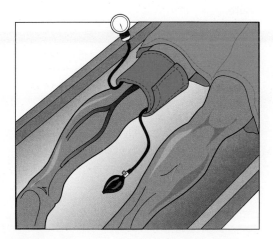

Figure 15-32 Measuring blood pressure in the patient's thigh – location of the popliteal artery and application of the cuff.

+ Locate the popliteal artery (see Figure 15-19 on page 351).
+ Wrap the cuff evenly around the midthigh with the compression bladder over the posterior aspect of the thigh and the bottom edge above the knee. *The bladder must be directly over the posterior popliteal artery if the reading is to be accurate.*
+ If this is the patient's initial examination, perform a preliminary palpatory determination of systolic pressure by palpating the popliteal artery.
+ In adults, the systolic pressure in the popliteal artery is usually 20-30 mm Hg higher than that in the brachial artery because of use of a larger bladder; the diastolic pressure is usually the same.

Variation: using an electronic indirect blood pressure monitoring device (Figure 15-28 on page 363)

+ Place the blood pressure cuff on the extremity according to the manufacturer's guidelines.
+ Turn on the blood pressure switch.
+ If appropriate, set the device for the desired number of minutes between blood pressure determinations.
+ When the device has determined the blood pressure reading, note the digital results.

CLINICAL ALERT

Electronic/automatic blood pressure cuffs can be left in place for many hours. Remove the cuff and check skin condition periodically.

10. Remove the cuff.
11. Wipe the cuff with an approved disinfectant. *Cuffs can become significantly contaminated.* Some clinical areas use disposable blood pressure cuffs. The patient uses it for the length of stay and then it is discarded. This decreases the risk of spreading infection through sharing of cuffs.
12. Document and report pertinent assessment data according to agency policy. Record two pressures in the form '130/80' where '130' is the systolic (phase 1) and '80' is the diastolic (phase 5) pressure. Record three pressures in the form '130/110/90', where '130' is the systolic, '110' is the first diastolic (phase 4) and '90' is the second diastolic (phase 5) pressure. Use the abbreviations *RA* or *RL* for right arm or right leg and *LA* or *LL* for left arm or left leg. Record a difference of greater than 10 mm Hg between the two arms or legs.

Evaluation

+ Relate blood pressure to other vital signs, to baseline data and health status.
+ Report any significant change in the patient's blood pressure. Also report these findings:
  • Systolic blood pressure (of an adult) above 140 mm Hg
  • Diastolic blood pressure (of an adult) above 90 mm Hg
  • Systolic blood pressure (of an adult) below 100 mm Hg
+ Conduct appropriate follow-up such as administration of medication. If the blood pressure is significantly higher or lower than usual, implement appropriate safety precautions.

LIFESPAN CONSIDERATIONS

Blood Pressure

Infants

+ Use a paediatric stethoscope with small diaphragm.
+ The lower edge of the blood pressure cuff can be closer to the antecubital space of an infant.
+ Use the palpation method if auscultation with a stethoscope or DUS is unsuccessful.
+ Arm and thigh pressures are equivalent in children under one year of age.
+ One quick way to determine the normal systolic blood pressure of a child is to use the following formula:

Normal systolic BP = 80 + (2 × child's age in years)

Children

+ Explain each step of the process and what it will feel like. Demonstrate on a doll.
+ Use the palpation technique for children under three years old.
+ Cuff bladder *width* should be 40% and *length* should be 80% to 100% of the arm circumference (see Figure 15-33).
+ Take the blood pressure prior to other uncomfortable procedures so that the blood pressure is not artificially elevated by the discomfort.
+ In children, the diastolic pressure is considered to be the onset of phase 4, where the sounds become muffled.
+ In children, the thigh pressure is about 10 mm Hg higher than the arm.

Older Adults

+ Skin may be very fragile. Do not allow cuff pressure to remain high any longer than necessary.
+ Determine if the patient is taking antihypertensives and, if so, when the last dose was taken.
+ Medications that cause vasodilation (antihypertensive medications) along with the loss of baroreceptor efficiency in the elderly place them at increased risk for having orthostatic hypotension. Measuring blood pressure while the patient is in the lying, sitting and standing positions, and noting any changes can determine this.
+ If the patient has arm contractures, assess the blood pressure by palpation, with the arm in a relaxed position. If this is not possible, take a thigh blood pressure.

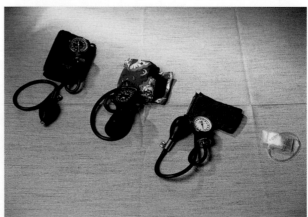

Figure 15-33 Paediatric blood pressure cuffs (with manometers).

Common Errors in Assessing Blood Pressure

The importance of the accuracy of blood pressure assessments cannot be overemphasised. Many judgements about a patient's health are made on the basis of blood pressure. It is an important indicator of the patient's condition and is used extensively as a basis for nursing interventions. Two possible reasons for blood pressure errors are haste on the part of the nurse and subconscious bias. For example, a nurse may be influenced by the patient's previous blood pressure measurements or diagnosis and 'hear' a value consonant with the practitioner's expectations. Some reasons for erroneous blood pressure readings are given in Table 15-5.

Procedure 15-6 provides guidelines for assessing blood pressure.

OXYGEN SATURATION

A **pulse oximeter** is a noninvasive device that measures a patient's arterial blood oxygen saturation (SaO_2) by means of a sensor attached to the patient's finger (see Figure 15-34), toe, nose, earlobe or forehead (or around the hand or foot of a neonate). The pulse oximeter can detect hypoxemia (low blood oxygen levels), before clinical signs and symptoms, such as dusky skin colour and dusky nailbeds colour develop. It is

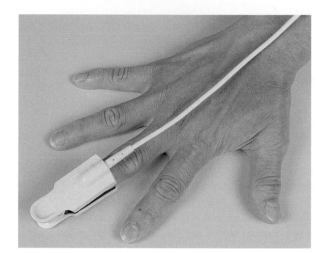

Figure 15-34 Finger tip oximeter sensor (adult).

especially important in patients with respiratory disease such as Chronic Obstructive Pulmonary Disease to detect deteriorating signs early.

The pulse oximeter's *sensor* has two parts: (a) two light-emitting diodes (LEDs) – one red the other infrared – that transmit light through nails, tissue, venous blood and arterial blood; and (b) a photodetector placed directly opposite the LEDs (e.g. the other side of the finger, toe or nose). The photodetector measures the amount of red and infrared light

Table 15-5 Selected Sources of Error in Blood Pressure Assessment

Error	Effect
Bladder cuff too narrow	Erroneously high
Bladder cuff too wide	Erroneously low
Arm unsupported	Erroneously high
Insufficient rest before the assessment	Erroneously high
Repeating assessment too quickly	Erroneously high systolic or low diastolic readings
Cuff wrapped too loosely or unevenly	Erroneously high
Deflating cuff too quickly	Erroneously low systolic and high diastolic readings
Deflating cuff too slowly	Erroneously high diastolic reading
Failure to use the same arm consistently	Inconsistent measurements
Arm above level of the heart	Erroneously low
Assessing immediately after a meal or while patient smokes or has pain	Erroneously high
Failure to identify auscultatory gap	Erroneously low systolic pressure and erroneously low diastolic pressure

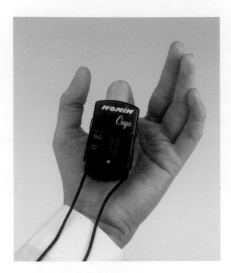

Figure 15-35 Finger tip oximeter sensor (cordless).
(Courtesy of Nonin Medical, Inc.)

absorbed by oxygenated and deoxygenated haemoglobin in arterial blood and reports it as SaO_2. Normal SaO_2 is 95% to 100% and an SaO_2 below 70% is life threatening.

Pulse oximeters with various types of sensors are available from several manufacturers. The *oximeter unit* consists of an inlet

connection for the sensor cable, a faceplate that indicates (a) the oxygen saturation measurement (expressed as a percentage) and (b) the pulse rate. Cordless units are also available (see Figure 15-35). A preset alarm system signals high and low SaO_2 measurements and a high and low pulse rate. The high and low SaO_2 levels are generally preset at 100% and 85%, respectively, for adults. The high and low pulse rate alarms are usually preset at 140 and 50 BPM for adults. These alarm limits can, however, be changed according to the manufacturer's directions.

Factors Affecting Oxygen Saturation Readings

+ *Haemoglobin*. If the haemoglobin is fully saturated with oxygen, the SaO_2 will appear normal even if the total haemoglobin level is low. Thus, the patient could be severely anaemic and have inadequate oxygen to supply the tissues but the pulse oximeter would return a normal value.
+ *Circulation*. The oximeter will not return an accurate reading if the area under the sensor has impaired circulation.
+ *Activity*. Shivering or excessive movement of the sensor site may interfere with accurate readings.

Procedure 15-7 outlines the steps in measuring oxygen saturation.

PROCEDURE 15-7 Measuring Oxygen Saturation

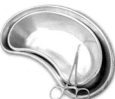

Purposes

+ To measure the arterial blood oxygen saturation (SaO_2)
+ To detect the presence of hypoemia before visible signs develop

---

Assessment

Assess

+ The best location for a pulse oximeter sensor based on the patient's age and physical condition
+ The patient's overall condition including risk factors for development of hypoxemia (e.g.

respiratory or cardiac disease) and haemoglobin level
+ Vital signs, skin and nail bed colour, and tissue perfusion of extremities as baseline data
+ Adhesive allergy

Planning

Many clinical areas have pulse oximeters readily available for use with other vital signs equipment (or even as an integrated part of the electronic blood pressure device).

Equipment

+ Nail polish remover as needed
+ Alcohol wipe
+ Sheet or towel
+ Pulse oximeter

Implementation

Preparation

Check that the oximeter equipment is functioning normally.

Performance

1. Explain to the patient what you are going to do, why it is necessary and how they can cooperate. Discuss how the results will be used in planning further care or treatments.
2. Observe appropriate infection control procedures.
3. Provide for patient privacy.
4. Choose a sensor appropriate for the patient's weight, size and desired location. Because weight limits of sensors overlap, a paediatric sensor could be used for a small adult.
   - If the patient is allergic to adhesive, use a clip or sensor without adhesive. If using an extremity, assess the proximal pulse and capillary refill at the point closest to the site.
   - If the patient has low tissue perfusion due to peripheral vascular disease or therapy using vasoconstrictive medications, use a nasal sensor or a reflectance sensor on the forehead. Avoid using lower extremities that have a compromised circulation and extremities that are used for infusions or other invasive monitoring.
5. Prepare the site.
   - Clean the site with an alcohol wipe before applying the sensor.
   - It may be necessary to remove a patient's nail polish/varnish or acrylic nails *since they can interfere with accurate measurements*.
6. Apply the sensor, and connect it to the pulse oximeter.
   - Make sure the LED and photodetector are accurately aligned, that is, opposite each other on either side of the finger, toe, nose or earlobe. Many sensors have markings to facilitate correct alignment of the LEDs and photodetector.
   - Attach the sensor cable to the connection outlet on the oximeter. Turn on the machine according to the manufacturer's directions. Appropriate connection will be confirmed by an audible beep indicating each arterial pulsation.
   - Ensure that the bar of light or waveform on the face of the oximeter fluctuates with each pulsation and reflects the pulse volume or strength.
7. Set and turn on the alarm.
   - Check the preset alarm limits for high and low oxygen saturation and high and low pulse rates. Change these alarm limits according to the manufacturer's directions as indicated. Ensure that the audio and visual alarms are on before you leave the patient. A tone will be heard and a number will blink on the faceplate.
8. Ensure patient safety.
   - Inspect and/or move or change the location of an adhesive toe or finger sensor every four hours and a spring-tension sensor every two hours.
   - Inspect the sensor site tissues for irritation from adhesive sensors.
9. Ensure the accuracy of measurement.
   - Minimise motion artefacts by using an adhesive sensor or immobilise the patient's monitoring site. *Movement of the patient's finger or toe may be misinterpreted by the oximeter as arterial pulsations*.
   - If indicated, cover the sensor with a sheet or towel to block large amounts of light from external sources (e.g. sunlight or procedure lamps). *Large amounts of outside light may be sensed by the photodetector and alter the SaO_2 value*.
10. Document the oxygen saturation on the appropriate record at designated intervals.

Evaluation

+ Compare the oxygen saturation to the patient's previous oxygen saturation level. Relate to pulse rate and other vital signs.

+ Conduct appropriate follow-up such as notifying the medical staff, adjusting oxygen therapy or providing breathing treatments.

LIFESPAN CONSIDERATIONS

Pulse Oximetry

Infants

+ If an appropriate-sized finger or toe sensor (see Figure 15-36) is not available, consider using an earlobe or forehead sensor.
+ The high and low SaO_2 levels are generally preset at 95% and 80% for neonates.
+ The high and low pulse rate alarms are usually preset at 200 and 100 for neonates.

Children

+ Instruct the child that the sensor does not hurt. Disconnect the probe whenever possible to allow for movement.

Older Adults

+ Use of vasoconstrictive medications, poor circulation or thickened nails may make finger or toe sensors inaccurate.

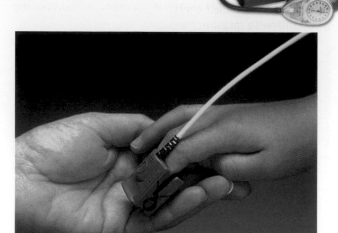

Figure 15-36 Finger tip oximeter sensor (child). (Courtesy of Nonin Medical, Inc.)

CRITICAL REFLECTION

Let us revisit the case study on page 336. Now that you have read this chapter what questions will you ask the patient at this time? After much discussion, Rosa agrees to let you take her blood pressure. After pumping up the cuff, you are unable to hear any sounds during release of the valve. What would you say to her? Once you are able to measure the blood pressure, your reading is 180/110. Before taking any action on this blood pressure, what do you need to know? The pulse oximeter on her finger reads 85%. Her skin is warm and has normal colour; she is awake and oriented, temperature is 37.1°C and apical pulse 78. What would be your next actions and why?

CHAPTER HIGHLIGHTS

+ Vital signs reflect changes in body function that otherwise might not be observed.
+ Body temperature is the balance between heat produced by the body and heat lost from the body.
+ Factors affecting body temperature include age, diurnal variations, exercise, hormones, stress and environmental temperatures.
+ Hypothermia involves three mechanisms: excessive heat loss, inadequate heat production by body cells and increasing impairment of hypothalamic thermoregulation.
+ Body temperature can be measured orally, tympanically, rectally or by axilla. The nurse selects the most appropriate site according to the patient's age and condition.
+ Pulse rate and volume reflect the stroke volume output, the compliance of the patient's arteries and the adequacy of blood flow.
+ Normally a peripheral pulse reflects the patient's heartbeat, but it may differ from the heartbeat in patients with certain cardiovascular diseases; in these instances, the nurse takes an apical pulse and compares it to the peripheral pulse.

+ Many factors may affect a person's pulse rate: age, gender, exercise, presence of fever, certain medications, hypovolaemia, stress, (in some situations) position changes and pathology.
+ Although the radial pulse is the site most commonly used, eight other sites may be used in certain situations.
+ Respirations are normally quiet, effortless and automatic, and are assessed by observing respiratory rate, depth, rhythm, quality and effectiveness.
+ Blood pressure reflects cardiac output, peripheral vascular resistance, blood volume and blood viscosity.
+ Among the factors influencing blood pressure are age, exercise, stress, race, gender, medications, obesity, diurnal variations and disease processes.
+ A blood pressure cuff too large or too small will give false readings.
+ During blood pressure measurement, the artery must be held at heart level.
+ A pulse oximeter measures the percentage of haemoglobin saturated with oxygen. A normal result is 95% to 100%.

REFERENCES

Bindler, R.C. and Ball, J.W. (2003) *Clinical skills manual for pediatric nursing: Caring for children* (3rd edn), Upper Saddle River, NJ: Prentice Hall Health.

DuBois, E.F. (1948) *Fever and the regulation of body temperature*, Springfield, IL: Charles C. Thomas.

Foster-Fitzpatrick, L., Ortiz, A., Sibilano, H., Marcantonio, R. and Braun, L.T. (1999) 'The effects of crossed leg on blood pressure measurement', *Nursing Research*, 48, 105–108.

Guyton, A.C. (1996) *Textbook of medical physiology* (9th edn), Philadelphia: W.B. Saunders.

Ladewig, P.W., London, M.L. and Olds, S.B. (1998) *Maternal–newborn nursing care: The nurse, the family, and the community* (4th edn), Menlo Park, CA: Addison Wesley Longman.

Lance, R., Link, M.E., Padua, M., Clavell, L.E., Johnson, G. and Knebel, E. (2000) 'Comparison of different methods of obtaining orthostatic vital signs', *Clinical Nursing Research*, 9, 479–491.

Marieb, E.N. (1998) *Human anatomy and physiology* (4th edn), Menlo Park, CA: Benjamin/Cummings.

National Institutes of Health, National Heart, Lung, and Blood Institute (1997) *The sixth report of the Joint National Committee on Prevention, Detection, Evaluation, and Treatment of High Blood Pressure* (NIH Publication #98-4080). Available from http://www.nhlbi.nih.gov/guidelines/hypertension/jnc6.pdf. (Accessed 26 December 2002.)

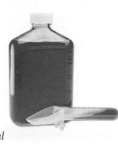

Chapter 16 Oxygenation

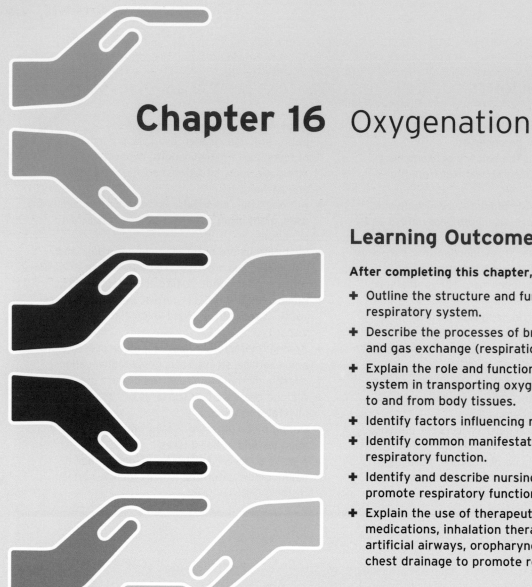

Learning Outcomes

After completing this chapter, you will be able to:

+ Outline the structure and function of the respiratory system.

+ Describe the processes of breathing (ventilation) and gas exchange (respiration).

+ Explain the role and function of the respiratory system in transporting oxygen and carbon dioxide to and from body tissues.

+ Identify factors influencing respiratory function.

+ Identify common manifestations of impaired respiratory function.

+ Identify and describe nursing measures to promote respiratory function and oxygenation.

+ Explain the use of therapeutic measures such as medications, inhalation therapy, oxygen therapy, artificial airways, oropharyngeal suction and chest drainage to promote respiratory function.

CASE STUDY

John is a 66-year-old who has been admitted to your clinical area with a history of chronic obstructive pulmonary disease (COPD). A new member of support staff on the ward asks you to describe and explain to them what this illness is and how the patient developed it.

You begin to explain he has worked in an industrial environment for 40 years that has a high dust exposure level as a bi-product and hazard. John, over-hearing your explanation, also explains to your colleague that during the early part of his career he was not issued with any respiratory protection such as a dust protection mask. You undertake a brief teaching session describing the structure and function of the respiratory system, how oxygen enters the body, is transported and how this delicate system can be damaged by environmental irritants such as dust. Your colleague then questions why John has supplemental oxygen to breathe.

As you explain further you show your colleague the various types of oxygen delivery devices and how they can be used for patients with varying types of respiratory problems such as John.

After you read this chapter you will be able to describe nursing measures to promote respiratory function and oxygenation.

PHYSIOLOGY OF THE RESPIRATORY SYSTEM

Oxygen, a clear, odourless gas that constitutes approximately 21% of the air we breathe, is necessary for all living cells. The absence of oxygen can lead to death. Although the delivery of oxygen to body tissues is affected at least indirectly by all body systems, the respiratory system is most directly involved in this process. Impaired function of the system can significantly affect our ability to breathe, transport gases and participate in everyday activities.

The function of the respiratory system is gas exchange. Oxygen from inspired air diffuses from alveoli in the lungs into the blood in pulmonary capillaries. Carbon dioxide produced during cell metabolism diffuses from the blood into the alveoli and is exhaled. The organs of the respiratory system facilitate this gas exchange and protect the body from foreign matter such as particulates (dust) and pathogens (diseases).

Structure of the Respiratory System

The respiratory system (see Figure 16-1) is divided structurally into the upper respiratory system and the lower respiratory system. The mouth, nose, pharynx and larynx compose the upper respiratory system. The lower respiratory system includes the trachea and lungs, with the bronchi, bronchioles, alveoli, pulmonary capillary network and pleural membranes.

Air enters through the nose, where it is warmed, humidified and filtered. Large particles in the air are trapped by the hairs at the entrance of the nares (nostrils), and smaller particles are

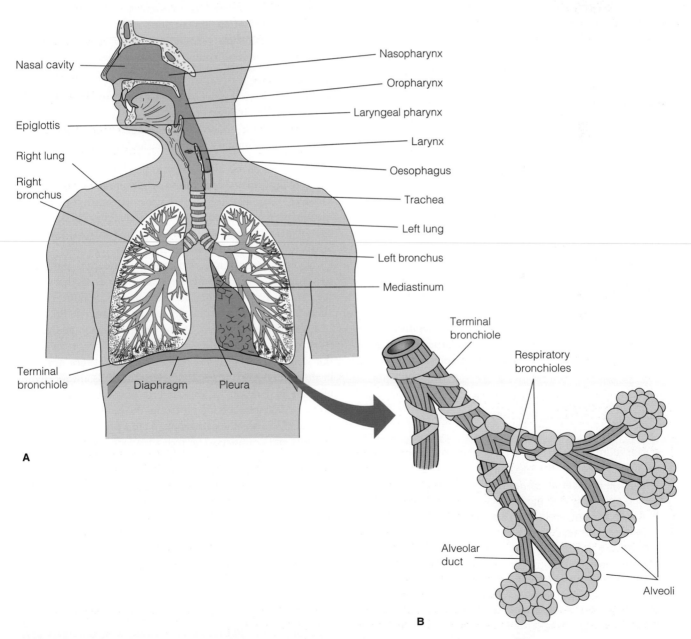

Figure 16-1 *A*, Organs of the respiratory tract. *B*, Respiratory bronchioles, alveolar ducts and alveoli.

filtered and trapped as air changes direction on contact with the nasal turbinates and septum. The sneeze reflex is initiated by irritants in nasal passages. A large volume of air rapidly exits through the nose and mouth during a sneeze, helping to clear nasal passages.

Inspired air passes from the nose through the pharynx. The pharynx is a shared pathway for air and food. It includes both the nasopharynx (upper part) and the oropharynx (lower part), which are richly supplied with lymphoid tissue that traps and destroys pathogens entering with the air.

The larynx is a cartilaginous structure that can be identified externally as the Adam's apple. In addition to its role in providing for speech, the larynx is important for maintaining airway clearance and protecting the lower airways from swallowed food and fluids. During swallowing, the inlet to the larynx (the epiglottis) closes, routing food to the oesophagus. The epiglottis is open during breathing, allowing air to move freely into the lower airways.

Below the larynx, the trachea leads to the right and left main bronchi (primary bronchi) and the conducting airways of the lungs. Within the lungs, the primary bronchi divide repeatedly into smaller and smaller bronchi, ending with the terminal bronchioles. Together these airways are known as the bronchial tree. The trachea and bronchi are lined with mucosal epithelium. These cells produce a thin layer of mucus, that traps pathogens and microscopic particulate matter. These foreign particles are then swept upward toward the larynx and throat by cilia, which are tiny hair-like projections on the epithelial cells. The cough reflex is triggered by irritants in the larynx, trachea or bronchi and is described in *Box 16-1*.

Until air passes through the terminal bronchioles and enters the respiratory bronchioles and alveoli, no gas exchange occurs. The respiratory zone of the lungs includes the respiratory bronchioles (which have scattered air sacs in their walls), the alveolar ducts and the alveoli (see Figure 16-1). Alveoli have very thin walls, composed of a single layer of epithelial cells covered by a thick mesh of pulmonary capillaries. The alveolar and capillary walls form the **respiratory membrane**, where gas exchange occurs between the air on the alveolar side and the blood on the capillary side. The airways move air to and from the alveoli; the right ventricle and pulmonary vascular system transport blood to the capillary side of the membrane.

The outer surface of the lungs is covered by a thin, double layer of tissue known as the pleura. The parietal pleura lines the thorax and surface of the diaphragm. It doubles back to form the visceral pleura, covering the external surface of the lungs. Between these pleural layers is a potential space that contains a small amount of pleural fluid, a serous lubricating solution. This fluid prevents friction during the movements of breathing and serves to keep the layers adherent through its surface tension.

Pulmonary Ventilation

Ventilation of the lungs is accomplished through the act of breathing: **inspiration (inhalation)** when air flows into the lungs and **expiration (exhalation)** as air moves out of the lungs. Adequate ventilation depends on several factors:

+ clear airways;
+ an intact central nervous system and respiratory centre in the medulla oblongata of the brain;
+ an intact thoracic cavity capable of expanding and contracting;
+ adequate pulmonary compliance and recoil.

A number of mechanisms including ciliary action and the cough reflex work to keep airways open and clear. In some cases, however, these defences may be overwhelmed. The inflammation, oedema and excess mucous production that occur with some types of pneumonia may clog small airways, impairing ventilation of distal alveoli.

The respiratory centres of the medulla and pons in the brain stem control breathing. Severe head injury or drugs that depress the central nervous system (e.g. opiates or barbiturates) can affect the respiratory centres, impairing the drive to breathe.

Expansion and recoil of the lungs occurs passively in response to changes in pressures within the thoracic cavity and the lungs themselves. The **intrapleural pressure** (pressure in the pleural cavity surrounding the lungs) is always slightly negative in relation to atmospheric pressure. This negative pressure is essential because it creates the suction that holds the visceral pleura and the parietal pleura together as the chest cage expands and contracts. The recoil tendency of the lungs is a major factor in creating this negative pressure. The intrapleural fluid also contributes by causing the pleura to adhere together, much as a film of water can cause two glass slides to adhere together.

The **intrapulmonary pressure** (pressure within the lungs) always equalises with atmospheric pressure. Inspiration occurs when the diaphragm and intercostal muscles contract, increasing the size of the thoracic cavity. The volume of the lungs increases, decreasing intrapulmonary pressure. Air then rushes into the lungs to equalise this pressure with atmospheric pressure. Conversely, when the diaphragm and intercostal muscles relax, the volume of the lungs decreases, intrapulmonary pressure rises, and air is expelled.

BOX 16-1 The Cough Reflex

+ Nerve impulses are sent through the vagus nerve (10th cranial) to the medulla.
+ A large inspiration of approximately 2.5 l occurs.
+ The epiglottis and glottis (vocal cords) close.
+ A strong contraction of abdominal and internal intercostal muscles dramatically raises the pressure in the lungs.
+ The epiglottis and glottis open suddenly.
+ Air rushes outward with great velocity.
+ Mucous and any foreign particles are dislodged from the lower respiratory tract and are propelled up and out.

The degree of chest expansion during normal breathing is minimal, requiring little energy expenditure. In adults, approximately 500 ml of air is inspired and expired with each breath. This is known as **tidal volume**. Breathing during strenuous exercise or some types of heart disease require greater chest expansion and effort. At this time, more than 1,500 ml of air may be moved with each breath. Accessory muscles of respiration, including the anterior neck muscles, intercostal muscles and muscles of the abdomen, are employed. Active use of these muscles and noticeable effort in breathing are seen in patients with obstructive pulmonary disease.

Diseases such as muscular dystrophy, or trauma such as spinal cord injury can affect the muscles of respiration, impairing the ability of the thoracic cavity to expand and contract. A penetrating wound or other trauma to the chest wall may allow intrapleural pressure to equalise with the atmosphere, causing the lung to collapse.

Lung compliance, the expansibility or stretchability of lung tissue, plays a significant role in the ease of ventilation. At birth, the fluid-filled lungs are stiff and resistant to expansion, much as a new balloon is difficult to inflate. With each subsequent breath, the alveoli become more compliant and easier to inflate, just as a balloon becomes easier to inflate after several tries. Lung compliance tends to decrease with ageing, making it more difficult to expand alveoli and increasing risk of **atelectasis**, or collapse of a portion of the lung.

In contrast to lung compliance is **lung recoil**, the continual tendency of the lungs to collapse away from the chest wall. Just as lung compliance is necessary for normal inspiration, lung recoil is necessary for normal expiration. Although elastic fibres in lung tissue contribute to lung recoil, the surface tension of fluid lining the alveoli has the greatest effect on recoil. Fluid molecules tend to draw together, reducing the size of alveoli. **Surfactant**, a lipoprotein produced by specialised alveolar cells, acts like a detergent, reducing the surface tension of alveolar fluid. Without surfactant, lung expansion is exceedingly difficult and the lungs collapse. Premature infants whose lungs are not yet capable of producing adequate surfactant develop respiratory distress syndrome.

Alveolar Gas Exchange

After the alveoli are ventilated, the second phase of the respiratory process – *the diffusion of* oxygen from the alveoli and into the pulmonary blood vessels – begins. **Diffusion** is the movement of gases or other particles from an area of greater pressure or concentration to an area of lower pressure or concentration.

Pressure differences in the gases on each side of the respiratory membrane obviously affect diffusion. When the pressure of oxygen is greater in the alveoli than in the blood, oxygen diffuses into the blood. The **partial pressure** (the pressure exerted by each individual gas in a mixture according to its concentration in the mixture) of oxygen (PO_2) in the alveoli is about 100 mm Hg (sometimes referred to as **torr** (unit of measure) which is the same as millimetres of mercury), whereas the PO_2 in the venous blood of the pulmonary arteries is about 60 mm Hg. These pressures rapidly equalise, however, so that the arterial oxygen pressure also reaches about 100 mm Hg. By contrast, carbon dioxide in the venous blood entering the pulmonary capillaries has a partial pressure of about 45 mm Hg (PCO_2), whereas that in the alveoli has a partial pressure of about 40 mm Hg. Therefore, carbon dioxide diffuses from the blood into the alveoli, where it can be eliminated with expired air. When referring to the pressure of oxygen in the arterial blood the abbreviation is PaO_2. When referring to partial pressure in venous blood there is no 'a', that is, PO_2.

Transport of Oxygen and Carbon Dioxide

The third part of the respiratory process involves the transport of respiratory gases. Oxygen needs to be transported from the lungs to the tissues, and carbon dioxide must be transported from the tissues back to the lungs. Normally most of the oxygen (97%) combines loosely with **haemoglobin** (oxygen-carrying red pigment) in the red blood cells and is carried to the tissues as **oxyhaemoglobin** (the compound of oxygen and haemoglobin). The remaining oxygen is dissolved and transported in the fluid of the plasma and cells.

Several factors affect the rate of oxygen transport from the lungs to the tissues:

+ cardiac output,
+ number of erythrocytes and blood haematocrit,
+ exercise.

The **haematocrit** is the percentage of the blood that is comprised of erythrocytes.

Any pathologic condition that decreases cardiac output (e.g. damage to the heart muscle, blood loss or pooling of blood in the peripheral blood vessels) diminishes the amount of oxygen delivered to the tissues. The heart compensates for inadequate output by increasing its pumping rate; however, with severe damage or blood loss, this compensatory mechanism may not restore adequate blood flow and oxygen to the tissues.

The second factor influencing oxygen transport is the number of **erythrocytes** (red blood cells, or RBCs) and the haematocrit. In men, the number of circulating erythrocytes normally averages about 5 million per cubic millilitre of blood, and in women, about $4^1/_2$ million per cubic millilitre. Normally the haematocrit is about 40% to 54% in men and 37% to 48% in women. Excessive increases in the blood haematocrit raise the blood viscosity, reducing the cardiac output and therefore reducing oxygen transport. Excessive reductions in the blood haematocrit, such as anaemia, reduce oxygen transport.

Exercise also has a direct influence on oxygen transport. In well-trained athletes, oxygen transport can be increased up to 20 times the normal rate, due in part to an increased cardiac output and to increased use of oxygen by the cells.

Carbon dioxide, continually produced in the processes of cell metabolism, is transported from the cells to the lungs in three ways. The majority (about 65%) is carried inside the red blood cells as bicarbonate (HCO_3^-) and is an important component of the bicarbonate buffer system. A moderate amount of carbon dioxide (30%) combines with haemoglobin as carboxyhaemoglobin for transport. Smaller amounts (5%) are transported in solution in the plasma and as carbonic acid (the compound formed when carbon dioxide combines with water).

RESPIRATORY REGULATION

Respiratory regulation includes both neurological and chemical controls to maintain the correct concentrations of oxygen, carbon dioxide and hydrogen ions in body fluids. The nervous system of the body adjusts the rate of alveolar ventilations to meet the needs of the body so that PO_2 and PCO_2 remain relatively constant. The body's 'respiratory centre' is actually a number of groups of neurons located in the medulla oblongata and pons of the brain.

A chemosensitive centre in the medulla oblongata is highly responsive to increases in blood CO_2 or hydrogen ion concentration. By influencing other respiratory centres, this centre can increase the activity of the inspiratory centre and the rate and depth of respirations. In addition to this direct chemical stimulation of the respiratory centre in the brain, special neural receptors sensitive to decreases in O_2 concentration are located outside the central nervous system in the carotid bodies (just above the bifurcation of the common carotid arteries) and aortic bodies. Decreases in arterial oxygen concentrations stimulate these chemoreceptors, and they in turn stimulate the respiratory centre to increase ventilation. Of the three blood gases (hydrogen, oxygen and carbon dioxide) that can trigger chemoreceptors, increased carbon dioxide concentration normally stimulates respiration most strongly.

However, in patients with certain chronic lung ailments such as **emphysema**, oxygen concentrations, not carbon dioxide concentrations, play a major role in regulating respiration. For such patients, decreased oxygen concentrations are the main stimuli for respiration. This is sometimes called the hypoxic drive. Increasing the concentration of oxygen depresses the respiratory rate. Thus, only low concentrations of supplemental oxygen are administered to these patients.

FACTORS AFFECTING RESPIRATORY FUNCTION

Factors that influence oxygenation affect the cardiovascular system as well as the respiratory system. These factors include age, environment, lifestyle, health status, medications and stress.

Age

Developmental factors are important influences on respiratory function. At birth, profound changes occur in the respiratory systems. The fluid-filled lungs drain, the PCO_2 rises and the neonate takes a first breath. The lungs gradually expand with each subsequent breath, reaching full inflation by two weeks of age. Changes of ageing that affect the respiratory system of older adults become especially important if the system is compromised by changes such as infection, physical or emotional stress, surgery, anaesthesia or other procedures. Changes are:

+ Chest wall and airways become more rigid and less elastic.
+ The amount of exchanged air is decreased.
+ The cough reflex and cilia action are decreased.
+ Mucous membranes become drier and more fragile.
+ Decreases in muscle strength and endurance occur.
+ If osteoporosis is present, adequate lung expansion may be compromised.
+ A decrease in efficiency of the immune system occurs.
+ Gastroesophageal reflux disease is more common in older adults and increases the risk of aspiration. The aspiration of stomach contents into the lungs often causes bronchospasm by setting up an inflammatory response.

LIFESPAN CONSIDERATIONS

Respiratory Development

Infants

+ Respiratory rates are highest and most variable in newborns. The respiratory rate of a neonate is 40-80 breaths per minute
+ Infant respiratory rates average about 30 per minute.
+ Because of rib cage structure, infants rely almost exclusively on diaphragmatic movement for breathing. This is seen as abdominal breathing, as the abdomen rises and falls with each breath.

Children

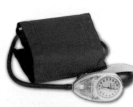

+ The respiratory rate gradually decreases, averaging around 25 per minute in the pre-school child and reaching the adult rate of 12-18 per minute by late adolescence.
+ During infancy and childhood, upper respiratory infections are common and, fortunately, usually not serious. Infants and pre-school children are also at risk for airway obstruction by foreign objects such as coins and small toys. Cystic fibrosis is a congenital disorder that affects the lungs, causing them to become congested with thick, tenacious

(sticky) mucus. Asthma is another chronic disease often identified in childhood. The airways of the asthmatic child respond to stimuli such as allergens, exercise or cold air by constricting, becoming oedematous and producing excessive mucus. Airflow is impaired, and the child may wheeze as air moves through narrowed air passages.

Older Adults

+ Older adults are at increased risk for acute respiratory diseases such as pneumonia and chronic diseases such as emphysema and chronic bronchitis. Chronic obstructive pulmonary disease (COPD) may affect older adults, particularly after years of exposure to cigarette smoke or industrial pollutants.
+ Pneumonia may not present with the usual symptoms of a fever, but will present with atypical symptoms, such as confusion, weakness, loss of appetite, and increase in heart rate and respirations.

Nursing interventions should be directed toward achieving optimal respiratory effort and gas exchange:

+ Always encourage wellness and prevention of disease by reinforcing the need for good nutrition, exercise and immunisations, such as for influenza and pneumonia.
+ Increase fluid intake, if not contraindicated by other problems, such as cardiac or renal impairment.
+ Correct positioning and frequent changing of positions allow for better lung expansion and air and fluid movement.
+ Teach patient to use breathing techniques for better air exchange.
+ Pace activities to conserve energy.
+ Encourage the patient to eat more frequent, smaller meals to decrease gastric distention, which can cause pressure on the diaphragm.
+ Teach patient to avoid extreme hot or cold temperatures that will further tax the respiratory system.
+ Explain actions and side effects of drugs, inhalers and treatments.

Environment

Altitude, heat, cold and air pollution affect oxygenation. The higher the altitude, the lower the PO_2 an individual breathes. As a result, the person at high altitudes has increased respiratory and cardiac rates and increased respiratory depth, which usually become most apparent when the individual exercises.

Healthy people exposed to air pollution, such as smog, often experience stinging of the eyes, headache, dizziness, coughing and choking. People who have a history of existing lung disease and altered respiratory function experience varying degrees of respiratory difficulty in a polluted environment. Some are unable to perform self-care in such an environment.

Lifestyle

Physical exercise or activity increases the rate and depth of respirations and hence the supply of oxygen in the body. Sedentary people, by contrast, lack the alveolar expansion and deep breathing patterns of people with regular activity and are less able to respond effectively to respiratory stressors.

Certain occupations predispose an individual to lung disease. For example, silicosis is seen more often in sandstone blasters and potters than in the rest of the population; asbestosis in asbestos workers; anthracosis in coal miners; and organic dust disease in farmers and agricultural employees who work with mouldy hay.

Health Status

In the healthy person, the respiratory system can provide sufficient oxygen to meet the body needs. Diseases of the respiratory system, however, can adversely affect the oxygenation of the blood.

Medications

A variety of medications can decrease the rate and depth of respirations. The most common medications with this effect are the benzodiazepine sedative-hypnotics and anti-anxiety drugs (e.g. diazepam (Valium), flurazepam, midazolam), barbiturates, and narcotics such as morphine. When administering these, the nurse must carefully monitor respiratory status, especially when the medication is begun or when the dose is increased. Although this is a safety concern, often the importance of the medication outweighs the risk of respiratory depression.

Stress

When stress and stressors are encountered, both psychological and physiological responses can affect oxygenation. Some people may hyperventilate in response to stress. When this occurs, arterial PO_2 rises and PCO_2 falls. The person may experience light-headedness and numbness and tingling of the fingers, toes and around the mouth as a result.

Physiologically, the sympathetic nervous system is stimulated and adrenaline is released. Adrenaline causes the bronchioles to dilate, increasing blood flow and oxygen delivery to active muscles. Although these responses are adaptive in the short term, when stress continues they can be destructive, increasing the risk of cardiovascular disease.

ALTERATIONS IN RESPIRATORY FUNCTION

Respiratory function can be altered by conditions that affect:

+ the movement of air into or out of the lungs;
+ the diffusion of oxygen and carbon dioxide between the alveoli and the pulmonary capillaries;
+ the transport of oxygen and carbon dioxide via the blood to and from the tissue cells.

Three major alterations in respiration are hypoxia, altered breathing patterns and obstructed or partially obstructed airway.

Hypoxia

Hypoxia is a condition of insufficient oxygen anywhere in the body, from the inspired gas to the tissues. It can be related to any of the parts of respiration – ventilation, diffusion of gases or transport of gases by the blood – and can be caused by any condition that alters one or more parts of the process.

Hypoventilation, that is, inadequate alveolar ventilation, can lead to hypoxia. Hypoventilation may occur because of diseases of the respiratory muscles, drugs or anesthesia. With hypoventilation, carbon dioxide often accumulates in the blood, a condition called **hypercarbia (hypercapnia)**.

Hypoxia can also develop when the diffusion of oxygen from alveoli into the arterial blood decreases, as with pulmonary oedema, or it can result from problems in the delivery of oxygen to the tissues (e.g. anaemia, heart failure and embolism). The term **hypoxaemia** refers to reduced oxygen in the blood and is characterised by a low partial pressure of oxygen in arterial blood or a low haemoglobin saturation. *Box 16-2* lists signs of hypoxia.

Cyanosis (bluish discoloration of the skin, nail beds and mucous membranes, due to reduced haemoglobin-oxygen saturation) may also be present. Cyanosis requires these two conditions: The blood must contain about 5 g or more of unoxygenated haemoglobin per 100 ml of blood, and the surface blood capillaries must be dilated. Factors that interfere with either of these conditions (e.g. severe anaemia or the administration of epinephrine/adrenaline) will eliminate cyanosis as a sign even if the patient is experiencing hypoxia.

BOX 16-2 Signs of Hypoxia

+ Rapid pulse
+ Rapid, shallow respirations and dyspnoea
+ Increased restlessness or light-headedness
+ Flaring of the nares
+ Substernal or intercostal retractions (sucking in of the chest)
+ Cyanosis

Adequate oxygenation is essential for cerebral functioning. The cerebral cortex can tolerate hypoxia for only 3–5 minutes before permanent damage occurs. The face of the acutely hypoxic person usually appears anxious, tired and drawn. The person usually assumes a sitting position, often leaning forward slightly to permit greater expansion of the thoracic cavity.

With chronic hypoxia, the patient often appears fatigued and is lethargic. The patient's fingers and toes may be clubbed as a result of long-term lack of oxygen in the arterial blood supply. With clubbing, the base of the nail becomes swollen and the ends of the fingers and toes increase in size. The angle between the nail and the base of the nail increases to more than 180 degrees.

Altered Breathing Patterns

Breathing patterns refer to the rate, volume, rhythm and relative ease or effort of respiration. Normal respiration (**eupnoea**) is quiet, rhythmic and effortless. **Tachyopnea** (rapid rate) is seen with fevers, metabolic acidosis, pain and with hypercapnia or hypoxemia. **Bradyopnea** is an abnormally slow respiratory rate, which may be seen in patients who have taken drugs such as morphine, who have metabolic alkalosis or who have increased intracranial pressure (e.g. from brain injuries). **Apnoea** is the cessation of breathing.

Hyperventilation, often called *alveolar hyperventilation*, is an increased movement of air into and out of the lungs. During hyperventilation, the rate and depth of respirations increase, and more CO_2 is eliminated than is produced. One particular type of hyperventilation that accompanies metabolic acidosis is **Kussmaul's breathing**, by which the body attempts to compensate (give off excess body acids) by blowing off the carbon dioxide through deep and rapid breathing. This may occur when there is a diabetic ketoacidosis or in severe renal failure. Hyperventilation can also occur in response to stress, as mentioned earlier.

Abnormal respiratory rhythms create an irregular breathing pattern. Two abnormal respiratory rhythms are:

1. **Cheyne-Stokes respirations**. Marked rhythmic waxing and waning of respirations from very deep to very shallow breathing and temporary apnoea; common causes include congestive heart failure, increased intracranial pressure and drug overdose
2. **Biot's (cluster) respirations**. Shallow breaths interrupted by apnoea; may be seen in patients with central nervous system disorders.

Orthopnoea is the inability to breathe except in an upright or standing position. Difficult or uncomfortable breathing is called **dyspnoea**. The dyspnoeic person often appears anxious and may experience *shortness of breath* (SOB), a feeling of being unable to get enough air (breathlessness). Often the nostrils are flared because of the increased effort of inspiration. The skin may appear dusky; heart rate is increased. Dyspnoea may have many causes, most of which stem from cardiac or respiratory disorders. It is a subjective feeling; that is, dyspnoea may not be directly observed or measured but is reported by the patient. Since treatment is aimed at removing the underlying cause, it is important for the nurse to conduct a thorough history of the onset, duration and precipitating and relieving factors of the patient's dyspnoea.

Obstructed Airway

A completely or partially obstructed airway can occur anywhere along the upper or lower respiratory passageways. An upper airway obstruction – that is, in the nose, pharynx or larynx – can arise because of a foreign object such as food, because the tongue falls back into the oropharynx when a person is unconscious, or when secretions collect in the passageways. In the latter instance, the respirations will sound gurgly or bubbly as the air attempts to pass through the secretions. Lower airway obstruction involves partial or complete occlusion of the passageways in the bronchi and lungs.

Maintaining an open (patent) airway is a nursing intervention, one that often requires immediate action. Partial obstruction of the upper airway passages is indicated by a low-pitched snoring sound during inhalation. Complete obstruction is indicated by extreme inspiratory effort that produces no chest movement. A patient in an effort to obtain air, may also exhibit marked sternal and intercostal retractions. Lower airway obstruction is not always as easy to observe. **Stridor**, a harsh, high-pitched sound, may be heard during inspiration. The patient may have altered arterial blood gas levels, restlessness, dyspnoea and **adventitious breath sounds** (abnormal breath sounds).

NURSING MANAGEMENT

ASSESSING

Nursing assessment of oxygenation status includes a history and review of relevant diagnostic data such as vital signs and oxygen saturation levels.

Patient History

A comprehensive patient history relevant to oxygenation status should include data about current and past respiratory problems; lifestyle; presence of cough, **sputum** (coughed-up material), pain; medications for breathing; and presence of risk factors for impaired oxygenation status. Examples of interview questions to elicit this information are shown in the *Assessment interview*.

Diagnostic Studies

The doctor may request various diagnostic tests to assess respiratory status, function and oxygenation. Included are sputum

ASSESSMENT INTERVIEW

Oxygenation

Current Respiratory Problems
+ Have you noticed any changes in your breathing pattern (e.g. shortness of breath, difficulty in breathing, need to be in upright position to breathe, or rapid and shallow breathing)?
+ If so, which of your activities might cause these symptom(s) to occur?
+ How many pillows do you use to sleep at night?

History of Respiratory Disease
+ Have you had colds, allergies, asthma, tuberculosis, bronchitis, pneumonia or emphysema?
+ How frequently have these occurred? How long did they last? And how were they treated?
+ Have you been exposed to any pollutants?

Lifestyle
+ Do you smoke? If so, how much? If not, did you smoke previously, and when did you stop?
+ Does any member of your family smoke?
+ Is there cigarette smoke or other pollutants (e.g. fumes, dust, coal, asbestos) in your workplace?
+ Do you use alcohol? If so, how many drinks (mixed drinks, glasses of wine or beers) do you usually have per day or per week?
+ Describe your exercise patterns. How often do you exercise and for how long?

Presence of Cough
+ How often and how much do you cough?
+ Is it productive, that is, accompanied by sputum, or nonproductive, that is, dry?

+ Does the cough occur during certain activity or at certain times of the day?

Description of Sputum
+ When is the sputum produced?
+ What is the amount, colour, thickness, odour?
+ Is it ever tinged with blood?

Presence of Chest Pain
+ Do you experience any pain with breathing or activity?
+ Where is the pain located?
+ Describe the pain. How does it feel?
+ Does it occur when you breathe in or out?
+ How long does it last, and how does it affect your breathing?
+ Do you experience any other symptoms when the pain occurs (e.g. nausea, shortness of breath or difficulty breathing, light-headedness, palpitations)?

+ What activities precede your pain?
+ What do you do to relieve the pain?

Presence of Risk Factors
+ Do you have a family history of lung cancer, cardiovascular disease (including strokes) or tuberculosis?
+ The nurse should also note the patient's weight, activity pattern and dietary assessment. Risk factors include obesity, sedentary lifestyle and diet high in saturated fats.

Medication History
+ Have you taken or do you take any over-the-counter or prescription medications for breathing (e.g. bronchodilator, inhalant, narcotic)?
+ If so, which ones? And what are the dosages, times taken and results, including side effects?

specimens, throat cultures, venous and arterial blood specimens, and pulmonary function tests.

Measurement of arterial blood gases is an important diagnostic procedure. Specimens of arterial blood are normally taken by specialty nurses or medical staff. Blood for these tests is taken directly from the radial, brachial or femoral arteries or from central catheters placed in large arteries. Because of the relatively great pressure of the blood in these arteries, it is important to prevent haemorrhaging by applying pressure to the puncture side for about five minutes after removing the needle.

Pulmonary Function Tests

Pulmonary function tests measure lung volume and capacity. Patients undergo pulmonary function tests, which are usually carried out by a respiratory physiologist. The patient breathes into a machine. The tests are painless, but the patient's cooperation is essential. Nurses need to explain the tests to the patient beforehand and help patients to get rest afterward because the tests are often tiring. Table 16-1 describes the measurements taken, and Figure 16-2 shows their relationships and normal adult values.

Table 16-1 Pulmonary Volumes and Capacities

Measurement	Description
Tidal volume (V_T)	Volume inhaled and exhaled during normal quiet breathing
Inspiratory reserve volume (IRV)	Maximum amount of air that can be inhaled over and above a normal breath
Expiratory reserve volume (ERV)	Maximum amount of air that can be exhaled following a normal exhalation
Residual volume (RV)	The amount of air remaining in the lungs after maximal exhalation
Total lung capacity (TLC)	The total volume of the lungs at maximum inflation; calculated by adding the V_T, IRV, ERV and RV
Vital capacity (VC)	Total amount of air that can be exhaled after a maximal inspiration; calculated by adding the V_T, IRV and ERV
Inspiratory capacity	Total amount of air that can be inhaled following normal quiet exhalation; calculated by adding the V_T and IRV
Functional residual capacity (FRC)	The volume left in the lungs after normal exhalation; calculated by adding the ERV and RV
Minute volume (MV)	The total volume or amount of air breathed in 1 minute

NURSING MANAGEMENT

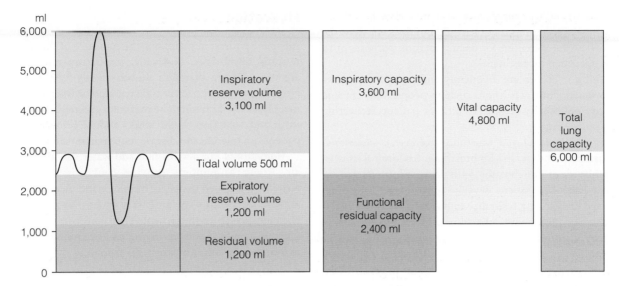

Figure 16-2 The relationship of lung volumes and capacities. Volumes (ml) shown are for an average adult male; female volumes are 20% to 25% smaller.

PLANNING

The overall goals for a patient with oxygenation problems are to:

+ Maintain a patent airway.
+ Improve comfort and ease of breathing.
+ Maintain or improve pulmonary ventilation and oxygenation.
+ Improve ability to participate in physical activities.
+ Prevent risks associated with oxygenation problems such as skin and tissue breakdown, syncope, acid–base imbalances, and feelings of hopelessness and social isolation.

Examples of nursing interventions to facilitate pulmonary ventilation may include ensuring a patent airway, positioning, encouraging deep breathing and coughing, and ensuring adequate hydration. Other nursing interventions helpful to ventilation are suctioning, lung inflation techniques, administration of analgesics before deep breathing and coughing, postural drainage, and percussion and vibration. Nursing strategies to facilitate the diffusion of gases through the alveolar membrane include encouraging coughing, deep breathing and suitable activity. A patient's nursing care plan should also include appropriate dependent nursing interventions such as oxygen therapy, tracheostomy care and maintenance of a chest drain.

IMPLEMENTING

Promoting Oxygenation

Most people in good health give little thought to their respiratory function. Changing position frequently, mobilising and exercising usually maintain adequate ventilation and gas exchange.

When people become ill, however, their respiratory functions may be inhibited for such reasons as pain and immobility. The result of inadequate chest expansion is pooling of respiratory secretions, which ultimately harbour micro-organisms and promote infection. This situation is often compounded by giving opiates for pain, which further depress the rate and depth of respiration.

Interventions by the nurse to maintain the normal respirations of patients include:

+ positioning the patient to allow for maximum chest expansion;
+ encouraging or providing frequent changes in position;
+ encouraging mobilisation;
+ implementing measures that promote comfort, such as giving pain medications.

The semi-Fowler's or high-Fowler's position allows maximum chest expansion in bed-confined patients, particularly dyspnoeic patients. In these positions the patient is semi-reclining with their knees bent and supported. The nurse should also encourage patients to turn from side to side frequently, so that alternate sides of the chest are permitted maximum expansion. Dyspnoeic patients often sit in bed and lean over their overbed tables (which are raised to a suitable height), usually with a pillow for support. This orthopnoeic position is an adaptation of the high-Fowler's position. It has a further advantage in that, unlike in high-Fowler's, the abdominal organs are not pressing on the diaphragm. Also, a patient in the orthopnoeic position can press the lower part of the chest against the table to help in exhaling.

Deep Breathing and Coughing

The nurse can facilitate respiratory functioning by encouraging deep breathing exercises and coughing to remove secretions from the airways. When coughing raises secretions high enough, the patient may either **expectorate** (spit out) or swallow them. Swallowing the secretions is not harmful but does not allow the nurse to view the secretions for documentation purposes or to obtain a specimen for testing.

Breathing exercises are frequently indicated for patients with restricted chest expansion, such as people with chronic obstructive pulmonary disease (COPD) or patients recovering from thoracic surgery.

A commonly employed breathing exercise is *abdominal (diaphragmatic)* and pursed-lip breathing. Abdominal breathing permits deep full breaths with little effort. Pursed-lip breathing helps the patient develop control over breathing. The pursed lips create a resistance to the air flowing out of the lungs, thereby prolonging exhalation and preventing airway collapse by maintaining positive airway pressure. The patient purses the lips as if about to whistle and breathes out slowly and gently, tightening the abdominal muscles to exhale more effectively. The patient usually inhales to a count of three and exhales to a count of seven.

Forceful coughing often is less effective than using controlled or huff coughing techniques. Instructions for abdominal (diaphragmatic) and pursed-lip breathing and coughing techniques are provided in *Teaching: patient care.*

Hydration

Adequate hydration maintains the moisture of the respiratory mucous membranes. Normally, respiratory tract secretions are thin and are therefore moved readily by ciliary action. However, when the patient is dehydrated or when the environment has a low humidity, the respiratory secretions can become thick and tenacious. Fluid intake should be as great as the patient can tolerate and disease management allows.

Humidifiers are devices that add water vapour to inspired air. Room humidifiers provide cool mist to room air. Nebulisers are used to deliver humidity and medications. They also are used with oxygen delivery systems to provide moistened air directly to the patient. Their purposes are to prevent mucous membranes from drying and becoming irritated and to loosen secretions for easier expectoration.

Medications

A number of types of medications can be used for patients with oxygenation problems. Bronchodilators, anti-inflammatory drugs, expectorants and cough suppressants are some medications that may be used to treat respiratory problems.

TEACHING: PATIENT CARE

Abdominal (Diaphragmatic) and Pursed-lip Breathing

+ Assume a comfortable semi-sitting position in bed or a chair or a lying position in bed with one pillow.
+ Flex your knees to relax the muscles of the abdomen.
+ Place one or both hands on your abdomen, just below the ribs.
+ Breathe in deeply through the nose, keeping the mouth closed.
+ Concentrate on feeling your abdomen rise as far as possible; stay relaxed, and avoid arching your back. If you have difficulty raising your abdomen, take a quick, forceful breath through the nose.
+ Then purse your lips as if about to whistle, and breathe out slowly and gently, making a slow 'whooshing' sound without puffing out the cheeks. This pursed-lip breathing creates a resistance to air flowing out of the lungs, increases pressure within the bronchi (main air passages), and minimises collapse of smaller airways, a common problem for people with COPD.
+ Concentrate on feeling the abdomen fall or sink, and tighten (contract) the abdominal muscles while

breathing out to enhance effective exhalation. Count to seven during exhalation.
+ Use this exercise whenever feeling short of breath, and increase gradually to 5-10 minutes four times a day. Regular practice will help you do this type of breathing without conscious effort. The exercise, once learned, can be performed when sitting upright, standing and walking.

Controlled and Huff Coughing

+ After using a bronchodilator treatment (if prescribed), inhale deeply and hold your breath for a few seconds.
+ Cough twice. The first cough loosens the mucus; the second expels secretions.
+ For huff coughing, lean forward and exhale sharply with a 'huff' sound. This technique helps keep your airways open while moving secretions up and out of the lungs.
+ Inhale by taking rapid short breaths in succession ('sniffing') to prevent mucus from moving back into smaller airways.
+ Rest.
+ Try to avoid prolonged episodes of coughing because these may cause fatigue and hypoxia.

Bronchodilators, including sympathomimetic drugs and beta two agonists, e.g. ventolin, reduce bronchospasm, opening tight or congested airways and facilitating ventilation. These drugs may be administered orally or intravenously, but the preferred route is by inhalation to prevent many systemic side-effects.

Since drugs used to dilate the bronchioles and improve breathing are usually drugs that enhance the sympathetic nervous system, patients must be monitored for side-effects of increased heart rate, blood pressure, anxiety and restlessness. This is especially important in older adults, who may also have cardiac problems.

Another class of drugs used is the *anti-inflammatory drugs*, such as glucocorticoids (steroids). They can be given orally, intravenously or by inhaler. They work by decreasing the oedema and inflammation in the airways and allowing a better air exchange. If both bronchodilators and anti-inflammatory drugs are prescribed by inhaler, the patient should be instructed to use the bronchodilator inhaler first and then the anti-inflammatory inhaler. If the bronchioles are dilated first, more tissue is exposed for the anti-inflammatory drugs to act upon.

Expectorants help 'break up' mucus, making it more liquid and easier to expectorate. When frequent or prolonged coughing interrupts sleep, a cough suppressant such as codeine may be prescribed.

Other medications can be used to improve oxygenation by improving cardiovascular function. The *digitalis glycosides* such as digoxin act directly on the heart to improve the strength of contraction and slow the heart rate. *Beta-adrenergic blocking agents* such as propranolol affect the sympathetic nervous system to reduce the workload of the heart. These drugs, however, can negatively affect people with asthma or COPD as they may constrict airways.

Incentive Spirometry

Incentive spirometers (see Figure 16-3), also referred to as *sustained maximal inspiration devices* (SMIs), measure the flow of air inhaled through the mouthpiece and are used to:

+ improve pulmonary ventilation;
+ counteract the effects of anaesthesia or hypoventilation;
+ loosen respiratory secretions;
+ facilitate respiratory gaseous exchange;
+ expand collapsed alveoli.

They offer an incentive to improve inhalation. When using an SMI, the patient should be assisted into a position, preferably an upright sitting position in bed or a chair, that facilitates maximum ventilation. *Teaching: patient care* (see page 388) lists instructions for patients in the use of incentive spirometers.

Percussion, Vibration and Postural Drainage

Percussion, vibration and postural drainage (PVD) are frequently performed by physiotherapists, however in some clinical areas may be formed by nursing staff. **Percussion**, sometimes called *clapping*, is forceful striking of the skin with cupped hands. Mechanical percussion cups and vibrators are also available but used less frequently. When the hands are used, the fingers and thumb are held together and flexed slightly to form a cup, as one would to scoop up water. Percussion over congested lung areas can mechanically dislodge tenacious secretions from the bronchial walls. Cupped hands trap the air against the chest. The trapped air sets up vibrations through the chest wall to the secretions.

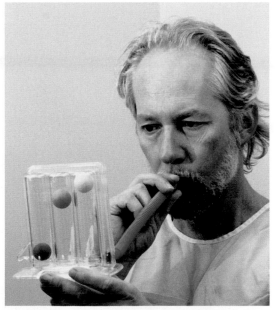

Figure 16-3 *A*, Flow-oriented SMI; *B*, volume-oriented SMI.

TEACHING: PATIENT CARE

Using an Incentive Spirometer

+ Hold or place the spirometer in an upright position. A tilted *flow-oriented* device requires less effort to raise the balls or discs; a *volume-oriented* device will not function correctly unless upright.
+ Exhale normally.
+ Seal the lips tightly around the mouthpiece.
+ Take in a slow, deep breath to elevate the balls or cylinder, and then hold the breath for two seconds initially, increasing to six seconds (optimum), to keep the balls or cylinder elevated if possible.
+ For a flow-oriented device, avoid brisk, low-volume breaths that snap the balls to the top of the chamber. Greater lung expansion is achieved with a very slow inspiration than with a brisk, shallow breath, even though it may not elevate the balls or keep them elevated while you hold your breath.

Sustained elevation of the balls or cylinder ensures adequate ventilation of the alveoli (lung air sacs).

+ If you have difficulty breathing only through the mouth, a nose clip can be used.
+ Remove the mouthpiece and exhale normally.
+ Cough after the incentive effort. Deep ventilation may loosen secretions, and coughing can facilitate their removal.
+ Relax and take several normal breaths before using the spirometer again.
+ Repeat the procedure several times and then four or five times hourly. Practise increases inspiratory volume, maintains alveolar ventilation and prevents atelectasis (collapse of the air sacs).
+ Clean the mouthpiece with water or as directed by the manufacturer and shake it dry.

To percuss a patient's chest, the nurse follows these steps:

+ Cover the area with a towel or gown to reduce discomfort.
+ Ask the patient to breathe slowly and deeply to promote relaxation.
+ Alternately flex and extend the wrists rapidly to slap the chest (see Figure 16-4).
+ Percuss each affected lung segment for 1-2 minutes.

When done correctly, the percussion action should produce a hollow, popping sound. Percussion is avoided over the breasts, sternum, spinal column and kidneys.

Vibration is a series of vigorous quiverings produced by hands that are placed flat against the patient's chest wall. Vibration is used after percussion to increase the turbulence of the exhaled air and thus loosen thick secretions. It is often done alternately with percussion.

To vibrate the patient's chest, the nurse follows these steps:

+ Place hands, palms down, on the chest area to be drained, one hand over the other with the fingers together and extended (see Figure 16-5). Alternatively, the hands may be placed side by side.

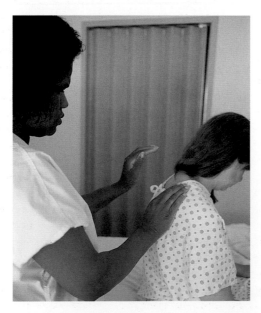

Figure 16-4 Percussing the upper posterior chest.

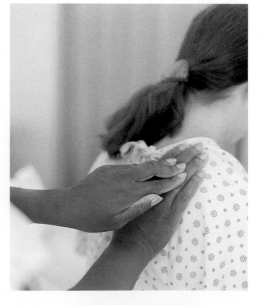

Figure 16-5 Vibrating the upper posterior chest.

- Ask the patient to inhale deeply and exhale slowly through the nose or pursed lips.
- During the exhalation, tense all the hand and arm muscles, and using mostly the heel of the hand, vibrate (shake) the hands, moving them downward. Stop the vibrating when the patient inhales.
- Vibrate during five exhalations over one affected lung segment.
- After each vibration, encourage the patient to cough and expectorate secretions into the sputum container.

Postural drainage is the drainage by gravity of secretions from various lung segments. Secretions that remain in the lungs or respiratory airways promote bacterial growth and subsequent infection. They also can obstruct the smaller airways and cause atelectasis. Secretions in the major airways, such as the trachea and the right and left main bronchi, are usually coughed into the pharynx, where they can be expectorated, swallowed or effectively removed by suctioning.

A wide variety of positions is necessary to drain all segments of the lungs, but not all positions are required for every patient. Only those positions that drain specific affected areas are used. The lower lobes require drainage most frequently because the upper lobes drain by gravity. Before postural drainage, the patient may be given a bronchodilator medication or nebulisation therapy to loosen secretions. Postural drainage treatments are usually performed two or three times daily, depending on the degree of lung congestion. The best times include before breakfast, before lunch, in the late afternoon, and before bedtime. It is best to avoid hours shortly after meals because postural drainage at these times can be tiring and can induce vomiting.

The nurse needs to evaluate the patient's tolerance of postural drainage by assessing the stability of the patient's vital signs, particularly the pulse and respiratory rates, and by noting signs of intolerance, such as pallor, diaphoresis, dyspnoea and fatigue. Some patients do not react well to certain drainage positions, and the nurse must make appropriate adjustments. For example, some become dyspnoeic in Trendelenburg's position (head of bed tilted lower than the feet), and require only a moderate tilt or a shorter time in that position.

The sequence for PVD is usually as follows: positioning, percussion, vibration and removal of secretions by coughing or suction. Each position is usually assumed for 10–15 minutes, although beginning treatments may start with shorter times and gradually increase.

Following PVD, the nurse should auscultate the patient's lungs, compare the findings to the baseline data, and document the amount, colour and character of expectorated secretions.

Oxygen Therapy

Patients who have difficulty ventilating all areas of their lungs, those whose gas exchange is impaired, or people with heart failure may require oxygen therapy to prevent hypoxia.

Oxygen therapy is a prescribed medication; the prescription should specify the concentration, method of delivery and litre flow per minute. The concentration is of more importance

BOX 16-3 Oxygen Therapy Safety Precautions

- For home oxygen use or when the facility permits smoking, teach family members to smoke only outside or in provided smoking rooms away from the patient.
- Place cautionary signs reading 'No Smoking: Oxygen in Use' on the oxygen equipment.
- Instruct the patient and visitors about the hazard of smoking with oxygen in use.
- Make sure that electric devices (such as razors, hearing aids, radios, televisions and heating pads) are in good working order to prevent the occurrence of short-circuit sparks.
- Avoid materials that generate static electricity, such as woollen blankets and synthetic fabrics.
- Avoid the use of volatile, flammable materials, such as oils, greases, alcohol and acetone (e.g. nail varnish remover), near patients receiving oxygen.
- Ground electric monitoring equipment, suction machines and portable diagnostic machines.
- Make known the location of fire extinguishers, and make sure personnel are trained in their use.

than the litre flow per minute. When administering oxygen is an emergency measure, the nurse may initiate the therapy without a prescription. For patients who have COPD, a low-flow oxygen system is essential.

Safety precautions are essential during oxygen therapy (see *Box 16-3*). Although oxygen by itself will not burn or explode, it does facilitate combustion. For example, a bed sheet ordinarily burns slowly when ignited in the atmosphere; however, if saturated with free-flowing oxygen and ignited by a spark, it will burn rapidly and explosively. The greater the concentration of oxygen, the more rapidly fires start and burn, and such fires are difficult to extinguish. Because oxygen is colourless, odourless and tasteless, people are often unaware of its presence.

Oxygen is supplied in several different ways. In hospitals and long-term care facilities, it is usually piped into wall outlets at the patient's bedside, making it readily available for use at all times. Tanks or cylinders of oxygen under pressure are also frequently available for use when wall oxygen either is unavailable or impractical (e.g. for transporting oxygen-dependent patients between clinical areas).

Patients who require oxygen therapy in the home may use small cylinders of oxygen or an oxygen concentrator. Portable oxygen delivery systems are available to increase the patient's independence. Home oxygen therapy services are readily available in communities. These services generally supply the oxygen and delivery devices, training for the patient and family, equipment maintenance and emergency services should a problem occur.

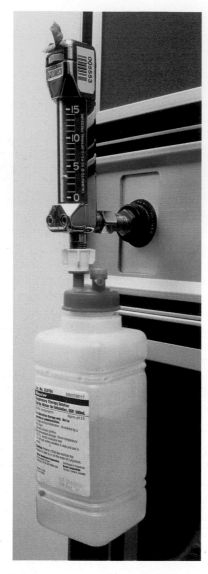

Figure 16-6 An oxygen humidifier attached to a wall outlet oxygen flow meter.

Oxygen administered from a cylinder or wall-outlet system is dry. Dry gases dehydrate the respiratory mucous membranes. Humidifying devices that add water vapour to inspired air are used as an adjunct of oxygen therapy in some patients; particularly for litre flows over 2 l per minute (see Figure 16-6). These devices provide 20% to 40% humidity. The oxygen passes through sterile distilled water or tap water and then along a line to the device through which the moistened oxygen is inhaled (e.g. a nasal cannula, or oxygen mask).

Humidifiers prevent mucous membranes from drying and becoming irritated and loosen secretions for easier expectoration. Oxygen passing through water picks up water vapour before it reaches the patient. The more bubbles created during this process, the more water vapour is produced. Very low litre flows (e.g. 1 to 2 l per minute by nasal cannula) do not require humidification.

Oxygen cylinders need to be handled and stored with caution and strapped securely in wheeled transport devices or stands to prevent possible falls and outlet breakages. They should be placed away from sources of heat.

To use an oxygen wall outlet, the nurse carries out these steps:

+ Attach the flow meter to the wall outlet, exerting firm pressure. The flow meter should be in the off position. (If not already inserted.)
+ Fill the humidifier bottle with distilled or tap water in accordance with local policy. This should be done before coming to the bedside. Some humidifier bottles come prefilled by the manufacturer.
+ Attach the humidifier bottle to the base of the flow meter.
+ Attach the prescribed oxygen tubing and delivery device to the humidifier.
+ Regulate the flow meter to the prescribed level.

Oxygen Delivery Systems

A number of systems are available to deliver oxygen to the patient. The choice of system depends on the patient's oxygen needs, comfort and developmental considerations. With many systems, the oxygen delivered mixes with room air before being inspired. The amount of oxygen delivered is determined by regulating its flow rate (e.g. 2–6 l per minute), and precise regulation of the percentage of inspired oxygen, or fraction of inspired oxygen (FiO_2), is not possible. When it is important to regulate the percentage of oxygen received by the patient more precisely, a device such as a Venturi mask may be used.

Cannula

The nasal cannula (nasal prongs) is the most common inexpensive device used to administer oxygen (see Figure 16-7).

The nasal cannula is easy to apply and does not interfere with the patient's ability to eat or talk. It also is relatively comfortable, permits some freedom of movement, and is well tolerated by the patient. It delivers a relatively low concentration of oxygen (24–45%) at flow rates of 2–6 l per minute. Above 6 l per minute, the patient tends to swallow air and the FiO_2 is not increased. Also at higher flow rates it causes nasal discomfort for the patient.

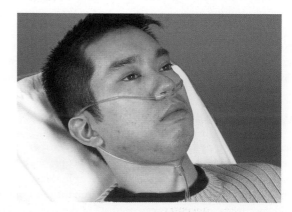

Figure 16-7 A nasal cannula.

Administering oxygen by cannula is detailed in *Procedure 16-1* on page 392).

Face Mask

Face masks that cover the patient's nose and mouth may be used for oxygen inhalation. Exhalation ports on the sides of the mask allow exhaled carbon dioxide to escape. A variety of oxygen masks are available from manufacturers:

+ The simple face mask delivers oxygen concentrations from 40–60% at litre flows of 5–8 l per minute, respectively (see Figure 16-8).
+ The partial rebreather mask delivers oxygen concentrations of 60–90% at litre flows of 6–15 l per minute, respectively. The oxygen reservoir bag that is attached allows the patient

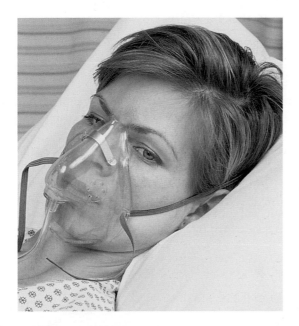

Figure 16-8 A simple face mask.

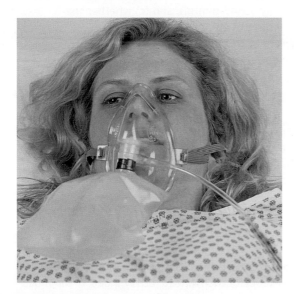

Figure 16-9 A partial rebreather mask.

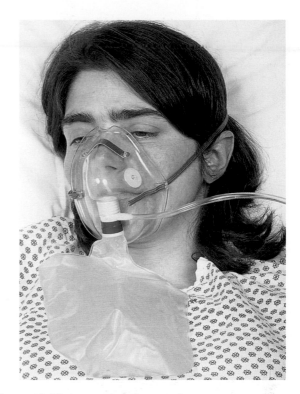

Figure 16-10 A nonrebreather mask.

to rebreathe about the first third of the exhaled air in conjunction with oxygen (see Figure 16-9). Thus, it increases the FiO_2 by recycling expired oxygen. The partial rebreather bag must not totally deflate during inspiration to avoid carbon dioxide buildup. If this problem occurs, the nurse increases the litre flow of oxygen.

+ The nonrebreather mask delivers the highest oxygen concentration possible (95–100%) by means other than intubation or mechanical ventilation, at litre flows of 10–15 l per minute. One-way valves on the mask and between the reservoir bag and the mask prevent the room air and the patient's exhaled air from entering the bag so only the oxygen in the bag is inspired (see Figure 16-10). To prevent carbon dioxide buildup, the nonrebreather bag must not totally deflate during inspiration. If it does, the nurse can correct this problem by increasing the litre flow of oxygen.
+ The Venturi mask delivers oxygen concentrations varying from 24–40% or 50% at litre flows of 4–10 l per minute (see Figure 16-11 on page 390). The Venturi mask has wide-bore tubing and colour-coded jet adapters that correspond to a precise oxygen concentration and litre flow. For example, a blue adapter delivers a 24% concentration of oxygen at 4 l per minute, and a green adapter delivers a 35% concentration of oxygen at 8 l per minute.

Initiating oxygen by mask is much the same as initiating oxygen by cannula, except that the nurse must find a mask of appropriate size. Smaller sizes are available for children and adults with small faces. Administering oxygen by mask or face tent is detailed in *Procedure 16-1* on page 390.

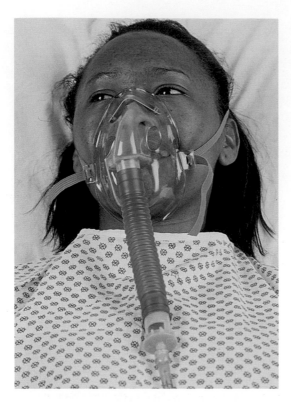

Figure 16-11 A Venturi mask.

Transtracheal Oxygen Delivery

Transtracheal oxygen delivery may be used for oxygen-dependent patients. Oxygen is delivered through a small,

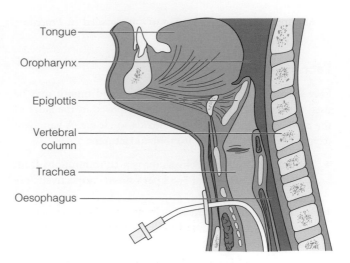

Figure 16-12 A transtracheal oxygen catheter in place.

narrow plastic cannula surgically inserted through the skin directly into the trachea (see Figure 16-12). A chain around the neck holds the catheter in place.

With this delivery system, the patient requires less oxygen (0.5–2 l per minute) because all of the flow delivered enters the lungs. The nurse/patient keeps the catheter patent by injecting 1.5 ml of normal saline into it, moving a cleaning rod in and out of it, and then injecting another 1.5 ml of saline solution. This is done two or three times a day.

PROCEDURE 16-1 Administering Oxygen by Cannula or Face Mask

Before administering oxygen, check (a) the prescription for oxygen, including the litre flow rate (l/min) or the percentage of oxygen; (b) the levels of oxygen (PO_2) and carbon dioxide ($PaCO_2$) in the patient's arterial blood (PaO_2 is normally 80-100 mm Hg; $PaCO_2$ is normally 35-45 mmHg); and (c) whether the patient has COPD.

Purposes

CANNULA

+ To deliver a relatively low concentration of oxygen when only minimal O_2 support is required
+ To allow uninterrupted delivery of oxygen while the patient ingests food or fluids

FACE MASK

+ To provide moderate O_2 support and a higher concentration of oxygen and/or humidity than is provided by cannula

ASSESSMENT

Assess

+ Skin and mucous membrane colour: Note whether cyanosis is present
+ Breathing patterns: Note depth of respirations and presence of tachypnoea, bradypnoea, orthopnoea

NURSING MANAGEMENT

+ Chest movements: Note whether there are any intercostal, substernal, suprasternal, supraclavicular or tracheal retractions during inspiration or expiration
+ Chest wall configuration (e.g. kyphosis)
+ Presence of clinical signs of hypoxemia: tachycardia, tachypnoea, restlessness, dyspnoea, cyanosis and confusion. Tachycardia and tachypnoea are often early signs. Confusion is a later sign of severe oxygen deprivation
+ Presence of clinical signs of hypercarbia (hypercapnia): restlessness, hypertension, headache, lethargy, tremor
+ Presence of clinical signs of oxygen toxicity: tracheal irritation and cough, dyspnoea and decreased pulmonary ventilation

Determine

+ Vital signs, especially pulse rate and quality, and respiratory rate, rhythm and depth
+ Whether the patient has COPD. A high carbon dioxide level in the blood is the normal stimulus to breathe. However, people with COPD may have a chronically high carbon dioxide level, and their stimulus to breathe is hypoxemia. Low flows of oxygen (2 l/min) stimulate breathing for such persons by maintaining slight hypoxemia. During continuous oxygen administration, arterial blood gas levels of oxygen (PO_2) and carbon dioxide (PCO_2) are measured periodically to monitor hypoxemia
+ Results of diagnostic studies
+ Haemoglobin, haematocrit, full blood count
+ Arterial blood gases
+ Pulmonary function tests

PLANNING

Equipment

CANNULA

+ Oxygen supply with a flow meter and adapter
+ Humidifier with distilled water or tap water according to agency protocol
+ Nasal cannula and tubing

FACE MASK

+ Oxygen supply with a flow meter and adapter
+ Humidifier with distilled water or tap water according to local policy
+ Face mask of the appropriate size

IMPLEMENTATION

Preparation

1. Determine the need for oxygen therapy, and verify the prescription for the therapy.
2. Prepare the patient.
   - Assist the patient to a semi-Fowler's position if possible. *This position permits easier chest expansion and hence easier breathing.*
   - Explain that oxygen is not dangerous when safety precautions are observed. Inform the patient about the safety precautions connected with oxygen use.

Performance

1. Explain to the patient what you are going to do, why it is necessary and how they can cooperate. Discuss how the effects of the oxygen therapy will be used in planning further care or treatments.
2. Wash hands and observe appropriate infection control procedures.
3. Provide for patient privacy, if appropriate.
4. Set up the oxygen equipment and the humidifier.
   - Attach the flow meter to the wall outlet or cylinder. The flow meter should be in the off position.
   - If needed, fill the humidifier bottle. (This can be done before coming to the bedside.)
   - Attach the humidifier bottle to the base of the flow meter.
   - Attach the prescribed oxygen tubing and delivery device to the humidifier.
5. Turn on the oxygen at the prescribed rate and ensure proper functioning.
   - Check that the oxygen is flowing freely through the tubing. There should be no kinks in the tubing, and the connections should be airtight. There should be bubbles in the humidifier as the oxygen flows through. You should feel the oxygen at the outlets of the cannula, or mask
   - Set the oxygen at the flow rate prescribed.
6. Apply the appropriate oxygen delivery device.
   #### CANNULA
   - Put the cannula over the patient's face, with the outlet prongs fitting into the nares and the elastic band around the head (see Figure 16-7 on page 388). Some models have a strap to adjust under the chin.
   - If the cannula will not stay in place, tape it at the sides of the face.
   - Pad the tubing and band over the ears and cheekbones as needed.

FACE MASK

- Guide the mask toward the patient's face, and apply it from the nose downward.
- Fit the mask to the contours of the patient's face (see Figure 16-8 earlier). *The mask should mould to the face, so that very little oxygen escapes into the eyes or around the cheeks and chin.*
- Secure the elastic band around the patient's head so that the mask is comfortable but snug.

7. Assess the patient regularly.
   - Assess the patient's vital signs, level of anxiety, colour and ease of respirations, and provide support while the patient adjusts to the device.
   - Assess the patient in 15–30 minutes, depending on the patient's condition, and regularly thereafter.
   - Assess the patient regularly for clinical signs of hypoxia, tachycardia, confusion, dyspnoea, restlessness and cyanosis. Review arterial blood gas results if they are available.

NASAL CANNULA

- Assess the patient's nares for encrustations and irritation. Apply a **water-soluble** lubricant as required to soothe the mucous membranes.

FACE MASK OR TENT

- Inspect the facial skin frequently for dampness or chafing, and dry and treat it as needed.

8. Inspect the equipment on a regular basis.
   - Check the litre flow and the level of water in the humidifier in 30 minutes and whenever providing care to the patient.
   - Make sure that safety precautions are being followed.

9. Document findings in the patient record using forms or checklists supplemented by narrative notes when appropriate.

EVALUATION

+ Perform follow-up based on findings that deviated from expected or normal for the patient. Relate findings to previous data if available.

+ Report significant deviations from normal to the medical staff.

LIFESPAN CONSIDERATIONS

Oxygen Delivery Equipment
Infants
Oxygen Hood
+ An oxygen hood is a rigid plastic dome that encloses an infant's head. It provides precise oxygen levels and high humidity.
+ The gas should not be allowed to blow directly into the infant's face, and the hood should not rub against the infant's neck, chin or shoulder.

Children
Oxygen Tent (see Figure 16-13)
+ The tent consists of a rectangular, clear, plastic canopy with outlets that connect to an oxygen or compressed air source and to a humidifier that moisturises the air or oxygen.
+ Because the enclosed tent becomes very warm, some type of cooling mechanism such as an ice chamber or a refrigeration unit is provided to maintain the temperature at 20–21°C.
+ Cover the child with a gown or a cotton blanket. A small towel may be wrapped around the head. *The child needs protection from chilling and from the dampness and condensation in the tent.*

+ Flood the tent with oxygen by setting the flow meter at 15 l/min for about five minutes. Then, adjust the flow meter according to orders (e.g. 10-15 l/min). *Flooding the tent quickly increases the oxygen to the desired level.*
+ The tent can deliver approximately 30% oxygen.

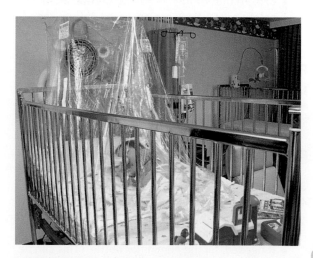

Figure 16-13 Paediatric oxygen tent.

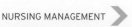

COMMUNITY CARE CONSIDERATIONS

Community Care Oxygen Equipment

Two major oxygen systems for home care use are available in most communities: cylinders or tanks of compressed gas and oxygen concentrators.

1. Cylinders: These are the system of choice for patients who need oxygen episodically (e.g. on a prn basis). Advantages are that cylinders deliver all litre flows (1–15 l/min). Disadvantages are that some cylinders are heavy and awkward to move, the supply company/community pharmacy must be notified when a refill is needed, and they are costly for the high-use patient (see Figure 16-14).

2. Oxygen concentrators: Concentrators are electrically powered systems that manufacture oxygen from room air. At 1 l/min, such a system can deliver a concentration of about 95% oxygen, but the concentration drops when the flow rate increases (e.g. 75% concentration at 4 l/min). Advantages are that they are more attractive in appearance, resembling furniture rather than medical equipment; they eliminate the need for regular delivery of oxygen or refilling of cylinders; because the supply of oxygen is constant, they alleviate the patient's anxiety about running out of oxygen; and they are the most economical system when continuous use is required. Major disadvantages of a concentrator are that it is expensive; lacks real portability; tends to be noisy; is powered by electricity (an emergency backup unit, for example, an oxygen cylinder, must be provided for patients for whom a power failure could be life threatening); and heat produced by the concentrator motor is a problem for those who live in small houses. The oxygen concentrator must also be checked periodically with an O_2 analyser to ensure that it is providing an adequate delivery of oxygen.

   Another type of oxygen concentrator is the *oxygen enricher*. It uses a plastic membrane that allows water vapour to pass through with the oxygen, thus eliminating the need for a humidifying device. It is also thought to filter out bacteria

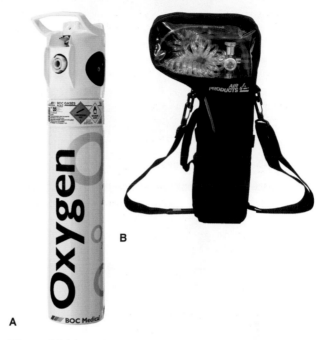

Figure 16-14 Typical oxygen cylinders without (a) and with (b) carrying case.

present in the air. The enricher provides an O_2 concentration of 40% at all flow rates, it tends to be quieter than the concentrator, there is less chance of combustion (since the gas is only 40% oxygen), it has only two moving parts (thus decreasing the risk of something going wrong), and a nebuliser can be operated off the enricher because of the high flow rate.

The nurse needs to ensure that the patient has an appropriate home oxygen supplier. Services furnished should include:

+ a 24-hour emergency service;
+ trained personnel to make the initial delivery and instruct the patient in safe, appropriate use of the oxygen and maintenance of the equipment;
+ at least monthly follow-up visits to check the equipment and reinstruct the patient as necessary.

Artificial Airways (see also Chapter 25)

Artificial airways are inserted to maintain a patent air passage for patients whose airway has become or may become obstructed. A patent airway is necessary so that air can flow to and from the lungs. Four of the more common types of airways are oropharyngeal, nasopharyngeal, endotracheal and tracheostomy.

Oropharyngeal and Nasopharyngeal Airways

Oropharyngeal and nasopharyngeal airways are used to keep the upper air passages open when they may become obstructed by secretions or the tongue. These airways are easy to insert and have a low risk of complications. Sizes vary and should be appropriate to the size and age of the patient. For nasopharyngeal

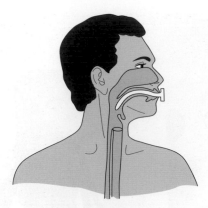

Figure 16-15 An oropharyngeal airway in place.

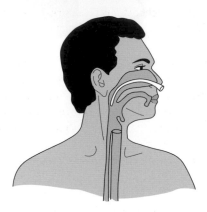

Figure 16-16 A nasopharyngeal airway in place.

airways the device should be well lubricated with water-soluble gel prior to inserting.

Oropharyngeal airways (see Figure 16-15) stimulate the gag reflex and are only used for patients with altered levels of consciousness (e.g. because of general anaesthesia, overdose or head injury) (see Chapter 25 for insertion technique).

Nasopharyngeal airways are tolerated better by alert patients. They are inserted through the nares, terminating in

CLINICAL ANECDOTE

The first time I used an oropharyngeal airway on a patient I was really nervous. The patient had come back from the operating theatre and I was checking their vital signs. Suddenly the patient stopped breathing. I opened the airway and they started again. I called for help; the patient was still unconscious, a support worker came in and brought me some oral airways. I sized them up and placed one in the patient's mouth and gave oxygen. When my mentor arrived she was really pleased with my actions but I was still shaking.

Joel, second-year student nurse

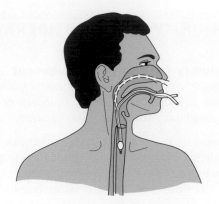

Figure 16-17 An endotracheal tube in place.

the oropharynx (see Figure 16-16). When caring for a patient with a nasopharyngeal airway, provide frequent oral and nares care, repositioning the airway in the other nostril every 8 hours or as directed to prevent necrosis of the mucosa.

Endotracheal Tubes

Endotracheal tubes are most commonly inserted for patients who have had general anaesthetics or for those in emergency situations where mechanical ventilation is required. An endotracheal tube is inserted by the practitioner with specialised education through either the mouth or the nose and into the trachea with the guide of a laryngoscope (see Figure 16-17). The tube terminates just superior to the bifurcation of the trachea into the bronchi. The tube may have an air-filled cuff to prevent air leakage around it. Because an endotracheal tube passes through the epiglottis and glottis, the patient is unable to speak while it is in place.

Tracheostomy

Patients who need long-term airway support may have a tracheostomy, a surgical incision in the trachea just below the larynx. A curved tracheostomy tube is inserted to extend through the stoma into the trachea (see Figure 16-18). Tracheostomy tubes may be either plastic or metal and are available in different sizes.

Tracheostomy tubes have an outer cannula that is inserted into the trachea and a flange that rests against the neck and allows the tube to be secured in place with tape or ties (see Figure 16-19). All tubes also have an obturator, used to insert the outer cannula and then removed. The obturator is kept at the patient's bedside in case the tube becomes dislodged and needs to be reinserted. Some tracheostomy tubes have an inner cannula that may be removed for periodic cleaning.

Cuffed tracheostomy tubes are surrounded by an inflatable cuff that produces an airtight seal between the tube and the trachea. This seal prevents aspiration of oropharyngeal secretions and air leakage between the tube and the trachea. Cuffed tubes are often used immediately after a tracheostomy and are essential when ventilating a tracheostomy patient with a mechanical ventilator. Children do not require cuffed tubes,

NURSING MANAGEMENT

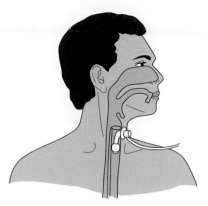

Figure 16-18 A tracheostomy tube in place.

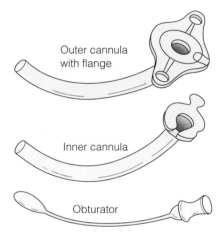

Outer cannula with flange

Inner cannula

Obturator

Figure 16-19 Components of a tracheostomy tube.

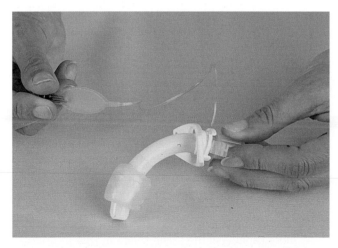

Figure 16-20 A tracheostomy tube with a low-pressure cuff.

because their tracheas are resilient enough to seal the air space around the tube.

Low-pressure cuffs (see Figure 16-20) are commonly used to distribute a low, even pressure against the trachea, thus decreasing the risk of tracheal tissue necrosis. They do not need to be deflated periodically to reduce pressure on the tracheal wall. Foam cuffed tracheostomy tubes (see Figure 16-21) do not require

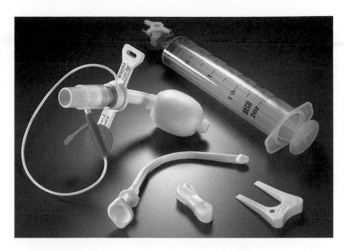

Figure 16-21 A tracheostomy tube with a foam cuff.
(Courtesy of Portex Inc., Keene, NH.)

injected air; instead, when the port is opened, ambient air enters the balloon, which then conforms to the patient's trachea. Air is removed from the cuff prior to insertion or removal of the tube.

The nurse provides tracheostomy care for the patient with a new or recent tracheostomy to maintain patency of the tube and reduce the risk of infection. Initially a tracheostomy may need to be suctioned (see the section on suctioning that follows) and cleaned as often as every one to two hours. After the initial inflammatory response subsides, tracheostomy care may only need to be done once or twice a day, depending on the patient. *Procedure 16-2* on page 396 describes tracheostomy care.

When the patient breathes through a tracheostomy, air is no longer filtered and humidified as it is when passing through the upper airways; therefore, special precautions are necessary. Humidity may be provided with a mist collar (see Figure 16-22). Patients with long-term tracheostomies may wear a light scarf or a 4-inch × 4-inch gauze held in place with a cotton tie over the stoma to filter air as it enters the tracheostomy.

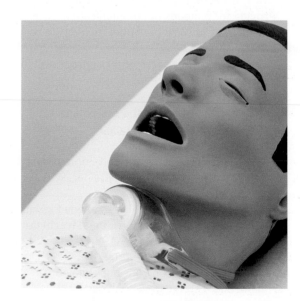

Figure 16-22 A tracheostomy mist collar.

NURSING MANAGEMENT >

PROCEDURE 16-2 Providing Tracheostomy Care

Purposes

+ To maintain airway patency
+ To maintain cleanliness and prevent infection at the tracheostomy site
+ To facilitate healing and prevent skin excoriation around the tracheostomy incision
+ To promote comfort

ASSESSMENT

Assess

+ Respiratory status including ease of breathing, rate, rhythm, depth and lung sounds
+ Pulse rate
+ Character and amount of secretions from tracheostomy site
+ Presence of drainage on tracheostomy dressing or ties
+ Appearance of incision (note any redness, swelling, purulent discharge or odour)

PLANNING

Equipment

+ Sterile disposable tracheostomy cleaning kit or supplies including sterile containers, sterile nylon brush and/or pipe cleaners, sterile applicators, gauze squares
+ Towel or drape to protect bed linens
+ Sterile suction catheter kit (suction catheter and sterile container for solution)
+ Sterile normal saline
+ Sterile gloves (two pairs)
+ Clean gloves
+ Moisture-proof bag
+ Commercially prepared sterile tracheostomy dressing or sterile 4 inch × 4 inch gauze dressing
+ Cotton ties
+ Clean sterile scissors

IMPLEMENTATION

Performance

1. Explain to the patient what you are going to do, why it is necessary and how they can cooperate. Provide for a means of communication, such as eye blinking or raising a finger, to indicate pain or distress.
2. Wash hands and observe other appropriate infection control procedures.
3. Provide for patient privacy.
4. Prepare the patient and the equipment.
   - Assist the patient into a position *to promote lung expansion.*
   - Open the tracheostomy kit or sterile basins. Pour sterile normal saline into container.
   - Establish a sterile field.
   - Open other sterile supplies as needed including sterile applicators, suction kit and tracheostomy dressing.
5. Suction the tracheostomy tube.
   - Put a clean glove on your non-dominant hand and a sterile glove on your dominant hand (or put on a pair of sterile gloves).
   - Suction the full length of the tracheostomy tube to remove secretions and ensure a patent airway (see *Procedure 16-3* on page 400).
   - Rinse the suction catheter and wrap the catheter around your hand, and peel the glove off so that it turns inside out over the catheter.
   - Using the gloved hand, unlock the inner cannula (if present) and remove it by gently pulling it out toward you in line with its curvature. Place the inner cannula in the saline solution. *This moistens and loosens dried secretions.*
   - Remove the soiled tracheostomy dressing. Place the soiled dressing in your gloved hand and peel the glove off so that it turns inside out over the dressing. Discard the glove and the dressing.
   - Put on sterile gloves. Keep your dominant hand sterile during the procedure.

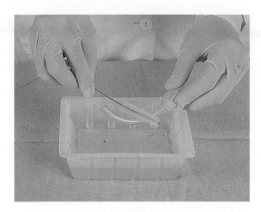

Figure 16-23 Cleaning the inner cannula with a brush.

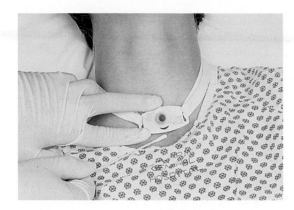

Figure 16-24 Using an applicator stick to clean the tracheostomy site.

6. Clean the inner cannula.
- Remove the inner cannula from the soaking solution.
- Clean the lumen and entire inner cannula thoroughly using the brush or pipe cleaners moistened with sterile normal saline (see Figure 16-23). Inspect the cannula for cleanliness by holding it at eye level and looking through it into the light.
- Rinse the inner cannula thoroughly in the sterile normal saline.
- After rinsing, gently tap the cannula against the inside edge of the sterile saline container. Use a pipe cleaner folded in half to dry only the inside of the cannula; do not dry the outside. *This removes excess liquid from the cannula and prevents possible aspiration by the patient, while leaving a film of moisture on the outer surface to lubricate the cannula for reinsertion.*
- Using sterile technique, suction the outer cannula. *Suctioning removes secretions from the outer cannula.*

7. Replace the inner cannula, securing it in place.
- Insert the inner cannula by grasping the outer flange and inserting the cannula in the direction of its curvature.
- Lock the cannula in place by turning the lock (if present) into position to secure the flange of the inner cannula to the outer cannula.

8. Clean the incision site and tube flange.
- Using sterile applicators or gauze dressings moistened with normal saline, clean the incision site (see Figure 16-24). Handle the sterile supplies with your dominant hand. Use each applicator or gauze dressing only once and then discard. *This avoids contaminating a clean area with a soiled gauze dressing or applicator.*

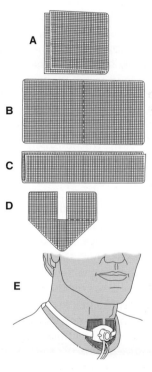

Figure 16-25 Folding a 4 inch × 4 inch gauze to make a tracheostomy dressing.

9. Apply a sterile dressing.
- Use a commercially prepared tracheostomy dressing of nonravelling material or open and refold a 4 inch × 4 inch gauze dressing into a V shape as shown in Figure 16-25 *A–D*. Avoid using cotton-filled gauze squares or cutting the 4 inch × 4 inch gauze. *Cotton lint or gauze fibres can be aspirated by the patient, potentially creating a tracheal abscess.*
- Place the dressing under the flange of the tracheostomy tube as shown in Figure 16-25 *E*.

- While applying the dressing, ensure that the tracheostomy tube is securely supported. *Excessive movement of the tracheostomy tube irritates the trachea.*

10. Change the tracheostomy ties.

TWO-STRIP METHOD

- Cut two unequal strips of twill tape, one approximately 25 cm (10 inch) long and the other about 50 cm (20 inch) long. *Cutting one tape longer than the other allows them to be fastened at the side of the neck for easy access and to avoid the pressure of a knot on the skin at the back of the neck.*
- Cut a 1 cm (0.5 inch) lengthwise slit approximately 2.5 cm (1 inch) from one end of each strip. To do this, fold the end of the tape back onto itself about 2.5 cm (1 inch), then cut a slit in the middle of the tape from its folded edge.
- Leaving the old ties in place, thread the slit end of one clean tape through the eye of the tracheostomy flange from the bottom side; then thread the long end of the tape through the slit, pulling it tight until it is securely fastened to the flange. *Leaving the old ties in place while securing the clean ties prevents inadvertent dislodging of the tracheostomy tube. Securing tapes in this manner avoids the use of knots, which can come untied or cause pressure and irritation.*
- If old ties are very soiled or it is difficult to thread new ties onto the tracheostomy flange with old ties in place, have an assistant put on a sterile glove and hold the tracheostomy in place while you replace the ties.
- Repeat the process for the second tie.
- Ask the patient to flex the neck. Slip the longer tape under the patient's neck, place two fingers between the tape and the patient's neck (see Figure 16-26), and tie the tapes together at the

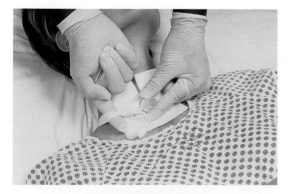

Figure 16-26 Placing a finger underneath the tie tape before tying it.

side of the neck. *Flexing the neck increases its circumference the way coughing does. Placing two fingers under the ties prevents making the ties too tight, which could interfere with coughing or place pressure on the jugular veins.*
- Tie the ends of the tapes using square knots. Cut off any long ends, leaving approximately 1 to 2 cm (0.5 inch). *Square knots prevent slippage and loosening. Adequate ends beyond the knot prevent the knot from inadvertently untying.*
- Once the clean ties are secured, remove the soiled ties and discard.

ONE-STRIP METHOD

- Cut a length of twill tape 2.5 times the length needed to go around the patient's neck from one tube flange to the other.
- Thread one end of the tape into the slot on one side of the flange.
- Bring both ends of the tape together, take them around the patient's neck, keeping them flat and untwisted.
- Thread the end of the tape next to the patient's neck through the slot from the back to the front.
- Have the patient flex the neck. Tie the loose ends with a square knot at the side of the patient's neck, allowing for slack by placing two fingers under the ties as with the two-strip method. Cut off long ends.

11. Tape and pad the tie knot.
- Place a folded 4 inch × 4 inch gauze square under the tie knot, and apply tape over the knot. *This reduces skin irritation from the knot and prevents confusing the knot with the patient's gown ties.*

12. Check the tightness of the ties.
- Frequently check the tightness of the tracheostomy ties and position of the tracheostomy tube. *Swelling of the neck may cause the ties to become too tight, interfering with coughing and circulation. Ties can loosen in restless patients, allowing the tracheostomy tube to extrude from the stoma.*

13. Document all relevant information.
- Record suctioning, tracheostomy care and the dressing change, noting your assessments.

VARIATION: USING A DISPOSABLE INNER CANNULA

- Check local policy for frequency of changing inner cannula *because standards vary among clinical areas.*
- Open a new cannula package.

- Using a gloved hand, unlock the current inner cannula (if present) and remove it by gently pulling it out toward you in line with its curvature.
- Check the cannula for amount and type of secretions and discard properly.

- Pick up the new inner cannula touching only the outer locking portion.
- Insert the new inner cannula into the tracheostomy.
- Lock the cannula in place by turning the lock (if present).

EVALUATION

+ Perform appropriate follow-up such as determining character and amount of secretions, drainage from the tracheostomy, appearance of the tracheostomy incision, pulse rate and respiratory status compared to baseline data, complaints of pain or discomfort at the tracheostomy site.

+ Relate findings to previous assessment data if available.

+ Report significant deviations from normal to the medical staff.

Suctioning

When patients have difficulty handling their secretions or an airway is in place, suctioning may be necessary to clear air passages. **Suctioning** is the aspiration of secretions through a catheter connected to a suction machine or wall suction outlet. Even though the upper airways (the oropharynx and nasopharynx) are not sterile, sterile technique is recommended for all suctioning to avoid introducing pathogens into the airways.

Suction catheters may be either open tipped or whistle tipped (see Figure 16-27 on page 400). The whistle-tipped catheter is less irritating to respiratory tissues, although the open-tipped catheter may be more effective for removing thick mucous plugs. An oral suction tube, or Yankauer device, is used to suction the oral cavity (see Figure 16-28 on page 400). Most suction catheters have a thumb port on the side to control the suction. The catheter is connected to suction tubing, which in turn is connected to a collection chamber and suction control gauge (see Figure 16-29 on page 400).

LIFESPAN CONSIDERATIONS

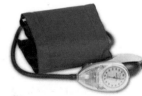

Tracheostomy Care

Infants and Children

+ An assistant should *always* be present while tracheostomy care is performed.
+ Always keep a sterile, packaged tracheostomy tube taped to the child's bed so that if the tube dislodges, a new one is available for immediate reintubation (Bindler and Ball, 2003: 95).

Older Adults

+ Older adult skin is more fragile and prone to breakdown. Care of the skin at the tracheostomy stoma is very important.

COMMUNITY CARE CONSIDERATIONS

Tracheostomy Care

+ For tracheostomies older than one month, clean technique is used for tracheostomy care and no asceptic (Humphrey, 1998).
+ Stress the importance of good hand washing technique to the caregiver/patient.
+ Tap water may be used for rinsing the inner cannula.

+ Teach the caregiver/patient the tracheostomy care procedure and observe a return demonstration.
+ Inform the caregiver/patient of the signs and symptoms that may indicate an infection of the stoma site or lower airway.
+ Names and telephone numbers of healthcare personnel who can be reached for emergencies or advice must be available to the patient and/or caregiver.

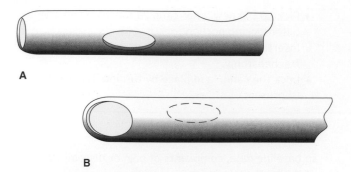

Figure 16-27 Types of suction catheters: *A*, open tipped; *B*, whistle tipped.

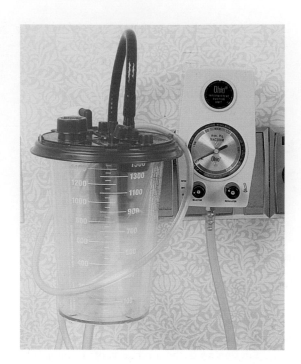

Figure 16-29 A wall suction unit.

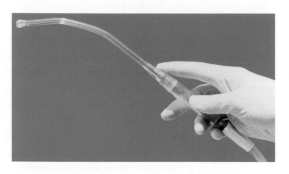

Figure 16-28 Oral (Yankauer) suction tube.

Oropharyngeal or nasopharyngeal suctioning removes secretions from the upper respiratory tract. Endotracheal suctioning is used to remove secretions from the trachea and bronchi. The nurse decides when suctioning is needed by assessing the patient for signs of respiratory distress or evidence that the patient is unable to cough up and expectorate secretions. Dyspnoea, bubbling or rattling breath sounds, poor skin colour (cyanosis), or decreased SaO_2 levels (also called O_2 sats) may indicate the need for suctioning. Good nursing judgement is necessary, because suctioning irritates mucous membranes and can increase secretions if performed too frequently. *Procedure 16-3* outlines oropharyngeal and nasopharyngeal suctioning.

PROCEDURE 16-3 Suctioning Oropharyngeal and Nasopharyngeal Cavities

Purposes

+ To remove secretions that obstruct the airway
+ To facilitate ventilation
+ To obtain secretions for diagnostic purposes

+ To prevent infection that may result from accumulated secretions

ASSESSMENT

Assess for clinical signs indicating the need for suctioning:

+ Restlessness
+ Gurgling sounds during respiration
+ Adventitious breath sounds when the chest is auscultated

+ Change in mental status
+ Skin colour
+ Rate and pattern of respirations
+ Pulse rate and rhythm

PLANNING

Equipment

+ Towel or moisture-resistant pad
+ Portable or wall suction machine with tubing and collection receptacle
+ Sterile disposable container for fluids
+ Sterile normal saline or water
+ Sterile gloves
+ Goggles or face shield, if appropriate
+ Sterile suction catheter kit (#12 to #18 Fr for adults; #8 to #10 Fr for children, and #5 to #8 Fr for

infants); if both the oropharynx and the nasopharynx are to be suctioned, one sterile catheter is required for each
+ Water-soluble lubricant (for nasopharyngeal suctioning)
+ Y-connector
+ Sterile gauzes
+ Moisture-resistant disposal bag
+ Sputum trap, if specimen is to be collected

IMPLEMENTATION

Performance

1. Explain to the patient what you are going to do, why it is necessary and how they can cooperate. Inform the patient that suctioning will relieve breathing difficulty and that the procedure is painless but may be uncomfortable and stimulate the cough, gag or sneeze reflex. *Knowing that the procedure will relieve breathing problems is often reassuring and enlists the patient's cooperation.*
2. Wash hands and observe other appropriate infection control procedures.
3. Provide for patient privacy.
4. Prepare the patient.
   • Position a conscious person who has a functional gag reflex in the semi-Fowler's position with the head turned to one side for oral suctioning or with the neck hyperextended for nasal suctioning. *These positions facilitate the insertion of the catheter and help prevent aspiration of secretions.*
   • Position an unconscious patient in the lateral position, facing you. *This position allows the tongue to fall forward, so that it will not obstruct the catheter on insertion. The lateral position also facilitates drainage of secretions from the pharynx and prevents the possibility of aspiration.*
   • Place the towel or moisture-resistant pad over the pillow or under the chin.
5. Prepare the equipment.
   • Set the pressure on the suction gauge in accordance with local policy, and turn on the suction.
   • Open the lubricant if performing nasopharyngeal suctioning.
   • Open the sterile suction package.
      (a) Set up container, touching only the outside.
      (b) Pour sterile water or saline into the container.

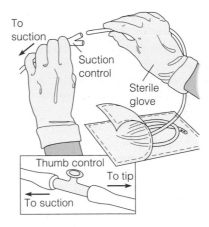

Figure 16-30 Attaching the catheter to the suction unit.

   (c) Put on the sterile gloves, or put on a nonsterile glove on the nondominant hand and then a sterile glove on the dominant hand. *The sterile gloved hand maintains the sterility of the suction catheter, and the unsterile glove prevents the transmission of the micro-organisms to the nurse.*
   • With your sterile gloved hand, pick up the catheter and attach it to the suction unit (see Figure 16-30).
6. Make an approximate measure of the depth for the insertion of the catheter and test the equipment.
   • Measure the distance between the tip of the patient's nose and the earlobe, or about 13 cm (5 inch) for an adult.
   • Mark the position on the tube with the fingers of the sterile gloved hand.
   • Test the pressure of the suction and the patency of the catheter by applying your sterile gloved finger or thumb to the port or open branch of the Y-connector (the suction control) to create suction.

7. Lubricate and introduce the catheter.
- For nasopharyngeal suction, lubricate the catheter tip with sterile water, saline or water-soluble lubricant; for oropharyngeal suction, moisten the tip with sterile water or saline. *This reduces friction and eases insertion.*

FOR OROPHARYNGEAL SUCTION

- Pull the tongue forward, if necessary, using gauze.
- Do not apply suction (that is, leave your finger off the port) during insertion. *Applying suction during insertion causes trauma to the mucous membrane.*
- Advance the catheter about 10-15 cm (4-6 inch) along one side of the mouth into the oropharynx. *Directing the catheter along the side prevents gagging.*

FOR NASOPHARYNGEAL SUCTION

- Without applying suction, insert the catheter the pre-measured or recommended distance into either nose and advance it along the floor of the nasal cavity. *This avoids the nasal turbinates.*
- Never force the catheter against an obstruction. If one nostril is obstructed, try the other.

8. Perform suctioning.
- Apply your finger to the suction control port to start suction, and gently rotate the catheter. *Gentle rotation of the catheter ensures that all surfaces are reached and prevents trauma to any one area of the respiratory mucosa due to prolonged suction.*
- Apply suction for 5–10 seconds while slowly withdrawing the catheter, then remove your finger from the control and remove the catheter.
- A suction attempt should last only 10 seconds. During this time, the catheter is inserted, the suction applied and discontinued, and the catheter removed.
- It may be necessary during oropharyngeal suctioning to apply suction to secretions that collect in the vestibule of the mouth and beneath the tongue.

9. Clean the catheter and repeat suctioning as above.
- Wipe off the catheter with sterile gauze if it is thickly coated with secretions. Dispose of the used gauze in a moisture-resistant bag.
- Flush the catheter with sterile water or saline.
- Relubricate the catheter, and repeat suctioning until the air passage is clear.
- Allow 20- to 30-second intervals between each suction and limit suctioning to five minutes in total. *Applying suction for too long may cause secretions to increase or decrease the patient's oxygen supply.*
- Alternate nares for repeat suctioning.

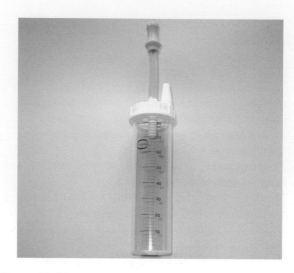

Figure 16-31 A sputum collection trap.

- Encourage the patient to breathe deeply and to cough between suctions. *Coughing and deep breathing help carry secretions from the trachea and bronchi into the pharynx, where they can be reached with the suction catheter.*

10. Obtain a sputum collection trap (see Figure 16.31).
- Attach the suction catheter to the tubing of the sputum trap.
- Attach the suction tubing to the sputum trap air vent.
- Suction the patient's nasopharynx or oropharynx. The sputum trap will collect the mucus during suctioning.
- Remove the catheter from the patient. Disconnect the sputum trap tubing from the suction catheter. Remove the suction tubing from the trap air vent.
- Connect the tubing of the sputum trap to the air vent. *This retains any micro-organisms in the sputum trap.*
- Connect the suction catheter to the tubing.
- Flush the catheter to remove secretions from the tubing.

11. Promote patient comfort.
- Offer to assist the patient with oral or nasal hygiene.
- Assist the patient to a position that facilitates breathing.

12. Dispose of equipment and ensure availability for the next suction.
- Dispose of the catheter, gloves, water and waste container. Wrap the catheter around your sterile gloved hand and hold the catheter as the glove is removed over it for disposal.
- Rinse the suction tubing as needed by inserting the end of the tubing into the

used water container. Empty and rinse the suction collection container as needed or indicated by protocol. Change the suction tubing and container daily.
- Ensure that supplies are available for the next suctioning (suction kit, gloves, water or normal saline).

13. Assess the effectiveness of suctioning.
- Observe skin colour, dyspnoea and level of anxiety.

14. Document relevant data.
- Record the procedure: the amount, consistency, colour and odour of sputum (e.g. foamy, white mucus; thick, green-tinged mucus; or blood-flecked mucus) and the patient's breathing status before and after the procedure.
- If the procedure is carried out frequently (e.g. every hour), it may be appropriate to record only once, at the end of the shift; however, the frequency of the suctioning must be recorded.

EVALUATION

✦ Conduct appropriate follow-up, such as appearance of secretions suctioned; breath sounds; respiratory rate, rhythm and depth; pulse rate and rhythm; and skin colour.

✦ Compare findings to previous assessment data if available.
✦ Report significant deviations from normal to the medical staff.

Following endotracheal intubation or a tracheostomy, the trachea and surrounding respiratory tissues are irritated and react by producing excessive secretions. Suctioning is necessary to remove these secretions and maintain a patent airway. The frequency of suctioning depends on the patient's health and how recently the intubation was done.

Suctioning is associated with several complications: hypoxemia, trauma to the airway, nosocomial infection and cardiac dysrhythmia, which is related to the hypoxemia. The following techniques are used to minimise or decrease these complications:

✦ **Hyperinflation.** This involves giving the patient breaths that are 1–1.5 times the tidal volume set on the ventilator through the ventilator circuit or via a manual resuscitation bag valve mask device. Three to five breaths are delivered before and after each pass of the suction catheter.

✦ **Hyperoxygenation.** This can be done with a manual resuscitation bag valve mask device or through the ventilator and is performed by increasing the oxygen flow (usually to 100%) before suctioning and between suction attempts.

For tracheostomy and endotracheal suctioning, the diameter of the suction catheter should be about half the inside diameter of the tracheostomy or endotracheal tube so that hypoxia can be prevented. The nurse uses sterile techniques to prevent infection of the respiratory tract (see *Procedure 16-4* on page 404). The traditional method of suctioning an endotracheal tube or tracheostomy is sometimes referred to as the *open method*. If a patient is connected to a ventilator, the nurse disconnects the patient from the ventilator, suctions the airway, reconnects the patient to the ventilator, and discards the suction catheter. Drawbacks to the open airway suction system include the nurse needing to wear personal protective equipment (e.g. goggles or face shield, gown) to avoid exposure to the patient's sputum and the potential cost of one-time catheter use, especially if the patient requires frequent suctioning.

With the alternative *closed airway/tracheal suction system (in-line suctioning)* (see Figure 16-32), the suction catheter attaches to the ventilator tubing and the patient does not need to be disconnected from the ventilator. The nurse is not exposed to any secretions because the suction catheter is enclosed in a

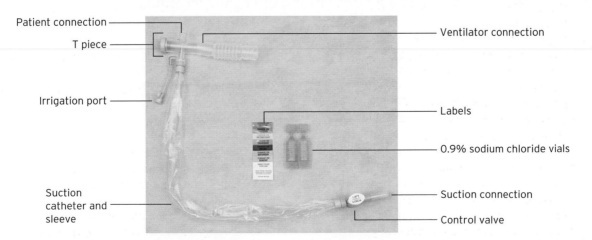

Figure 16-32 A closed airway suction (in-line) system.

plastic sheath. The catheter can be reused as many times as necessary until the system is changed. Manufacturers recommend changing closed suction catheter systems on a daily basis. Some studies, however, challenge this recommendation with showing no difference in specified factors such as ventilator-associated pneumonia and length of hospital stay for patients who had the closed system changed daily versus once a week (Hess, 1999) or the system changed on an as-needed basis (Little, 1998). The closed catheter system costs many times more than a conventional suction catheter. However, closed suctioning is becoming more common in some healthcare settings given the benefit of using the catheter multiple times along with other recent studies indicating a cost saving with weekly or as-needed changing of the system.

LIFESPAN CONSIDERATIONS

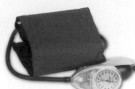

Suctioning

Infants

+ A bulb syringe may be used to remove secretions from an infant's nose or mouth. Care needs to be taken to avoid stimulating the gag reflex.

Children

+ A catheter is used to remove secretions from an older child's mouth or nose.

COMMUNITY CARE CONSIDERATIONS

Suctioning

+ Teach patients and families that the most important aspect of infection control is frequent hand washing.
+ Airway suctioning in the home is considered a clean procedure (Humphrey, 1998).
+ The catheter or Yankauer should be flushed by suctioning recently boiled or distilled water to rinse away mucus, followed by the suctioning of air through the device to dry the internal surface and, thus, discourage bacterial growth. The outer surface of the device may be wiped with alcohol or hydrogen peroxide. The suction catheter or Yankauer should be allowed to dry and then be stored in a clean, dry area.
+ Suction catheters treated in the manner described above may be reused. It is recommended that catheters be discarded after 24 hours.

PROCEDURE 16-4 Suctioning a Tracheostomy or Endotracheal Tube

Purposes

+ To maintain a patent airway and prevent airway obstructions
+ To promote respiratory function (optimal exchange of oxygen and carbon dioxide into and out of the lungs)
+ To prevent pneumonia that may result from accumulated secretions

ASSESSMENT

Assess the patient for the presence of congestion of the thorax. Note the patient's ability or inability to remove the secretions through coughing.

PLANNING

Equipment

+ Resuscitation bag (bag valve mask device) connected to 100% oxygen
+ Sterile towel (optional)
+ Equipment for suctioning (see *Procedure 16-3* on page 400)

+ Goggles and mask if necessary
+ Gown (if necessary)
+ Sterile gloves
+ Moisture-resistant bag

IMPLEMENTATION

Preparation

Determine if the patient has been suctioned previously and, if so, review the documentation of the procedure. This information can be very helpful in preparing the nurse for both the physiological and psychological impact of suctioning on the patient.

Performance

1. Explain to the patient what you are going to do, why it is necessary and how they can cooperate. Inform the patient that suctioning usually causes some intermittent coughing and that this assists in removing the secretions.
2. Wash hands and observe other appropriate infection control procedures (e.g. gloves, goggles).
3. Provide for patient privacy.
4. Prepare the patient.
   - If not contraindicated because of health, place the patient in the semi-Fowler's position to promote deep breathing, maximum lung expansion and productive coughing. *Deep breathing oxygenates the lungs, counteracts the hypoxic effects of suctioning, and may induce coughing. Coughing helps to loosen and move secretions.*
   - If necessary, provide analgesia before suctioning. Endotracheal suctioning stimulates the cough reflex, which can cause pain for patients who have had thoracic or abdominal surgery or who have experienced traumatic injury. *Pre-medication can increase the patient's comfort during the suctioning procedure.*
5. Prepare the equipment.
   - Attach the resuscitation apparatus to the oxygen source (see Figure 16-33). Adjust the oxygen flow to 100% flush.
   - Open the sterile supplies in readiness for use.
   - Place the sterile towel, if used, across the patient's chest below the tracheostomy.
   - Turn on the suction, and set the pressure in accordance with local policy. For a wall unit, a pressure setting of about 100-120 mm Hg is

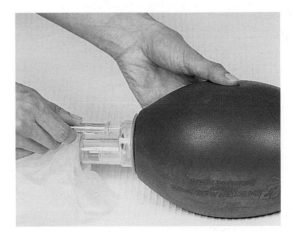

Figure 16-33 Attaching the resuscitation apparatus to the oxygen source.

normally used for adults, 50-95 mm Hg for infants and children.
   - Put on goggles, mask and gown if necessary.
   - Put on sterile gloves. Some clinical policies recommend putting a sterile glove on the dominant hand and an unsterile glove on the nondominant hand to protect the nurse.
   - Holding the catheter in the dominant hand and the connector in the nondominant hand, attach the suction catheter to the suction tubing (see Figure 16-30 on page 401).
6. Flush and lubricate the catheter.
   - Using the dominant hand, place the catheter tip in the sterile saline solution.
   - Using the thumb of the nondominant hand, occlude the thumb control and suction a small amount of the sterile solution through the catheter. *This determines that the suction equipment is working properly and lubricates the outside and the lumen of the catheter. Lubrication eases insertion and reduces tissue trauma during insertion. Lubricating the lumen also helps prevent secretions from sticking to the inside of the catheter.*

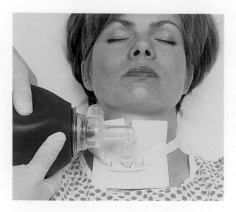

Figure 16-34 Attaching the resuscitator to the tracheostomy.

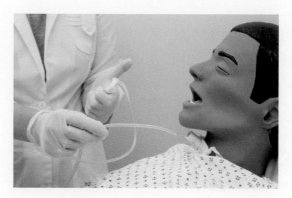

Figure 16-35 Inserting the catheter into the trachea through the tracheostomy tube. *Note:* Suction is not applied while inserting the catheter.

7. If the patient does not have copious secretions, hyperventilate the lungs with a resuscitation bag before suctioning.
   - Summon an assistant, if one is available, for this step.
   - Using your nondominant hand, turn on the oxygen to 12-15 l/min.
   - If the patient is receiving oxygen, disconnect the oxygen source from the tracheostomy tube using your nondominant hand.
   - Attach the resuscitator to the tracheostomy or endotracheal tube (see Figure 16-34).
   - Compress the bag valve mask device three to five times, as the patient inhales. This is best done by a second person who can use both hands to compress the bag, thus, providing a greater inflation volume.
   - Observe the rise and fall of the patient's chest to assess the adequacy of each ventilation.
   - Remove the resuscitation device and place it on the bed or the patient's chest with the connector facing up.

VARIATION - USING A VENTILATOR TO PROVIDE-HYPERVENTILATION.

If the patient is on a ventilator, use the ventilator for hyperventilation and hyperoxygenation. Newer models have a mode that provides 100% oxygen for two minutes and then switches back to the previous oxygen setting as well as a manual breath or sigh button. *The use of ventilator settings provides more consistent delivery of oxygenation and hyperinflation than a resuscitation device.*

8. If the patient has copious secretions, do not hyperventilate with a resuscitator. *Instead:*
   - Keep the regular oxygen delivery device on and increase the litre flow or adjust the FiO₂ to 100% for several breaths before suctioning. *Hyperventilating a patient who has copious*

secretions can force the secretions deeper into the respiratory tract.

9. Quickly but gently insert the catheter *without* applying any suction.
   - With your nondominant thumb off the suction port, quickly but gently insert the catheter into the trachea through the tracheostomy tube (see Figure 16-35). *To prevent tissue trauma and oxygen loss, suction is not applied during insertion of the catheter.*
   - Insert the catheter about 12.5 cm for adults, less for children, or until the patient coughs or you feel resistance. *Resistance usually means that the catheter tip has reached the bifurcation of the trachea. To prevent damaging the mucous membranes at the bifurcation, withdraw the catheter about 1-2 cm (0.4-0.8 inch) before applying suction.*

10. Perform suctioning.
    - Apply intermittent suction for 5-10 seconds by placing the nondominant thumb over the thumb port. *Suction time is restricted to 10 seconds or less to minimise oxygen loss.*
    - Rotate the catheter by rolling it between your thumb and forefinger while slowly withdrawing it. *This prevents tissue trauma by minimising the suction time against any part of the trachea.*
    - Withdraw the catheter completely, and release the suction.
    - Hyperventilate the patient.
    - Then suction again.

11. Reassess the patient's oxygenation status and repeat suctioning.
    - Observe the patient's respirations and skin colour. Check the patient's pulse if necessary, using your nondominant hand.
    - Encourage the patient to breathe deeply and to cough between suctions.

- Allow 2–3 minutes between suctions when possible. *This provides an opportunity for reoxygenation of the lungs.*
- Flush the catheter and repeat suctioning until the air passage is clear and the breathing is relatively effortless and quiet.
- After each suction, pick up the resuscitation bag with your nondominant hand and ventilate the patient with no more than three breaths.

12. Dispose of equipment and ensure availability for the next suction.
- Flush the catheter and suction tubing.
- Turn off the suction and disconnect the catheter from the suction tubing.
- Wrap the catheter around your sterile hand and peel the glove off so that it turns inside out over the catheter.

- Discard the glove and the catheter in the moisture-resistant bag.
- Replenish the sterile fluid and supplies so that the suction is ready for use again. *Patients who require suctioning often require it quickly, so it is essential to leave the equipment at the bedside ready for use.*

13. Provide for patient comfort and safety.
- Assist the patient to a comfortable, safe position that aids breathing. If the person is conscious, a semi-Fowler's position is frequently indicated. If the person is unconscious, Sims' position aids in the drainage of secretions from the mouth.

14. Document relevant data.
- Record the suctioning, including the amount and description of suction returns and any other relevant assessments.

Evaluation

+ Perform a follow-up assessment of the patient to determine the effectiveness of the suctioning (e.g. respiratory rate, depth and character; breath sounds; colour of skin and nail beds; character and amount of secretions suctioned; changes in vital signs).

+ Relate findings to previous assessment data if available.
+ Report significant deviations from normal to the medical staff.

LIFESPAN CONSIDERATIONS

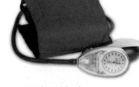

Suctioning a Tracheostomy or Endotracheal Tube

Infants and Children
+ Have an assistant gently support the child to keep the child's hands out of the way. The assistant will need to keep the child's head in the midline position (Bindler and Ball, 2003: 107).

Older Adults
+ Older adult often have cardiac and/or pulmonary disease, thus increasing their susceptibility to hypoxemia related to suctioning. Watch closely for signs of hypoxemia. If noted, stop suctioning and hyperoxygenate.
+ Do a thorough lung assessment before and after suctioning to determine effectiveness of suctioning and to be aware of any special problems.

COMMUNITY CARE CONSIDERATIONS

Suctioning a Tracheostomy or Endotracheal Tube
+ Whenever possible, the patient should be encouraged to clear the airway by coughing.
+ Patients may need to learn to suction their secretions if they cannot cough effectively.
+ Clean gloves should be used when endotracheal suctioning is performed in the home environment.

+ The nurse needs to instruct the caregiver on how to determine the need for suctioning and the correct process of suctioning to avoid potential complications of suctioning.
+ Stress the importance of adequate hydration as it thins secretions, which can aid in the removal of secretions by coughing or suctioning.

RESEARCH NOTE

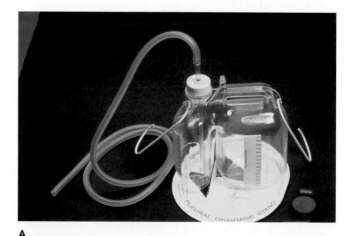

How Well Do Nurses Use Current Knowledge about Closed-System Suctioning Techniques?

The purposes of a study by Paul-Allen and Ostrow (2000) were to determine the frequency of use of closed and open suctioning systems and the nurses' knowledge about proper techniques for using the closed system. Critical care nurses were surveyed and 120 responses analysed. Almost all of the nurses reported using the closed system all or some of the time. The majority of the nurses who used the closed system reported using hyperoxygenation although a few of those only used it before the first catheter insertion or between passes rather than before, between and after. Only about half of the nurses used hyperinflation and, again, some used it only before or after suctioning rather than at both times.

Implications

In this sample, more than half of the nurses never use the open system of suctioning. It suggests that this may be a trend that will continue. However, not all of the nurses properly oxygenated their patients. More research is needed to quantify the suspected positive impact of hyperoxygenation and hyperinflation as well as the potential negative effects. In addition, the best mechanism for informing practising nurses of this evidence must be established.

Note: From 'Survey of Nursing Practices with Closed-System Suctioning,' by J. Paul-Allen and C.L. Ostrow, 2000, *American Journal of Critical Care*, 9(1), pp. 9–17.

Chest Tubes and Drainage Systems

If the thin, double-layered pleural membrane is disrupted by lung disease, surgery or trauma, the negative pressure between the pleural layers may be lost. The lung then collapses because it is no longer drawn outward as the diaphragm and intercostal muscles contract during inhalation. When air collects in the pleural space, it is known as a **pneumothorax**. Blood or fluid in the pleural space, a **haemothorax**, places pressure on lung tissue and interferes with lung expansion. Chest tubes may be inserted into the pleural cavity to restore negative pressure and drain collected fluid or blood. Because air rises, chest tubes for pneumothorax often are placed in the upper anterior thorax, whereas chest tubes used to drain fluid generally are placed in the lower lateral chest wall.

When chest tubes are inserted, they must be connected to a sealed drainage system or a one-way valve that allows air and fluid to be removed from the chest cavity but prevents air from entering from the outside. Sterile disposable drainage systems are used to prevent outside air from entering the chest tube. These systems typically have a closed collection chamber for drainage that is connected to a wet or dry seal chamber (see Figure 16-36). With the water-seal system, when the patient inhales, the water prevents air from entering the system from the atmosphere. During exhalation, however, air can exit the chest cavity, bubbling up through the water. Suction can be added to the system to facilitate removing air and secretions from the chest cavity. The drainage system should always be kept below the level of the patient's chest to prevent fluid and drainage from being drawn back into the chest cavity.

A Heimlich valve or comparable system may be used for mobile patients who have a pneumothorax. These valves allow

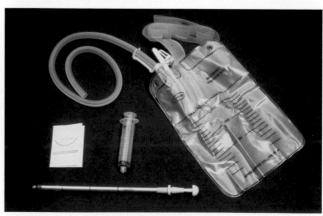

A

B

Figure 16-36 Chest drainage systems.

 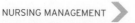

air to escape from the chest cavity, but they close during inhalation to prevent air from entering.

Chest tube insertion and removal require sterile technique and must be done without introducing air or micro-organisms into the pleural cavity.

Nursing responsibilities regarding drainage systems include the following:

+ Monitor and maintain the patency and integrity of the drainage system.
+ Assess the patient's vital signs, oxygen saturation, cardiovascular status and respiratory status.
+ Keep chest tube clamps and a sterile occlusive dressing near the patient. If the tube becomes disconnected from the collecting system, submerge the end in 5 cm of sterile saline or water *to maintain the seal*. If the chest tube is inadvertently pulled out, the wound should be immediately covered with a dry sterile dressing. If you can hear air leaking out of the site, ensure that the dressing is not occlusive. *If the air cannot escape, this would lead to pneumothorax.*
+ Use standard precautions and personal protective equipment while manipulating the system and assisting with insertion or removal.
+ Observe the dressing site at least every four hours. Inspect the dressing for excessive and abnormal drainage, such as bleeding or foul-smelling discharge. Palpate around the dressing site, and listen for a crackling sound indicative of subcutaneous emphysema. *Subcutaneous emphysema can result from a poor seal at the chest tube insertion site.*
+ Determine level of discomfort with and without activity and administer analgesia as required.
+ Encourage deep breathing and coughing exercises every two hours (this may be contraindicated in patients who have had a lung removed). Have the patient sit upright to perform the exercises, and splint the chest around the tube insertion site with a pillow or with a hand to minimise discomfort.
+ Reposition the patient every two hours. When the patient is lying on the affected side, place rolled towels beside the tubing. *Frequent position changes promote drainage, prevent complications and provide comfort. Rolled towels prevent occlusion of the chest tube by the patient's weight.*
+ Assist the patient with range-of-motion exercises of the affected shoulder three times per day to maintain joint mobility.
+ When moving and mobilising the patient:
  (a) Attach chest drain forceps to the patient's gown/clothing for emergency use.
  (b) Keep the water-seal unit below chest level and upright.
  (c) Disconnect the drainage system from the suction apparatus before moving the patient and make sure the air vent is open.

Removal of a chest tube is a brief but quite painful procedure. Administer analgesia before the removal. Remove the dressing around the tube and prepare the dressing that will cover the insertion site. This will be an occlusive dressing if there is no purse-string suture around the insertion site to prevent air from entering the chest. Generally, the medical staff perform the removal but, in some areas, specially trained nurses may be permitted to do so.

EVALUATING

Using the goals and desired outcomes identified in the planning stage of the nursing process, the nurse collects data to evaluate the effectiveness of interventions. If outcomes are not achieved, the nurse and patient need to explore the reasons before modifying the care plan.

CRITICAL REFLECTION

Let us revisit the case study on page 374. Now that you have read this chapter why is it important to monitor John's respiratory rate? What would be the danger of giving John high concentration oxygen? What is the best oxygen delivery device to use for John?

CHAPTER HIGHLIGHTS

+ Respiration is the process of gas exchange between the individual and the environment.
+ The respiratory system contributes to effective respiration through pulmonary ventilation (the movement of air between the atmosphere and the lungs) and the diffusion of oxygen and carbon dioxide across the pulmonary membrane.
+ Alveoli and the capillaries that surround them form the respiratory membrane, where gas exchange between the lungs and the blood occurs.
+ Effective pulmonary ventilation, or breathing, requires clear airways, an intact central nervous system and respiratory centre, an intact thoracic cavity and musculature, and adequate pulmonary compliance (stretch) and recoil.
+ Gas exchange occurs by diffusion, as gas molecules move from an area of higher concentration to an area of lower concentration. At the respiratory membrane, oxygen moves from the alveolus into the blood, while carbon dioxide moves from the blood into the alveolus.
+ Respiratory rates normally are highest in neonates and infants, gradually slowing to adult ranges.
+ Ageing affects the respiratory system: the chest wall becomes more rigid and lungs less elastic.
+ Other factors affecting oxygenation include the environment, lifestyle, health status, narcotic analgesics, and stress and coping.
+ Hypoxia, insufficient oxygen in the tissues, can result from impaired ventilation (hypoventilation) or diffusion, or from impaired oxygen transportation to the tissues because of anaemia or decreased cardiac output.
+ Airway obstruction interferes with ventilation. A low-pitched snoring sound, stridor and abnormal breath sounds may accompany partial airway obstruction. Extreme inspiratory effort with no chest movement indicates complete upper airway obstruction.
+ The patient history includes questions about current or past respiratory problems and about lifestyle, presence of symptoms such as cough or shortness of breath, smoking and other risk factors, and medications.
+ Nursing interventions to promote oxygenation include promoting healthy breathing and a healthy heart, deep breathing and coughing, and hydration; administering medications; implementing measures to clear secretions (e.g. incentive spirometry, percussion, vibration and postural drainage); initiating and monitoring oxygen therapy; initiating or assisting with procedures to maintain the airway (e.g. artificial airways and suctioning); providing tracheostomy care; and monitoring chest drainage systems.
+ The effectiveness of nursing interventions is evaluated by using the goals and desired outcomes identified in the planning stage of the nursing process. If a goal is not met, the nurse asks pertinent questions to assess the reason for not meeting the goal.

REFERENCES

Bindler, R.C. and Ball, J.W. (2003) *Clinical skills manual for pediatric nursing: Caring for children* (3rd edn), Upper Saddle River, NJ: Prentice Hall Health.

Hess, D.R. (1999) 'Managing the artificial airway', *Respiratory Care*, 44, 759–776.

Humphrey, C.J. (1998) *Home care nursing handbook* (3rd edn), Gaithersburg, MD: Aspen.

Little, K. (1998) 'As needed in line suction catheter changes were as safe as and less expensive than daily scheduled catheter changes during mechanical ventilation', *Evidence Based Nursing*, 1(3), 82.

Paul-Allen, J. and Ostrow, C.L. (2000) 'Survey of nursing practices with closed-system suctioning', *American Journal of Critical Care*, 9(1), 9–17.

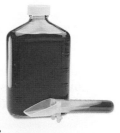

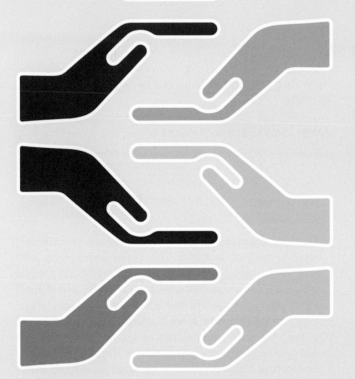

Chapter 17 Nutrition

Learning Outcomes

After completing this chapter, you will be able to:

+ Identify essential nutrients and dietary sources of each.

+ Explain essential aspects of energy balance.

+ Discuss body weight and the body mass index.

+ Identify factors influencing nutrition.

+ Identify developmental nutritional considerations.

+ Evaluate a diet using the tilted plate.

+ Discuss essential components and purposes of nutritional screening and nutritional assessment.

+ Identify risk factors for and clinical signs of malnutrition.

+ Describe nursing interventions to promote optimal nutrition.

+ Discuss nursing interventions to treat patients with nutritional problems.

CASE STUDY

'Size zero' is attractive according to a *New Woman* magazine 2007 poll but is it healthy?

Size zero (US) is equivalent to a size 4 in the UK and has been inextricably linked to the fashion world. But with eating disorders being the third most common chronic condition in adolescent girls (Viner and Booy, 2005) resulting in outcries from the media, government and public alike, the British Fashion Council has now advised the fashion industry only to use models who look 'healthy', but have not banned the use of size zero models. However Spain and Italy have banned using models with a body mass index (BMI) less than 18 (underweight).

After reading this chapter you will be able to reflect on the importance of nutrition and understand the components of a healthy diet.

INTRODUCTION

According to the British Association for Parenteral and Enteral Nutrition (BAPEN, 2003), a charitable organisation that aims to increase the profile of nutrition within the UK, malnourishment costs the UK more than £7.3 billion a year. Malnourishment leads to prolonged hospital admissions, increased risk of infection and more GP and outpatient visits. Approximately 30% of people admitted to hospital and care homes are 'at nutritional risk' with more than 10% of over-65s suffering from nutritional problems.

Food is fundamental for survival. It is needed for cellular and tissue growth and repair, and for the regulating of body processes. The body requires an adequate and balanced intake of carbohydrates, proteins, fats, vitamins and minerals. Foods differ greatly in their **nutritional value**, and no one food provides all essential nutrients.

In order to survive, human beings will eat almost anything to ensure their hunger is satisfied. However, when survival is guaranteed a number of factors can affect the type, quantity and nutritional quality of foods that will be eaten, for example, age, culture, taste preferences, mobility and nutritional knowledge.

CLINICAL ANECDOTE

As the student nurse on the ward, I'm usually the one who feeds the patients. I don't mind, but why don't qualified nurses do it as well. I think it is one of the most important things we can do in nursing – to make sure that our patients are having adequate food and water.

John James, student nurse

MACRONUTRIENTS

Carbohydrates

Carbohydrates can be divided into two major groups: simple carbohydrates (sugars) and complex carbohydrates (starch).

Sugars, the simplest of all carbohydrates, are water soluble and are produced naturally by both plants and animals. Sugars may be **monosaccharides** (single molecules, e.g. glucose and fructose) or **disaccharides** (two monosaccharides, e.g. maltose). There is no real practical difference between these two types of sugars and it certainly does not mean that a monosaccharide is easier to digest that a disaccharide.

Most sugars are produced naturally by plants, especially fruits, sugar cane and sugar beets. Processed or refined sugars (e.g. table sugar) are those that have been extracted and concentrated from natural sources and are added to foods such as biscuits.

Starches are the insoluble, nonsweet forms of carbohydrate. They are **polysaccharides**; that is, they are composed of branched chains of dozens, sometimes hundreds, of monosaccharide molecules. Like sugars, nearly all starches exist naturally in plants, such as grains, legumes and potatoes.

Proteins

Protein is found in every cell of the human body and is required for growth and wound healing. The protein in the human body is essentially the same as the protein that is eaten, except it is structurally different. Basically proteins are made up of chains of amino acids that are chemical compound made up of carbon, hydrogen, oxygen and nitrogen and can be combined together to form different structures within the body. There are 22 different amino acids all of which the body needs. These are divided into:

+ Fourteen **nonessential amino acids** that can be manufactured by the body and do not have to be derived from food sources. Examples of nonessential amino acids are glycine, which is a neurotransmitter within the spine, and alanine, which plays an important part in the metabolism of glucose.
+ Eight **essential amino acids** that cannot be manufactured in the body and therefore must be ingested in the diet. For example arginine, which has a role in the immune system, and leucine, which is necessary for tissue growth and maintenance, can only be derived from food.

Proteins are found in meat, fish, eggs, soya, tofu, nuts and pulses. Eating too much protein can result in ill health as it puts excess strain on the liver and kidneys. Also the body is unable to store protein so it is digested into glucose and then used up as energy or stored as fat. Therefore eating too much protein can result in obesity.

Eating too little protein can also have detrimental health effects. Protein is lost every day in the form of skin cells and hair. If we do not replenish protein this can result in skin problems and make the individual tired, stunt their growth and could lead to poor mental health.

Fats

Fats are organic substances that are greasy and insoluble in water and are found in solid fats, liquid oils and dairy products. It is important that fat is contained in a healthy diet as it helps the body absorb some fat soluble vitamins; it provides energy and is a good source of fatty acids. However a diet rich in fat can lead to obesity as excess fat is stored underneath the dermis (skin).

There are three major dietary fats – fatty acids, triglycerides and cholesterol.

Fatty acids are the basic structural units of all fats and fall into three groups:

1. **Saturated fatty acids** are mainly of animal origin and when eaten can increase cholesterol levels thereby increasing the risk of heart disease.
2. **Unsaturated fatty acids**:
   - **Monounsaturated fatty acids** are found in olive oil and increase 'healthy' (high density lipoprotein – HDL) cholesterol in the blood, which helps to remove fat from the walls of arteries, transporting it to the liver for breakdown.
   - **Polyunsaturated fatty acids** are found in nuts, grains and seeds and are important for maintaining cell membranes. They can lower the levels of both the bad cholesterol (low density lipoprotein – LDL) and the 'healthy' cholesterol (HDL). Polyunsaturated fatty acids therefore are a good source of fat.
   - **Trans-fats** are polyunsaturated fats that have been artificially hardened by the process of hydrogenation of vegetable oil. Hydrogenation is a chemical process that turns liquid oil into solid fat. A by-product of this process is trans-fats, which are as unhealthy as saturated fats.

Triglyceride fats are found in food such as meat, dairy products and cooking oils. Triglycerides are made up of three fatty acids and account for more than 90% of the fat in food and in the body. Triglycerides may contain saturated or unsaturated fatty acids. Excess dietary fat is stored as triglyceride fats in the body.

Cholesterol is a waxy substance that is both produced by the body and found in foods of animal origin. It is made up of fat and protein and is synthesised in the liver; however, some is absorbed from the diet (e.g. from milk, egg yolk and organ meats). Cholesterol is needed to create bile acids and to synthesise steroid hormones. It can be divided into two groups:

1. **High density lipoprotein (HDL)** is mostly made up of protein with a small amount of fat and is known as the 'good' cholesterol because it helps to lower the low density lipoprotein (LDL).
2. **Low density lipoprotein (LDL)** is mostly made up of fat with a small amount of protein and is known as the 'bad' cholesterol as it has been linked to fatty deposits being laid down in the arteries (atherosclerosis), which can lead to coronary heart disease and cerebrovascular accidents (CVA or stroke).

Micro-nutrients

Micro-nutrients are substances that are found in small amounts in food such as vitamins and minerals.

Vitamins

A **vitamin** is an organic compound that cannot be manufactured by the body and is needed in small quantities to catalyse metabolic processes. Thus, when vitamins are lacking in the diet, metabolic deficits result. Vitamins are generally classified as follows:

+ **Water-soluble vitamins** include C and the B-complex vitamins: B_1 (thiamine), B_2 (riboflavin), B_3 (niacin or nicotinic acid), B_6 (pyridoxine), B_9 (folic acid), B_{12} (cobalamin), pantothenic acid, and biotin. The body cannot store water-soluble vitamins; thus, people must get a daily supply in the diet. Water-soluble vitamins can be affected by food processing, storage and preparation.
+ **Fat-soluble vitamins** include A, D, E and K. The body can store these vitamins, although there is a limit to the amounts of vitamin E and K the body can store. Therefore, a daily supply of fat-soluble vitamins is not absolutely necessary. Vitamin content is highest in fresh foods that are consumed as soon as possible after harvest.

Minerals

Minerals are inorganic compounds such as sodium, calcium and iron. These molecules cannot be broken down, changed or destroyed by the body in any way. Calcium and phosphorus make up 80% of all mineral elements in the body. There are two categories of minerals:

1. **Macro-minerals** are those that people require daily in amounts over 100 mg. They include calcium, phosphorus, sodium, potassium, magnesium, chloride and sulphur.
2. **Microminerals** are those that people require daily in amounts less than 100 mg. They include iron, zinc, manganese, iodine, fluoride, copper, cobalt, chromium and selenium.

Common problems associated with the lack of mineral nutrients are iron deficiency resulting in anaemia, and osteoporosis resulting from loss of bone calcium.

ENERGY BALANCE

Energy balance is the relationship between the energy derived from food and the energy used by the body. The body obtains energy in the form of calories from carbohydrates, protein and fat. The body uses energy for voluntary activities such as walking and talking and for involuntary activities such as breathing and secreting enzymes. A person's energy balance is determined by comparing their energy intake with energy output.

Energy Intake

The amount of energy that nutrients or foods supply to the body is their **caloric value**. A **calorie (c, cal and kcal)** is a unit of heat energy. One calorie is the amount of heat required to raise the temperature of 1 gram of water 1°C and one **kilocalorie (Kcal)** is the amount needed to raise 1 kg of water by 1°C. The energy liberated from the metabolism of food has been determined to be:

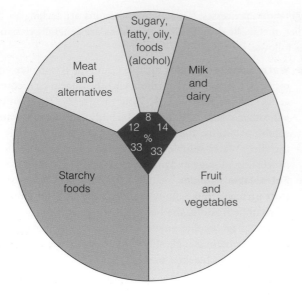

Figure 17-1 Tilted plate (from Hogston and Simpson, 2002).

+ 4 calories/gram of carbohydrates
+ 4 calories/gram of protein
+ 9 calories/gram of fat.

Energy Output

Metabolism refers to all biochemical and physiological processes by which the body grows and maintains itself. Metabolic rate is normally expressed in terms of the rate of heat liberated during these chemical reactions. The **basal metabolic rate (BMR)** is the rate at which the body metabolises food to maintain the energy requirements of a person who is awake and at rest. The energy in food maintains the basal metabolic rate of the body and provides energy for activities such as running and walking.

HEALTHY DIET

It can be difficult to establish if a patient is eating a 'balanced' diet. In order to help the healthcare professional, Penelope Simpson (in Hogston and Simpson, 2002), a nurse lecturer in the University of Southampton, has developed a tilted plate that shows the percentages of food groups that a healthy individual should aim to eat in a day (see Figure 17-1). The tilted plate demonstrates the percentages of food groups needed for a balanced diet. A healthy diet needs to gain most of its calories from starchy foods such as potatoes and rice, and fruit and vegetables. It is important that sugary, fatty and oily foods are kept to a minimum.

Vegetarian Diets

People may become vegetarians for many reasons. There are two basic vegetarian diets: those that use only plant foods (vegan) and those that include milk, eggs or dairy products. Some people eat fish and poultry but not beef, lamb or pork; others eat only fresh fruit, juices and nuts; and still others eat plant foods and dairy products but not eggs.

Vegetarian diets can be nutritionally sound if they include a wide variety of foods and if proper protein, vitamin and mineral supplementation are provided. Proteins found in plant foods are incomplete proteins (made up of amino acids that are different to body protein), therefore vegetarians must eat complementary protein foods (proteins that are similar to body protein) to obtain all the essential amino acids. For example, eating two different foods such as beans on toast with butter will ensure that the individual is receiving the amino acids required for health. Simpson (in Hogston and Simpson, 2002) adapted the tilted plate for vegetarians (see Figure 17-2) and demonstrates the fine balance that needs to be made between the different food groups.

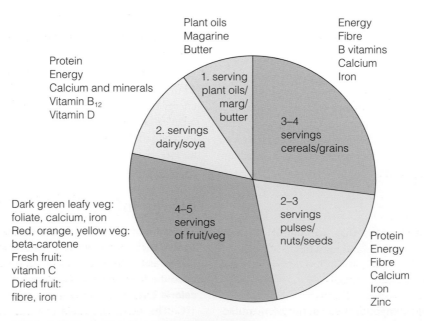

Figure 17-2 Vegetarian tilted plate (from Hogston and Simpson, 2002).

BODY WEIGHT

Maintaining a health body weight requires a balance between the expenditure of energy and the intake of nutrients. Generally, when energy requirements of an individual equate with the daily calorie intake, the body weight remains stable.

The **body mass index (BMI)** has been used for many years by healthcare professionals as a means of reliably indicating a healthy weight for a person. However it is not infallible: for instance it is possible for a healthy, muscular athlete with very low body fat to be classified obese using the BMI formula.

For people older than 18 years, the BMI is an indicator of changes in body fat stores and whether a person's weight is appropriate for height, and may provide a useful estimate of malnutrition. To calculate the BMI:

✦ Measure the person's height in metres (e.g. 1.5 m) (1 metre = 3.3 feet, or 39.6 inches)
✦ Measure the weight in kilograms (e.g. 60 kg) (1 kg = 2.2 lb)
✦ Calculate the BMI using the following formula

$$BMI = \frac{\text{Weight in kilograms}}{(\text{Height in metres})^2}$$

or

$$\frac{60 \text{ kilograms}}{1.5 \times 1.5 \text{ (metres)}^2} = 26.6$$

Box 17-1 provides an interpretation of the results.

BOX 17-1 Guide for BMI Evaluation

<16	Malnourished
16-19	Underweight
20-25	Normal
26-30	Overweight
31-40	Moderately to severely obese
>40	Morbidly obese

Note: From 'Know How: Nutritional Assessment,' by E. Walters, 1998, *Nursing Times*, 94(8), pp. 68-69. Copyright Emap Healthcare, reproduced with permission.

FACTORS AFFECTING NUTRITION

Although the nutritional content of food is an important consideration when planning a diet, an individual's food preferences and habits are often a major factor affecting actual food intake. Habits about eating are influenced by developmental considerations, gender, ethnicity and culture, beliefs about food, personal preferences, religious practices, lifestyle, medications and therapy, health, alcohol consumption, advertising and psychological factors.

Gender

Nutrient requirements are different for men and women because of body composition and reproductive functions. The larger muscle mass of men translates into a greater need for calories and proteins. Also, prior to the menopause, women require more iron than men due to menstruation and pregnant and breast feeding women need a higher calorie and fluid intake.

Ethnicity and Culture

Ethnicity often determines food preferences. Traditional foods (e.g. rice for Asians, and pasta for Italians) can be eaten as long as there is variety in the diet to ensure that all the macronutrients (e.g. protein, fat and carbohydrate) and micronutrients, vitamins and minerals are eaten.

It is also important to recognise that food preferences differ from individual to individual within the same culture: for example, not all Italians like pasta.

Beliefs about Food

Beliefs about effects of foods on health and well-being can affect food choices. Many people acquire their beliefs about food from television, magazines and other media.

Personal Preferences

People develop likes and dislikes based on associations with a typical food. Individual likes and dislikes can also be related to familiarity. Preferences in the tastes, smells, flavours (blends of taste and smell), temperatures, colours, shapes, textures and sizes of food influence a person's food choices.

Religious Practices

Religious practice also affects diet. Some Roman Catholics avoid meat on certain days, and some Protestant faiths prohibit meat, tea, coffee or alcohol. Both Orthodox Judaism and Islam prohibit pork. Orthodox Jews observe kosher customs, eating certain foods only if they are inspected by a rabbi and prepared according to dietary laws. The nurse must be sensitive to such religious dietary practices.

Lifestyle

Certain lifestyles are linked to food-related behaviours. People who are always in a hurry probably buy convenience grocery items or eat restaurant meals. People who spend many hours at home may take time to prepare more meals 'from scratch'. Individual differences also influence lifestyle patterns (e.g. cooking skills, concern about health). Some people work at different times, such as evening or night shifts. They might need to adapt their eating habits to this and also make changes in their medication schedules if they are related to food intake.

What, how much and how often a person eats are frequently affected by socioeconomic status. For example, people with limited income, including some older people, may not be able to afford meat and fresh vegetables. In contrast, people with higher incomes may purchase more proteins and fats and fewer complex carbohydrates.

Medications and Therapy

The effects of drugs on nutrition vary considerably. They may alter appetite, disturb taste perception or interfere with nutrient absorption or excretion. Nurses need to be aware of the nutritional effects of specific drugs when evaluating a patient for nutritional problems.

Health

An individual's health status greatly affects eating habits and nutritional status. The lack of teeth, ill-fitting teeth or a sore mouth makes chewing food difficult. Difficulty swallowing (**dysphagia**) due to a painfully inflamed throat or a stricture of the oesophagus can prevent a person from obtaining adequate nourishment. Disease processes and surgery of the gastrointestinal tract can affect digestion, absorption, metabolism and excretion of essential nutrients. Gastrointestinal and other diseases also create anorexia (loss of appetite), nausea, vomiting and diarrhoea, all of which can adversely affect a person's appetite and nutritional status.

Alcohol Consumption

Excessive alcohol use contributes to nutritional deficiencies in a number of ways. Alcohol may replace food in a person's diet and it can depress the appetite. Excessive alcohol can have a toxic effect on the intestinal mucosa, thereby decreasing the absorption of nutrients. The need for vitamin B increases, because it is used in alcohol metabolism. Alcohol can impair the storage of nutrients and increase nutrient catabolism (break down or metabolism) and excretion.

Psychological Factors

Although some people overeat when stressed, depressed or lonely, others eat very little under the same conditions. Anorexia and weight loss can indicate severe stress or depression. Anorexia nervosa and bulimia are severe psychophysiological conditions seen most frequently in female adolescents probably as a result of puberty and the unhealthy images of thin models in the media.

Changing Nutritional Requirements Among Different Age Groups

According to the Department of Health (DoH, 1991) nutritional requirements is influenced by a number of factors including growth. However, as there are so many other factors

Table 17-1 Physical Activity Level (PAL) for Adults

PAL level	Gender	Description
1.4	Male/Female	Very little activity at work and in leisure time
1.6	Female	Moderate activity at work/leisure
1.7	Male	Moderate activity at work/leisure
1.8	Female	High levels of activity at work/leisure
1.9	Male	High levels of activity at work/leisure

Source: Adapted from Hogston and Simpson (2002).

that can affect nutritional needs in an individual it is impossible to identify the specific needs of each age group.

Growth has great energy demands: for example, a baby has half the energy requirements of an older adult but is probably less than a third of the older person's weight. This energy is required not only for growth but for activities such as crying and sucking. According to Hogston and Simpson (2002) the peak of energy requirements is between the ages of 15 and 18 years, usually associated with a growth spurt around the time of puberty.

A relatively accurate way of estimating nutritional energy requirement is to use the following formula, which allows the healthcare professional to work out the individual's calorie intake to maintain their body weight:

$$BMR \times PAL = EAR$$

Where:

+ BMR is the basal metabolic rate that is measured at rest, after sleeping and 12 hours after eating. Basal metabolic rate depends on gender, height, weight and age. For example the basal metabolic rate for a female aged 40 who is 5 feet 3 inches tall and weighs 10 stone is 1364.7 compared with a male aged 40 who is 6 feet tall and weighs 14 stone whose BMR is 1926.4.
+ PAL is the physical activity level calculated according to Table 17-1.
+ EAR is the estimated average requirements.

Therefore, for a female aged 40, who is 5 feet 3 inches tall, weighs 10 stone and has moderate activity, the estimated average requirements would be $1364.7 \times 1.6 = 2183.52$ calories to maintain her body weight.

ALTERED NUTRITION

Malnutrition is commonly defined as the lack of necessary or appropriate food substances but in practice includes both undernutrition and overnutrition. **Overnutrition** refers to a caloric intake in excess of daily energy requirements, resulting in storage of energy in the form of adipose tissue. As the amount of stored fat increases, the individual becomes overweight or obese.

Undernutrition refers to an intake of nutrients insufficient to meet daily energy requirements because of inadequate food intake or improper digestion and absorption of food. An inadequate food intake may be caused by the inability to acquire and prepare food, inadequate knowledge about essential nutrients and a balanced diet, discomfort during or after eating, dysphagia, **anorexia** (loss of appetite), nausea or vomiting, and so on. Improper digestion and absorption of nutrients may be caused by an inadequate production of hormones or enzymes or by medical conditions resulting in inflammation or obstruction of the gastrointestinal tract.

Inadequate nutrition is associated with marked weight loss, generalised weakness, altered functional abilities, delayed wound healing, increased susceptibility to infection, immuno-suppression, impaired pulmonary function and prolonged length of hospitalisation. In response to undernutrition, carbohydrate reserves, stored as liver and muscle glycogen, are mobilised. However, these reserves can only meet energy requirements for a short time (e.g. 24 hours) and then body protein is mobilised which results in depletion of protein reserves (muscle mass).

Protein energy malnutrition (PEM), once associated with the manifestation of malnutrition seen in starving children of third world countries, is now recognised as a significant problem of patients with long-term deficiencies in caloric intake (e.g. those with cancer and chronic disease). Characteristics of PEM are depressed visceral proteins (proteins that are in blood, e.g. albumin), weight loss and visible muscle and fat wasting.

NURSING MANAGEMENT

ASSESSING

The purpose of a nutritional assessment is to identify patients at risk of malnutrition and those with poor nutritional status. In most healthcare environments, the responsibility for nutritional assessment and support is shared by the doctor, the dietitian and the nurse. Generally, nurses perform a nutritional screen. A comprehensive nutritional assessment is often performed by a nutritionist or a dietitian. Components of a nutritional assessment are shown in Table 17-2.

Nutritional Screening

A nutritional screen is an assessment performed to identify patients at risk for malnutrition or those who are malnourished. Nutritional screening is performed by nurses as part of the holistic assessment of the patient. In order to facilitate the assessment of a patient's nutritional and hydration state, nurses can use a nutritional screening tool. Many nutritional screening tools have been developed over the years when choosing a tool it is important to select one that is appropriate for the patient or patient group.

In 2003, the Malnutrition Advisory Group (MAG) of the British Association of Parenteral and Enteral Nutrition (BAPEN) developed a nutritional screening tool for adults called the Malnutrition Universal Screening Tool (MUST) which is based on Body Mass Index (BMI), unintentional weight loss and the effect of acute illness on the nutritional state of the patient (see Figure 17-3 on page 418). The aim of the screening tool is to standardise nutritional screening in an easy, reliable and valid manner. The simplicity of the tool means that it is quick to complete and is acceptable to both patients and healthcare professionals.

Following screening of the patient with the tool it is important that a nutrition plan is developed to meet the needs of the patient. Those patients considered to be at low risk of malnutrition may require little or no action or may need to be reassessed at a later time. Those patients considered to be at medium risk may require food supplements such as fortified

Table 17-2 Components of a Nutritional Assessment

	Screening data
Body measurements	+ Height + Weight + Ideal body weight + Usual body weight + Body mass index
Biochemical data	+ Haemoglobin - a complex protein-iron compound that carries oxygen and is found in red blood cells + Serum albumin - protein found in blood that helps to maintain blood volume + Total lymphocyte count - number of white cells in the blood. White cells are primarily made of protein
Clinical	+ Skin + Hair and nails + Mucous membranes + Activity level
Dietary data	+ 24-hour food recall + Food frequency record

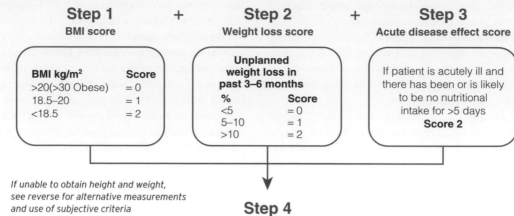

Figure 17-3 The Malnutrition Universal Screening Tool (from BAPEN http://www.bapen.org.uk/the-must.htm).

(The MUST Report – nutritional screening of adults: a multi-disciplinary responsibility. Development and use of the 'Malnutrition Universal Screening Tool' (MUST) for aduts. Editor: Professor Marinos Elia. BAPEN, 2003, ISBN 1 899467 70 X. Copies of the full report are available from the BAPEN Office, Secure Hold Business Centre, Studley Road, Redditch, WORCS B98 7LG; tel: +44 (0) 1527 457850.)

BOX 17-2 Summary of Risk Factors for Nutritional Problems

+ Chewing or swallowing difficulties (including ill-fitting dentures, dental caries and missing teeth)
+ Inadequate food budget
+ Inadequate food intake
+ Inadequate food preparation facilities
+ Inadequate food storage facilities
+ Living and eating alone
+ Physical disabilities
+ Alcohol or substance abuse
+ Conditions that cause increased metabolism such as burns or trauma
+ Chronic illness: end-stage renal disease, liver disease, HIV, pulmonary disease (COPD), cancer
+ Fluid and electrolyte imbalance
+ Gastrointestinal problems: anorexia, dysphagia (inability to swallow), nausea, vomiting, diarrhoea, constipation
+ Neurological or cognitive impairment
+ Oral and gastrointestinal surgery

a problem with eating and drinking. See the summary of risk factors in *Box 17-2*.

A patient history will also establish the patient's usual eating patterns and habits; food preferences, allergies and intolerances; frequency, types and quantities of foods consumed; and social, economic, ethnic or religious factors influencing nutrition. Factors that may affect nutrition and hydration may include, but are not limited to, living and eating alone, ability to purchase and prepare food, availability of refrigeration and cooking facilities, income and effect of religion and ethnicity on food choices.

A **food diary** or chart can hold useful information regarding the patient's choice of food and the patient's pattern of eating. However, it is important that these records are updated regularly and the findings are acted upon.

Physical Examination

A physical examination of the patient can also reveal nutritional deficiencies. Clinical signs associated with malnutrition are provided in Table 17-3. To confirm malnutrition, clinical findings need to be substantiated with laboratory tests and dietary information.

Body Measurements

Changes in body composition can be established by measuring certain parts of the body. These techniques are not routinely used in nursing practice but may be used if there is significant weight gain or loss. On such measurement used to determine fat stores is the **skinfold measurement**. The most common site for skinfold measurement is the triceps (the area at the back of the upper arm) skinfold. The fold of skin measured includes subcutaneous (fat) tissue but not the underlying muscle. It is measured in millimetres using special calipers. To measure the triceps skinfold (TSF), locate the midpoint of the upper arm, then

drinks like *Fortisip* and will need further monitoring to ensure there is no deterioration in the patient's nutritional state. Those patients considered to be at high risk will require a more detailed assessment and referral to a dietitian.

Patient History

As mentioned earlier, nurses obtain considerable patient information during the routine admission process. This information can indicate to the nurse if the patient may have

Table 17-3 Clinical Signs of Malnutrition

Area of examination	Signs associated with malnutrition
General appearance	Apathetic, listless, looks tired, easily fatigued
Weight	Overweight or underweight
Skin	Dry, flaky or scaly; pale or pigmented; presence of petechiae (bruising); lack of subcutaneous fat
Hair	Dry, dull, sparse, loss of colour, brittle
Eyes	Pale or red conjunctiva, dryness, soft cornea, dull cornea
Lips	Swollen, red cracks at side of mouth, vertical fissures
Tongue	Swollen, beefy red or magenta coloured; smooth appearance; decrease or increase in size
Gums	Spongy, swollen, inflamed; bleed easily
Muscles	Underdeveloped, flaccid, wasted, soft
Gastrointestinal system	Anorexia, indigestion, diarrhoea, constipation, enlarged liver
Nervous system	Decreased reflexes, sensory loss, burning and tingling of hands and feet, mental confusion or irritability

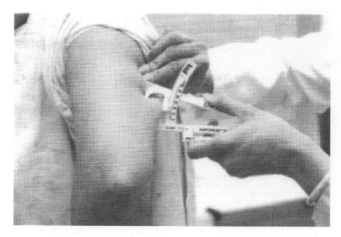

Figure 17-4 Measuring the triceps skinfold.

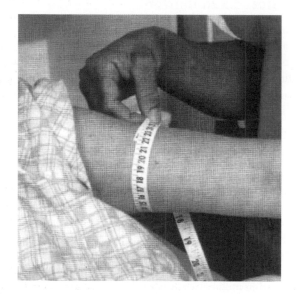

Figure 17-5 Measuring the mid-arm circumference.

grasp the skin on the back of the upper arm (see Figure 17-4). Placing the calipers 1 cm below the fingers, measure the thickness of the fold to the nearest millimetre.

The **midarm circumference (MAC)** is a measure of fat, muscle and skeleton. To measure the MAC, ask the patient to sit or stand with the arm hanging freely and the forearm flexed to horizontal. Measure the circumference at the midpoint of the arm, recording the measurement in centimetres, to the nearest millimetre (e.g. 24.6 cm) (see Figure 17-5).

Standard values for body measurements for adults are shown in Table 17-4.

Changes in body measurements often occur slowly and reflect chronic rather than acute changes in nutritional status. They are, therefore, used to monitor the patient's progress for months to years rather than days to weeks. Ideally, initial and subsequent measurements need to be taken by the same healthcare professional to ensure similar measurements, and measurements obtained need to be interpreted with caution.

Table 17-4 Standard Values for Anthropometric Measurements for Adults

Measurement	Male	Female
Triceps skinfold (mm)	12.5	16.5
Midarm circumference (cm)	29.3	28.5

Note: From *Nutrition Handbook for Nursing Practice*, 3rd edn (p. 239), by S.G. Dudek, 1997, Philadelphia: Lippincott. Adapted with permission.

Fluctuations in hydration status that often occur during illness can influence the accuracy of results. In addition, normal standards often do not account for normal changes in body composition such as those that occur with ageing.

Laboratory Data

Laboratory tests provide objective data to the nutritional assessments, but because many factors can influence these tests, no single test specifically predicts nutritional risk or measures the presence or degree of a nutritional problem. The tests most commonly used are serum proteins, urinary urea nitrogen and creatinine, and total lymphocyte count.

Serum Proteins

Serum protein (proteins in the plasma) levels provide an estimate of protein stores within the body. Tests commonly include haemoglobin, albumin and transferrin. **Haemoglobin** is a complex protein-iron compound that is found in red blood cells and carries oxygen from the lungs to the tissues. A low haemoglobin level may be evidence of iron deficiency anaemia (shortage of red blood cells caused by iron deficiency). However, iron deficiencies can be caused by an insufficiency in the diet but it may also be caused by blood loss and some illnesses such as gastrointestinal cancer.

Albumin, a protein made in the liver which is found in blood and maintains blood volume, accounts for more than 50% of the total serum proteins (proteins in the blood), has been traditionally used as an indicator of nutritional status (Gupta *et al.*, 2004). However albumin can be affected by nonnutritional factors (Gupta *et al.*, 2004) such as altered liver function, hydration and albumin losses from wounds and burns. Also albumin is not broken down very quickly in the body which makes it difficult to assess short-term nutritional problems (Gupta *et al.*, 2004).

Another protein traditionally used as part of nutritional assessment is **transferrin** which is a protein that binds and carries iron from the intestine through the blood. Transferrin is broken down much quicker than albumin therefore if the patient has a poor nutritional status testing for transferrin will show a more accurate picture of short-term nutritional problems. Transferrin levels below normal indicate protein loss, iron deficiency anaemia, pregnancy, hepatitis and liver dysfunction.

Prealbumin, also referred to as thyroxine-binding albumin and transthyretin, is the best indicator of nutritional deficiencies as it is broken down the quickest within the body. However this test is rarely performed in the UK as a result of its cost.

Urinary Tests

Certain urine tests can be performed to measure the breakdown (catabolism) of proteins within the body. These tests include urinary urea nitrogen and urinary creatinine. **Urea** is a waste product of protein metabolism which is excreted in urine. Urea concentrations in the blood and urine, therefore, directly reflect the intake and breakdown of dietary protein, the rate of urea production in the liver, and the rate of urea removal by the kidneys.

Creatinine, which is also a waste product of protein metabolism which is excreted in urine, is an indicator of a person's total muscle mass. The greater the muscle mass, the greater the excretion of creatinine. As skeletal muscle atrophies during malnutrition, creatinine excretion decreases. Urinary creatinine is also influenced by protein intake, exercise, age, renal function and thyroid function.

Total Lymphocyte Count

Certain nutrient deficiencies and forms of protein energy malnutrition (PEM) can depress the immune system. The total number of lymphocytes decreases as protein depletion occurs.

PLANNING

Major goals for patients with or at risk for nutritional problems include:

+ Maintain or restore optimal nutritional status.
+ Promote healthy nutritional practices.
+ Prevent complications associated with malnutrition.
+ Decrease weight.
+ Regain specified weight.
+ Prevent associated risks (tissue breakdown).

Obviously, goals will vary according to the diagnosis and defining characteristics for each individual. Appropriate preventive and corrective nursing interventions that relate to these must be identified.

IMPLEMENTING

Nursing interventions to promote optimal nutrition for patients are often provided in collaboration with the multidisciplinary team. The nurse's role is to create an atmosphere that encourages eating, provide assistance with eating, monitor the patient's appetite and food intake, administer enteral and parenteral feedings, and consults with the multidisciplinary team about nutritional problems that arise.

Assisting with Special Diets

Some patients require changes to their diet. This may be due to a disease process such as diabetes mellitus, to increase or decrease weight, to restore nutritional deficits or to allow an organ to rest and promote healing. Diets can be modified in a number of ways including: change in texture, change in amount of calories in food, specific nutrients, seasonings and consistency.

It is important to include the patient in any decisions made regarding diet alterations as they are more likely to concord with the treatment if their needs and wishes have been considered.

Stimulating an Appetite

Physical illness, unfamiliar or unpalatable food, environmental and psychological factors, and physical discomfort or pain may depress the appetites of many patients. A short-term decrease in food intake usually is not a problem for adults; over time, however, it leads to weight loss, decreased strength and stamina, and other nutritional problems. A decreased food intake is often accompanied by a decrease in fluid intake, which may cause fluid and electrolyte problems. Stimulating a person's appetite requires the nurse to determine the reason for the lack of appetite and then deal with the problem. Some interventions for improving the patient's appetite are summarised in *Box 17-3* on page 422.

Assisting Patients with Eating

Within most healthcare environments, meals are brought to the patient either at the bedside or in a day room facility. Some hospitals provide hostesses who serve the food to the patient while in other hospitals the food is served onto plates in a central kitchen, delivered to the wards/units by porters and served to the patient by nursing and support staff. Guidelines for providing meals to patients are summarised in *Box 17-4* on page 422.

As part of the assessment process it is important to identify any actual or potential problems that could affect nutritional intake, such as patients with disabilities that affect their hands, e.g. arthritis. The nursing care plan should indicate the type of assistance the patient requires at mealtimes.

When nursing a patient who has difficulties with eating, it is important that the nurse is sensitive to the patient's feelings. Often they may feel embarrassment, resentment, loss of autonomy and can become depressed as a result of needing help with eating. Whenever possible, it is important that the nurse helps those patients who may have difficulties with eating to feed themselves rather than feed them. Although feeding a patient is time consuming, nurses should try to appear unhurried and convey that they have ample time. Sitting at the bedside is one way to convey this impression.

When feeding a patient, ask in which order the patient would like to eat the food. If the patient cannot see, tell the patient which food is being given. Always allow ample time for the patient to chew and swallow the food before offering more. Also, provide fluids as requested or, if the patient is unable to

BOX 17-3 Improving Appetite

+ Provide familiar food that the person likes. Often the relatives of patients are pleased to bring food from home but may need some guidance about special diet requirements.
+ Select small portions rather than larger portions as this can be daunting for the patient with very little appetite.
+ Avoid unpleasant or uncomfortable treatments immediately before or after a meal.
+ Provide a tidy, clean environment that is free of unpleasant sights and odours. A soiled dressing, a used bedpan, an uncovered irrigation set or even used dishes can negatively affect the appetite.
+ Encourage or provide oral hygiene before mealtime. This improves the patient's ability to taste.
+ Relieve illness symptoms that depress appetite before mealtime; for example, give an analgesic for pain or an antipyretic for a fever or allow rest for fatigue.
+ Reduce psychological stress. A lack of understanding of therapy, the anticipation of an operation and fear of the unknown can cause anorexia. Often, the nurse can help by discussing feelings with the patient, giving information and assistance, and allaying fears.

BOX 17-4 Providing Patient Meals

+ Offer the patient help with hand washing and oral hygiene before a meal.
+ Most people sit during a meal; if the patient's condition permits, assist them into a comfortable position in bed or in a chair, whichever is appropriate.
+ Ensure that the correct meal is served to the patient; this is particularly important for patients on specific diets such as those with diabetes.
+ If the patient is blind, it is useful to identify the placement of food as you would describe the time on a clock (see Figure 17-6). For instance, the nurse might say, 'The potatoes are at eight o'clock, the chicken at 12 o'clock and the green beans at 4 o'clock.'
+ Following mealtime observe how much and what the patient has eaten and the amount of fluid taken. Record fluid intake and quantity of food eaten as required.
+ If the patient is on a special diet or is having problems eating, record the amount of food eaten and any pain, fatigue or nausea experienced.
+ If the patient is not eating, document this so that changes can be made, such as rescheduling the meals, providing smaller, more frequent meals or obtaining special self-feeding aids.

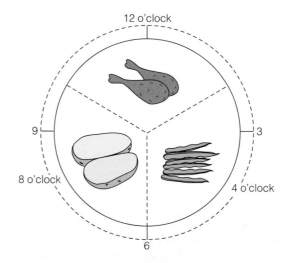

Figure 17-6 For a patient who is blind, the nurse can use the clock system to describe the location of food on the plate.

communicate, offer fluids after every three or four mouthfuls of solid food.

Although normal utensils should be used whenever possible, special utensils may be needed to assist a patient to eat. For patients who have difficulty drinking from a cup or glass, a straw often permits them to obtain liquids with less effort and less spillage although straws should not be used for patients with swallowing difficulties. Special drinking cups are also available. One model has a spout; another is specially designed to permit drinking with less tipping of the cup than is normally required.

Many adaptive feeding aids are available to help patient maintain independence including knives, forks and spoons with widened handles, plates with rims and plastic or metal plate guards enable the patient to pick up the food by first pushing it against this raised edge. Figures 17-7 and 17-8 show some of these aids.

Enteral Nutrition

Enteral nutrition (through the gastrointestinal system) is an alternative feeding method to ensure adequate nutrition. Enteral nutrition (EN) is provided when the patient is unable to ingest foods or the upper gastrointestinal tract is impaired and the transport of food to the small intestine is interrupted. Enteral feedings are administered through nasogastric and small-bore feeding tubes or through gastrostomy or jejunostomy tubes.

A **nasogastric tube** is inserted through one of the nostrils, down the nasopharynx, and into the alimentary tract. Nasogastric

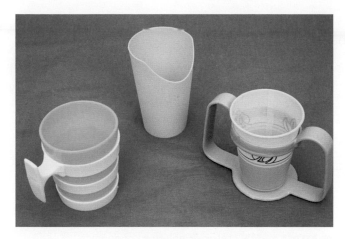

Figure 17-7 Left to right: glass holder, cup with hole for nose, two-handled cup holder.

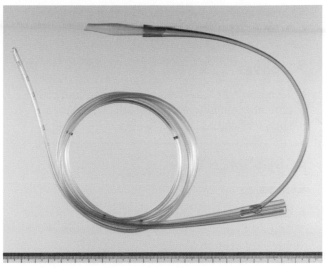

A

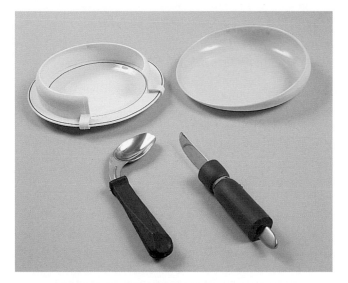

Figure 17-8 Dinner plate with guard attached and lipped plate facilitate scooping; wide-handled spoon and knife facilitate grip.

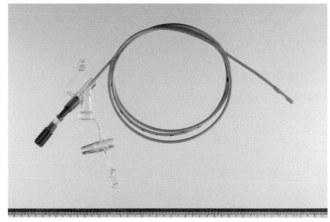

B

Figure 17-9 Left: Wide bore nasogastric tube (from http://www.yuyumedical.com/medidis1.asp). Right: fine bore nasogastric tube with stylet and Y-Port connector for administration of medication (from http://www.silmag.com/Imagenes/Productos/394_c.jpg).

tubes are available in a number of different sizes and designs, the choice of which should be based on the patient's needs. Traditional firm, large-bore nasogastric tubes (i.e. those larger than 12 Fr in diameter) are placed in the stomach and should be considered for short-term use whereas the softer, more flexible and less irritating small bore tubes (smaller than 12 Fr in diameter) should be considered for longer-term use (see Figure 17-9).

Nasogastric tubes are used for patients who have intact gag and cough reflexes, who have adequate gastric emptying, and who require short-term feedings. It is important to note that in some trusts nurses are not allowed to insert nasogastric tubes without further training. *Procedure 17-1* on page 424 provides guidelines for inserting a nasogastric tube. *Procedure 17-2* on page 426 outlines the steps for removing a nasogastric tube.

CLINICAL ANECDOTE

Making sure patients are adequately nourished is important. I don't particularly like inserting nasogastric tubes and I'm sure the patients don't particularly like it. How- ever, I know that the patient needs it so I feel that it's for the best.
Anonymous ward nurse, Swansea

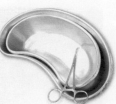

PROCEDURE 17-1 Inserting a Nasogastric Tube

Purposes

+ To administer tube feedings and medications to patients unable to eat by mouth or swallow a sufficient diet

+ To establish a means for suctioning stomach contents to prevent gastric distention, nausea and vomiting

ASSESSMENT

Assess

+ Check patency of nostrils and intactness of nasal tissues. Check for history of nasal surgery or deviated septum.

+ Determine presence of gag reflex.
+ Assess mental status or ability to cooperate with procedure.

PLANNING

Before inserting a nasogastric tube, determine the size of tube to be inserted and whether or not the tube is to be attached to a free drainage bag.

Equipment

+ Large- or small-bore tube
+ Guidewire or stylet for small-bore tube
+ Nonallergenic adhesive tape
+ Clean gloves
+ Water-soluble lubricant
+ Tissues
+ Glass of water
+ 50 ml catheter tip syringe
+ Receiver
+ pH indicator strips
+ Stethoscope
+ Disposable pad or towel
+ Free drainage bag if required.
+ Spigot

IMPLEMENTATION

Preparation

Assist the patient to a sitting position if their condition permits. *It is often easier to swallow in this position and gravity helps the passage of the tube.*

Place a towel or disposable pad across the chest.

Performance

1. Explain to the patient what you plan to do. The passage of a gastric tube is not painful, but it is unpleasant because the gag reflex is activated during insertion. Establish a method for the patient to indicate distress and a desire for you to pause the insertion. Raising a finger or hand is often used for this.
2. Wash hands and observe other appropriate infection control procedures (e.g. clean gloves and apron).
3. Provide for patient privacy.
4. Assess the patient's nostrils.
   - Ask the patient to hyperextend the head and, using a flashlight, observe the intactness of the tissues of the nostrils, including any irritations or abrasions.
   - Examine the nostrils for any obstructions or deformities by asking the patient to breathe through one nostril while occluding the other.
   - Select the nostril that has the greater airflow.
5. Determine how far to insert the tube.
   - Use the tube to mark off the distance from the tip of the patient's nose to the tip of the earlobe and then from the tip of the earlobe to the tip of the xiphoid (see Figure 17-10). *This length approximates the distance from the nostril to the stomach. This distance varies among individuals.*
   - Note this length on the tubes graduated marks.
6. Insert the tube.
   - Put on gloves.
   - Lubricate the tip of the tube well with water-soluble lubricant or water to ease insertion. A water-soluble lubricant dissolves if the tube accidentally enters the lungs. An oil-based lubricant, such as petroleum jelly, will not dissolve and could cause respiratory complications if it enters the lungs.

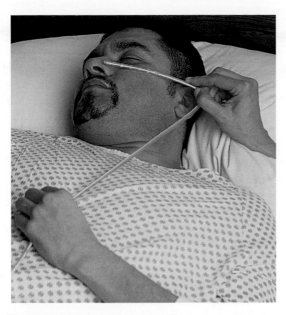

Figure 17-10 Measuring the appropriate length to insert a nasogastric tube.

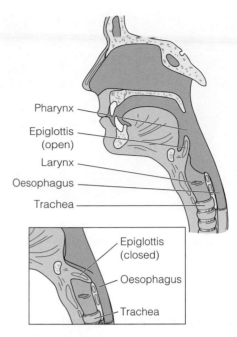

Pharynx
Epiglottis (open)
Larynx
Oesophagus
Trachea

Epiglottis (closed)
Oesophagus
Trachea

Figure 17-11 Swallowing closes the epiglottis.

- Insert the tube, with its natural curve toward the patient, into the selected nostril. Ask the patient to hyperextend the neck, and gently advance the tube toward the nasopharynx. *Hyperextension of the neck reduces the curvature of the nasopharyngeal junction.*
- Direct the tube along the floor of the nostril and toward the ear on that side.
- Slight pressure is sometimes required to pass the tube into the nasopharynx and some patients' eyes may water at this point. *Tears are a natural body response.* Provide the patient with tissues as needed.
- If the tube meets resistance, withdraw it, relubricate it and insert it in the other nostril. *The tube should never be forced against resistance because of the danger of injury.*
- Once the tube reaches the oropharynx (throat), the patient will feel the tube in the throat and may gag and retch. Ask the patient to tilt the head forward, and encourage the patient to drink and swallow. *Tilting the head forward facilitates passage of the tube into the posterior pharynx and oesophagus rather than into the larynx; swallowing moves the epiglottis over the opening to the larynx* (see Figure 17-11).
- If the patient gags, stop passing the tube momentarily. Have the patient rest, take a few breaths and take sips of water to calm the gag reflex.
- In cooperation with the patient, pass the tube 5–10 cm with each swallow, until the indicated length is inserted.

- If the patient continues to gag and the tube does not advance with each swallow, withdraw it slightly, and inspect the throat by looking through the mouth. *The tube may be coiled in the throat.* If so, withdraw it until it is straight, and try again to insert it.

7. Ascertain correct placement of the tube according to local policy.
   - Aspirate stomach contents, and check the pH, which should be acidic.
   - Depending on local policy the position of the tube can be checked by x-ray. However this should not be routinely performed. It is important when using a small-bore tube that the guidewire is left in place when x-ray is performed.
   - If the signs do not indicate placement in the stomach, advance the tube 5 cm, and repeat the tests.

8. Secure the tube by taping it to the bridge of the patient's nose.
   - If the patient has oily skin, wipe the nose first with alcohol.
   - Cut 7.5 cm of tape, and split it lengthwise at one end, leaving a 2.5 cm tab at the end.
   - Place the tape over the bridge of the patient's nose, and bring the split ends either under and around the tubing, or under the tubing and back up over the nose (see Figure 17-12 on page 426). *Taping in this manner prevents the tube from pressing against and irritating the edge of the nostril.*

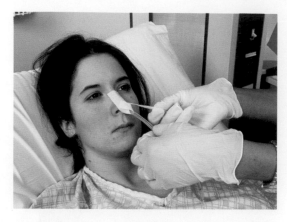

Figure 17-12 Taping a nasogastric tube to the bridge of the nose.

9. Attach the tube to the feeding apparatus or free drainage as required as ordered, or clamp the end of the tubing.
10. Document relevant information: the insertion of the tube, the means by which correct placement was determined and patient responses (e.g. discomfort or abdominal distention).
11. Establish a plan for providing daily nasogastric tube care.
    - Inspect the nostril for discharge and irritation.
    - Clean the nostril and tube.
    - Apply water-soluble lubricant to the nostril if it appears dry or encrusted.
    - Change the adhesive tape as required.
    - Give frequent mouth care as the patient may breathe through the mouth.

EVALUATION

The patient's tolerance of the nasogastric tube, the correct placement of the nasogastric tube in the stomach, the patient's understanding of restrictions, the colour and amount of gastric contents if attached to free drainage, or the stomach contents aspirated, needs to be regularly evaluated according to local policy.

PROCEDURE 17-2 Removing a Nasogastric Tube

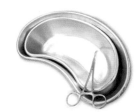

ASSESSMENT

Assess

+ For the presence of bowel sounds.

+ For the absence of nausea or vomiting when tube is clamped.

PLANNING

Equipment

+ Disposable pad
+ Tissues
+ Clean gloves

+ 50 ml syringe (optional)
+ Clinical waste bag

IMPLEMENTATION

Preparation

+ Ensure that patient's condition permits removal of nasogastric tube.
+ Assist the patient to a sitting position if condition permits.
+ Place the disposable pad across the patient's chest to collect any spillage of mucous and gastric secretions from the tube.
+ Provide tissues to the patient to wipe the nose and mouth after tube removal.

Performance

1. Explain to the patient what you are going to do, why it is necessary and how they can cooperate. Explain that the procedure will cause no discomfort.
2. Wash hands and observe other appropriate infection control procedures (e.g. clean gloves and apron).
3. Provide for patient privacy.

4. Detach the tube.
   - Disconnect the nasogastric tube from the feeding apparatus.
   - Remove the adhesive tape securing the tube to the nose.
5. Remove the nasogastric tube.
   - Put on disposable gloves.
   - Ask the patient to take a deep breath and to hold it. *This closes the glottis, thereby preventing accidental aspiration of any gastric contents.*
   - Pinch the tube with the gloved hand. *Pinching the tube prevents any contents inside the tube from draining into the patient's throat.*
   - Quickly and smoothly withdraw the tube.
   - Place the tube in the clinical waste bag. *Placing the tube immediately into the bag prevents the transference of micro-organisms from the tube to other articles or people.*
   - Observe the intactness of the tube.
6. Ensure patient comfort.
   - Provide mouth care if desired.
   - Assist the patient as required to blow the nose. *Excessive secretions may have accumulated in the nasal passages.*
7. Dispose of the equipment appropriately.
8. Document all relevant information.
   - Record the removal of the tube, the amount and appearance of any drainage and any relevant assessments of the patient.

EVALUATION

✚ Perform a follow-up examination, such as presence of bowel sounds, absence of nausea or vomiting when tube is removed, and intactness of tissues of the nostrils.

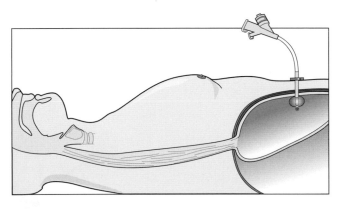

Figure 17-13 Percutaneous endoscopic gastrostomy (PEG) tube.

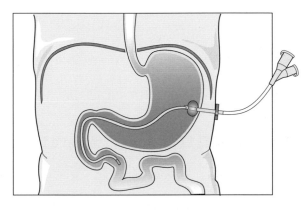

Figure 17-14 Percutaneous endoscopic jejunostomy (PEJ) tube.

Gastrostomy and **jejunostomy** devices are used for long-term nutritional support, generally more than 6–8 weeks. Conventional tubes are placed surgically or by laparoscopy through the abdominal wall into the stomach (gastrostomy) or into the jejunum (jejunostomy).

A **percutaneous endoscopic gastrostomy (PEG)** (see Figure 17-13) or **percutaneous endoscopic jejunostomy (PEJ)** (see Figure 17-14) is created by using an endoscope to visualise the inside of the stomach, making a puncture through the skin and subcutaneous tissues of the abdomen into the stomach, and inserting the PEG or PEJ catheter through the puncture. The catheter has internal and external bumpers and an inflatable retention balloon to maintain placement. Once the opening has healed, replacement tubes can be inserted without the use of endoscopy.

Enteral Feedings

The frequency of feedings and amounts to be administered are usually prescribed by the doctor or dietician. Liquid feeding mixtures are available commercially or may be prepared by the dietary department in accordance with the patient's individual needs. A standard formula provides protein, fat, carbohydrate, minerals and vitamins in specified proportions.

Enteral feedings can be given intermittently or continuously. Intermittent feedings are the administration of 300–500 ml of enteral formula several times per day. The stomach is the preferred site for these feedings, which are usually administered over at least 30 minutes. Bolus intermittent feedings are those that use a syringe to deliver the formula into the stomach. Because the formula is delivered rapidly by this method, it is not usually recommended but may be used in long-term situations if the patient tolerates them. These feedings must be given only into the stomach; the patient must be monitored closely for distention and aspiration.

Continuous feedings are generally administered over a 24-hour period using an infusion pump that guarantees a constant flow rate (see Figure 17-15). Continuous feedings are essential when feedings are administered in the small bowel. They are also used when smaller bore gastric tubes are in place or when gravity flow is insufficient to instil the feeding.

Cyclic feedings are continuous feedings that are administered in less than 24 hours (e.g. 12–16 hours). These feedings, often administered at night and referred to as nocturnal feedings, allow the patient to attempt to eat regular meals through the day. Because nocturnal feedings may use higher nutrient densities and higher infusion rates than the standard continuous feeding, particular attention needs to be given to monitoring fluid status and circulating volume overload.

Procedure 17-3 provides the essential steps involved in administering a tube feeding, and *Procedure 17-4* on page 430 indicates the steps involved in administering a gastrostomy or jejunostomy tube feeding.

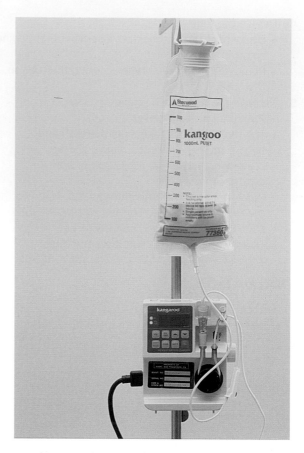

Figure 17-15 An enteric feeding pump.

PROCEDURE 17-3 Administering a Continuous Tube Feed

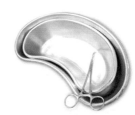

Purposes

+ To restore or maintain nutritional and hydration status

ASSESSMENT

Assess

+ For any clinical signs of malnutrition or dehydration.
+ Check for allergies to any food in the feeding.
+ For the presence of bowel sounds.

+ Note any problems that suggest lack of tolerance of previous feedings (e.g. delayed gastric emptying, abdominal distention, constipation or dehydration).

PLANNING

Before commencing a nasogastric feed, determine the type, amount and frequency of feedings and tolerance of previous feedings.

Equipment

+ Correct amount of feeding solution
+ Receiver
+ Clean gloves
+ pH test strip
+ Water (at room temperature)
+ Feeding pump as required

IMPLEMENTATION

Preparation

Assist the patient to sitting position in a bed or a chair, the normal position for eating. However if the patient cannot sit up they should be placed with their head tilted upwards at a 30-40 degree angle. *These positions enhance the gravitational flow of the solution and prevent aspiration of fluid into the lungs.*

Performance

1. Explain to the patient what you are going to do, why it is necessary and how they can cooperate. Inform the patient that the feeding should not cause any discomfort but may cause a feeling of fullness.
2. Wash hands and observe appropriate infection control procedures (e.g. clean gloves).
3. Provide privacy for this procedure if the patient desires it.
4. Assess tube placement.
   - Check graduations on the nasogastric tube.
   - Ensure that there are no signs that the tube has been dislodged such as coughing, gagging, retching.
5. Assess residual feeding contents.
   - Aspirate all stomach contents and measure the amount before administering the feeding. *This is done to evaluate absorption of the last feeding; that is, whether undigested formula from a previous feeding remains.*
   - If 100 ml (or more than half the last feeding) is withdrawn, check with the nurse in charge or refer to local policy before proceeding.
   - Reinstil the gastric contents into the stomach if this is the local policy. *Removal of the contents could disturb the patient's electrolyte balance.*
   - If the patient is on a continuous feeding regimen, check the gastric residual every 4-6 hours or according to local protocol.
6. Administer the feeding.
   - Before administering feeding: check the expiration date of the feeding; and warm the feeding to room temperature. *An excessively cold feeding may cause cramps.*
   - Remove the screw-on cap from the container and attach the administration set with the drip chamber and tubing (see Figure 17-16).
   - Close the clamp on the tubing.
   - Hang the container on an intravenous pole about 30 cm above the tube's insertion point into the patient. *At this height, the formula should run at a safe rate into the stomach or intestine.*

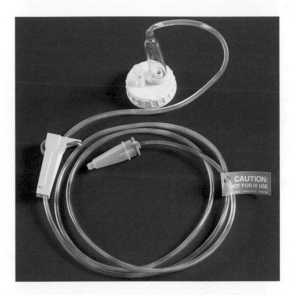

Figure 17-16 Feeding set tubing with drip chamber. (Ross Products Division, Abbott Laboratories. Used with permission.)

   - Squeeze the drip chamber to fill it to one-third to one-half of its capacity.
   - Open the tubing clamp, run the formula through the tubing, and reclamp the tube. *The formula will displace the air in the tubing, thus preventing the instillation of excess air.*
   - Attach the feeding set tubing to the feeding tube and regulate the drip rate to deliver the feeding over the desired length of time.
7. Rinse the feeding tube immediately before all of the formula has run through the tubing.
   - Instil water through the feeding tube according to prescription. Water flushes the lumen of the tube, preventing future blockage by sticky formula.
8. Ensure patient comfort and safety.
   - Ask the patient to remain sitting upright in sitting position or in a slightly elevated right lateral position for at least 30 minutes. *These positions facilitate digestion and movement of the feeding from the stomach along the alimentary tract, and prevent the potential aspiration of the feeding into the lungs.*
   - Check local policy on the frequency of changing the nasogastric tube and the use of smaller lumen tubes if a large-bore tube is in place. *These measures prevent irritation and erosion of the pharyngeal and oesophageal mucous membranes.*

9. Dispose of equipment appropriately.
   • Change the equipment every 24 hours or according to local policy.
10. Document all relevant information.
    • Document the amount of gastric contents aspirated, the amount and kind of feed given, duration of the feeding and assessments of the patient.

   • Record the volume of the feeding and water administered on the patient's intake and output record.
12. Monitor the patient for possible problems.
    • Carefully assess patients receiving tube feedings for problems.
    • To prevent dehydration, give the patient supplemental water in addition to the prescribed tube feeding as ordered.

EVALUATION

Perform a follow-up examination of the following:

+ Tolerance of feeding
+ Regurgitation and feelings of fullness after feedings
+ Weight gain or loss
+ Faecal elimination pattern (e.g. diarrhoea, flatulence, constipation)

+ Skin turgor
+ Urine output

Relate findings to previous assessment data if available. Report significant changes.

PROCEDURE 17-4 Administering a Gastrostomy or Jejunostomy Feeding

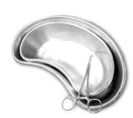

Purposes

See *Procedure 17-3* on page 428.

ASSESSMENT

See *Procedure 17-3* on page 428.

PLANNING

Before commencing a gastrostomy or jejunostomy feeding, determine the type and amount of feeding to be instilled, frequency of feedings and any pertinent information about previous feedings (e.g. the positioning which the patient best tolerates the feeding).

Equipment

+ Pump
+ Appropriate giving set
+ 50 ml syringe
+ Sterile water
+ Cap

IMPLEMENTATION:

Preparation

See *Procedure 17-3* on page 428.

Performance

1. Explain to the patient what you are going to do, why it is necessary and how they can cooperate.
2. Wash hands and observe other appropriate infection control procedures.

3. Provide for patient privacy.
4. Assess and prepare the patient. See *Procedure 17-3* on page 428.
5. Check the patency of a tube.
   • Administering 50 ml of sterile water via the tube.
   • If the water does not flow freely, notify the nurse in charge and/or physician.

7. Check for residual formula, if required by local policy.
   - Attach the syringe to the end of the feeding tube, and withdraw and measure the stomach or jejunal contents.
   - For continuous feedings, check the residual every 4-6 hours and hold feedings according to local policy. The doctor and/or dietician should be notified if a large residual persists.

8. Administer the feeding.
   - Before administering feeding: check the expiration date of the feeding; and warm the feeding to room temperature. *An excessively cold feeding may cause cramps.*
   - Remove the screw-on cap from the container and attach the administration set with the drip chamber and tubing.
   - Close the clamp on the tubing.
   - Hang the container on an intravenous pole about 30 cm above the tube's insertion point into the patient. *At this height, the formula should run at a safe rate into the stomach or intestine.*
   - Squeeze the drip chamber to fill it to one-third to one-half of its capacity.
   - Open the tubing clamp, run the formula through the tubing, and reclamp the tube. *The formula will displace the air in the tubing, thus preventing the instillation of excess air.*
   - Attach the feeding set tubing to the feeding tube and regulate the drip rate to deliver the feeding over the desired length of time.

9. Ensure patient comfort and safety.
   - After the feeding, ask the patient to remain in the sitting position or head is elevated at 30-40 degrees for at least 30 minutes. *This minimises the risk of aspiration.*

- Assess status of peristomal skin. Gastric or jejunal drainage contains digestive enzymes that can irritate the skin. Document any redness and broken skin areas.
- Check orders about cleaning the peristomal skin, applying a skin protectant and applying appropriate dressings. Generally, the peristomal skin is washed with mild soap and water at least once daily.
- Observe for common complications of enteral feedings: aspiration, hyperglycemia, abdominal distention, diarrhoea and faecal impaction. Report findings to the doctor and/or dietician. Often, a change in formula or rate of administration can correct problems.
- When appropriate, teach the patient how to administer feedings and when to notify the healthcare provider concerning problems.

VARIATION: PERCUTANEOUS ENDOSCOPIC GASTROSTOMY (PEG)

A PEG is kept in place with a short crosspiece or bolster near the skin level at the stoma.

- Clean the stoma daily with soap and water using a cotton swab or small piece of gauze in a circular motion.
- Rotate the tube 360° and clean the skin under it.
- After cleaning, allow the skin to air dry.
- Report any signs of redness, pain, soreness, swelling or drainage to the healthcare provider.
- Do not apply a dressing over the PEG. *A dressing and tape may result in skin excoriation and breakdown.*

10. Document all assessments and interventions.

EVALUATION

See *Procedure 17-3* on page 428.

Before administering a tube feeding, the nurse must determine any food allergies of the patient and assess tolerance to previous feedings. Table 17-5 on page 432 lists essential assessments to conduct before administering tube feedings. The nurse must also check the expiration date on a commercially prepared formula or the preparation date and time of locally-prepared solution, discarding any formula that has passed the expiration date or solution more than 24 hours old.

Parenteral Nutrition

Parenteral nutrition (PN), also referred to as total parenteral nutrition (TPN), is provided when the gastrointestinal tract is non-functional because of an interruption in its continuity or because its absorptive capacity is impaired. **Parenteral** nutrition is administered intravenously such as through a central venous catheter into the superior vena cava.

Table 17-5 Assessing Patients Receiving Tube Feedings

Assessments	Rationale
Allergies to any food in the feeding	Common allergenic foods include milk, sugar, water, eggs and vegetable oil.
Bowel sounds before each feeding or, for continuous feedings, every 4–8 hours	To determine intestinal activity.
Correct placement of tube, before feedings	To prevent aspiration of feedings
Presence of regurgitation and feelings of fullness after feedings	May indicate delayed gastric emptying, need to decrease quantity or rate of the feeding, or high fat content of the formula.
Abdominal distention, at least daily. Measure abdominal girth at the umbilicus	Abdominal distention may indicate intolerance to a previous feeding.
Diarrhoea, constipation or flatulence	The lack of bulk in liquid feedings may cause constipation. The presence of hypertonic or concentrated ingredients may cause diarrhoea and flatulence.
Urine for sugar and acetone	Hyperglycaemia may occur if the sugar content is too high.
Haematocrit	Increases as a result of dehydration.

Parenteral feedings are solutions of dextrose, water, fat, proteins, electrolytes, vitamins and trace elements; they provide all needed calories. Because TPN solutions are hypertonic (highly concentrated in comparison to the solute concentration of blood), they are injected only into high-flow central veins, where they are diluted by the patient's blood.

TPN is a means of giving nutrition and fluid to patient such as those with severe malnutrition, severe burns, bowel disease disorders (e.g. ulcerative colitis or enteric fistula), acute renal failure, hepatic failure, metastatic cancer, or major surgeries where nothing may be taken by mouth for more than five days.

TPN is not risk free. Infection control is of utmost importance during TPN therapy. The nurse must always observe surgical aseptic technique when changing solutions, tubing, dressings and filters. Patients are at increased risk of fluid, electrolyte and glucose imbalances, and require frequent evaluation and modification of the TPN mixture.

Enteral or parenteral feedings may be continued beyond hospital care in the patient's home or may be initiated in the home.

Food and water are vital in maintaining life and are essential elements of care (RCN, 2007). A new clinical campaign launched by the Royal College of Nursing (2007) sets out guidelines for nurses working with patients with or without nutritional problems, clearly stating that all members of the nursing team are responsible for assessing, planning, implementing and evaluating the nutritional needs of patients.

CRITICAL REFLECTION

Let us revisit the case study on page 411. Now that you have read this chapter how would you assess a patient who looks underweight? What information would you give this patient and their family?

CHAPTER HIGHLIGHTS

+ Although people are bombarded with information about what to eat and what not to eat, each person is responsible for selecting foods that provide essential nutrients. Nurses assist people to evaluate the information they receive about nutrients.

+ Essential nutrients are grouped into six categories: water, carbohydrates, fats, proteins, vitamins and minerals.

+ Nutrients serve three basic purposes: forming body structures (such as bones and blood), providing energy, and helping to regulate the body's biochemical reactions.

+ Energy balance is the relationship between the energy derived from food and the energy used by the body.

+ The amount of energy that nutrients or foods supply to the body is their caloric value.

+ A person's state of energy balance can be determined by comparing caloric intake with caloric expenditure.

+ Body mass index (BMI) or percentage body fat are indicators of changes in body fat stores, whether a person's weight is appropriate for height, and may provide a useful estimate of nutrition.

+ Factors influencing a person's nutrition include development, gender, ethnicity and culture, beliefs about foods, personal preferences, religious practices, lifestyle, medications and medical therapy, health status, alcohol abuse, advertising, and psychological factors such as stress, isolation and depression.

+ Nutritional needs vary considerably according to age, growth and energy requirements. Adolescents have high energy requirements due to their rapid growth. Middle-aged adults and older adults often need to reduce their caloric intake because of decreases in metabolic rate and activity levels.

+ A well-balanced diet includes a healthy balance of the different food groups and fluid. The tilted plate can show the patient the correct portions of the different food groups. The vegetarian tilted plate can be used for all types of vegetarians.

+ Both inadequate and excessive intakes of nutrients result in malnutrition. The effects of malnutrition can be general or specific, depending on which nutrients and what level of deficiency or excess are involved.

+ Some of the long-range effects of certain nutrient excesses are among the many factors involved in certain diseases, such as coronary artery disease and cancer.

+ Assessment of nutritional status may involve all or some of the following: patient history, nutritional screening, physical examination, calculation of the percentage of weight loss, a dietary history, anthropometric measurements and laboratory tests.

+ Major goals for patients with or at risk for nutritional problems include the following: maintain or restore optimal nutritional status, decrease or regain specified weight, promote healthy nutritional practices and prevent complications associated with malnutrition.

+ Assisting and supporting patients with therapeutic diets is a function shared by the nurse and the dietitian. The nurse reinforces the dietitian's instructions, assists the patient to make beneficial changes and evaluates the patient's response to planned changes.

+ Because many hospitalised patients have poor appetites, a major responsibility of the nurse is to provide nursing interventions that stimulate their appetites.

+ Whenever possible, the nurse should help incapacitated patients to feed themselves; a number of self-feeding aids help patients who have difficulty handling regular utensils.

+ Enteral feedings, administered through nasogastric, nasointestinal, gastrostomy or jejunostomy tubes, are provided when the patient is unable to ingest foods or the upper gastrointestinal tract is impaired.

+ A nasogastric or nasointestinal tube is used to provide enteral nutrition for short-term use (less than six weeks) while a gastrostomy or jejunostomy tube can be used to supply nutrients via the enteral route for long-term use.

+ Parenteral nutrition (PN), provided when the gastrointestinal tract is nonfunctional (e.g. absorptive capacity impaired), is given intravenously into a large central vein (e.g. the superior vena cava).

REFERENCES

BAPEN (2003) *The Malnutrition Universal Screening Tool.* Available from http://www.bapen.org.uk/the-must.htm.

DoH (Department of Health) (1991) *Dietary reference values for food energy and nutrients for the UK. Report of the Panel on Dietary Reference Values of the Committee on Medical Aspects of Food Policy*, London: HMSO.

Dudek, S.G. (1997) *Nutrition handbook for nursing practice* (3rd edn), Philadelphia: Lippincott.

Gupta, D., Lis, C.G., Dahlk, S.L., Vashi, P.G., Grutsch, J.F. and Lammerfeld, C.A. (2004) 'Biochemical impedence phase angle as a prognostic indicator in advanced pancreatic cancer', *British Journal of Nutrition*, 92, 957–962.

Hogston, R. and Simpson, P.M. (Eds) (2002) *Foundations of nursing practice: Making the difference*, Basingstoke: Palgrave Macmillan.

RCN (2007) *Nutrition now*, London: RCN. Available from http://www2.rcn.org.uk/campaigns/nutritionnow. (Accessed on 30 April 2007.)

Viner, R. and Booy, R. (2005) 'Epidemiology of health and illness', *British Medical Journal*, 330, 411–414.

Walters, E. (1998) 'Know how: Nutritional assessment', *Nursing Times*, 94(8), 68–69.

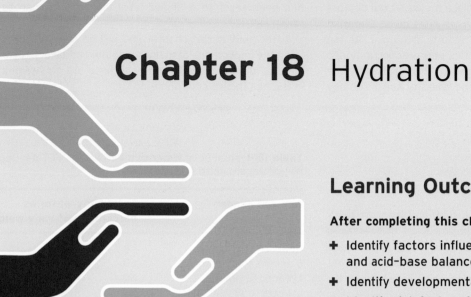

Chapter 18 Hydration

Learning Outcomes

After completing this chapter, you will be able to:

+ Identify factors influencing hydration, electrolyte and acid-base balance.

+ Identify developmental hydration considerations.

+ Identify risk factors for and clinical signs of dehydration.

+ Describe nursing interventions to alter fluid, electrolyte or acid-base imbalances.

+ Teach patients measures to maintain fluid and electrolyte balance.

+ Implement measures to correct imbalances of fluids and electrolytes or acids and bases such as enteral or parenteral replacements.

+ Evaluate the effect of nursing interventions on the patient's fluid, electrolyte or acid-base balance.

CASE STUDY

In 2005, a West Midlands couple were convicted of killing their three-year-old foster son Christian by forcing him to eat a significant amount of salt. Christian collapsed and died of a brain haemorrhage in 2002. Post-mortem results showed that Christian's blood contained high levels of salt that the court heard was the result of a high intake of salt. The prosecution claimed that the couple had force fed Christian six teaspoons of salt as punishment.

According to the Department of Health (2007) adults should consume less than 6 g of salt each day and children aged 1-3 years should only be eating 2 g per day. High salt intake is known to increase blood pressure (the pressure within the arteries), which increases the risk of

a stroke (cerebrovascular accident (CVA)) - a clot or haemorrhage (bleeding) in the brain. This in turn can cause paralysis of one side of the body and a heart attack (myocardial infarction (MI)), which is a clot in one of the arteries in the heart.

In 2007, based on new evidence, the couple's original conviction was quashed and a retrial ordered. In March 2007 the couple were cleared of manslaughter and child cruelty based on medical evidence. The court heard that Christian had suffered with a condition known as diabetes insipidis (salt diabetes) which causes the body to lose too much water thereby increasing the levels of salt in the blood. One treatment for someone presenting with diabetes insipidis is to replace the water, but doctors treating Christian found that even after giving Christian water his salt levels did not return to normal. At the trial Professor Ashley Grossman, neuro-endocrinologist at St Bartholomew's Hospital, said that maybe the part of the brain controlling the levels of salt in the boy had been reset to a higher level leading Christian to retain salt.

After reading this chapter you will be able to reflect upon the importance of maintaining fluid and electrolyte balance within the body and how these are maintained in the healthcare environment.

BODY FLUIDS AND ELECTROLYTES

In good health, fluids, electrolytes, acids and bases are finely balanced, a condition known as physiological **homoeostasis** (stability). This balance depends on a number of physiological processes that regulate fluid intake and output, and the movement of water and the substances dissolved in it between the body compartments.

Almost every illness has the potential to threaten this balance. Even in daily living, excessive temperatures or vigorous activity can disturb the balance if adequate water and salt intake is not maintained. Medical and nursing interventions used to treat the patient, such as use of diuretics (medications used to make the patient urinate more) or aspiration of a nasogastric tube (see Chapter 17) can also affect this balance.

Body Fluids

Survival is based on the rule of three; humans can survive three minutes without oxygen, three days without water and three weeks without food. Water is fundamental for survival and vital as it is:

+ a medium for metabolic reactions within cells;
+ a transporter for nutrients, waste products and other substances;
+ a lubricant;
+ an insulator and shock absorber;
+ a means of regulating and maintaining body temperature.

Water makes up 50–70% of the human body (see Table 18-1), and without regular intake of water many bodily functions would be affected. Age, sex and body fat affect total body water. For example, infants have the highest proportion of water, accounting for 70–80% of their body weight, but the proportion of body water decreases with ageing. In people older than 60, it decreases to approximately 50%.

On average an adult needs to drink between 1.5 and 2.0 litres of fluid a day in order to function efficiently. Children however need differing amounts of fluid according to their body weight (see *Box 18-1*).

Approximately 9 litres of fluid passes through an adult's gastrointestinal tract every day but 7.7 litres are reabsorbed in the small intestine. Hydration status can be assessed by checking the patient's urine output. An adult should pass 0.5 millilitres of urine for every kilogram of body weight every hour: for

Table 18-1 Total Body Water as a Percentage of Total Body Weight According to Age and Gender

Age and gender	Total body water as percentage of body weight
Newborn to 6 months	74
6 months to 1 year	60
1 year to 12 years	60
12 years to 18 years (Male)	59
12 years to 18 years (Female)	56
19 years to 50 years (Male)	59
19 years to 50 years (Female)	50
51+ years (Male)	56
51+ years (Female)	47

BOX 18-1 Fluid Requirements for Children

Body weight	Fluid requirements
1-10 kg	100 ml/kg
11-20 kg	1,000 ml plus 50 ml/kg over 10 kg
<20 kg	1,500 ml
>20 kg	1,500 ml plus 20 ml/kg over 20 kg

Source: Hogston, R. and Simpson P.M. (Eds) (2002) *Foundations of Nursing Practice: Making the Difference.* Basingstoke: Palgrave Macmillan.

example, an adult weighing 70 kg should pass 35 ml of urine every hour. However, it is important to note that an individual's urine output may be reduced if they are sweating profusely or have a pyrexia (high temperature).

Distribution of Body Fluids

The body's fluid is divided into two major compartments: intracellular (inside the cells) and extracellular (outside the cells). **Intracellular fluid** is found within the cells of the body. It constitutes approximately two-thirds of the total body fluid in adults. While **extracellular fluid** is found outside the cells and accounts for about one-third of total body fluid.

The extracellular fluids comprise of:

+ **Intravascular fluid** or **plasma**, which is found within the vascular system (arteries, capillaries and veins).
+ **Interstitial fluid** which surrounds the cells.

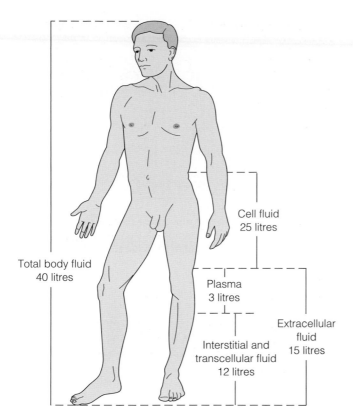

Figure 18-1 Total body fluid represents 40 litres in an adult male weighing 70 kg.

+ **Lymph** which carries lymphocytes and is transported through the lymphatic system. Lymph forms part of the body's immune system.
+ **Transcellular fluid** include cerebrospinal, pericardial, pancreatic, pleural, intraocular, biliary, peritoneal and synovial fluids (see Figure 18-1). The trancellular fluid is often termed the 'third space' (see later in the chapter).

Intracellular fluid is vital to normal cell functioning. It contains solutes such as oxygen, electrolytes and glucose, and it provides a medium in which metabolic processes of the cell take place.

Although extracellular fluid is in the smaller of the two compartments, it is vital to the transport system of the body. Extracellular fluid carries nutrients to and waste products away from the cells. For example, plasma carries oxygen from the lungs to the capillaries of the vascular system. From there, the oxygen moves across the capillary membranes into the interstitial spaces and then across the cellular membranes into the cells. The opposite route is taken for waste products, such as carbon dioxide going from the cells to the lungs. Interstitial fluid transports wastes from the cells by way of the lymph system as well as directly into the blood plasma through capillaries.

Composition of Body Fluids

Extracellular and intracellular fluids contain oxygen from the lungs, dissolved nutrients from the gastrointestinal tract, excretory products of metabolism such as carbon dioxide, and **electrolytes** such as sodium (Na^+).

Electrolytes are charged ions that when dissolved in water can conduct electricity. They form as a result of a salt breaking up in water, for example the salt sodium chloride breaks up into one ion of sodium (Na^+) and one ion of chloride (Cl^-).

The composition of fluids varies from one body compartment to another.

+ Extracellular fluid have ↑ sodium, chloride and bicarbonate and ↓ potassium, calcium and magnesium, and interstitial fluid also contains ↑ protein.
+ Intracellular fluid have ↑ potassium, magnesium, phosphate and sulphate and ↓ sodium, chloride and bicarbonate.

While

+ Intravascular fluid (plasma) contains ↑ protein (albumin).
+ Interstitial fluid have ↓ protein (albumin).

Maintaining a balance of fluid volumes and electrolyte compositions in the fluid compartments of the body is essential to health. Normal and unusual fluid and electrolyte losses must be replaced if homoeostasis is to be maintained.

Other body fluids such as gastric and intestinal secretions also contain electrolytes. This is of particular concern when these fluids are lost from the body (e.g. in severe vomiting or diarrhoea or when gastric suction removes the gastric secretions). Fluid and electrolyte imbalances can result from excessive losses through these routes.

Movement of Body Fluids and Electrolytes

The body fluid compartments are separated from one another by cell membranes and the capillary membranes. These membranes allow substances across them at different rates and are described as **selectively permeable**. These membranes almost act like a sieve. Small particles such as electrolytes, oxygen and carbon dioxide easily move across these membranes, but larger molecules like glucose and proteins have more difficulty moving between fluid compartments.

Solutes, which are substances dissolved in liquid such as electrolytes, oxygen and protein, and water, move across these membranes by a number of different methods: osmosis, diffusion, filtration and active transport.

Osmosis

Osmosis is the movement of water across cell membranes, from the less concentrated solution to the more concentrated solution (Figure 18-2 on page 438). In other words, water moves toward the higher concentration of solute in an attempt to equalise the concentrations.

For example, a marathon runner loses a significant amount of water through perspiration, increasing the concentration of solutes in the plasma because of water loss. This higher solute concentration draws water from the interstitial space and cells into the vascular compartment to equalise the concentration of

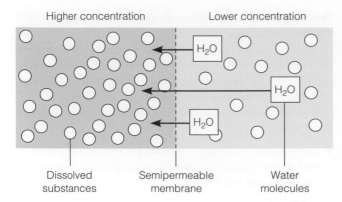

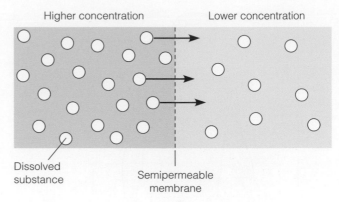

Higher concentration   Lower concentration

Dissolved substances   Semipermeable membrane   Water molecules

Figure 18-2 Osmosis: water molecules move from the less concentrated area to the more concentrated area in an attempt to equalise the concentration of the solutions on two sides of a membrane.

Higher concentration   Lower concentration

Dissolved substance   Semipermeable membrane

Figure 18-3 Diffusion: the movement of molecules through a semipermeable membrane from an area of higher concentration to an area of lower concentration.

solutes in all fluid compartments. Osmosis is an important mechanism for maintaining homoeostasis and fluid balance.

The concentration of solutes in body fluids is usually expressed as the **osmolality (tonicity)** and is reported as milliosmols per kilogram (mOsm/kg). Sodium is the best determinant of plasma osmolality (concentration of solutes in the blood) otherwise known as *serum osmolality*, while potassium, glucose and urea are primary contributors to the osmolality of intracellular fluid. Serum osmolality can be checked easily by taking a blood sample from a vein in the arm. However intracellular osmolality is far more difficult to test.

It is important that the nurse understands osmolality (tonicity) particularly when giving patients intravenous fluids (fluids straight into the vein). Most intravenous fluid administered are termed as **isotonic** solutions, which means they have the same osmolality as body fluids, for example 0.9% sodium chloride is an isotonic solution. Other fluids that are administered are **hypertonic** solutions which have a higher osmolality than body fluids such as 3% sodium chloride is a hypertonic solution and **hypotonic** solutions which have a lower osmolality than body fluids such as 0.45% sodium chloride.

Infusing a hypertonic intravenous solution such as 3% sodium chloride will draw fluid out of red blood cells (RBCs), causing them to shrink. On the other hand, a hypotonic solution administered intravenously will cause the RBCs to swell as water is drawn into the cells.

Diffusion

Diffusion is spontaneous intermingling (spreading) of particles. Diffusion can be demonstrated by adding high coloured solution (squash) to a clear fluid (water), the squash intermingles with the water until the final solution is a mixture of the squash and water. The process of diffusion occurs even when two substances are separated by a thin membrane. In the body, diffusion of water, electrolytes and other substances occurs through the capillary membranes.

The rate of diffusion of substances varies according to (a) the size of the molecules, (b) the concentration of the solution

and (c) the temperature of the solution. Larger molecules move less quickly than smaller ones because they require more energy to move about. With diffusion, the molecules move from a solution of higher concentration to a solution of lower concentration (see Figure 18-3). Increases in temperature increase the rate of motion of molecules and therefore the rate of diffusion.

Filtration

Filtration is a process whereby fluid and solutes move together across a membrane from one compartment to another. The movement is from an area of higher pressure to one of lower pressure. An example of filtration is the movement of fluid and nutrients from the capillaries of the arterioles to the interstitial fluid around the cells.

Active Transport

Substances can move across cell membranes from a less concentrated solution to a more concentrated one by **active transport** (see Figure 18-4). This process differs from diffusion and osmosis in that energy is required for this process. In active transport, a substance combines with a carrier on the outside surface of the cell membrane, and they move to the inside surface of the cell membrane. Once inside, they separate, and the substance is released to the inside of the cell.

Regulating Body Fluids

In a healthy person, fluid intake and fluid loss are balanced, however illness can upset this balance so that the body has too little or too much fluid.

Fluid Intake

Fluid intake comes from a number of sources:

+ fluids such as water, squash, pop and coffee,
+ food such as fruit, vegetables,
+ metabolism.

Intracellular fluid   Extracellular fluid

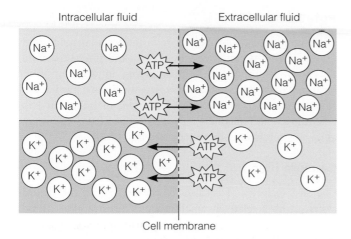

Cell membrane

Figure 18-4 An example of active transport. Energy ATP is used to move sodium molecules and potassium molecules across a semipermeable membrane against sodium's and potassium's concentration gradients (i.e. from areas of lesser concentration to areas of greater concentration).

A moderately active adult requires approximately 2.5 l of fluid each day. However the average adult normally drinks about 1.5 l of fluid each day which is insufficient to maintain health. The outstanding fluid comes from food and the metabolism of food. The water content of food is relatively large and accounts for approximately 750 ml of fluid each day. While the metabolism of food, the physical and chemical processes used to breakdown the food, makes up the remaining fluid volume required (see Table 18-2).

The body's thirst mechanism is main regulator of fluid intake. The thirst centre is located in the hypothalamus of the brain and is stimulated by volume of fluid in the vascular system and angiotensin (a hormone released in response to decreased blood flow to the kidneys). For example, a long-distance runner loses significant amounts of water through perspiration and rapid breathing during a race, increasing the concentration of solutes of body fluids. This stimulates the thirst centre causing the runner to experience the sensation of thirst and the desire to drink to replace lost fluids.

Table 18-2 Average Daily Fluid Requirements by Age and Weight

	Approximate age ml/24 hr	Body weight (kg)
3 days	3.0	250 to 300
1 year	9.5	1,150 to 1,300
2 years	11.8	1,350 to 1,500
6 years	20.0	1,800 to 2,000
10 years	28.7	2,000 to 2,500
14 years	45.0	2,200 to 2,700
18 years (adult)	54.0	2,200 to 2,700

Note: From: *Nelson Textbook of Pediatrics* (p. 107), by R.E. Behrman, 1992, Philadelphia: Saunders. Adapted with permission.

Table 18-3 Average Daily Fluid Output for an Adult

Route	Amount (ml)
Urine	1,400 to 1,500
Insensible losses	
Lungs	350 to 400
Skin	350 to 400
Sweat	100
Faeces	100 to 200
Total	2,300 to 2,600

Thirst however is not a reliable indicator of hydration status as the body is already dehydrated before the thirst mechanism is stimulated. It is also important to note that the thirst mechanism can be affected by a number of factors including the patient's age. In particular reduced thirst has been noted in older adults (Mangoni and Jackson, 2003).

Fluid Output

Fluid losses from the body counterbalance the adult's 2.5 l average daily intake of fluid, as shown in Table 18-3. There are three main routes of fluid output:

1. urine,
2. insensible loss through the skin as perspiration and through the lungs as water vapour in the expired air,
3. loss through the intestines in faeces.

Urine.   Urine formed by the kidneys and excreted from the urinary bladder is the major avenue of fluid output. Normal urine output for an adult is 1,400 to 1,500 ml per 24 hours, or at least 0.5 ml per kilogram per hour. In healthy people, urine output may vary noticeably from day to day. Urine volume automatically increases as fluid intake increases. If fluid loss through perspiration is large, however, urine volume decreases to maintain fluid balance in the body.

Insensible losses.   **Insensible fluid loss** occurs through the skin, in the form of perspiration and lungs, as water vapour. It is not noticeable and therefore cannot be measured. Insensible losses can increase and decrease according to the climate, activity and any skin losses such as a burn or abrasion.

Faeces.   Partly digested food or chime contains water and electrolytes. Approximately 1.5 l of chime enter the large intestine in an adult, however only 100 ml is reabsorbed.

Maintaining Homoeostasis

The volume and composition of body fluids is regulated by a number of body systems including the kidneys, the endocrine system, the cardiovascular system, the lungs and the gastrointestinal system.

Kidneys.   The kidneys are the primary regulator of body fluids and electrolyte balance. The kidneys adjust the amount of water reabsorbed from the plasma (extracellular fluid) and therefore regulate how much fluid is excreted as urine. Approximately 1.5 l of urine is excreted daily by the average adult. The kidneys also select which and how much electrolytes are excreted.

Antidiuretic hormone (ADH). Antidiuretic hormone regulates water excretion from the kidney. When serum osmolality rises (plasma electrolytes increase), ADH is produced and causes the kidneys to reabsorb more water back into the plasma. This results in urine output falling. Conversely if serum osmolality decreases (plasma electrolytes decrease), ADH is suppressed and the urine output increases.

Rennin-angiotensin-aldosterone system. Specialised receptors in the kidneys respond to changes in renal perfusion (the amount of blood passing through the kidneys for filtration) and initiate the **rennin-angiotensin-aldosterone system**. If blood flow to the kidney decreases, rennin, an enzyme, is released. Rennin causes the conversion of angiotensinogen to angiotensin I, which is then converted to angiotensin II by angiotensin-converting enzyme. Angiotensin II acts directly on the kidneys to promote sodium and water retention. In addition, it stimulates the release of aldosterone from the adrenal cortex. Aldosterone also promotes sodium retention in the distal kidneys. The net effect of the rennin-angiotensin-aldosterone system is to restore blood volume (and renal perfusion) by sodium and water retention.

Regulating Electrolytes

Electrolytes are present in all body fluids and fluid compartments. Just as maintaining the fluid balance is vital to normal body function, so is maintaining electrolyte balance. Although the concentration of specific electrolytes differs between fluid compartments, a balance of cations (positively charged ions) and anions (negatively charged ions) always exists. Electrolytes are important for:

+ maintaining fluid balance;
+ contributing to acid–base regulation;
+ facilitating enzyme reactions;
+ transmitting neuromuscular reactions.

Most electrolytes enter the body through dietary intake and are excreted in the urine. Some electrolytes, such as sodium and chloride, are not stored by the body and must be consumed daily to maintain normal levels. Potassium and calcium, on the other hand, are stored in the cells and bone, respectively. The regulatory mechanisms and functions of the major electrolytes are summarised in Table 18-4.

Sodium (Na⁺)

Sodium is the most abundant electrolyte in extracellular fluid. Sodium's main function is to control and regulate water balance. Sodium is found in many foods, such as bacon, ham, processed cheese and table salt.

Potassium (K⁺)

Potassium is the major electrolyte in intracellular fluids, with only a small amount found in plasma and interstitial fluid. Potassium is important in maintaining intracellular water balance. Potassium is a vital electrolyte for skeletal, cardiac and smooth muscle activity. It is involved in maintaining acid–base balance as well. Potassium is found in many fruits and vegetables, meat, fish and other foods (see *Box 18-2*).

Calcium (Ca²⁺)

The vast majority of calcium in the body is in the skeletal system, with a relatively small amount in extracellular fluid. Calcium is important in the development of bones, regulating muscle contraction and relaxation and cardiac function. Extracellular calcium is regulated by the parathyroid hormone, calcitonin and calcitriol (derived from vitamin D). When extracellular calcium falls the parathyroid hormone and calcitriol cause calcium to be released from the bones and when there is a rise in extracellular calcium calcitonin stimulates the deposition of calcium in bones.

With ageing, more calcium is excreted by the kidneys causing osteoporosis (brittle bones) increasing the risk of fractures of the bones. Milk and milk products are the richest sources of calcium, with other foods such as dark green leafy vegetables and canned salmon containing smaller amounts.

BOX 18-2 Potassium-Rich Foods

Vegetables
Avocado
Raw carrot
Baked potato
Raw tomato
Spinach

Meats and Fish
Beef
Cod
Pork
Veal

Fruits
Dried fruits (e.g. raisins and dates)
Banana
Apricot
Cantaloupe
Orange

Beverages
Milk
Orange juice
Apricot nectar

Table 18-4 Regulation and Functions of Electrolytes

Electrolyte	Regulation	Function
Sodium (Na⁺)	<ul><li>Reabsorbed or excreted by kidneys</li></ul>	<ul><li>Regulating extracellular fluid volume</li><li>Maintaining blood volume</li><li>Transmitting nerve impulses and contracting muscles</li></ul>
Potassium (K⁺)	<ul><li>Excreted or conserved by the kidneys. Renal excretion and conservation</li><li>Movement into cells from plasm by insulin</li><li>Movement out of cells when cells are damaged or if there is acidosis (see later in chapter)</li></ul>	<ul><li>Maintaining intracellular osmolality</li><li>Transmitting nerve and other electrical impulses</li><li>Regulating cardiac impulse transmission and muscle contraction</li><li>Skeletal and smooth muscle function</li><li>Regulating acid–base balance</li></ul>
Calcium (Ca²⁺)	<ul><li>Redistribution between bones and extracellular fluid</li><li>Parathyroid hormone and calcitriol increase serum Ca²⁺ levels; calcitonin decreases serum levels</li></ul>	<ul><li>Forming bones and teeth</li><li>Transmitting nerve impulses</li><li>Regulating muscle contractions</li><li>Maintaining cardiac pacemaker (automaticity)</li><li>Blood clotting</li><li>Activating enzymes such as pancreatic lipase and phospholipase</li></ul>
Magnesium (Mg²⁺)	<ul><li>Conservation and excretion by kidneys</li><li>Intestinal absorption increased by vitamin D and parathyroid hormone</li></ul>	<ul><li>Intracellular metabolism</li><li>Operating sodium-potassium pump</li><li>Relaxing muscle contractions</li><li>Transmitting nerve impulses</li><li>Regulating cardiac function</li></ul>
Chloride (Cl⁻)	<ul><li>Excreted and reabsorbed along with sodium in the kidneys</li><li>Aldosterone increases chloride reabsorption with sodium</li></ul>	<ul><li>HCl production</li><li>Regulating ECF balance and vascular volume</li><li>Regulating acid-base balance</li><li>Buffer in oxygen-carbon dioxide exchange in RBCs</li></ul>
Phosphate (PO₄⁻)	<ul><li>Excretion and reabsorption by the kidneys</li><li>Parathyroid hormone decreases serum levels by increasing renal excretion</li><li>Reciprocal relationship with calcium: increasing serum calcium levels decrease phosphate levels; decreasing serum calcium increases phosphate</li></ul>	<ul><li>Forming bones and teeth</li><li>Metabolising carbohydrate, protein and fat</li><li>Cellular metabolism; producing ATP and DNA</li><li>Muscle, nerve and RBC function</li><li>Regulating acid-base balance</li><li>Regulating calcium levels</li></ul>
Bicarbonate (HCO₃⁻)	<ul><li>Excretion and reabsorption by the kidneys</li><li>Regeneration by kidneys</li></ul>	<ul><li>Major body buffer involved in acid-base regulation</li></ul>

Magnesium (Mg²⁺)

Magnesium is primarily found in the skeleton and in intracellular fluid. It is important for intracellular metabolism, being particularly involved in the production and use of ATP (Adenosine Triphosphate) which gives the cells energy. Magnesium also is necessary for protein and Deoxyribonucleic Acid (DNA) synthesis within the cells. Extracellular magnesium is involved in neuromuscular and cardiac function. Maintaining and ensuring adequate magnesium levels is an important part of care of patients with heart problems. Cereal grains, nuts, dried fruit, legumes and green leafy vegetables are good sources of magnesium in the diet, as are dairy products, meat and fish.

Chloride (Cl⁻)

Chloride is found in extracellular fluid and is regulated by the kidneys. Chloride is a major component of gastric juice as hydrochloric acid (HCl) and is involved in regulating acid–base balance. Chloride is found in the same foods as sodium.

Phosphate PO₄⁻

Phosphate is found in intracellular fluid, extracellular fluid, bone, muscle and nerve tissue. Phosphate is involved in many chemical actions of the cell; it is essential for functioning of muscles, nerves and red blood cells. It is also involved in the metabolism of protein, fat and carbohydrate. Phosphate is absorbed from the intestine and is found in many foods such as meat, fish, poultry, milk products and legumes.

Bicarbonate HCO₃⁻

Bicarbonate is present in both intracellular and extracellular fluids. Its primary function is regulating acid–base balance. Extracellular bicarbonate levels are regulated by the kidneys:

Bicarbonate is excreted when too much is present; if more is needed, the kidneys both regenerate and reabsorb bicarbonate. Unlike other electrolytes that must be consumed in the diet, adequate amounts of bicarbonate are produced through metabolic processes to meet the body's needs.

ACID-BASE BALANCE

An important part of regulating the chemical balance or homoeostasis of body fluids is regulating their acidity or alkalinity. An **acid** is a substance that releases hydrogen ions (H+) in solution while **bases** or *alkalis* have a low hydrogen ion concentration and can accept hydrogen ions in solution. The relative acidity or alkalinity of a solution is measured as **pH**. The pH reflects the hydrogen ion concentration of the solution: The higher the hydrogen ion concentration (and the more acidic the solution), the lower the pH. Water has a pH of 7 and is neutral; that is, it is neither acidic in nature nor is it alkaline; solutions with a pH lower than 7 are acidic; those with a pH higher than 7 are alkaline.

Regulation of Acid-Base Balance

Body fluids are maintained within a narrow range that is slightly alkaline. The normal pH of arterial blood is between 7.35 and 7.45 (Figure 18-5). Acids are continually produced during metabolism. Several body systems, including buffers, the respiratory system and the renal system, are actively involved in maintaining the narrow pH range necessary for optimal function.

Buffers

Buffers prevent excessive changes in pH by removing or releasing hydrogen ions. If excess hydrogen ion is present in body fluids, buffers bind with the hydrogen ion, minimising the change in pH. When body fluids become too alkaline, buffers can release hydrogen ion, again minimising the change in pH. The action of a buffer is immediate, but limited in its capacity to maintain or restore normal acid–base balance.

The major buffer system in extracellular fluids is the bicarbonate HCO_3^- and carbonic acid (H_2CO_3) system. So when an acid, for example hydrochloric acid, is added it will cause a condition called acidosis, this acid combines with the bicarbonate which prevents the pH from dropping too much. When a base (alkali), for example sodium hydroxide, is added it combines with carbonic acid which prevents the pH from rising too much. If a strong acid is added to extracellular fluid the bicarbonate is used up quickly to try to neutralise the acid. This causes a drop in the pH and causes a condition known as **acidosis**. If a strong base is added to extracellular fluid carbonic acid is depleted quickly causing the pH to rise causing a condition known as **alkalosis**.

Respiratory Regulation

The lungs help regulate acid–base balance by eliminating or retaining carbon dioxide (CO_2) which is a potential acid. When carbon dioxide combines with water carbonic acid is formed. Working together with the bicarbonate–carbonic acid buffer system, the lungs regulate acid–base balance and pH by altering the rate and depth of respirations. The response of the respiratory system to changes in pH is rapid, occurring within minutes.

When carbon dioxide and carbonic acid rises in the blood, the respiratory centre of the brain is stimulated; this increases the rate and depth of respirations. Carbon dioxide is exhaled, and carbonic acid levels fall. By contrast, when bicarbonate levels are excessive, the rate and depth of respirations are reduced. This causes carbon dioxide to be retained, carbonic acid levels to rise, and the excess bicarbonate to be neutralised.

Carbon dioxide levels in the blood are measured as the PCO_2, or partial pressure of the dissolved gas in the blood. PCO_2 refers to the pressure of carbon dioxide in venous blood. $PaCO_2$ refers to the pressure of carbon dioxide in arterial blood. The normal $PaCO_2$ is 35 to 45 mm Hg.

Renal Regulation

Although buffers and the respiratory system can compensate for changes in pH, the kidneys are the ultimate long-term regulator of acid–base balance. They are slower to respond to changes, requiring hours to days to correct imbalances, but their response is more permanent and selective than that of the other systems.

The kidneys maintain acid–base balance by selectively excreting or conserving bicarbonate and hydrogen ions. When excess hydrogen ion is present and the pH falls (acidosis), the kidneys reabsorb and regenerate bicarbonate and excrete hydrogen ion. In the case of alkalosis and a high pH, excess bicarbonate is excreted and hydrogen ion is retained. The normal serum bicarbonate level is 22 to 26 mmol/l.

FACTORS AFFECTING BODY FLUID, ELECTROLYTES AND ACID-BASE BALANCE

The ability of the body to adjust fluids, electrolytes and acid–base balance is influenced by age, gender and body size, environmental temperature and lifestyle.

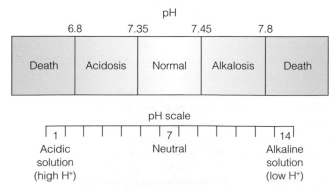

Figure 18-5 Body fluids are normally slightly alkaline, between a pH of 7.35 and 7.45.

Age

Infants and growing children have a much higher metabolic rate than adults which increases fluid loss. Infants lose more fluid through the kidneys because immature kidneys are less able to conserve water than adult kidneys. In addition, infants respirations are more rapid and the body surface area is proportionately greater than that of adults, increasing insensible fluid losses. This rapid turnover of fluid and an increase in losses, such as fever, associated with illness can create critical fluid imbalances in children far more rapidly than in adults.

In older people, the normal ageing process may affect fluid balance. The thirst response often is blunted (Mangoni and Jackson, 2003). This added to the fact that the kidneys are less able to conserve water increases the risk of dehydration.

Gender and Body Size

Total body water also is affected by gender and body size (see Table 18-1 earlier). Because fat cells contain little or no water and lean tissue has a high water content, people with a higher percentage of body fat have less body fluid. Women have proportionately more body fat and less body water than men.

Environmental Temperature

People with an illness and those participating in strenuous activity are at risk of fluid and electrolyte imbalances when the environmental temperature is high. Fluid losses through sweating are increased in hot environments as the body attempts to dissipate heat. These losses are even greater in people who have not been acclimatised to the environment.

Both salt and water are lost through sweating. When only water is replaced, salt depletion is a risk. The person who is salt depleted may experience fatigue, weakness, headache and gastrointestinal symptoms such as anorexia (loss of appetite) and nausea. If water is not replaced, body temperature rises, and the person is at risk for heat exhaustion or heatstroke.

Drinking adequate amounts of cool liquids, particularly during strenuous activity, reduces the risk of adverse effects from heat. Balanced electrolyte solutions and carbohydrate-electrolyte solutions such as sports drinks are recommended because they replace both water and electrolytes lost through sweat.

Lifestyle

Other factors such as diet, exercise and stress affect fluid, electrolyte and acid–base balance.

The intake of fluids and electrolytes is affected by the diet. For example people with anorexia nervosa or bulimia are at risk of severe fluid and electrolyte imbalances because of inadequate intake, induced vomiting and use of diuretics and laxatives.

Stress can increase production of ADH, which decreases urine production. The overall response of the body to stress is to increase the blood volume.

Other lifestyle factors can also affect fluid, electrolyte and acid–base balance. Heavy alcohol consumption affects electrolyte balance, increasing the risk of low calcium, magnesium and phosphate levels. The risk of acidosis associated with breakdown of fat tissue also is greater in the person who drinks large amounts of alcohol.

DISTURBANCES IN FLUID VOLUME, ELECTROLYTE AND ACID-BASE BALANCES

Hypovolaemia

Hypovolaemia or decreased blood volume occurs when the body loses both water and electrolytes. Hypovolaemia generally occurs as a result of (a) abnormal losses through the skin, gastrointestinal tract or kidney; (b) decreased intake of fluid; (c) bleeding; or (d) movement of fluid into a third space. See the section on third space syndrome that follows.

For the risk factors and clinical signs related to hypovolaemia, see Table 18-5.

Table 18-5 Hypervolaemia

Risk factors	Clinical manifestations	Nursing interventions
Excess intake of sodium-containing intravenous fluids	Weight gain	Assess for clinical manifestations of hypervolaemia.
Excess ingestion of sodium in diet or medications (e.g. sodium bicarbonate antacids such as Alka-Seltzer or hypertonic enema solutions such as Fleet's)	Fluid intake greater than output	Monitor weight and vital signs.
	Moist mucous membranes	Assess for oedema.
	Full, bounding pulse; tachycardia	Assess breath sounds.
Impaired fluid balance regulation related to	Increased blood pressure and central venous pressure	Monitor fluid intake and output.
✚ heart failure	Distended neck and peripheral veins; slow vein emptying	Monitor laboratory findings.
✚ renal failure	Moist crackles in lungs; dyspnoea, shortness of breath	Place in Fowler's position.
✚ cirrhosis of the liver	Mental confusion	Administer diuretics as ordered.
		Restrict fluid intake as indicated.
		Restrict dietary sodium as ordered.
		Implement measures to prevent skin breakdown.

Third space syndrome

Third space syndrome is caused by movement of fluid from the vascular space (plasma) into an area where it is not readily accessible as extracellular fluid. This fluid remains in the body but is essentially unavailable for use. The fluid may be found in the bowel, in the interstitial space as oedema, in inflamed tissue, or in potential spaces such as the peritoneal or pleural cavities.

Oedema

Oedema is excess interstitial fluid caused by increased water and sodium content. Oedema typically is most apparent in areas where the tissue pressure is low, such as around the eyes.

Oedema can be caused by several different mechanisms.

✦ Pressure building within the capillaries pushes fluid into the tissues. This is mainly found in the feet, ankles and sacrum and is mainly due to gravity.

✦ Low levels of protein in the plasma as a result of malnutrition can also cause oedema because fluid is not drawn out of the tissues into the capillaries.

✦ Tissue trauma and some disorders such as allergic reactions, cause the capillaries to become more permeable, allowing fluid to escape into interstitial tissues.

✦ Obstructed lymph flow impairs the movement of fluid from interstitial tissues back into the vascular compartment, resulting in oedema.

Pitting oedema is oedema that leaves a small depression or pit after finger pressure is applied to the swollen area. The pit is caused by movement of fluid to adjacent tissue, away from the point of pressure (see Figure 18-6). Within 10 to 30 seconds the pit normally disappears.

Dehydration

Dehydration occurs when water is lost from the body without significant loss of electrolytes. Because water is lost while electrolytes, particularly sodium, are retained, the serum osmolality (concentration of sodium in the blood) increase. Water is drawn into the vascular compartment from the interstitial space and cells, resulting in cells becoming dehydrated. Older adults are at particular risk for dehydration because of decreased thirst sensation (Mangoni and Jackson, 2003). This type of water deficit also can affect patients who are hyperventilating or have prolonged fever.

Overhydration

Overhydration also known as *water intoxication*, occurs when water is gained in excess of electrolytes, resulting in low serum osmolality (concentration of sodium in the blood). Water is drawn into the cells, causing them to swell. In the brain this can lead to cerebral oedema and impaired neurological function. Water intoxication often occurs when both fluid and electrolytes are lost, for example, through excessive sweating, but only water is replaced. It can also result from the syndrome of inappropriate antidiuretic hormone (SIADH), a disorder that can occur with some malignant tumours, AIDS, head injury or administration of certain drugs such as barbiturates or anaesthetics.

Electrolyte Imbalances

The most common and most significant electrolyte imbalances involve sodium, potassium, calcium, magnesium, chloride and phosphate.

Sodium

Sodium (Na^+), the most abundant electrolyte in the extracellular fluid, is found in most body secretions, for example, saliva, gastric and intestinal secretions, bile and pancreatic fluid, therefore, continuous excretion of any of these fluids, such as vomiting, can result in a sodium deficit.

Hyponatraemia is a sodium deficit, or serum sodium level of less than 135 mmol/l. As a result water is drawn out of the vascular compartment into interstitial tissues and the cells (see Figure 18-7, A), causing the clinical manifestations associated with this disorder.

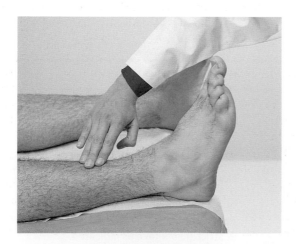

Figure 18-6 Evaluation of oedema. Palpate for oedema over the tibia as shown here and behind the medial malleolus, and over the dorsum of each foot.

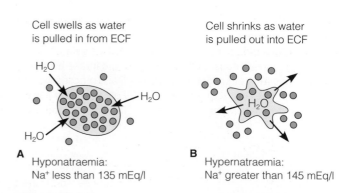

Figure 18-7 The extracellular sodium level affects cell size. *A,* In hyponatraemia, cells swell; *B,* in hypernatraemia, cells shrink in size.

Hypernatraemia is excess sodium, or a serum sodium of greater than 145 mmol/l. As a result fluid moves out of the cells into the extracellular fluid (see Figure 18-7, B) and the cells become dehydrated.

Table 18-6 on page 446 lists risk factors and clinical signs for hyponatraemia and hypernatraemia.

Potassium

Although the amount of potassium (K^+) in extracellular fluid is small, it is vital to normal neuromuscular and cardiac function. Potassium is usually excreted by the kidneys. However, the kidneys do not regulate potassium excretion as effectively as they do sodium excretion. Therefore, an acute potassium deficiency can develop rapidly. Of the body's secretions, the gastrointestinal secretions are high in potassium.

Hypokalaemia is a potassium deficit or a serum potassium level of less than 3.5 mmol/l. Gastrointestinal losses of potassium through vomiting and gastric suction are common causes of hypokalaemia, as are the use of potassium-wasting diuretics, such as thiazide diuretics or loop diuretics (e.g. frusemide).

Hyperkalaemia is a potassium excess or a serum potassium level greater than 5.0 mmol/l and is less common than hypokalaemia and rarely occurs in patients with normal renal (kidney) function. It is, however, more dangerous than hypokalaemia, and can lead to cardiac arrest. Table 18-6 lists risk factors and clinical signs for hypokalaemia and hyperkalaemia.

CLINICAL ALERT

Potassium may be given intravenously for severe hypokalemia. It must always be diluted appropriately and never given in a bolus. Potassium that is to be given IV should be mixed in the pharmacy and double checked prior to administration by two nurses. The usual concentration of IV potassium is 20 to 40 mmol/l.

Calcium

Regulating levels of calcium (Ca^{2+}) in the body is more complex than the other major electrolytes so calcium balance can be affected by many factors. Imbalances of this electrolyte are relatively common.

Hypocalcaemia is a calcium deficit, or a total serum calcium level of less than 8.5 mg/dl. Severe depletion of calcium can cause muscle spasms and paresthesias (abnormal sensation such as pins and needles) and can lead to convulsions. Low serum magnesium levels (hypomagnesaemia) and chronic alcoholism also increase the risk of hypocalcaemia.

Hypercalcemia, or serum calcium levels greater than 10.5 mg/dl, most often occurs when calcium is mobilised from the bony skeleton. This may be due to malignancy or prolonged immobilisation.

The risk factors and clinical manifestations related to calcium imbalances are found in Table 18-6.

Magnesium

Magnesium (Mg^{2+}) imbalances are relatively common in hospitalised patients, although they may be unrecognised. **Hypomagnesaemia** or deficiency in magnesium occurs more frequently than hypermagnesaemia. Chronic alcoholism is the most common cause of hypomagnesaemia. Magnesium deficiency also may aggravate the manifestations of alcohol withdrawal, such as delirium tremens (DTs). **Hypermagnesaaemia** is present when the serum magnesium level rises. It is due to increased intake or decreased excretion. It is often iatrogenic, that is, a result of overzealous magnesium therapy.

Table 18-6 lists risk factors and manifestations for patients with altered magnesium balance.

Chloride

Because of the relationship between sodium ions and chloride ions (Cl^-), imbalances of chloride commonly occur in conjunction with sodium imbalances. **Hypochloraemia** is a decreased serum chloride level and is usually related to excess losses of chloride through the GI tract, kidneys or sweating. Hypochloremic patients are at risk for alkalosis and may experience muscle twitching, tremors or tetany.

Conditions that cause sodium retention also can lead to a high serum chloride level or **hyperchloraemia**. Excess replacement of sodium chloride or potassium chloride is additional risk factors for high serum chloride levels. The manifestations of hyperchloraemia include acidosis, weakness and lethargy, with a risk of dysrhythmias and coma.

Phosphate

The phosphate anion PO_4^- is found both in intracellular and extracellular fluid. Most of the phosphorus (P^+) in the body exists as PO_4^-. Phosphate is critical for cellular metabolism because it is a major component of adenosine triphosphate (ATP).

Phosphate imbalances frequently are related to therapeutic interventions for other disorders. Glucose and insulin administration and total parenteral nutrition can cause phosphate to shift into the cells from extracellular fluid compartments, leading to **hypophosphataemia**, a low serum phosphate. Alcohol withdrawal, acid–base imbalances, and the use of antacids that bind with phosphate in the GI tract are other possible causes of low serum phosphate levels. Manifestations of hypophosphataemia include paresthesias, muscle weakness and pain, mental changes, and possible seizures.

Hyperphosphataemia occurs when phosphate shifts out of the cells into extracellular fluids (e.g. due to tissue trauma or chemotherapy for malignant tumours), in renal failure, or when excess phosphate is administered or ingested. Infants who are fed cow's milk are at risk for hyperphosphataemia, as are people using phosphate-containing enemas or laxatives. Patients who have high serum phosphate levels may experience numbness and tingling around the mouth and in the fingertips, muscle spasms and tetany.

Table 18-6 Electrolyte Imbalances

Risk factors	Clinical manifestations	Nursing interventions
Hyponatraemia		
Loss of sodium	Lethargy, confusion, apprehension	Assess clinical manifestations.
+ Gastrointestinal fluid loss	Muscle twitching	Monitor fluid intake and output.
+ Sweating	Abdominal cramps	Monitor laboratory data (e.g. serum sodium).
+ Use of diuretics	Anorexia, nausea, vomiting	Assess patient closely if administering hypertonic
Gain of water	Headache	saline solutions.
+ Hypotonic tube feedings	Seizures, coma	Encourage food and fluid high in sodium if permitted
+ Drinking water	*Laboratory findings:*	(e.g. table salt, bacon, ham, processed cheese).
+ Excess Intravenous infusion of	Serum sodium below 135 mmol/l	Limit water intake as indicated.
dextrose in water administration	Serum osmolality below 280	
Syndrome of inappropriate ADH	mOsm/kg	
(SIADH)		
+ Head injury		
+ AIDS		
+ Malignant tumours		
Hypernatraemia		
Loss of fluids	Thirst	Monitor fluid intake and output.
+ Insensible water loss	Dry, sticky mucous membranes	Monitor behaviour changes (e.g. restlessness,
(hyperventilation or fever)	Tongue red, dry, swollen	disorientation).
+ Diarrhoea	Weakness	Monitor laboratory findings (e.g. serum sodium).
Water deprivation	Postural hypotension, dyspnoea	Encourage fluids as ordered.
Excess salt intake	Severe hypernatraemia:	Monitor diet as ordered (e.g. restrict intake of salt and
+ Parenteral administration of	+ Fatigue, restlessness	foods high in sodium).
saline solutions	+ Decreasing level of consciousness	
+ Hypertonic tube feedings	+ Disorientation	
without adequate water	+ Convulsions	
+ Excessive use of table salt	*Laboratory findings:*	
Conditions such as	Serum sodium above 145 mmol/l	
+ Diabetes insipidus	Serum osmolality above 300	
+ Heat stroke	mOsm/kg	
Hypokalaemia		
Loss of potassium	Muscle weakness, leg cramps	Monitor heart rate and rhythm.
+ Vomiting and gastric suction	Fatigue, lethargy	Monitor patients receiving digitalis (e.g. digoxin) closely,
+ Diarrhoea	Anorexia, nausea, vomiting	because hypokalemia increases risk of digitalis toxicity.
+ Heavy perspiration	Decreased bowel sounds, decreased	Administer oral potassium as ordered with food or fluid
Use of potassium-wasting drugs	bowel motility	to prevent gastric irritation.
(e.g. diuretics)	Cardiac dysrhythmias	Administer IV potassium solutions at a rate no faster
Poor intake of potassium (as with	Depressed deep-tendon reflexes	than 10–20 mmol/h; never administer undiluted
debilitated patients, alcoholics,	*Laboratory findings:*	potassium intravenously. For patients receiving IV
anorexia nervosa)	Serum potassium below 3.5 mmol/l	potassium, monitor for pain and inflammation at the
Hyperaldosteronism	Arterial blood gases (ABGs) may	injection site.
	show alkalosis	Teach patient about potassium-rich foods.
	T wave flattening and ST segment	Teach patients how to prevent excessive loss
	depression on ECG	of potassium (e.g. through abuse of diuretics
		and laxatives).
Hyperkalaemia		
Decreased potassium excretion	Gastrointestinal hyperactivity,	Closely monitor cardiac status and ECG.
+ Renal failure	diarrhoea	Administer diuretics and other medications such as
+ Hypoaldosteronism	Irritability, apathy, confusion	glucose and insulin as ordered.
+ Potassium-conserving diuretics	Cardiac dysrhythmias or arrest	Hold potassium supplements and K+ conserving
High potassium intake	Muscle weakness, areflexia	diuretics.
+ Excessive use of K+ containing	(absence of reflexes)	
salt substitutes	Paresthesias and numbness in	Monitor serum K+ levels carefully; a rapid drop may
+ Excessive or rapid IV infusion of	extremities	occur as potassium shifts into the cells.
potassium	*Laboratory findings:*	Teach patients to avoid foods high in potassium and
Potassium shift out of the	Serum potassium above 5.0 mmol/l	salt substitutes.
tissue cells into the plasma	Peaked T wave, widened QRS on ECG	
(e.g. infections, burns, acidosis)		

Table 18-6 (*continued*)

Risk factors	Clinical manifestations	Nursing interventions
Hypocalcaemia *Surgical removal of the parathyroid glands* Conditions such as ✚ Hypoparathyroidism ✚ Acute pancreatitis ✚ Hyperphosphataemia ✚ Thyroid carcinoma *Inadequate vitamin D intake* ✚ Malabsorption ✚ Hypomagnesaemia ✚ Alkalosis ✚ Sepsis ✚ Alcohol abuse	Numbness, tingling of the extremities and around the mouth Muscle tremors, cramps; if severe can progress to tetany and convulsions Cardiac dysrhythmias; decreased cardiac output Confusion, anxiety, possible psychoses *Laboratory findings:* Serum calcium less than 8.5 mg/dL or 4.5 mmol/l (total)	Closely monitor respiratory and cardiovascular status. Take precautions to protect a confused patient. Administer oral or parenteral calcium supplements as ordered. When administering intravenously, closely monitor cardiac status and ECG during infusion. Teach patients at high risk for osteoporosis about ✚ Dietary sources rich in calcium ✚ Recommendation for 1,000–1,500 mg of calcium per day ✚ Calcium supplements ✚ Regular exercise ✚ Oestrogen replacement therapy for postmenopausal women.
Hypercalcaemia Prolonged immobilisation Conditions such as ✚ Hyperparathyroidism ✚ Malignancy of the bone ✚ Paget's disease	Lethargy, weakness Depressed deep-tendon reflexes Anorexia, nausea, vomiting Constipation Polyuria, hypercalciuria Flank pain secondary to urinary calculi Dysrhythmias, possible heart block *Laboratory findings:* Serum calcium greater than 10.5 mg/dL or 5.5 mmol/l (total)	Increase patient movement and exercise. Encourage oral fluids as permitted to maintain a dilute urine. Teach patients to limit intake of food and fluid high in calcium. Encourage ingestion of fibre to prevent constipation. Protect a confused patient; monitor for pathologic fractures in patients with long-term hypercalcemia. Encourage intake of acid-ash fluids (e.g. prune or cranberry juice) to counteract deposits of calcium salts in the urine.
Hypomagnesaemia Excessive loss from the gastrointestinal tract (e.g. from nasogastric suction, diarrhoea, fistula drainage) Long-term use of certain drugs (e.g. diuretics, aminoglycoside antibiotics) Conditions such as ✚ Chronic alcoholism ✚ Pancreatitis ✚ Burns	Neuromuscular irritability with tremors Increased reflexes, tremors, convulsions Tachycardia, elevated blood pressure, dysrhythmias Disorientation and confusion Vertigo *Laboratory findings:* Serum magnesium below 1.5 mmol/l	Assess patients receiving digitalis for digitalis toxicity. Hypomagnesemia increases the risk toxicity. Take protective measures when there is a possibility of seizures. ✚ Assess the patient's ability to swallow water prior to initiating oral feeding. ✚ Initiate safety measures to prevent injury during seizure activity. ✚ Carefully administer magnesium salts as ordered. Encourage patients to eat magnesium-rich foods if permitted (e.g. whole grains, meat, seafood and green leafy vegetables). Refer patients to alcohol treatment programmes as indicated.
Hypermagnesaemia Abnormal retention of magnesium, as in ✚ Renal failure ✚ Adrenal insufficiency Treatment with magnesium salts	Peripheral vasodilation, flushing Nausea, vomiting Muscle weakness, paralysis Hypotension, bradycardia Depressed deep-tendon reflexes Lethargy, drowsiness Respiratory depression, coma Respiratory and cardiac arrest if hypomagnesaemia is severe *Laboratory findings:* Serum magnesium above 2.5 mmol/l Electrocardiogram showing prolonged QT interval; an AV block may occur	Monitor vital signs and level of consciousness when patients are at risk. If patellar reflexes are absent, notify the physician. Advise patients who have renal disease to contact their care provider before taking over-the-counter drugs.

Table 18-7 Acid–Base Imbalances

Risk factors	Clinical manifestations	Nursing interventions
Respiratory acidosis Acute lung conditions that impair alveolar gas exchange (e.g. pneumonia, acute pulmonary oedema, aspiration of foreign body, near-drowning) Chronic lung disease (e.g. asthma, cystic fibrosis or emphysema) Overdose of narcotics or sedatives that depress respiratory rate and depth Brain injury that affects the respiratory centre	Increased pulse and respiratory rates Headache, dizziness Confusion, decreased level of consciousness (LOC) Convulsions Warm, flushed skin **Chronic:** Weakness Headache *Laboratory findings:* Arterial blood pH less than 7.35 $PaCO_2$ above 45 mm Hg HCO_3^- normal or slightly elevated in acute; above 26 mmol/l in chronic	Frequently assess respiratory status and lung sounds. Monitor airway and ventilation; insert artificial airway and prepare for mechanical ventilation as necessary. Administer pulmonary therapy measures such as inhalation therapy, percussion and postural drainage, bronchodilators and antibiotics as ordered. Monitor fluid intake and output, vital signs and arterial blood gases. Administer narcotic antagonists as indicated. Maintain adequate hydration (2–3 l of fluid per day).
Respiratory alkalosis Hyperventilation due to + Extreme anxiety + Elevated body temperature + Overventilation with a mechanical ventilator + Hypoxia + Salicylate overdose	Complaints of shortness of breath, chest tightness Light-headedness with circumoral paresthesias and numbness and tingling of the extremities Difficulty concentrating Tremulousness, blurred vision *Laboratory findings (in uncompensated respiratory alkalosis):* Arterial blood pH above 7.45 $PaCO_2$ less than 35 mm Hg	Monitor vital signs and ABGs. Assist patient to breathe more slowly. Help patient breathe in a paper bag or apply a rebreather mask (to inhale CO_2).
Metabolic acidosis Conditions that increase nonvolatile acids in the blood (e.g. renal impairment, diabetes mellitus, starvation) Conditions that decrease bicarbonate (e.g. prolonged diarrhoea) Excessive infusion of chloride-containing IV fluids (e.g. NaCl)	Kussmaul's respirations (deep, rapid respirations) Lethargy, confusion Headache Weakness Nausea and vomiting *Laboratory findings:* Arterial blood pH below 7.35 Serum bicarbonate less than 22 mmol/l $PaCO_2$ less than 38 mm Hg with respiratory compensation	Monitor ABG values, intake and output, and LOC. Administer IV sodium bicarbonate carefully if ordered. Treat underlying problem as ordered.
Metabolic alkalosis Excessive acid losses due to + Vomiting + Gastric suction Excessive use of potassium-losing diuretics Excessive adrenal corticoid hormones due to + Cushing's syndrome + Hyperaldosteronism Excessive bicarbonate intake from + Antacids + Parenteral $NaHCO_3$	Decreased respiratory rate and depth Dizziness Circumoral paresthesias, numbness and tingling of the extremities Hypertonic muscles, tetany *Laboratory findings:* Arterial blood pH above 7.45 Serum bicarbonate greater than 26 mmol/l $PaCO_2$ higher than 45 mm Hg with respiratory compensation	Monitor intake and output closely. Monitor vital signs, especially respirations, and LOC. Administer ordered IV fluids carefully. Treat underlying problem.

Acid-Base Imbalances

Acid–base imbalances generally are classified as *respiratory* or *metabolic* by the general or underlying cause of the disorder. Carbonic acid levels are normally regulated by the lungs through the retention or excretion of carbon dioxide, and problems of regulation lead to respiratory acidosis or alkalosis. Bicarbonate and hydrogen ion levels are regulated by the kidneys, and problems of regulation lead to metabolic acidosis or alkalosis. Healthy regulatory systems will attempt to correct acid–base imbalances, a process called **compensation**.

Respiratory Acidosis

Hypoventilation and carbon dioxide retention cause carbonic acid levels to increase and the pH to fall below 7.35, a condition known as **respiratory acidosis**. Serious lung diseases such as asthma and COPD are common causes of respiratory acidosis. Central nervous system depression due to anaesthesia or a narcotic overdose can sufficiently slow the respiratory rate so that carbon dioxide is retained. When respiratory acidosis occurs, the kidneys retain bicarbonate to restore the normal carbonic acid to bicarbonate ratio. Recall, however, that the kidneys are relatively slow to respond to changes in acid–base balance, so this compensatory response may require hours to days to restore the normal pH.

Respiratory Alkalosis

When a person hyperventilates, more carbon dioxide than normal is exhaled, carbonic acid levels fall, and the pH rises to greater than 7.45. This condition is termed **respiratory alkalosis**. Psychogenic or anxiety-related hyperventilation is a common cause of respiratory alkalosis. Other causes include fever and respiratory infections. In respiratory alkalosis, the kidneys will excrete bicarbonate to return the pH to within the normal range. Often, however, the cause of the hyperventilation is eliminated and the pH returns to normal before renal compensation occurs.

Metabolic Acidosis

When bicarbonate levels are low in relation to the amount of carbonic acid in the body, the pH falls and **metabolic acidosis** develops. This may develop because of renal failure and the inability of the kidneys to excrete hydrogen ion and produce bicarbonate. It also may occur when too much acid is produced in the body, for example, in diabetic ketoacidosis or starvation when fat tissue is broken down for energy. Metabolic acidosis stimulates the respiratory centre, and the rate and depth of respirations increase. Carbon dioxide is eliminated and carbonic acid levels fall, minimising the change in pH. This respiratory compensation occurs within minutes of the pH imbalance.

Metabolic Alkalosis

In **metabolic alkalosis**, the amount of bicarbonate in the body exceeds normal values. Ingestion of bicarbonate of soda as an antacid is one cause of metabolic alkalosis. Another cause is prolonged vomiting with loss of hydrochloric acid from the stomach. The respiratory centre is depressed in metabolic alkalosis, and respirations slow and become shallower. Carbon dioxide is retained and carbonic acid levels increase, helping balance the excess bicarbonate.

The risk factors and manifestations for acid–base imbalances are listed in Table 18-7.

NURSING MANAGEMENT

ASSESSING

Assessing a patient's fluid, electrolyte and acid–base balance and imbalances is an important nursing function. Components of the assessment include (a) the patient history, (b) physical assessment of the patient, (c) clinical measurements and (d) review of laboratory test results.

Patient History

The patient history is particularly important for identifying patients who are at risk for fluid, electrolyte and acid–base imbalances. The current and past medical history may reveal conditions such as chronic lung disease or diabetes mellitus that can disrupt normal balances. Medications prescribed to treat acute or chronic conditions (e.g. diuretic therapy for

hypertension) also may place the risk of fluid, electrolyte and acid base disturbances.

Common risk factors are listed in *Box 18-3* on page 450.

When obtaining the patient history, the nurse needs to not only recognise risk factors but also elicit data about the patient's food and fluid intake, fluid output, and the presence of signs or symptoms suggestive of altered fluid and electrolyte balance, such as headaches, lethargy and nausea and vomiting.

Physical Assessment

Physical assessment of the patient will usually focus on the skin, oral cavity, heart, lungs, muscles and neurological status. The findings from the physical assessment is used to expand and verify information taken when taking the patient history of

> **BOX 18-3** Common Risk Factors for Fluid, Electrolyte and Acid–Base Imbalances
>
> ### Chronic Diseases and Conditions
> + Chronic lung disease (COPD, asthma, cystic fibrosis)
> + Heart failure
> + Kidney disease
> + Diabetes mellitus
> + Cushing's syndrome or Addison's disease
> + Cancer
> + Malnutrition, anorexia nervosa, bulimia
> + Ileostomy (an operation that involves bringing the end of the ileum to the surface of the skin and a stoma formed)
>
> ### Acute Conditions
> + Acute gastroenteritis
> + Bowel obstruction
> + Head injury or decreased level of consciousness
> + Trauma such as burns or crushing injuries
> + Surgery
> + Fever, draining wounds, fistulas (an abnormal opening between two organs)
>
> ### Medications
> + Diuretics
> + Corticosteroids
> + Nonsteroidal anti-inflammatory drugs
>
> ### Treatments
> + Chemotherapy
> + IV therapy and total parenteral nutrition
> + Nasogastric suction
> + Enteral feedings
> + Mechanical ventilation
>
> ### Other Factors
> + Age: Very old or very young
> + Inability to access food and fluids independently

the patient. Table 18-8 expands on the physical assessment of the patient. You may also want to refer to Tables 18-6 and 18-7 for possible abnormal findings related to specific imbalances.

Clinical Measurements

Three simple clinical measurements that can be initiated by the nurse to detect signs of fluid and nutritional problems.

Daily Weights

Daily weight measurements provide a relatively accurate assessment of a patient's fluid status. Significant changes in weight over a short time (e.g. days to a week or two) are indicative of

acute fluid changes. Each kilogram (2.2 lb) of weight gained or lost is equivalent to 1 litre of fluid gained or lost. Such fluid gains or losses indicate changes in total body fluid volume rather than in any specific compartment, such as the intravascular compartment. Rapid losses or gains of 5–8% of total body weight indicate moderate to severe fluid volume deficits or excesses.

To obtain accurate weight measurements, the nurse should weigh the patient (a) at the same time each day (e.g. before breakfast), (b) wearing the same or similar clothing, and (c) on the same scale. The type of scale (i.e. standing, bed, chair) should be documented.

Vital Signs

Changes in the vital signs may indicate, or in some cases precede, fluid, electrolyte and acid–base imbalances. For example, elevated body temperature may be a result of dehydration or a cause of increased body fluid losses.

Respiratory rate is the clearest indicator that the patient is having some difficulty with fluid, electrolyte and/or acid–base balances. The 'Patient at risk' scoring system, a means of assessing the patient's stability, is currently being widely used within the UK as a means of identifying those patients at risk of deterioration. One of the vital signs that this scoring system focuses on is respiratory rate as this is one of the first indicators of potential health problems.

Tachycardia is an early sign of hypovolaemia. Pulse volume will decrease in hypovolaemia and increase in hypervolaemia. Irregular pulse rates may occur with electrolyte imbalances. Changes in respiratory rate and depth may cause respiratory acid–base imbalances or act as a compensatory mechanism in metabolic acidosis or alkalosis.

Blood pressure, a sensitive measure to detect blood volume changes, may fall significantly with hypovolaemia or increase with hypervolaemia. Postural, or orthostatic, hypotension may also occur with hypovolaemia.

To assess for orthostatic hypotension, measure the patient's blood pressure and pulse in a supine position. Allow the patient to remain in that position for 3–5 minutes, leaving the blood pressure cuff on the arm. Stand the patient up and immediately reassess the blood pressure and pulse. A drop of 10–15 mm Hg in the systolic blood pressure with a corresponding drop in diastolic pressure and an increased pulse rate (by 10 or more beats per minute) is indicative of orthostatic or postural hypotension.

Fluid Intake and Output

The measurement and recording of all fluid intake and output (I and O) during a 24-hour period provides important data about the patient's fluid and electrolyte balance.

The unit used to measure intake and output is the millilitre (ml). Most hospitals have a form for recording fluid balance, usually a bedside record on which the nurse lists all items measured and the quantities per shift (see Figure 18-8 on page 452). Some agencies have another form for recording the specifics of

Table 18-8 Focused Physical Assessment for Fluid, Electrolyte or Acid–Base Imbalances

System	Assessment focus	Technique	Possible abnormal findings
Skin	Colour, temperature, moisture	Inspection, palpation	Flushed, warm, very dry Moist or diaphoretic Cool and pale
	Turgor	Gently pinch up a fold of skin over sternum or inner aspect of thigh for adults, on the abdomen or medial thigh for children	Poor turgor: Skin remains tented for several seconds instead of immediately returning to normal position
	Oedema	Inspect for visible swelling around eyes, in fingers and in lower extremities Compress the skin over the dorsum of the foot, around the ankles, over the tibia, in the sacral area	Skin around eyes is puffy, lids appear swollen; rings are tight; shoes leave impressions on feet Depression remains (pitting): see scale for describing oedema in Figure 18-6
Mucous membranes	Colour, moisture	Inspection	Mucous membranes dry, dull in appearance; tongue dry and cracked
Eyes	Firmness	Gently palpate eyeball with lid closed	Eyeball feels soft to palpation
Fontanels (soft spot on the top of an infant's head)	Firmness, level	Inspect and gently palpate anterior fontanel	Fontanel bulging, firm Fontanel sunken, soft
Cardiovascular system	Heart rate	Auscultation, cardiac monitor	Tachycardia, bradycardia; irregular; dysrhythmias
	Peripheral pulses	Palpation	Weak and thready; bounding
	Blood pressure	Auscultation of Korotkoff's sounds BP assessment lying and standing	Hypotension Postural hypotension
	Capillary refill	Palpation	Slowed capillary refill
	Venous filling	Inspection of jugular veins and hand veins	Jugular venous distention; flat jugular veins, poor venous refill
Respiratory system	Respiratory rate and pattern	Inspection	Increased or decreased rate and depth of respirations
	Lung sounds	Auscultation	Crackles or moist rales
Neurological	Level of consciousness (LOC)	Observation, stimulation	Decreased LOC, lethargy, stupor or coma
	Orientation, cognition	Questioning	Disoriented, confused; difficulty concentrating
	Motor function	Strength testing	Weakness, decreased motor strength
	Reflexes	Deep-tendon reflex (DTR) testing	Hyperactive or depressed DTRs
	Abnormal reflexes	*Chvostek's sign*: Tap over facial nerve about 2 cm anterior to tragus of ear *Trousseau's sign*: Inflate a blood pressure cuff on the upper arm to 20 mm Hg greater than the systolic pressure, leave in place for 2–5 minutes	Facial muscle twitching including eyelids and lips on side of stimulus Carpal spasm: contraction of hand and fingers on affected side

intravenous fluids, such as the type of solution, additives, time started, amounts absorbed and amounts remaining per shift.

It is important to inform patients, family members and all caregivers that accurate measurements of the patient's fluid intake and output are required, explaining why and emphasising the need to use a bedpan, urinal or commode. Instruct the patient not to put toilet tissue into the container with urine. Patients who wish to be involved in recording fluid intake measurements need to be taught how to compute the values and what foods are considered fluids.

To measure fluid intake, the nurse records on the fluid balance form each fluid item taken (if the patient has not already done so), specifying the time and type of fluid. All of the following fluids need to be recorded:

+ Oral fluids
+ Water
+ Milk
+ Juice
+ Soft drinks

Fluid balance chart

Hospital/Ward:			Date:			
Hospital number:						
Surname:						
Forenames:						
Date of birth:						
Sex:						

	Fluid intake			Fluid output		
Time (hrs)	Oral	IV	Other (specify route)	Urine	Vomit	Other (specify)
01.00						
02.00						
03.00						
04.00						
05.00						
06.00						
07.00						
08.00						
09.00						
10.00						
11.00						
12.00						
13.00						
14.00						
15.00						
16.00						
17.00						
18.00						
19.00						
20.00						
21.00						
22.00						
23.00						
24.00						
TOTAL						

Figure 18-8 Fluid balance chart (from Nicol *et al.* (2000) *'Essential Nursing Skills'*, Mosby).

+ Coffee or tea
+ Cream
+ Soup
+ Any other beverages including water taken with medications
+ Foods that are or tend to become liquid at room temperature, including ice cream, sherbet, custard and gelatine
+ Do not measure foods that are pureed, because purees are simply solid foods prepared in a different form
+ Tube feedings. Remember to include the water flushes at the end of intermittent feedings or during continuous feedings
+ Parenteral fluids (intravenous fluids). The exact amount of intravenous fluid administered is to be recorded, since some fluid containers may be overfilled. Blood transfusions are included
+ Intravenous medications. Intravenous medications that are prepared with solutions such as normal saline (NS) and are administered as an intermittent or continuous infusion must also be included
+ Catheter or tube irrigants. Fluid used to irrigate urinary catheters, nasogastric tubes and intestinal tubes must be measured and recorded if not immediately withdrawn.

To measure fluid output, measure the following fluids (remember to observe appropriate infection control precautions):

+ Urinary output. Following each voiding, pour the urine into a measuring container, observe the amount, and record it and the time of voiding on the fluid balance form.
+ For patients with retention catheters, empty the drainage bag into a measuring container at the end of the shift (or at prescribed times if output is to be measured more often). Note and record the amount of urine output.
+ In intensive care areas, urine output often is measured hourly.
+ If the patient is incontinent of urine, estimate and record these outputs. For example, for an incontinent patient the nurse might record 'Incontinent × 3' or 'Drawsheet soaked in 12 inch diameter'. A more accurate estimate of the urine output of infants and incontinent patients may be obtained by first weighing nappies or incontinent pads that are dry, and then subtracting this weight from the weight of the soiled items. Each gram of weight left after subtracting is equal to 1 ml of urine. If urine is frequently soiled with faeces, the number of voidings may be recorded rather than the volume of urine.
+ Vomitus and liquid faeces. The amount and type of fluid and the time need to be specified.
+ Tube drainage, such as gastric or intestinal drainage.
+ Wound drainage and draining fistulas. Wound drainage may be recorded by documenting the type and number of dressings or linen saturated with drainage or by measuring the exact amount of drainage collected in a vacuum drainage or gravity drainage system.

Fluid intake and output measurements are totalled at the end of the shift (every 8–12 hours), and the totals are recorded in the patient's permanent record. In intensive care areas, the nurse may record intake and output hourly. Usually the staff on night shift totals the amounts of input and output recorded for each shift and records the 24-hour total.

To determine whether the fluid output is proportional to fluid intake or whether there are any changes in the patient's fluid status, the nurse (a) compares the total 24-hour fluid output measurement with the total fluid intake measurement and (b) compares both to previous measurements. Urinary output is normally equivalent to the amount of fluids ingested; the usual range is 1.5–2 litres in 24 hours, or 40–80 ml in 1 hour (0.5 ml/kg/hour). Patients whose output substantially exceeds intake are at risk for fluid volume deficit. By contrast, patients whose intake substantially exceeds output are at risk for fluid volume excess. In assessing the patient's fluid balance it is important to consider additional factors that may affect intake and output. The patient who is extremely diaphoretic (excess perspiration) or who has rapid, deep respirations has fluid losses that cannot be measured but must be considered in evaluating fluid status.

When there is a significant discrepancy between intake and output or when fluid intake or output is inadequate (e.g. a urine output of less than 500 ml in 24 hours or less than 0.5 ml per kilogram per hour in an adult), this information should be reported to the charge nurse or doctor immediately.

Laboratory Tests

Laboratory tests provide objective information about the patient's fluid, electrolyte and acid-base balance.

Full Blood Count (FBC)

The full blood count, another basic screening test, includes information about the haematocrit (Hct). The **haematocrit** measures the volume (percentage) of whole blood that is composed of red blood cells (RBC) in relation to plasma. Therefore haematocrit is affected by changes in plasma volume. Normal haematocrit values are 40–54% in men and 37–47% in women. With severe dehydration haematocrit increases and conversely severe overhydration decreases haematocrit.

Osmolality

Serum osmolality is a measure of the solute concentration of the blood and is used primarily to evaluate fluid balance. Normal values are 280–300 mOsm/kg. An increase in serum osmolality indicates a fluid volume deficit; a decrease reflects a fluid volume excess.

Serum Electrolytes

Serum electrolyte levels are often routinely ordered for any patient admitted to hospital as a screening test for electrolyte and acid–base imbalances. Serum electrolytes also are routinely assessed for patients at risk in the community, for example, patients who are being treated with a diuretic for hypertension or heart failure. The most commonly ordered serum tests are for sodium, potassium, chloride, magnesium and bicarbonate ions. Normal values of commonly measured electrolytes are shown in *Box 18-4*.

Urine pH

Measurement of urine pH may be obtained by laboratory analysis or by using a dipstick on a fresh urine specimen. Because the kidneys play a critical role in regulating acid–base balance,

---

BOX 18-4 Normal Electrolyte Values for Adults*

Venous blood

Sodium	135-145 mmol/l
Potassium	3.5-5.0 mmol/l
Chloride	95-105 mmol/l
Calcium (total)	4.5-5.5 mmol/l or 8.5-10.5 mg/dl
Magnesium	1.5-2.5 mmol/l or 1.6-2.5 mg/dl
Phosphate (phosphorus)	1.8-2.6 mmol/l
Serum osmolality	280-300 mOsm/kg water

Normal laboratory values vary from trust to trust.

assessment of urine pH can be useful in determining whether the kidneys are responding appropriately to acid–base imbalances. Normally the pH of the urine is relatively acidic, averaging about 6.0, but a range of 4.6–8.0 is considered normal. In metabolic acidosis, urine pH should decrease as the kidneys excrete hydrogen ions; in metabolic alkalosis, the pH should increase.

Urine Specific Gravity

Specific gravity is an indicator of urine concentration that can be performed quickly and easily by nursing staff. Normal specific gravity ranges from 1.005 to 1.030 (usually 1.010 to 1.025). When the concentration of solutes in the urine is high, the specific gravity rises; in very dilute urine with few solutes, it is abnormally low.

Arterial Blood Gases

Arterial blood gases (ABGs) are performed to evaluate the patient's acid–base balance and oxygenation. Arterial blood is used because it provides a truer reflection of gas exchange in the pulmonary system than venous blood. Blood gases may be drawn by nurses with specialised skills and can be taken by inserting a needle into the artery or by taking blood from a line that has already been inserted into the artery which is commonly found in critical care areas.

Six measurements are commonly used to interpret arterial blood gas tests:

1. pH, a measure of the relative acidity or alkalinity of the blood
2. PaO_2, the pressure exerted by oxygen dissolved in the plasma of arterial blood; an indirect measure of blood oxygen content
3. $PaCO_2$, the partial pressure of carbon dioxide in arterial plasma; the respiratory component of acid–base determination

4. Bicarbonate HCO_3^- a measure of the metabolic component of acid–base balance
5. Base excess (BE), a calculated value of bicarbonate levels, also reflective of the metabolic component of acid–base balance
6. Oxygen saturation (SaO_2), the percentage of haemoglobin saturated (combined) with oxygen.

Normal ABG values are listed in *Box 18-5* and changes seen in common acid–base imbalances are summarised in Table 18-9. However, please note that although the PaO_2 and SaO_2 are important for assessing respiratory status, they generally do not provide useful information for assessing acid–base balance and so are not included in this table.

When evaluating ABG results to determine acid–base balance, it is important to use a systematic approach such as the one outlined in *Box 18-6*. Nurses need to assess each measurement individually, then look at the interrelationships to determine what type of acid–base imbalance may be present.

BOX 18-5 Normal Values of Arterial Blood Gases*

pH	7.35-7.45
PaO_2	80-100 mm Hg
$PaCO_2$	35-45 mm Hg
HCO_3^-	22-26 mmol/l
Base excess	–2 to +2 mmol/l
O_2 saturation	95-98%

Some normal values will vary according to the kind of test carried out in the laboratory. Nurses are advised to use the normal values issued by the trust when interpreting laboratory results.

Table 18-9 Arterial Blood Gas Values in Common Acid-Base Disorders

Disorder		ABG values
Respiratory acidosis	pH	<7.35
	$PaCO_2$	>45 mm Hg (excess CO_2 and carbonic acid)
	HCO_3^-	Normal; >26 mmol/l with renal compensation
Respiratory alkalosis	pH	>7.45
	$PaCO_2$	<35 mm Hg (inadequate CO_2 and carbonic acid)
	HCO_3^-	Normal; <22 mmol/l with renal compensation
Metabolic acidosis	pH	<7.35
	$PaCO_2$	Normal; <35 mm Hg with respiratory compensation
	HCO_3^-	<22 mmol/l
	BE	<–2 mmol/l
Metabolic alkalosis	pH	<7.45
	$PaCO_2$	Normal; >45 mm Hg with respiratory compensation
	HCO_3^-	>26 mmol/l (excess bicarbonate)
	BE	>+2 mmol/l

BOX 18-6 Interpreting ADGs

1. Look at the pH:
   a. If the pH is less than 7.35, the problem is acidosis.
   b. If the pH is greater than 7.45, the problem is alkalosis.
2. Look at the $PaCO_2$:
   a. If the $PaCO_2$ is less than 35 mm Hg, more carbon dioxide is being exhaled than normal.
   b. If the $PaCO_2$ is greater than 45 mm Hg, less carbon dioxide is being exhaled than normal.
3. Assess the pH and $PaCO_2$ relationship for a possible respiratory problem:
   a. If the pH is less than 7.35 (acidosis), and the $PaCO_2$ is greater than 45 mm Hg, retained carbon dioxide is causing **respiratory acidosis**.

   b. If the pH is greater than 7.45 (alkalosis), and the $PaCO_2$ is less than 35 mm Hg, lack of carbon dioxide is causing **respiratory alkalosis**.
4. Look at the bicarbonate:
   a. If the HCO_3 is less than 22 mmol/l, bicarbonate levels are lower than normal.
   b. If the HCO_3^- is greater than 26 mmol/l, bicarbonate levels are higher than normal.
5. Assess pH, HCO_3^- and base excess (BE) values for a possible metabolic problem:
   a. If the pH is less than 7.35 and the bicarbonate is less than 22 mmol/l, and the BE is less than -2 mmol/l this is **metabolic acidosis**.
   b. If the pH is more than 7.45 (alkalosis) and the bicarbonate is greater than 26 mmol/l, and the BE is greater $+2$ mmol/l this is **metabolic alkalosis**.

PLANNING

Major goals for patients with or at risk for nutritional and hydration problems include:

+ Maintain or restore normal fluid balance.
+ Maintain or restore normal balance of electrolytes in the intracellular and extracellular compartments.
+ Maintain or restore pulmonary ventilation and oxygenation.
+ Prevent associated risks (tissue breakdown, decreased cardiac output, confusion, other neurologic signs).

Obviously, goals will vary according to the diagnosis and defining characteristics for each individual. Appropriate preventive and corrective nursing interventions that relate to these must be identified.

IMPLEMENTING

Promoting Wellness

Most people rarely think about their fluid, electrolyte or acid–base balance. They know it is important to drink adequate fluids and consume a balanced diet, but they may not understand the potential effects when this is not done. Nurses can promote patients' health by providing education that will help them maintain fluid and electrolyte balance.

Enteral Fluid and Electrolyte Replacement

Fluids and electrolytes can be provided orally in the hospital and the home if the patient's health permits, that is, if the patient is not vomiting, has not experienced an excessive fluid loss, and has an intact gastrointestinal tract and gag and swallow reflexes. Patients who are unable to ingest solid foods may be able to ingest fluids.

Modifications to Fluid

Increased fluids are often prescribed for patients with actual or potential fluid volume deficits arising, for example, from mild diarrhoea or mild to moderate fevers. Guidelines for helping patients increase fluid intake are shown in the *Practice guidelines* on page 456.

Restricted fluids may be necessary for patients who have fluid retention (fluid volume excess) as a result of renal failure, congestive heart failure, SIADH or other disease processes. Fluid restrictions vary from 'nothing by mouth' to a precise amount ordered by a doctor. The restriction of fluids can be difficult for some patients, particularly if they are experiencing thirst. Guidelines for helping patients restrict fluid intake are shown in the *Practice guidelines* on page 456.

Dietary Changes

Specific fluid and electrolyte imbalances may require simple dietary changes. For example, patients receiving potassium-depleting diuretics need to be informed about foods with a high potassium content (e.g. bananas, oranges and leafy greens). Some patients with fluid retention need to avoid foods high in sodium. Most healthy patients can benefit from foods rich in calcium.

Oral Electrolyte Supplements

Some patients can benefit from oral supplements of electrolytes, particularly when a medication is prescribed that affects electrolyte balance, when dietary intake is inadequate

PRACTICE GUIDELINES

Facilitating Fluid Intake

+ Explain to the patient the reason for the required intake and the specific amount needed. This provides a rationale for the requirement and promotes compliance.
+ Set short-term goals that the patient can realistically meet. Examples include drinking a glass of fluid every hour while awake or a pitcher of water by 12 noon.
+ Identify fluids the patient likes and make available a variety of those items, including fruit juices, soft drinks and milk (if allowed). Remember that beverages such as coffee and tea have a diuretic effect, so their consumption should be limited.
+ Help patients to select foods that tend to become liquid at room temperature (e.g. ice cream, sherbet, custard), if these are allowed.
+ For patients who are confined to bed, supply appropriate cups and glasses to facilitate appropriate fluid intake and keep the fluids within easy reach.
+ Make sure fluids are served at the appropriate temperature: hot fluids hot and cold fluids very cold.
+ Encourage patients when possible to participate in maintaining the fluid intake record. This assists them to evaluate the achievement of desired outcomes.
+ Be alert to any cultural implications of food and fluids. Some cultures may restrict certain foods and fluids and view others as having healing properties.

PRACTICE GUIDELINES

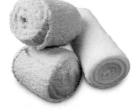

Helping Patients Restrict Fluid Intake

+ Explain the reason for the restricted intake and how much and what types of fluids are permitted orally. Many patients need to be informed that ice cubes, gelatin and ice cream, for example, are considered fluid.
+ Identify fluids or fluidlike substances the patient likes and make sure that these are provided, unless contraindicated.
+ Set short-term goals that make the fluid restriction more tolerable. For example, schedule a specified amount of fluid at one- or two-hourly intervals between meals. Some patients may prefer fluids only between meals if the food provided at mealtime helps relieve thirst.
+ Place allowed fluids in small containers.
+ Periodically offer the patient ice cubes as an alternative to water, because ice cubes when melted are approximately half of the frozen volume.
+ Provide frequent mouth care and rinses to reduce the thirst sensation.
+ Instruct the patient to avoid eating salty or sweet foods because these foods tend to produce thirst. Sugarless gum may be an alternative for some patients.
+ Encourage the patient when possible to participate in maintaining the fluid intake record.

for a specific electrolyte, or when fluid and electrolyte losses are excessive as a result of, for example, excessive perspiration.

Parenteral Fluid and Electrolyte Replacement

Intravenous (IV) fluid therapy is essential when patients are unable to take food and fluids orally. It is an efficient and effective method of supplying fluids directly into the intravascular fluid compartment and replacing electrolyte losses. Intravenous fluid therapy is prescribed by a doctor. The nurse is responsible for administering and maintaining the therapy, and also monitoring the patient receiving the therapy.

Intravenous Solutions

Intravenous solutions can be classified as isotonic, hypotonic or hypertonic. Most IV solutions are *isotonic*, having the same concentration of solutes as blood plasma. Isotonic solutions are often used to restore blood volume. *Hypertonic* solutions have a greater concentration of solutes than plasma; *hypotonic* solutions have a lesser concentration of solutes. Table 18-10 provides examples of IV solutions and nursing implications.

Table 18-10 Selected Intravenous Solutions

Type/examples	Comments/nursing Implications
Isotonic solutions 0.9% NaCl (normal saline) Lactated Ringer's (a balanced electrolyte solution) 5% dextrose in water (D5W)	Isotonic solutions such as normal saline and lactated Ringer's initially remain in the vascular compartment, expanding vascular volume. Assess patients carefully for signs of hypervolaemia such as bounding pulse and shortness of breath. D5W is isotonic on initial administration but provides free water when dextrose is metabolised, expanding intracellular and extracellular fluid volumes.
Hypotonic solutions 0.45% NaCl (half normal saline) 0.33% NaCl (one-third normal saline)	Hypotonic solutions are used to provide free water and treat cellular dehydration. These solutions promote waste elimination by the kidneys.
Hypertonic Solutions 5% dextrose in normal saline (D5NS) 5% dextrose in 0.45% NaCl (D5 1/2NS) 5% dextrose in lactated Ringer's (D5LR)	Hypertonic solutions draw fluid out of the cells and interstitial compartments into the vascular compartment, expanding vascular volume. Do not administer to patients with kidney or heart disease or patients who are dehydrated. Watch for signs of hypervolaemia.

Volume expanders or colloids are used to increase the blood volume following severe loss of blood (e.g. from haemorrhage) or loss of plasma (e.g. from severe burns, which draw large amounts of plasma from the bloodstream to the burn site). Examples of expanders are fresh frozen plasma, blood and albumin.

Venepuncture Sites

The site chosen for venepuncture varies with the patient's age, the length of time the infusion is to run, the type of solution used and the condition of veins. For adults, veins in the hand and arm are commonly used; for infants, veins in the scalp and dorsal foot veins are often used. Larger veins are preferred for infusions that need to be given rapidly and for solutions that could be irritating (e.g. certain medications).

The metacarpal, basilic and cephalic veins are commonly used for intermittent or continuous infusions (see Figure 18-9, B). The ulna and radius act as natural splints at these sites, and the patient has greater freedom of arm movements for activities such as eating. Although the basilic and median cubital veins in the antecubital space are convenient sites for venepuncture, they are usually used for blood sampling, and insertion sites for a peripherally inserted central catheter line (see Figure 18-9, A).

When long-term IV therapy or parenteral nutrition is anticipated or the patient is receiving IV medications that are damaging to vessels (e.g. chemotherapy), a central venous catheter may be inserted. **Central venous catheters** usually are inserted into the subclavian or jugular vein, with the distal tip of the catheter resting in the superior vena cava just above the right atrium (see Figure 18-10 on page 458). They may be inserted at the patient's bedside or, for longer-term access, surgically inserted. Subclavian central venous catheters permit freedom of movement for ambulation; however, there is a risk of pneumothorax on catheter insertion. Assess the patient closely for manifestations such as shortness of breath, chest pain, cough, hypotension, tachycardia and anxiety after the insertion procedure.

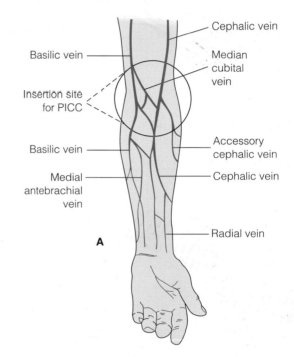

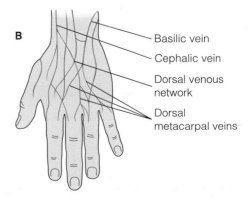

Figure 18-9 Commonly used venepuncture sites of the *A*, arm; *B*, hand. *A* also shows the site used for a peripherally inserted central catheter (PICC).

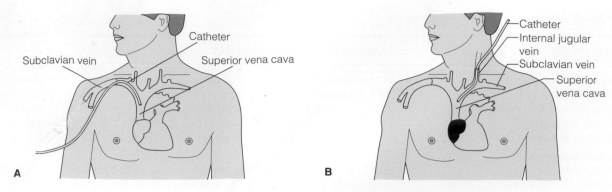

Figure 18-10 Central venous lines with *A*, subclavian vein insertion and *B*, left jugular insertion.

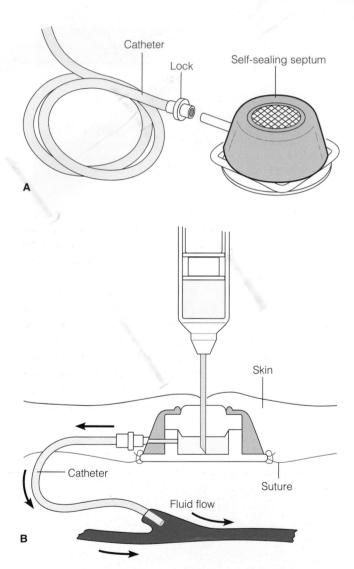

Figure 18-11 An implantable venous access device: *A*, components; *B*, the device in place.

With a **peripherally inserted central venous catheter (PICC)**, the catheter is inserted in the basilic or cephalic vein just above or below the antecubital space of the right arm. The tip of the catheter rests in the superior vena cava. The risk

of pneumothorax is eliminated with PICC. These catheters frequently are used for long-term intravenous access when the patient will be managing IV therapy at home.

Implantable venous access devices or ports (see Figure 18-11, A and B) are used for patients with chronic illness who require long-term IV therapy (e.g. intermittent medications such as chemotherapy, total parenteral nutrition and frequent blood samples). The device is designed to provide repeated access to the central venous system, avoiding the trauma and complications of multiple venepunctures. Using local anaesthesia, implantable ports are surgically placed into a small subcutaneous pocket, usually on the upper chest. The distal end of the catheter is placed in the subclavian or jugular vein. There are different kinds of implantable venous access devices and they may be tunnelled or nontunnelled.

Special precautions need to be taken with all central lines and venous access ports to ensure asepsis and catheter patency. Nursing care of patients with these devices is outlined in *Practice guidelines* on page 460.

Intravenous Equipment

Because equipment varies according to the manufacturer, the nurse must become familiar with the equipment used in each particular hospital or care environment and receive appropriate training on the equipment.

Most solutions are currently dispensed in plastic bags (see Figure 18-12). However, glass containers may need to be used if the administered medications are incompatible with plastic such as albumin infusions. Glass containers require an air vent so that air can enter the bottle and replace the fluid that enters the patient's vein. Air vents usually have filters to prevent contamination from the air that enters the container. Air vents are not required for plastic solution containers, because plastic bags collapse under atmospheric pressure when the solution enters the vein.

Avoid selecting a container whose volume is greater than the volume ordered. For example, if 750 ml 5% Dextrose has been prescribed, the nurse should use one 500 ml container and one 250 ml container, which total 750 ml. Do not obtain a 1,000 ml container with the intention of stopping the solution after 750 ml has been administered. Too often, the incorrect amount can be instilled unless an electronic device is used to regulate

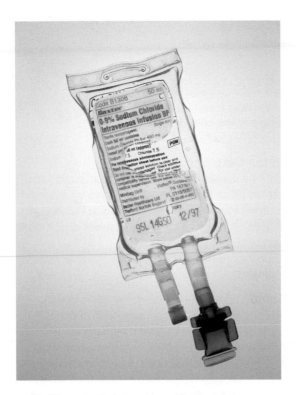

Figure 18-12 A plastic intravenous fluid container.

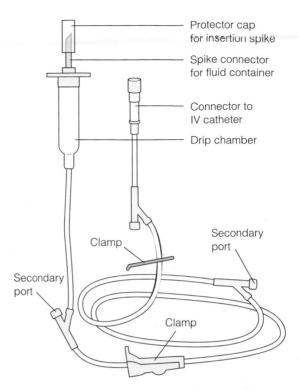

Protector cap
for insertion spike

Spike connector
for fluid container

Connector to
IV catheter

Drip chamber

Clamp

Secondary
port

Secondary
port

Clamp

Figure 18-13 A standard IV administration set.

the volume. If a 1,000 ml solution container must be used, remove 250 ml before starting the infusion.

It is essential that the solution be sterile and clear. Cloudiness, evidence that the container has been opened previously or leaks indicate possible contamination. Always check the expiration date on the label. Return any questionable or contaminated solutions to pharmacy.

Infusion sets usually include an insertion spike, a drip chamber, a roller valve, tubing with secondary ports and a protective cap over the needle adapter (see Figure 18-13). The insertion spike is kept sterile and inserted into the solution container when the equipment is set up and ready to start. The drip chamber permits a predictable amount of fluid to be

delivered. The roller valve or screw clamp, which compresses the lumen of the tubing, controls the rate of the flow. The protective cap over the needle adapter maintains the sterility of the end of the tubing so that it can be attached to a sterile venous cannula inserted in the patient's vein.

Most infusion sets include one or more injection ports for administering IV medications or secondary infusions. Needleless systems are increasingly used because they reduce the risk of needlestick injury and contamination of the intravenous line. With a needleless system, a blunt cannula is inserted into a special injection port or adapter on the IV tubing to administer medications or secondary infusions (see Figure 18-14). Many infusion sets include an in-line filter to trap air, particulate

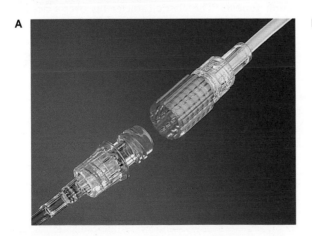

A

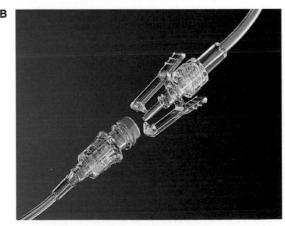

B

Figure 18-14 Cannulae used to connect the tubing of additive sets to primary infusions: *A*, threaded-lock cannula; *B*, lever-lock cannula. (Photographs reprinted courtesy of (BD) Becton, Dickinson and Company and courtesy of Baxter Healthcare Corporation. All rights reserved.)

PRACTICE GUIDELINES

Caring for Patients with a Venous Access Device

+ On insertion, document the date; the site; the brand, gauge and catheter length; the location of the catheter tip (verified by x-ray); and the length of the external segment. Do not utilise the access device until correct placement has been verified by x-ray.

Site Care

+ Use strict aseptic technique when caring for central lines and long-term venous access devices.
+ The frequency of dressing changes may vary from every 1 to 5 days, depending on the site. Dressings also should be changed when loose or soiled.
+ Assess the site for any redness, swelling, tenderness or drainage. Compare the length of the external portion of the catheter with its documented length to assess for possible displacement. Obtain a chest x-ray to determine the catheter tip's position if in doubt. Report and document any position changes or signs of infection.
+ Follow local protocol for cleaning solutions and types of dressings. Some protocols recommend using saline to clean the site while others recommend solutions such as Chlorhexadine.
+ Before using the port it should be cleaned using an alcohol swab, starting at the centre of the port site, moving outwards. Allow the site to air dry.

+ Secure the catheter, and cover the entry site and external portion of the catheter with a transparent occlusive dressing.

Catheter Care and Flushing

+ Flush the port with normal saline, a heparin flush solution (10 units/ml or 100 units/ml), or as local protocol recommends for the specific type of port being used. After infusing medications or solutions, again flush the port with saline.
+ Remember to flush all lumens for multiple-lumen catheters.

Teaching

Provide patients with the following instructions:
+ Do not allow anyone to take a blood pressure on the arm in which a PICC line is inserted.
+ For a PICC, you do not need to restrict activities, except do not immerse the arm in water. Showering is allowed if the site and catheter are covered by an occlusive dressing.
+ For an implanted venous port there are no activity restrictions, but remember that the port or catheter tip can become dislodged. Signs of a dislodged catheter tip include pain in the neck or ear on the affected side, swishing or gurgling sounds, or palpitations. Free movement of the port, swelling or difficulty accessing the port may indicate port dislodgement. Notify the physician should any of these occur or if symptoms of infection develop.

Note: From 'Getting a Line on Central Vascular Access Devices,' by S. Masoorli and T. Angeles, 2002, *Nursing*, 32(4), pp. 36-43. Adapted with permission.

matter and microbes. A special infusion set may be required if the IV flow rate will be regulated by an infusion pump.

Catheters and needles are commonly used for intravenous infusions. Over-the-needle catheters are commonly used for adult patients. The plastic catheter fits over a needle used to pierce the skin and vein wall (see Figure 18-15). Once inserted into the vein, the needle is withdrawn and discarded, leaving the catheter in place. IV catheters allow the patient more

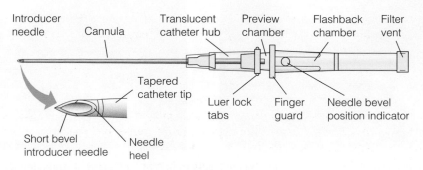

Figure 18-15 An over-the-needle catheter.

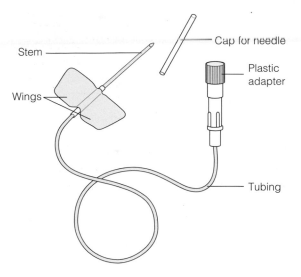

Figure 18-16 Schematic of a butterfly needle with adapter.

mobility and rarely infiltrate, that is, become dislodged from the vein and allow fluid to flow into interstitial spaces.

Butterfly, or wing-tipped, needles with plastic flaps attached to the shaft are sometimes used (see Figure 18-16). The flaps are held tightly together to hold the needle securely during insertion; after insertion, they are flattened against the skin and secured with tape.

IV poles are used to hang the solution container. Some poles are attached to hospital beds; others stand on the floor or hang from the ceiling. The height of most poles is adjustable. The higher the solution container, the greater the force of the solution as it enters the patient and the faster the rate of flow.

Starting an Intravenous Infusion

Although the doctor is responsible for prescribing IV therapy for patients, nurses initiate, monitor and maintain the prescribed IV infusion. This is true not only in hospitals and long-term care facilities but increasingly in community-based settings such as clinics and patients' homes.

Before starting an infusion, the nurse determines the following:

+ The type and amount of solution to be infused
+ The exact amount (dose) of any medications to be added to a compatible solution
+ The rate of flow or the time over which the infusion is to be completed.

If solutions are prepared by the pharmacy or another department, the nurse must verify that the solution supplied exactly matches that which the doctor has prescribed. The nurse needs to understand the purpose for the infusion in order to assess the patient effectively.

To start an intravenous infusion, see *Procedure 18-1*.

EVALUATING

The goals established in the planning phase are evaluated according to specific desired outcomes. If the outcomes are not achieved, the nurse should explore the reasons.

Management of patients with fluid, electrolyte and acid-base disturbances is a vital role within nursing. It is important to note that all nurses should be able to manage a patient's fluid and electrolyte balance however not all nurses are able to administer intravenous fluids or medications without further often formal education. The safe administration of intravenous medications and fluid requires knowledge and experience.

PROCEDURE 18-1 Starting an Intravenous Infusion

Before preparing the infusion, the nurse first checks the prescription chart. The nurse needs to know the type of solution required, the amount to be administered, the rate of flow of the infusion and any patient allergies.

Purposes

+ To supply fluid when patients are unable to take in an adequate volume of fluids by mouth
+ To provide salts needed to maintain electrolyte balance
+ To provide glucose (dextrose), the main fuel for metabolism
+ To provide medications

NURSING MANAGEMENT

ASSESSMENT

+ Vital signs (pulse, respiratory rate and blood pressure) for baseline data
+ Skin turgor
+ Allergy to tape or iodine

PLANNING

Prior to initiating the IV infusion, consider how long the patient is likely to have the IV, what kinds of fluids will be infused, mobility and any physical constraints.

Equipment

+ Infusion set
+ Container of sterile parenteral solution
+ IV pole
+ Adhesive or nonallergenic tape
+ Clean gloves
+ Alcohol swabs
+ Electronic infusion device or pump. (The nurse decides what device is needed as appropriate to the patient's condition.)

IMPLEMENTATION

Preparation

1. Prepare the patient.
   • Explain the need for the intravenous therapy to the patient.
   • Make sure that the patient's clothing or gown can be removed over the IV apparatus if necessary.

Performance

1. Wash your hands. Open and prepare the infusion set.
   • Remove tubing from the container and straighten it out.
   • Slide the tubing clamp along the tubing until it is just below the drip chamber to facilitate its access.
   • Close the clamp.
   • Leave the ends of the tubing covered with the plastic caps until the infusion is started. *This will maintain the sterility of the ends of the tubing.*
2. After checking that it is the correct solution and the expiry date, spike the solution container.
   • Remove the protective cover from the entry site of the bag.
   • Remove the cap from the spike and insert the spike into the insertion site of the bag or bottle (see Figure 18-17). Follow the manufacturer's instructions.
3. Apply a medication label to the solution container if a medication is added.
4. Hang the solution container on the pole.
   • Adjust the pole so that the container is suspended about 1 m (3 feet) above the patient's head. *This height is needed to enable gravity to overcome venous pressure and facilitate flow of the solution into the vein.*

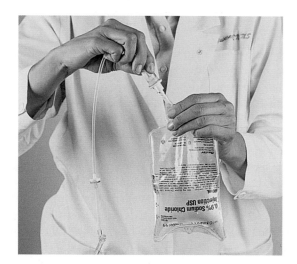

Figure 18-17 Inserting the spike.

5. Partially fill the drip chamber with solution.
   • Squeeze the chamber gently until it is half full of solution (see Figure 18-18).
6. Prime the tubing.
   • Remove the protective cap and hold the tubing over a container. Maintain the sterility of the end of the tubing and the cap.
   • Release the clamp and let the fluid run through the tubing until all bubbles are removed. Tap the tubing if necessary with your fingers to help the bubbles move. *The tubing is primed to prevent the introduction of air into the patient.* Air bubbles smaller than 0.5 ml usually do not cause problems in peripheral lines.
   • Reclamp the tubing and replace the tubing cap, maintaining sterile technique.

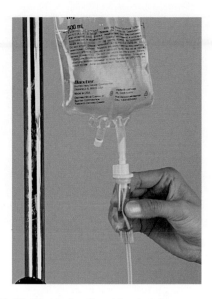

Figure 18-18 Squeezing the drip chamber.

- If an infusion control pump, electronic device or controller is being used, follow the manufacturer's directions for inserting the tubing and setting the infusion rate.
7. Clean port of venous catheter with alcohol swab and allow to dry.
8. Flush venous access with sodium chloride to ensure the line is patent.
9. Attach infusion line to venous catheter and commence infusion according to the prescription.
10. Document relevant data, including assessments.
    - Record the start of the infusion on the patient's chart. Include the date and time of commencement of infusion; amount and type of solution used, including any additives (e.g. kind and amount of medications); fluid batch number; flow rate; and the patient's general response.

EVALUATION

+ Skin status at IV site (warm temperature and absence of pain, redness and swelling)
+ Status of dressing
+ IV flow rate consistent with that prescribed

+ Ability to perform self-care activities; understanding of any mobility limitations
+ Vital signs compared to baseline level

Regulating and Monitoring Intravenous Infusions

Orders for IV infusions may take several forms: '3,000 ml over 24 hours'; '1,000 ml every 8 hours × 3 bags'; '125 ml/h until oral intake is adequate'. The nurse initiating the IV calculates the correct flow rate, regulates the infusion and monitors the patient's responses. Unless an infusion control device is used, the nurse manually regulates the drops per minute of flow using the roller clamp to ensure that the prescribed amount of solution will be infused in the correct time span. If the flow is incorrect, problems such as hypervolaemia, hypovolaemia or inadequate medication administration can result.

The number of drops delivered per millilitre of solution varies with different brands and types of infusion sets. This rate, called the **drop factor**, generally is printed on the package of the infusion set. Commonly infusion giving sets have drop factors of 10, 12, 15 or 20 drops/ml.

To calculate flow rates, the nurse must know the volume of fluid to be infused and the specific time for the infusion. Two commonly used methods of indicating flow rates are designating the number of millilitres to be administered in 1 hour (ml/h) and the number of drops to be given in 1 minute (drops/min).

Millilitres per Hour

Hourly rates of infusion can be calculated by dividing the total infusion volume by the total infusion time in hours. For example, if 3,000 ml is infused in 24 hours, the number of millilitres per hour is

$$\frac{3{,}000 \text{ ml (total infusion volume)}}{24 \text{ h (total infusion time)}} = 125 \text{ ml/h}$$

Nurses need to check infusions at least every hour to ensure that the indicated millilitres per hour have infused and that IV patency is maintained.

DROPS PER MINUTE. The nurse initiating and monitoring an infusion via a gravity set (not using a pump) must regulate the drops per minute to ensure that the prescribed amount of solution will infuse. Drops per minute are calculated by the following formula:

$$\text{Drops per minute} = \frac{\text{Total infusion volume} \times \text{drop factor}}{\text{Total time of infusion in } \textit{minutes}}$$

If the requirements are 1,000 ml in 8 hours and the drop factor is 20 drops/ml, the drops per minute should be

$$\frac{1{,}000 \text{ ml} \times 20}{8 \times 60 \text{ min (480 min)}} = 41 \text{ drops/min}$$

Approximating this rate as 40 drops/min, the nurse regulates the drops per minute by tightening or releasing the IV tubing clamp and counting the drops for 1 minute. A number of factors influence flow rate (see *Box 18-7* on page 464).

BOX 18-7 Factors Influencing Flow Rates

✚ The position of the forearm. Sometimes a change in the position of the patient's arm decreases flow. Bending of the arm can also alter the flow rate.

✚ The position and patency of the tubing. Tubing can be obstructed by the patient's weight, a kink or a clamp closed too tightly. The flow rate also diminishes when part of the tubing dangles below the puncture site.

✚ The height of the infusion bag. Elevating the height of the infusion bag a few inches can speed the flow by creating more pressure.

✚ Possible infiltration or fluid leakage. Swelling, a feeling of coldness and tenderness at the venepuncture site may indicate infiltration.

✚ Size of the venous catheter, a narrow catheter will slow infusion rates.

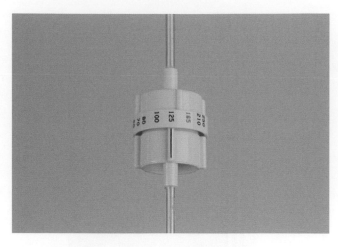

Figure 18-19 The Dial-A-Flo in-line device.

Devices to Control Infusions

A number of devices are used to control the rate of an infusion. *Electronic infusion devices* regulate the infusion rate at preset limits. They also have an alarm that is triggered when the solution in the IV bag is low, when there is air in the tubing, or when the tubing is not high enough. The *Dial-A-Flo* in-line device (see Figure 18-19) is a regulator that controls the amount of fluid to be administered. Hospitals may stock the Dial-A-Flo for use in situations where a pump is not required, but prevention of fluid overload is important. It is preset at the volume to be infused and can be attached at the time the infusion is set up or when the tubing is changed. Another variation is a *volume-control set*, which is used if the volume of fluid administered is to be carefully controlled.

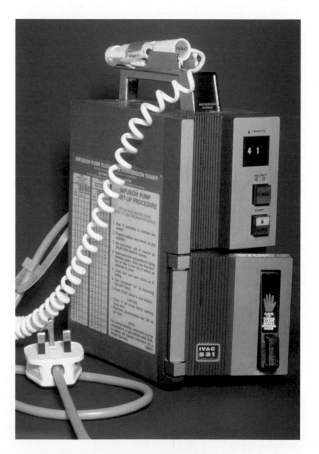

Figure 18-20 Intravenous infusion pump.
(From http://www.medcatalog.com/images/medequip2.jpg.)

An infusion pump (see Figure 18-20) delivers fluids intravenously by exerting positive pressure on the tubing or on the fluid. In situations where the fluid flow is unrestricted, the pump pressure is comparable to that of gravity flow. However, if restrictions develop (increased venous resistance), the pump can maintain the fluid flow by increasing the pressure applied to the fluid.

Procedure 18-2 outlines the steps involved in monitoring an intravenous infusion.

PROCEDURE 18-2 Monitoring an Intravenous Infusion

Purposes

+ To maintain the prescribed flow rate

+ To prevent complications associated with IV therapy

ASSESSMENT

+ Appearance of infusion site; patency of system
+ Type of fluid being infused and rate of flow

+ Response of the patient

PLANNING

Review the type of equipment needed away from the patient's bedside.

IMPLEMENTATION

Preparation

Gather the relevant information.

+ From the prescription chart, determine the type and sequence of solutions to be infused.
+ Determine the rate of flow and infusion regimen.

Performance

1. Ensure that the correct solution is being infused.
   • If the solution in incorrect stop the infusion immediately and flush the intravenous catheter to maintain patency of the cannula.
   • Change the solution to the correct one. Document and report the error according to local protocol.
2. Observe the rate of flow every hour.
   • Compare the rate of flow regularly, for example, every hour, against the prescription chart. *Infusions that are infusing incorrectly can be harmful to a patient.*
   • If the rate is too fast, slow it so that the infusion will be completed at the planned time. *Solution administered too quickly may cause a significant*

increase in circulating blood volume. Hypervolaemia may result in pulmonary oedema and cardiac failure. Assess the patient for manifestations of hypervolaemia and its complications, including dyspnoea; rapid, laboured breathing; cough; crackles in the lung bases; tachycardia; and bounding pulses.
   • If the rate is too slow adjust the flow to the specified rate in the prescription chart. *Solution that is administered too slowly can supply insufficient fluid, electrolytes or medication for a patient's needs.*
3. Inspect the patency of the IV tubing and needle.
   • Observe the position of the solution container and readjust height if needed. *If the container is too low, the solution may not flow into the vein because there is insufficient gravitational pressure to overcome the pressure of the blood within the vein.*
   • Observe the drip chamber. If it is less than half full, squeeze the chamber to allow the correct amount of fluid to flow in.

- Inspect the tubing for pinches or kinks or obstructions to flow. Arrange the tubing so that it is lightly coiled and under no pressure. Sometimes the tubing becomes caught under the patient's body and the weight blocks the flow.
- Observe the position of the tubing. *The solution may not flow upward into the vein against the force of gravity.*
- If there is leakage, locate the source. If the leak is at the catheter connection, tighten the tubing into the catheter. If the leak cannot be stopped, slow the infusion as much as possible without stopping it, and replace the tubing with a new sterile set. Estimate the amount of solution lost, if it was substantial.

4. Inspect the insertion site for fluid infiltration.
   - When an IV needle becomes dislodged from the vein, fluid flows into interstitial tissues, causing swelling. This is known as *infiltration* and is manifested by localised swelling, coolness, pallor and discomfort at the IV site.
   - If an infiltration is present, stop the infusion and remove the catheter. Restart the infusion at another site.
   - Apply a warm compress to the site of the infiltration. *Warmth promotes comfort and vasodilation, facilitating absorption of the fluid from interstitial tissues.*

5. If infiltration is not evident but the infusion is not flowing, determine whether the needle is dislodged from the vein.
   - Use a sterile syringe of saline to withdraw fluid from the port. If blood does not return, discontinue the intravenous solution.

6. Inspect the insertion site for phlebitis (inflammation of a vein).

- Inspect and palpate the site at least every eight hours. Phlebitis can occur as a result of injury to a vein, for example, because of mechanical trauma or chemical irritation. Chemical injury to a vein can occur from intravenous electrolytes (especially potassium and magnesium) and medications. The clinical signs are redness, warmth and swelling at the intravenous site and burning pain along the course of a vein.
- If phlebitis is detected, discontinue the infusion, and apply warm compresses to the venepuncture site. Do not use this injured vein for further infusions.

7. Inspect the intravenous site for bleeding.
   - Oozing or bleeding into the surrounding tissues can occur while the infusion is freely flowing but is more likely to occur after the needle has been removed from the vein.
   - Observation of the venepuncture site is extremely important for patients who bleed readily, such as those receiving anticoagulants.

8. Teach the patient ways to maintain the infusion system, for example:
   - Avoid sudden twisting or turning movements of the arm with the needle or catheter.
   - Avoid stretching or placing tension on the tubing.
   - Try to keep the tubing from dangling below the level of the needle.
   - Notify a nurse if:
     (a) The flow rate suddenly changes or the solution stops dripping.
     (b) The solution container is nearly empty.
     (c) There is blood in the IV tubing.
     (d) Discomfort or swelling is experienced at the IV site.

9. Document all relevant information.

EVALUATION

- ✚ Amount of fluid infused according to the schedule
- ✚ Intactness of IV system
- ✚ Appearance of IV site (e.g. dry, tissue infiltration, discomfort)
- ✚ Urinary output compared to urinary intake
- ✚ Tissue turgor; specific gravity of urine
- ✚ Vital signs and lung sounds compared to baseline data

Changing Intravenous Containers, Tubing and Dressings

Intravenous solution containers are changed when only a small amount of fluid remains in the neck of the container and fluid still remains in the drip chamber. However, all IV bags should be changed every 24 hours, regardless of how much solution remains, to minimise the risk of contamination. *Procedure 18-3* provides guidelines for changing an IV solution container, tubing and the IV site dressing.

PROCEDURE 18-3 Changing an Intravenous Container, Tubing and Dressing

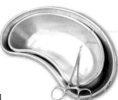

Purposes

+ To maintain the flow of required fluids
+ To maintain sterility of the IV system and decrease the incidence of phlebitis and infection
+ To maintain patency of the IV tubing
+ To prevent infection at the IV site

ASSESSMENT

+ Presence of fluid infiltration, bleeding or phlebitis at IV site
+ Allergy to tape or other substances
+ Infusion rate
+ Blockages in IV system
+ Appearance of the dressing for integrity, moisture and need for change
+ The date and the time of the previous dressing change

PLANNING

Review prescription chart for changes in fluid administration.

Equipment

+ Container with the correct type and amount of sterile solution
+ Administration set

FOR THE DRESSING

+ Sterile gloves
+ Transparent dressing
+ Sodium chloride or other solution for cleaning puncture site
+ Alcohol swabs
+ Tape
+ Sterile dressing pack

IMPLEMENTATION

Preparation

1. Obtain the correct solution container.
   - Read the label of the new container.
   - Verify that you have the correct solution, correct patient, correct additives (if any) and correct dose (number of bags or total volume ordered).

Performance

1. Wash your hands.
2. Set up the intravenous equipment with the new bag of fluid. See *Procedure 18-1* earlier.
   - Prime the tubing.
3. Prepare the IV catheter site.
   - Open all equipment: swabs, cleansing fluid and dressing. *This facilitates access to supplies after gloves have been put on.*
   - Place a towel under the extremity. *This prevents soiling of bed linens.*
   - Apply sterile gloves.
4. Remove the soiled dressing and all tape, except the tape holding the catheter or IV needle in place.

   - Remove tape and gauze from the old dressing one layer at a time. *This prevents dislodgement of the catheter or needle in case tubing becomes entangled between layers of dressing.*
   - Remove adhesive dressings in the direction of the patient's hair growth when possible. *This minimises discomfort when adhesive is removed from the skin.*
   - Discard the used dressing materials in the appropriate container.
5. Assess the IV site.
   - Inspect the IV site for the presence of infiltration or inflammation. *Inflammation or infiltration necessitates removal of the IV needle or catheter to avoid further trauma to the tissues.*
6. Disconnect the used tubing.
   - Place a sterile swab under the hub of the catheter. *This absorbs any leakage that might occur when the tubing is disconnected.*
   - Clamp the tubing.

- Holding the hub of the catheter with the nondominant hand, loosen the tubing with the dominant hand, using a twisting, pulling motion. *Holding the catheter firmly but gently maintains its position in the vein.*
- Remove the used IV tubing.
- Place the end of the tubing in the basin or other receptacle.

7. Connect the new tubing, and re-establish the infusion.
- Continue to hold the catheter and grasp the new tubing with the dominant hand.
- Remove the protective tubing cap and, maintaining sterility, insert the tubing end securely into the needle hub. Twist it to secure it.
- Open the clamp to start the solution flowing.

8. Remove the tape securing the needle or catheter.
- When removing this tape and while cleaning the site, stabilise the needle or catheter hub with one hand. *This prevents inadvertent dislodgement of the needle or catheter.*

9. Clean the IV site.
- Use appropriate cleansing fluid such as sodium chloride or chlorhexidine (as per local policy). Clean the site, beginning at the catheter or needle and cleaning outward in an 8-cm diameter. *Cleaning in this manner prevents contamination of the IV site from bacteria on the peripheral skin areas. Antiseptics reduce the number of micro-organisms present at the site, thus reducing the risk of infection.*

10. Retape the needle or catheter.
11. Apply the dressing.
- Apply a sterile transparent dressing over the site.
- Remove gloves.

12. Secure IV tubing with additional tape as required.
13. Regulate the rate of flow of the solution according to the prescription chart.
14. Document all relevant information.
- Record the change of the solution container, tubing and/or dressing in the appropriate place on the patient's chart. Also record the fluid intake according to local practice. Also record your assessments.

EVALUATION

+ Status of IV site
+ Patency of IV system

+ Accuracy of flow

When an IV infusion is no longer necessary to maintain the patient's fluid intake or to provide a route for medication administration, the infusion is either discontinued and the catheter removed or the catheter is left in place and converted to a saline or heparin lock. Guidelines for discontinuing an IV infusion are outlined in *Procedure 18-4*.

PROCEDURE 18-4 Discontinuing an Intravenous Infusion

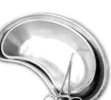

Purpose

To discontinue an intravenous infusion when the therapy is complete or when the IV site needs to be changed.

ASSESSMENT

+ Appearance of the venepuncture site
+ Any bleeding from the infusion site

+ Amount of fluid infused
+ Appearance of IV catheter

PLANNING

Review prescription chart.

Equipment

+ Clean gloves
+ Gauze swabs
+ Small sterile dressing and tape

IMPLEMENTATION

Performance

1. Prepare the equipment.
   - Clamp the infusion tubing. *Clamping the tubing prevents the fluid from flowing out of the needle onto the patient or bed.*
   - Loosen the tape at the venepuncture site while holding the needle firmly and applying countertraction to the skin. *Movement of the needle can injure the vein and cause discomfort to the patient. Countertraction prevents pulling the skin and causing discomfort.*
   - Put on clean gloves and hold a sterile gauze above the venepuncture site.
2. Withdraw the needle or catheter from the vein.
   - Withdraw the needle or catheter by pulling it out along the line of the vein. *Pulling it out in line with the vein avoids injury to the vein.*
   - Immediately apply firm pressure to the site, using sterile gauze, for 2–3 minutes. *Pressure helps stop the bleeding and prevents haematoma formation.*
   - Hold the patient's arm or leg above the body if any bleeding persists. *Raising the limb decreases blood flow to the area.*
3. Examine the catheter removed from the patient.
   - Check the catheter to make sure it is intact. *If a piece of tubing remains in the patient's vein it could move centrally (toward the heart or lungs) and cause serious problems.*
   - Report a broken catheter to the nurse in charge or doctor immediately.
   - If a broken piece can be palpated, apply a tourniquet above the insertion site. *Application of a tourniquet decreases the possibility of the piece moving until a doctor is notified.*
4. Cover the venepuncture site.
   - Apply the sterile dressing. *The dressing continues the pressure and covers the open area in the skin, preventing infection.*
   - Discard the IV solution container properly, if infusions are being discontinued, and discard the used supplies appropriately.
5. Document all relevant information.
   - Record the amount of fluid infused on the intake and output record and on the chart, according to local practice. Include the container number, type of solution used, time of discontinuing the infusion and the patient's response.

EVALUATION

+ Appearance of the venepuncture site
+ The pulse
+ Respirations, skin colour, oedema, sputum, cough and urine output
+ And how the person feels physically and psychologically.

CRITICAL REFLECTION

Let us revisit the case study on page 435. Now that you have read this chapter what tests do you think were performed to ascertain Christian's sodium levels? What part does sodium play in the stability of the body? What other tests do you think would have been performed on Christian?

CHAPTER HIGHLIGHTS

+ Factors influencing a person's hyd (hydration) ration include development, gender, ethnicity and culture, beliefs about foods, personal preferences, religious practices, lifestyle, medications and medical therapy, health status, alcohol abuse, advertising, and psychological factors such as stress, isolation and depression.

+ A balance of fluids, electrolytes, acids and bases in the body is necessary for health and life.

+ Some of the long-range effects of certain nutrient excesses are among the many factors involved in certain diseases, such as coronary artery disease and cancer.

+ Assessment of hydration status may involve all or some of the following: patient history, nutritional screening, physical examination, calculation of the percentage of weight loss, a dietary history, anthropometric measurements and laboratory tests.

+ In healthy adults, measurable fluid intake and output should balance (about 1,500 ml per day). The output of urine normally approximates the oral intake of fluids. Water from food and oxidation is balanced by fluid loss through the skin, respiratory process and faeces.

+ Fluid imbalances include
  (a) hypovolaemia
  (b) hypervolaemia
  (c) dehydration, a deficit in water only
  (d) overhydration, an excess of water only.

+ The most common electrolyte imbalances are deficits or excesses in sodium, potassium and calcium.

+ The acid-base balance (pH range) of body fluids is maintained within a precise range of 7.35 to 7.45.

+ Acid-base balance is regulated by buffers that neutralise excess acids or bases; the lungs, which eliminate or retain carbon dioxide, a potential acid; and the kidneys, which excrete or conserve bicarbonate and hydrogen ions.

+ Acid-base imbalance occurs when the normal 20-to-1 ratio of bicarbonate to carbonic acid is upset. Imbalances may be either respiratory or metabolic in origin; either can result in acidosis or alkalosis.

+ Fluid, electrolyte and acid-base imbalance is most accurately determined through laboratory examination of blood plasma.

+ For patients with fluid retention, fluids may need to be restricted; a schedule and short-term goals that make the fluid restriction more tolerable need to be developed.

+ For patients experiencing excessive fluid losses, the administration of fluids and electrolytes intravenously is necessary. Meticulous aseptic technique is required when caring for patients with intravenous infusions.

+ Preventing complications such as infiltration, phlebitis, hypervolaemia (circulatory overload), and infection are an important aspect of intravenous therapy.

REFERENCES

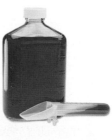

Behrman, R.E. (1992) *Nelson text book of pediatrics*, Philadelphia: Saunders.

Department of Health (DoH) (2007) *Salt*. London: DoH. Available from http://www.dh.gov.uk/en/Policyandguidance/Healthandsocialtopics/Bloodsafety/Bloodpressure/DH_4084299. (Accessed on 28 April 2007.)

Mangoni, A.A. and Jackson, H.D. (2003) 'Age-related changes in pharmacokinetics and pharmacodynamics: Basic principles and practical application', *British Journal of Clinical Pharmacology*, 57(1), 6–14.

Masoorli, S. and Angeles, T. (2002). 'Getting a line on central vascular access devices', *Nursing*, 32(4), 36–43.

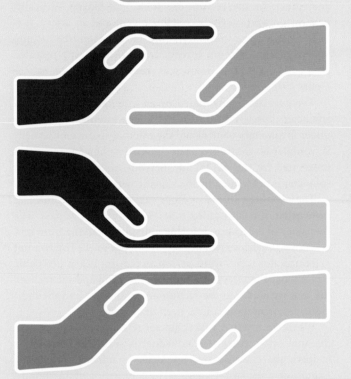

Chapter 19 Bowel Elimination

Learning Outcomes

After completing this chapter, you will be able to:

+ Understand the physiology of defecation.

+ Identify factors that influence bowel elimination.

+ Distinguish normal from abnormal characteristics and constituents of faeces.

+ Describe the assessment of bowel elimination.

+ Identify common causes and effects of selected bowel elimination problems.

+ Identify measures that maintain normal elimination patterns.

+ Describe essentials of bowel stoma care for patients with ostomies.

CASE STUDY

Cases of Clostridium difficile are on the rise according to recent news headlines (Lawrence, 2006; Carvel, 2005). Much of the media attention up until now has been on methicillin resistant staphylococcus aureus (MRSA), however there is a growing awareness that *Clostridium difficile* can pose serious health risks to patients. Reported cases have risen from 1,172 in 1990 to 46,501 in 2004.

Clostridium difficile is a bacterium that causes diarrhoea. It is a hospital acquired infection that can cause colitis (inflammation of the lining of the intestine) and even death. Certain groups of people are at particular risk of developing *Clostridium difficile* including older patients and children. The main cause of *Clostridium*

difficile is antibiotics which disturb the balance of 'normal' bacteria in the gut making the patient more susceptible to infection with *Clostridium difficile*.

Clostridium difficile produces offensive diarrhoea and many patients become faecally incontinent as a result of the bacteria. It can cause abdominal pain and is wholly unpleasant as patients usually are nursed in single rooms (isolation). The nurse's role is to ensure that this infection is not spread from patient to patient and to promote continence where possible.

After reading this chapter you will be able to discuss ways in which continence can be promoted and understand the process of defecation.

PHYSIOLOGY OF DEFECATION

Elimination of waste products is a necessity for maintaining health and is a very personal, private and independent act (Pellatt, 2007). However, nurses frequently are consulted or involved in assisting patients with elimination problems. These problems can be embarrassing to patients and can cause considerable discomfort. Nurses need to have an understanding of the normal physiology of defecation and ways in which associated problems can be managed.

Elimination of the waste products of digestion from the body is essential to health. The excreted waste products are referred to as **faeces** or **stool**.

The large intestine extends from the ileocaecal (ileocolic) valve, which lies between the small and large intestines, to the anus. The colon (large intestine) in the adult is generally about 125–150 cm (50–60 inches) long. It has seven parts: the caecum; ascending, transverse and descending colons; sigmoid colon; rectum; and anus (see Figure 19-1).

The large intestine is a muscular tube lined with mucous membrane. The muscle fibres are both circular and longitudinal, permitting the intestine to enlarge and contract in both width and length. The longitudinal muscles are shorter than the colon and therefore cause the large intestine to form pouches or **haustra**.

The colon's main functions are the absorption of water and nutrients, the mucal protection of the intestinal wall and bowel elimination. The contents of the colon normally represent foods ingested over the previous four days, although most of the waste products are excreted within 48 hours of **ingestion** (the act of taking food). The waste products leaving the stomach through the small intestine and then passing through the ileocaecal valve are called **chyme**. As much as 1,500 ml of chyme passes into the large intestine daily, and all but about 100 ml is reabsorbed in the proximal half of the colon. The 100 ml of fluid is excreted in the faeces.

The colon also serves a protective function in that it secretes mucus. This mucus contains large amounts of bicarbonate ions and serves to protect the wall of the large intestine from trauma by the acids formed in the faeces, and it serves as an adherent for holding the faecal material together. Mucus also protects the intestinal wall from bacterial activity.

The products of digestion are flatus and faeces. **Flatus** is largely air and the by-products of the digestion of carbohydrates. Flatus and faeces are propelled along the intestines by wavelike movements produced by the circular and longitudinal muscle fibres of the intestinal walls, known as **peristalsis**.

The faeces and flatus pass along the intestine towards the rectum and anal canal. The rectum in the adult is usually 10–15 cm long; the most distal portion, 2.5–5 cm long, is the anal canal. In the rectum are folds that extend vertically. Each of the vertical folds contains a vein and an artery. It is believed that these folds help retain faeces within the rectum. When the veins become distended, as can occur with repeated pressure, a condition known as **haemorrhoids** occurs (see Figure 19-2).

The anal canal is bounded by an internal and an external sphincter muscle (see Figure 19-3). The internal sphincter is under involuntary control and the external sphincter normally is voluntarily controlled. The internal sphincter muscle is innervated by the autonomic nervous system; the external sphincter is innervated by the somatic nervous system.

The expulsion of faeces from the anal canal is known as **defecation**. It is also called a *bowel movement or motion*. The frequency of defecation is highly individual, varying from several times per day to two or three times per week. The amount defecated also varies from person to person. When peristaltic waves move the faeces into the sigmoid colon and the rectum, the sensory nerves in the rectum are stimulated and the individual becomes aware of the need to defecate.

When the internal anal sphincter relaxes, faeces move into the anal canal. After the individual is seated on a toilet or bedpan, the external anal sphincter is relaxed voluntarily. Expulsion of the faeces is assisted by contraction of the abdominal muscles and the diaphragm, which increases abdominal

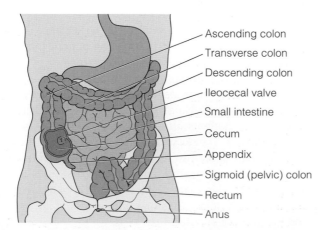

Figure 19-1 The large intestine and rectum.

Ascending colon
Transverse colon
Descending colon
Ileocecal valve
Small intestine
Cecum
Appendix
Sigmoid (pelvic) colon
Rectum
Anus

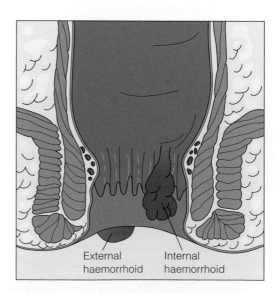

Figure 19-2 Internal and external haemorrhoids.

External haemorrhoid   Internal haemorrhoid

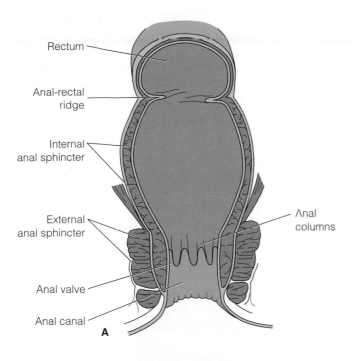

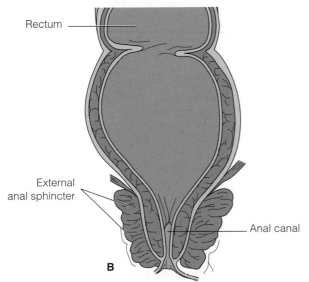

Figure 19-3 The rectum, anal canal and anal sphincters: *A*, open; *B*, closed.

pressure, and by contraction of the muscles of the pelvic floor, which moves the faeces through the anal canal. Normal defecation is facilitated by (a) thigh flexion, which increases the pressure within the abdomen, and (b) a sitting position, which increases the downward pressure on the rectum.

If the defecation reflex is ignored, or if defecation is consciously inhibited by contracting the external sphincter muscle, the urge to defecate normally disappears for a few hours before occurring again. Repeated inhibition of the urge to defecate can result in expansion of the rectum to accommodate accumulated faeces and eventual loss of sensitivity to the need to defecate. Constipation can be the ultimate result.

The faeces that are expelled from the anal canal are made of about 75% water and 25% solid materials. They are soft but formed. If the faeces are propelled very quickly along the large intestine, there is not time for most of the water in the chyme to be reabsorbed and the faeces will be more fluid, containing perhaps 95% water. Normal faeces require a normal fluid intake; faeces that contain less water may be hard and difficult to expel.

Faeces are normally brown, chiefly due to the presence of stercobilin and urobilin, which are derived from bilirubin (a red pigment in bile). Another factor that affects faecal colour is the action of bacteria such as *Escherichia coli* or staphylococci, which are normally present in the large intestine. The action of micro-organisms on the chyme is also responsible for the odour of faeces. Table 19-1 on page 474 lists the characteristics of normal and abnormal faeces.

An adult usually forms 7–10 l of flatus (gas) in the large intestine every 24 hours. The gases include carbon dioxide, methane, hydrogen, oxygen and nitrogen. Some are swallowed with food and fluids taken by mouth, others are formed through the action of bacteria on the chyme in the large intestine, and other gas diffuses from the blood into the gastrointestinal tract.

FACTORS THAT AFFECT DEFECATION

There are a number of factors that can affect defaecation. **Developmental stage** is a major factor for defecation as it dictates the stage of maturity of the intestine and the body's ability to cope with ageing. For example, some older adults suffer with constipation as a result of reduced activity levels, poor diet and fluid intake and muscle weakness whereas infants tend to have soft stools due to the immaturity of the intestine and the inability to reabsorb water.

Diet and fluid intake can also affect defecation, as a low fibre diet creates insufficient residue of waste products to stimulate the reflex of defecation and a reduced fluid intake leads to the chyme becomes drier than normal, both of which can cause constipation.

Activity stimulates peristalsis, thus facilitating the movement of chyme along the colon; therefore patients who are confined to bed often suffer with constipation.

The **psychological state** can also affect defecation. For example, some people who are anxious or angry experience increased peristaltic activity and subsequent nausea or diarrhoea, while people who are depressed may experience slowed intestinal motility, resulting in constipation.

Early bowel training may establish the **habit** of defecating at a regular time. Many people defecate after breakfast, when the gastrocolic reflex causes mass peristaltic waves in the large intestine. However, it should be recognised that each individual's bowel habits are different.

Some **medications** have side-effects that can interfere with normal bowel elimination. Some cause diarrhoea; others, such

Table 19-1 Characteristics of Normal and Abnormal Faeces

Characteristic	Normal	Abnormal	Possible cause
Colour	Adult: brown	Clay or white	Absence of bile pigment (bile obstruction); diagnostic study using barium
	Infant: yellow	Black or tarry	Drug (e.g. iron); bleeding from upper gastrointestinal tract (e.g. stomach, small intestine); diet high in red meat and dark green vegetables (e.g. spinach)
		Red	Bleeding from lower gastrointestinal tract (e.g. rectum); some foods (e.g. beets)
		Pale	Malabsorption of fats; diet high in milk and milk products and low in meat
		Orange or green	Intestinal infection
Consistency	Formed, soft, semisolid, moist	Hard, dry	Dehydration; decreased intestinal motility resulting from lack of fibre in diet, lack of exercise, emotional upset, laxative abuse
		Diarrhoea	Increased intestinal motility (e.g. due to irritation of the colon by bacteria)
Shape	Cylindrical (contour of rectum) about 2.5 cm (1 inch) in diameter in adults	Narrow, pencil-shaped, or string like stool	Obstructive condition of the rectum
Amount	Varies with diet (about 100-400 g per day)		
Odour	Aromatic: affected by ingested food and person's own bacterial flora	Pungent	Infection, blood
Constituents	Small amounts of undigested roughage, sloughed dead bacteria and epithelial cells, fat, protein, dried constituents of digestive juices (e.g. bile pigments, inorganic matter)	Pus Mucus Parasites Blood Large quantities of fat Foreign objects	Bacterial infection Inflammatory condition Gastrointestinal bleeding Malabsorption Accidental ingestion

as large doses of certain tranquillisers and repeated administration of morphine and codeine, cause constipation because they decrease gastrointestinal activity through their action on the central nervous system. Some medications are meant to directly affect bowel elimination (e.g. laxatives).

Patients who experience discomfort when defecating (e.g. following haemorrhoid surgery) often suppress the urge to defecate to avoid the pain. Such patients can experience constipation as a result.

BOWEL ELIMINATION PROBLEMS

Four common problems are related to bowel elimination: constipation, diarrhoea, bowel incontinence and flatulence.

Constipation may be defined as fewer than three bowel movements per week. This infers the passage of dry, hard stool or the passage of no stool. It occurs when the movement of faeces through the large intestine is slow, thus allowing time for additional reabsorption of fluid from the large intestine. Many causes and factors contribute to constipation including insufficient fibre intake, insufficient fluid intake, inactivity or immobility and some medications. See *Box 19-1*.

BOX 19-1 Sample Defining Characteristics for Constipation

+ Decreased frequency of defecation
+ Hard, dry, formed stools
+ Straining at stool; painful defecation
+ Reports of rectal fullness or pressure or incomplete bowel evacuation
+ Abdominal pain, cramps or distention
+ Use of laxatives
+ Decreased appetite
+ Headache

Table 19-2 Major Causes of Diarrhoea

Cause	Physiologic effect
Psychological stress (e.g. anxiety)	Increased intestinal motility and mucus secretion
Medications	
Antibiotics	Inflammation and infection of mucosa due to overgrowth of pathogenic intestinal micro-organisms
Iron	Irritation of intestinal mucosa
Cathartics	Irritation of intestinal mucosa
Allergy to food, fluid, drugs	Incomplete digestion of food or fluid
Intolerance of food or fluid	Increased intestinal motility and mucus secretion
Diseases of the colon (e.g.	
malabsorption syndrome	Reduced absorption of fluids
Crohn's disease)	Inflammation of the mucosa often leading to ulcer formation

Faecal impaction is a mass or collection of hardened faeces in the folds of the rectum. Impaction results from prolonged retention and accumulation of faecal material. In severe impactions the faeces accumulate and extend well up into the sigmoid colon and beyond. Faecal impaction can be recognised by the passage of liquid faecal seepage (diarrhoea) and no normal stool. The liquid portion of the faeces seeps out around the impacted mass. The causes of faecal impaction are usually poor defecation habits and constipation.

Diarrhoea refers to the passage of liquid faeces and an increased frequency of defecation. It is the opposite of constipation and results from rapid movement of faecal contents through the large intestine. Diarrhoea is generally the result of increased stool water content (Watson, 1999) and can be acute, chronic or iatrogenic, as with Clostridium difficile (see the *Case study* at the start of this chapter). Rapid passage of chyme reduces the time available for the large intestine to reabsorb water and electrolytes. Some people pass stool with increased frequency, but diarrhoea is not present unless the stool is relatively unformed and excessively liquid. The person with diarrhoea finds it difficult or impossible to control the urge to defecate for very long. Table 19-2 lists some of the major causes of diarrhoea and the physiologic responses of the body.

The nurse's role in managing patients with diarrhoea is to:

+ Obtain a stool specimen to identify if there are any infective cause for the diarrhoea.
+ Observe the stool for blood, or other abnormalities such as pale, offensive stools which indicate infection (Watson, 1999).
+ Take a history of onset, frequency and duration of diarrhoea.
+ Observe and assess for any other symptoms such as pain or nausea and vomiting.
+ Check past medical history including any medications.
+ Check hydration status (Dougherty and Lister, 2004).

Bowel incontinence, also called **faecal incontinence**, refers to the loss of voluntary ability to control faecal and flatus discharges through the anal sphincter (Watson, 1999). Powell and Rigby (2000) suggest that 1% of the adult population in the UK is affected by faecal incontinence but state that this is probably an underestimation as the condition is embarrassing. Faecal incontinence may occur at specific times, such as after meals, or it may occur irregularly. It is generally associated with impaired functioning of the anal sphincter or its nerve supply, such as in some neuromuscular diseases, spinal cord trauma, and tumours of the external anal sphincter muscle.

Faecal incontinence is an emotionally distressing problem that can ultimately lead to social isolation. However, several surgical procedures are used for the treatment of faecal incontinence including repair of the sphincter and faecal diversion or colostomy.

Flatulence is the presence of excessive flatus in the intestines and leads to stretching and inflation of the intestines (intestinal distention). Flatulence can occur in the colon from a variety of causes, such as foods (e.g. cabbage, onions), abdominal surgery or narcotics. If the gas is propelled by increased colon activity before it can be absorbed, it may be expelled through the anus. If excessive gas cannot be expelled through the anus, it may be necessary to insert a rectal tube to remove it.

BOWEL DIVERSION OSTOMIES

Bowel diversion ostomies are openings from the gastrointestinal tract onto the skin surface. The purpose of bowel ostomies is to divert and drain faecal material and is often classified according to (a) their status as permanent or temporary, (b) their anatomic location, and (c) the construction of the **stoma**, the opening created in the abdominal wall by the ostomy.

Colostomies open into the colon and can be either temporary or permanent. Colostomies can be further classified according to anatomical position. An ascending colostomy empties from the ascending colon, a transverse colostomy from the transverse colon, a descending colostomy from the descending colon, and a sigmoidostomy from the sigmoid colon (see Figure 19-4 on page 476).

The location of the colostomy influences the character of the faeces. Ascending colostomies tend to produce liquid stool which cannot be regulated. A transverse colostomy produces a

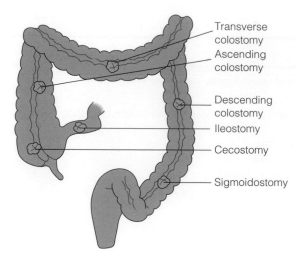

Figure 19-4 The locations of bowel diversion ostomies.

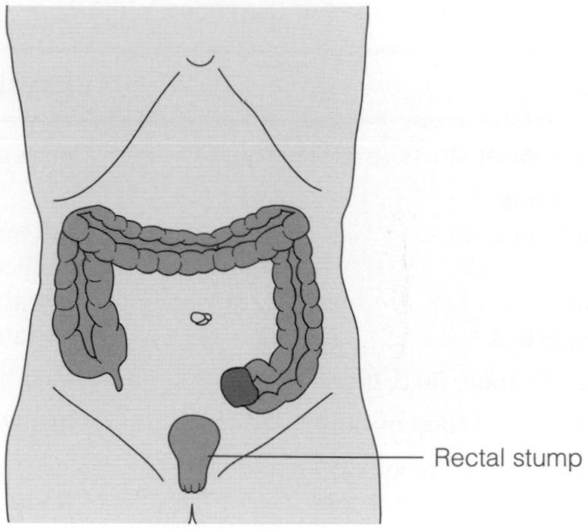

Transverse colostomy
Ascending colostomy
Descending colostomy
Ileostomy
Cecostomy
Sigmoidostomy

Rectal stump

Figure 19-5 End colostomy: the diseased portion of bowel is removed and a rectal pouch remains.

malodorous, mushy drainage because some of the liquid has been reabsorbed which cannot usually be controlled. A descending colostomy produces increasingly solid faecal drainage and a sigmoidostomy produces faeces that are of normal or formed consistency, and the frequency of discharge can be regulated. People with a sigmoidostomy may not have to wear an appliance at all times, and odours can usually be controlled.

Temporary colostomies are generally performed for traumatic injuries or inflammatory conditions of the bowel. They allow the distal diseased portion of the bowel to rest and heal. Permanent colostomies are performed to provide a means of elimination when the rectum or anus is nonfunctional as a result of a birth defect or a disease such as cancer of the bowel.

Ileostomies are openings into the ileum and generally empty from the distal end of the small intestine producing liquid faecal drainage. Drainage is constant and cannot be regulated. Ileostomy drainage contains some digestive enzymes, which are damaging to the skin. For this reason, ileostomy patients must wear an appliance continuously and take special precautions to prevent skin breakdown. Compared to colostomies, however, odour is minimal because fewer bacteria are present.

The length of time that an ostomy is in place also helps to determine the consistency of the stool, particularly with transverse and descending colostomies. Over time, the stool becomes more formed because the remaining functioning portions of the colon tend to compensate by increasing water reabsorption.

Colostomies are constructed by different techniques and are described as single, loop, divided or double-barrelled colostomies. The *single* stoma is created when one end of the bowel is brought out through an opening onto the anterior abdominal wall. This is referred to as an *end* or *terminal colostomy*; the stoma is permanent (see Figure 19-5).

In the *loop colostomy*, a loop of bowel is brought out onto the abdominal wall and supported by a plastic bridge, a glass

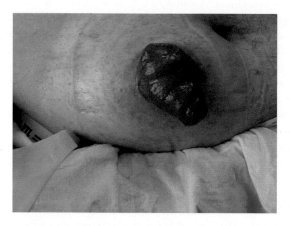

Figure 19-6 Loop colostomy. (Courtesy of Cory Patrick Hartley, San Ramon Regional Medical Center, San Ramon, CA.)

rod or a piece of rubber tubing (see Figure 19-6). A loop stoma has two openings: the proximal or afferent end, which is active, and the distal or efferent end, which is inactive. The loop colostomy is usually performed in an emergency procedure and is often situated on the right transverse colon. It is a bulky stoma that is more difficult to manage than a single stoma.

The *divided colostomy* consists of two edges of bowel brought out onto the abdomen but separated from each other (see Figure 19-7). The opening from the digestive or proximal end is the colostomy. The distal end in this situation is often referred to as a mucous fistula, since this section of bowel continues to secrete mucus. The divided colostomy is often used in situations where spillage of faeces into the distal end of the bowel needs to be avoided.

The *double-barrelled colostomy* resembles a double-barrelled shotgun (see Figure 19-8). In this type of colostomy, the proximal and distal loops of bowel are sutured together for about 10 cm (4 inches) and both ends are brought up onto the abdominal wall.

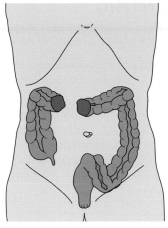

Figure 19-7 Divided colostomy with two separated stomas.

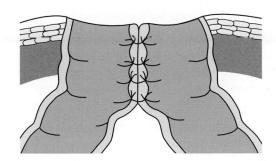

Figure 19-8 Double-barrelled colostomy.

NURSING MANAGEMENT

ASSESSING

Assessment of bowel elimination includes taking a patient history; physically examining the patient; and inspecting the faeces. The nurse also should review any data obtained from relevant diagnostic tests.

Patient History

A patient history for bowel elimination helps the nurse ascertain the patient's normal pattern. The nurse elicits a description of usual faeces and any recent changes and collects information about any past or current problems with elimination, the presence of an ostomy and factors influencing the elimination pattern.

When obtaining information about the patient's defecation pattern, the nurse needs to understand that the time of defecation and the amount of faeces expelled are as individual as the frequency of defecation. Often, the patterns individuals follow depend largely on childhood training and on convenience.

Physical Examination

Physical examination of the abdomen in relation to bowel elimination problems includes inspection, listening for bowel sounds and palpation with specific reference to the intestinal tract. They should always listen for bowel sounds before palpation as palpation can alter peristalsis. Examination of the rectum and anus includes inspection and palpation; this may be done by medical staff or nursing staff who have been specifically trained in rectal examinations (see also Chapter 26).

Inspecting the Faeces

Observe the patient's stool for colour, consistency, shape, amount, odour and the presence of abnormal constituents. Table 19-1 on page 476 summarises normal and abnormal characteristics of stool and possible causes.

CLINICAL ANECDOTE

If anyone had told me that I would be inspecting faeces before coming into nursing I probably would have run a mile. But it's not that bad. You just get used to it. At the end of the day it's part of my job and although it's not that pleasant it's something that I need to do as part of my job as a nurse.

Claire Jones, staff nurse, medical ward

Diagnostic Studies

Diagnostic studies of the gastrointestinal tract include direct visualisation techniques, indirect visualisation techniques and laboratory tests for abnormal constituents (see Chapter 26).

PLANNING

Following the assessment of the patient the nurse must identify any problems and plan realistic and achievable goals for the patient. The major goals for patients with bowel elimination problems are to:

+ Maintain or restore normal bowel elimination pattern.
+ Maintain or regain normal stool consistency.
+ Prevent associated risks such as fluid and electrolyte imbalance, skin breakdown, abdominal distention and pain.

Appropriate interventions need to be implemented in order to achieve these goals.

IMPLEMENTING

Promoting Regular Defecation

The nurse can help patients achieve regular defecation by (a) ensuring privacy, (b) offering toileting at specific times which are usually individual to the patient, for example after food, (c) encouraging nutrition and fluids, (d) encouraging mobilisation and exercise, and (e) positioning appropriate for defecation (see the *Practice guidelines* for use of bedpan). See *Teaching: wellness care* for healthy habits related to bowel elimination.

TEACHING: WELLNESS CARE

Healthy Defecation
+ Establish a regular exercise regimen.
+ Include high-fibre foods, such as vegetables, fruits and whole grains, in the diet.
+ Maintain fluid intake of 2,000 to 3,000 ml a day.

+ Do not ignore the urge to defecate.
+ Allow time to defecate, preferably at the same time each day.
+ Avoid over-the-counter medications to treat constipation and diarrhoea.

TEACHING: PATIENT CARE

Managing Diarrhoea
+ Drink at least eight glasses of water per day to prevent dehydration.
+ Ingest foods with sodium and potassium. Most foods contain sodium. Potassium is found in meats, and many vegetables and fruits, especially tomatoes, potatoes, bananas, peaches and apricots.
+ Increase foods containing soluble fibre, such as oatmeal and skinless fruits and potatoes.
+ Avoid alcohol and beverages with caffeine, which aggravate the problem.
+ Limit foods containing insoluble fibre, such as whole-wheat and whole-grain breads and cereals, and raw fruits and vegetables.

+ Limit fatty foods.
+ Thoroughly clean and dry the perineal area after passing stool to prevent skin irritation and breakdown. Use soft toilet tissue to clean and dry the area. Apply a moisture-barrier cream or ointment, such as zinc oxide or petrolatum, as needed.
+ If possible, discontinue medications that cause diarrhoea.
+ When diarrhoea has stopped, re-establish normal bowel flora by taking fermented dairy products, such as yoghurt or buttermilk.

Administering Enemas

An **enema** is a solution introduced into the rectum and large intestine. The action of an enema is to distend the intestine and sometimes to irritate the intestinal mucosa, thereby increasing peristalsis and the excretion of faeces and flatus. The most common type of enema used is the cleansing enema which is used to remove faeces and is given chiefly for constipation, or for bowel preparation prior to surgery or certain diagnostic tests.

CLINICAL ALERT

Some patients may wish to administer their own enemas. If this is appropriate, the nurse checks the patient's knowledge of correct technique and assists as needed.

PRACTICE GUIDELINES

Giving and Removing a Bedpan

+ Provide privacy.
+ Wear disposable gloves.
+ If the bedpan is metal, warm it by rinsing it with warm water.
+ Adjust the bed to a height appropriate to prevent back strain.
+ Elevate the side rail on the opposite side to prevent the patient from falling out of bed.
+ Ask the patient to assist by flexing the knees, resting the weight on the back and heels, and raising the buttocks, or by using a trapeze bar, if present.
+ Help lift the patient as needed by placing one hand under the lower back, resting your elbow on the mattress, and using your forearm as a lever.
+ Place a regular bedpan so that the patient's buttocks rest on the smooth, rounded rim. Place a slipper pan with the flat, low end under the patient's buttocks (see Figure 19-9).
+ For the patient who cannot assist, obtain the assistance of another nurse to help move the patient onto the bedpan or place the patient on his or her side, place the bedpan against the buttocks (see Figure 19-10), and roll the patient back onto the bedpan.
+ To provide a more normal position for the patient's lower back, elevate the patient's bed to a semi-Fowler's position, if permitted. If elevation is contraindicated, support the patient's back with pillows as needed to prevent hyperextension of the back.
+ Cover the patient with bed linen to maintain comfort and self-dignity.

+ Provide toilet tissue, place the call light within reach, lower the bed to the low position, elevate the side rail if indicated, and leave the patient alone.
+ Answer the call bell promptly.
+ When removing the bedpan, return the bed to the position used when giving the bedpan, hold the bedpan steady to prevent spillage of its contents, cover the bedpan and place it on the adjacent chair.
+ If the patient needs assistance, don gloves and wipe the patient's perineal area with several layers of toilet tissue. If a specimen is to be collected, discard the soiled tissue into a moisture-proof receptacle other than the bedpan. For female patients, clean from the urethra toward the anus to prevent transferring rectal micro-organisms into the urinary meatus.
+ Wash the perineal area of dependent patients with soap and water as indicated and thoroughly dry the area.
+ For all patients, offer warm water, soap, a washcloth and a towel to wash the hands.
+ Assist the patient to a comfortable position, empty and clean the bedpan, and return it to the bedside.
+ Remove and discard your gloves and wash your hands.
+ Spray the room with air freshener as needed to control odour unless contraindicated because of respiratory problems or allergies.
+ Document colour, odour, amount and consistency of urine and faeces, and the condition of the perineal area.

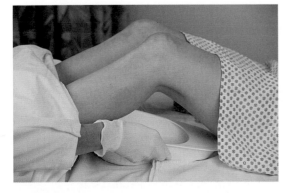

Figure 19-9 Placing a slipper pan under the buttocks.

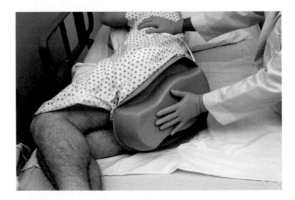

Figure 19-10 Placing a regular bedpan against the patient's buttocks.

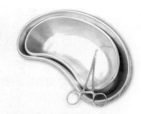

PROCEDURE 19-1 Administering an Enema

Purposes

+ To achieve one or more of the actions described above

ASSESSMENT

Assess

+ When the patient last had a bowel movement and the amount, colour and consistency of the faeces
+ Presence of abdominal distention (the distended abdomen appears swollen and feels firm rather than soft when palpated)
+ Whether the patient has sphincter control
+ Whether the patient can use a toilet or commode or must remain in bed and use a bedpan

---

PLANNING

Before administering an enema, determine whether the enema needs to be prescribed. Manufacturer's instruction should be read to ensure correct administration.

Equipment

+ Incontinence sheet or pad
+ Sheet
+ Bedpan or commode
+ Clean gloves
+ Water-soluble lubricant if tubing not prelubricated
+ Gauze swab
+ Enema solution

IMPLEMENTATION

Preparation

1. Explain to the patient what you are going to do, why it is necessary and how they can cooperate.
2. Wash hands, apply clean gloves and observe universal precautions.
3. Ensure privacy.
4. Warm the enema to body temperature to prevent intestinal cramping.
5. Position the patient lying on the left hand side as this ease the flow of the fluid into the rectum by following the anatomy of the colon (see Figure 19-11).

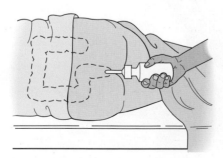

Figure 19-11 Assuming a left lateral position for an enema. Note the commercially prepared enema.

   The patient should flex their knees as this will aid the passage of the nozzle of the enema container through the anal canal.
6. Place the incontinence sheet or pad under the buttocks.
7. Expel any air from the enema container, as introducing air into the colon can cause distention and discomfort.
8. Lubricate the tip of the container nozzle.
9. Insert the tip smoothly and slowly into the rectum, directing it toward the umbilicus. *The angle follows the normal contour of the rectum. Slow insertion prevents spasm of the sphincter.*
10. If pain or resistance is felt at any time during the procedure, stop and seek medical advice.
11. Squeeze the fluid gently into the rectum from the base of the container to prevent back flow (see Figure 19-12).
12. Slowly withdraw the container nozzle to avoid reflux emptying of the rectum.
13. Clean the perineal area and make the patient comfortable.

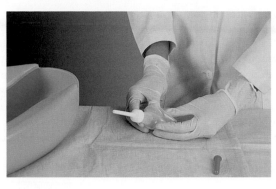

Figure 19-12 Rolling up a commercial enema container.

14. Ask the patient to retain the enema according to manufacturer's instructions.
15. The patient should remain lying down with access to a call bell.
16. Dispose of equipment, remove gloves and apron and wash hands thoroughly.
17. Document that the enema has been administered.
18. Monitor the patient and record the effects of the enema.
19. Offer handwashing facilities and perineal hygiene if the patient is unable to walk to the toilet.

EVALUATION

✛ Perform a detailed follow-up based on findings that deviated from expected or normal for the patient. Relate findings to previous assessment data if available. Report significant deviations from expected to the physician.

Digital Evacuation of Faeces

Digital evacuation of faeces is viewed as a last resort in the management of patients with constipation and is only used when all other methods for relief of constipation have failed. However for some patients this procedure is a vital part of the bowel management (RCN, 2004). For example patients with spinal cord injury may not be able to pass faeces without digital evacuation as they have lost sensation for defecation (Ash, 2005). It involves breaking up the faecal mass digitally and removing it in portions. Nurses should not attempt this without first receiving formal teaching as there is a risk of damage to the bowel mucosa.

CLINICAL ANECDOTE

The first time I ever saw a nurse using digital evacuation of faeces was with a patient who had fallen down the stairs five years previously. He sustained a neck injury and was unable to feel or move anything below his neck. The only way that he could open his bowels was by digital evacuation. As a student nurse I didn't realise that this procedure ever took place but after speaking to my mentor afterwards she told me that if she did not manually remove the faeces he would suffer with hypertension (high blood pressure) which could result in a brain haemorrhage and cardiac arrest.

Diane, staff nurse, Swansea

Bowel Training Programmes

For patients who have chronic constipation, frequent impactions or faecal incontinence, some NHS trusts offer bowel training programmes. These programmes aim to establish normal defecation by implemented a range of interventions and techniques. These programmes generally consist of:

✛ A full assessment of the patient's usual bowel habits and factors that help and hinder normal defecation.
✛ Designing a plan with the patient that includes the following:
  • Fluid intake of about 2,500 to 3,000 ml per day
  • Increase in fibre in the diet
  • Intake of hot drinks, especially just before the usual defecation time
  • Increase in exercise.
✛ Following a routine that includes the administration of a cathartic suppository (a capsule that is inserted into the rectum that aids evacuation of faeces); assisting the patient to the toilet, commode or onto a bedpan; providing the patient with privacy; educating the patient to lean forward at the hips and to apply pressure to the abdomen with the hands while defecating; and providing positive feedback when the patient successfully defecates.

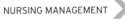

Faecal Incontinence Pouch

To collect and contain large volumes of faeces, the nurse may place a faecal incontinence pouch (rectal pouch) around the anal area. The purpose of the pouch is to prevent progressive perineal skin irritation and breakdown and frequent linen changes necessitated by incontinence.

A rectal pouch is secured around the anal opening and may or may not be attached to drainage. Pouches are best applied before the perineal skin becomes excoriated. If perineal skin excoriation is present, the nurse either (a) applies a moisture-barrier cream to the skin to protect it from faeces until it heals and then applies the pouch or (b) applies a protective powder, skin barrier or hydrocolloid wafer such as Duoderm underneath the pouch to achieve the best possible seal.

Nursing responsibilities for patients with a rectal pouch include (a) regular assessment and documentation of the perineal skin status, (b) changing the bag every 72 hours or sooner if there is leakage, (c) maintaining the drainage system and (d) providing explanations and support to the patient and support people.

Some patients may be treated surgically for faecal incontinence with surgical repair of a damaged sphincter or an artificial bowel sphincter. The artificial sphincter consists of three parts: a cuff around the anal canal, a pressure-regulating balloon and a pump that inflates the cuff (see Figure 19-13). The cuff is inflated to close the sphincter, maintaining continence. To have a bowel movement, the patient deflates the cuff. The cuff automatically reinflates in 10 minutes.

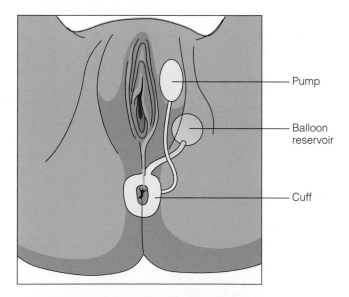

— Pump

— Balloon reservoir

— Cuff

Figure 19-13 Inflatable artificial sphincter.

Ostomy Management

Patients with bowel diversions (ostomies) need considerable psychological support, instruction and physical care however, here only physical interventions of stoma assessment, application of an appliance to collect faeces, and promotion of predictable evacuation with colostomy irrigation are discussed. Many NHS trusts have stoma nurses who work alongside other healthcare professionals, providing care to patients with stomas.

Stoma and Skin Care

Care of the stoma and skin is important for all patients who have ostomies. The faecal material from a colostomy or ileostomy is irritating to the peristomal skin. This is particularly true of ileal effluent, which contains digestive enzymes. It is important to assess the peristomal skin for irritation each time the appliance is changed. Any irritation or skin breakdown needs to be treated immediately. The skin is kept clean by washing with warm water and dried thoroughly. Specially formulated barrier creams and gels are available to protect the skin from excoriation. See *Procedure 19-2* for changing a bowel diversion ostomy appliance.

Colostomy Irrigation

Colostomy irrigation is a method of mechanically cleaning the colon of faeces by instilling water through the stoma. The water stimulates peristalsis resulting in evacuation of faeces. Colostomy irrigation aims to allow the patient some control over the evacuation of faeces from the stoma.

For most patients, a relatively small amount of fluid (300–500 ml) stimulates evacuation. For others, up to 1,000 ml may be needed because a colostomy has no sphincter and the fluid tends to return as it is instilled.

EVALUATING

The goals established during the planning phase are evaluated according to specific desired outcomes, also established in that phase. If outcomes are not achieved, the nurse should explore the reasons and modify the nursing care plan as appropriate.

Empathy and sensitivity is required when dealing with bowel elimination. Nurses need to be aware that patients may be embarrassed about their bowel habits and may be reluctant to discuss this with the nurse as it is considered 'dirty'. The nurse needs to effectively communicate with the patient in order to implement appropriate interventions and evaluate their effectiveness.

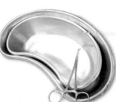

PROCEDURE 19-2 Changing a Bowel Diversion Ostomy Appliance

Purposes

+ To assess and care for the peristomal skin
+ To collect effluent for assessment of the amount and type of output
+ To minimise odours for the patient's comfort and self-esteem

ASSESSMENT

Determine

+ The kind of ostomy and its placement on the abdomen. Surgeons often draw diagrams when there are two stomas. If there is more than one stoma, it is important to confirm which is the functioning stoma.
+ The type and size of appliance currently used and the special barrier substance applied to the skin, according to the nursing care plan.
+ Any allergies.

Assess

+ Stoma colour: the stoma should appear red, similar in colour to the mucosal lining of the inner cheek. Very pale or darker-coloured stomas with a bluish or purplish hue indicate impaired blood circulation to the area.
+ Stoma size and shape: most stomas protrude slightly from the abdomen. New stomas normally appear swollen, but swelling generally decreases over two or three weeks or for as long as six weeks.

Failure of swelling to recede may indicate a problem, for example, blockage.
+ Stomal bleeding: Slight bleeding initially when the stoma is touched is normal, but other bleeding should be reported.
+ Status of peristomal skin: Any redness and irritation of the peristomal skin – the 5-13 cm of skin surrounding the stoma – should be noted. Transient redness after removal of adhesive is normal.
+ Amount and type of faeces. Inspect for abnormalities, such as pus or blood.
+ Complaints: complaints of burning sensation under the base plate may indicate skin breakdown. The presence of abdominal discomfort and/or distention also needs to be determined.
+ The patient's and family members' learning needs regarding the ostomy and self-care.
+ The patient's emotional status, especially strategies used to cope with the ostomy.

PLANNING

Review features of the appliance to ensure that all parts are present and function correctly.

Equipment

+ Clean gloves
+ Suitable container to empty appliance contents into
+ Cleaning materials, including tissues, warm water, mild soap (optional), washcloth or cotton balls, towel
+ Tissue or gauze pad
+ Skin barrier (paste, powder, water or liquid skin sealant)
+ Stoma measuring guide
+ Pen or pencil and scissors
+ Clean ostomy appliance
+ Deodorant (liquid or tablet) for a nonodour-proof colostomy bag

IMPLEMENTATION

Preparation

1. Determine the need for an appliance change.
   • Assess the used appliance for leakage of effluent. *Effluent can irritate the peristomal skin.*
   • Ask the patient about any discomfort at or around the stoma. *A burning sensation may indicate breakdown beneath the faceplate of the pouch.*
   • Assess the fullness of the pouch. *The weight of an overly full bag may loosen the faceplate and separate it from the skin, causing the effluent to leak and irritate the peristomal skin.*
2. If there is pouch leakage or discomfort at or around the stoma, change the appliance.

3. Select an appropriate time to change the appliance.
- Avoid times close to meal or visiting hours. *Ostomy odour and effluent may reduce appetite or embarrass the patient.*
- Avoid times immediately after meals or the administration of any medications that may stimulate bowel evacuation. *It is best to change the pouch when drainage is least likely to occur.*

Procedure

1. Explain to the patient what you are going to do, why it is necessary and how they can assist.

2. Make the patient comfortable and ensure privacy.

3. Wash hands, apply clean gloves and observe appropriate infection control procedures.

4. Empty and remove the ostomy appliance.
- Empty the contents of the pouch through the bottom opening into a bedpan. *Emptying before removing the pouch prevents spillage of effluent onto the patient's skin.*
- Assess the consistency and the amount of effluent.
- The appliance is then gently removed from the top, using slight pressure with the fingers on the surrounding skin to prevent pulling or tearing.
- If the appliance is disposable, discard according to local policy.

5. Clean and dry the peristomal skin and stoma.
- Use toilet tissue to remove excess stool.
- Use warm water, mild soap (optional) and soft tissues or wipes to clean the skin and stoma (see Figure 19-14).
- Dry the area thoroughly by patting with soft tissues. *Excess rubbing can abrade the skin.*

6. Assess the stoma and peristomal skin.
- Inspect the stoma for colour, size, shape and bleeding.

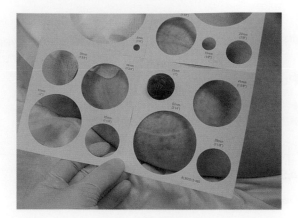

Figure 19-15 A guide for measuring the stoma. (Cory Patrick Hartley, San Ramon Regional Medical Center, San Ramon, CA. Reprinted with permission.)

- Inspect the peristomal skin for any redness, ulceration or irritation. Transient redness after the removal of adhesive is normal.

7. Apply skin barrier cream or gel if needed.

8. The stoma should be measured regularly using a guide (see Figure 19-15) and 3 mm clearance allowed between the stoma edge and the appliance. *This allows space for the stoma to expand slightly when functioning and minimises the risk of effluent contacting peristomal skin.*

9. If the stoma is irregular in shape or oval, the adhesive plate of some appliances can be cut to shape.

10. Cut out the traced stoma pattern to make an opening that is the appropriate size and shape.

11. Remove the backing to expose the sticky adhesive side.

12. Centre the skin barrier over the stoma, and gently press it onto the patient's skin, smoothing out any wrinkles or bubbles (see Figure 19-16).

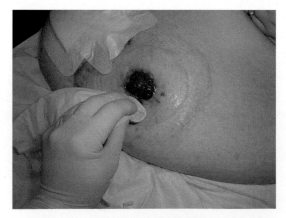

Figure 19-14 Cleaning the skin. (Cory Patrick Hartley, San Ramon Regional Medical Center, San Ramon, CA. Reprinted with permission.)

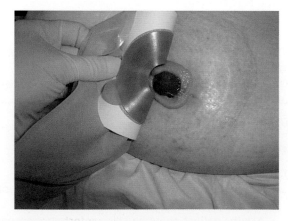

Figure 19-16 Centring the skin barrier over the stoma. (Cory Patrick Hartley, San Ramon Regional Medical Center, San Ramon, CA. Reprinted with permission.)

13. Document the procedure in the patient record using forms or checklists supplemented by narrative notes when appropriate. Report and record the patient assessment and any interventions implemented.

It is important that any changes in size, colour and skin irritation are documented. A change in stoma colour could be indicative of circulatory impairment and should be reported to the doctor immediately.

EVALUATION

+ Relate findings to previous information if available. Adjust the nursing care plan as needed.

+ Perform detailed follow-up based on findings if appropriate and report and significant changes to the doctor.

CRITICAL REFLECTION

Let us revisit the case study on page 471. Now that you have read this chapter, reflect on the priorities of caring for a patient with bowel problems. How can the nurse promote bowel continence?

CHAPTER HIGHLIGHTS

+ Primary functions of the large intestine are the excretion of digestive waste products and the maintenance of fluid balance.
+ Patterns of bowel elimination vary greatly among people, but a regular pattern of bowel elimination with formed, soft stools is essential to health and a sense of well-being.
+ A variety of factors affects defecation: developmental level, diet, fluid intake, activity and exercise, psychological factors, medications and pathologic conditions.
+ Normal defecation is often facilitated in both well and ill patients by providing privacy, teaching patients to attend to defecation urges promptly, assisting patients to normal sitting positions whenever possible, encouraging appropriate food and fluid intake, and scheduling regular exercise.
+ Common bowel elimination problems include constipation, diarrhoea, bowel incontinence and flatulence.
+ Lack of exercise, irregular defecation habits, low fibre diets and overuse of laxatives are all thought to contribute to constipation. Sufficient fluid and fibre intake are required to keep faeces soft.
+ An adverse effect of prolonged diarrhoea is fluid and electrolyte imbalance.

+ Assessment relative to bowel elimination includes a patient history; physical examination of the abdomen, rectum and anus; and in some situations, visualisation studies and inspection and analysis of stool for abnormal constituents such as blood.
+ A patient history includes data about the patient's defecating pattern, description of faeces and any changes, problems associated with elimination, and data about possible factors altering bowel elimination.
+ When inspecting the patient's stool, the nurse must observe its colour, consistency, shape, amount, odour and the presence of abnormal constituents.
+ Nursing strategies include administering laxatives and antidiarrheals; administering cleansing enemas; applying protective skin agents; monitoring fluid and electrolyte balance; and instructing patients in ways to promote normal defecation.
+ Manual evacuation can only be performed once the practitioner has received appropriate training.
+ Patients who have bowel diversion ostomies require special care, with attention to psychological adjustment, diet, and stoma and skin care. A variety of stomal management methods is available to these patients, depending on the type and position of the ostomy.

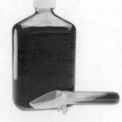

REFERENCES

Ash, D. (2005) 'Sustaining safe and acceptable bowel care in spinal cord injured patients', *Nursing Standard*, 20(8), 55–64.

Carvel, J. (2005) '45,000 patients infected with hospital superbug', *The Guardian*, 27 August 2005.

Dougherty, L. and Lister, S. (2004) *Royal Marsden Hospital manual of clinical nursing procedures*, Oxford: Blackwell Publishing.

Lawrence, J. (2006) 'Deaths from "dirty hospital bug" double in five years', *The Independent*, 26 May 2006.

Pellatt, G.C. (2007) 'Clinical skills: bowel elimination and management of complications', *British Journal of Nursing*, 16(6), 351–355.

Powell, M. and Rigby, D. (2000) 'Management of bowel dysfunction: evacuation difficulties', *Nursing Standard*, 14(47), 47–54.

Royal College of Nursing (2004) *Digital rectal examination and manual removal of faeces: Guidance for nurses*, London: RCN.

Watson, A. (1999) 'Diarrhoea' in D. Jones (Ed.) *ABC of colorectal diseases*, London: BMJ Books.

Chapter 20 Urinary Elimination

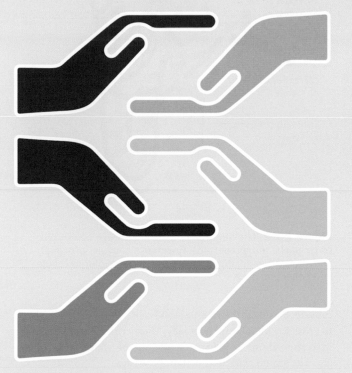

Learning Outcomes

After completing this chapter, you will be able to:

+ Understand the physiology of urination.
+ Identify factors that influence urinary elimination.
+ Identify common causes of selected urinary problems.
+ Describe the assessment of urinary elimination.
+ Identify measures that maintain normal elimination patterns.
+ Explain the care of patients with indwelling catheters or urinary diversions.

CASE STUDY

Imagine every time you sneeze, cough or laugh you pass urine involuntarily. Well this is what thousands of men and women face on a daily basis. In a study performed by Roe and Doll (2000) 23% of the respondents had experienced urinary incontinence. This same study also found that significantly more women than men were incontinent and that incontinence became more problematic with age (Roe and Doll, 2000).

In fact women are three times more likely to develop urinary incontinence than men as a result of pregnancy. It is estimated that urinary incontinence affects five million women over the age of 20 in England and Wales (BBC News, 2006). In response to these statistics the National Institute for Health and Clinical Excellence (NICE) has published guidance for healthcare professionals treating women with urinary incontinence (NICE, 2006). These guidelines recommend a range of treatments for urinary incontinence including behavioural techniques such as reducing caffeine intake, losing weight and doing regular pelvic floor exercises, medication and surgery for severe cases.

After reading this chapter you will be able to discuss ways in which continence can be promoted and understand the process of urination.

PHYSIOLOGY OF URINARY ELIMINATION

Elimination from the urinary tract is a private, independent function that is usually taken for granted. Control of urinary elimination is usually developed by the age of six (Carr, 1996). Only when a problem arises do most people become aware of their urinary habits and any associated symptoms. However, nurses frequently are consulted or involved in assisting patients with elimination problems. These problems can be embarrassing to patients and can cause considerable discomfort. Nurses need to have an understanding of the normal physiology of urination and ways in which associated problems can be managed.

Urinary elimination depends on effective functioning of four urinary tract organs: kidneys, ureters, bladder and urethra (see Figure 20-1).

The paired kidneys are situated on either side of the spinal column, behind the peritoneal cavity. They are the primary regulators of fluid and acid–base balance in the body. The functional units of the kidneys, the nephrons, filter the blood and remove metabolic wastes. In the average adult 1,200 ml of blood, or about 21% of the cardiac output, passes through the kidneys every minute. Each kidney contains approximately 1 million nephrons. Each nephron has a **glomerulus**, a tuft of capillaries surrounded by Bowman's capsule (see Figure 20-2). The endothelium of glomerular capillaries is porous, allowing fluid and solutes to readily move across this membrane into the

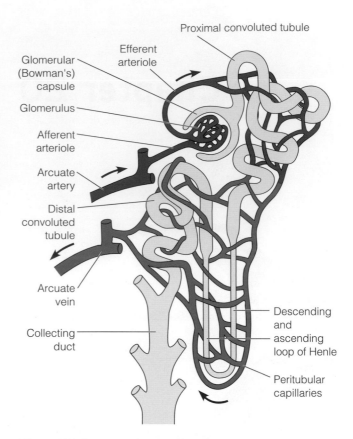

Figure 20-2 The nephrons of the kidney are composed of six parts: the glomerulus, Bowman's capsule, proximal convoluted tubule, loop of Henle, distal convoluted tubule and collecting duct.

capsule. Plasma proteins and blood cells, however, are too large to cross the membrane normally. Glomerular filtrate is similar in composition to plasma, made up of water, electrolytes, glucose, amino acids and metabolic wastes.

From Bowman's capsule the filtrate moves into the tubule of the nephron. In the proximal convoluted tubule, most of the water and electrolytes are reabsorbed. Solutes such as glucose are reabsorbed in the loop of Henle, but in the same area, other substances are secreted into the filtrate, concentrating the urine. In the distal convoluted tubule, additional water and sodium are reabsorbed under the control of hormones such as antidiuretic hormone (ADH) and aldosterone. This controlled reabsorption allows fine regulation of fluid and electrolyte balance in the body. When fluid intake is low or the concentration of solutes in the blood is high, ADH is released from the anterior pituitary, more water is reabsorbed in the distal tubule, and less urine is excreted. By contrast, when fluid intake is high or the blood solute concentration is low, ADH is suppressed. Without ADH, the distal tubule becomes impermeable to water, and more urine is excreted. Aldosterone also affects the tubule. When aldosterone is released from the adrenal cortex, sodium and water are reabsorbed in greater quantities, increasing the blood volume and decreasing urinary output.

Once the urine is formed in the kidneys, it moves through the collecting ducts into the calyces of the renal pelvis and from

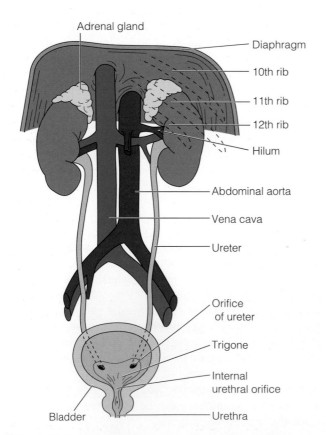

Figure 20-1 Anatomic structures of the urinary tract.

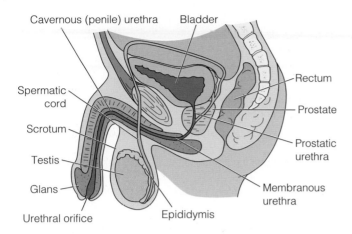

Figure 20-3 labels:
Cavernous (penile) urethra — Bladder — Rectum — Prostate — Prostatic urethra — Membranous urethra — Epididymis — Urethral orifice — Glans — Testis — Scrotum — Spermatic cord

Figure 20-3 The male urogenital system.

there into the ureters. The ureters are from 25–30 cm long in the adult and about 1.25 cm in diameter. The upper end of each ureter is funnel shaped as it enters the kidney. The lower ends of the ureters enter the bladder at the posterior corners of the floor of the bladder (see Figure 20-1). At the junction between the ureter and the bladder, a flaplike fold of mucous membrane acts as a valve to prevent **reflux** (backflow) of urine up the ureters.

The urinary bladder is a hollow, muscular organ that serves as a reservoir for urine and as the organ of excretion. When empty, it lies behind the symphysis pubis. In men, the bladder lies in front of the rectum and above the prostate gland (see Figure 20-3); in women it lies in front of the uterus and vagina (see Figure 20-4). The wall of the bladder is made up of four layers: (a) an inner mucous layer, (b) a connective tissue layer, (c) three layers of smooth muscle fibres, some of which extend lengthwise, some obliquely, and some more or less circularly, and (d) an outer serous layer. The smooth muscle layers are collectively called the **detrusor muscle**. The **trigone** at the base of the bladder is a triangular area marked by the ureter openings at the posterior corners and the opening of the urethra at the anterior inferior corner.

The bladder is capable of considerable distention because of rugae (folds) in the mucous membrane lining and because of the elasticity of its walls. When full, the dome of the bladder

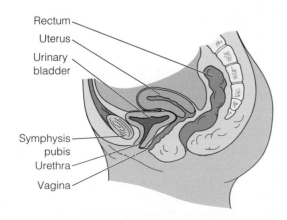

Figure 20-4 labels:
Rectum — Uterus — Urinary bladder — Symphysis pubis — Urethra — Vagina

Figure 20-4 The female urogenital system.

may extend above the symphysis pubis; in extreme situations, it may extend as high as the umbilicus.

The urethra extends from the bladder to the urinary **meatus** (opening). In the adult woman, the urethra lies directly behind the symphysis pubis, anterior to the vagina, and is about 3.7 cm long (see Figure 20-4). The urethra serves only as a passageway for the elimination of urine. The urinary meatus is located between the labia minora, in front of the vagina and below the clitoris. The male urethra is about 20 cm long and serves as a passageway for semen as well as urine (see Figure 20-3). The meatus is located at the distal end of the penis.

The internal sphincter muscle situated at the base of the urinary bladder is under involuntary control. The external sphincter muscle is under voluntary control, allowing the individual to choose when urine is eliminated.

In both men and women, the urethra has a mucous membrane lining that is continuous with the bladder and the ureters. Thus, an infection of the urethra can extend through the urinary tract to the kidneys. Women are particularly prone to urinary tract infections because of their short urethra and the proximity of the urinary meatus to the vagina and anus.

URINATION

Micturition, voiding and **urination** all refer to the process of emptying the urinary bladder. Urine collects in the bladder until pressure stimulates special sensory nerve endings in the bladder wall called stretch receptors. This occurs when the adult bladder contains 250–450 ml of urine. In children, a considerably smaller volume, 50–200 ml, stimulates these nerves.

The stretch receptors transmit impulses to the spinal cord, specifically to the voiding reflex centre located at the level of the second to fourth sacral vertebrae, causing the internal sphincter to relax and stimulating the urge to void. If the time and place are appropriate for urination, the conscious portion of the brain relaxes the external urethral sphincter muscle and urination takes place. If the time and place are inappropriate, the micturition reflex usually subsides until the bladder becomes more filled and the reflex is stimulated again.

Voluntary control of urination is possible only if the nerves supplying the bladder and urethra, the neural tracts of the cord and brain, and the motor area of the cerebrum are all intact. The individual must be able to sense that the bladder is full. Injury to any of these parts of the nervous system – for example, by a cerebral haemorrhage or spinal cord injury above the level of the sacral region – results in intermittent involuntary emptying of the bladder. Older adults whose cognition is impaired may not be aware of the need to urinate or able to respond to this urge by seeking toilet facilities.

FACTORS AFFECTING VOIDING

Numerous factors affect the volume and characteristics of the urine produced and the manner in which it is excreted. An

Table 20-1 Changes in Urinary Elimination through the Life Span

Stage	Variations
Foetuses	The foetal kidney begins to excrete urine between the 11th and 12th week of development.
Infants	Ability to concentrate urine is minimal; therefore, urine appears light yellow. Because of neuromuscular immaturity, voluntary urinary control is absent.
Children	Kidney function reaches maturity between the first and second year of life; urine is concentrated effectively and appears a normal amber colour. Between 20 and 24 months of age, the child starts to recognise bladder fullness and is able to hold urine beyond the urge to void. At approximately $2\frac{1}{2}$ to 3 years of age, the child can perceive bladder fullness, hold urine after the urge to void, and communicate the need to urinate. Full urinary control usually occurs at age 4 or 5 years; daytime control is usually achieved by age 3 years. The kidneys grow in proportion to overall body growth.
Adults	The kidneys reach maximum size between 35 and 40 years of age. After 50 years, the kidneys begin to diminish in size and function. Most shrinkage occurs in the cortex of the kidney as individual nephrons are lost.
Older adults	An estimated 30% of nephrons are lost by age 80. Renal blood flow decreases because of vascular changes and a decrease in cardiac output. The ability to concentrate urine declines. Bladder muscle tone diminishes, causing increased frequency of urination and nocturia (awakening to urinate at night). Diminished bladder muscle tone and contractibility may lead to residual urine in the bladder after voiding, increasing the risk of bacterial growth and infection. Urinary incontinence may occur due to mobility problems or neurological impairments.

individual's age can have an effect on the characteristics of urine output. Table 20-1 summaries developmental changes that affect urine output.

Psychosocial factors can also affect voiding particularly as many people require certain conditions in order to stimulate the micturition reflex. These conditions include privacy, normal position, sufficient time and, occasionally, running water. Circumstances that counter the patient's accustomed conditions may produce anxiety and muscle tension. As a result, the person is unable to relax abdominal and perineal muscles and the external urethral sphincter and voiding is inhibited.

In order to maintain a normal micturition the body maintains a balance between the amount of fluid ingested and the amount of fluid eliminated. When the amount of fluid intake increases, the urine output normally increases. Certain fluids, such as alcohol, increase fluid output by inhibiting the production of antidiuretic hormone. By contrast, food and fluids high in sodium can cause fluid retention because water is retained to maintain the normal concentration of electrolytes.

Many medications can also affect micturition, particularly those affecting the autonomic nervous system, interfere with the normal urination process and may cause retention (see *Box 20-1*). **Diuretics** (e.g. frusemide) increase urine formation by preventing the reabsorption of water and electrolytes from the tubules of the kidney into the bloodstream. Some medications may also alter the colour of the urine.

Good muscle tone is important to maintain the stretch and contractility of the detrusor muscle so the bladder can fill

BOX 20-1 Medications that May Cause Urinary Retention

+ Anticholinergic and antispasmodic medications, such as atropine and papaverine
+ Antidepressant and antipsychotic agents, such as phenothiazines and MAO inhibitors
+ Antihistamine preparations, such as pseudoephedrine (Actifed and Sudafed)
+ Antihypertensives, such as hydralazine (Apresoline) and methyldopa (Aldomet)
+ Antiparkinsonism drugs, such as levodopa, trihexyphenidyl (Artane) and benztropine mesylate (Cogentin)
+ Beta-adrenergic blockers, such as propranolol (Inderal)
+ Opioids, such as hydrocodone (Vicodin)

adequately and empty completely. Patients who require an indwelling catheter for a long period may have poor bladder muscle tone because continuous drainage of urine prevents the bladder from filling and emptying normally. Abdominal muscle contraction also assists in bladder emptying while pelvic muscle tone is a factor in being able to retain urine voluntarily once the urge to urinate is perceived.

Some diseases and pathologies can affect the formation and excretion of urine. Diseases of the kidneys may affect the ability of the nephrons to produce urine. Abnormal amounts of protein or blood cells may be present in the urine, or the kidneys may virtually stop producing urine altogether, a condition known as renal failure. Heart and circulatory disorders such as heart failure, shock or hypertension can affect blood flow to the kidneys, interfering with urine production. If abnormal amounts of fluid are lost through another route (e.g. vomiting or high fever), water is retained by the kidneys and urinary output falls.

Processes that interfere with the flow of urine from the kidneys to the urethra affect urinary excretion. A urinary stone (calculus) may obstruct a ureter, blocking urine flow from the kidney to the bladder. Hypertrophy of the prostate gland, a common condition affecting older men, may obstruct the urethra, impairing urination and bladder emptying.

Some surgical and diagnostic procedures can affect the passage of urine and the urine itself. The urethra may swell following a cystoscopy, and surgical procedures on any part of the urinary tract may result in some post-operative bleeding; as a result, the urine may be red or pink tinged for a time.

Also, spinal anaesthetics can affect the passage of urine because they decrease the patient's awareness of the need to void. Surgery on structures adjacent to the urinary tract (e.g. the uterus) can also affect voiding because of swelling in the lower abdomen.

URINARY ELIMINATION PROBLEMS

Although people's patterns of elimination are highly individual, most people urinate about five times a day. Table 20-2 shows the average urinary output per day at different ages.

Table 20-2 Average Daily Urine Output by Age

Age	Amount (ml)
1 to 2 days	15-60
3 to 10 days	100-300
10 days to 2 months	250-450
2 months to 1 year	400-500
1 to 3 years	500-600
3 to 5 years	600-700
5 to 8 years	700-1,000
8 to 14 years	800-1,400
14 years through adulthood	1,500
Older adulthood	1,500 or less

There are a number of problems associated with the urinary system. **Polyuria** (or **diuresis**) is the production of abnormally large amounts of urine by the kidneys and is associated with excessive fluid intake, diabetes mellitus and chronic nephritis.

Oliguria and **anuria** are terms used to describe decreased urinary output. **Oliguria** is low urine output, usually less than 500 ml a day or 30 ml an hour and is associated with poor fluid intake or impaired blood flow to the kidneys, while **anuria** refers to a lack of urine production.

Urinary frequency means urinating at frequent intervals, that is, more often than usual. An increased intake of fluid causes some increase in the frequency of voiding. Conditions such as urinary tract infection, stress and pregnancy can cause frequent voiding of small quantities (50–100 ml) of urine.

Nocturia, on the other hand is a term used to describe the need to urinate two or more times a night.

Urgency is the feeling that the person must urinate. There may or may not be a great deal of urine in the bladder, but the person feels a need to urinate immediately. It is common in young children who have poor external sphincter control.

CLINICAL ANECDOTE

I remember a patient who was only 17 years of age and was in our ward after having an appendectomy (removal of appendix). He came back from theatre and was relatively well. We put him in bed and after about 15 minutes he told us he was 'bursting for a pee'. We gave him a urinal bottle, drew the curtains and told him to call us when he was finished. After 10 minutes I went to check on him and he told me that he couldn't pass urine. I asked if he felt that he needed to go and he answered yes. I called for help to stand him as I thought gravity might help. My colleague came along and we stood with him while he tried to urinate in a bottle. I can't imagine how he felt with two young nurses standing by his side while he tried to urinate. In the end we had to pass a catheter into his bladder to drain the urine as it was becoming very painful for him.

Margaret Thomas, staff nurse, surgical ward

Dysuria means voiding that is either painful or difficult. It can accompany a stricture (decrease in calibre) of the urethra, urinary infections and injury to the bladder and urethra. Often patients will say they have to push to void or that burning accompanies or follows voiding. Often, **urinary hesitancy** (a delay and difficulty in initiating voiding) is associated with dysuria.

Enuresis is involuntary urination in children beyond the age when voluntary bladder control is normally acquired, usually four or five years of age. **Nocturnal enuresis** often is irregular in occurrence and affects boys more often than girls. **Diurnal** (daytime) **enuresis** may be persistent and pathologic in origin. It affects women and girls more frequently.

Urinary incontinence, or involuntary urination, is a symptom, not a disease. It can have a significant impact on the patient's life, creating physical problems such as skin breakdown and possibly leading to psychosocial problems such as embarrassment, isolation and social withdrawal. Although incontinence is sometimes common in older adults, it is not a normal consequence of ageing and can often be treated. All patients should be asked about their voiding patterns. If incontinence is described, a thorough history and assessment is indicated. Treatment may include surgery, medication or behavioural therapies.

Urinary retention refers to accumulated urine in the bladder which becomes over distended. Overdistention (overstretching) of the bladder causes poor contractility of the detrusor muscle, further impairing urination. Common causes of urinary retention include prostatic hypertrophy (enlargement), surgery and some medications.

Neurogenic bladder refers to an impairment of the neurological function interfering with the normal mechanisms of urine elimination. The patient with a neurogenic bladder does not perceive bladder fullness and is unable to control the urinary sphincters. The bladder may become flaccid and distended or spastic, with frequent involuntary urination.

A number of factors can be associated with altered urinary elimination (see Table 20-3).

Managing Urinary Elimination

Managing urinary elimination is a key role within nursing. Nurses need to be sensitive, empathetic and use effective communication skills to manage elimination problems (Baillie and Arrowsmith, 2005). As indicated on the following pages, assessment is vital to effective management of patients with urinary problems and the nurse needs to have knowledge of normal physiology as well as altered physiology and associated problems in order to implement effective interventions.

Table 20-3 Selected Factors Associated with Altered Urinary Elimination

Pattern	Selected associated factors
Polyuria	Ingestion of fluids containing caffeine or alcohol Prescribed diuretic Presence of thirst, dehydration and weight loss History of diabetes mellitus, diabetes insipidus or kidney disease
Oliguria, anuria	Decrease in fluid intake Signs of dehydration Presence of hypotension, shock or heart failure History of kidney disease Signs of renal failure such as elevated blood urea nitrogen (BUN) and serum creatinine, oedema, hypertension
Frequency or nocturia	Pregnancy Increase in fluid intake Urinary tract infection
Urgency	Presence of psychological stress Urinary tract infection
Dysuria	Urinary tract inflammation, infection or injury Hesitancy, haematuria, pyuria (pus in the urine) and frequency
Enuresis	Family history of enuresis Difficult access to toilet facilities Home stresses
Incontinence	Bladder inflammation or other disease Difficulties in independent toileting (mobility impairment) Leakage when coughing, laughing, sneezing Cognitive impairment
Retention	Distended bladder on palpation and percussion Associated signs, such as pubic discomfort, restlessness, frequency and small urine volume Recent anaesthesia Recent perineal surgery Presence of perineal swelling Medications prescribed Lack of privacy or other factors inhibiting micturition

NURSING MANAGEMENT

ASSESSING

A complete assessment of a patient's urinary function includes the following:

+ Patient history
+ Physical assessment of the genitourinary system, hydration status and examination of the urine
+ Relating the data obtained to the results of any diagnostic tests and procedures.

Patient History

The nurse determines the patient's normal voiding pattern and frequency, appearance of the urine and any recent changes, any past or current problems with urination, the presence of an ostomy and factors influencing the elimination pattern.

Physical Assessment

Complete physical assessment of the urinary tract usually includes percussion of the kidneys to detect areas of tenderness. Palpation and percussion of the bladder are also performed. If the patient's history or current problems indicate a need for it, the urethral meatus of both male and female patients is inspected for swelling, discharge and inflammation.

Because problems with urination can affect the elimination of wastes from the body, it is important that the nurse assess the skin for colour, texture and tissue turgor as well as the presence of oedema. If incontinence, dribbling or dysuria is noted in the history, the skin of the perineum should be inspected for irritation because contact with urine can excoriate the skin.

Assessing Urine

Normal urine consists of 96% water and 4% solutes. Organic solutes include urea, ammonia, creatinine and uric acid. Urea is the chief organic solute. Inorganic solutes include sodium, chloride, potassium, sulphate, magnesium and phosphorus. Sodium chloride is the most abundant inorganic salt.

Urinalysis is an important diagnostic test used to assess patients for conditions such as urinary tract infections and renal calculi (kidney stones). Urine is collected midstream or from a catheter using sterile equipment (Beynon and Nicholls, 2004) and tested immediately as any delay may result in unreliable results (Simerville *et al.*, 2005). The urine can be tested in a laboratory and/or using reagent strips (dipsticks). If used according to manufacturer's guidelines these strips are relatively accurate.

Another important diagnostic test used to assess patients' urinary function is a **24-hour urine collection**. This test looks for sodium, creatinine and protein (Beynon and Nicholls, 2004)

and involves collecting urine from the patient over a 24-hour period. Description of other tests related to urinary functions such as collecting urine specimens, measuring specific gravity and visualisation procedures are described in Chapter 26.

Characteristics of normal and abnormal urine are shown in Table 20-4 on page 494.

> ## CLINICAL ANECDOTE
>
> I work in intensive care where we monitor patients' urine hourly to ensure adequate urine output. The weirdest urine that I ever saw was luminous green. I couldn't understand how someone could have bright green urine until someone told me it was a side-effect of a sedative drug that we use.
>
> *Robert Francis,*
> *staff nurse, intensive care unit*

Measuring Urinary Output

Normally, the kidneys produce urine at a rate of approximately 0.5 ml per kg of body weight and is affected by many factors, including fluid intake, body fluid losses through other routes such as perspiration, and the cardiovascular and renal status of the individual. Urine outputs below 0.5 ml per kg of body weight may indicate low blood volume or kidney malfunction and must be reported.

In order to measure urine output the following procedure should be followed. Universal precautions should be implemented as urine can carry a number of infections. Once the patient has passed urine into a clean urinal, bedpan or commode the nurse should pour the urine into a measuring jug or if appropriate weigh the urine by weighing the container plus the urine, then weighing the container without the urine and subtract the two weights to determine the volume of urine: 1 gram = 1 millilitre. Once the volume of urine has been established this information should be recorded on a fluid balance chart which is usually kept at the bedside. The fluid intake and output are then calculated at the end of each shift and at the end of 24 hours.

When measuring urine output from a patient with an indwelling urinary catheter, a similar procedure can be carried out. However, it is important that the spout of the catheter bag does not come into contact with the container used to collect the urine, as there is a high risk of infection.

Table 20-4 Characteristics of Normal and Abnormal Urine

Characteristic	Normal	Abnormal	Nursing considerations
Amount in 24 hours (adult)	1,200–1,500 ml	Under 1,200 ml A large amount over intake	Urinary output normally is approximately equal to fluid intake. Output of less than 30 ml/hr may indicate decreased blood flow to the kidneys and should be immediately reported.
Colour, clarity	Straw, amber Transparent	Dark amber Cloudy Dark orange Red or dark brown Mucous plugs, viscid, thick	Concentrated urine is darker in colour. Dilute urine may appear almost clear or very pale yellow. Some foods and drugs may colour urine. Red blood cells in the urine (haematuria) may be evident as pink, bright red or rusty brown urine. Menstrual bleeding can also colour urine but should not be confused with haematuria. White blood cells, bacteria, pus or contaminants such as prostatic fluid, sperm or vaginal drainage may cause cloudy urine.
Odour	Faint aromatic	Offensive	Some foods (e.g. asparagus) cause a musty odour; infected urine can have a fetid odour; urine high in glucose has a sweet odour.
Sterility	No micro-organisms present	Micro-organisms present	Urine specimens may be contaminated by bacteria from the perineum during collection.
pH	4.5–8	Over 8 Under 4.5	Freshly voided urine is normally somewhat acidic. Alkaline urine may indicate a state of alkalosis, urinary tract infection or a diet high in fruits and vegetables. More acidic urine (low pH) is found in starvation, diarrhoea or with a diet high in protein foods or cranberries.
Specific gravity	1.010–1.025	Over 1.025 Under 1.010	Concentrated urine has a higher specific gravity; diluted urine has a lower specific gravity.
Glucose	Not present	Present	Glucose in the urine indicates high blood glucose levels (>180 mg/dl) and may be indicative of undiagnosed or uncontrolled diabetes mellitus.
Ketone bodies (acetone)	Not present	Present	Ketones, the end product of the breakdown of fatty acids, are not normally present in the urine. They may be present in the urine of patients who have uncontrolled diabetes mellitus, are in a state of starvation or who have ingested excessive amounts of aspirin.
Blood	Not present	Occult (microscopic) Bright red	Blood may be present in the urine of patients who have urinary tract infection, kidney disease or bleeding from the urinary tract.

Measuring Residual Urine

Residual urine (urine remaining in the bladder following the voiding) is normally not present or amounts to only a few millilitres. However, a bladder outlet obstruction (e.g. enlargement of the prostate gland) or loss of bladder muscle tone may interfere with complete emptying of the bladder during urination. Residual urine is measured to assess the amount of retained urine after voiding and determine the need for interventions (e.g. medications to promote detrusor muscle contraction).

To measure residual urine, the nurse catheterises the patient immediately after voiding. The amount of urine voided and the amount obtained by catheterisation are measured and recorded. An indwelling catheter may be inserted if the residual urine exceeds a specified amount.

PLANNING

The goals established will vary according to the diagnosis and defining characteristics. Examples of overall goals for patients with urinary elimination problems may include the following:

+ Maintain or restore a normal voiding pattern.
+ Regain normal urine output.
+ Prevent associated risks such as infection, skin breakdown, fluid and electrolyte imbalance, and lowered self-esteem.
+ Perform toilet activities independently with or without assistive devices.

Appropriate preventive and corrective nursing interventions that relate to these must be identified. Specific nursing activities associated with each of these interventions can be selected to meet the patient's individual needs.

IMPLEMENTING

Maintaining Normal Urinary Elimination

Most interventions to maintain normal urinary elimination are independent nursing functions. These include promoting adequate fluid intake, maintaining normal voiding habits and assisting with toileting.

Promoting Fluid Intake

Increasing fluid intake increases urine production, which in turn stimulates the micturition reflex. A normal daily intake averaging 1,500 ml of measurable fluids is adequate for most adult patients.

Many patients have increased fluid requirements, necessitating a higher daily fluid intake. For example, patients who are perspiring excessively (have diaphoresis) or who are experiencing abnormal fluid losses through vomiting, gastric suction, diarrhoea or wound drainage require fluid to replace these losses in addition to their normal daily intake requirements.

Patients who are at risk of urinary tract infection or urinary calculi (stones) should consume 2,000 to 3,000 ml of fluid daily. Dilute urine and frequent urination reduce the risk of urinary tract infection as well as stone formation.

Increased fluid intake may be contraindicated for some patients such as people with kidney failure or heart failure. For these patients, a fluid restriction may be necessary to prevent fluid overload and oedema.

Maintaining Normal Voiding Habits

Prescribed medical therapies often interfere with a patient's normal voiding habits. When a patient's urinary elimination pattern is adequate, the nurse helps the patient adhere to normal voiding habits as much as possible (see the *Practice guidelines*).

Assisting with Toileting

Patients who are weakened by a disease process or impaired physically require assistance to toilet. The nurse should assist these patients to the bathroom and remain with them if the patient is at risk for falling. The bathroom should contain an easily accessible call signal to summon help if needed. Patients also need to be encouraged to use handrails placed near the toilet.

PRACTICE GUIDELINES

Maintaining Normal Voiding Habits

Positioning
+ Assist the patient to a normal position for voiding: standing for male patients; for female patients, squatting or leaning slightly forward when sitting. These positions enhance movement of urine through the tract by gravity.
+ If the patient is unable to ambulate to the bathroom, use a bedside commode for females and a urinal for males standing at the bedside.
+ If necessary, encourage the patient to push over the pubic area with the hands or to lean forward to increase intra-abdominal pressure and external pressure on the bladder.

Relaxation
+ Provide privacy for the patient. Many people cannot void in the presence of another person.
+ Allow the patient sufficient time to void.
+ Suggest the patient read or listen to music.
+ Provide sensory stimuli that may help the patient relax. Pour warm water over the perineum of a female or have the patient sit in a warm bath to promote muscle relaxation. Applying a hot water bottle to the lower abdomen of both men and women may also foster muscle relaxation.

+ Turn on running water within hearing distance of the patient to stimulate the voiding reflex and to mask the sound of voiding for people who find this embarrassing.
+ Provide ordered analgesics and emotional support to relieve physical and emotional discomfort to decrease muscle tension.

Timing
+ Assist patients who have the urge to void immediately. Delays only increase the difficulty in starting to void, and the desire to void may pass.
+ Offer toileting assistance to the patient at usual times of voiding, for example, on awakening, before or after meals and at bedtime.

For Bed-confined Patients
+ Warm the bedpan. A cold bedpan may prompt contraction of the perineal muscles and inhibit voiding.
+ Elevate the head of the patient's bed to Fowler's position, place a small pillow or rolled towel at the small of the back to increase physical support and comfort, and have the patient flex the hips and knees. This position simulates the normal voiding position as closely as possible.

For patients unable to use bathroom facilities, the nurse provides urinary equipment close to the bedside (e.g. urinal, bedpan or commode) and provides the necessary assistance to use them.

Preventing Urinary Tract Infections

Infections of the urinary tract are very common. Most women will have at least one urinary tract infection in their lives; however it is more unusual in men as they have longer urethras. Most urinary tract infections (UTI) are caused by bacteria common to the intestinal environment (e.g. *Escherichia coli*). These gastrointestinal bacteria can colonise the perineal area and move into the urethra, especially when there is urethral trauma, irritation or manipulation.

For women who have experienced a UTI, nurses need to provide instructions about ways to prevent a recurrence. Marchiondo (1998) suggests a number of ways to prevent recurrence of infection:

+ Drink two litres of water per day to flush bacteria out of the urinary system.
+ Avoid use of harsh soaps, bubble bath, powder or sprays in the perineal area.
+ Avoid tight-fitting pants or other clothing and wear cotton underwear.
+ Girls and women should always wipe the perineal area from front to back following urination or defecation in order to prevent introduction of gastrointestinal bacteria into the urethra.
+ Increase the acidity of urine through regular intake of vitamin C and drinking two to three glasses of cranberry juice daily.

Managing Urinary Incontinence

It is important to remember that urinary incontinence is not a normal part of ageing and often is treatable. Independent nursing interventions for patients with urinary incontinence (UI) include (a) a behaviour-oriented continence training programme that may consist of bladder training, habit training, prompted voiding, pelvic muscle exercises and positive reinforcement; (b) meticulous skin care; and (c) for males, application of an external drainage device (condom-type catheter device).

Promoting Continence

Promoting continence requires the involvement of the patient, the patient's family and the multidisciplinary team, in order for an individualised programme to be designed. The programme may include the following:

+ **Education** of the patient and their family.
+ **Bladder training**, involves the patient postponing voiding, resisting the sensation of urgency and voiding according to a timetable rather than according to the urge to void. Over the course of the programme the patient will be required to lengthen the intervals between urination with the ultimate goal of bladder stabilisation and diminished urgency. This form of training may be used for patients who have bladder instability and urge incontinence.
+ **Habit training**, also referred to as timed voiding or scheduled toileting, attempts to keep patients dry by having them void at regular intervals. With habit training, there is no attempt to motivate the patient to delay voiding if the urge occurs.
+ **Prompted voiding** supplements habit training by encouraging the patient to try to use the toilet (prompting) and reminding the patient when to void.

Pelvic Floor Exercises

Pelvic floor exercises strengthen pelvic floor muscles in women and can reduce episodes of incontinence. The patient can identify perineal muscles by stopping urination midstream or by tightening the anal sphincter as if to hold a bowel movement.

Pelvic floor exercises can be performed anytime, anywhere, sitting or standing – even when voiding. Specific patient instructions for performing pelvic floor exercises are summarised in *Teaching: patient care.*

Maintaining Skin Integrity

Skin that is continually moist becomes macerated (softened). Urine that accumulates on the skin is converted to ammonia, which is very irritating to the skin. Because both skin irritation and maceration predispose the patient to skin breakdown and

---

TEACHING: PATIENT CARE

Pelvic Floor Exercises
+ First, sit or stand with the legs apart.
+ Pull your rectum, urethra and vagina up inside, and hold for a count of 3–5 seconds. The pull should be felt at the cleft of your buttocks.
+ Initially perform each contraction 10 times, five times daily.

+ Develop a schedule that will help remind you to do these exercises.
+ Try to start and stop your stream of urine.
+ To control episodes of stress incontinence squeeze the pelvic floor muscles when doing any activity that increases intra-abdominal pressure, such as coughing, laughing, sneezing or lifting.

NURSING MANAGEMENT

ulceration, the incontinent person requires meticulous skin care. To maintain skin integrity, the nurse washes the patient's perineal area with soap and water after episodes of incontinence, rinses it thoroughly, dries it gently and thoroughly, and provides clean, dry clothing or bed linen. If the skin is irritated, the nurse applies barrier creams such as zinc oxide ointment to protect it from contact with urine. If it is necessary to pad the patient's clothes for protection, the nurse should use products that absorb wetness and leave a dry surface in contact with the skin.

Specially designed incontinence sheets are double layered, quilted and have a waterproof backing on its underside. The design of the sheet allows fluid (i.e. urine) to pass through the upper quilted layer and is absorbed, leaving the quilted surface dry to the touch. This absorbent sheet helps maintain skin integrity; it does not stick to the skin when wet and reduces odour.

Applying External Urinary Drainage Devices

The application of a condom or external catheter connected to a urinary drainage system is commonly prescribed for incontinent males. Use of a condom appliance is preferable to insertion of an indwelling catheter because the risk of urinary tract infection is minimal. *Procedure 20-1 on page 502* describes how to apply and remove an external catheter.

Managing Urinary Retention

Interventions that assist the patient to maintain a normal voiding pattern, discussed earlier, also apply when dealing with urinary retention. Patients who have a **flaccid** bladder (weak, soft and lax bladder muscles) may use manual pressure on the bladder to promote bladder emptying. This is known as **Credé's manoeuvre** or Credé's method, which is normally only used for patients who have lost and are not expected to regain voluntary bladder control. When all measures fail to initiate voiding, urinary catheterisation may be necessary to empty the bladder completely. An indwelling Foley catheter may be inserted until the underlying cause is treated. Alternatively, intermittent catheterisation (every 3–4 hours) may be performed because the risk of urinary tract infection may be less than with an indwelling catheter.

Urinary Catheterisation

Urinary catheterisation is the introduction of a catheter through the urethra into the urinary bladder. This is usually performed only when absolutely necessary, because the danger exists of introducing micro-organisms into the bladder. Patients who are immunocompromised are at the greatest risk. Once an infection is introduced into the bladder, it can ascend the ureters and eventually involve the kidneys. The hazard of infection remains after the catheter is in place because normal defence mechanisms such as intermittent flushing of

micro-organisms from the urethra through voiding are bypassed. Therefore urinary catheters have to be inserted under strict asepsis.

Another hazard is trauma, particularly in the male patient, whose urethra is longer and more tortuous. It is important to insert a catheter along the normal contour of the urethra. Damage to the urethra can occur if the catheter is forced through strictures or at an incorrect angle. In males, the urethra is normally curved, but it can be straightened by elevating the penis to a position perpendicular to the body.

Catheters are commonly made of rubber or plastics although they may be made from latex, silicone or polyvinyl chloride (PVC). They are sized by the diameter of the lumen using the French (Fr) scale: the larger the number, the larger the lumen. Some catheters are designed for intermittent catheterisation whereby the tube is inserted, the bladder drained and the tube is removed or catheters that are designed to remain within the bladder: indwelling catheters.

There are two basic types of catheters available for intermittent catheterisation, uncoated and coated PVC Nelaton. They both come in various sizes from 10–14 Charrier (ch) and come in female or male lengths. The uncoated catheter requires separate lubrication in order to enter the urethra easily and prevent discomfort and can be reused while the coated catheters are single use only and do not require separate lubrication to be inserted.

The indwelling, or Foley, catheter is a double-lumen catheter. The larger lumen drains urine from the bladder. A second, smaller lumen is used to inflate a balloon near the tip of the catheter to hold the catheter in place within the bladder (see Figure 20-5). Patients who require continuous or intermittent bladder irrigation may have a three-way Foley catheter (see Figure 20-6 on page 498). The three-way catheter has a

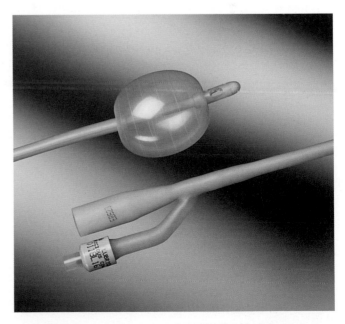

Figure 20-5 A retention (Foley) catheter with the balloon inflated. (Courtesy of C.R. Bard Inc.)

NURSING MANAGEMENT >

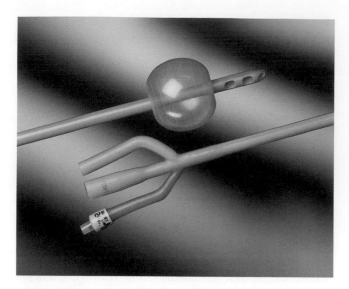

Figure 20-6 A three-way Foley catheter. (Courtesy of C.R. Bard Inc.)

third lumen through which sterile irrigating fluid can flow into the bladder. The fluid then exits the bladder through the drainage lumen, along with the urine.

The balloons of indwelling catheters are various sizes; paediatric catheters hold 2.5–5 ml while adult catheters hold 10–50 ml depending on the manufacturer. *Box 20-2* provides guidelines for catheter selection.

Indwelling catheters are connected via tubing to a gravity drainage system. This system consists of a drainage tube and a collecting bag for the urine and depend on the force of gravity to drain urine from the bladder to the collecting bag. *Procedure 20-2* (see page 504) describes catheterisation of females and males, using straight and retention catheters.

Nursing Interventions for Patients with Indwelling Catheters

Nursing care of the patient with an indwelling catheter and continuous drainage is largely directed toward preventing infection of the urinary tract and encouraging urinary flow through the drainage system.

The patient with an indwelling catheter should drink up to 3,000 ml per day if permitted. Large amounts of fluid ensure a large urine output, which keeps the bladder flushed out and decreases the likelihood of urinary stasis and subsequent infection. Large volumes of urine also minimise the risk of sediment or other particles obstructing the drainage tubing.

Acidifying the urine of patients with an indwelling catheter may reduce the risk of urinary tract infection and calculus formation. Foods such as eggs, cheese, meat and poultry, whole grains, cranberries, plums, prunes and tomatoes tend to increase the acidity of urine. Conversely, most fruits and vegetables, legumes and milk and milk products result in alkaline urine.

No special cleaning other than routine hygienic care is necessary for patients with retention catheters, nor is special meatal care recommended. Local policy regarding catheter care should be adhered to.

Routine changing of catheter and tubing is not recommended. A collection of sediment in the catheter or tubing or impaired urine drainage are indicators for changing the catheter and drainage system. When this occurs, the catheter and drainage system are removed and discarded, and a new sterile catheter is inserted and attached to a new drainage system.

Guidelines to prevent catheter-associated urinary tract infections are given in the *Practise guidelines*. Ongoing assessment of patients with indwelling catheters is a high priority (see *Box 20-3*).

BOX 20-2 Selecting an Appropriate Catheter

+ Select the type of material in accordance with the estimated length of the catheterisation period.
  (a) Use polyvinyl chlorine or plastic catheters for short periods only (e.g. one week or less), because they are inflexible.
  (b) Use plain latex catheters for periods of 2–3 weeks. Latex may be used for patients with no known latex allergy. However, because of these allergies, latex is being phased out of healthcare products.
  (c) Use polytetrafluorothylene (PTFE) for up to four weeks.
  (d) Use silicone elastomer catheters for long-term use (e.g. 2–3 months) because they create less encrustation at the urethral meatus. However, they are expensive.

  (e) Use hydrogel catheters for periods of up to 12 weeks.
  (f) Use polymer hydromer for up to 12 weeks.
  (g) Use pure silicone catheters for patients who have latex allergies and can be left in place for up to 12 weeks.
+ Determine appropriate catheter length by the patient's gender. For adult female patients, use a 22 cm catheter; for adult male patients, a 40 cm catheter.
+ Determine appropriate catheter size by the size of the urethral canal. Use sizes such as #8 or #10 for children, #14 or #16 for adults. Men frequently require a larger size than women, for example, #18.

BOX 20-3 Ongoing Assessment of Patients with Indwelling Catheters

+ Ensure that there are no obstructions in the drainage. Check that there are no kinks in the tubing, the patient is not lying on the tubing, and the tubing is not clogged with mucus or blood.
+ Check that there is no tension on the catheter or tubing.
+ Ensure that gravity drainage is maintained. Make sure there are no loops in the tubing below its entry to the drainage receptacle and that the drainage receptacle is below the level of the patient's bladder.
+ Ensure that the drainage system is well sealed and that there are no leaks at the connection sites.
+ Observe the flow of the urine as indicated by the patient's condition, and note colour, odour and any abnormal constituents. If sediment is present, check the catheter more frequently to ascertain whether it is plugged.

Removing Indwelling Catheters

Indwelling catheters are removed when clinically indicated. If the catheter has been in place for a short time (e.g. a few days), the patient usually has little difficulty regaining normal urinary elimination patterns. Swelling of the urethra, however, may initially interfere with voiding, so the nurse should regularly assess the patient for urinary retention until voiding is re-established.

Patients who have had an indwelling catheter for a prolonged period may require bladder retraining to regain bladder muscle tone. With an indwelling catheter in place, the bladder muscle does not stretch and contract regularly as it does when the bladder fills and empties by voiding. A few days before removal, the catheter may be clamped for specified periods of time (e.g. 2–4 hours), then released to allow the bladder to empty. This allows the bladder to distend and stimulates its musculature. Check local policy regarding bladder training procedures.

PRACTICE GUIDELINES

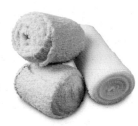

Preventing Catheter-associated Urinary Infections

+ Have an established infection control programme.
+ Catheterise patients only when necessary, by using aseptic technique and sterile equipment.
+ Do not disconnect the catheter and drainage tubing unless absolutely necessary.
+ Remove the catheter as soon as possible.
+ Follow and reinforce good hand washing technique.
+ Provide routine perineal hygiene.
+ Prevent contamination of the catheter with faeces in the incontinent patient.

To remove a retention catheter, the nurse follows these steps:

+ Obtain a receptacle for the catheter (e.g. a disposable basin); a clean, disposable towel; clean gloves; and a sterile syringe to deflate the balloon. The syringe should be large enough to withdraw all the solution in the catheter balloon. The size of the balloon is indicated on the label at the end of the catheter.
+ Ask the patient to assume a supine position as for a catheterisation.
+ Put on clean gloves and place the towel between the legs of the female patient or over the thighs of the male.
+ Insert the syringe into the injection port of the catheter, and withdraw the fluid from the balloon.
+ Do not pull the catheter while the balloon is inflated; doing so may injure the urethra.
+ After all of the fluid is withdrawn from the balloon, gently withdraw the catheter and place it in the waste receptacle.
+ It may be necessary, if clinically indicated, to send the tip of the catheter to the pathology laboratory. The tip should be removed using a sterile scissors and placed in an appropriate sterile container which is labelled with the patient's details.
+ Dry the perineal area with a towel.
+ Remove gloves.
+ Measure the urine in the drainage bag, and record the removal of the catheter. Include in the recording (a) the time the catheter was removed; (b) the amount, colour and clarity of the urine; (c) the intactness of the catheter; and (d) instructions given to the patient.
+ Following removal of the catheter, determine the time of the first voiding and the amount voided during the first eight hours. Compare this output to the patient's intake.

 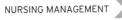

Clean Intermittent Self-catheterisation

Clean intermittent self-catheterisation (CISC) is performed by many patients who have some form of neurogenic bladder dysfunction, such as that caused by spinal cord injury. Clean or medical aseptic technique is used. Intermittent self-catheterisation:

+ Enables the patient to retain independence and gain control of the bladder.
+ Reduces incidence of urinary tract infection.
+ Protects the upper urinary tract from reflux.
+ Allows normal sexual relations without incontinence.
+ Reduces the use of aids and appliances.
+ Frees the patient from embarrassing dribbling.

The procedure for self-catheterisation is similar to that used by the nurse to catheterise a patient. Essential steps are outlined in the *Teaching: Patient care*. Because the procedure requires physical and mental preparation, patient assessment is important. The patient should have:

+ Sufficient manual dexterity to manipulate a catheter
+ Sufficient mental ability
+ Motivation and acceptance of the procedure

+ For women, reasonable agility to access the urethra
+ Bladder capacity greater than 100 ml.

Before teaching CISC, the nurse should establish the patient's voiding patterns, the volume voided, fluid intake and residual amounts. CISC is easier for males to learn because of the visibility of the urinary meatus. Females need to learn initially with the aid of a mirror but eventually should perform the procedure by using only the sense of touch (as described in *Teaching: Patient care*).

Urinary Diversions

A urinary diversion is the surgical rerouting of urine from the kidneys to a site other than the bladder. Urinary diversions are usually created when the bladder must be removed, for example, because of cancer or trauma. The most common urinary diversion is the ileal conduit or ileal loop (see Figure 20-7). In this procedure, a segment of the ileum is removed and the intestinal ends are reattached. One end of the portion removed is closed with sutures to create a pouch, and the other end is brought out through the abdominal wall to create a stoma. The ureters are implanted into the ileal pouch and urine drains continuously.

TEACHING: PATIENT CARE

Clean Intermittent Self-catheterisation
+ Catheterise as often as needed to maintain. At first, catheterisation may be necessary every 2-3 hours, increasing to 4-6 hours.
+ Attempt to void before catheterisation; insert the catheter to remove residual urine if unable to void or if amount voided is insufficient (e.g. less than 100 ml).
+ Assemble all needed supplies ahead of time. Good lighting is essential, especially for women.
+ If a woman, remove a tampon before catheterising. *A tampon can inhibit catheterisation.*
+ Wash your hands.
+ Clean the urinary meatus with either a flannel or soapy washcloth, and then rinse with a wet washcloth. Women should clean the area from front to back.
+ Assume a position that is comfortable and that facilitates passage of the catheter, such as a semi-reclining position in bed or sitting on a chair or the toilet. Men may prefer to stand over the toilet; women may prefer to stand with one foot on the side of the bathtub.
+ Apply lubricant to the catheter tip (2.5 cm) for women; (5-15 cm) for men).
+ Insert the catheter until urine flows through.
  (a) If a woman, locate the meatus using a mirror or other aid, or use the 'touch' technique as follows:

  - Place the index finger of the nondominant hand on the clitoris.
  - Place the third and fourth fingers at the vagina.
  - Locate the meatus between the index and third fingers.
  - Direct the catheter through the meatus and then upward and forward.
  (b) If a man, hold the penis with a slight upward tension at a 60- to 90-degree angle to insert the catheter. Return the penis to its natural position when urine starts to flow.
+ Hold the catheter in place until all urine is drained.
+ Withdraw the catheter slowly *to ensure complete drainage of urine*.
+ Wash the catheter with soap and water; store in a clean container. Replace the catheter when it becomes difficult to clean, or too soft or hard to insert easily.
+ The patient should be told to inform their general practitioner if their urine becomes cloudy or contains sediment; if there is bleeding, difficulty or pain when passing the catheter; or if the patient has a fever.
+ Drink at least 2,000 to 2,500 ml of fluid a day *to ensure adequate bladder filling and flushing.*

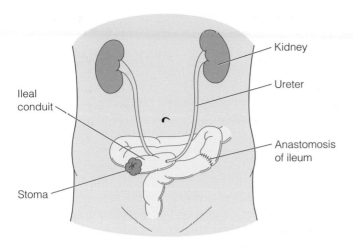

Figure 20-7 An ileal conduit.

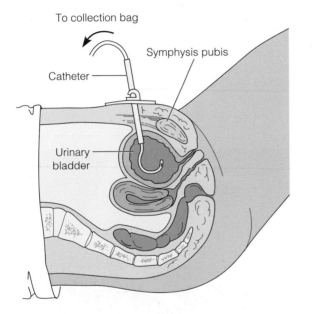

Figure 20-8 A suprapubic catheter in place.

When caring for patients with a urinary diversion, the nurse must accurately assess intake and output, note any changes in urine colour, odour or clarity (mucous shreds are commonly seen in the urine of patients with an ileal diversion), and frequently assess the condition of the stoma and surrounding skin. Patients who must wear a urine collection appliance are at risk for impaired skin integrity because of irritation by urine.

Well-fitting appliances are vital. The nurse should consult with a stoma nurse and continence nurse to identify the most appropriate appliance for the patient's needs.

Patients with urinary diversions may experience problems with their body image and sexuality and may require assistance in coping with these changes and managing the stoma. Most patients are able to resume their normal activities and lifestyle.

Suprapubic Catheter Care

A **suprapubic catheter** is inserted through the abdominal wall above the symphysis pubis into the urinary bladder (see Figure 20-8). It is inserted using local anaesthesia or during bladder or vaginal surgery. The catheter may be secured in place with sutures if a retention balloon is not used. The suprapubic catheter may be placed for temporary bladder drainage until the patient is able to resume normal voiding or may be a permanent device.

Care of patients with a suprapubic catheter includes regular assessments of the patient's urine, fluid intake, and comfort; maintenance of a patent drainage system; skin care around the insertion site; and periodic clamping of the catheter preparatory to removing it if it is not a permanent appliance. If the catheter is temporary, orders generally include leaving the catheter open to drainage for 48–72 hours, then clamping the catheter for three- to four-hour periods during the day until the patient can void satisfactory amounts. Satisfactory voiding is determined by measuring the patient's residual urine after voiding.

Care of the catheter insertion site involves sterile technique. Dressings around the newly placed suprapubic catheter are changed whenever they are soiled with drainage to prevent bacterial growth around the insertion site and reduce the potential for infection. For catheters that have been in place for an extended period, no dressing may be needed and the healed insertion tract enables removal and replacement of the catheter as needed. The nurse assesses the insertion area at regular intervals. Any redness or discharge at the skin around the insertion site must be reported.

EVALUATING

+ Using the overall goals and desired outcomes identified in the planning stage, the nurse collects data to evaluate the effectiveness of nursing activities. If the desired outcomes are not achieved, explore the reasons before modifying the care plan.

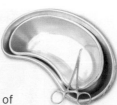

PROCEDURE 20-1 Applying an External Catheter

Purposes

+ To collect urine and control urinary incontinence
+ To permit the patient physical activity without fear of embarrassment because of leaking urine

+ To prevent skin irritation as a result of urine incontinence

Assessment

+ Review the patient record to determine a pattern to voiding and other pertinent data.

+ Apply clean gloves and examine the patient's penis for swelling or excoriation that would contraindicate use of the condom catheter.

Planning

Determine if the patient has had an external catheter previously and any difficulties with it. Perform any procedures that are best completed without the catheter in place, for example, weighing the patient would be easier without the tubing and bag. Ensure that the correct size of external catheter is ordered.

Equipment

+ Leg drainage bag with tubing or urinary drainage bag with tubing
+ Condom sheath
+ Clean gloves
+ Basin of warm water and soap
+ Washcloth and towel
+ Elastic tape or Velcro strap

Implementation

Preparation

+ Assemble the leg drainage bag or urinary drainage bag for attachment to the condom sheath.
+ Roll the condom outward onto itself to facilitate easier application (see Figure 20-9). On some models, an inner flap will be exposed. This flap is applied around the urinary meatus to prevent the reflux of urine.
+ Position the patient in either a supine or a sitting position.

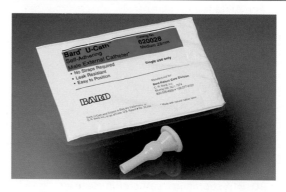

Figure 20-9 Before application, roll the condom outward onto itself. (Courtesy of C.R. Bard Inc.)

Performance

1. Explain to the patient what you are going to do, why it is necessary and how he can cooperate.
2. Discuss if using a condom catheter will impact further care or treatments.
3. Wash hands, apply clean gloves and observe appropriate infection control procedures.
4. Provide for patient privacy.
   • Drape the patient appropriately with the bath blanket, exposing only the penis.

5. Inspect and clean the penis.
   • Clean the genital area and dry it thoroughly. *This minimises skin irritation and excoriation after the condom is applied.*
6. Apply and secure the condom.
   • Roll the condom smoothly over the penis, leaving 2.5 cm between the end of the penis and the rubber or plastic connecting tube (see Figure 20-10). *This space prevents irritation of the tip of the penis and provides for full drainage of urine.*

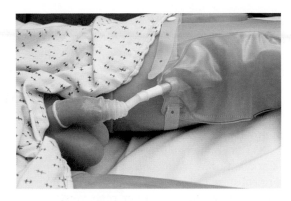

Figure 20-10 The condom rolled over the penis.

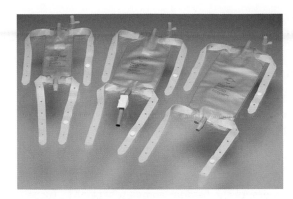

Figure 20-11 Urinary drainage leg bags. (Courtesy of C.R. Bard Inc.)

- Secure the condom firmly, but not too tightly, to the penis. Some condoms have an adhesive inside the proximal end that adheres to the skin of the base of the penis. Many condoms are packaged with special tape. If neither is present, use a strip of elastic tape or Velcro around the base of the penis over the condom. Ordinary tape is contraindicated because it is not flexible and can stop blood flow.
7. Securely attach the urinary drainage system.
   - Make sure that the tip of the penis is not touching the condom and that the condom is not twisted. *A twisted condom could obstruct the flow of urine.*
   - Attach the urinary drainage system to the condom.
   - Remove the gloves and wash your hands.
   - If the patient is to remain in bed, attach the urinary drainage bag to the bed frame.
   - If the patient is ambulatory, attach the bag to the patient's leg (see Figure 20-11). *Attaching the drainage bag to the leg helps control the movement of the tubing and prevents twisting of the thin material of the condom appliance at the tip of the penis.*

8. Teach the patient about the drainage system.
   - Instruct the patient to keep the drainage bag below the level of the condom and to avoid loops or kinks in the tubing.
9. Inspect the penis 30 minutes following the condom application, and check urine flow. Document these findings.
   - Assess the penis for swelling and discoloration, *which indicates that the condom is too tight*.
   - Assess urine flow if the patient has voided. Normally, some urine is present in the tube if the flow is not obstructed.
10. Change the condom daily and provide skin care.
    - Remove the elastic or Velcro strip, apply clean gloves and roll off the condom.
    - Wash the penis with soapy water, rinse and dry it thoroughly.
    - Assess the foreskin for signs of irritation, swelling and discoloration.
    - Reapply a new condom.
11. Document in the patient record using forms or checklists supplemented by narrative notes when appropriate. Record the application of the condom, the time, and pertinent observations, such as irritated areas on the penis.

Evaluation

+ Perform a detailed follow-up based on findings that deviated from expected or normal for the patient. Relate findings to previous assessment data if available.

+ Report significant deviations from normal to the primary care provider.

PROCEDURE 20-2 Performing Urinary Catheterisation

Purposes

+ To relieve discomfort due to bladder distention or to provide gradual decompression of a distended bladder
+ To assess the amount of residual urine if the bladder empties incompletely
+ To obtain a urine specimen
+ To empty the bladder completely prior to surgery
+ To facilitate accurate measurement of urinary output for critically ill patients whose output needs to be monitored hourly
+ To provide for intermittent or continuous bladder drainage and irrigation
+ To prevent urine from contacting an incision after perineal surgery
+ To manage incontinence when other measures have failed

Assessment

+ Determine the most appropriate method of catheterisation based on the purpose and any criteria specified in the order such as total amount of urine to be removed or size of catheter to be used.
+ Assess the patient's overall condition. Determine if the patient is able to cooperate during the procedure and if the patient can be positioned supine with head relatively flat.
+ Determine when the patient last voided or was last catheterised.
+ Palpate the bladder to check for fullness or distension.

Planning

Allow adequate time to perform the catheterisation. Although the entire procedure can require as little as 15 minutes, several sources of difficulty could result in a much longer time. If possible, it should not be performed just prior to or after the patient eats.

Equipment

+ Sterile catheter of appropriate size. (An extra catheter should also be at hand.)
+ Catheterisation kit (see Figure 20-12) or individual sterile items:
  • foil bowl
  • cotton wool balls
  • gauze swabs
  • forceps
  • cardboard tray
  • small gallipot
  • paper towels
  • paper sheet
  • sterile gloves
  • cleansing fluid as in local policy
+ For an indwelling catheter:
  • Syringe and sterile water to fill balloon.
  • Collection bag and tubing
  • Antiseptic, lubricant gel containing lignocaine hydrochloride 2%
  • Bath blanket or sheet for draping the patient
  • Adequate lighting. (Obtain a flashlight or lamp if necessary.)

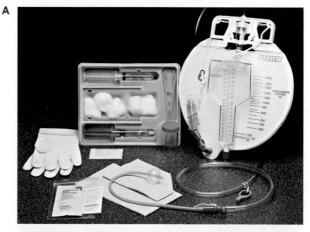

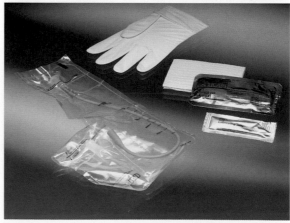

Figure 20-12 Catheter insertion kits: *A*, indwelling; *B*, straight. (Courtesy of C.R. Bard Inc.)

Implementation

Preparation

If using a catheterisation kit check the expiry date.

Performance

1. Explain to the patient what you are going to do, why it is necessary and how they can cooperate. Explain that catheter insertion causes the sensation of voiding and, possibly, a burning feeling. Discuss how the results of the catheterisation will be used in planning further care or treatments.
2. Provide for patient privacy.
3. Place the patient in the appropriate position and drape all areas except the perineum.
   (a) Female: supine with knees flexed and externally rotated.
   (b) Male: supine, legs slightly abducted.
4. Establish adequate lighting. Stand on the patient's right if you are right-handed, on the patient's left if you are left-handed.
5. Wash hands and dry hands and observe appropriate infection control procedures.
6. Prepare a sterile field and equipment using an aseptic technique.
7. If using a collecting bag and it is not contained within the catheterisation kit, open the drainage package and place the end of the tubing within reach. *Since one hand is needed to hold the catheter once it is in place, open the package while two hands are still available.*
8. Repeat handwashing, then dry hands and put on sterile gloves.
9. Arrange sterile towels to cover the surrounding area and fill the syringe with the sterile water and attach to the indwelling catheter inflation hub and test the balloon. *If the balloon malfunctions, it is important to replace it prior to use.*
10. Cleanse the meatus. *Note*: The nondominant hand is considered contaminated once it touches the patient's skin.
    (a) *Women*: Use your nondominant hand to spread the labia. Establish a firm but gentle position. The antiseptic may make the tissues slippery but the labia must not be allowed to return over the cleaned meatus. Pick up a cleansing ball with the forceps in your dominant hand and wipe one side of the labia majora in an anteroposterior direction (see Figure 20-13). Use great care that wiping the patient does not contaminate this sterile hand. Use a new ball for the opposite side. Repeat for the labia minora. Use the last ball to cleanse directly over the meatus.

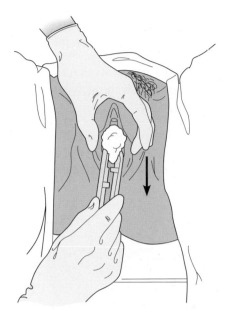

Figure 20-13 When cleaning the urinary meatus, move the swab downward.

   (b) *Men*: Use your nondominant hand to grasp the penis just below the glans. If necessary, retract the foreskin. Hold the penis firmly upright, with slight tension. *Lifting the penis in this manner helps straighten the urethra.* Pick up a cleansing ball with the forceps in your dominant hand and wipe from the centre of the meatus in a circular motion around the glans. Use great care that wiping the patient does not contaminate this sterile hand. Use a new ball and repeat three more times. The antiseptic may make the tissues slippery but the foreskin must not be allowed to return over the cleaned meatus nor the penis be dropped.
11. Break the seal on the local anaesthetic gel (2% lignocaine hydrochloride) according to manufacturer's instructions.
12. Gently insert the nozzle of the local anaesthetic gel into the urethral meatus and apply enough gel to achieve surface anaesthesia (e.g. 10-15 ml in men).
13. Wait 3-4 minutes for the anaesthetic gel to take effect.
14. Wash and dry hands and put on a new pair of sterile gloves.
15. Place the collecting tray on paper towel close to the patient in order to collect urine once the catheter has been inserted.
16. Open the catheter on the sterile field so that it is ready to use.

17. Insert the catheter.
    - Grasp the catheter firmly 4–6 cm from the tip. Ask the patient to take a slow deep breath and insert the catheter as the patient exhales. Slight resistance is expected as the catheter passes through the sphincters. If necessary, twist the catheter or hold pressure on the catheter until the sphincter relaxes.
    - Advance the catheter 4 cm further after the urine begins to flow through it; *to be sure it is fully in the bladder*.
    - If the catheter accidentally contacts the labia or slips into the vagina, it is considered contaminated and a new, sterile catheter must be used. The contaminated catheter may be left in the vagina until the new catheter is inserted to help avoid mistaking the vaginal opening for the urethral meatus. For an indwelling catheter, inflate the retention balloon with the designated volume.
    - Without releasing the catheter, hold the inflation valve between two fingers of your nondominant hand while you attach the syringe (if not left attached earlier when testing the balloon) and inflate with your dominant hand. If the patient complains of discomfort, immediately withdraw the instilled fluid, advance the catheter further, and attempt to inflate the balloon again.
    - Pull gently on the catheter until resistance is felt to ensure that the balloon has inflated and to place it in the trigone of the bladder (see Figure 20-14, *A* and *B*).

20. For intermittent catheterisation, when the urine flow stops remove the catheter. For an indwelling catheter, secure the collecting tubing to the bed linens and hang the bag below the level of the bladder. No tubing should fall below the top of the bag (see Figure 20-15).

23. Wipe the perineal area of any remaining antiseptic or lubricant. Replace the foreskin if retracted earlier. Return the patient to a comfortable position.

23. Discard all used supplies appropriately and wash your hands.

24. Document the catheterisation procedure including catheter size and results in the patient's notes.

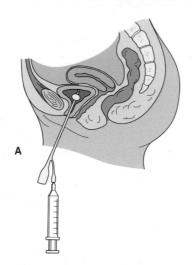
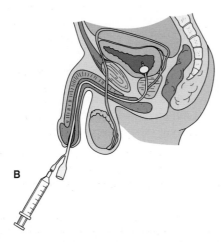

Figure 20-14 Placement of retention catheter and inflated balloon in *A*, female patient; and *B*, male patient.

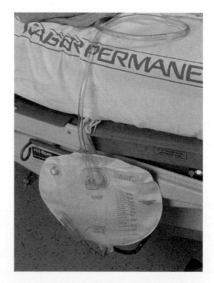

Figure 20-15 Correct position for urine drainage bag and tubing.

Evaluation

Perform a detailed follow-up based on findings that deviated from expected or normal for the patient. Relate findings to previous assessment data if available.

Teach the patient how to care for the indwelling catheter, to drink more fluids, and other appropriate instructions.

CRITICAL REFLECTION

Let us revisit the case study on page 487. Now that you have read this chapter reflect on the process of urination and the impact incontinence can have on the individual. How would you assess a patient with urinary incontinence? What interventions would you implement to promote continence?

CHAPTER HIGHLIGHTS

+ Urinary elimination depends on normal functioning of the urinary, cardiovascular and nervous systems.
+ Urine is formed in the nephron, the functional unit of the kidney, through a process of filtration, reabsorption and secretion. Hormones such as antidiuretic hormone (ADH) and aldosterone affect the reabsorption of sodium and water, thus affecting the amount of urine formed.
+ The normal process of urination is stimulated when sufficient urine collects in the bladder to stimulate stretch receptors. Impulses from stretch receptors are transmitted to the spinal cord and the brain, causing relaxation of the internal sphincter (unconscious control) and, if appropriate, relaxation of the external sphincter (conscious control).
+ In the adult, urination generally occurs after 250-450 ml of urine has collected in the bladder.
+ Many factors influence a person's urinary elimination including growth and development, fluid intake, stress, activity, medications and various diseases.
+ Alterations in urine production and elimination include polyuria, oliguria, anuria, frequency, nocturia, urgency, dysuria, enuresis, haematuria, incontinence and retention. Each may have various influencing and associated factors that need to be identified.
+ Assessment of a patient's urinary function includes (a) patient history that identifies voiding patterns, recent changes, past and current problems with urination, and factors influencing the elimination pattern; (b) a physical assessment of the genitourinary system; (c) inspection of the urine for amount, colour, clarity and odour; and, if indicated, (d) testing of urine for specific gravity, pH and the presence of glucose, ketone bodies, protein and occult blood.
+ Incontinence can be physically and emotionally distressing to patients because it is considered socially unacceptable.
+ Bladder training can often reduce episodes of incontinence.
+ Patients with urinary retention not only experience discomfort but also are at risk of urinary tract infection.
+ The most common cause of urinary tract infection is invasive procedures such as catheterisation and cystoscopic examination. Women in particular are prone to ascending urinary tract infections because of their short urethras.
+ Goals for the patient with problems with urinary elimination include maintaining or restoring normal elimination patterns and preventing associated risks such as skin breakdown.
+ Nursing interventions related to urinary elimination are generally directed toward facilitating the normal functioning of the urinary system or toward assisting the patient with particular problems.
+ Interventions include (a) assisting the patient to maintain an appropriate fluid intake, (b) assisting the patient to maintain normal voiding patterns, (c) monitoring the patient's daily fluid intake and output, and (d) maintaining cleanliness of the genital area.
+ Urinary catheterisation is frequently required for patients with urinary retention but is only performed when all other measures to facilitate voiding fail. Sterile technique is essential to prevent ascending urinary infections.
+ Care of patients with indwelling catheters is directed toward preventing infection of the urinary tract and encouraging urinary flow through the drainage system.
+ Patients with urinary retention may be taught to perform clean intermittent self-catheterisation to enhance their independence, reduce the risk of infection and eliminate incontinence.
+ When the urinary bladder is removed, a urinary diversion is formed to allow urine to be eliminated from the body. The ileal conduit or ileal loop is the most common diversion and requires that the patient wear a urine collection device continually over the stoma.

REFERENCES

BBC News (2006) 'Incontinence care plan launched'. Available from http://news.bbc.co.uk/1/hi/health/6080884.stm . (Accessed on 21 July 2007.)

Baillie, L. and Arrowsmith, V. (2005) 'Meeting elimination needs' in L. Baillie (Ed.) *Developing practical nursing skills*, London: Hodder Arnold.

Beynon, M. and Nicholls, C. (2004) 'Urological investigations' in S. Fillingham and J. Douglas (Eds), *Urological nursing*, London: Bailliere Tindall.

Carr, B. (1996) 'Assessing incontinence', *Practise Nursing*, 7(2), 19–23.

Marchiondo, K. (1998) 'A new look at urinary tract infection', *American Journal of Nursing*, 98(3), 34–39.

NICE (2006) *Urinary incontinence: The management of urinary incontinence in women*, London: NICE.

Roe, B. and Doll, H. (2000) 'Prevalence of urinary incontinence and its relationship with health status', *Journal of Clinical Nursing*, 9, 178–188.

Simerville, J., Maxted, W. and Palura, J. (2005) 'Urinalysis: a comprehensive review', *American Family Physician*, 71(6), 1153–1162.

Chapter 21 Administration of Medication

Learning Outcomes

After completing this chapter, you will be able to:

+ Define selected terms related to the administration of medications.

+ Describe legal aspects of administering medications.

+ Describe various routes of medication administration.

+ Recognise systems of measurement that are used in the administration of medications.

+ List six essential steps to follow when administering medication.

+ State the six 'rights' to accurate medication administration.

+ Describe physiological changes in older adults that alter medication administration and effectiveness.

+ Outline steps required to administer medications via various routes safely.

CASE STUDY

Barbara is a 52-year-old who has recently been diagnosed with cancer of the oesophagus and is suffering from increasing pain. Originally she had been taking oral medication but is now finding it hard to swallow even liquids.

Following a full assessment of her care needs using the nursing process and a model of care you discuss her pain management options for her medication. One of the suggestions made is the use of transdermal medication patches or to have subcutaneous injections of pain medication.

Barbara is unsure which of the routes to adopt for her medication and asks you to explain to her family how each would work. Eventually Barbara decides she would like to try transdermal medication and asks you to explain to her family how this will work.

After reading this chapter you will be able to discuss the nurse's role in administering medication to patients.

INTRODUCTION

A **medication** is a substance administered for the diagnosis, cure, treatment or relief of a symptom or for prevention of disease. In the healthcare context, the words medication and drug are generally used interchangeably. The term drug also has the potential meaning of an illegally obtained substance such as heroin, cocaine or amphetamines. The development of medication for the treatment of illness can be charted over many centuries; originally drugs, such as opium, castor oil and vinegar were used. During the past 300 years the number of drugs available has increased greatly, and knowledge about these drugs has become correspondingly more accurate and detailed.

Within the UK medications may be prescribed by doctors, dentists or by a practitioner trained and authorised as a supplementary prescriber. Supplementary prescribers may include nurses with extended skills, community nurses, health visitors or pharmacists. The written direction for the preparation and administration of a drug is called a **prescription**. A medication may also be known by various kinds of names: its generic name, official name, chemical name and trademark or brand name. The generic name is given before a drug becomes official. The official name is the name under which it is listed in one of the official publications (e.g. the *British National Formulary* or *The Association of the British Pharmaceutical Industry data sheet compendium*). The chemical name is the name by which a chemist knows it; this name describes the constituents of the drug precisely. The trademark, or brand name, is the name given by the drug manufacturer. Because one drug may be manufactured by several companies, it can have several trade names; for example, the drug salbutamol (official name) is known by the trade names salamol and ventolin.

Medications are often available in a variety of forms (see Table 21-1).

Terms frequently used when referring to medications in a clinical context include **pharmacology**, which is the study of the effect of drugs on living organisms. All drugs will have their own unique **pharmacodynamics**, the particular effect they have on the systems of the body. **Pharmacy** may be defined as the art of preparing, compounding and dispensing drugs. The word also refers to the place where drugs are prepared and dispensed.

Table 21-1 Types of Drug Preparation

Type	Description
Aerosol spray or foam	A liquid, powder or foam deposited in a thin layer on the skin by air pressure
Aqueous solution	One or more drugs dissolved in water
Aqueous suspension	One or more drugs finely divided in a liquid such as water
Caplet	A solid form, shaped like a capsule, coated and easily swallowed
Capsule	A gelatinous container to hold a drug in powder, liquid or oil form
Cream	A non-greasy, semisolid preparation used on the skin
Elixir	A sweetened and aromatic solution of alcohol used as a vehicle for medicinal agents
Extract	A concentrated form of a drug made from vegetables or animals
Gel or jelly	A clear or translucent semisolid that liquefies when applied to the skin
Liniment	A medication mixed with alcohol, oil or soapy emollient and applied to the skin
Lotion	A medication in a liquid suspension applied to the skin
Lozenge	A flat, round or oval preparation that dissolves and releases a drug when held in the mouth
Ointment	A semisolid preparation of one or more drugs used for application to the skin and mucous membrane
Paste	A preparation like an ointment, but thicker and stiff, that penetrates the skin less than an ointment
Pill	One or more drugs mixed with a cohesive material, in oval, round or flattened shapes
Powder	A finely ground drug or drugs; some are used internally, others externally
Suppository	One or several drugs mixed with a firm base such as gelatin and shaped for insertion into the body (e.g. the rectum); the base dissolves gradually at body temperature, releasing the drug
Syrup	An aqueous solution of sugar often used to disguise unpleasant-tasting drugs
Tablet	A powdered drug compressed into a hard small disc; some are readily broken along a scored line; others are enteric coated to prevent them from dissolving in the stomach
Tincture	An alcoholic or water-and-alcohol solution prepared from drugs derived from plants
Transdermal patch	A semi-permeable membrane shaped in the form of a disc or patch that contains a drug to be absorbed through the skin over a long period of time

DRUG STANDARDS

Drugs may have natural (e.g. plant, mineral and animal) sources, or they may be synthesised in the laboratory. For example, digitalis and opium are plant derived, iron and sodium chloride are minerals, insulin and vaccines have animal or human sources, and the sulphonamides (trimethoprim an antibacterial drug) are the products of laboratory synthesis. Early drugs were derived from the three natural sources only. More and more drugs, however, are being produced synthetically.

Drugs vary in strength and activity. Drugs derived from plants, for example, vary in strength according to the age of the plant, the variety, the place in which it is grown and the method by which it is preserved. Drugs must be pure and of uniform strength if drug dosages are to be predictable in their effect. Drug standards have therefore been developed to ensure uniform quality. In the UK, official drugs are those regulated by the government. These drugs are officially listed in the British National Formulary (BNF) and the Association of the British Pharmaceutical Industry data sheet compendium (ABPI). Both publications include the drug name, licensed indication for the drug, normal dose range, contraindications and side-effects.

When administering any medication that the nurse is not familiar with it is advisable that the practitioner should become familiar with the drug prior to administration. It is important to be aware of potential side-effects that the patient may need to be made aware of or be monitored, and also ensure the dosage of the drug is appropriate. Prior to administering medication the nurse should always have available an up-to-date copy of the BNF or ABPI.

LEGAL ASPECTS OF DRUG ADMINISTRATION

The administration of drugs is controlled by law. Key legislation is included in *Box 21-1*.

The Nursing Midwifery Council (2004) standards for the administration of medicines establish the standards that all registered nurses are expected to work to when administering drugs. This is regulatory body guidance and standards that state the registered nurse is accountable for any action or omission relating to drug administration in their practice. The nurse must know the therapeutic uses of the medicine to be administered, its normal dosage, side effects, precautions and contraindications. The nurse must be certain of the identity of the patient to whom the medicine is to be administered and be aware of the patient's care plan. The nurse must also check the prescription, or the label on the medicine dispensed by a pharmacist, which must be clearly written and unambiguous. Consideration should also be given to the dosage, method of administration, route and timing of the administration in the context of the condition of the patient and any co-existing therapies. The expiry date of the medicine to be administered must also be checked.

In hospitals, controlled substances as defined under the Misuse of Drugs Act 1971 are kept in a locked cupboard within

> **BOX 21-1** Key Legislation Relating to the Administration of Medication
>
> + Medicines Act 1968 - established three legal categories of drugs; prescription only medicines (POM); pharmacy medicines (P), sold on the authority of a pharmacist; and general sales list medicines (GSL).
>   The Act also states no person shall administer other than to himself any such medicinal product unless he is an appropriate practitioner or a person acting in accordance with the directions of an appropriate practitioner.
> + Misuse of Drugs Act 1971 - established the categories of drugs that may be misused from their therapeutic purposes such as opiate analgesics (morphine). The Act established recommended practices for the supply and storage of controlled drugs.
> + Medicinal Products: Prescription by Nurses etc Act 1992 - established nurse prescribing for trained specialist community health practitioners.
> + Nurse Midwives and Health Visitors Act 1997 - extended nurse prescribing to additionally trained registered nurses other than community health specialists.
> + Consumer Protection Act 1987 - established a protection mechanism for the sale of over-the-counter preparations that may be used as medical treatments.

a locked cupboard. Clinical areas may have special log books/registers for recording the use of controlled substances. The information required usually includes the name of the patient, the date and time of administration, the name of the drug, the dosage, and the signature of the person who prepared, checked and gave the drug. Before removing a controlled substance to administer, the nurse must verify the unit quantity of drug actually available with the number indicated within the controlled substance record book. If the number is not the same, the nurse must investigate and correct the discrepancy before proceeding in accordance with local policy.

Included on the record are the controlled substances wasted during preparation. When a portion or all of a controlled substance dose is discarded, the nurse must ask a second registered nurse to witness the discarding. Both nurses must sign the control inventory record.

In most clinical areas, counts of controlled substances are taken at the end of each shift or as a minimum once every 24 hours. The count total should tally with the total at the end of the last shift minus the number used. If the totals do not tally and the discrepancy cannot be resolved, it must be reported immediately in accordance with local policy.

EFFECTS OF DRUGS

The therapeutic effect of a drug is the primary effect intended, and is the reason the drug is prescribed. For example, the therapeutic effect of morphine sulphate is analgesia (pain relief), and the therapeutic effect of diazepam is relief of anxiety. See Table 21-2 for kinds of therapeutic actions.

A **side-effect**, or secondary effect, of a drug is one that is unintended. Side-effects are usually predictable and may be either harmless or potentially harmful. For example, digitalis increases the strength of myocardial contractions (desired effect), but it can have the side-effect of inducing nausea and vomiting. Some side-effects are tolerated for the drug's therapeutic effect; more severe side-effects, also called **adverse effects**, may justify the discontinuation of a drug.

Drug toxicity (adverse effects of a drug on an organism or tissue) results from overdosage, ingestion of a drug intended for external use and build up of the drug in the blood because of impaired metabolism or excretion (cumulative effect). Some toxic effects are apparent immediately; some are not apparent for weeks or months. Fortunately, most drug toxicity is avoidable if careful attention is paid to dosage and monitoring for toxicity. An example of a toxic effect is respiratory depression due to the cumulative effect of morphine sulphate in the body.

A drug allergy is an immunologic reaction to a drug. When a patient is first exposed to a foreign substance (antigen), the body may react by producing antibodies. A patient can react to a drug as to an antigen and thus develop symptoms of an allergic reaction.

Allergic reactions can be either mild or severe. A mild reaction has a variety of symptoms, from skin rashes to diarrhoea (see Table 21-3). An allergic reaction can occur any time from a few minutes to two weeks after the administration of the drug. A severe allergic reaction usually occurs immediately after the administration of the drug and is called an anaphylactic reaction. This response can be fatal if the symptoms are not noticed immediately and treatment is not obtained promptly. The earliest symptoms are acute shortness of breath, wheezing, rash, acute hypotension and tachycardia.

Drug tolerance exists in a person who has an unusually low physiological response to a drug and who requires increases in the dosage to maintain a given therapeutic effect. Drugs that commonly produce tolerance are opiates, barbiturates and tobacco. A cumulative effect is the increasing response to repeated doses of a drug that occurs when the rate of administration exceeds the rate of metabolism or excretion. As a result, the amount of the drug builds up in the patient's body unless the dosage is adjusted. Toxic symptoms may occur. An

Table 21-2 Therapeutic Actions of Drugs

Drug type	Description	Examples
Palliative	Relieves the symptoms of a disease but does not affect the disease itself.	Morphine sulphate, Fentanyl for pain
Curative	Cures a disease or condition.	Antibiotics for infection
Supportive	Supports body function until other treatments or the body's response can take over.	Paracetamol for high body temperature
Substitutive	Replaces body fluids or substances.	Thyroxine for hypothyroidism, insulin for diabetes mellitus
Chemotherapeutic	Destroys malignant cells.	Mitomycin for bladder cancer
Restorative	Returns the body to health.	Vitamin, mineral supplements

Table 21-3 Common Mild Allergic Responses

Symptom	Description/rationale
Skin rash	Either an intraepidermal vesicle rash or a rash typified by an urticarial wheal or macular eruption; rash is usually generalised over the body
Pruritus	Itching of the skin with or without a rash
Angioedema	Oedema due to increased permeability of the blood capillaries
Rhinitis	Excessive watery discharge from the nose
Lacrimal tearing	Excessive tearing
Nausea, vomiting	Stimulation of these centres in the brain
Wheezing and dyspnoea	Shortness of breath and wheezing on inhalation and exhalation due to accumulated fluids and swelling of the respiratory tissues
Diarrhoea/abdominal pain	Irritation of the mucosa of the large intestine

idiosyncratic effect is unexpected and individual. Under-response and over-response to a drug may be idiosyncratic. Also, the drug may have a completely different effect from the normal one or cause unpredictable and unexplainable symptoms in a particular patient.

A drug interaction occurs when the administration of one drug before, at the same time as, or after another drug alters the effect of one or both drugs. The effect of one or both drugs may be either increased (potentiating or synergistic effect) or decreased (inhibiting effect). Drug interactions may be beneficial or harmful. Two analgesics, such as paracetamol and codeine, are often given together because together they provide greater pain relief (additive effect). In this example of paracetamol and codeine, using a combination of drugs often decreases the total dose of narcotics needed. In addition, certain foods may interact adversely with a medication: for example, cranberry may affect the action of certain anticoagulants.

Iatrogenic disease (disease caused unintentionally by medical therapy) can be due to drug therapy. Hepatic toxicity resulting in biliary obstruction, renal damage and malformations of the foetus as a result of specific drugs taken during pregnancy are examples.

DRUG MISUSE

Drug misuse is the improper use of common medications in ways that lead to acute and chronic toxicity. Both over-the-counter drugs and prescription drugs may be misused. Laxatives, antacids, vitamins, headache remedies and cough and cold medications are often self-prescribed and overused. Most people suffer no harmful effects from these drugs, but some people do. A persistent cough may go undiagnosed until the underlying problem becomes serious and advanced, for example if the patient has an undiagnosed lung cancer.

Drug abuse is inappropriate intake of a substance, either continually or periodically. By definition, drug use is abusive when society considers it abusive. For example, the intake of alcohol at work may be considered alcohol abuse, but intake at a social gathering may not. Drug abuse has two main facets, drug dependence and habituation. Drug dependence is a person's reliance on or need to take a drug or substance. The two types of dependence, physiological and psychological, may occur separately or together. **Physiological dependence** is due to biochemical changes in body tissues, especially the nervous system. These tissues come to require the substance for normal functioning. A dependent person who stops using the drug experiences withdrawal symptoms. **Psychological dependence** is emotional reliance on a drug to maintain a sense of well-being, accompanied by feelings of need or cravings for that drug. There are varying degrees of psychological dependence, ranging from mild desire to craving and compulsive use of the drug.

Drug habituation denotes a mild form of psychological dependence. The individual develops the habit of taking the substance and feels better after taking it. The habituated individual tends to continue the habit even though it may be injurious to health.

Illicit drugs, also called street drugs, are those sold illegally. Illicit drugs are of two types: (a) drugs unavailable for purchase under any circumstances, such as cannabis, and (b) drugs normally available with prescriptions that are being obtained through illegal channels. Illicit drugs often are taken because of their mood-altering effect; that is, they make the person feel happy or relaxed.

ACTIONS OF DRUGS ON THE BODY

The action of a drug in the body can be described in terms of its half-life, the time interval required for the body's elimination processes to reduce the concentration of the drug in the body by one-half. For example, if a drug's half-life is eight hours, then the amount of drug in the body is as follows:

+ initially: 100%
+ after 8 hours: 50%
+ after 16 hours: 25%
+ after 24 hours: 12.5%
+ after 32 hours: 6.25%.

Because the purpose of most drug therapy is to maintain a constant drug level in the body, repeated doses are required to maintain that level. When an orally administered drug is absorbed from the gastrointestinal tract into the blood plasma, its concentration in the plasma increases until the elimination rate equals the rate of absorption. This point is known as the peak plasma level (see Figure 21-1). Unless the patient receives another dose of the drug, the concentration steadily decreases. Key terms related to drug actions are as follows:

+ **Onset of action**: the time after administration when the body initially responds to the drug.

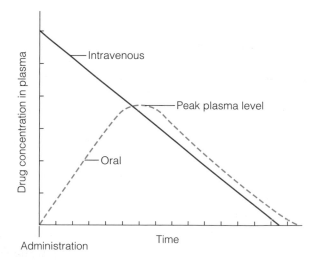

Figure 21-1 A graphic plot of drug concentration in the blood plasma following a single dose.

+ **Peak plasma level**: the highest plasma level achieved by a single dose when the elimination rate of a drug equals the absorption rate.
+ **Drug half-life (elimination half-life)**: the time required for the elimination process to reduce the concentration of the drug to one-half what it was at initial administration.
+ **Plateau**: a maintained concentration of a drug in the plasma during a series of scheduled doses.

Pharmacodynamics

Pharmacodynamics is the process by which a drug alters cell physiology. One of the mechanisms is the drug interaction with a cellular receptor to produce a response known as an agonist. Drugs that have no special pharmacological action of their own but that inhibit or prevent the action of an agonist are called specific antagonists. Drugs may also produce a response by stimulating enzyme activity or hormone production. They have a syngeristic effect.

Pharmacokinetics

Pharmacokinetics is the study of the absorption, distribution, biotransformation and excretion of drugs.

Absorption

Absorption is the process by which a drug passes into the bloodstream. Unless the drug is administered directly into the bloodstream, absorption is the first step in the movement of the drug through the body. For absorption to occur, the correct form of the drug must be given by the route intended.

The rate of absorption of a drug in the stomach is variable. Food, for example, can delay the dissolution and absorption of some drugs as well as their passage into the small intestine, where most drug absorption occurs. Food can also combine with molecules of certain drugs, thereby changing their molecular structure and subsequently inhibiting or preventing their absorption. Another factor that affects the absorption of some drugs is the acid medium in the stomach. Acidity can vary according to the time of day, foods ingested and the age of the patient. Some drugs do not dissolve or have limited ability to dissolve in the gastrointestinal fluids, decreasing their absorption into the bloodstream. Some drugs are absorbed by tissues before they reach the stomach. For example, glyceryl trinitrate is administered under the tongue, where it is absorbed into the blood vessels that carry it directly to the heart, the intended site of action. If swallowed, this drug will be absorbed into the bloodstream and carried to the liver, where it will be destroyed.

A drug administered directly into the bloodstream, that is, intravenously, is immediately in the vascular system without having to be absorbed. This, then, is the route of choice for rapid action. Because subcutaneous tissue has a poorer blood supply than muscle tissue, absorption from subcutaneous tissue is slower. The rate of absorption of a drug can be accelerated by the application of heat, which increases blood flow to the area;

conversely, absorption can be slowed by the application of cold. In addition, the injection of a vasoconstrictor drug such as epinephrine/adrenaline into the tissue can slow absorption of other drugs. Some drugs intended to be absorbed slowly are suspended in a low-solubility medium, such as oil. The absorption of drugs from the rectum into the bloodstream tends to be unpredictable. Therefore, this route is normally used when other routes are unavailable or when the intended action is localised to the rectum or sigmoid colon.

Distribution

Distribution is the transportation of a drug from its site of absorption to its site of action. When a drug enters the bloodstream, it is carried to the most vascular organs – that is, liver, kidneys and brain. Body areas with lower blood supply – that is, skin and muscles – receive the drug later. The chemical and physical properties of a drug largely determine the area of the body to which the drug will be attracted. For example, fat-soluble drugs will accumulate in fatty tissue, whereas other drugs may bind with plasma proteins.

Biotransformation

Biotransformation, also called detoxification or metabolism, is a process by which a drug is converted to a less active form. Most biotransformation takes place in the liver, where many drug-metabolising enzymes in the cells detoxify the drugs. The products of this process are called metabolites. There are two types of metabolites: active and inactive. An active metabolite has a pharmacological action itself, whereas an inactive metabolite does not.

Biotransformation may be impaired if a person is older or has an unhealthy liver. Nurses must be alert to the accumulation of the active drug in these patients and to subsequent toxicity.

Excretion

Excretion is the process by which metabolites and drugs are eliminated from the body. Most metabolites are eliminated by the kidneys in the urine; however, some are excreted in the faeces, the breath, perspiration, saliva and breast milk. Certain drugs, such as general anaesthetic agents, are excreted in an unchanged form via the respiratory tract. The efficiency with which the kidneys excrete drugs and metabolites diminishes with age. Older people may require smaller doses of a drug because the drug and its metabolites may accumulate in the body.

FACTORS AFFECTING MEDICATION ACTION

A number of factors other than the drug itself can affect its action. A person may not respond in the same manner to successive doses of a drug. In addition, the identical drug and dosage may affect different patients differently.

Developmental Factors

During pregnancy women must be very careful about taking medications. Drugs taken during pregnancy pose a risk throughout the pregnancy, but pose the highest risk during the first trimester, due to the formation of vital organs and functions of the foetus during this time. Most drugs are contraindicated because of the possible adverse effects on the foetus.

Infants usually require small dosages because of their body size and the immaturity of their organs, especially the liver and kidneys. They often do not have all of the enzymes required for drug metabolism and therefore may require different medications than adults. In adolescence or adulthood, allergic reactions may occur to drugs formerly tolerated.

Older adults have different responses to medications due to physiological changes that accompany ageing. These changes include decreased liver and kidney function, which can result in the accumulation of the drug in the body. In addition, the older person may be on multiple drugs and incompatibilities may occur.

Older adults often experience decreased gastric mobility and decreased gastric acid production and blood flow, which can impair drug absorption. Increased adipose tissue and decreased total body fluid proportionate to the body mass can increase the possibility of drug toxicity. Older adults may also experience a decreased number of protein-binding sites and changes in the blood–brain barrier. The latter permits fat-soluble drugs to move readily to the brain, often resulting in dizziness and confusion. This is particularly evident with beta blockers.

Gender

Differences in the way men and women respond to drugs are chiefly related to the distribution of body fat and fluid and hormonal differences. Because most drug research is done on men, more research on women is required to reflect the effects of hormonal changes on drug actions in women.

Cultural, Ethnic and Genetic Factors

A patient's response to a drug is influenced by age, gender, size and body composition. This variation in response is called drug polymorphism (Kudzma, 1999). Research studies indicate that ethnicity may contribute to differences in responses to medication. Kudzma (1999) points out that drug metabolism is genetically determined and, as a result, race may affect a drug response. This is called genetic polymorphism. The genes that control liver metabolism vary and some patients may have slow metabolism, whereas others are rapid metabolisers. Research has shown that certain medication may work well at usual therapeutic dosages for certain ethnic groups but be toxic for others. Kudzma (1999) provides the example of antipsychotic and antianxiety drugs being effective for African Americans, Caucasians and Hispanics; however, patients of Asian descent may need a lower dosage because of slower metabolism of that drug classification, which results in them being more prone to an adverse reaction. Cultural factors and practices (e.g. values

and beliefs) can also affect a drug's action. For example, an herbal remedy (e.g. the Chinese herb ginseng) may speed up or slow down the metabolism of prescribed medications.

Diet

Nutrients can affect the action of a medication. For example, vitamin K found in green leafy vegetables can counteract the effect of an anticoagulant such as warfarin.

Environment

The patient's environment can affect the action of drugs, particularly those used to alter behaviour and mood. Therefore, nurses assessing the effects of a drug need to consider the drug in the context of the patient's personality.

Environmental temperature may also affect drug activity. When environmental temperature is high the peripheral blood vessels dilate, thus intensifying the action of vasodilators. In contrast, a cold environment and the consequent vasoconstriction inhibit the action of vasodilators but enhance the action of vasoconstrictors. A patient who takes a sedative or analgesic in a busy, noisy environment may not benefit as fully as if the environment were quiet and peaceful.

Psychological Factors

A patient's expectations about what a drug can do can affect the response to the medication. For example, a patient who believes that codeine is ineffective as an analgesic may experience no relief from pain after it is given.

Illness and Disease

Illness and disease can also affect the action of drugs. For example, Paracetamol can reduce the body temperature of a feverish patient but has no effect on the body temperature of a patient without fever. Drug action is altered in patients with circulatory, liver or kidney dysfunction.

Time of Administration

The time of administration of oral medications affects the relative speed with which they act. Orally administered medications are absorbed more quickly if the stomach is empty. Thus oral medications taken two hours before meals act faster than those taken after meals. However, some medications, for example iron preparations, irritate the gastrointestinal tract and need to be given after a meal, when they will be better tolerated. A patient's sleep–wake rhythm may affect the action of a drug. Circadian variations in urine output and blood circulation, for example, may affect a patient's response to a drug.

ROUTES OF ADMINISTRATION

Pharmaceutical preparations are generally designed for one or two specific routes of administration (see Table 21-4 on page 516). The route of administration should be indicated

Table 21-4 Routes of Administration

Route	Advantages	Disadvantages
Oral	Most convenient Usually least expensive Safe, does not break skin barrier Administration usually does not cause stress	Inappropriate for patients with nausea or vomiting Drug may have unpleasant taste or odour Inappropriate when gastrointestinal tract has reduced motility Inappropriate if patient cannot swallow or is unconscious Cannot be used before certain diagnostic tests or surgical procedures Drug may discolour teeth, harm tooth enamel Drug may irritate gastric mucosa Drug can be aspirated by seriously ill patients
Sublingual	Same as for oral, *plus* Drug can be administered for local effect More potent than oral route because drug directly enters the blood and bypasses the liver	If swallowed, drug may be inactivated by gastric juice Drug must remain under tongue until dissolved and absorbed Drug is rapidly absorbed into the bloodstream
Buccal	Same as for sublingual	Same as for sublingual
Rectal	Can be used when drug has objectionable taste or odour Drug released at slow, steady rate	Dose absorbed is unpredictable
Vaginal	Provides a local therapeutic effect	Limited use
Topical	Provides a local effect Few side-effects	May be messy and may soil clothes Drug can enter body through abrasions and cause systemic effects
Transdermal	Prolonged systemic effect Few side-effects Avoids gastrointestinal absorption problems	Leaves residue on the skin that may soil clothes
Subcutaneous	Onset of drug action faster than oral	Must involve sterile technique because breaks skin barrier More expensive than oral Can administer only small volume Slower than intramuscular administration Some drugs can irritate tissues and cause pain Can produce anxiety
Intramuscular	Pain from irritating drugs is minimised Can administer larger volume than subcutaneous Drug is rapidly absorbed	Breaks skin barrier Can produce anxiety
Intradermal	Absorption is slow (this is an advantage in testing for allergies)	Amount of drug administered must be small Breaks skin barrier
Intravenous	Rapid effect	Limited to highly soluble drugs Drug distribution inhibited by poor circulation
Inhalation	Introduces drug throughout respiratory tract Rapid localised relief Drug can be administered to unconscious patient	Drug intended for localised effect can have systemic effect Of use only for the respiratory system

when the drug is prescribed. When administering a drug, the nurse should ensure that the pharmaceutical preparation is appropriate for the route specified.

Oral

Oral administration is the most common, least expensive and most convenient route for most patients. In oral administration,

the drug is swallowed. Because the skin is not broken as it is for an injection, oral administration is also a safe method.

The major disadvantages are possibly unpleasant taste of the drugs, irritation of the gastric mucosa, irregular absorption from the gastrointestinal tract, slow absorption and, in some cases, harm to the patient's teeth. For example, the liquid preparation of ferrous sulphate (iron) can stain the teeth.

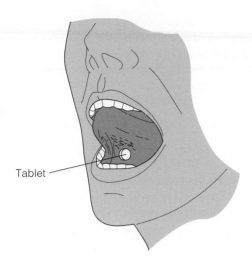

Figure 21-2 Sublingual administration of a tablet.

Sublingual

In **sublingual** administration a drug is placed under the tongue, where it dissolves (see Figure 21-2). In a relatively short time, the drug is largely absorbed into the blood vessels on the underside of the tongue. The medication should not be swallowed. Glyceryl trinitrate is one example of a drug commonly given in this manner.

Buccal

Buccal means 'pertaining to the cheek'. In buccal administration, a medication (e.g. a tablet) is held in the mouth against the mucous membranes of the cheek until the drug dissolves (see Figure 21-3). The drug may act locally on the mucous membranes of the mouth or systemically when it is swallowed in the saliva.

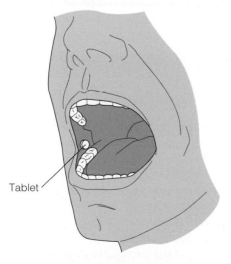

Figure 21-3 Buccal administration of a tablet.

Parenteral

The **parenteral** route is defined as other than through the alimentary or respiratory tract; that is, by needle. The following are some of the more common routes for parenteral administration:

+ **subcutaneous** – into the subcutaneous tissue, just below the skin;
+ **intramuscular** – into a muscle;
+ **intradermal** – under the epidermis (into the dermis);
+ **intravenous** – into a vein.

Some of the less commonly used routes for parenteral administration are intra-arterial (into an artery), intracardiac (into the heart muscle), intraosseous (into a bone), **intrathecal** or **intraspinal** (into the spinal canal), intrapleural (into the pleural space), **epidural** (into the epidural space) and intra-articular (into a joint). Sterile equipment and sterile drug solution are essential for all parenteral therapy. The main advantage is fast absorption.

Topical

Topical applications are those applied to a circumscribed surface area of the body. They affect only the area to which they are applied. Topical applications include the following:

+ dermatologic preparations – applied to the skin;
+ instillations and irrigations – applied into body cavities or orifices, such as the urinary bladder, eyes, ears, nose, rectum or vagina;
+ inhalations – administered into the respiratory tract by a nebuliser or positive pressure breathing apparatus. Air, oxygen and vapour are generally used to carry the drug into the lungs.

MEDICATION PRESCRIPTIONS AND CHARTS

A physician usually determines the patient's medication needs and prescribes medications, although in some settings nurse practitioners and supplementary prescribers now prescribe some drugs. The prescription chart is written, although telephone and verbal orders are acceptable in some instances, but a written prescription should also be completed as soon as possible.

Frequently abbreviations may be used on medication charts; wherever possible these should be avoided as they may have different meanings in different clinical areas (see Table 21-5 on page 518).

Types of Medication Prescriptions

Four common medication prescriptions are the stat, the single once only, the regular daily and the prn prescription.

+ A stat prescription indicates that the medication is to be given immediately and only once (e.g. Aspirin 300 mg orally stat).
+ The single or one once only is for medication to be given once at a specified time (e.g. Cefuroxime 750 mg iv before surgery).

Table 21-5 Common Abbreviations Used on Medication Charts

Abbreviation	Explanation	Example of administration time
ac	before meals	0700, 1100 and 1700 hours
ad lib	freely, as desired	
aq	water	
bd	twice a day	0900 and 2100 hours
b	with	
cap	capsule	
dil	dissolve, dilute	
elix	elixir	
g	gram	
gtt	drop	
h	an hour	
nocte	at bedtime (hour of sleep)	
ID	intradermal	
IM	intramuscular	
IV	intravenous	
Kg	kilogram	
L	litre	
M or m	mix	
mcg or μg	microgram	
mg	milligram	
OD	once daily	
po or PO	by mouth	
prn	when needed	
q	every	
qAM	every morning	1000 hours
qh (q1h)	every hour	
q2h	every 2 hours	0800, 1,000, 1200 hours, and so on
q3h	every 3 hours	0900, 1,200, 1500 hours, and so on
q4h	every 4 hours	1000, 1400, 1800 hours, and so on
q6h	every 6 hours	0600, 1200, 1800 2400 hours
qds	four times a day	1000, 1400, 1800 2200 hours
qs	sufficient quantity	
Rx	take	
sc or Sc	subcutaneous	
stat	at once	
sup or supp	suppository	
susp	suspension	
tab	tablet	
tds	three times a day	1000, 1400, and 1800 hours
Tr or tinct	tincture	

+ The regular daily may or may not have a termination date and is administered until the medication chart is reviewed.

+ A prn or as needed prescription, permits the nurse to give a medication when, in the nurse's judgement, the patient requires it (e.g. Co-Codamol 30/500 two prn 6 hourly). The nurse must use good judgement about when the medication is needed and when it can be safely administered.

Essential Parts of a Prescription Chart

The drug chart has seven essential parts, as listed in *Box 21-2*. In addition, unless it is a regular administration section it should state the number of doses or the number of days the drug is to be administered.

The patient's full name, that is, the first and last names and middle initials or names, should always be used to avoid confusion between two patients who have the same last name. Some hospitals imprint the patient's name, address, date of birth and identification number on all forms while some areas use stickers with similar information.

The name of the drug to be administered must be clearly written. In some settings only generic names are permitted; however, trade names are widely used in hospitals and clinical areas.

The dosage of the drug includes the amount, the times or frequency of administration, and in many instances the strength; for example, tetracycline 250 mg (amount) four times a day (frequency); potassium chloride 10% (strength) 5 ml (amount) three times a day with meals (time and frequency).

Also included on the chart is the route of administration of the drug. This part of the prescription, like other parts, is frequently abbreviated. It is not unusual for a drug to have several possible routes of administration; therefore, it is important that the route be included in the prescription.

The signature of the prescriber makes the drug chart a legal document. An unsigned chart has no validity, and the ordering prescriber needs to be notified if the chart is unsigned. A pharmacist should also check all in-patient prescriptions within 24 hours of admission or according to local policy.

Medication administration records (see Figure 21-4) vary in form, but all include the patient's name, identification number,

---

BOX 21-2 Essential Parts of a Drug Prescription

+ Should be written legibly in black ink
+ Full name and address of the patient
+ Patient's hospital/record/NHS number
+ Date and time the drug is written
+ Name of the drug to be administered
+ Dosage of the drug
+ Frequency of administration
+ Route of administration
+ Signature of the person prescribing

IN-PATIENT MEDICATION ADMINISTRATION RECORD

NHS WALES GIG CYMRU

HOSPITAL NO: _____
SURNAME: _____
FIRST NAMES: _____
ADDRESS: _____
_____
_____

DATE OF BIRTH: _____

HOSPITAL: _____

WARD: _____

CONSULTANT: _____

DATE OF ADMISSION	WEIGHT	HEIGHT	B.S.A.
	kg	cm	m²

SUPPLEMENTARY/MULTIPLE MEDICATION CHARTS (Specify)

Drug Allergies THIS SECTION MUST BE COMPLETED

YES
Specify Drugs ....   Specify Allergy Type ....
Signature ....   Date ....

NONE KNOWN
Signature ....   Date ....

PRESCRIPTION FOR ONCE-ONLY and PRE-ANAESTHETIC MEDICATION

DATE	MEDICINE (APPROVED NAME)	DOSE	ROUTE	TIME TO BE GIVEN	DOCTOR'S SIGNATURE	PHARMACY	DATE	TIME GIVEN	GIVEN BY	CHECKED BY
					bleep No.					
					bleep No.					
					bleep No.					
					bleep No.					
					bleep No.					
					bleep No.					
					bleep No.					
					bleep No.					
					bleep No.					
					bleep No.					

OXYGEN THERAPY: Tick one box to select device and enter % or flow rate of oxygen as appropriate. Oxygen delivered by any other device should be clearly prescribed on the regular prescription section. Nurse to sign at least every 12 hours.

		Change 1	date	time	sign	date	time	sign	date	time	sign	date	time	sign
Venturi mask	❏ ..... %	❏ ..... %												
Nasal Cannula	❏ ..... L/min	❏ ..... L/min												
Humidified (circle)	Yes/No	Yes/No												
MC Mask	❏ ..... L/min	❏ ..... L/min												
Duration/Continuous Instructions														
Doctor's signature														
Date														

NON-ADMINISTRATION OF MEDICINES
When a patient does not receive a prescribed dose, the nurse should enter one of the code numbers given below in the administration box, to explain the reason for non-administration. Please attempt to obtain any unavailable medicines.

X. Doctor's request
2. Patient not on ward.
3. Patient unable to receive medicines/or no access.
4. Patient refused medicine.
5. Medicine unavailable.
6. See Notes.

IN-PATIENT MEDICATION ADMINISTRATION RECORD

Figure 21-4 Sample medication administration record.
Courtesy of Welsh Chief Pharmacists. This chart is only used in Wales and will be Current up to December 2007.

clinical area name; drug name and dose; and times and method of administration.

The nurse should always question the prescriber about any chart that is ambiguous, unusual (e.g. an abnormally high dosage of a medication) or contraindicated by the patient's condition. When the nurse judges a prescribed medication inappropriate, the following actions are required:

✦ Contact the prescriber and discuss the rationale for believing the medication or dosage to be inappropriate.

✦ Document in the patient notes the following: when the prescriber was notified, what was conveyed to the prescriber and how the prescriber responded.

✦ If the prescriber cannot be reached, document all attempts to contact the prescriber and the reason for withholding the medication.

✦ Contact an appropriate member of medical staff responsible for the care of the patient.

✦ If someone else gives the medication, document data about the patient's condition before and after the medication.

✦ If an incident report is indicated, clearly document factual information in accordance with local policy.

SYSTEMS OF MEASUREMENT: METRIC SYSTEM

The metric system, devised by the French in the latter part of the 18th century, is the system prescribed by law in most European countries. The metric system is logically organised into units of 10; it is a decimal system. Basic units can be multiplied or divided by 10 to form secondary units. Multiples are calculated by moving the decimal point to the right, and division is accomplished by moving the decimal point to the left.

Basic units of measurement are the metre, the litre and the gram. Prefixes derived from Latin designate subdivisions of the basic unit: deci (1/10 or 0.1), centi (1/100 or 0.01) and milli (1/1,000 or 0.001). Multiples of the basic unit are designated by prefixes derived from Greek: deka (10), hecto (100) and kilo (1,000). Only the measurements of volume (the litre) and of weight (the gram) are discussed in this chapter. These are the measures used in medication administration (see Figure 21-5). In nursing practice, the kilogram (kg) is the only multiple of the gram used, and the milligram (mg) and microgram (mcg or μg) are subdivisions. Fractional parts of the litre are usually expressed in millilitres (ml), for example, 600 ml; multiples of the litre are usually expressed as litres or millilitres, for example, 2.5 l or 2,500 ml.

Converting Weights within the Metric System

It is relatively simple to arrive at equivalent units of weight within the metric system because the system is based on units of 10. Only three metric units of weight are used for drug dosages, the gram (g), milligram (mg) and microgram (mcg or μg): 1,000 mg or 1,000,000 mcg equals 1 g. Equivalents are

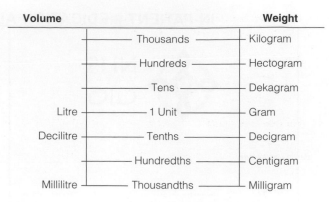

Figure 21-5 Basic metric measurements of volume and weight.

computed by dividing or multiplying; for example, to change milligrams to grams, the nurse divides the number of milligrams by 1,000. The simplest way to divide by 1,000 is to move the decimal point three places to the left:

500 mg = ? g

Move the decimal point three places to the *left:*

Answer = 0.5 g

Conversely, to convert grams to milligrams, multiply the number of grams by 1,000 or move the decimal point three places to the right:

0.006 g = ? mg

Move the decimal point three places to the *right:*

Answer = 6 mg

Calculating Dosages

Several formulas can be used to calculate drug dosages. One formula uses ratios:

$$\frac{\text{Dose available}}{\text{Quantity available}} = \frac{\text{Desired dose}}{\text{Quantity desired } (x)}$$

For example, erythromycin 500 mg is prescribed. It is supplied in a liquid form containing 250 mg in 5 ml. To calculate the dosage, the nurse uses the formula

$$\frac{\text{Dose available (250 mg)}}{\text{Quantity available (5 ml)}} = \frac{\text{Desired dose (500 mg)}}{\text{Quantity desired } (x)}$$

Then the nurse cross-multiplies:

$$250 \, x = 5 \text{ ml} \times 500 \text{ mg}$$

$$x = \frac{5 \text{ ml} \times 500 \text{ mg}}{250 \text{ mg}}$$

$$x = 10 \text{ ml}$$

Therefore, the dose prescribed is 10 ml. The nurse can also use this formula to calculate dosages:

Amount to administer (x)

$$= \frac{\text{Desired dose}}{\text{Dose available}} \times \text{Quantity available}$$

For example, heparin sodium mucous is often distributed in vials in prepared dilutions of 10,000 units per millilitre. If 5,000 units is prescribed, the nurse can use the preceding formula to calculate

$$x = \frac{5,000}{10,000} \times 1$$

$$x = {}^{1}\!/_{2}\ \text{ml}$$

Therefore, the nurse injects 0.5 ml for a 5,000-unit dose.

Dosages for Children

Although dosage is stated in the medication prescription, nurses must understand something about the safe dosage for children. Unlike adult dosages, children's dosages are not always standard. Body size significantly affects dosage.

Body Surface Area

Body surface area is determined by using a nomogram and the child's height and weight. This is considered to be the most accurate method of calculating a child's dose. Standard nomograms give a child's body surface area according to weight and height (see Figure 21-6 on page 522). The formula is the ratio of the child's body surface area to the surface area of an average adult (1.7 square metres, or 1.7 m²), multiplied by the normal adult dose of the drug:

Child's dose

$$= \frac{\text{Surface area of child (m}^2)}{1.7\ \text{m}^2} \times \text{Normal adult dose}$$

For example, a child who weighs 10 kg and is 50 cm tall has a body surface area of 0.4 m². Therefore, the child's dose of tetracycline corresponding to an adult dose of 250 mg would be as follows:

$$\text{Child's dose} = \frac{0.4\ \text{m}^2}{1.7\ \text{m}^2} \times 250\ \text{mg} = 0.23 \times 250$$

$$= 58.82\ \text{mg}$$

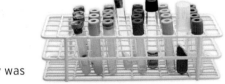

RESEARCH NOTE

Are Nursing Students Mathematically Prepared?

Nurses need to be competent in mathematics to prevent drug administration errors. Brown (2002) reviewed studies, conducted at degree nursing programmes, that found a large percentage of nursing students could not pass a basic arithmetic test on entry to the programme.

The purpose of this study was to identify the weak links in computational mathematical abilities. The population group consisted of first-semester associate degree nursing students from universities in the USA. The students were administered a standard basic mathematic ability test for which each item had four response choices. There was no time limit and no calculators were allowed.

In addition, nursing faculty were asked to review the maths test and indicate what percentage of the nursing students should be able to answer all items correctly. The mean student score was 75% and the mean score expected by faculty was 87.9%.

Examination of individual test items provided more information, however, than just the group means. At least 70% could calculate maths problems dealing with whole numbers. When the items dealt with fractions, decimals and percentages, however, the correct response rate dropped between 30% and 65%. One of the lowest correct response rate was 1/400 — (change to a decimal), which is common in medication administration.

Implications

Nursing students are mathematically underprepared. The author stressed the importance of the ability to calculate medication dosages correctly and suggested the following strategies: Require students to take a maths placement test, provide maths remedial courses and administer a maths skills test each semester.

Note: From 'Does 1 + 1 Still Equal 2? A Study of the Mathematic Competencies of Associate Degree Nursing Students' by D.L. Brown, 2002, *Nurse Educator, 27*(3), pp. 132–135.

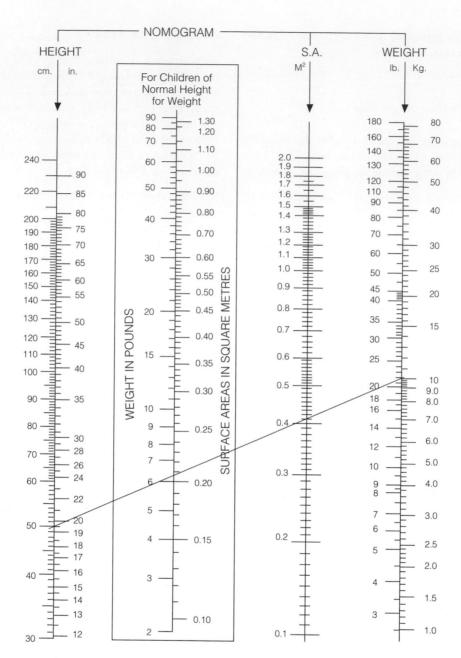

Figure 21-6 Nomogram with estimated body surface area. A straight line is drawn between the child's height (on the left) and the child's weight (on the right). The point at which the line intersects the surface area column is the estimated body surface area.

ADMINISTERING MEDICATIONS SAFELY

The nurse should always assess a patient's health status and obtain a medication history prior to giving any medication. This may be done as part of the nursing process (see Chapter 9). The extent of the assessment depends on the patient's illness or current condition, the intended drug and the route of administration. For example, if a patient has dyspnoea, the nurse should assess respirations carefully before administering any medication that might affect breathing. It is important to determine whether the route of administration is suitable. For example,

a patient who is nauseated may not be able to tolerate a drug taken orally. In general, the nurse assesses the patient prior to administering any medication to obtain baseline data by which to evaluate the effectiveness of the medication.

The medication history includes information about the drugs the patient is taking currently or has taken recently. This includes prescription drugs; over-the-counter drugs such as antacids, alcohol and tobacco; and non-sanctioned drugs such as marijuana. Sometimes an incompatibility with one or more of these drugs affects the choice of a new medication.

Older adults often take vitamins, herbs, food supplements and/or use complementary remedies that they do not list in their medication history. Because many of these have unknown or unpredictable actions and side-effects, they need to be noted, with attention paid to possible incompatibilities with other prescribed medications.

An important part of the history is patient's knowledge of their drug allergies. Some patients can tell a nurse, 'I am allergic to penicillin, adhesive tape, and eggs.' Other patients may not be sure about allergic reactions. An illness occurring after a drug was taken may not be identified as an allergy, but the patient may associate the drug with an illness or unusual reaction. The patient's general practitioner can often give information about allergies. During the history, the nurse tries to elicit information about drug dependencies. How often drugs are taken and the patient's perceived need for them are measures of dependence.

Also included in the history are the patient's normal eating habits. Sometimes the medication regimen needs to be coordinated with mealtimes or the ingestion of foods. Where a medication must be taken with food on a specified time scale, patients can often adjust their mealtime or have a snack (e.g. with a bedtime medication). In addition, certain foods are incompatible with certain medications, for example, milk is incompatible with tetracycline.

Any problems the patient may have in self-administering a medication must also be identified. A patient with poor eyesight, for example, may require special labels for the medication container; elderly patients with unsteady hands may not be able to hold a syringe or to inject themselves or another person. Obtaining information as to how and where the patient stores their medications is also important. If the patient has difficulty opening certain containers, they may change containers but leave old labels on, which increases the risk of medication errors.

Socioeconomic factors need to be considered for all patients, but especially for older adults. Common problems are lack of transportation to obtain medications although this is overcome by some community pharmacies arranging a home delivery service. If the nurse is aware of these problems, proper resources can be obtained for the patient.

PRACTICE GUIDELINES

Administering Medications

+ Nurses who administer medications are responsible for their own actions. Question any prescription that is illegible or that you consider incorrect. Call the person who prescribed the medication for clarification.
+ Be knowledgeable about the medications you administer. You need to know why the patient is receiving the medication. Look up the necessary information if you are not familiar with the medication.
+ Use only medications that are in a clearly labelled container.
+ Do not use liquid medications that are cloudy or have changed colour.
+ Calculate drug doses accurately. If you are uncertain, ask another nurse to double check your calculations.
+ Administer only medications personally prepared.

+ Before administering a medication, identify the patient correctly using the appropriate means of identification, such as checking the identification bracelet, asking a patient to state his or her name, or both.
+ Do not leave medications at the bedside, with certain exceptions (e.g. nitroglycerin, cough syrup). Check local clinical policy.
+ If a patient vomits after taking an oral medication, report this to the nurse in charge and document.
+ Take special precautions when administering certain medications, for example, have another nurse check the dosages of anticoagulants, insulin and certain IV preparations.
+ When a medication is omitted for any reason, record the fact together with the reason.
+ When a medication error is made, report it immediately to the nurse in charge, the medical staff, and follow local incident reporting policy.

Process of Administering Medications

When administering any drug, regardless of the route of administration, the nurse must do the following:

1. *Identify the patient.* Errors can and do occur, usually because one patient gets a drug intended for another. In hospitals, all patients wear some sort of identification, such as a wristband with name and hospital identification number. Before giving the patient any drug, always check the patient's identification band. As a double check, the nurse can ask the alert patient to state his or her name.

2. *Inform the patient.* If the patient is unfamiliar with the medication, the nurse should explain the intended action as well as any side-effects or adverse effects that might occur.

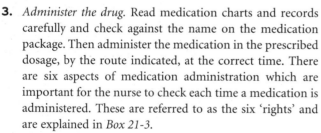

BOX 21-3 Six 'Rights' of Medication Administration

Right Medication
+ The medication given was the medication prescribed.

Right Dose
+ The dose prescribed is appropriate for the patient.
+ Give special attention if the calculation indicates multiple pills/tablets or a large quantity of a liquid medication.
+ Double check calculations that appear questionable.
+ Know the usual dosage range of the medication.
+ Question a dose outside of the usual dosage range.

Right Time
+ Give the medication at the right frequency and at the time prescribed according to local policy.
+ Medications given within 30 minutes before or after the scheduled time are considered to meet the right time standard.

Right Route
+ Give the medication by the prescribed route.
+ Make certain that the route is safe and appropriate for the patient.

Right Patient
+ Medication is given to the intended patient.
+ Check the patient's identification band with each administration of a medication.
+ Know the clinical area name alert procedure when patients with the same or similar last names are on the nursing unit. This may be a sticky label on the chart or a patient warning arm band.

Right Documentation
+ Document medication administration after giving it, not before.
+ If time of administration differs from prescribed time, note the time on the chart and explain reason and follow-through activities (e.g. pharmacy states medication will be available in two hours) in nursing notes.
+ If a medication is not given, follow local policy for documenting the reason why.

3. *Administer the drug.* Read medication charts and records carefully and check against the name on the medication package. Then administer the medication in the prescribed dosage, by the route indicated, at the correct time. There are six aspects of medication administration which are important for the nurse to check each time a medication is administered. These are referred to as the six 'rights' and are explained in *Box 21-3.*

4. *Provide adjunctive interventions as indicated.* Patients may need help when receiving medications. They may require physical assistance, for instance, in assuming positions for intramuscular injections, or they may need guidance about measures to enhance drug effectiveness and prevent complications, such as drinking fluids. Some patients convey fear about their medications. The nurse can allay fears by listening carefully to patients' concerns and giving correct information.

5. *Record the drug administered.* The facts recorded on the chart in ink are name of the drug, dosage, method of administra-

tion, specific relevant data such as pulse rate (taken in most settings prior to the administration of digitalis) and any other pertinent information. The record should also include the exact time of administration and the signature of the nurse providing the medication. Often, medications that are given regularly are recorded on a special flow record. PRN (as needed) or stat (at once) medications are recorded separately.

6. *Evaluate the patient's response to the drug.* The kinds of behaviour that reflect the action or lack of action of a drug and its untoward effects (both minor and major) are as variable as the purposes of the drugs themselves. The anxious patient may show the desired effects of a tranquilliser by behaviour that reflects a lowered stress level (e.g. slower speech or fewer random movements). The effectiveness of a sedative can often be measured by how well a patient slept, and the effectiveness of an antispasmodic by how much pain the patient feels. In all nursing activities, nurses need to be aware of the medications that a patient is taking and record their effectiveness as assessed by the patient and the nurse on the patient's chart.

CLINICAL ANECDOTE

Last week I was administering medications under the supervision of my mentor. When we went to one patient, John Smith, the address and date of birth on the medication chart did not match the one he gave. When we checked there was another patient by the name of John Smith on the ward. This incident will always remind me to check for the rest of my career. I dread to think what the effects could have been if we gave the wrong medication to the wrong patient.

Danni, third-year student nurse

Developmental Considerations

It is important for the nurse to be aware of how growth and development impacts administration of medications for all age groups, particularly the very young and the very old.

Infants and Children

Knowledge of growth and development is essential for the nurse administering medications to children. Oral medications for children are usually prepared in sweetened liquid form to make them more palatable. The parents may provide suggestions about what method is best for their child. Necessary foods such as milk or orange juice should not be used to mask the taste of medications, because the child may develop unpleasant associations and refuse that food in the future.

Children tend to fear any procedure in which a needle is used because they anticipate pain or because the procedure is unfamiliar and threatening. The nurse needs to acknowledge that the child will feel some pain; denying this fact only deepens the child's distrust. After the injection, the nurse (or the parent) can cuddle and speak softly to the infant and give the child a toy to dispel the child's association of the nurse only with pain.

Older Adults

Older adults can have special problems, most of which are related to physiological changes, to past experiences and to established attitudes toward medications. The physiological changes in older adults that may affect the administration and effectiveness of medications are listed in *Box 21-4*.

Many of these changes enhance the possibility of cumulative effects and toxicity. For example, impaired circulation delays the action of medications given intramuscularly or subcutaneously. Digitalis, which is frequently taken by older adults, can accumulate to toxic levels and be lethal. It is not uncommon for older adults to take several different medications daily.

The possibility of error increases with the number of medications taken, whether self-administered at home or administered in a hospital. The greater number of medications also compounds the problem of drug interactions. A general rule to follow is that older adults should take as few medications as possible.

Older adults usually require smaller dosages of drugs, especially sedatives and other central nervous system depressants. Reactions of older adults to medications, particularly sedatives, are unpredictable and often bizarre. It is not uncommon to see irritability, confusion, disorientation, restlessness and incontinence as a result of sedatives. Nurses therefore need to observe patients carefully for untoward reactions. Physicians often follow the unwritten rule to 'start low and go slow' when prescribing medications for older adults. The initial prescribed dosage will often be low and then be gradually increased with careful monitoring of actions and side-effects of the drug.

Attitudes of older adults toward medical care and medications vary, they tend to believe in the wisdom of the physician more readily than younger people. Some older people are bewildered by the prescription of several medications and may passively accept their medications from nurses but not swallow them, spitting out tablets or capsules after the nurse leaves the room. For this reason, the nurse is advised to stay with patients until they have swallowed the medications. Others may be suspicious of medications and actively refuse them.

Older adults are mature and capable of reasoning. Therefore, the nurse needs to explain the reasons for and the effects of medications. This education can prevent patients from continuing to take a medication long after there is a need for it or discontinuing a drug too quickly. For example, patients should know that diuretics will cause them to urinate more frequently and may reduce ankle oedema. Instructions about medications need to be given to all patients. These instructions should include when to take the drugs, what effects to expect, and when to consult a healthcare professional.

BOX 21-4 Physiological Changes Associated with Ageing That Influence Medication Administration and Effectiveness

+ Altered memory
+ Less acute vision
+ Decrease in renal function, resulting in slower elimination of drugs and higher drug concentrations in the bloodstream for longer periods
+ Less complete and slower absorption from the gastrointestinal tract
+ Increased proportion of fat to lean body mass, which facilitates retention of fat-soluble drugs and increases potential for toxicity

+ Decreased liver function, which hinders biotransformation of drugs
+ Decreased organ sensitivity, which means that the response to the same drug concentration in the vicinity of the target organ is less in older people than in the young
+ Altered quality of organ responsiveness, resulting in adverse effects becoming pronounced before therapeutic effects are achieved
+ Decrease in manual dexterity due to arthritis and/or decrease in flexibility

Because some patients are required to take several medications daily and because visual acuity and memory may be impaired, the nurse needs to develop simple, realistic plans for patients to follow at home. For example, remembering to take drugs can be difficult for most people, including the elderly. If medications are scheduled to be taken with meals or at bedtime, patients are not as likely to forget. Some patients may take their medications and then an hour later not remember whether they took them. One solution to forgetfulness is to use a special container or glass strictly for medications. An empty glass or container indicates that the person took the pills. Loss of visual acuity presents problems that can be overcome by writing out the plan in block letters large enough to be read. In some situations the help of a friend or relative can be enlisted.

ORAL MEDICATIONS

The oral route is the most common route by which medications are given. As long as a patient can swallow and retain the drug in the stomach, this is the route of choice (see *Procedure 21-1*). Oral medications are contraindicated when a patient is vomiting, has gastric or intestinal suction, or is unconscious and unable to swallow. Patients in this group are usually 'Nil by Mouth'.

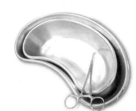

PROCEDURE 21-1 Administering Oral Medications

Purpose

+ To provide a medication that has systemic effects or local effects on the gastrointestinal tract or both (see specific drug action).

Assessment

Assess

+ Allergies to medication(s)
+ Patients ability to swallow the medication
+ Presence of vomiting or diarrhoea that would interfere with the ability to absorb the medication
+ Specific drug action, side-effects, interactions and adverse reactions
+ Patient's knowledge of and learning needs about the medication

Perform appropriate assessments (e.g. vital signs, check laboratory results) specific to the medication.

Determine if the assessment data influence administration of the medication (i.e. is it appropriate to administer the medication or does the medication need to be withheld and the physician notified?).

Planning

Equipment

+ Medication trolley/key to bedside drug locker
+ Disposable medication cups: small paper or plastic cups for tablets and capsules, plastic calibrated medication cups for liquids
+ Prescription chart

+ Pill crusher
+ Straws to administer medications that may discolour the teeth or to facilitate the ingestion of liquid medication for certain patients
+ Drinking glass and water

Implementation

Preparation

1. Know the reason why the patient is receiving the medication, the drug classification, contraindications, usual dosage range, side-effects and nursing considerations for administering and evaluating the intended outcomes for the medication.

2. Check the medication prescription chart.
    • Check the chart for the drug name, dosage, frequency, route of administration and expiration date for administering the medication, if appropriate. *Certain medications (e.g. antibiotics)*

have a specified time frame at which they expire and need to be re-prescribed.
- If the chart is unclear or pertinent information is missing, report any discrepancies to the prescriber and withhold medication until issues are clarified.

3. Verify the patient's ability to take medication orally.
   - Determine whether the patient can swallow, is NBM, is nauseated or vomiting or has gastric suction.

4. Organise the supplies.
   - Assemble the chart(s) for each patient together so that medications can be prepared for one patient at a time. *Organisation of supplies saves time and reduces the chance of error.*

Performance

1. Wash hands and observe other appropriate infection control procedures.
2. Unlock the medication trolley/locker.
3. Obtain appropriate medication.
   - Read the medication chart and take the appropriate medication from the shelf or locker. The medication may be dispensed in a bottle, box or unit-dose package.
   - Compare the label of the medication container or unit-dose package against the chart (see Figure 21-7). *This is a safety check to ensure that the right medication is given.* If these are not identical, recheck the patient's chart. If there is still a discrepancy, check with the nurse in charge or the pharmacist.
   - Check the expiration date of the medication. Return expired medications to the pharmacy. *Outdated medications are not safe to administer.*
   - Use only medications that have clear, legible labels *to ensure accuracy.*

4. Prepare the medication.
   - Calculate medication dosage accurately.
   - Prepare the correct amount of medication for the required dose, without contaminating the medication. *Aseptic technique maintains drug cleanliness (see Chapter 14).*
   - While preparing the medication, recheck each prepared drug and container with the chart again. *This second safety check reduces the chance of error.*

Tablets or Capsules

- Place packaged unit-dose capsules or tablets directly into the medicine cup. Do not remove the medication from the wrapper until at the bedside. *The wrapper keeps the medication clean. Not removing the medication from the wrapper facilitates identification of the medication in the event the patient refuses the drug or assessment data indicate the drug should be withheld. Unopened unit-dose packages can usually be returned to the medication trolley/locker.*
- If using a stock container, pour the required number into the bottle cap, and then transfer the medication to the disposable cup without touching the tablets.
- Keep medications that require specific assessments, such as pulse measurements, respiratory rate or depth, or blood pressure, separate from the others. *This reminds the nurse to complete the needed assessment(s) in order to decide whether to give the medication or to withhold the medication if indicated.*
- Break only scored tablets if necessary to obtain the correct dosage. Use a file or cutting device if needed (see Figure 21-8). Check local policy as to whether unused portions of a medication can be discarded and, if so, how they are to be discarded.

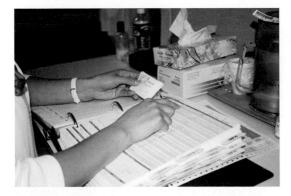

Figure 21-7 Compare the medication label to the medication chart.

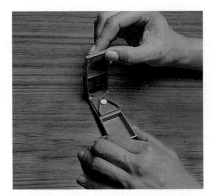

Figure 21-8 A cutting device can be used to divide tablets.

- If the patient has difficulty swallowing, crush the tablets to a fine powder with a pill crusher if permitted by local policy and the manufacturer of the drug recommends this. Some medications should not be crushed. An example of tablets that should not be crushed is naproxen, a slow release anti-inflammatory, which normally lasts 12 hours after administration. If the tablet is crushed, the patient gets a surge of action in the first two hours, then may start having severe pain again in 4–6 hours, as the effects wear off too soon. The crushing of these tablets causes an uneven effect and the 'continuous' pain control is lost. It may also cause an overdose or other adverse side-effects with some medication.

Liquid Medication

- Thoroughly mix the medication before pouring. Discard any medication that has changed colour or turned cloudy.
- Remove the cap and place it upside down *to avoid contaminating the inside of the cap.*
- Hold the bottle so the label is next to your palm and pour the medication away from the label (see Figure 21-9). *This prevents the label from becoming soiled and illegible as a result of spilled liquids.*
- Hold the medication cup at eye level and fill it to the desired level, using the bottom of the **meniscus** (crescent-shaped upper surface of a column of liquid) to align with container scale (see Figure 21-10). *This method ensures accuracy of measurement.*
- Before capping the bottle, wipe the lip with a paper towel. *This prevents the cap from sticking.*
- When giving small amounts of liquids (e.g. < 5 ml), prepare the medication in a sterile syringe without the needle.
- Keep unit-dose liquids in their package and open them at the bedside.

All Medications

- Avoid leaving prepared medications unattended. *This precaution prevents potential mishandling errors.*

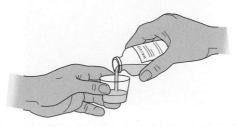

Figure 21-9 Pouring a liquid medication from a bottle.

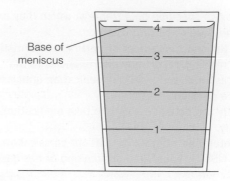

Base of meniscus

Figure 21-10 The *bottom* of the meniscus is the measuring guide.

- Lock the medication trolley/locker before leaving a patient's room. This is a *safety measure because medication stores are not to be left open when unattended.*

5. Provide for patient privacy.
6. Prepare the patient.
   - Check the patient's identification band. *This ensures that the right patient receives the medication.*
   - Assist the patient to a sitting position or, if not possible, to a side-lying position. *These positions facilitate swallowing and prevent aspiration.*
   - If not previously assessed, take the required assessment measures, such as pulse and respiratory rates or blood pressure. Take the apical pulse rate before administering digitalis preparations. Take blood pressure before giving antihypertensive drugs. Take the respiratory rate prior to administering narcotics. *Narcotics depress the respiratory centre.* If any of the findings are above or below the predetermined parameters, consult the physician before administering the medication.
7. Explain the purpose of the medication and how it will help, using language that the patient can understand. Include relevant information about effects; for example, tell the patient receiving a diuretic to expect an increase in urine output. *Information facilitates acceptance of and compliance with the therapy.*
8. Administer the medication at the correct time.
   - Take the medication to the patient within the time frame of 30 minutes before or after the scheduled time.
   - Give the patient sufficient water or preferred liquid to swallow the medication. Before using juice, check for any food and medication incompatibilities. *Fluids ease swallowing and facilitate absorption from the gastrointestinal tract.* Liquid medications other than antacids or cough preparations are generally diluted with 15 ml ($^{1}/_{2}$ oz) of water to facilitate absorption.

- If the patient is unable to hold the pill cup, use the pill cup to introduce the medication into the patient's mouth, and give only one tablet or capsule at a time. *Putting the cup to the patient's mouth maintains the cleanliness of the nurse's hands. Giving one medication at a time eases swallowing.*
- If an older child or adult has difficulty swallowing, ask the patient to place the medication on the back of the tongue before taking the water. *Stimulation of the back of the tongue produces the swallowing reflex.*
- If the medication has an objectionable taste, ask the patient to suck a few ice cubes beforehand, or give the medication with juice, if there are no contraindications. *The cold of the ice cubes will desensitise the taste buds, and juices can mask the taste of the medication.*
- If the patient says that the medication you are about to give is different from what the patient has been receiving, do not give the medication without first checking the original prescription.

Most patients are familiar with the appearance of medications taken previously. Unfamiliar medications may signal a possible error.
- Stay with the patient until all medications have been swallowed. *The nurse must see the patient swallow the medication before the drug administration can be recorded.*

9. Document each medication given.
   - Record the medication given, dosage, time, any complaints or assessments of the patient and your signature.
   - If medication was refused or omitted, record this fact on the appropriate record; document the reason, when possible, and the nurse's actions according to local policy.
10. Dispose of all supplies appropriately.
    - Replenish stock (e.g. medication cups).
    - Discard used disposable supplies.
11. Evaluate the effects of the medication.
    - Return to the patient when the medication is expected to take effect (usually 30 minutes) to evaluate the effects of the medication on the patient.

Evaluation

+ Conduct appropriate follow-up.
+ Desired effect (e.g. relief of pain or decrease in body temperature)
+ Any adverse effects or side-effects (e.g. nausea, vomiting, skin rash, change in vital signs)

+ Relate to previous findings, if available.
+ Report significant deviations from normal to the physician.

LIFESPAN CONSIDERATIONS

Administering Oral Medications

Infants

+ A syringe provides the best control for administering medications.
+ Place small amounts of liquid along the side of the infant's mouth. To prevent aspiration or spitting out, wait for the infant to swallow before giving more (Bindler and Ball, 2003).
+ If using a spoon, retrieve and re-feed medication that is thrust outward by the infant's tongue.

Children

+ Knowledge of growth and development is essential for the nurse administering medications to children.
+ Whenever possible, give children a choice between the use of a spoon or syringe.

+ Dilute the oral medication, if indicated, with a small amount of water. Many oral medications are readily swallowed if they are diluted with a small amount of water. If large quantities of water are used, the child may refuse to drink the entire amount and receive only a portion of the medication.
+ Oral medications for children are usually prepared in sweetened liquid form to make them more palatable.
+ Necessary foods such as milk or orange juice should not be used to mask the taste of medications because the child may develop unpleasant associations and refuse that food in the future.
+ Disguise disagreeable-tasting medications with sweet-tasting substances mentioned previously. However, present any altered medication to the child honestly and not as a food or treat.

+ Place the young child or toddler on your lap or a parent's lap in a sitting position.
+ Administer the medication slowly with a measuring spoon, plastic syringe or medicine cup.
+ To prevent nausea, pour a carbonated beverage over finely crushed ice and give it before or immediately after the medication is administered.
+ Follow medication with a drink of water, juice or a soft drink. This removes any unpleasant aftertaste.
+ For children who take sweetened medications on a long-term basis, follow the medication administration with oral hygiene. These children are at high risk of dental caries.

Older Adults

+ The physiological changes associated with ageing influence medication administration and effectiveness. Examples include altered memory, less acute vision, decrease in renal function, less complete and slower absorption from the gastrointestinal tract, and decreased liver function. Many of these changes enhance the possibility of cumulative effects and toxicity.
+ Older adults usually require smaller dosages of drugs, especially sedatives and other central nervous system depressants.
+ Older adults are mature adults capable of reasoning. The nurse, therefore, needs to explain the reasons for and the effects of the patient's medications.
+ Socioeconomic factors such as lack of transportation and decreased finances may influence obtaining medications when needed.
+ An increase in marketing and availability of vitamins, herbs and supplements alerts the nurse to include this information in a medication history.

COMMUNITY CARE CONSIDERATIONS

Administering Medications

Instruct the patient to:

+ Learn the names of the medications as well as their actions and possible adverse effects.
+ Keep all medications out of reach of children and pets.
+ If using a syringe to administer the medication to an infant or child, remove and dispose of the plastic cap that fits on the end of the syringe. Infants and small children have been known to choke on these caps.
+ Take the medications only as prescribed. Immediately consult the nurse, pharmacist or physician about any problems with the medication.
+ Always check the medication label to make sure the correct medication is being taken.
+ Request labels printed with larger type on medication containers if there is difficulty reading the label.

+ Check the expiration date and discard outdated medications.
+ Ask the pharmacist to substitute childproof caps with ones that are more easily opened, as necessary.
+ If a dose or more is missed, do not take two or more doses; ask the pharmacist or physician for directions.
+ Do not crush or cut a tablet or capsule without first checking with the physician or pharmacist. Doing so may affect the medication's absorption.
+ Never stop taking the medication without the prescriber's permission.
+ Always check with the pharmacist before taking any non-prescription medications. Some over-the-counter medications can interact with the prescribed medication.
+ Set up a medication plan day schedule. Weekly pill containers (available at pharmacies) or a written plan may be helpful.

NASOGASTRIC AND GASTROSTOMY MEDICATIONS

For patients who cannot take anything by mouth (NBM) and have **nasogastric tubes** or a **gastrostomy tube** in place, an alternative route for administering medications is through the nasogastric or gastrostomy tube. A nasogastric (NG) tube is inserted by way of the nasopharynx and is placed into the patient's stomach for the purpose of feeding the patient or to remove gastric secretions. A gastrostomy tube is surgically placed directly into the patient's stomach and provides another route for administering medications and nutrition. Guidelines for administering medications by nasogastric tubes and gastrostomy tubes are shown in the *Practice guidelines* overleaf.

PRACTICE GUIDELINES

Administering Medications by Nasogastric or Gastrostomy Tube

✚ Always check with the pharmacist to see if the patient's medications come in a liquid form because these are less likely to cause tube obstruction.

✚ If medications do not come in liquid form, check to see if they may be crushed. (Note that enteric-coated, sustained action, buccal and sublingual medications should never be crushed.)

✚ Crush a tablet into a fine powder and dissolve in at least 30 ml of warm water. Cold liquids may cause patient discomfort. Use only water for mixing and flushing.

✚ Read medication labels carefully before opening a capsule. Open capsules and mix the contents with water only with the pharmacist's advice.

✚ Do not administer whole or undissolved medications because they will clog the tube.

✚ When administering the medication(s):

  • Remove the plunger from the syringe and connect the syringe to a pinched or kinked tube. Pinching or kinking the tube prevents excess air from entering the stomach and causing distension.

• Put 15 to 30 ml (5 to 10 ml for children) of water into the syringe barrel to flush the tube before administering the first medication. Raise or lower the barrel of the syringe to adjust the flow as needed. Pinch or clamp the tubing before all the water is instilled to avoid excess air entering the stomach.

• Pour liquid or dissolved medication into syringe barrel and allow to flow by gravity into the enteral tube.

• If you are giving several medications, administer each one separately and flush with at least 15 to 30 ml (5 ml for children) of tap water between each medication.

• When you have finished administering all medications, flush with another 15 to 30 ml (5 to 10 ml for children) of warm water to clear the tube.

• If the tube is connected to suction, disconnect the suction and keep the tube clamped for 20-30 minutes after giving the medication to enhance absorption.

PARENTERAL MEDICATIONS

Parenteral administration of medications is a common nursing procedure. Nurses give parenteral medications intradermally (ID), subcutaneously (SC), intramuscularly (IM) or intravenously (IV). Because these medications are absorbed more quickly than oral medications and are irretrievable once injected, the nurse must prepare and administer them carefully and accurately. Administering parenteral drugs requires the same nursing knowledge as for oral and topical drugs; however, because injections are invasive procedures, aseptic technique must be used to minimise the risk of infection.

Equipment

To administer parenteral medications, nurses use syringes and needles to withdraw medication from ampoules and vials.

Syringes

Syringes have three parts: the tip, which connects with the needle; the barrel, or outside part, on which the scales are printed; and the plunger, which fits inside the barrel (see Figure 21-11). When handling a syringe, the nurse may touch the outside of the barrel and the handle of the plunger; however, the nurse

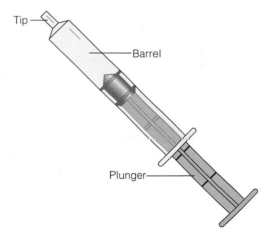

Figure 21-11 The three parts of a syringe.

must *avoid letting any unsterile object contact the tip or inside of the barrel, the shaft of the plunger or the shaft or tip of the needle.*

There are several kinds of syringes, differing in size, shape and material. The three most commonly used types are the standard hypodermic syringe, the insulin syringe and the tuberculin syringe (see Figure 21-12 on page 532). A **hypodermic syringe** comes in 2, 2.5 and 3 ml sizes. The syringe usually

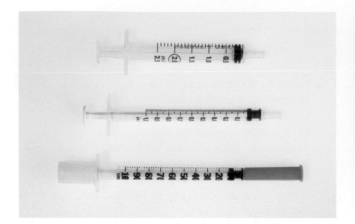

Figure 21-12 Three kinds of syringes: *A*, hypodermic syringe marked in tenths (0.1) of millilitres and in minims; *B*, insulin syringe marked in 100 units; *C*, tuberculin syringe marked in tenths and hundredths (0.01) of cubic millimetres and in minims.

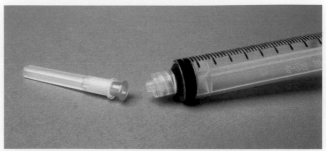

A

B

Figure 21-13 Tips of syringes: *A*, Luer-Lok syringe (note threaded tip); *B*, non-Luer-Lok syringe (note the smooth graduated tip).

has the millilitre scale or international units marked on it. The millilitre scale is the one normally used; the international unit scale is used for very small dosages.

An **insulin syringe** is similar to a hypodermic syringe, but the scale is specially designed for insulin: a 100-unit calibrated scale intended for use with U-100 insulin. Several low-dose insulin syringes are also available and frequently have a non-removable needle. All insulin syringes are calibrated on the 100-unit scale. The correct choice of syringe is based on the amount of insulin required.

The **tuberculin syringe** was originally designed to administer tuberculin. It is a narrow syringe, calibrated in tenths and hundredths of a millilitre (up to 1 ml). This type of syringe can also be useful in administering other drugs, particularly when small or precise measurement is indicated (e.g. paediatric dosages).

Syringes are made in other sizes as well (e.g. 5, 10, 20 and 50 ml). These are not generally used to administer drugs directly but can be useful for adding medications to intravenous solutions or for irrigating wounds. The tip of a syringe varies and is classified as either a Luer-Lock or non-Luer-Lock. A Luer-Lock syringe has a tip that requires the needle to be twisted onto it to avoid accidental removal of the needle (see Figure 21-13). The non-Luer-Lock syringe has a smooth graduated tip onto which needles are slipped. The non-Luer-Lock syringe is often used for irrigation purposes (e.g. wounds, tubes).

Most syringes used today are made of plastic, are individually packaged for sterility in a paper wrapper or a rigid plastic container (see Figure 21-14), and are disposable. The syringe and needle may be packaged together or separately. Needleless systems are also available in which the needle is replaced by a plastic cannula.

Injectable medications are frequently supplied in disposable **prefilled unit-dose systems**. These are available as (a) prefilled syringes ready for use or (b) prefilled sterile cartridges and needles that require the attachment of a reusable holder

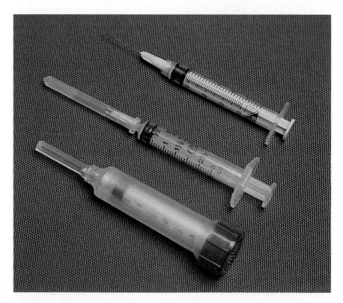

Figure 21-14 Disposable plastic syringes and needles: *Top*, with syringe and needle exposed; *Middle*, with plastic cap over the needle; *Bottom*, with plastic case over the needle and syringe.

(injection system) before use (see Figure 21-15). Examples of the latter system are the Clexane injection systems. The manufacturers provide specific directions for use. Because most prefilled cartridges are overfilled, excess medication must be ejected before the injection to ensure the right dosage. Because the needle is fused to the syringe, the nurse cannot change the gauge or length of the needle. The nurse, however, can transfer the

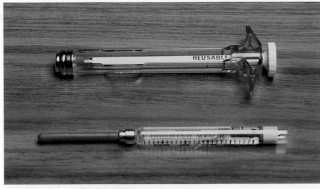

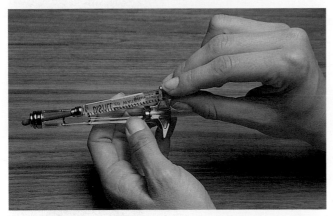

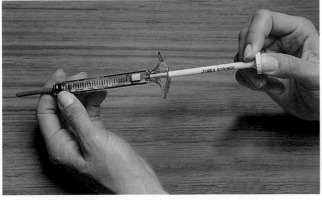

Figure 21-15 *A,* Syringe and prefilled sterile cartridge with needle; *B,* assembling the device; *C,* the cartridge slides into the syringe barrel, turns and locks at the needle end. The plunger then screws into the cartridge end.

medication into a regular syringe if the assessment of the patient necessitates a different needle gauge or length.

Needles

Needles are made of stainless steel, and most are disposable. Reusable needles (e.g. for special procedures) need to be sharpened periodically before re-sterilisation because the points

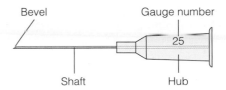

Figure 21-16 The parts of a needle.

become dull with use and are occasionally damaged or acquire burrs on the tips. A dull or damaged needle should *never* be used.

A needle has three discernible parts: the **hub**, which fits onto the syringe; the **cannula** or **shaft**, which is attached to the hub; and the **bevel**, which is the slanted part at the tip of the needle (see Figure 21-16). A disposable needle has a plastic hub. Needles used for injections have three variable characteristics:

1. *Slant or length of the bevel.* The bevel of the needle may be short or long. Longer bevels provide the sharpest needles and cause less discomfort. They are commonly used for subcutaneous and intramuscular injections. Short bevels are used for intradermal and intravenous injections because a long bevel can become occluded if it rests against the side of a blood vessel.
2. *Length of the shaft.* The shaft length of commonly used needles varies from 1-5 cm. The appropriate needle length is chosen according to the patients' muscle development, the patient's weight and the type of injection.
3. **Gauge** *(or diameter) of the shaft.* The gauge varies from #18 to #28. The larger the gauge number, the smaller the diameter of the shaft. Smaller gauges produce less tissue trauma, but larger gauges are necessary for viscous medications, such as penicillin.

For an adult requiring a subcutaneous injection, it is appropriate to use a needle of #24 to #26 gauge and 0.5 to 2 cm long. Obese patients may require a 2.5 cm needle. For intramuscular injections, a longer needle with a larger gauge (e.g. #20 to #22 gauge) is used. Slender adults and children usually require a shorter needle. The nurse must assess the patient to determine the appropriate needle length.

Preventing Needlestick Injuries

One of the most potentially hazardous procedures that healthcare personnel face is using and disposing of needles and sharps. Needlestick injuries present a major risk for infection with hepatitis B virus, human immunodeficiency virus (HIV) and many other pathogens. Standards have been set by the Royal College of Nursing and Department of Health to prevent such injuries. Some of these are summarised in *Box 12-6* on page 534. If an accidental needlestick injury occurs, the nurse needs to follow specific steps outlined by local policy.

Safety syringes have been designed in recent years to protect healthcare workers. Safety devices are categorised as either *passive* or *active.* The nurse does not need to activate the passive safety device. For example, for some syringes, after injection, the needle retracts immediately into the barrel

BOX 21-6 Avoiding Puncture Injuries

+ Use appropriate puncture-proof disposal containers to dispose of uncapped needles and sharps. These are provided in all patient areas (see Figure 21-17). Never throw sharps in clinical waste bags or bins. Sharps include any items that can cut or puncture skin such as:

Needles
Surgical blades
Lancets
Razors
Broken glass
Broken capillary pipettes
Exposed dental wires
Reusable items (e.g. large-bore needles, hooks, rasps, drill points)
ANY SHARP INSTRUMENT!

+ Never bend or break needles before disposal.
+ Never recap used needles except under specified circumstances (e.g. when transporting a syringe to the laboratory for an arterial blood gas or blood culture).
+ When recapping a needle:
  • Use a safety mechanical device that firmly grips the needle cap and holds it in place until it is ready to recap.
  • Use a one-handed 'scoop' method. This is performed by (a) placing the needle cap and syringe with needle horizontally on a flat surface, (b) inserting the needle into the cap, using one hand (see Figure 21-18), and then (c) using your other hand to pick up the cap and tighten it to the needle hub.

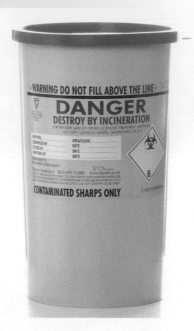

Figure 21-17 A disposal container for contaminated needles and other sharps.

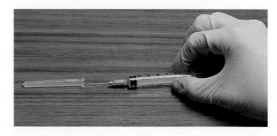

Figure 21-18 Recapping a used needle using the one-handed scoop method.

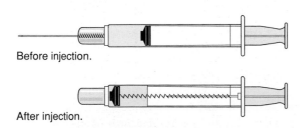

Before injection.

After injection.

Figure 21-19 Passive safety device. The needle retracts immediately into the barrel after injection.

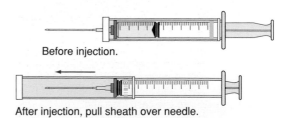

Before injection.

After injection, pull sheath over needle.

Figure 21-20 Active safety device. The nurse manually pulls the sheath or guard over the needle after injection.

(see Figure 21-19). In contrast, the active safety device requires the nurse to manually activate the safety feature. For example, the nurse activates a mechanism to retract the needle into the syringe barrel or the nurse, after injection, manually pulls a plastic sheath or guard over the needle (see Figure 21-20).

Preparing Injectable Medications

Injectable medications can be prepared by withdrawing the medication from an ampoule or vial into a sterile syringe, using prefilled syringes, or using needleless injection systems.

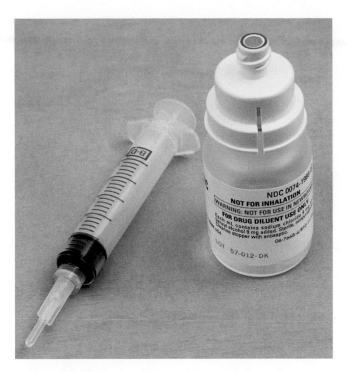

Figure 21-21 A needleless system can extract medication from a vial.

Figure 21-21 shows an example of a needleless system used to access medication from a vial.

Ampoules and Vials

Ampoules and vials (see Figure 21-22) are frequently used to package sterile parenteral medications. An **ampoule** is a glass container usually designed to hold a single dose of a drug. It is made of clear glass and has a distinctive shape with a constricted neck. Ampoules vary in size from 1–20 ml or more. Most ampoule necks have coloured marks around them, indicating where they are pre-scored for easy opening.

To access the medication in an ampoule, the ampoule must be broken at its constricted neck. Traditionally, files have been used to score the ampoule. Today ampoule openers are available that prevent injury from broken glass. The device consists of a plastic cap that fits over the top of an ampoule and a cutter within the cap that scores the neck of the ampoule when rotated. The head of the ampoule, when broken, remains inside the cap where it can then be ejected into a sharps container. If an ampoule opener is not available, the neck should be held with a small swab, then broken off at that point. Once the ampoule is broken, the fluid is aspirated into a syringe using a small gauge needle. This prevents aspiration of any glass particles.

A **vial** is a small glass bottle with a sealed rubber cap. Vials come in different sizes, from single to multidose vials. They usually have a metal or plastic cap that protects the rubber seal. To access the medication in a vial, the vial must be pierced with a needle. In addition, air must be injected into a vial before the medication can be withdrawn. Failure to inject air before withdrawing the medication leaves a vacuum within the vial that makes withdrawal difficult.

Several drugs (e.g. penicillin) are dispensed as powders in vials. A liquid (solvent or diluent) must be added to a powdered medication before it can be injected. The technique of adding a solvent to a powdered drug to prepare it for administration is called **reconstitution**. Powdered drugs usually have printed instructions (enclosed with each packaged vial) that describe the amount and kind of solvent to be added. Commonly used solvents are sterile water or sterile normal saline. Some preparations are supplied in individual-dose vials; others come in multidose vials. The following are two examples of the preparation of powdered drugs:

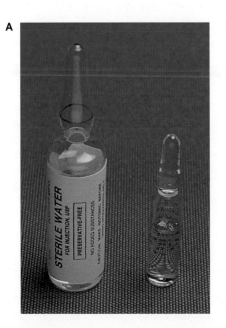

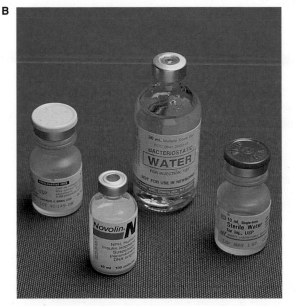

Figure 21-22 *A*, Ampoules; *B*, Vials.

1. *Single-dose vial*: Instructions for preparing a single-dose vial direct that 1.5 ml of sterile water be added to the sterile dry powder, thus providing a single dose of 2 ml. The volume of the drug powder was 0.5 ml. Therefore, the 1.5 ml of water plus the 0.5 ml of powder results in 2 ml of solution. In other instances, the addition of a solution does not increase the volume. Therefore, it is important to follow the manufacturer's directions.

2. *Multidose vial*: A dose of 750 mg of a certain drug is ordered for a patient. Available is a 10-g multidose vial. The directions for preparation read: 'Add 8.5 ml of sterile water, and each millilitre will contain 1.0 g or 1,000 mg.' To determine the amount to inject, the nurse calculates as follows:

$$1 \text{ ml} = 1,000 \text{ mg}$$
$$x \text{ ml} = 750 \text{ mg}$$
$$(\text{cross multiply})$$
$$x = \frac{750 \times 1}{1,000}$$
$$x = 0.75$$

The nurse will thus give 0.75 ml of the medication.

Glass and rubber particulate have been found in medications withdrawn from ampoules and vials using a regular needle. As a result, it is strongly recommended that the nurse use a small gauge needle when withdrawing medications from ampoules and vials to prevent withdrawing glass and rubber particles. After drawing the medication into the syringe, the filter needle is replaced with the regular needle for injection. This prevents tracking of the medication through the patient's tissues during the insertion of the needle, which minimises discomfort.

Procedures 21-2 and *21-3* describe how to prepare medications from ampoules and vials. Additionally, it is important to remember that when powdered drugs have been reconstituted, the date and time should be written on the label of the vial. Many of these drugs have to be used immediately, so nurses need to know the expiration time after it has been reconstituted.

PROCEDURE 21-2 Preparing Medications from Ampoules

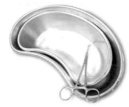

Planning

Equipment

+ Medication chart
+ Ampoule of sterile medication
+ If ampoule is not scored, small gauze square

+ Antiseptic swabs
+ Needle and syringe
+ Filler needle

Implementation

Preparation

1. Check the medication administration chart.
   - Check the label on the ampoule carefully against the chart to make sure that the correct medication is being prepared.
   - Follow the three checks for administering medications. Read the label on the medication (1) when it is taken from the medication store, (2) before withdrawing the medication and (3) after withdrawing the medication.
2. Organise the equipment.

Performance

1. Wash hands and observe other appropriate infection control procedures.
2. Prepare the medication ampoule for drug withdrawal.
   - Flick the upper stem of the ampoule several times with a fingernail or, holding the upper stem of the ampoule, shake the ampoule similar to shaking down a mercury thermometer. *This will bring all medication down to the main portion of the ampoule.*
   - Partially file the neck of the ampoule, if necessary, to start a clean break.
   - Place a piece of sterile gauze between your thumb and the ampoule neck or around the ampoule neck, and break off the top by bending it toward you (see Figure 21-23). *The sterile gauze protects the fingers from the broken glass and any glass fragments will spray away from the nurse.*
     or
   - Place the antiseptic wipe packet over the top of the ampoule before breaking off the top. *This method ensures that all glass fragments fall into the packet and reduces the risk of cuts.*
   - Dispose of the top of the ampoule in the sharps container.

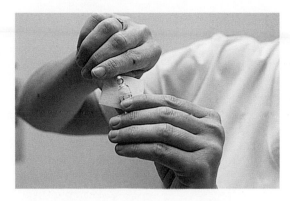

Figure 21-23 Breaking the neck of an ampoule.

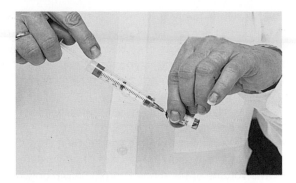

Figure 21-24 Withdrawing a medication from an ampoule.

3. Withdraw the medication.
   - Place the ampoule on a flat surface.
   - Using a filler needle to withdraw the medication, disconnect the regular needle, leaving its cap on and attach the filler needle to the syringe. *The filter needle prevents glass particles from being withdrawn with the medication.*
   - Remove the cap from the filter needle and insert the needle into the centre of the ampoule. Do not

touch the rim of the ampoule with the needle tip or shaft. *This will keep the needle sterile.* Withdraw the amount of drug required for the dosage.
   - With a single-dose ampoule, hold the ampoule slightly on its side, if necessary, to obtain all medication (see Figure 21-24).
   - Replace the filler needle with a regular needle and tighten the cap at the hub of the needle before injecting the patient.

PROCEDURE 21-3 Preparing Medications from Vials

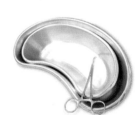

Planning

Equipment

+ Medication chart
+ Vial of sterile medication
+ Antiseptic swabs
+ Needle and syringe

+ Filler needle
+ Sterile water or normal saline, if drug is in powdered form

---

Implementation

Preparation

+ Same preparation as described in Procedure 21-2.

Performance

1. Wash hands and observe other appropriate infection control procedures.
2. Prepare the medication vial for drug withdrawal.
   - Mix the solution, if necessary, by rotating the vial between the palms of the hands, not by shaking. *Some vials contain aqueous suspensions, which*

settle when they stand. In some instances, shaking is contraindicated because it may cause the mixture to foam.
   - Remove the protective cap, or clean the rubber cap of a previously opened vial with an antiseptic wipe by rubbing in a circular motion. *The antiseptic cleans the cap of dust or grease and reduces the number of micro-organisms.*

3. Withdraw the medication.

- Attach a filler needle, as agency practice dictates, to draw up premixed liquid medications from multidose vials. *Using the filter needle prevents any solid particles from being drawn up through the needle.*
- Ensure that the needle is firmly attached to the syringe.
- Remove the cap from the needle, then draw up into the syringe the amount of air equal to the volume of the medication to be withdrawn.
- Carefully insert the needle into the upright vial through the centre of the rubber cap, maintaining the sterility of the needle.
- Inject the air into the vial, keeping the bevel of the needle above the surface of the medication (see Figure 21-25). *The air will allow the medication to be drawn out easily because negative pressure will not be created inside the vial. The bevel is kept above the medication to avoid creating bubbles in the medication.*
- Withdraw the prescribed amount of medication using either of the following methods:

  (a) Hold the vial down (i.e. with the base lower than the top), move the needle tip so that it is below the fluid level, and withdraw the medication (see Figure 21-26). Avoid drawing up the last drops of the vial. *Proponents of this method say that keeping the vial in the upright position while withdrawing the*

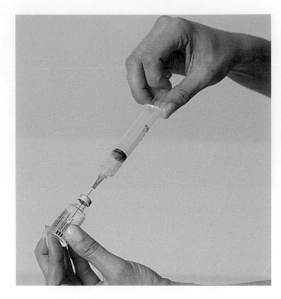

Figure 21-26 Withdrawing a medication from a vial that is held with the base down.

medication allows particulate matter to precipitate out of the solution. Leaving the last few drops reduces the chance of withdrawing foreign particles.
or

  (b) Invert the vial; ensure the needle tip is *below* the fluid level; and gradually withdraw the medication (see Figure 21-27). *Keeping the tip of the needle below the fluid level prevents air from being drawn into the syringe.*

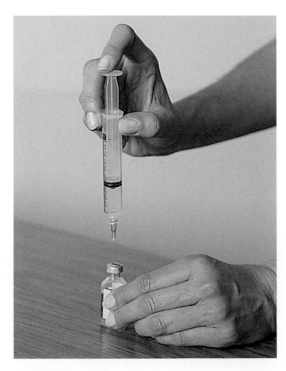

Figure 21-25 Injecting air into a vial.

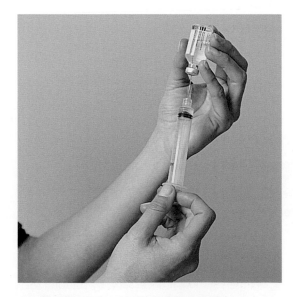

Figure 21-27 Withdrawing a medication from an inverted vial.

- Hold the syringe and vial at eye level to determine that the correct dosage of drug is drawn into the syringe. Eject air remaining at the top of the syringe into the vial.
- When the correct volume of medication is obtained, withdraw the needle from the vial, and replace the cap over the needle using the scoop method, thus maintaining its sterility.
- If necessary, tap the syringe barrel to dislodge any air bubbles present in the syringe. *The tapping motion will cause the air bubbles to rise to the top of the syringe where they can be ejected out of the syringe.*
- Replace the filler needle, if used, with a regular needle and cover of the correct gauge and length before injecting the patient.

Variation: Preparing and Using Multidose Vials

+ Read the manufacturer's directions.
+ Withdraw an equivalent amount of air from the vial before adding the dilution, unless otherwise indicated by the directions.
+ Add the amount of sterile water or saline indicated in the directions.
+ If a multidose vial is reconstituted, label the vial with the date and time it was prepared, the amount of drug contained in each millilitre of solution and your initials. *Time is an important factor to consider in the expiration of these medications.*
+ Once the medication is reconstituted, store it in a refrigerator or as recommended by the manufacturer.

Mixing Medications in One Syringe

Frequently, patients need more than one drug injected at the same time. To spare the patient the experience of being injected twice, two drugs (if compatible) are often mixed in one syringe and given as one injection. It is common, for instance, to combine two types of insulin in this manner or to combine injectable pre-operative medications such as morphine with atropine. Drugs can also be mixed in intravenous solutions. When uncertain about drug compatibilities, the nurse should consult a pharmacist or check a compatibility chart before mixing the drugs.

The nurse must also exercise caution when mixing short- and long-acting insulins, because they vary in content. Chemically, insulin is a protein that, when hydrolysed in the body, yields a number of amino acids. Some insulin preparations contain an additional modifying protein, such as globulin or protamine that slows absorption. This fact is particularly relevant to mixing two insulin preparations for injection because many insulin syringes have needles that cannot be changed. A vial of insulin that does not have the added protein (i.e. regular insulin) should *never* be contaminated with insulin that does have the added protein (i.e. Lente or NPH insulin). *Procedure 21-4* describes how to mix medications in one syringe.

PROCEDURE 21-4 Mixing Medications Using One Syringe

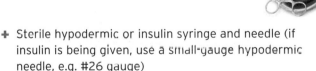

Planning

Equipment

+ Medication chart.
+ Two vials of medication; one vial and one ampoule; two ampoules; or one vial or ampoule and one cartridge
+ Antiseptic swabs

+ Sterile hypodermic or insulin syringe and needle (if insulin is being given, use a small-gauge hypodermic needle, e.g. #26 gauge)
+ Additional sterile subcutaneous or intramuscular needle (optional)

Implementation

Preparation

1. Check the medication chart.
   - Check the label on the medications carefully against the medication chart to make sure that the correct medication is being prepared.
   - Follow the three checks for administering medications. Read the label on the medication

   (1) when it is taken from the medication store, (2) before withdrawing the medication and (3) after withdrawing the medication.
   - Before preparing and combining the medications, ensure that the total volume of the injection is appropriate for the injection site.
2. Organise the equipment.

Performance

1. Wash hands and observe other appropriate infection control procedures.
2. Prepare the medication ampoule or vial for drug withdrawal.
   - See Procedure 21-2, step 2, page 536 for an ampoule.
   - Inspect the appearance of the medication for clarity. Some medications are always cloudy. *Preparations that have changed in appearance should be discarded.*
   - If using insulin, thoroughly mix the solution in each vial prior to administration. Rotate the vials between the palms of the hands and invert the vials. *Mixing ensures an adequate concentration and thus an accurate dose. Shaking insulin vials can make the medication frothy, making precise measurement difficult.*
   - Clean the tops of the vials with antiseptic swabs.
3. Withdraw the medications.

Mixing Medications from Two Vials

+ Take the syringe and draw up a volume of air equal to the volume of medications to be withdrawn from both vials A *and* B.
+ Inject a volume of air equal to the volume of medication to be withdrawn into vial A. Make sure the needle does not touch the solution. *This prevents cross-contamination of the medications.*
+ Withdraw the needle from vial A and inject the remaining air into vial B.
+ Withdraw the required amount of medication from vial B. *The same needle is used to inject air into and withdraw medication from the second vial. It must not be contaminated with the medication in vial A.*
+ Using a newly attached sterile needle, withdraw the required amount of medication from vial A. Avoid pushing the plunger as that will introduce medication B into vial A. If using a syringe with a fused needle, withdraw the medication from vial A. The syringe now contains a mixture of medications from vials A and B. *With this method, neither vial is contaminated by micro-organisms or by medication from the other vial.* Be careful to withdraw only the ordered amount and to not create air bubbles. *The syringe now contains two medications and an excess amount cannot be returned to the vial.*

See also the Variation later in this procedure.

Mixing Medications from One Vial and One Ampule

+ First prepare and withdraw the medication from the vial. *Ampoules do not require the addition of air prior to withdrawal of the drug.*
+ Then withdraw the required amount of medication from the ampoule.

Mixing Medications from One Cartridge and One Vial or Ampoule

+ First ensure that the correct dose of the medication is in the cartridge. Discard any excess medication and air.
+ Draw up the required medication from a vial or ampoule into the cartridge. Note that when withdrawing medication from a vial, an equal amount of air must first be injected into the vial.
+ If the total volume to be injected exceeds the capacity of the cartridge, use a syringe with sufficient capacity to withdraw the desired amount of medication from the vial or ampoule, and transfer the required amount from the cartridge to the syringe.

Variation: Mixing Insulins

The following is an example of mixing 10 units of regular insulin and 30 units of neutral protamine Hagedorn (NPH) insulin, which contains protamine.

+ Inject 30 units of air into the NPH vial and withdraw the needle. (There should be no insulin in the needle.) The needle should not touch the insulin (see Figure 21-28, step 1).
+ Inject 10 units of air into the regular insulin vial and immediately withdraw 10 units of regular insulin (see Figure 21-28, steps 2 and 3). Always withdraw the regular insulin first *to minimise the possibility of contamination.*
+ Reinsert the needle into the NPH insulin vial and withdraw 30 units of NPH insulin (see Figure 21-28, step 4). (The air was previously injected into the vial.) Be careful to withdraw only the ordered amount and to not create air bubbles. *The syringe now contains two medications, and an excess amount cannot be returned to the vial.*

By using this method, you avoid adding NPH insulin to the regular insulin.

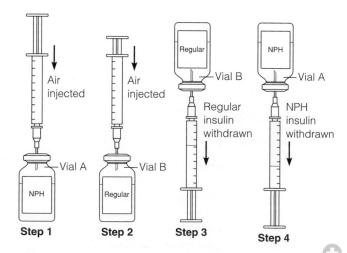

Figure 21-28 Mixing two types of insulin.

CLINICAL ALERT

One way to determine which insulin to withdraw first is to remember the saying 'Clear before cloudy'.

Intradermal Injections

An **intradermal (ID) injection** is the administration of a drug into the dermal layer of the skin just beneath the epidermis. Usually only a small amount of liquid is used, for example, 0.1 ml. This method of administration is frequently used for allergy testing and tuberculosis (TB) screening. Common sites for intradermal injections are the inner lower arm, the upper chest and the back beneath the scapulae (see Figure 21-29). The left arm is commonly used for TB screening and the right arm is used for all other tests. The steps for administering an intradermal are described in *Procedure 21-5*.

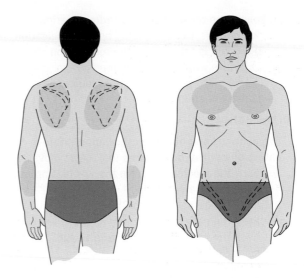

Figure 21-29 Body sites commonly used for intradermal injections.

PROCEDURE 21-5 Administering an Intradermal Injection

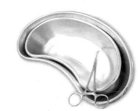

Purpose

+ To provide a medication that the patient requires for allergy testing and TB screening

---

Assessment

Assess

+ Appearance of injection site
+ Specific drug action and expected response
+ Patient's knowledge of drug action and response

Check local protocol about sites to use for skin tests.

Planning

Equipment

+ Vial or ampoule of the correct medication
+ Sterile 1-ml syringe calibrated into hundredths of a millilitre (i.e. tuberculin syringe) and a # 25- to # 27-gauge needle
+ Alcohol swabs
+ 5 cm × 5 cm sterile gauze square (optional)

+ Clean gloves (according to local protocol)
+ Bandage (optional)
+ Epinephrine/Adrenaline (a bronchodilator and antihistamine) on hand for allergic reactions. As per local policy.

Implementation

Preparation

1. Check the medication chart.
   • Check the label on the medication carefully against the chart to make sure that the correct medication is being prepared.

- Follow the three checks for administering medications. Read the label on the medication (1) when it is taken from the medication store, (2) before withdrawing the medication and (3) after withdrawing the medication.

2. Organise the equipment.

Performance

1. Wash hands and observe other appropriate infection control procedures (e.g. clean gloves).

2. Prepare the medication from the vial or ampoule for drug withdrawal.
   - See Procedures 21-2 and 21-3 earlier.

3. Prepare the patient.
   - Check the patient's identification band. *This ensures that the right patient receives the medication.*

4. Explain to the patient that the medication will produce a small weal/swelling. A *weal* is a small raised area, like a blister. The patient will feel a slight prick as the needle enters the skin. Some medications are absorbed slowly through the capillaries into the general circulation, and the swelling gradually disappears. Other drugs remain in the area and interact with the body tissues to produce redness and induration (hardening), which will need to be interpreted at a particular time (e.g. in 24 or 48 hours). This reaction will also gradually disappear. *Information facilitates acceptance of and compliance with the therapy.*

5. Provide for patient privacy.

6. Select and clean the site.
   - Select a site (e.g. the forearm about a hand's width above the wrist and three or four fingerwidths below the antecubital space).
   - Avoid using sites that are tender, inflamed or swollen and those that have lesions.
   - Put on gloves as indicated by agency policy.
   - Cleanse the skin at the site using a firm circular motion starting at the centre and widening the circle outward. Allow the area to dry thoroughly.

7. Prepare the syringe for the injection.
   - Remove the needle cap while waiting for the antiseptic to dry.
   - Expel any air bubbles from the syringe. Small bubbles that adhere to the plunger are of no consequence. *A small amount of air will not harm the tissues.*
   - Grasp the syringe in your dominant hand, holding it between thumb and forefinger. Hold the needle almost parallel to the skin surface, with the bevel of the needle up. *The possibility of the medication entering the subcutaneous tissue increases when using an angle greater than 15 degrees or if the bevel is down.*

8. Inject the fluid.
   - With the non-dominant hand, pull the skin at the site until it is taut. For example, if using the ventral forearm, grasp the patient's dorsal forearm and gently pull it to tighten the ventral skin. *Taut skin allows for easier entry of the needle and less discomfort for the patient.*
   - Insert the tip of the needle far enough to place the bevel through the epidermis into the dermis (see Figure 21-30, *A*). The outline of the bevel should be visible under the skin surface.
   - Stabilise the syringe and needle, inject the medication carefully and slowly so that it produces a small weal on the skin (see Figure 21-30, *B, C*). *This verifies that the medication entered the dermis.*

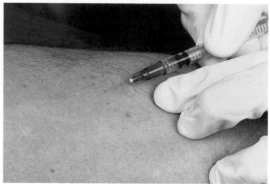

A

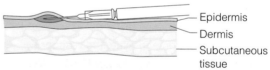

Epidermis
Dermis
Subcutaneous tissue

B

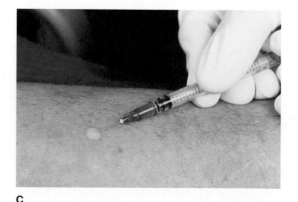

C

Figure 21-30 For an intradermal injection: *A*, the needle enters the skin at a 5- to 15-degree angle; *B, C*, the medication forms a bleb under the epidermis.

- Withdraw the needle quickly at the same angle at which it was inserted. Apply a dressing if indicated.
- Do not massage the area. *Massage can disperse the medication into the tissue or out through the needle insertion site.*
- Dispose of the syringe and needle safely. *Do not recap the needle in order to prevent needlestick injuries.*

- Remove gloves.
- Circle the injection site with ink to observe for redness or induration (hardening), as per local policy if indicated.

9. Document all relevant information.
   - Record the testing material given, the time, dosage, route and site.

Evaluation

+ Evaluate the patient's response to the testing substance. *Some medications used in testing may cause allergic reactions.* An antidote drug (e.g. epinephrine) may need to be used.

+ Evaluate the condition of the site in 24 or 48 hours, depending on the test. Measure the area of redness and induration in millimetres at the largest diameter and document findings.

LIFESPAN CONSIDERATIONS

Administering an Intradermal Injection

Children

+ A small child or infant will need to be gently restrained during the procedure. *This prevents injury from sudden movement.*

+ Make sure the child understands that the procedure is not a punishment.

+ Ask the child not to rub or scratch the injection site. Place a stockinet or gauze dressing over the site if needed. *Rubbing the site can interfere with test results by irritating the underlying tissue.*

Subcutaneous Injections

Among the many kinds of drugs administered subcutaneously (just beneath the skin) are vaccines, pre-operative medications, narcotics, insulin and heparin. Common sites for subcutaneous (SC) injections are the outer aspect of the upper arms and the anterior aspect of the thighs. These areas are convenient and normally have good blood circulation. Other areas that can be used are the abdomen, the scapular areas of the upper back and the upper ventrogluteal and dorsogluteal areas (see Figure 21-31 on page 546). Only small doses (0.5 to 1 ml) of medication are usually injected via the subcutaneous route.

The type of syringe used for subcutaneous injections depends on the medication to be given. Generally a 2 ml syringe is used for most SC injections. However, if insulin is being administered, an insulin syringe is used; and if heparin is being administered, a prefilled cartridge may be used.

Needle sizes and lengths are selected based on the patient's body mass, the intended angle of insertion and the planned site. Generally a #25-gauge is used for adults of normal weight and the needle is inserted at a 45-degree angle; an insulin needle is used at a 90-degree angle.

One method nurses use to determine length of needle is to pinch the tissue at the site and select a needle length that is half the width of the skinfold. To determine the angle of insertion, a general rule to follow relates to the amount of tissue that can be bunched or grasped at the site. A 45-degree angle is used when 2.5 cm of tissue can be grasped at the site; a 90-degree angle is used when 5 cm of tissue can be grasped.

When administering insulin to adults, the current standard needle gauge is #30 gauge. Most patients prefer the shorter and thinner needles because they are less painful. The risk of injecting into the muscle is lessened with the shorter needle.

Subcutaneous injection sites need to be rotated in an orderly fashion to minimise tissue damage, aid absorption and avoid discomfort. This is especially important for patients who must receive repeated injections, such as diabetics. Because insulin is absorbed at different rates at different parts of the body, the diabetic patient's blood glucose levels can vary when various sites are used. Insulin is absorbed most quickly when injected into the abdomen than into the arms, and most slowly when injected into the thighs and buttocks. Current recommendations include rotating injections within an anatomical area (Fleming, 1999).

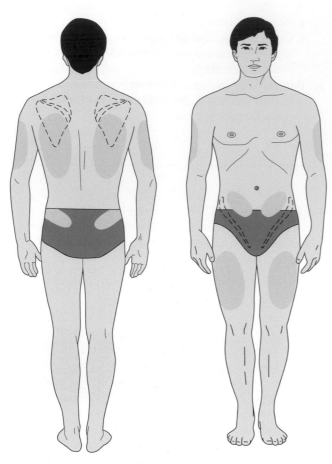

Figure 21-31 Body sites commonly used for subcutaneous injections.

Nurses have traditionally been taught to aspirate by pulling back on the plunger after inserting the needle and before injecting the medication. The nurse could then determine whether the needle had entered a blood vessel. Absence of blood was believed to indicate that the needle was in subcutaneous tissue and not in the more vascular muscular tissue. Fleming challenges the traditional practice of aspiration for insulin subcutaneous injections because it 'is cumbersome, rarely yields blood, and isn't a reliable indicator of correct needle placement, and there are no clinical studies confirming or rejecting it' (1999: 73). As a result, the practice of aspirating subcutaneous injections varies among nurses.

The steps for administering a subcutaneous injection are described in *Procedure 21-6*.

CLINICAL ANECDOTE

Last week I gave a patient an injection for the first time. I was really nervous and did not want to tell the patient it was the first injection I had ever given. I felt really bad when I lied to him when he asked if I had given lots of injections. I just laughed and said that I had given loads before, after the injection the patient said he didn't feel anything. When we went from the patient's bed side my mentor told me that I had done well and it was right to not tell the patient it was my first injection. If I had, the patient may have been more anxious and felt the needle go into the skin more.

Jayne, first-year student nurse

PROCEDURE 21-6 Administering a Subcutaneous Injection

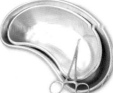

Purposes

+ To provide a medication the patient requires (see specific drug action)

+ To allow slower absorption of a medication compared with either the intramuscular or intravenous route

Assessment

Assess

+ Allergies to medication
+ Specific drug action, side-effects and adverse reactions
+ Patient's knowledge and learning needs about the medication

+ Status and appearance of subcutaneous site for lesions, erythemia, swelling, ecchymosis, inflammation and tissue damage from previous injections
+ Ability of patient to cooperate during the injection
+ Previous injection sites used

Planning

Equipment

+ Patient medication prescription chart
+ Vial or ampoule of the correct sterile medication
+ Syringe and needle (e.g. 2-ml syringe, #25 gauge needle)

+ Antiseptic swabs
+ Dry sterile gauze for opening an ampoule (optional)
+ Clean gloves

Implementation

Preparation

1. Check the medication chart
   - Check the label on the medication carefully against the chart to make sure that the correct medication is being prepared.
   - Follow the three checks for administering medications. Read the label on the medication (1) when it is taken from the medication store, (2) before withdrawing the medication and (3) after withdrawing the medication.
2. Organise the equipment.

Performance

1. Wash hands and observe other appropriate infection control procedures (e.g. clean gloves).
2. Prepare the medication from the ampoule or vial for drug withdrawal.
   - See Procedure 21-2, page 536 (ampoule) or 21-3, page 537 (vial).
3. Provide for patient privacy.
4. Prepare the patient.
   - Check the patient's identification band for name, address, date of birth and hospital number. *This ensures that the right patient receives the medication.*
   - Assist the patient to a position in which the arm, leg or abdomen can be relaxed, depending on the site to be used. *A relaxed position of the site minimises discomfort.*
   - Obtain assistance in holding an uncooperative patient. *This prevents injury due to sudden movement after needle insertion.*
5. Explain the purpose of the medication and how it will help, using language that the patient can understand. Include relevant information about effects of the medication. *Information facilitates acceptance of and compliance with the therapy.*
6. Select and clean the site.
   - Select a site free of tenderness, hardness, swelling, scarring, itching, burning or localised inflammation. Select a site that has not been used frequently. *These conditions could hinder the absorption of the medication and also increase the likelihood of injury and discomfort at the injection site.*
   - Put on clean gloves.
   - As local policy indicates, clean the site with an antiseptic swab. Start at the centre of the site and clean in a widening circle to about 5 cm. Allow the area to dry thoroughly. *The mechanical action of swabbing removes skin secretions, which contain micro-organisms.*
   - Place and hold the swab between the third and fourth fingers of the nondominant hand, or position the swab on the patient's skin above the intended site. *Using this technique keeps the swab readily accessible when the needle is withdrawn.*
7. Prepare the syringe for injection.
   - Remove the needle cap while waiting for the antiseptic to dry. Pull the cap straight off to avoid contaminating the needle by the outside edge of the cap. *The needle will become contaminated if it touches anything but the inside of the cap, which is sterile.*
8. Inject the medication.
   - Grasp the syringe in your dominant hand by holding it between your thumb and fingers. With palm facing to the side or upward for a 45-degree angle insertion, or with the palm downward for a 90-degree angle insertion, prepare to inject (see Figure 21-32 on page 546).
   - Using the nondominant hand, spread the skin at the site, and insert the needle using the dominant hand and a firm steady push (see Figure 21-33 on page 546). Recommendations vary about whether to pinch or spread the skin and at what angle to administer subcutaneous injections. The most important consideration is the depth of the subcutaneous tissue in the area to be injected. If the patient has more than 2 cm of adipose tissue in the injection site, it would be safe to administer the injection at a 90-degree angle with the skin spread. If the patient is thin or lean and lacks adipose tissue, the subcutaneous injection should be given with the skin pinched and at a 45- to 60-degree angle.

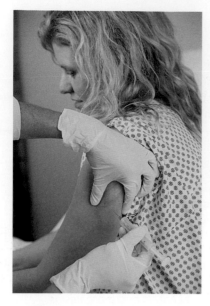

Figure 21-32 Administering a subcutaneous injection into pinched tissue.

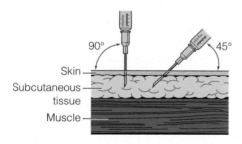

Figure 21-33 Inserting a needle into the subcutaneous tissue using 90- and 45-degree angles.

- When the needle is inserted, move your nondominant hand to the end of the plunger. Some nurses find it easier to move the nondominant hand to the barrel of the syringe and the dominant hand to the end of the plunger.
- Dependent upon personal choice *and* type of medication, aspirate by pulling back on the plunger. If blood appears in the syringe, withdraw the needle, discard the syringe and prepare a new injection. If blood does not appear, continue to administer the medication. *This allows the nurse to determine whether the needle has entered a blood vessel. Subcutaneous medications may be dangerous if placed directly into the bloodstream; they are intended for the subcutaneous tissues, where the absorption time is greater.* See the Variation for administering a heparin injection.

- Inject the medication by holding the syringe steady and depressing the plunger with a slow, even pressure. *Holding the syringe steady and injecting the medication at an even pressure minimises discomfort for the patient.*
9. Remove the needle.
   - Remove the needle slowly and smoothly, pulling along the line of insertion while depressing the skin with your nondominant hand. *Depressing the skin places countertraction on it and minimises the patient's discomfort when the needle is withdrawn.*
   - If bleeding occurs, apply pressure to the site with dry sterile gauze until it stops. *Bleeding rarely occurs after subcutaneous injection.*
10. Dispose of supplies appropriately.
    - Discard the uncapped needle and attached syringe into designated receptacles. *Proper disposal protects the nurse and others from injury and contamination. The RCN recommends re-sheathing the needle before disposal to reduce the risk of needlestick injuries.*
    - Remove gloves. Wash hands.
11. Document all relevant information.
    - Document the medication given, dosage, time, route and any assessments.
12. Assess the effectiveness of the medication at the time it is expected to act.

Variation: Administering a Heparin Injection

The subcutaneous administration of heparin requires special precautions because of the drug's anticoagulant properties.

+ Select a site on the abdomen 3–5 cm away from the umbilicus and above the level of the iliac crests. Some clinical areas support the practice of subcutaneous injection of heparin in the thighs or arms as alternate sites to the abdomen.
+ Use a #25- or #26-gauge needle, and insert it at a 90-degree angle. If a patient is very lean or wasted, use a shorter needle and insert it at a 45-degree angle. The arms or thighs may be used as alternate sites.
+ Do *not* aspirate when giving heparin by subcutaneous injection. *Aspiration can possibly damage the surrounding tissue and cause bleeding as well as bruising.*
+ Do not massage the site after the injection. *Massaging could cause bleeding and ecchymoses (bruises) and hasten drug absorption.*
+ Alternate the sites of subsequent injections.

Evaluation

+ Conduct appropriate follow-up such as desired effect (e.g. relief of pain, sedation, lowered blood sugar, a prothrombin time within pre-established limits), any adverse effects (e.g.

nausea, vomiting, skin rash), and clinical signs of side-effects.
+ Relate to previous findings if available.
+ Report deviations from normal to the physician.

COMMUNITY CARE CONSIDERATIONS

Subcutaneous Injections

+ If the patient has impaired vision, consider prefilling syringes and storing them in an appropriate environment (e.g. the refrigerator).
+ For frequent injections, develop a plan for site rotation with the patient.
+ For cost-saving measures, teach able patients to safely reuse disposable syringes where appropriate. Diabetic patients in the home can safely use disposable syringes until the needles become dull, which can vary from 2–10 times (Fleming, 1999).

Any patient reusing syringes should have the ability to safely and correctly recap needles. Patients with poor personal hygiene, acute concurrent illness, open wounds on the hands or decreased resistance to infection should be discouraged from reusing syringes.
+ For insulin-dependent patients, ensure that at least one knowledgeable relative/friend can correctly inject insulin in an emergency situation and recognise and treat hypoglycaemia.

Intramuscular Injections

Injections into muscle tissue, or **intramuscular (IM) injections**, are absorbed more quickly than subcutaneous injections because of the greater blood supply to the body muscles. Muscles can also take a larger volume of fluid without discomfort than subcutaneous tissues can, although the amount varies among individuals, chiefly with muscle size and condition and with the site used. An adult with well-developed muscles can usually safely tolerate up to 5 ml of medication in the gluteus medius and gluteus maximus muscles (see Figure 21-34). A volume of 1–2 ml is usually recommended for adults with less developed muscles. In the deltoid muscle, volumes of 0.5–1 ml are recommended.

Usually a 2–5 ml syringe is needed. The size of syringe used depends on the amount of medication being administered. The standard prepackaged intramuscular needle is 3 cm and #21 or #22 gauge. Several factors indicate the size and length of the needle to be used:

+ the muscle;
+ the type of solution;
+ the amount of adipose tissue covering the muscle;
+ the age of the patient.

For example, a smaller needle such as a #23- to #25-gauge needle is commonly used for the deltoid muscle. More viscous solutions require a larger gauge (e.g. #20 gauge). Very obese patients may require a needle longer than 4 cm and emaciated patients may require a shorter needle (e.g. 2 cm).

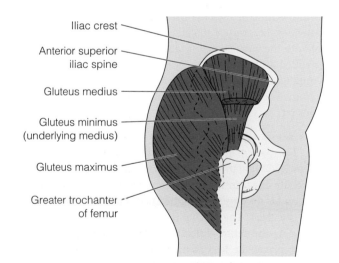

Figure 21-34 Lateral view of the right buttock showing the three gluteal muscles used for intramuscular injections.

A major consideration in the administration of intramuscular injections is the selection of a safe site located away from large blood vessels, nerves and bone. Several body sites can be used for intramuscular injections. These sites are discussed in detail next. Contraindications for using a specific site include tissue injury and the presence of nodules, lumps, abscesses, tenderness or other pathology.

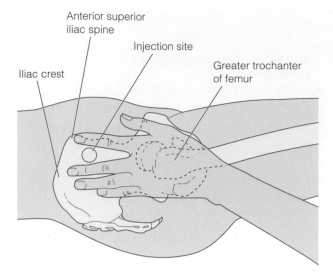

Anterior superior
iliac spine

Injection site

Greater trochanter
of femur

Iliac crest

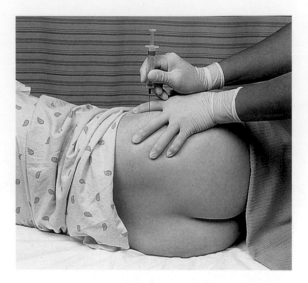

Figure 21-35 Landmarks for the ventrogluteal site for an intramuscular injection.

Figure 21-36 Administering an intramuscular injection into the ventrogluteal site.

Ventrogluteal Site

The ventrogluteal site is in the gluteus medius muscle, which lies over the gluteus minimus (see Figure 21-35). The ventrogluteal site is the *preferred* site for intramuscular injections because the area:

+ contains no large nerves or blood vessels;
+ provides the greatest thickness of gluteal muscle consisting of both the gluteus medius and gluteus minimus;
+ is sealed off by bone;
+ contains consistently less fat than the buttock area, thus eliminating the need to determine the depth of subcutaneous fat.

This site is suitable for children over seven months and adults. The patient position for the injection can be a back, prone or side-lying position. The side-lying position, however, helps locate the ventrogluteal site more easily. Position the patient on his or her side with the knee bent and raised slightly toward the chest. The trochanter will protrude, which facilitates locating the ventrogluteal site. To establish the exact site, the nurse places the heel of the hand on the patient's greater trochanter, with the fingers pointing toward the patient's head. The right hand is used for the left hip, and the left hand for the right hip. With the index finger on the patients's anterior superior iliac spine, the nurse stretches the middle finger dorsally (toward the buttocks), palpating the crest of the ilium and then pressing below it. The triangle formed by the index finger, the third finger and the crest of the ileum is the injection site (see Figures 21-35 and 21-36).

Vastus Lateralis Site

The vastus lateralis muscle is usually thick and well developed in both adults and children. It is recommended as the site of choice for intramuscular injections for infants seven months

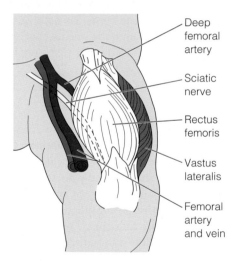

Deep
femoral
artery

Sciatic
nerve

Rectus
femoris

Vastus
lateralis

Femoral
artery
and vein

Figure 21-37 The vastus lateralis muscle of an infant's upper thigh, used for intramuscular injections.

and younger. Because there are no major blood vessels or nerves in the area, it is desirable for infants whose gluteal muscles are poorly developed. It is situated on the anterior lateral aspect of the infant's thigh (see Figure 21-37). The middle third of the muscle is suggested as the site. In the adult, the landmark is established by dividing the area between the greater trochanter of the femur and the lateral femoral condyle into thirds and selecting the middle third (see Figures 21-38 and 21-39). The patient can assume a back-lying or a sitting position for an injection into this site.

Dorsogluteal Site

The dorsogluteal site is composed of the thick gluteal muscles of the buttocks (see Figure 21-34 earlier). The dorsogluteal site can be used for adults and for children with well-developed

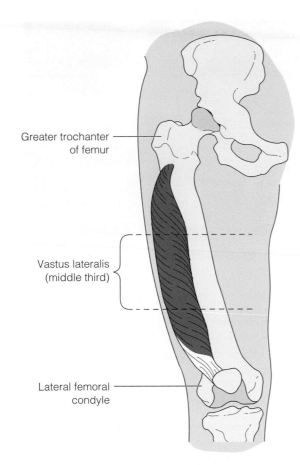

Greater trochanter of femur

Vastus lateralis (middle third)

Lateral femoral condyle

Figure 21-38 Landmarks for the vastus lateralis site of an adult's right thigh, used for an intramuscular injection.

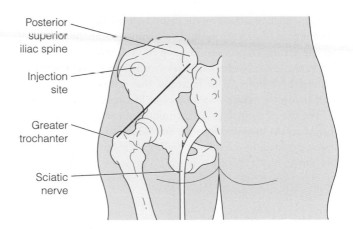

Posterior superior iliac spine

Injection site

Greater trochanter

Sciatic nerve

Figure 21-40 Landmarks for the dorsogluteal site for an intramuscular injection.

gluteal muscles. Because these muscles are developed by walking, this site should not be used for children under three unless the child has been walking for at least a year. The nurse must choose the injection site carefully to avoid striking the sciatic nerve, major blood vessels or bone.

The nurse palpates the posterior superior iliac spine, then draws an imaginary line to the greater trochanter of the femur.

This line is lateral to and parallel to the sciatic nerve. The injection site is lateral and superior to this line (see Figure 21-40). Palpating the ilium and the trochanter is important; visual calculations alone can result in an injection that is placed too low and injures other structures.

The patient needs to assume a prone position with the toes pointed inward or a side-lying position with the upper knee flexed and in front of the lower leg. These positions promote muscle relaxation and therefore minimise discomfort from the injection.

Deltoid Site

The deltoid muscle is found on the lateral aspect of the upper arm. It is not used often for intramuscular injections because it is a relatively small muscle and is very close to the radial nerve and radial artery. It is sometimes considered for use in adults because of rapid absorption from the deltoid area, but no more than 1 ml of solution can be administered. This site is recommended for the administration of hepatitis B vaccine in adults.

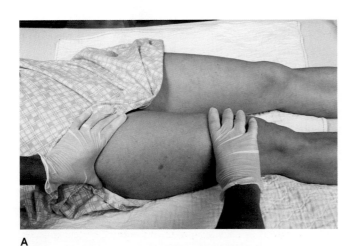

A

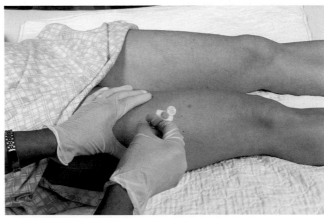

B

Figure 21-39 *A*, Determining landmarks and *B*, Administering an intramuscular injection into the vastus lateralis site.

The upper landmark for the deltoid site is located by the nurse placing four fingers across the deltoid muscle with the first finger on the acromion process. The top of the axilla is the line that marks the lower border landmark (see Figure 21-41). A triangle within these boundaries indicates the deltoid muscle about 5 cm below the acromion process (see Figures 21-42 and 21-43).

The use of a pinch-grasp technique can reduce the discomfort of an IM injection into the deltoid muscle. This technique involves grasping the muscle, pulling it about 2–3 cm toward the nurse, and applying a pinching pressure hard enough to

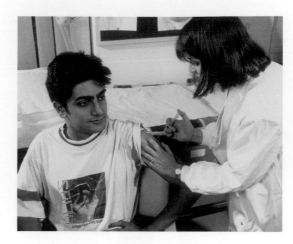

Figure 21-43 Administering an intramuscular injection into the deltoid site.

cause mild discomfort. The injection is given at a 90-degree angel (McCaffery and Pasero, 1999). It is important for the nurse to inform the patient about pinching the skin and explain the purpose.

Rectus Femoris Site

The rectus femoris muscle, which belongs to the quadriceps muscle group, is used only occasionally for intramuscular injections. It is situated on the anterior aspect of the thigh (see Figure 21-44). Its chief advantage is that patients who administer

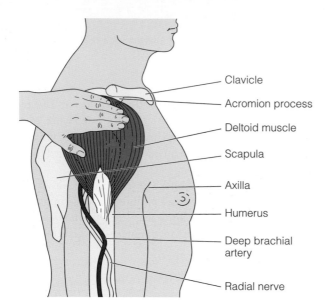

- Clavicle
- Acromion process
- Deltoid muscle
- Scapula
- Axilla
- Humerus
- Deep brachial artery
- Radial nerve

Figure 21-41 A method of establishing the deltoid muscle site for an intramuscular injection.

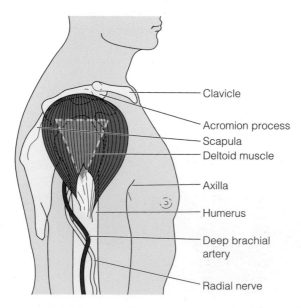

- Clavicle
- Acromion process
- Scapula
- Deltoid muscle
- Axilla
- Humerus
- Deep brachial artery
- Radial nerve

Figure 21-42 Landmarks for the deltoid muscle of the upper arm, used for intramuscular injections.

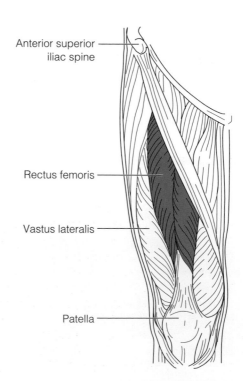

- Anterior superior iliac spine
- Rectus femoris
- Vastus lateralis
- Patella

Figure 21-44 Landmarks for the rectus femoris muscle of the upper right thigh, used for intramuscular injections.

their own injections can reach this site easily. Its main disadvantage is that an injection here may cause considerable discomfort for some people.

IM Injection Technique

Procedure 21-7 describes how to administer an intramuscular injection using the Z-track technique, which is recommended for any intramuscular injection. The Z-track method has been found to be less painful than the traditional injection technique. It involves stretching the skin with two fingers before the needle goes into the skin. Once the needle is through the skin and into the desired structure the stretching can be released. This prevents any of the administered drugs leaking from the site through the track the needle originally took (McCaffery and Pasero, 1999).

PROCEDURE 21-7 Administering an Intramuscular Injection

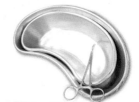

Purpose

+ To provide a medication the patient requires (see specific drug action)

Assessment

Assess

+ Patient allergies to medication(s)
+ Specific drug action, side-effects and adverse reactions
+ Patient's knowledge of and learning needs about the medication
+ Tissue integrity of the selected site
+ Patient's age and weight to determine site and needle size
+ Patient's ability or willingness to cooperate

Determine whether the size of the muscle is appropriate to the amount of medication to be injected. An average adult's deltoid muscle can usually absorb 0.5-1 ml of medication, although some authorities believe 1-2 ml can be absorbed by a well-developed deltoid muscle. The gluteus medius muscle can often absorb 1-4 ml, although 4 ml may be very painful.

Planning

Equipment

+ Medication chart
+ Sterile medication (usually provided in an ampoule or vial)

+ Syringe and needle of a size appropriate for the amount of solution to be administered
+ Antiseptic swabs
+ Clean gloves

Implementation

Preparation

1. Check the medication chart.
   • Check the label on the medication carefully against the chart to make sure that the correct medication is being prepared.
   • Follow the three checks for administering the medication and dose. Read the label on the medication (1) when it is taken from the medication store, (2) before withdrawing the medication and (3) after withdrawing the medication.
   • Confirm that the dose is correct.
2. Organise the equipment.

Performance

1. Wash hands and observe other appropriate infection control procedures (e.g. clean gloves).
2. Prepare the medication from the ampoule or vial for drug withdrawal.
   • See Procedure 21-2, page 536 (ampule) or 21-3, page 537 (vial).
   • Whenever feasible, change the needle on the syringe before the injection. *Because the outside of a new needle is free of medication, it does not irritate subcutaneous tissues as it passes into the muscle.*
   • Invert the syringe needle uppermost and expel all excess air.

3. Provide for patient privacy.
4. Prepare the patient.
   - Check the patient's identification band. *This ensures that the right patient receives the medication.*
   - Assist the patient to a supine, lateral, prone or sitting position, depending on the chosen site. If the target muscle is the gluteus medius (ventrogluteal site), have the patient in the supine position flex the knee(s); in the lateral position, flex the upper leg; and in the prone position, toe in. *Appropriate positioning promotes relaxation of the target muscle.*
   - Obtain assistance in supporting an uncooperative patient. *This prevents injury due to sudden movement after needle insertion.*
5. Explain the purpose of the medication and how it will help, using language that the patient can understand. Include relevant information about effects of the medication. *Information facilitates acceptance of and compliance with the therapy.*
6. Select, locate and clean the site.
   - Select a site free of skin lesions, tenderness, swelling, hardness or localised inflammation and one that has not been used frequently.
   - If injections are to be frequent, alternate sites. Avoid using the same site twice in a row. *This is to reduce the discomfort of intramuscular injections.* If necessary, discuss with the prescriber an alternative method of providing the medication.
   - Locate the exact site for the injection.
   - Put on clean gloves.
   - Clean the site with an antiseptic swab. Using a circular motion, start at the centre and move outward about 5 cm.
   - Transfer and hold the swab between the third and fourth fingers of your nondominant hand in readiness for needle withdrawal, or position the swab on the patient's skin above the intended site. Allow skin to dry prior to injecting medication *because this will help reduce the discomfort of the injection.*
7. Prepare the syringe for injection.
   - Remove the needle cover without contaminating the needle.
   - If using a prefilled unit-dose medication, take caution to avoid dripping medication on the needle prior to injection. If this does occur, wipe the medication off the needle with a sterile gauze. *Medication left on the needle can cause pain when it is tracked through the subcutaneous tissue.*
8. Inject the medication using a Z-track technique.
   - Use the ulnar side of the nondominant hand to pull the skin approximately 2.5 cm to the side (see Figure 21-45). Under some circumstances, such as for an emaciated patient or an infant, the muscle may be pinched. *Pulling the skin and subcutaneous tissue or pinching the muscle makes it firmer and facilitates needle insertion.*
   - Holding the syringe between the thumb and forefinger (as if holding a pencil), pierce the skin quickly and smoothly at a 90-degree angle (see Figure 21-36, page 548), and insert the needle into the muscle. *Using a quick motion lessens the patient's discomfort.*
   - Hold the barrel of the syringe steady with your nondominant hand and aspirate by pulling back on the plunger with your dominant hand. Aspirate for 5 seconds. *If the needle is in a small blood vessel, it takes time for the blood to appear.* If blood appears in the syringe, withdraw the needle, discard the syringe and prepare a new injection. *This step determines whether the needle has been inserted into a blood vessel.*

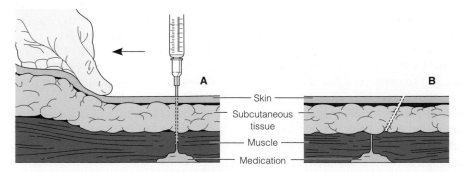

Figure 21-45 Inserting an intramuscular needle at a 90-degree angle using the Z-track method: *A*, skin pulled to the side; *B*, skin released. *Note:* When the skin returns to its normal position after the needle is withdrawn, a seal is formed over the intramuscular site. This prevents seepage of the medication into the subcutaneous tissues and subsequent discomfort.

- If blood does not appear, inject the medication steadily and slowly (approximately 10 seconds per millilitre) while holding the syringe steady. *Injecting medication slowly promotes comfort and allows time for tissue to expand and begin absorption of the medication. Holding the syringe steady minimises discomfort.*
- After injection, wait 10 seconds *to permit the medication to disperse into the muscle tissue, thus decreasing the patient's discomfort.*

9. Withdraw the needle.
   - Withdraw the needle smoothly at the same angle of insertion. *This minimises tissue injury.*

- Apply gentle pressure at the site with dry gauze. Do not massage the site. *Massaging the site can increase discomfort of the injection and can result in tissue irritation.*
- If bleeding occurs, apply pressure with dry sterile gauze until it stops.

10. Discard the uncapped needle and attached syringe into the proper receptacle.
    - Remove gloves. Wash hands.
11. Document all relevant information.
    - Include the time of administration, drug name, dose and route.
    Assess effectiveness of the medication at the time it is expected to act.

Evaluation

+ Conduct appropriate follow-up, such as
  - Desired effect (e.g. relief of pain or vomiting)
  - Any adverse reactions or side-effects
  - Local skin or tissue reactions at injection site (e.g. redness, swelling, pain or other evidence of tissue damage)

+ Relate to previous findings, if available
+ Report significant deviation from normal to medical staff

LIFESPAN CONSIDERATIONS

Intramuscular Injections

Infants

+ The ventrogluteal site cannot be used for children under seven months.
+ The vastus lateralis site is recommended as the site of choice for intramuscular injections for infants seven months and younger. Because there are no major blood vessels or nerves in the area, it is desirable for infants whose gluteal muscles are poorly developed. It is situated on the anterior lateral aspect of the thigh (see Figure 21-37 earlier).
+ Obtain assistance to immobilise an infant or young child. The parent may hold the infant or young child. This prevents accidental injury during the procedure.

Children

+ Infants and young children usually require smaller, shorter needles (#22 to #25 gauge) for intramuscular injection.
+ The gluteal muscles are developed by walking. Therefore, the dorsogluteal site should not be used for children under three unless the child has been walking for at least a year.

Older Adults

+ Older patients may have a decreased muscle mass or muscle atrophy. A shorter needle may be needed. Assessment of appropriate injection site is critical. Absorption of medication may occur more quickly than expected.

Intravenous Medications

Because intravenous (IV) medications enter the patient's bloodstream directly by way of a vein, they are appropriate when a rapid effect is required. This route is also appropriate when medications are too irritating to tissues to be given by other routes. When an intravenous line is already established, this route is desirable because it avoids the discomfort of other parenteral routes. Medications are administered intravenously by the following methods:

+ large-volume infusion of intravenous fluid;
+ intermittent intravenous infusion (piggyback or tandem setups);
+ volume-controlled infusion (often used for children);
+ intravenous bolus;
+ intermittent injection ports (device).

In all of these methods, the patent has an existing intravenous line or an IV access site such as a PICC line which is a peripheral intravenous central catheter. A tube is placed through a vein and goes directly into the vena cava. All clinical areas have procedures and policies about who may administer an IV medication, in the majority only the registered nurse is permitted to do so.

With all IV medication administration it is very important to observe patients closely for signs of adverse reactions. Because the drug enters the bloodstream directly and acts immediately, there is no way it can be withdrawn or its action terminated. Therefore, the nurse must take special care to avoid any errors about the preparation of the drug and the calculation of the dosage. When the drug being administered is particularly potent, an antidote to the drug should be available. In addition, the vital signs are assessed before, during and after infusion of the drug.

Before adding any medications to an existing intravenous infusion, the nurse must check for the six 'rights' and check compatability of the drug and the existing intravenous fluid. Be aware of any incompatabilities of the drug and the fluid that is

infusing. For example, the drug amiodarone is incompatible with saline and will form a precipitate if injected through a port in an intravenous line with saline infusing.

Large-Volume Infusions

Mixing a medication into a large-volume IV fluid bag is the safest and easiest way to administer a drug intravenously. The drugs are diluted in volumes of 1,000 ml or 500 ml of compatible fluids or as per directions. It may be necessary to consult a pharmacist to confirm compatibility. Fluids such as IV normal saline or 5% glucose are frequently used. Commonly added drugs are potassium chloride and vitamins. See *Procedure 21-8.*

The main danger of infusing a large volume of fluid is circulatory overload (hypervolaemia).

The medication should be added to the fluid container before it is attached and infusing.

PROCEDURE 21-8 Adding Medications to Intravenous Fluid Containers

Purposes

+ To provide and maintain a constant level of a medication in the blood
+ To administer well-diluted medications at a continuous and slow rate

Assessment

+ Inspect and palpate the intravenous insertion site for signs of infection, infiltration or a dislocated cannula.
+ Inspect the surrounding skin for redness, pallor or swelling.
+ Palpate the surrounding tissues for coldness and the presence of oedema, which could indicate leakage of the IV fluid into the tissues.
+ Take vital signs for baseline data if the medication being administered is particularly potent.
+ Determine if the patient has allergies to the medication(s).
+ Check the compatibility of the medication(s) and IV fluid.

Planning

Equipment

+ Medication chart
+ Correct sterile medication
+ Dilutent/solvent for medication in powdered form (see manufacturer's instructions)
+ Correct solution container, if a new one is to be attached
+ Antiseptic or alcohol swabs
+ Sterile syringe of appropriate size (e.g. 5 or 10 ml) and a #20- or #21-gauge sterile needle or equivalent from needleless system
+ IV additive label

Implementation

Preparation

1. Check the medication chart.
   • Check the label on the medication carefully against the medication chart to make sure that the correct medication is being prepared.

- Follow the three checks for administering medications. Read the label on the medication (1) when it is taken from the medication store, (2) before withdrawing the medication and (3) after withdrawing the medication.
- Confirm that the dosage and route is correct.
- Verify which infusion solution is to be used with the medication.
- Consult a pharmacist, if required, to confirm compatibility of the drugs and solutions being mixed.

2. Organise the equipment.

Performance

1. Wash hands and observe other appropriate infection control procedures.
2. Prepare the medication ampoule or vial for drug withdrawal.
   - See Procedure 21-2, page 536 (ampoule) or 21-3, page 537 (vial).
3. Add the medication.

   To New IV Container/Fluid Bag
   - Locate the injection port and carefully remove its cover. Clean the port with the antiseptic or alcohol swab. *This reduces the risk of introducing micro-organisms into the container when the needle is inserted.*
   - Remove the needle cap from the syringe, insert the needle through the centre of the injection port, and inject the medication into the bag or bottle (see Figure 21-46).

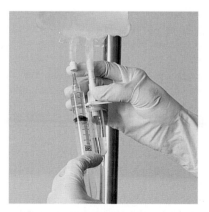

Figure 21-46 Inserting a medication through the injection port of an infusing container.

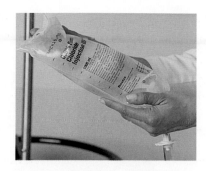

Figure 21-47 *Rotating an intravenous bag to distribute a medication.*

- Mix the medication and solution by gently rotating the bag or bottle (see Figure 21-47). *This should disperse the medication throughout the solution.*
- Complete the IV additive label with name and dose of medication, date, time and nurse's initials. Attach it upside down on the bag or bottle (see Figure 21-48). *This documents that medication has been added to the solution. When the label is attached upside down, it is easily read when the bag is hanging up.*
- Clamp the IV tubing. Spike the bag or bottle with IV administration set and hang the fluid. *Clamping prevents rapid infusion of the solution.*
- Regulate infusion rate as prescribed.

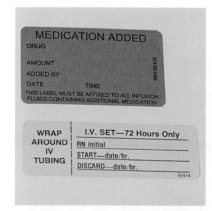

Figure 21-48 *Top,* label indicating a medication added to an IV infusion; *Bottom,* label indicating time for IV tubing change.

Intermittent Intravenous Infusions

An intermittent infusion is a method of administering a medication mixed in a small amount of IV solution, such as 50 or 100 ml (see Figure 21-49 on page 556). The drug is administered at regular intervals, such as every four hours, with the drug being infused for a short period of time such as 30–60 minutes. Two commonly used additive or secondary IV setups are the **tandem** and the **piggyback**.

Another method of intermittently administering an IV medication is by a syringe pump. The medication is mixed in a syringe that is connected to an intravenous cannula and administered at a controlled administration rate (see Figure 21-50 on page 556).

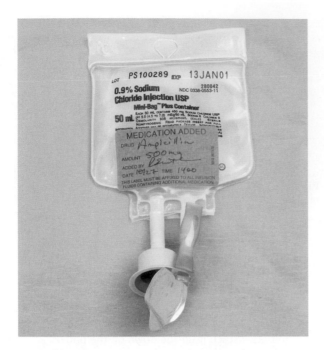

Figure 21-49 Medication in a labelled infusion bag.

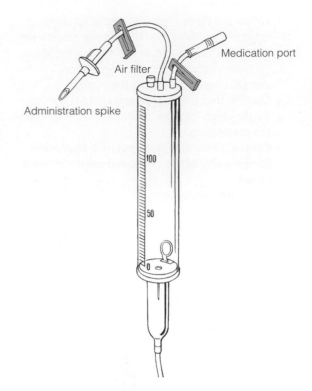

Figure 21-51 A volume-control infusion set.

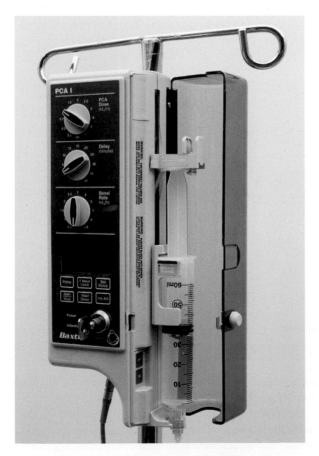

Figure 21-50 Syringe pump or mini-infuser for administration of IV medications.

Volume-Control Infusions

Intermittent medications may also be administered by a **volume-control infusion set** such as Buretrol, Soluset, Volutrol and Pediatrol (see Figure 21-51). Although increasingly this system is being replaced with the more accurate administration of fluids and medications via infusion pumps. They are small fluid containers (100–150 ml in size) attached below the primary infusion container so that the medication is administered through the patient's IV cannula. Volume-control sets are frequently used to infuse solutions into children and older patients when the volume administered is critical and must be carefully monitored, usually when infusion pumps are unavailable.

Intravenous Bolus

Intravenous bolus is the intravenous administration of a drug directly into the systemic circulation. It is used when a medication is not diluted or in an emergency. An IV bolus can be introduced directly into a vein by venipuncture or into an existing IV line through a cannula.

There are two major disadvantages to this method of drug administration: any error in administration cannot be corrected after the drug has entered the patient, and the drug may be irritating to the lining of the blood vessels. Before administering a bolus, the nurse should look up the maximum concentration recommended for the particular drug and the rate of administration. The administered medication takes effect immediately (see *Procedure 21-9*).

PROCEDURE 21-9 Administering Intravenous Medications Using IV Bolus

Purpose

+ To achieve immediate and maximum effects of a medication

Assessment

+ Inspect and palpate the IV insertion site for signs of infection, infiltration or a dislocated cannula.
+ Inspect the surrounding skin for redness, pallor or swelling.
+ Palpate the surrounding tissues for coldness and the presence of oedema, which could indicate leakage of the IV fluid into the tissues.
+ Take vital signs for baseline data if the medication being administered is particularly potent.

+ Determine if the patient has allergies to the medication(s).
+ Check the compatibility of the medication(s) and IV fluid.
+ Determine specific drug action, side-effects, normal dosage, recommended administration time and peak action time.
+ Check patency of IV line by assessing flow rate.

Planning

Equipment

IV Bolus for an Existing Line

+ Medication in a vial or ampoule
+ Sterile syringe (size dependent upon volume of drug) (to prepare the medication)

+ Sterile needles #21 to #25 gauge, 2.5 cm or equivalent from a needleless system
+ Antiseptic swabs
+ Watch with a digital readout or second hand
+ Clean gloves

Implementation

Preparation

1. Check the medication chart.
   - Check the label on the medication carefully against the chart to make sure that the correct medication is being prepared.
   - Follow the three checks for correct medication and dose. Read the label on the medication (1) when it is taken from the medication store, (2) before withdrawing the medication and (3) after withdrawing the medication.
   - Calculate medication dosage accurately.
   - Confirm that the route is correct.
2. Organise the equipment.

Performance

1. Wash hands and observe other appropriate infection control procedures.
2. Prepare the medication.
   - Prepare the medication according to the manufacturer's direction. *It is important to have the correct dose and the correct dilution.*

   a. Flushing with saline
      - Prepare two syringes, each with 2.5 ml of sterile normal saline.
   b. Flushing with heparin and saline
      - Prepare one syringe with 2.5 ml of heparin flush solution.
      - Prepare two syringes with 2.5 ml each of sterile, normal saline.
      - Draw up the medication into a syringe.
3. Put a small-gauge needle on the syringe if using a needle system through a bung.
4. Wash hands and put on clean gloves. *This reduces the transmission of micro-organisms and reduces the likelihood of the nurse's hands contacting the patient's blood.*
5. Provide for patient privacy.
6. Prepare the patient.
   - Check the patient's identification band. *This ensures that the right patient receives the medication.*

- If not previously assessed, take the appropriate assessment measures necessary for the medication. If any of the findings are above or below the predetermined parameters, consult the prescriber before administering the medication.

7. Explain the purpose of the medication and how it will help, using language that the patient can understand. Include relevant information about the effects of the medication.
8. Administer the medication by IV bolus slowly in accordance with manufacturer advice for rate of adminstration.

IV Cannula

- Remove the protective cap from the cannula port.
- Insert syringe containing normal saline into the lock.

- Flush the lock with 2.5 ml sterile saline. *This clears the lock of blood.*
- Remove the syringe.
- Insert the syringe containing the medication into the valve of the cannula.
- Inject the medication following the precautions described previously.
- Withdraw the syringe.
- Repeat injection of 2.5 ml of saline.
- Replace cap on cannula.

9. Dispose of equipment according to local policy. *This reduces needlestick injuries and spread of micro-organisms.*
10. Remove and dispose of gloves. Wash hands.
11. Observe the patient closely for adverse reactions.
12. Document all relevant information.
    - Record the date, time, drug, dose and route; patient response; and assessments of infusion or cannula site if appropriate.

Evaluation

+ Conduct appropriate follow-up such as desired effect of medication, any adverse reactions or side-effects, or change in vital signs.

+ Reassess status of IV cannula site and patency of IV infusion, if running.
+ Relate to previous findings, if available.
+ Report significant deviations from normal.

Topical Medications

A topical medication is applied locally to the skin or to mucous membranes in areas such as the eye, external ear canal, nose, vagina and rectum. Most topical applications used therapeutically are not absorbed well, completely or predictably when applied to intact skin because the skin's thick outer layer serves as a natural barrier to drug diffusion. This route of absorption through the skin, called percutaneous, can be increased if the skin is altered by a laceration, burn or some other problem. However, if high concentrations or large amounts of a topical medication are applied to the skin, especially if it is done repeatedly, sufficient amounts of the drug can enter the bloodstream to cause systemic effects, usually undesirable ones.

A particular type of topical or dermatologic medication delivery system is the transdermal patch. This system administers sustained-action medications (e.g. nitroglycerin, oestrogen, fentanyl and nicotine) via multilayered films containing the drug and an adhesive layer. The rate of delivery of the drug is controlled and varies with each product (e.g. from 12 hours to one week). Generally, the patch is applied to a hairless, clean area of skin that is not subject to excessive movement or wrinkling (i.e. the trunk or lower abdomen). It may also be applied on the side, lower back or buttocks. Patches should not be applied to areas with cuts, burns or abrasions, or on distal parts of extremities (e.g. the forearms). If hair is likely to interfere with patch adhesion or removal, clipping may be necessary before application.

Reddening of the skin with or without mild local itching or burning, as well as allergic contact dermatitis, may occasionally occur. Upon removal of the patch, any slight reddening of the skin usually disappears within a few hours. All applications should be changed regularly to prevent local irritation, and each successive application should be placed on a different site. All patients need to be assessed for allergies to the drug and to materials in the patch before the patch is applied. If a patient has a transdermal patch on and develops a fever, the medication may be absorbed and metabolise at a faster rate than normal. The patient will need to be monitored for changes in effects of the medication.

When transdermal patches are removed, care needs to be taken as to how and where they are discarded. In the home environment, if they are simply discarded into normal refuse, pets or children can be exposed to them, causing effects from any drug remaining on the patch. When removed, they should be folded with the medication side to the inside, put into a closed container and kept out of reach of children and pets.

CLINICAL ALERT

The nurse should always wear gloves when applying a transdermal patch to avoid getting any of the medication on their skin, which can result in receiving the effect of the medication.

Skin Applications

Topical skin or dermatologic preparations include ointments, pastes, creams, lotions, powders, sprays and patches (see Table 21-1 on page 510). See *Practice guidelines* for applying topical medications. Before applying a dermatologic preparation, thoroughly clean the area with soap and water and dry it with a patting motion. Skin encrustations harbour microorganisms and these as well as previously applied applications can prevent the medication from coming in contact with the area to be treated. Nurses should wear gloves when administering skin applications and always use surgical asepsis when an open wound is present.

Ophthalmic Medications

Medications may be administered to the eye using irrigations or instillations. Eye irrigation is administered to wash out the conjunctival sac to remove secretions or foreign bodies or to remove chemicals that may injure the eye. Medications for the eyes, called ophthalmic medications, are instilled in the form of liquids or ointments. Eye drops are packaged in single drip plastic containers that are used to administer the preparation. Ointments are usually supplied in small tubes. All containers must state that the medication is for ophthalmic use. Sterile preparations and sterile technique are indicated. Prescribed liquids are usually dilute, for example, less than 1% strength.

Procedure 21-10 illustrates how to administer ophthalmic instillations.

PRACTICE GUIDELINES

Applying Skin Preparations

Powder
Make sure the skin surface is dry. Spread apart any skin folds, and sprinkle the site until the area is covered with a fine *thin* layer. Cover the site with a dressing if ordered.

Suspension-based Lotion
Shake the container before use to distribute suspended particles. Put a little lotion on a small gauze dressing or pad, and apply the lotion to the skin by stroking it evenly in the direction of the hair growth.

Creams, Ointments, Pastes and Oil-based Lotions
Warm and soften the preparation in gloved hands to make it easier to apply and to prevent chilling (if a large area is to be treated). Smear it evenly over the skin using long strokes that follow the direction of the hair growth. Explain that the skin may feel somewhat greasy after application. Apply a sterile dressing if necessary.

Aerosol Spray
Shake the container well to mix the contents. Hold the spray container at the recommended distance from the area (usually about 15-30 cm (check the label)). Cover the patient's face with a towel if the upper chest or neck is to be sprayed. Spray the medication over the specified area.

Transdermal Patches
Select a clean, dry area that is free of hair and matches the manufacturer's recommendations. Remove the patch from its protective covering, holding it without touching the adhesive edges, and apply it by pressing firmly with the palm of the hand for about 10 seconds. Advise the patient to avoid using a heating pad over the area to prevent an increase in circulation and the rate of absorption. Remove the patch at the appropriate time, folding the medicated side to the inside so it is covered.

PROCEDURE 21-10 Administering Ophthalmic Instillations

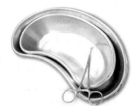

Purpose

+ To provide an eye medication the patient requires (e.g. an antibiotic) to treat an infection or for other reasons (see specific drug action)

Assessment

In addition to the assessment performed by the nurse related to the admininstration of any medication, prior to applying ophthalmic medications, assess:

+ Appearance of eye and surrounding structures for lesions, exudate, erythema or swelling

+ The location and nature of any discharge, lacrimation, and swelling of the eyelids or of the lacrimal gland
+ Patient complaints (e.g. itching, burning pain, blurred vision and photophobia)

+ Patient behaviour (e.g. squinting, blinking excessively, frowning or rubbing the eyes)

Determine if assessment data influence administration of the medication.

Planning

Equipment

+ Clean gloves
+ Sterile absorbent gauze soaked in sterile normal saline
+ Medication
+ Sterile eye dressing (pad) as needed and paper eye tape to secure it

For irrigation, add:

+ Irrigating solution (e.g. normal saline) and irrigating syringe or tubing
+ Dry sterile gauze swabs
+ Moisture-resistant towel
+ Basin (e.g. kidney basin)

Implementation

Preparation

1. Check the medication chart.
   - Check the chart for the drug name, dose and strength. Also confirm the prescribed frequency of the instillation and which eye is to be treated.
2. Know the reason why the patient is receiving the medication, the drug classification, contraindications, usual dose range, side-effects, and nursing considerations for administering and evaluating the intended outcomes of the medication.

Performance

1. Compare the label on the medication tube or bottle with the medication chart and check the expiration date.
2. If necessary, calculate the medication dosage.
3. Explain to the patient what you are going to do, why it is necessary and how they can cooperate. The administration of an ophthalmic medication is not usually painful. Ointments are often soothing to the eye, but some liquid preparations may sting initially. Discuss how the results will be used in planning further care or treatments.
4. Wash hands and observe appropriate infection control procedures.
5. Provide for patient privacy.
6. Prepare the patient.
   - Check the patient's identification band and ask the patient's name. This ensures that the right patient receives the medication.
   - Assist the patient to a comfortable position, either sitting or lying.
7. Clean the eyelid and the eyelashes.
   - Put on clean gloves.

- Use sterile gauze moistened with sterile irrigating solution or sterile normal saline, and wipe from the inner canthus to the outer canthus. *If not removed, material on the eyelid and lashes can be washed into the eye. Cleaning toward the outer canthus prevents contamination of the other eye and the lacrimal duct.*
8. Administer the eye medication.
   - Check the ophthalmic preparation for the name, strength and number of drops if a liquid is used. *Checking medication data is essential to prevent a medication error.* Draw the correct number of drops into the shaft of the dropper if a dropper is used. If ointment is used, discard the first bead. *The first bead of ointment from a tube is considered to be contaminated.*
   - Instruct the patient to look up to the ceiling. Give the patient dry sterile absorbent gauze. *The person is less likely to blink if looking up. While the patient looks up, the cornea is partially protected by the upper eyelid. A gauze swab is needed to press on the nasolacrimal duct after a liquid instillation or to wipe excess ointment from the eyelashes after an ointment is instilled.*
   - Expose the lower conjunctival sac by placing the thumb or fingers of your nondominant hand on the patient's cheekbone just below the eye and gently drawing down the skin on the cheek. If the tissues are oedematous, handle the tissues carefully to avoid damaging them. *Placing the fingers on the cheekbone minimises the possibility of touching the cornea, avoids putting any pressure on the eyeball, and prevents the person from blinking or squinting.*

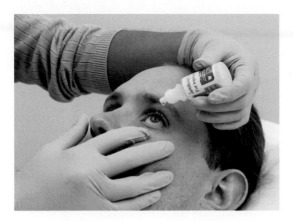

Figure 21-52 Instilling an eyedrop into the lower conjunctival sac.

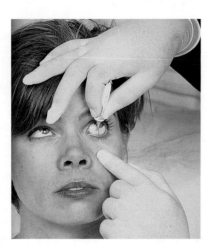

Figure 21-53 Instilling an eye ointment into the lower conjunctival sac.

- Approach the eye from the side and instill the correct number of drops onto the outer third of the lower conjunctival sac. Hold the dropper 1-2 cm above the sac (see Figure 21-52). *The patient is less likely to blink if a side approach is used. When instilled into the conjunctival sac, drops will not harm the cornea as they might if dropped directly on it. The dropper must not touch the sac or the cornea.*

  or

- Holding the tube above the lower conjunctival sac, squeeze 2 cm of ointment from the tube into the lower conjunctival sac from the inner canthus outward (see Figure 21-53).
- Instruct the patient to close the eyelids but not to squeeze them shut. *Closing the eye spreads the medication over the eyeball. Squeezing can injure the eye and push out the medication.*
- For liquid medications, press firmly or have the patient press firmly on the nasolacrimal duct for at least 30 seconds (see Figure 21-54). *Pressing*

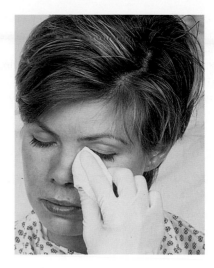

Figure 21-54 Pressing on the nasolacrimal duct.

on the nasolacrimal duct prevents the medication from running out of the eye and down the duct.

Variation: Irrigation

- Place absorbent pads under the head, neck and shoulders. Place a kidney basin next to the eye to catch drainage. Some eye medications cause systemic reactions such as confusion or a decrease in heart rate and blood pressure if the eye drops go down the nasolacrimal duct and get into the systemic circulation.
- Expose the lower conjunctival sac. Or, to irrigate in stages, first hold the lower lid down, then hold the upper lid up. Exert pressure on the bony prominences of the cheekbone and beneath the eyebrow when holding the eyelids. *Separating the lids prevents reflex blinking. Exerting pressure on the bony prominences minimises the possibility of pressing the eyeball and causing discomfort.*
- Fill and hold the eye irrigator about 2.5 cm above the eye. *At this height the pressure of the solution will not damage the eye tissue, and the irrigator will not touch the eye.*
- Irrigate the eye, directing the solution onto the lower conjunctival sac and from the inner canthus to the outer canthus. *Directing the solution in this way prevents possible injury to the cornea and prevents fluid and contaminants from flowing down the nasolacrimal duct.*
- Irrigate until the solution leaving the eye is clear (no discharge is present) or until all the solution has been used.
- Instruct the patient to close and move the eye periodically. *Eye closure and movement help to move secretions from the upper to the lower conjunctival sac.*

9. Clean and dry the eyelids as needed. Wipe the eyelids gently from the inner to the outer canthus to collect excess medication.
10. Apply an eye pad if needed, and secure it with paper eye tape.
11. Assess the patient's response immediately after the instillation or irrigation and again after the medication should have acted.
12. Document all relevant assessments and interventions. Include the name of the drug or irrigating solution, the strength, the number of drops if a liquid medication, the time, and the response of the patient.

Evaluation

+ Perform follow-up based on findings of the effectiveness of the administration or outcomes that deviated from expected or normal for the patient. Relate findings to previous data if available.

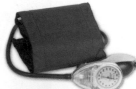

LIFESPAN CONSIDERATIONS

Administering Ophthalmic Medications

Infants/Children

+ Explain the technique to the parents of an infant or child.
+ For a young child or infant, obtain assistance to immobilise the arms and head. The parent may hold the infant or young child. *This prevents accidental injury during medication administration.*
+ For a young child, use a doll to demonstrate the procedure. *This facilitates cooperation and decreases anxiety.*
+ An intravenous (IV) bag and tubing may be used to deliver irrigating fluid to the eye (see Figure 21-55).

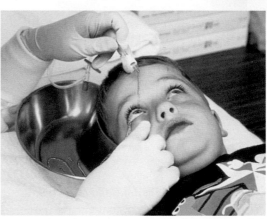

Figure 21-55 Eye irrigation using IV tubing.

Otic Medications

Instillations or irrigations of the external auditory canal are referred to as **otic** and are generally carried out for cleaning purposes. Sometimes applications of heat and antiseptic solutions are prescribed. Irrigations performed in a hospital require aseptic technique so that micro-organisms will not be introduced into the ear. Sterile technique is used if the eardrum is perforated. The position of the external auditory canal varies with age. In the child under three, it is directed upward. In the adult, the external auditory canal is an S-shaped structure about 2.5 cm long.

Procedure 21-11 explains how to administer otic instillations.

PROCEDURE 21-11 Administering Otic Instillations

Purpose

+ To soften earwax so that it can be readily removed at a later time

+ To provide local therapy to reduce inflammation, destroy infective organisms in the external ear canal, or both
+ To relieve pain

Assessment

In addition to the assessment performed by the nurse related to the administration of any medications, prior to applying otic medications, assess:

+ Appearance of the pinna of the ear and meatus for signs of redness and abrasions

+ Type and amount of any discharge

Determine if assessment data influence administration of the medication.

Planning
Equipment

+ Clean gloves
+ Correct medication bottle with a dropper
+ Flexible rubber tip (optional) for the end of the dropper, which prevents injury from sudden motion, for example, by a disoriented patient
+ Cotton wool

For irrigation, add:

+ Moisture-resistant towel
+ Basin (e.g. kidney basin)
+ Irrigating solution at the appropriate temperature, about 500 ml (container for the irrigating solution)

Implementation
Preparation

1. Check the medication chart.
   • Check the chart for the drug name, strength, number of drops and prescribed frequency.
   • If the chart is unclear or pertinent information is missing check with the prescriber
2. Know the reason why the patient is receiving the medication, the drug classification, contraindications, usual dose range, side-effects and nursing considerations for administering and evaluating the intended outcomes of the medication.

Performance

1. Compare the label on the medication container with the medication chart and check the expiration date.
2. If necessary, calculate the medication dosage.
3. Explain to the patient what you are going to do, why it is necessary and how they can cooperate. The administration of an otic medication is not usually painful. Discuss how the results will be used in planning further care or treatments.

4. Wash hands and observe appropriate infection control procedures.
5. Provide for patient privacy.
6. Prepare the patient.
   • Check the patient's identification band, and ask the patient's name. *This ensures that the right patient receives the medication.*
   • Assist the patient to a comfortable position for eardrops, lying with the ear being treated uppermost.
7. Clean the pinna of the ear and the meatus of the ear canal.
   • Put on gloves if infection is suspected.
   • Use a gauze swab and solution to wipe the pinna and auditory meatus. *This removes any discharge present before the instillation so that it won't be washed into the ear canal.*
8. Administer the ear medication.
   • Warm the medication container in your hand, or place it in warm water for a short time. *This promotes patient comfort.*
   • Partially fill the ear dropper with medication.

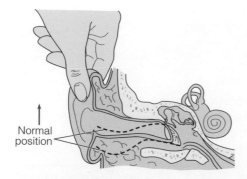

Figure 21-56 Straightening the adult ear canal by pulling pinna upward and backward.

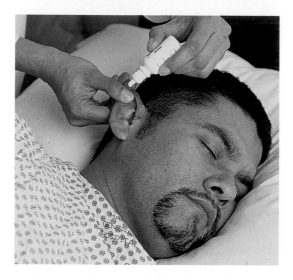

Figure 21-57 Instilling eardrops.

- Straighten the auditory canal. Pull the pinna upward and backward (see Figure 21-56). *The auditory canal is straightened so that the solution can flow the entire length of the canal.*
- Instill the correct number of drops along the side of the ear canal (see Figure 21-57).
- Press gently but firmly a few times on the tragus of the ear (the cartilaginous projection in front of the exterior meatus of the ear). *Pressing on the tragus assists the flow of medication into the ear canal.*
- Ask the patient to remain in the side-lying position for about five minutes. *This prevents the drops from escaping and allows the medication to reach all sides of the canal cavity.*
- Insert a small piece of cotton wool loosely at the meatus of the auditory canal for 15–20 minutes.

Do not press it into the canal. *The cotton helps retain the medication when the patient is up. If pressed tightly into the canal, the cotton would interfere with the action of the drug and the outward movement of normal secretions.*

Variation: Ear Irrigation

- Explain that the patient may experience a feeling of fullness, warmth and, occasionally, discomfort when the fluid comes in contact with the tympanic membrane.
- Assist the patient to a sitting or lying position with head turned toward the affected ear. *The solution can then flow from the ear canal to a basin.*
- Place the moisture-resistant towel around the patient's shoulder under the ear to be irrigated, and place the basin under the ear to be irrigated.

or

- Hang up the irrigating container, and run solution through the tubing and the nozzle. *Solution is run through to remove air from the tubing and nozzle.*
- Straighten the ear canal.
- Insert the tip of the syringe into the auditory meatus, and direct the solution gently upward against the top of the canal. *The solution will flow around the entire canal and out at the bottom. The solution is instilled gently because strong pressure from the fluid can cause discomfort and damage the tympanic membrane.*
- Continue instilling the fluid until all the solution is used or until the canal is cleaned, depending on the purpose of the irrigation. Take care not to block the outward flow of the solution with the syringe.
- Assist the patient to a side-lying position on the affected side. *Lying with the affected side down helps drain the excess fluid by gravity.*
- Place a cotton wool in the auditory meatus to absorb the excess fluid.

9. Assess the patient's response and the character and amount of discharge, appearance of the canal, discomfort, and so on, immediately after the instillation and again when the medication is expected to act. Inspect the cotton wool for any drainage.

10. Document all nursing assessments and interventions relative to the procedure. Include the name of the drug or irrigating solution, the strength, the number of drops if a liquid medication, the time, and the response of the patient.

Evaluation

✚ Perform follow-up based on findings of the effectiveness of the administration or outcomes that deviated from expected or normal for the patient. Relate findings to previous data if available.

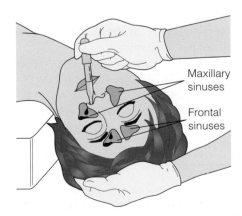

LIFESPAN CONSIDERATIONS

Administering Otic Medications

Infants/Children

+ Obtain assistance to immobilise an infant or young child. This prevents accidental injury due to sudden movement during the procedure.
+ Because in infants and children under three, the ear canal is directed upward, to administer medication, gently pull the pinna down and back (see Figure 21-58). For a child *older* than three, pull the pinna upward and backward (see Figure 21-56).

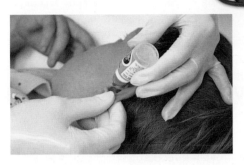

Figure 21-58 Straightening the ear canal of a child by pulling the pinna down and back.

Nasal Medications

Nasal instillations (nose drops and sprays) usually are instilled for their astringent effect (to shrink swollen mucous membranes), to loosen secretions and facilitate drainage or to treat infections of the nasal cavity or sinuses. Nasal decongestants are the most common nasal instillations. Many of these products are available without a prescription. Patients need to be taught to use these agents with caution. Chronic use of nasal decongestants may lead to a rebound effect, that is, an increase in nasal congestion. If excess decongestant solution is swallowed, serious systemic effects may also develop, especially in children. Saline drops are safer as a decongestant for children.

Usually patients self-administer sprays. In the supine position with the head tilted back, the patient holds the tip of the container just inside the nares and inhales as the spray enters the nasal passages. For patients who use nasal sprays repeatedly, the nares need to be assessed for irritation. In children, nasal sprays are given with the head in an upright position to prevent excess spray from being swallowed.

Nasal drops are used to treat sinus infections. Patients need to learn ways to position themselves to effectively treat the affected sinus:

+ To treat the ethmoid and sphenoid sinuses, instruct the patient to lie back with the head over the edge of the bed or a pillow under the shoulders so that the head is tipped backward (see Figure 21-59).
+ To treat the maxillary and frontal sinuses, instruct the patient to assume the same back-lying position, with the head turned toward the side to be treated (see Figure 21-60). The patient should also be instructed to (a) breathe through the mouth to prevent aspiration of medication into the trachea and bronchi, (b) remain in a back-lying position for at least a minute so that the solution will come into contact with all of the nasal surface, and (c) avoid blowing the nose for several minutes.

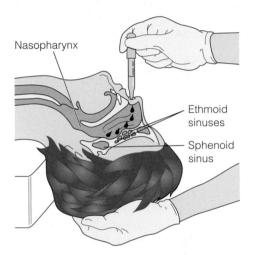

Figure 21-59 Position of the head to instill drops into the ethmoid and sphenoid sinuses.

Figure 21-60 Position of the head to instill drops into the maxillary and frontal sinuses.

Vaginal Medications

Vaginal medications or instillations, are inserted as creams, jellies, foams or pessaries to treat infection or to relieve vaginal discomfort (e.g. itching or pain). Medical aseptic technique is usually used. Vaginal creams, jellies and foams are applied by using a tubular applicator with a plunger. Suppositories are inserted with the index finger of a gloved hand. Suppositories are designed to melt at body temperature, so they are generally stored in the refrigerator to keep them firm for insertion. See *Procedure 21-12* for administering vaginal instillations.

PROCEDURE 21-12 Administering Vaginal Instillations

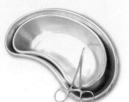

Purpose

+ To treat or prevent infection
+ To reduce inflammation

+ To relieve vaginal discomfort

Assessment

In addition to the assessment performed by the nurse related to the administration of any medications, prior to applying vaginal medications, assess:

+ The vaginal orifice for inflammation; amount, character and odour of vaginal discharge

+ For complaints of vaginal discomfort (e.g. burning or itching)

Determine if assessment data influence administration of the medication (i.e. is it appropriate to administer the medication or does the medication need to be reviewed).

Planning

Equipment

+ Drape/ patient bed sheet
+ Correct vaginal suppository or cream
+ Applicator for vaginal cream
+ Clean gloves
+ Lubricant for a suppository
+ Disposable towel
+ Clean perineal pad

For an irrigation, add:

+ Moisture-proof pad
+ Vaginal irrigation set (these are often disposable) containing a nozzle, tubing and a clamp, and a container for the solution
+ IV drip stand
+ Irrigating solution

Implementation

Preparation

1. Check the medication chart.
   • Check the chart for the drug name, strength and prescribed frequency.
2. Know the reason why the patient is receiving the medication, the drug classification, contraindications, usual dose range, side-effects and nursing considerations for administering and evaluating the intended outcomes of the medication.

Performance

1. Compare the label on the medication container with the medication chart and check the expiration date.

2. If necessary, calculate the medication dosage.
3. Explain to the patient what you are going to do, why it is necessary and how she can cooperate. Explain to the patient that a vaginal instillation is normally a painless procedure, and in fact may bring relief from itching and burning if an infection is present. Many people feel embarrassed about this procedure, and some may prefer to perform the procedure themselves if instruction is provided. Discuss how the results will be used in planning further care or treatments.
4. Wash hands and observe appropriate infection control procedures.
5. Provide for patient privacy.

6. Prepare the patient.
- Check the patient's identification band, and ask the patient's name. *This ensures that the right patient receives the medication.*
- Ask the patient to void urine. *If the bladder is empty, the patient will have less discomfort during the treatment, and the possibility of injuring the vaginal lining is decreased.*
- Assist the patient to a back-lying position with the knees flexed and the hips rotated laterally.
- Cover the patient appropriately so that only the perineal area is exposed.

7. Prepare the equipment.
- Unwrap the suppository, and put it on the opened wrapper.

or

- Fill the applicator with the prescribed cream, jelly or foam. Directions are provided with the manufacturer's applicator.

8. Assess and clean (according to local policy) the perineal area.
- Put on gloves. *Gloves prevent contamination of the nurse's hands from vaginal and perineal micro-organisms.*
- Inspect the vaginal orifice, note any odour of discharge from the vagina and ask about any vaginal discomfort.
- Provide perineal care to remove micro-organisms. *This decreases the chance of moving micro-organisms into the vagina.*

9. Administer the vaginal suppository, cream, foam, jelly or irrigation.

Suppository
- Lubricate the rounded (smooth) end of the suppository, which is inserted first. *Lubrication facilitates insertion.*

- Lubricate your gloved index finger.
- Expose the vaginal orifice by separating the labia with your nondominant hand.
- Insert the suppository about 8–10 cm along the posterior wall of the vagina, or as far as it will go (see Figure 21-61). *The posterior wall of the vagina is about 2.5 cm longer than the anterior wall because the cervix protrudes into the uppermost portion of the anterior wall.*
- Ask the patient to remain lying in the supine position for 5–10 minutes following insertion. The hips may also be elevated on a pillow. *This position allows the medication to flow into the posterior fornix after it has melted.*

Vaginal Cream, Jelly or Foam
- Gently insert the applicator about 5 cm.
- Slowly push the plunger until the applicator is empty (see Figure 21-62).
- Remove the applicator and place it on the towel. *The applicator is put on the towel to prevent the spread of micro-organisms.*
- Discard the applicator if disposable or clean it according to the manufacturer's directions.
- Ask the patient to remain lying in the supine position for 5–10 minutes following the insertion.

Irrigation
- Place the patient on a bedpan.
- Clamp the tubing. Hang the irrigating container on the IV drip stand so that the base is about 30 cm above the vagina. *At this height, the pressure of the solution should not be great enough to injure the vaginal lining.*
- Run fluid through the tubing and nozzle into the bedpan. *Fluid is run through the tubing to remove air and to moisten the nozzle.*

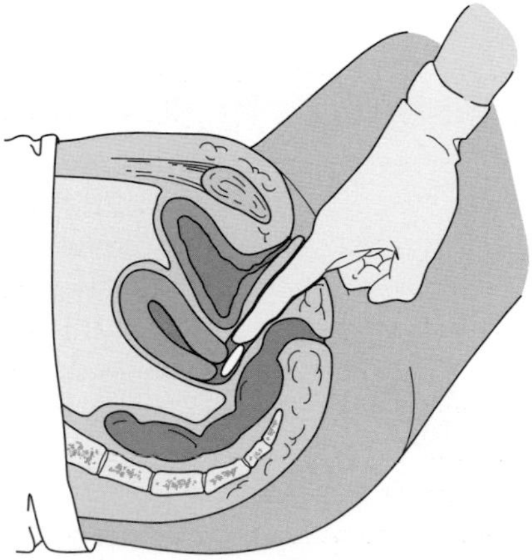

Figure 21-61 Instilling a vaginal suppository.

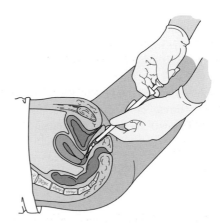

Figure 21-62 Using an applicator to instill a vaginal cream.

- Insert the nozzle carefully into the vagina. Direct the nozzle toward the sacrum, following the direction of the vagina.
- Insert the nozzle about 7–10 cm, start the flow and rotate the nozzle several times. *Rotating the nozzle irrigates all parts of the vagina.*
- Use all of the irrigating solution, permitting it to flow out freely into the bedpan.
- Remove the nozzle from the vagina.

- Assist the patient to a sitting position on the bedpan. *Sitting on the bedpan will help drain the remaining fluid by gravity.*
10. Ensure patient comfort.
    - Dry the perineum with tissues as required.
    - Apply a clean perineal pad if there is excessive drainage.
11. Document all nursing assessments and interventions relative to the procedure. Include the name of the drug or irrigating solution, the strength, the time, and the response of the patient.

Evaluation

+ Perform follow-up based on findings of the effectiveness of the administration or outcomes that deviated from expected or normal for the patient. Relate findings to previous data if available.

A vaginal irrigation (douche) is the washing of the vagina by a liquid at a low pressure. Vaginal irrigations are not necessary for ordinary female hygiene but are used to prevent infection by applying an antimicrobial solution that discourages the growth of micro-organisms, to remove an offensive or irritating discharge, and to reduce inflammation or prevent haemorrhage by the application of heat or cold. In hospitals, sterile supplies and equipment are used; in a home, sterility is not usually necessary because people are accustomed to the micro-organisms in their environments. Sterile technique, however, is indicated if there is an open wound.

Rectal Medications

Insertion of medications into the rectum in the form of suppositories is a frequent practice. Rectal administration is a convenient and safe method of giving certain medications. Advantages include the following:

+ It avoids irritation of the upper gastrointestinal tract in patients who encounter this problem.
+ It is advantageous when the medication has an objectionable taste or odour.
+ The drug is released at a slow but steady rate.
+ Rectal suppositories are thought to provide higher bloodstream levels (titres) of medication because the venous blood from the lower rectum is not transported through the liver.

To insert a rectal suppository:

+ Assist the patient to a left lateral position, with the upper leg flexed.
+ Fold back the top bedclothes to expose the buttocks.
+ Put on a glove on the hand used to insert the suppository.
+ Unwrap the suppository and lubricate the smooth rounded end, or see manufacturer's instructions. The rounded end is usually inserted first and lubricant reduces irritation of the mucosa.

+ Lubricate the gloved index finger.
+ Encourage the patient to relax by breathing through the mouth. This usually relaxes the external anal sphincter.
+ Insert the suppository gently into the anal canal, rounded end first (or according to manufacturer's instructions), along the rectal wall using the gloved index finger. For an adult, insert the suppository beyond the internal sphincter (i.e. 10 cm) (see Figure 21-63).
+ Avoid embedding the suppository in faeces in order for the suppository to be absorbed effectively.
+ Press the patient's buttocks together for a few minutes.
+ Ask the patient to remain in the left lateral or supine position for at least 5 minutes to help retain the suppository. The suppository should be retained for at least 30–40 minutes or according to manufacturer's instructions.

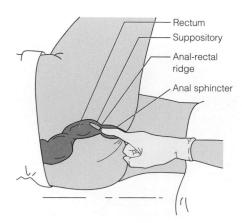

Rectum
Suppository
Anal-rectal ridge
Anal sphincter

Figure 21-63 Inserting a rectal suppository beyond the internal sphincter and along the rectal wall.

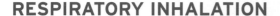

LIFESPAN CONSIDERATIONS

Administering Rectal Medications

Infants/Children

+ Obtain assistance to immobilise an infant or young child. This prevents accidental injury due to sudden movement during the procedure.

+ For a child or infant, insert a suppository 5 cm or less. Rectal medication is not routinely administered to children other routes are used in preference.

RESPIRATORY INHALATION

Nebulisers deliver most medications administered through the inhaled route. A nebuliser is used to deliver a fine spray (fog or mist) of medication or moisture to a patient. There are two kinds of nebulisation: *atomisation* and *aerosolisation*. In atomisation, a device called an *atomiser* produces rather large droplets for inhalation. In aerosolisation, the droplets are suspended in a gas, such as oxygen. The smaller the droplets, the further they can be inhaled into the respiratory tract. When a medication is intended for the nasal mucosa, it is inhaled through the nose; when it is intended for the trachea, bronchi and/or lungs, it is inhaled through the mouth.

A large-volume nebuliser can provide a heated or cool mist. It is used for long-term therapy, such as that following a tracheostomy. The ultrasonic nebuliser (see Figure 21-64) provides 100% humidity and can provide particles small enough to be inhaled deeply into the respiratory tract.

The **metered-dose inhaler (MDI)**, a handheld nebuliser, (see Figure 21-65), is a pressurised container of medication that can be used by the patient to release the medication through a nosepiece or mouthpiece. The force with which the air moves through the nebuliser causes the large particles of medicated solution to break up into finer particles, forming a mist or fine spray.

To ensure correct delivery of the prescribed medication by MDIs, nurses need to instruct patients to use aerosol inhalers correctly. The patient compresses the medication canister by hand to release medication through a mouthpiece. An extender or spacer may be attached to the mouthpiece to facilitate medication absorption for better results (see Figure 21-66). Spacers

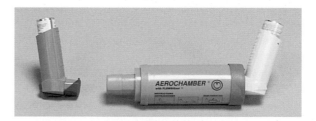

Figure 21-65 Metred-dose inhaler.

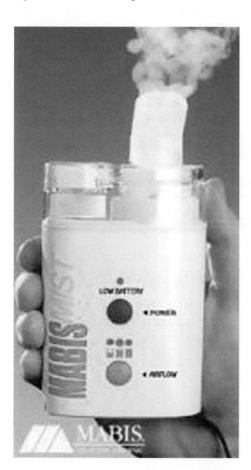

Figure 21-64 Ultrasonic nebuliser. (Courtesy of Mabis Healthcare, Inc.)

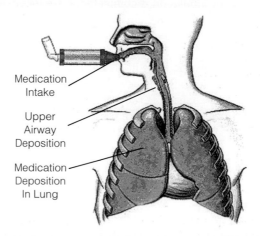

Medication Intake

Upper Airway Deposition

Medication Deposition In Lung

Figure 21-66 Delivery of medication to the lungs using a metered-dose inhaler extender. (Courtesy of Trudell Medical International.)

are holding chambers into which the medication is fired and from which the patient inhales, so that the dose is not lost by exhalation. *Teaching: patient care* provides instructions for patients about using an MDI. Newer breath-activated MDIs are being produced in which inhalation triggers the release of a pre-measured dose of medication.

TEACHING: PATIENT CARE

Using a Metered-dose Inhaler
+ Make sure the canister is firmly and fully inserted into the inhaler.
+ Remove the mouthpiece cap and, holding the inhaler upright, shake the inhaler vigorously for 3-5 seconds to mix the medication evenly.
+ Exhale comfortably (as in a normal full breath).
+ Hold the canister upside down.
+ Put the mouthpiece far enough into the mouth with its opening toward the throat. Close the lips tightly around the mouthpiece. An MDI with a spacer or extender is always placed in the mouth (see Figure 21-67).

Administering the Medication
+ Press down *once* on the MDI canister (which releases the dose) and inhale slowly and deeply through the mouth.
+ Hold your breath for 10 seconds. *This allows the aerosol to reach deeper airways.*
+ Remove the inhaler from or away from the mouth.
+ Exhale slowly through *pursed* lips. *Controlled exhalation keeps the small airways open during exhalation.*
+ Repeat the inhalation if ordered. Wait 20-30 seconds between inhalations of bronchodilator medications *so the first inhalation has a chance to work and the subsequent dose reaches deeper into the lungs.*
+ After the inhalation is completed, rinse mouth with tap water to remove any remaining medication and reduce irritation and risk of infection.
+ Clean the MDI mouthpiece after each use. Use mild soap and water, rinse it, and let it air dry before replacing it on the device.
+ Store the canister at room temperature. Avoid extremes of temperature.

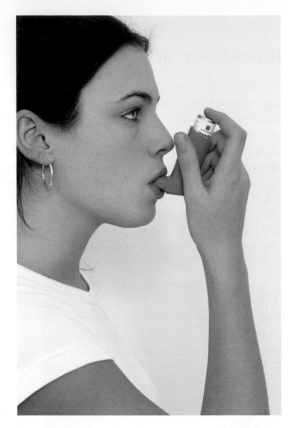

Figure 21-67 Inhaler positioned away from the open mouth.

+ Report adverse reactions such as restlessness, palpitations, nervousness or rash to the prescriber.
+ Many MDIs contain steroids for an anti-inflammatory effect. Prolonged use increases the risk of fungal infections in the mouth.

SUMMARY

Medication can be administered by several routes including the oral, parenteral and topical routes. Each route has its own procedure and equipment with which the nurse should be familiar.

CRITICAL REFLECTION

Revisit the case study on page 509. Now that you have read this chapter, by which route are medications absorbed the fastest-oral, transdermal or subcutaneous? Could any other routes be used for administering Barbara's medication? What must always be checked when administering any medication?

Finally, how might you notice a patient is having an allergic reaction to a medication?

CHAPTER HIGHLIGHTS

+ Medications have several names. Nurses need to know the generic and trade names of a medication and be aware of both its therapeutic and side-effects.
+ Adverse effects of medications include drug toxicity, drug allergy, drug tolerance, idiosyncratic effect and drug interactions.
+ Various routes are used to administer medications: oral, sublingual, buccal, parenteral, topical or via a nasogastric or gastrostomy tube. When administering a medication, the nurse must ensure that it is appropriate for the route specified.
+ Nurses must always assess a patient's physical status before giving any medication and obtain a medication history.
+ When administering medications the nurse observes the six rights to ensure accurate administration. When preparing medications, the nurse checks the medication container label against the medication administration record (MAR).
+ The nurse who prepares the medication administers it and must never leave a prepared medication unattended.
+ The nurse always identifies the patient appropriately before administering a medication and stays with the patient until the medication is taken.

+ Medications, once given, are documented as soon as possible after administration.
+ Medications given parenterally act more quickly than those given orally or topically and must be prepared using sterile technique.
+ Proper site selection is essential for an intramuscular injection to prevent tissue, bone and nerve damage. The nurse should always palpate anatomic landmarks when selecting a site.
+ The Z-track method for intramuscular injection is recommended to prevent discomfort caused by seepage of the medication into subcutaneous tissues.
+ Patients receiving a series of injections should have the injection sites rotated.
+ After use, needles should not be recapped but must be placed in puncture-resistant containers.
+ Topical medications are applied to the skin and mucous membranes primarily for their local effects, although some systemic effects may occur.
+ A metered-dose inhaler (MDI) is a handheld nebuliser that can be used by patients to self-administer measured doses of an aerosol medication. To ensure correct delivery of the prescribed medication by MDIs, nurses need to instruct patients to use aerosol inhalers correctly.

REFERENCES

Bindler, R.C. and Ball, J.W. (2003) *Clinical skills manual for pediatric nursing: Caring for children* (3rd edn), Upper Saddle River, NJ: Prentice Hall.

Brown, D.L. (2002) 'Does 1 + 1 still equal 2? A study of the mathematic competencies of associate degree nursing students', *Nurse Educator*, 27(3), 132–135.

Fleming, D.R. (1999). 'Challenging traditional insulin injection practices', *American Journal of Nursing*, 99(2), 72–74.

Kudzma, E.C. (1999). 'Culturally competent drug administration', *American Journal of Nursing*, 99(8), 46–51.

McCaffery, M. and Pasero, C. (1999) *Pain clinical manual* (2nd edn), St. Louis, MO: Mosby.

Nursing Midwifery Councl (2004) *Standards for the administration of medicines*, London: NMC.

GUIDANCE

For the full text of Acts and Regulations mentioned in this chapter see www.legislation.hmso.gov.uk.

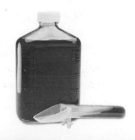

Chapter 22 Pain Management

Learning Outcomes

After completing this chapter, you will be able to:

+ Identify types and categories of pain according to location, aetiology and duration.

+ Differentiate pain threshold from pain tolerance.

+ Describe the four processes involved in nociception and how pain interventions can work during each process.

+ Outline the gate control theory and its application to nursing care.

+ Identify subjective and objective data to collect and analyse when assessing pain.

+ Identify barriers to effective pain management.

+ Describe pharmacological interventions for pain.

+ Describe the World Health Organization's ladder step approach to cancer pain.

+ Identify rationales for using various analgesic delivery routes.

+ Describe nonpharmacological pain control interventions.

+ Evaluate the effectiveness of pain relief.

CASE STUDY

A 'one-in-a-billion boy', that is how Ben Whittaker is being hailed by the British press (*Daily Mail*, 2005). Ben, a 17-month-old boy from Yorkshire, is the 33rd person in the world to be diagnosed with a rare genetic disorder known as congenital analgesia or congenital indifference to pain which means that he cannot feel any pain.

Although being unable to feel pain sounds appealing, it is in fact extremely dangerous and life-threatening. Pain after all is a protective warning sign that the body is being damaged. Therefore a person with congenital analgesia may be caused serious injury without being aware of it.

This chapter will aim to explore the concept of pain and the importance of pain in protecting the body.

INTRODUCTION

Pain is an unpleasant and personal sensation that cannot be shared with others. It can be all-consuming, occupying a person's thinking and being. Yet pain is a difficult concept for an individual to communicate. McCaffery defines **pain** as 'whatever the experiencing person says it is, existing whenever he (or she) says it does' (McCaffery and Pasero, 1999: 5). McCaffery's definition of pain hints at the subjective nature of pain and the importance of believing the patient.

People experience and react to pain differently and as nurses we cannot feel what the patient feels yet we have a duty to maintain the individual's dignity and where possible relieve their pain and promote comfort. Indeed pain management is an important aspect of nursing care.

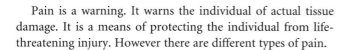

CLINICAL ANECDOTE

On one of my first placements in a hospital I was looking after a patient who had returned from theatre after having a laparoscopy. She was having pain relief via a patient controlled analgesia (PCA) pump but when I went to check on her she was complaining of pain. I went to see my mentor who said that the patient couldn't possibly be in that much pain after such a small operation. I couldn't believe my ears, and the first thing that came into my mind was McCaffery's definition of pain.

A student nurse

Pain is a warning. It warns the individual of actual tissue damage. It is a means of protecting the individual from life-threatening injury. However there are different types of pain.

TYPES OF PAIN

Clear distinctions cannot always be made between the different types of pain. The more simplified classification of pain are (1) acute, (2) chronic malignant or cancer pain or (3) chronic non-malignant pain. However other methods of classifying pain exist such as those according to inferred pathophysiology: (1) nociceptive and (2) neuropathic. Pain can also be classified according to its location: (1) superficial, (2) deep and (3) referred. In order to classify the type of pain the patient is experiencing the nurse needs to have knowledge of each type of pain, possible location, duration, severity and sensation. Table 22-1 on page 574 compares each of these classifications of pain.

CONCEPTS ASSOCIATED WITH PAIN

Nursing patients with pain requires knowledge of pain and its related concepts. A number of terms are used in relation to pain such as **pain threshold**, which refers to the amount of painful stimulation that an individual requires in order to feel pain. A number of research studies have looked at this concept over the past six decades. The study by Hardy *et al.* (1943) suggested that everyone perceives the same intensity of pain from the same stimuli, meaning that we all have the same pain threshold. However later studies have proved that this is not the case (Beecher, 1956). Indeed pain threshold and intensity varies from person to person as in the case of someone with **hyperalgesia** who is extremely sensitive to pain compared to another person with **congenital analgesia** who feel no pain.

Another common term heard in nursing is **pain tolerance**. Pain tolerance is the maximum amount and duration of pain that an individual is willing to endure. Some patients are unable to tolerate even the slightest pain, whereas others are willing to endure severe pain rather than be treated for it. Like pain threshold, pain tolerance varies from person to person and is widely influenced by psychological and sociocultural factors.

In order to understand the nursing management of a patient in pain, we must first understand the physiology of pain.

PHYSIOLOGY OF PAIN

Transmission and perception of pain is still not fully understood. A number of pain theories have been proposed over the past few decades including the Gate Control Theory (Melzack and Wall, 1965). However McCaffery and Pasero (1999) suggest that there are four processes involved in nociception (no-si-sep-shon), a term used to describe the point at which an individual becomes conscious of pain: (1) transduction, (2) transmission, (3) perception and (4) modulation (Paice, 2002) (see Figure 22-2 on page 576).

Transduction

Transduction is the first process involved in nociception and begins with tissue injury. This injury is sensed by nociceptors (no-si-sep-tors, the nerve endings that sense pain). These trigger the release of chemical substances (e.g. prostagladins, bradykinin, serotonin, histamine, substance P) that help the

Table 22-1 Types of Pain

Type of pain	Location/severity/duration	Sensation	Examples
Superficial	Skin and mucous membranes. Short duration, mild to severe pain depending on cause. Can be acute, chronic, nociceptive or neuropathic in nature.	Burning or pricking sensation.	First degree burn (superficial burn minimal damage to skin).
Deep	Muscles, joints and body organs. Short to long lasting depending on cause. Mild to severe pain depending on cause. Can be acute, chronic, nociceptive or neuropathic in nature.	Aching, not easily localised.	Sprain, bowel obstruction.
Referred	Felt at a site other than the injured site. Mild to severe pain depending on cause. Usually short duration. Usually acute or nociceptive in nature.	Aching pain.	Pain in left arm during myocardial infarction (heart attack). 'Brain freeze' – when cold food hits the roof of the mouth the vagus nerve is chilled and causes referred pain in the forehead. See Figure 22-1 for common sites for referred pain.
Acute	Anywhere in the body. Sudden onset and foreseeable end. Mild to severe pain depending on cause. Relatively short duration. The patient will display fight or flight responses (see Table 22-2). Can be superficial, deep, referred or nociceptive in nature.	Sharp, burning, pricking, aching pains noted.	Pain following surgery.
Chronic	Anywhere in the body. Usually lasts longer than six months. Moderate to severe pain depending on the cause.	Sharp, burning, pricking, aching pains noted.	Arthritis, back pain, cancer pain.
Nociceptive	Results from injury to the skin, mucous membranes, bones, muscles or organs of the body. Short or long lasting. Mild to severe depending on cause. Can be acute, chronic, superficial, deep or referred in nature.	Sharp, burning, pricking, aching pains noted.	Sprains, fractures, inflammation (such as arthritis) and obstructions.
Neuropathic	Caused by injury or malfunction of the peripheral or central nervous system.	Sharp, burning, pricking, aching pains noted.	Post-herptic zoster pain (pain felt after having shingles), phantom pain following amputation of a limb.

pain impulse travel from the periphery to the spinal cord (see Figure 22-2). The process of transduction can be stimulated by different types of pain stimuli (see Table 22-3 on page 576). Certain analgesic (pain) medications have been developed to work during transduction, such as ibuprofen which blocks the production of prostaglandin.

Transmission

The second process of nociception, transmission of pain, includes three segments (McCaffery and Pasero, 1999).

1. The pain impulse travels from the peripheral nerve fibres to the spinal cord.
2. Transmission of the pain impulse by neurotransmitters from the spinal cord to the brain stem and thalamus (see Figure 22-2).
3. Transmission of pain impulse between the thalamus and the cortex where pain perception occurs.

Pain control can take place during the second segment of transmission. For example, opioids (morphine) block the release of neurotransmitters which stops the pain at the spinal level.

Perception

The third process, perception, is when the patient becomes conscious of the pain. It is not known where the precise location for perception is in the brain. However it is believed that pain perception occurs in the cortical structures of the brain. It is here that non-pharmacological interventions can be used to relieve pain including distractions such as watching television, talking and guided imagery, which use the power of the imagination to relieve pain.

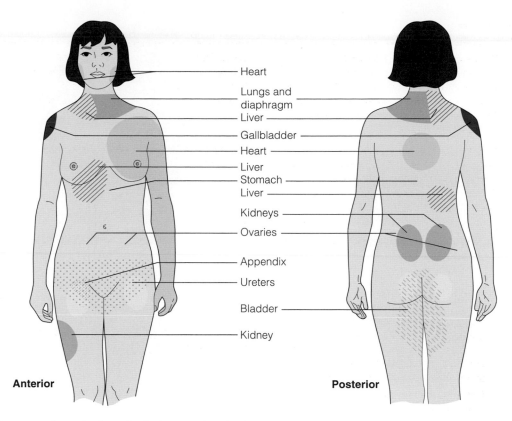

Figure 22-1 Common sites of referred pain from various body organs.

Table 22-2 Comparison of Acute and Chronic Pain

Acute pain	Chronic pain
Mild to severe	Mild to severe

Sympathetic nervous system responses:
   Increased pulse rate
   Increased respiratory rate
   Elevated blood pressure
   Diaphoresis
   Dilated pupils
	Parasympathetic nervous system responses:
	   Vital signs normal
	
	   Dry, warm skin
	   Pupils normal or dilated

Related to tissue injury; resolves with healing	Continues beyond healing
Patient appears restless and anxious	Patient appears depressed and withdrawn
Patient reports pain	Patient often does not mention pain unless asked
Patient exhibits behaviour indicative of pain: crying, rubbing area, holding area	Pain behaviour often absent

Modulation

Modulation is the fourth process involved in nociception. During this process, nerves in the brain stem send signals back down to the spinal cord (Paice, 2002: 75), releasing substances that act as natural painkillers such as endorphins and serotonin. These substances do not last long in the body and therefore their painkilling use is limited. However patients with chronic pain may be prescribed medications such as tricyclic antidepressants which inhibit (stop) the body from absorbing the endorphins and serotonin thereby increasing their painkilling effect.

Gate Control Theory

Melzack and Wall (1965) proposed an alternative notion for the perception and treatment of pain. Their theory is based on the fact that pain impulses are normally carried to the spinal cord from the peripheries in small nerve fibres. Large nerve

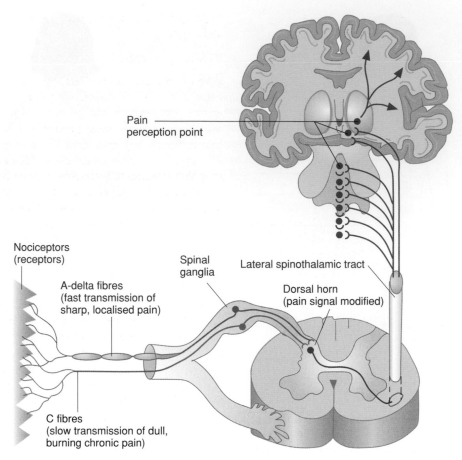

Figure 22-2 Physiology of pain perception.

Table 22-3 Types of Pain Stimuli

Stimulus type	Physiological basis of pain
Mechanical	
1. Trauma to body tissues (e.g. surgery)	Tissue damage; direct irritation of the pain receptors; inflammation
2. Alterations in body tissues (e.g. oedema)	Pressure on pain receptors
3. Blockage of a body duct	Distention (swelling) of the lumen (hole) of the duct
4. Tumour	Pressure on pain receptors; irritation of nerve endings
5. Muscle spasm	Stimulation of pain receptors (also see chemical stimuli)
Thermal	
Extreme heat or cold (e.g. burns)	Tissue destruction; stimulation of thermo sensitive pain receptors
Chemical	
1. Tissue ischemia (e.g. blocked coronary artery)	Stimulation of pain receptors because of accumulated lactic acid (and other chemicals, such as bradykinin and enzymes) in tissues
2. Muscle spasm	Tissue ischemia secondary to mechanical stimulation (see above)

fibres, on the other hand, carry non-nociceptive stimuli such as touch, warmth, massage, vibration, etc. According to Melzack and Wall (1965) impulses travelling through the large fibres can block the impulses travelling through the small fibres at a 'gate', which is situated at the spinal cord (see Figure 22-3). They therefore suggest that skin stimulation following injury can block the pain impulses from the injury. For example, if you bang your head what is the first thing you do; rub it.

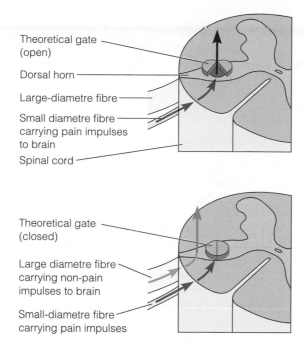

Figure 22-3 A schematic illustration of the gate control theory.

Responses to Pain

Response to pain varies from person to person. Some patients may show little response to pain as they have developed coping strategies to distract themselves. Others may verbalise their pain, or shout or scream with pain.

The body's response to pain is a complex process that incorporates physiological and psychosocial aspects. When pain is initially felt, the sympathetic nervous system responds, resulting in the fight or flight response, which explains the dilation of the pupils and an increased heart and respiratory rate. As pain continues, the body adapts as the parasympathetic nervous system takes over, reversing many of the initial physiological responses so blood pressure decreases and heart rate and respiratory rate return to normal. This adaptation to pain occurs after several hours or days of pain. The actual pain receptors adapt very little and continue to transmit the pain message. The person may learn to cope with the pain through cognitive and behavioural activities, such as diversions, imagery and excessive sleeping.

A proprioceptive reflex also occurs with the stimulation of pain receptors. Impulses travel along sensory pain fibres to the spinal cord. There they synapse with motor neurons, and the impulses travel back via motor fibres to a muscle near the site of the pain. The muscle then contracts in a protective action. For example, when a person touches a hot stove the hand reflexively draws back from the heat even before the person is aware of the pain.

Factors Affecting the Pain Experience

There are a number of factors that can affect a person's perception of and reaction to pain such as developmental stage, previous pain experiences, cultural beliefs, anxiety and stress.

Ethnic and Cultural Values

Ethnic background and cultural heritage have long been recognised as factors that influence both a person's reaction to pain and the expression of that pain. Behaviour related to pain is a part of the socialisation process. For example, individuals in one culture may have learned to be expressive about pain, whereas individuals from another culture may have learned to keep those feelings to themselves and not bother others.

Although there appears to be little variation in pain threshold, cultural background can affect the level of pain that an individual is willing to tolerate. In some Middle Eastern and African cultures, self-infliction of pain is a sign of mourning or grief. In other groups, pain may be anticipated as part of the ritualistic practices, and therefore tolerance of pain signifies strength and endurance. Additionally, there are significant variations in the expression of pain. Studies have shown that individuals of northern European descent tend to be more stoic and less expressive of their pain than individuals from southern European backgrounds.

Nurses must realise they have their own attitudes and expectations about pain. Andrews and Boyle (2003) point out that healthcare has been dominated by white Anglo-Saxon Protestants and most nurses have been influenced by these values and beliefs. For example, nurses may place a higher value on silent suffering or self-control in response to pain. Nurses expect people to be objective about pain and to be able to provide a detailed description of the pain. Nurses may deny or downplay the pain they observe in others. Therefore, identifying your own personal attitude about pain and creating an effective nurse–patient relationship is imperative for providing culturally competent care for patients in pain.

Developmental Stage

The age and developmental stage of a patient is an important variable that will influence both the reaction to and the expression of pain. Age variations and related nursing interventions are presented in Table 22-4 on page 578.

The field of pain management for infants and children has grown significantly. It is now accepted that anatomic, physiological and biochemical elements necessary for pain transmission are present in newborns, regardless of their gestational age. Physiological indicators may vary in infants, so behavioural observation is recommended for pain assessment (Ball and Bindler, 2003). Children may be less able than an adult to articulate their experience or needs related to pain, which may result in their pain being under treated.

Older adults constitute a major portion of the individuals within the healthcare system. The prevalence of pain in the older population is generally higher due to both acute and chronic disease conditions. Pain threshold does not appear to change with ageing, although the effect of analgesics may increase due to physiological changes related to drug metabolism and excretion (Eliopoulos, 2001).

Table 22-4 Age Variations in the Pain Experience

Age group	Pain perception and behaviour	Selected nursing interventions
Infant	Perceives pain. Responds to pain with increased sensitivity. Older infant tries to avoid pain; for example, turns away and physically resists.	Use tactile stimulation. Play music or tapes of a heartbeat.
Toddler and preschooler	Develops the ability to describe pain and its intensity and location. Often responds with crying and anger because child perceives pain as a threat to security. Reasoning with child at this stage is not always successful. May consider pain a punishment. Feels sad. Tends to hold someone accountable for the pain.	Distract the child with toys, books, pictures. Involve the child in blowing bubbles as a way of 'blowing away the pain'. Appeal to the child's belief in magic by using a 'magic' blanket or glove to take away pain. Hold the child to provide comfort. Explore misconceptions about pain.
School-age child	Tries to be brave when facing pain. Rationalises in an attempt to explain the pain. Responsive to explanations. Can usually identify the location and describe the pain. With persistent pain, may regress to an earlier stage of development.	Use imagery to turn off 'pain switches'. Provide a behavioral rehearsal of what to expect and how it will look and feel. Provide support and nurturing.
Adolescent	May be slow to acknowledge pain. Recognising pain or 'giving in' may be considered weakness. Wants to appear brave in front of peers and not report pain.	Provide opportunities to discuss pain. Provide privacy. Present choices for dealing with pain. Encourage music or TV for distraction.
Adult	Behaviours exhibited when experiencing pain may be gender-based behaviours learned as a child. May ignore pain because to admit it is perceived as a sign of weakness or failure. Fear of what pain means may prevent some adults from taking action.	Deal with any misconceptions about pain. Focus on the patient's control in dealing with the pain. Allay fears and anxiety when possible.
Older adult	May have multiple conditions presenting with vague symptoms. May perceive pain as part of the ageing process. May have decreased sensations or perceptions of the pain. Lethargy, anorexia and fatigue may be indicators of pain. May withhold complaints of pain because of fear of the treatment, of any lifestyle changes that may be involved, or of becoming dependent. May describe pain differently, that is, as 'ache', 'hurt' or 'discomfort'. May consider it unacceptable to admit or show pain.	Thorough history and assessment is essential. Spend time with the patient and listen carefully. Clarify misconceptions. Encourage independence whenever possible.

Environmental Factors and Support People

A number of environmental factors can compound pain, such as a strange environment (e.g. hospital and loneliness). An individual who is without a support network may perceive pain as severe, whereas an individual who is surrounded by supportive family and friends may perceive less pain.

Expectations of significant others can affect a person's perceptions of and responses to pain. In some situations, for example, girls may be permitted to express pain more openly than boys. Family role can also affect how a person perceives or responds to pain. For instance, a single mother supporting three children may ignore pain because of her need to stay on the job.

Past Pain Experiences

Previous pain experiences alter a patient's sensitivity to pain. People who have personally experienced pain or who have been exposed to the suffering of someone close are often more threatened by anticipated pain than people without a pain experience. In addition, the success or lack of success of pain relief measures influences a person's expectations for relief. For example, a person who has tried several pain relief measures without success may have little hope about the helpfulness of nursing interventions.

Meaning of Pain

Some patients may accept pain more readily than others, depending on the circumstances and the patient's interpretation of its significance. A patient who associates the pain with a positive outcome may withstand the pain amazingly well. For example, a woman giving birth to a child or an athlete undergoing knee surgery to prolong his career may tolerate pain better because of the benefit associated with it. These patients may view the pain as a temporary inconvenience rather than a potential threat or disruption to daily life.

By contrast, patients with unrelenting chronic pain may suffer more intensely. They may respond with despair, anxiety and depression because they cannot attach a positive significance or purpose to the pain. In this situation, the pain may be looked on as a threat to body image or lifestyle and as a sign of possible impending death.

Anxiety and Stress

Anxiety often accompanies pain. The threat of the unknown and the inability to control the pain or the events surrounding it often augment the pain perception. Fatigue also reduces a person's ability to cope, thereby increasing pain perception. When pain interferes with sleep, fatigue and muscle tension often result and increase the pain; thus a cycle of pain–fatigue–pain develops. People in pain who believe that they have control of their pain have decreased fear and anxiety, which decreases their pain perception. A perception of lacking control or a sense of helplessness tends to increase pain perception. Patients who are able to express pain to an attentive listener and participate in pain management decisions can increase a sense of control and decrease pain perception.

NURSING MANAGEMENT

ASSESSING

Accurate pain assessment is essential for effective pain management. Pain is subjective and experienced uniquely by each individual; therefore nurses need to assess all factors affecting the pain experience – physiological, psychological, behavioural, emotional and sociocultural.

The extent and frequency of the pain assessment varies according to the situation. For patients experiencing acute or severe pain, the nurse may focus only on location, quality, severity and early intervention. Patients with less severe or chronic pain can usually provide a more detailed description of the experience. Frequency of pain assessment usually depends on the pain control measures being used and the clinical circumstances. Following pain management interventions, pain intensity should be reassessed at an interval appropriate for the intervention. For example, following the intravenous administration of morphine, the severity of pain should be reassessed in 20–30 minutes.

Because it has been found that many people will not voice their pain unless asked about it, pain assessments must be initiated by the nurse. Some of the many reasons patients may be reluctant to report pain are listed in *Box 22-1*. It is also essential that nurses listen to and rely on the patient's perceptions of pain. Believing the person experiencing and conveying the perceptions is crucial in establishing a sense of trust.

Pain assessments consist of two major components: (a) a history of the pain to obtain facts from the patient and (b) direct observation of behavioural and physiological responses of the patient. The goal of assessment is to gain an objective understanding of a subjective experience. *Box 22-2* on page 580 provides helpful mnemonics to make a complete pain assessment.

> **BOX 22-1** Why Patients May Be Reluctant to Report Pain
>
> + Unwillingness to trouble staff who are perceived as busy
> + Fear of the injectable route of analgesic administration
> + Belief that pain is to be expected as part of the recovery process
> + Belief that pain is a normal part of ageing or a necessary part of life – older adults in particular
> + Belief that expressions of pain reveal weakness
> + Difficulty expressing personal discomfort
> + Concern about risks associated with opioid drugs (e.g. addiction)
> + Fear about the cause of pain
> + Concern about unwanted side-effects, especially of opioid drugs
> + Concern that use of drugs now will render the drug inefficient if or when the pain becomes worse

BOX 22-2 Mnemonics for Pain Assessment

OLDCART mnemonic

O – onset
L – location
D – duration
C – characteristic
A – aggravating factors
R – radiation
T – treatment (what was previously ineffective and what has alleviated the pain)

PQRST mnemonic

P – provoked (what brought about pain)
Q – quality
R – region/radiation
S – severity
T – timing

Note: From 'Undertreated Pain: Could It Land You in Court?' by S. LaDuke, 2002, *Nursing, 32*, p. 18. Reprinted with permission.

Pain History

While questioning the patient about the pain it is important that the nurse provides an opportunity for the patient to express in their own words how they view the pain and the situation. This will help the nurse understand what the pain means to the patient and how the patient is coping with it. Remember that each person's pain experience is unique and that the patient is the best interpreter of the pain experience. This history should be geared to the specific patient: for example, questions asked of an accident victim would be different from those asked of a post-operative patient or one suffering from chronic pain. The initial pain assessment for someone in severe acute pain may consist of only a few questions before intervention occurs. In addition, the nurse may focus on the following:

+ Previous pain treatment and effectiveness
+ When and what analgesics were last taken
+ Other medications being taken
+ Allergies to medications.

For the person with chronic pain, the nurse may focus on the patient's coping mechanisms, effectiveness of current pain management, and ways in which the pain has affected activities of daily living (ADLs).

Information needed include pain location, intensity/severity, quality, patterns, precipitating factors, alleviating factors, associated symptoms, effect on activities of daily living (ADLs), past pain experiences, meaning of the pain to the person, coping mechanisms and emotional responses.

Location

To ascertain the specific location of the pain, ask the individual to point to the site of the discomfort or ask the patient to mark the location of the pain on a chart consisting of drawings of the body. This tool can be especially effective with patients who have more than one source of pain.

When assessing the location of a child's pain, the nurse needs to understand the child's vocabulary. For example, *tummy* might refer either to the abdomen or to part of the chest. Asking the child to point to the pain helps clarify where the pain is located. Again the use of figure drawings can assist in identifying pain locations. Parents can also be helpful in interpreting the meaning of a child's words.

Pain Intensity or Rating Scales

The single most important indicator of the existence and intensity of pain is the patient's report of pain. In practice, however, McCaffery *et al.* (2000) found that nurses tend to use less reliable measures for assessing pain. The top factors used to identify the level of pain in a patient were facial expressions, verbalisation (what the patient reports) and request for pain relief. In addition, studies have shown that healthcare professionals may underrate or overrate the pain intensity (Bergh and Sjostrom, 1999). The use of pain intensity scales is an easy and reliable method of determining the patient's pain intensity. Such scales provide consistency for nurses to communicate with the patient and other healthcare providers. Most scales use either a 0–5 or 0–10 range with 0 indicating 'no pain' and the highest number indicating the 'worst pain possible' for that individual. A 10-point rating scale is shown in Figure 22-4. These scales also include words such as 'no pain' or 'severe pain' to assist patients who find it difficult to apply a number level to their pain. The patient is asked to indicate the scale point that best represents the pain intensity.

CLINICAL ALERT

Perception is reality. The patient's self-report of pain is what must be used to determine pain intensity. If you do not believe the patient, you are not acting in the patient's best interests.

When noting pain intensity it is important to determine any related factors that may be affecting the pain. If there is a change in the intensity of the pain, the nurse needs to consider possible causes. Several factors affect the perception of intensity: (1) the amount of distraction or the patient's concentration on another event; (2) the patient's state of consciousness; (3) the level of activity; and (4) the patient's expectations.

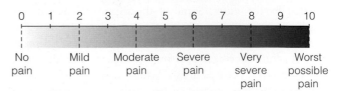

Figure 22-4 A 10-point pain intensity scale with word modifiers.

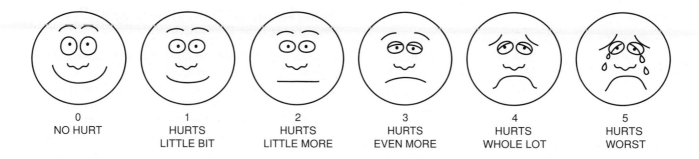

0	1	2	3	4	5
NO HURT	HURTS LITTLE BIT	HURTS LITTLE MORE	HURTS EVEN MORE	HURTS WHOLE LOT	HURTS WORST

Explain to the person that each face is for a person who feels happy because he has no pain (hurt) or sad because he has some or a lot of pain. Face 0 is very happy because he doesn't hurt at all. Face 1 hurts just a little bit. Face 2 hurts a little more. Face 3 hurts even more. Face 4 hurts a whole lot. Face 5 hurts as much as you can imagine, although you don't have to be crying to feel this bad. Ask the person to choose the face that best describes how he is feeling.

Rating scale is recommended for persons age 3 years and older.

Brief word instructions: Point to each face using the words to describe the pain intensity. Ask the child to choose the face that best describes own pain and record the appropriate number.

Figure 22-5 The Wong-Baker FACES Rating Scale. (*Note: From Wong's Essentials of Pediatric Nursing*, 6th edn (p. 1301), by D.L. Wong M. Hockenserry-Eaton, D. Wilson, M.L. Winkelstein, and P. Schwartz, 2001, St. Louis, MO: Mosby. Reprinted with permission.)

Not all patients can understand or relate to numerical pain intensity scales. These include children who are unable to communicate discomfort verbally, older patients with impairments in cognition or communication, and people who do not speak English. For these patients the Wong-Baker FACES Rating Scale (see Figure 22-5) may be easier to use (Wong *et al.*, 2001). The face scale includes a number scale in relation to each expression so that the pain intensity can be documented. When it is not possible to use any kind of rating scale with a patient, the nurse must rely on observation of behaviour and any physiological cues discussed later in this section. The input of the patient's significant others, such as parents or caregivers, can assist the nurse in interpreting the observations. An objective description of the patient's behaviour and any physiological observations such as an increase in blood pressure should then be documented.

CLINICAL ALERT

A guideline based on studies: on a scale of 0-10, a pain rating of 3 or greater signals a need to revise the pain treatment plan (e.g. higher dose or different analgesia). A rating of 6 or more demands immediate attention (McCaffery and Pasero, 1999: 74-75).

Pain Quality

Descriptive adjectives help people communicate the quality of pain. A headache may be described as 'hammerlike' or an abdominal pain as 'piercing like a knife'. Sometimes patients have difficulty describing pain because they have never experienced any sensation like it. Some of the terms commonly used to describe pain are listed in Table 22-5.

Table 22-5 Commonly Used Pain Descriptors

Term	Sensory words	Affective words
Pain	Searing	Unbearable
	Scalding	Killing
	Sharp	Intense
	Piercing	Torturing
	Drilling	Agonising
	Wrenching	Terrifying
	Shooting	Exhausting
	Burning	Suffocating
	Crushing	Frightful
	Penetrating	Punishing
		Miserable
Hurt	Hurting	Heavy
	Pricking	
	Pressing	
	Tender	Throbbing
Ache	Numb	Annoying
	Cold	Nagging
	Flickering	Tiring
	Radiating	Troublesome
	Dull	Gnawing
	Sore	Uncomfortable
	Aching	Sickening
	Cramping	Tender

Nurses need to record the exact words patients use to describe pain. A patient's words are more accurate and descriptive than an interpretation in the nurse's words. Exact information can be significant in both the diagnosis of the cause of the pain and in the treatment choices made.

NURSING MANAGEMENT

Pattern

The pattern of pain includes time of onset, duration and recurrence or intervals without pain. The nurse therefore determines when the pain began; how long the pain lasts; whether it recurs and, if so, the length of the interval without pain; and when the pain last occurred.

Precipitating Factors

Certain activities sometimes precede pain. For example, physical exertion may precede chest pain or abdominal pain may occur after eating. These observations can help prevent pain and determine its cause.

Environmental factors such as extreme cold or heat and extremes of humidity can affect some types of pain. For example, sudden exercise on a hot day can cause muscle spasm.

Physical and emotional stressors can also precipitate pain. Emotional tension frequently brings on a migraine headache. Intense fear or physical exertion can cause angina.

Alleviating Factors

Nurses must ask patients to describe anything that they have done to alleviate the pain (e.g. home remedies such as herbal teas, medications, rest, applications of heat or cold, prayer or distractions like TV). It is important to explore the effect any of these measures had on the pain, whether or not relief was obtained, or whether the pain became worse.

Associated Symptoms

Also included in the clinical appraisal of pain are associated symptoms such as nausea, vomiting, dizziness and diarrhoea. These symptoms may relate to the onset of the pain or they may result from the presence of the pain.

Effect on Activities of Daily Living (ADLs)

Knowing how ADLs, such as ability to maintain hygiene needs, are affected by chronic pain helps the nurse understand the patient's perspective on the pain's severity.

Coping Mechanisms

Each individual will exhibit personal ways of coping with pain. Strategies may relate to earlier pain experiences or the specific meaning of the pain; some may reflect religious or cultural influences. Nurses can encourage and support the patient's use of methods known to have helped in alleviating or relieving the pain. Strategies may include withdrawal, distraction, prayer or other religious practices, and support from significant others.

Emotional Responses

Emotional responses vary according to the situation, the degree and duration of pain, the interpretation of it and many other factors. The nurse needs to explore the patient's feelings of anxiety, fear, exhaustion, depression or a sense of failure. Because many people with chronic pain become depressed and potentially suicidal, it may also be necessary to assess the patient's suicide risk.

Observation of Behavioural and Physiological Responses

There are wide variations in nonverbal responses to pain. For patients who are very young, aphasic (apha-sic, an inability to use or understand language), confused or disoriented, nonverbal expressions may be the only means of communicating pain. Facial expression is often the first indication of pain and it may be the only one. Clenched teeth, tightly shut eyes, biting of the lower lip and other facial grimaces may be indicative of pain. The patient may also moan, groan, cry or scream when in pain.

Immobilising the body or a part of the body may also indicate pain. The patient with chest pain often holds the left arm across the chest. A person with abdominal pain may assume the position of greatest comfort, often with the knees and hips flexed, and move reluctantly. Purposeless body movements can also indicate pain – for example, tossing and turning in bed or flinging the arms about.

Rhythmic body movements or rubbing may indicate pain. An adult or child may assume a foetal position and rock back and forth when experiencing abdominal pain. During labour a woman may massage her abdomen rhythmically with her hands.

It is important to note that behavioural responses can be controlled and so may not be very revealing. When pain is chronic the patient may not show any visible signs of being in pain as they will have developed personal coping mechanisms for dealing with the pain.

Physiological responses vary with the origin and duration of the pain. Early in the onset of acute pain the sympathetic nervous system is stimulated, resulting in increased blood pressure, pulse rate, respiratory rate, pallor, diaphoresis and pupil dilation. The body does not sustain the increased sympathetic function over a prolonged period of time and, therefore, the sympathetic nervous system adapts, making the physiological responses less evident or even absent. Physiological responses are most likely to be absent in people with chronic pain because of central nervous system (CNS) adapts to the pain. Thus, it is important that the nurse assess more than only physiological responses, because they may be poor indicators of pain.

Daily Pain Diary

For patients who experience chronic pain, a daily diary may help the patient and nurse identify pain patterns and factors that exacerbate or mediate the pain experience. In the community, the family or other carer can be taught to complete the diary. The record can include:

+ Time or onset of pain
+ Activity before pain
+ Pain-related positions or behaviours
+ Pain intensity level
+ Use of analgesics or other relief measures
+ Duration of pain
+ Time spent in relief activities.

Recorded data can provide the basis for developing or modifying the care plan. For this tool to be effective, it is important that the nurse educate the patient and family about the value and use of the diary in achieving effective pain control. Determining the patient's abilities to use the diary is essential.

PLANNING

The established goals for the patient will vary according to the diagnosis and its defining characteristics. Specific nursing interventions can be selected to meet the individual needs of the patient.

PRACTICE GUIDELINES

Individualising Care for Patients with Pain

+ Establish a trusting relationship through effective communication.
+ Consider the patient's ability and willingness to participate actively in pain relief measures. Some patients who are excessively fatigued are sedated; those who have altered levels of consciousness are less able to participate actively.
+ Use a variety of pain relief measures. It is thought that using more than one measure has an additive effect in relieving pain.
+ Provide measures to relieve pain before it becomes severe. For example, providing an analgesic before the onset of pain is preferable to waiting for the patient to complain of pain, when a larger dose may be required.
+ Use pain-relieving measures that the patient believes are effective unless it is known to be harmful.
+ Base the choice of pain relief measure on the patient's report of the severity of the pain.
+ If a pain relief measure is ineffective, encourage the patient to try it once or twice more before

abandoning it. Anxiety may diminish the effects of a pain measure, and some approaches, such as distraction strategies, require practice before they are effective.

+ Maintain an open mind about what may relieve the pain. New ways to relieve pain are continually being developed. It is not always possible to explain pain relief measures; however, measures should be supported unless they are harmful.
+ Keep trying. Do not ignore a patient because pain persists in spite of measures. In these circumstances, reassess the pain, and consider other ways of relieving the pain.
+ Prevent harm to the patient. Pain therapy should not increase discomfort or harm the patient. Some pain relief measures may have adverse untoward effects, such as drowsiness, but they should not disable the patient.
+ Educate the patient and support people about pain. Patients and their families need to be informed about possible causes of pain, precipitating and alleviating factors, and alternatives to drug therapy. Misconceptions also need to be corrected.

Planning Independent of Setting

When planning, nurses need to choose pain relieving measures appropriate for the patient, based on the assessment. Nursing interventions may include a variety of pharmacological and nonpharmacological interventions. Developing a plan that incorporates a wide range of strategies is usually most effective. Whether in acute care or in the community, it is important for everyone involved in pain management to understand the plan of care.

IMPLEMENTING

Pain management is the alleviation of pain or a reduction in pain to a level of comfort that is acceptable to the patient. It includes two basic types of nursing interventions: pharmacological and nonpharmacological. Management of pain requires

input from the multidisciplinary team in conjunction with the patient.

Generally speaking, a combination of strategies is best for the patient in pain. Sometimes strategies need to be tried and changed until the patient obtains effective pain relief. See the *Practice guidelines* for individualising care for patients with pain.

Barriers to Pain Management

Misconceptions and biases can affect pain management. These may involve attitudes of the nurse or the patient as well as knowledge deficits. Patients respond to pain experiences based on their culture, personal experiences and the meaning the pain has for them. For many people, pain is expected and accepted as a normal aspect of illness. Patients and their families may lack knowledge of the effects of pain and the use of analgesia. Common misconceptions are shown in Table 22-6 on page 584.

Table 22-6 Common Misconceptions about Pain

Misconception	Correction
Patients experience severe pain only when they have had major surgery.	Even after minor surgery, patients can experience intense pain.
The nurse or other healthcare professionals are the authorities on a patient's pain.	The person who experiences the pain is the only authority on its existence and nature.
Administering analgesia regularly for pain will lead to addiction.	Patients are unlikely to become addicted to analgesia provided to treat pain.
The amount of tissue damage is directly related to the amount of pain.	Pain is a subjective experience, and the intensity and duration of pain vary considerably among individuals.
Visible physiological or behavioural signs accompany pain and can be used to verify its existence.	Even with severe pain, periods of physiologic and behavioural adaptation can occur.

Key Factors in Pain Management

Key factors in reducing pain include acknowledging and accepting the patient's pain, assisting family and friends, reducing misconceptions about pain, reducing fear and anxiety, and preventing pain.

Acknowledging and Accepting Patient's Pain

Basic to all strategies for reducing pain is that nurses convey to patient that they believe the patient is having pain. This can be done by:

1. Verbally acknowledging the presence of the pain. 'I understand your leg is very painful. How do you feel about the pain?'
2. Listening attentively to what the patient says about the pain.
3. Conveying that you are assessing the patient's pain to understand it better, not to determine whether the pain is real, for example, 'How does your pain feel now?' or 'Tell me how it feels compared to an hour ago.'
4. Attending to the patient's needs promptly.

Assisting Family and Friends

Family and friends of the patient often need assistance to respond positively to the patient experiencing pain. Nurses can help by giving them accurate information about the pain and providing opportunities for them to discuss their emotional reactions, which may include anger, fear, frustration and feelings of inadequacy. Enlisting the aid of family members in providing pain relief to the patient, such as massaging the patient's back, may diminish their feelings of helplessness and foster a more positive attitude toward the patient's pain experience.

Reducing Misconceptions about Pain

Reducing a patient's misconceptions about the pain and its treatment will often avoid intensifying the pain. The nurse should explain to the patient that pain is a highly individual experience and that it is only the patient who really experiences the pain, although others can understand and empathise. Misconceptions are also dealt with when nurse and patient discuss why the pain has increased or decreased at certain times. For example, a patient whose pain increases in the evening may mistakenly think this is the result of eating dinner rather than fatigue.

Reducing Fear and Anxiety

It is important to help relieve the emotional component, that is, anxiety or fear, associated with the pain. When patients have no opportunity to talk about their pain and associated fears, their perceptions and reactions to the pain can be intensified. The patient may become angry or complain about the nurse's care when the problem really is a belief that the pain is not being treated. If the nurse is honest and sincere and promptly attends to the patient's needs, the patient is much more likely to know that the nurse does believe the patient is in pain.

By providing accurate information, the nurse can also reduce many of the patient's fears, such as a fear of addiction or a fear that the pain will always be present. It also helps many patients to have privacy when they are experiencing pain.

Preventing Pain

A preventive approach to pain management involves the provision of measures to treat the pain before it occurs or before it becomes severe. **Pre-emptive analgesia** is the administration of analgesics prior to an invasive or operative procedure in order to treat pain before it occurs. For example, treating patients pre-operatively with local infiltration of an anaesthetic or parenteral administration of an opioid can reduce post-operative pain. Nurses can also use a pre-emptive approach by providing an analgesic around the clock (ATC), rather than as needed (prn).

Pharmacological Pain Management

Pharmacological pain management involves the use of opioids (narcotics), nonopioids/nonsteroidal anti-inflammatory drugs (NSAIDS), and adjuvants, or coanalgesic drugs (see *Box 22-3*).

BOX 22-3 Categories and Examples of Analgesics

Opioid Analgesics
+ Fentanyl (Sublimaze)
+ Hydromorphone hydrochloride (Palladone)
+ Codeine
+ Morphine sulphate
+ Diamorphine hydrochloride
+ Dihyrocodeine tartrate (DF118)

Nonopioid Analgesics/NSAIDs
+ Paracetamol
+ Acetylsalicylic acid (aspirin)
+ Diclofenac sodium (Voltarol)
+ Ibuprofen
+ Naproxen (Naprosyn)
+ Piroxicam (Feldene)

Adjuvant Analgesics
+ Amitriptyline (Elavil)
+ Chlorpromazine (Thorazine)
+ Diazepam (Valium)
+ Hydroxyzine (Atarax)

Opioid Analgesia

Opioid analgesia include opium derivatives, such as morphine and codeine, relieving pain and providing a sense of euphoria. Changes in mood and attitude and feelings of well-being make the person feel more comfortable even though the pain persists.

When administering any analgesia, the nurse must review side-effects. All opioids result in some initial drowsiness when first administered, but with regular administration, this side-effect tends to decrease. Opioids also may cause nausea, vomiting, constipation and respiratory depression. Opioids must be used cautiously in patients with respiratory problems.

CLINICAL ALERT

Constipation is an almost universal adverse effect of opioid use and as such all patients receiving opioids should receive laxatives, unless contraindicated. Inform patients about the following options to prevent constipation: increasing fibre intake, using a mild laxative (e.g. milk of magnesia) regularly, taking oral laxatives at bedtime, and using rectal suppositories if absolutely necessary.

If the patient experiences significant respiratory depression or is overly sedated, the dosage is excessive. The nurse needs to assess a patient's level of alertness and respiratory rate for baseline data before administering opioid analgesia. An increasing sedation level can be an early warning sign of impending respiratory depression (Pasero and McCaffery, 2002). The nurse should assess and document the patient's level of sedation at the same time respiratory status is checked. Early recognition of an increasing level of sedation or respiratory depression will enable the nurse to implement appropriate measures promptly (e.g. reducing the opioid dosage). *Box 22-4 on page 586 provides suggested measures to prevent and treat side-effects of opioid analgesia.*

CLINICAL ALERT

Assessing for sedation and respiratory status is critical during the first 12-24 hours after starting opioid therapy. The longer the patient receives opioids, the wider the safety margin as the patient develops a tolerance to the sedative and respiratory depressive effects of the drug.

Older patients are particularly sensitive to the analgesic properties of opioids and often require less medication than younger patients. This sensitivity may be related to reduced excretion of the drug in elderly patients.

Nonopioids/NSAIDs

Nonopioids include paracetamol and **nonsteroidal anti-inflammatory drugs (NSAIDs)** such as ibuprofen. NSAIDs have anti-inflammatory, analgesic and antipyretic effects, whereas acetaminophen has only analgesic and antipyretic effects.

The most common side-effect of nonopioid analgesics is gastrointestinal, such as heartburn or indigestion. Patients should be taught to take NSAIDs with food or a glass of water. Most NSAIDs also interfere with platelet aggregation. Paracetamol, on the other hand, does not affect platelet function and rarely causes gastrointestinal distress. It can, however, cause hepatotoxicity (liver toxicity) and should be used cautiously in patients with liver problems.

The NSAIDs reduce the dose of opioids needed when the drugs are given together and provide better pain relief than use of either type separately. There are advantages to giving combination drugs such as NSAIDS and opioids for pain management but close attention must be paid to the amount that the patient takes in a 24-hour period. Opioids have no ceiling, so the codeine could be gradually increased as needed for pain management. A change in medication or dosage may be needed to provide pain relief while maintaining safe, nontoxic levels.

Pharmacological management of mild to moderate pain should begin with NSAIDs, unless there is a specific contraindication (USDHHS, 1992: 16). NSAIDs are contraindicated, for example, in patients with impaired blood clotting or those on warfarin, gastrointestinal bleeding or ulcer risk, renal disease, thrombocytopenia and possibly infection (because NSAIDs will obscure fever). NSAIDS are also contraindicated

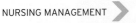

BOX 22-4 Common Opioid Side Effects, Preventive and Treatment Measures

Constipation
+ Increase fluid intake (e.g. 6–8 glasses daily).
+ Increase fibre and bulk-forming agents to the diet (e.g. fresh fruits and vegetables).
+ Increase exercise regimen.
+ Administer stool softeners and if necessary provide a mild laxative.

Nausea and Vomiting
+ Inform patient that tolerance to this emetic effect generally develops after several days of opiate therapy.
+ Provide an antiemetic as required.
+ Change the analgesic as indicated.

Sedation
+ Inform patient that tolerance usually develops over 3–5 days.
+ Administer a stimulant each morning to patients who receive opiate therapy for chronic pain and do not develop tolerance.

Respiratory Depression
+ Administer an opioid antagonist, such as naloxone hydrochloride (Narcan) until respirations return to an acceptable rate. Administer the medication slowly by intravenous route with 10 ml of saline. Monitor the patient, and repeat the procedure as required.
+ If the patient is receiving intravenous patient-controlled analgesia, stop or slow the infusion.

Pruritus (proo-RY-tuss = Itching)
+ Apply cool packs, lotion and diversional activity.
+ Administer an antihistamine (e.g. diphenhydramine hydrochloride (Benadryl)).
+ Inform the patient that tolerance also develops to pruritus.

Urinary Retention
+ May need to catheterise patient.
+ Administer narcotic antagonist (naloxone hydrochloride (Narcan)).

Table 22-7 Misconceptions about Nonopioids

Misconception	Correction
Regular daily use of NSAIDs is much safer than taking opioids.	Side-effects from long-term use of NSAIDs are considerably more severe and life threatening than the side-effects from daily doses of oral morphine or other opioids. The most common side-effect from long-term use of opioids is constipation, whereas NSAIDs can cause gastric ulcers, increased bleeding time and renal insufficiency. Paracetamol can cause hepatotoxicity.
A nonopioid should not be given at the same time as an opioid.	It is safe to administer a nonopioid and opioid at the same time. Giving a dose of nonopioid at the same time as a dose of opioid poses no more danger than giving the doses at different times.
Administering antacids with NSAIDs is an effective method of reducing gastric distress.	Administering antacids with NSAIDs can lessen distress but may be counterproductive. Antacids reduce the absorption and therefore the effectiveness of the NSAID by releasing the drug in the stomach rather than in the small intestine where absorption occurs.
Nonopioids are not useful analgesics for severe pain.	Nonopioids alone are rarely sufficient to relieve severe pain, but they are an important part in achieving pain relief. One of the basic principles of analgesic therapy is: whenever pain is severe enough to require an opioid, adding a nonopioid should be considered.
Gastric distress (e.g. abdominal pain) is indicative of NSAID-induced gastric ulceration.	Most patients with gastric lesions have no symptoms until bleeding or perforation occurs.

Note: From *Pain: Clinical Manual*, 2nd edn, by M. McCaffery and C. Pasero, 1999, St. Louis, MO: Mosby. Reprinted with permission from Elsevier Science.

for patients with asthma. Table 22-7 lists common misconceptions about nonopioids. Some NSAIDs have also been linked to an increased risk of coronary heart disease (Hippisley-Cox and Coupland, 2005), however doctors have warned patients not to stop taking these drugs as the risk is small in most cases.

Adjuvant Analgesics

An **adjuvant analgesic** is a medication that was developed for a use other than analgesia but has been found to reduce chronic pain and sometimes acute pain, in addition to its

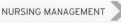

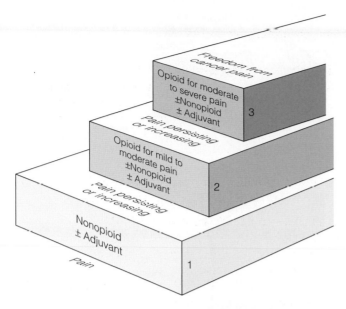

Figure 22-6 The WHO three-step analgesic ladder.
(*Note:* From *Cancer Pain Relief*, 2nd edn, by World Health Organization, 1996, Geneva: Author. Reprinted with permission.)

primary action. For example, mild sedatives or tranquillisers may help reduce anxiety, stress and tension so that the patient can obtain a good night's sleep. Antidepressants are used to treat underlying depression or mood disorders but may also enhance other pain strategies. Anticonvulsants, usually prescribed to treat seizures (fits), can be useful in controlling painful neuropathies (abnormal functioning of the nerves) such as herpes zoster (shingles) and diabetic neuropathies.

WHO Three-Step Ladder Approach

The World Health Organization (WHO) recommends a three-step ladder approach to manage chronic cancer pain (see Figure 22-6). This approach focuses on the intensity of the pain, and patients do not necessarily progress through the three steps. Step 1 of the analgesic ladder suggests a nonopioid analgesic and the possibility of an adjuvant analgesic. If the patient receives the maximum recommended dose of nonopioids and continues to experience pain, step 2 recommends adding an opioid. It appears that there is no difference between steps 2 and 3; however, in practice the difference is in the choice of analgesic. For example, opioid analgesics at step 3 should be available by a variety of routes (e.g. oral, rectal, subcutaneous). They should also have a short half-life in order to increase the dosage for severe, escalating (increasing) pain (McCaffery and Pasero, 1999: 117).

Routes for Opiate Delivery

Opioids have traditionally been administered by oral, subcutaneous, intramuscular and intravenous routes. In addition, newer methods of delivering opiates have been developed such as transdermal drug therapy (patches), continuous subcutaneous infusions and epidural infusion.

Oral

Oral administration of opiates remains the preferred route of delivery because of ease of administration. Patients who require regular opiates for chronic pain can be prescribed long-acting or sustained-release forms of morphine. However they may need doses of immediate release analgesia such as fentanyl lozenges, for acute breakthrough pain.

Transdermal

Transdermal drug therapy is advantageous in that it delivers a relatively stable plasma drug level and is non-invasive. Fentanyl is an opioid currently available as a skin patch with various dosages. It provides drug delivery for up to 72 hours.

Rectal

Several opiates are now available in suppository form. The rectal route is particularly useful for patients who have dysphagia (difficulty swallowing) or nausea and vomiting.

Subcutaneous

Although the subcutaneous (SC) route has been used extensively to deliver opioids, another technique uses subcutaneous catheters and infusion pumps to provide continuous subcutaneous infusion (CSCI) of narcotics. CSCI is particularly helpful for patients (a) whose pain is poorly controlled by oral medications, (b) who are experiencing dysphagia or gastrointestinal obstruction or (c) who have a need for prolonged use of parenteral narcotics. CSCI involves the use of a small, light, battery-operated pump that administers the drug through a #23- or #25-gauge butterfly needle. The needle can be inserted into the anterior chest, the subclavicular region, the abdominal wall, the outer aspects of the upper arms or the thighs.

Intramuscular

The intramuscular (IM) route is the least desirable route for opioid administration because of variable absorption, pain involved with administration, and the need to repeat administration every 3–4 hours.

Intravenous

The intravenous (IV) route provides rapid and effective pain relief with few side-effects. The analgesic can be administered by IV bolus or by continuous infusion controlled by the patient using a patient-controlled analgesia (PCA) machine at the bedside (see the discussion of PCA later in this chapter).

Intraspinal

An increasingly popular method of delivery is the infusion of opiates into the epidural or intrathecal (subarachnoid) space

 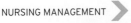

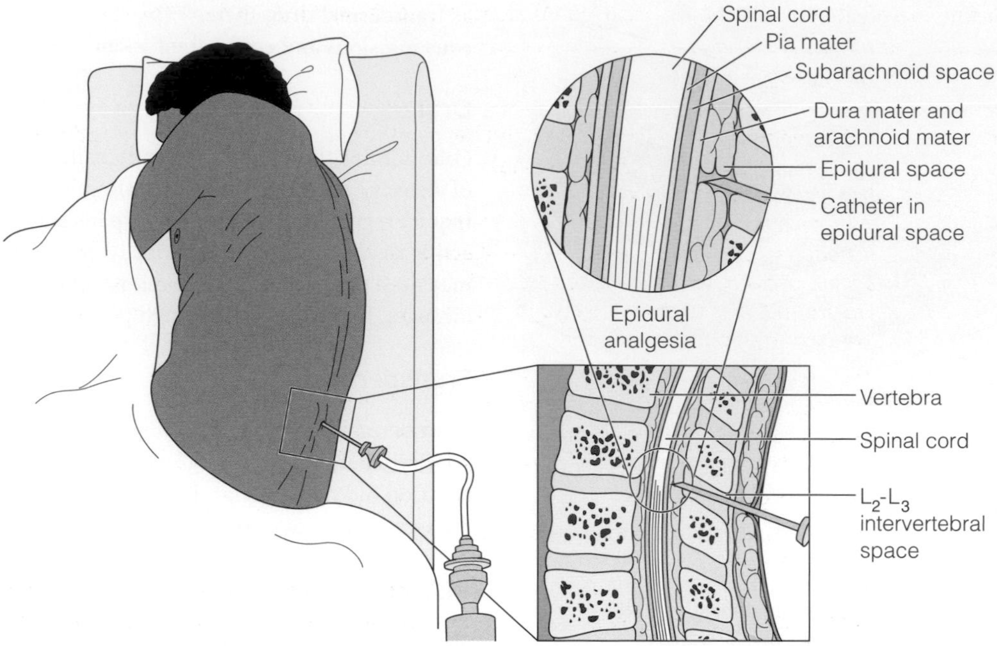

Figure 22-7 Placement of intraspinal catheter in the epidural space.

(see Figure 22-7). Intraspinal analgesia acts directly on opiate receptors in the dorsal horn of the spinal cord. Two commonly used medications are morphine sulphate and fentanyl. The major benefit of intraspinal drug therapy is that it exerts a lesser sedative effect than do systemic opiates. The epidural space is most commonly used because the dura mater acts as a protective barrier against infection, including meningitis. Because the epidural catheter is in a space and not a blood vessel, a continuous epidural infusion may be stopped for hours and restarted without concern that the catheter has become occluded (blocked) (McCaffery and Pasero, 1999: 37).

Intraspinal analgesia can be administered by three methods:

1. *Bolus.* For some surgical procedures (e.g. caesarean section), a single bolus may provide sufficient pain control for up to 24 hours. After this time, the patient may be given oral or IV analgesia.
2. *Continuous infusion administered by pump.* The pump may be external (for acute or chronic pain) or implanted (for chronic pain).
3. *Patient-controlled epidural analgesia (PCEA).* Patient-controlled epidural analgesia is administered by the patient using a pump. This is similar to patient-controlled analgesia in which a basal rate may meet the patient's analgesic needs. If not, the patient can push a button to deliver a preset dose. PCEA is often used to manage acute post-operative pain, chronic pain and intractable cancer pain.

Temporary catheters, used for short-term acute pain management, are usually placed at the lumbar or thoracic vertebral level and often removed after 2–4 days. Permanent catheters, for patients with chronic pain, may be tunnelled subcutaneously through the skin and exit at the patient's side. Tunnelling of the catheter reduces the risk of infection and displacement of the catheter. After the catheter is inserted, the nurse is responsible for monitoring the infusion and assessing the patient. Nursing care of patients with intraspinal infusions is summarised in Table 22-8.

A common misconception is that there is a higher incidence of respiratory depression when opioids are administered by the epidural route and, therefore, patients receiving epidural analgesia should be monitored in an intensive care setting. The fact is that respiratory depression occurs less often with epidural analgesia than by the IM route (McCaffery and Pasero, 1999: 224). Patients who are receiving epidural analgesia do not require intensive care monitoring. The nurse who is outside the intensive care setting can safely monitor the respiratory and sedation status of a patient receiving epidural analgesia.

> **CLINICAL ALERT**
>
> *As a precaution, have naloxone (Narcan), sodium chloride 0.9% diluent, and injection equipment on hand for each patient receiving an opioid-containing epidural infusion (Cox, 2001), as this will reverse the effects of the opioid.*

Continuous Local Anaesthetics

Continuous subcutaneous administration of long-acting local anaesthetics into or near the surgical site is a technique being used to provide post-operative pain control. This technique is being used for a variety of surgical procedures including knee

Table 22-8 Nursing Interventions for Patients Receiving Analgesics through an Epidural Catheter

Nursing goals	Interventions
Maintain patient safety	Label the tubing, the infusion bag and the front of the pump with tape marked EPIDURAL to prevent confusion with similar-looking IV lines.
	Secure all connections with tape.
	If there is no continuous infusion, apply tape over all injection ports on the epidural line to avoid the injection of substances intended for IV administration into the epidural catheter.
	Do not use alcohol in any care of catheter or insertion site as it can be neurotoxic.
	Ensure that any solution injected or infused intraspinally is sterile, preservative free and safe for intraspinal administration.
Maintain catheter placement	Secure temporary catheters with tape.
	Assist patient in repositioning or moving out of bed.
	Teach patient to avoid tugging on the catheter.
	Assess insertion site for leakage with each bolus dose or at least every 8-12 hours.
Prevent infection	Use strict aseptic techniques with all epidural-related procedures.
	Maintain sterile occlusive dressing over insertion site.
	Assess insertion site for signs of infection.
	Assess for increasing diffuse back pain or tenderness and/or paresthesia (pins and needles) on intraspinal injection because these are cardinal signs of intraspinal infection (McCaffery and Pasero, 1999: 234).
Maintain urinary and bowel function	Monitor intake and output.
	Assess for bowel and bladder distention.
Prevent respiratory depression	Assess sedation level and respiratory status regularly.
	Do not administer other opioids or central nervous system depressants unless ordered.
	Keep an ampoule of naloxone hydrochloride (0.4 mg) at the bedside.
	Notify the nurse in charge or doctor if the respiratory rate falls below 8 per minute or if the patient is difficult to rouse.

arthroplasty, abdominal hysterectomy, hernia repair and mastectomy (Pasero, 2000: 22).

The surgeon inserts a catheter under the subcutaneous tissue and on top of the muscle near or in the surgical wound site. A transparent dressing secures the catheter. The patient is given a loading dose of local anaesthetic before the continuous infusion is started. The catheter is connected to an infusion pump that is set at the rate as per prescription.

Nursing interventions for the patient with infusion of a continuous local anaesthetic include:

+ Conduct pain assessment and documentation every 2–4 hours while the patient is awake.
+ Check the dressing every shift for intactness. The dressing is not usually changed in order to avoid dislodging the catheter.
+ Check the site of the catheter. It should be clean and dry.
+ Assess the patient for signs of local anaesthetic toxicity (e.g. dizziness; ringing in the ears; a metallic taste; tingling or numbness of the lips, gums or tongue) (Pasero, 2000: 22–23) and notify the doctor if any of the signs are noted.

Patient-controlled Analgesia

Patient-controlled analgesia (PCA) is an interactive method of pain management that permits patients to treat their pain by self-administering analgesia (McCaffery and Pasero, 1999).

The oral route for PCA is most common, but the subcutaneous, intravenous and epidural routes are increasingly being used. The PCA mode of therapy minimises the roller-coaster effect of peaks of sedation and valleys of pain that occur with the traditional method of 'as required' dosing. With the parenteral routes, the patient administers a predetermined dose of an opioid by an electronic infusion pump. This allows the patient to maintain a more constant level of relief yet need less medication for pain relief. Patient-controlled analgesia can be effectively used for patients with acute pain related to a surgical incision, traumatic injury, or labour and delivery, and for chronic pain as with cancer.

Regardless of the setting the nurse is responsible for the initial instruction regarding use of the PCA and for the ongoing monitoring of the therapy. The patient's pain must be assessed at regular intervals and the use of the analgesia should be documented in the patient's record.

Patient-controlled analgesia pumps are designed with built-in safety mechanisms to prevent patient overdosage, abusive use and narcotic theft. The most significant adverse effects are respiratory depression and hypotension; however, they occur rarely. Although PCA pumps vary in design, they all have the same protective features. The line of the PCA pump, a syringe-type pump, is usually introduced into the injection port of a primary IV fluid line (see Figure 22-8 on page 590). When patients want a dose of analgesia, they can push a button attached to the

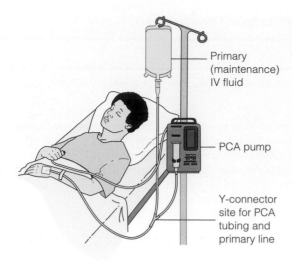

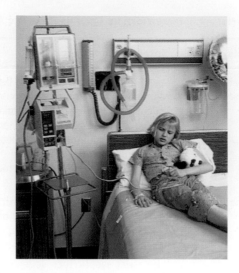

Figure 22-8 PCA line introduced into the injection port of a primary line.

Figure 22-9 The older child is able to regulate a PCA pump.

infusion pump and the preset dose is delivered (see Figure 22-9). A programmable lockout interval (usually 10–15 minutes) follows the dose, when an additional dose cannot be given even if the patient activates the button. It is also possible to programme the maximum dose that can be delivered over a period of hours. Many pumps are capable of delivering a low continuous infusion, to provide sustained analgesia during times of rest and sleep.

PCA is suitable for patients:

+ With moderate to severe pain who cannot tolerate oral analgesia
+ Who are able to understand the concept of PCA
+ Who are willing to control their own pain relief
+ Who are physically able to use the equipment.

TEACHING: PATIENT CARE

Patient Self-management of Pain

Choose a time to teach the patient about pain management when the pain is controlled so that the patient is able to focus on the teaching.

Teaching the patient about self-management of pain can include the following:

+ Demonstrate the operation of the PCA pump and explain that the patient can safely push the button without fear of overmedicating.
+ Describe the use of the pain scale and encourage the patient to respond in order to demonstrate understanding.
+ Explain to the patient the need to notify staff when ambulation is desired (e.g. for bathroom use).

LIFESPAN CONSIDERATIONS

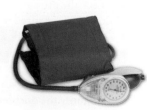

PCA Pump

Children
+ Include the parents in teaching.
+ Assess the child's ability to use the patient control button.

Older Adults
+ Carefully monitor for drug side-effects.
+ Use cautiously for individuals with impaired pulmonary or renal function.
+ Assess the patient's cognitive and physical ability to use the patient control button.

Nonpharmacological Pain Management

Nonpharmacological pain management consists of a variety of physical and cognitive-behavioural pain management strategies. Physical interventions include cutaneous stimulation, immobilisation, transcutaneous electrical nerve stimulation (TENS) and acupuncture. Mind–body (cognitive-behavioural) interventions include distraction activities, relaxation techniques, imagery (using imagination), meditation, hypnosis and therapeutic touch.

Physical Interventions

The goals of physical intervention include providing comfort, altering physiological responses, and reducing fears associated with pain-related immobility or activity restriction.

Cutaneous Stimulation

Cutaneous stimulation can provide effective temporary pain relief. It distracts the patient and focuses attention on the tactile stimulation and, away from the painful sensations, thus reducing pain perception. Cutaneous stimulation techniques include the following:

+ Massage
+ Application of heat or cold
+ Acupressure.

Cutaneous stimulation can be applied directly to the painful area, proximal (near) to the pain, distal (away from) to the pain and contralateral (opposite side) to the pain. Cutaneous stimulation is contraindicated in areas of skin breakdown.

Massage

Massage is a comfort measure that can aid relaxation, decrease muscle tension and may ease anxiety because the physical contact communicates caring. It can also decrease pain intensity by increasing superficial circulation to the area. Massage can involve the back and neck, hands and arms, or feet. The use of ointments or liniments may provide localised pain relief with joint or muscle pain. Massage is contraindicated in areas of skin breakdown.

Heat and Cold Applications

A warm bath, heating pads, ice bags, ice massage, hot or cold compresses and warm or cold baths in general relieve pain and promote healing of injured tissues.

Acupressure

Acupressure developed from the ancient Chinese healing system of acupuncture. The therapist applies finger pressure to points that correspond to many of the points used in acupuncture.

Immobilisation

Immobilising or restricting the movement of a painful body part (e.g. arthritic joint, traumatised limb) may help to manage episodes of acute pain. Splints or supportive devices should hold

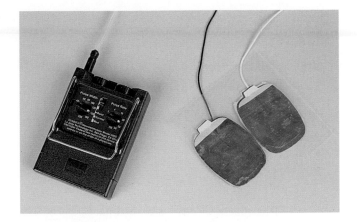

Figure 22-10 A transcutaneous electric nerve stimulator.

joints in the position of optimal function and should be removed regularly in accordance with agency protocol to provide range-of-motion exercises. Prolonged immobilisation can result in joint contracture (distortion), muscle atrophy (shrinking) and cardiovascular problems such as an increased risk of thrombosis (clot formation). Therefore, patients should be encouraged to participate in self-care activities and remain as active as possible.

Transcutaneous Electrical Nerve Stimulation

Transcutaneous electrical nerve stimulation (TENS) is a method of applying low-voltage electrical stimulation directly over identified pain areas, at an acupressure point, along peripheral nerve areas that innervate the pain area or along the spinal column. The TENS unit consists of a portable, battery-operated device with lead wire and electrode pads that are applied to the chosen area of skin (see Figure 22-10). Cutaneous stimulation from the TENS unit is thought to activate large-diameter fibres and close the pain 'gate', resulting in pain relief. The use of TENS is contraindicated for patients with pacemakers, arrhythmias or in areas of skin breakdown.

Distraction

Distraction draws the person's attention away from the pain and lessens the perception of pain. In some instances, distraction can make a patient completely unaware of pain. For example, a patient recovering from surgery may feel no pain while watching a football game on television, yet feel pain again when the game is over. Different types of distractions are shown in *Box 22-5* on page 592.

Nonpharmacological Invasive Therapies

A **nerve block** is a chemical interruption of a nerve pathway, affected by injecting a local anaesthetic into the nerve. Nerve blocks are widely used during dental work. The injected drug blocks nerve pathways from the painful tooth, thus stopping the transmission of pain impulses to the brain. Nerve blocks are often used to relieve the pain of whiplash injury, lower back disorders and cancer.

BOX 22-5 Types of Distraction

Visual Distraction
+ Reading or watching TV
+ Watching a football match
+ Guided imagery (using imagination)

Auditory Distraction
+ Humour
+ Listening to music

Tactile Distraction
+ Slow, rhythmic breathing
+ Massage
+ Holding or stroking a pet or toy

Intellectual Distraction
+ Crossword puzzles
+ Card games (e.g. bridge)
+ Hobbies (e.g. stamp collecting, writing a story)

COMMUNITY CARE CONSIDERATIONS

Pain Management
+ Teach patient to keep a pain diary to monitor pain onset, activity before pain, pain intensity, use of analgesia or other relief measures, and so on.
+ Instruct patient to contact a healthcare professional if planned pain control measures are ineffective.
+ Teach the use of preferred and selected nonpharmacological techniques such as relaxation, guided imagery, distraction, music therapy, massage, and so on.
+ Instruct the patient to use pain control measures before the pain becomes severe.
+ Inform the patient of the effects of untreated pain.
+ Provide appropriate information about how to access community resources, home care agencies, and associations that offer self-help groups and educational materials.

EVALUATING

The goals established in the planning phase are evaluated according to specific desired outcome. To assist in the evaluation process, nurse documentation or a patient diary may be helpful.

If outcomes are not achieved, the nurse and patient need to explore the reasons before modifying the care plan. The nurse might consider the following questions:

+ Is adequate analgesia being given? Would the patient benefit from a change in dose or in the time interval between doses?

+ Were the patient's beliefs and values about pain therapy considered?
+ Did the patient understate the pain experience for some reason?
+ Were appropriate instructions provided to allay misconceptions about pain management?
+ Did the patient and their family understand the instructions about pain management techniques?
+ Is the patient receiving adequate support from significant others?
+ Has the patient's physical condition changed, necessitating modifications in interventions?
+ Should selected intervention strategies be reevaluated?

CRITICAL REFLECTION

Let us revisit the case study on page 572. Now that you have read this chapter what do you feel are the nursing priorities for nursing a patient such as Ben? What information would you give Ben's parents?

NURSING MANAGEMENT

CHAPTER HIGHLIGHTS

+ Pain is a subjective sensation to which no two people respond in the same way. It can directly impair health and prolong recovery from surgery, disease and trauma.

+ Pain can be categorised according to its origin as superfical, deep or referred – or according to its duration as acute pain or chronic pain.

+ Pain threshold is generally similar in all people, but pain tolerance and response vary considerably.

+ For pain to be perceived, nociceptors must be stimulated. Three types of pain stimuli are mechanical, thermal and chemical.

+ Nociception is comprised of the physiological processes related to pain perception. It involves four processes: transduction, transmission, perception and modulation.

+ According to the gate control theory, small nerve fibres which carry pain impulses to the spinal cord can be blocked by stimulation of the large nerve fibres at a 'gate'.

+ Numerous factors influence a person's perception and reaction to pain: ethnic and cultural values, developmental stage, environmental factors and support people, earlier pain experiences, meaning of pain, and anxiety and stress.

+ Pain is subjective, and the most reliable indicator of the presence or intensity of pain is the patient's self-report. Assessment of a patient who is experiencing pain should include a comprehensive pain history.

+ Overall patient goals include preventing, modifying or eliminating pain so that the patient is able to partly or completely resume usual daily activities and to cope more effectively with the pain experience.

+ When planning, nurses need to choose pain relief measures appropriate for the patient.

+ Pain management includes two basic types of nursing interventions: pharmacological and nonpharmacological.

+ Scheduling measures to prevent pain is far more supportive of the patient than trying to deal with pain once it is established.

+ Major nursing strategies for all patients are to acknowledge and convey belief in the patient's pain, assist family, reduce misconceptions about pain, prevent pain, and reduce fear and anxiety associated with the pain.

+ Pharmacological interventions, prescribed by the doctor, include the use of opioids, nonopioids/NSAIDs and adjuvant drugs.

+ The World Health Organization recommends a three-step ladder approach to manage chronic cancer pain.

+ Analgesic medication can be delivered through a variety of routes and methods to meet the specific needs of the patient. These routes include oral, rectal, transdermal, topical, subcutaneous or intravenous with a continuous infusion or a bolus dose, and intraspinal.

+ Patient-controlled analgesia enables the patient to exercise control and treat the pain by self-administering doses of analgesics.

+ Physical nonpharmacological pain interventions include such cutaneous stimulation as hot and cold applications, massage and acupressure; transcutaneous electrical nerve stimulation; immobilisation; and acupuncture.

+ Cognitive-behavioural interventions include distraction techniques, relaxation techniques, guided imagery, therapeutic touch and hypnosis.

REFERENCES

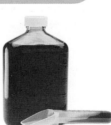

Andrews, M.M. and Boyle, J.S. (2003) *Transcultural concepts in nursing care* (4th edn), Philadelphia: Lippincott Williams and Wilkins.

Ball, J.W. and Bindler, R.C. (2003) *Pediatric nursing: Caring for children* (3rd edn), Upper Saddle River, NJ: Prentice Hall.

Beecher, H.K. (1956) 'Limiting factors in experimental pain', *Journal of Chronic Disease*, 4, 11–22.

Bergh, I. and Sjostrom, B. (1999) 'A comparative study of nurses' and elderly patients' ratings of pain and pain tolerance', *Journal of Gerontological Nursing*, 25(5), 30–36.

Cox, F. (2001) 'Clinical care of patients with epidural infusions', *The Professional Nurse*, 16, 1429–1432.

Daily Mail (2005) 'The one-in-a-billion boy who feels no pain'. London: *Daily Mail*. Available from: http://www.dailymail.co.uk/pages/live/articles/health/womenfamily.html?in_article_id=334924&in_page_id=1799&in_a_source. (Accessed on 28 February 2007.)

Eliopoulos, C. (2001) *Gerontological nursing* (5th edn), Philadelphia: Lippincott.

Hardy, J.D., Wolff, H.G. and Goodell, H. (1943) 'Pain threshold in man', *Association of Research into Nervous Mental Diseases*, 23, 1.

Hippisley-Cox, J. and Coupland, C. (2005) 'Risk of myocardial infarction in patients taking cyclo-oxygenase-2 inhibitors or conventional non-steroidal anti-inflammatory drugs: population based nested case-control analysis', *British Medical Journal*, 330. Available from http://www.bmj.com/cgi/reprint/330/7504/1366. (Accessed on 19 April 2007.)

LaDuke, S. (2002) 'Undertreating pain: Could it land you in court?', *Nursing*, 32, 18.

McCaffery, M., Ferrell, B.R. and Pasero, C. (2000) 'Nurses' personal opinions about patients' pain and their effect on recorded assessments and titration of opioid doses', *Pain Management Nursing*, 1(3), 79–87.

McCaffery, M. and Pasero, C. (1999) *Pain: Clinical manual* (2nd edn), St. Louis, MO: Mosby.

Melzack, R. and Wall, P.D. (1965) 'Pain mechanisms: A new theory', *Science*, 150, 971–979.

Paice, J.A. (2002) 'Controlling pain. Understanding nociceptive pain', *Nursing*, 32(3), 74–75.

Pasero, C. (2000) 'Continuous local anaesthetics', *American Journal of Nursing*, 100(8), 22–23.

Pasero, C. and McCaffery, M. (2002) 'Pain control: Monitoring sedation', *American Journal of Nursing*, 102(2), 67–68.

US Department of Health and Human Services (1992) *Clinical practice guidelines: Acute pain management in adults – operative procedures: A quick reference guide for clinicians*. Rockville, MD: Public Health Services Agency in Health Care Policy and Research.

WHO (1996) *Cancer pain relief* (2nd edn), Geneva: WHO.

Wong, D.L., Hockenberry-Eaton, M., Wilson, D., Winkelstein, M.L. and Schwartz, P. (2001) *Essentials of paediatric nursing* (6th edn), St. Louis, MO: Mosby.

Chapter 23 Activity and Exercise

Learning Outcomes

After completing this chapter, you will be able to:

+ Describe four basic elements of normal movement.
+ Differentiate isotonic, isometric, isokinetic, aerobic and anaerobic exercise.
+ Compare the effects of exercise and immobility on body systems.
+ Identify factors influencing a person's body alignment and activity.
+ Assess activity-exercise pattern, alignment, mobility capabilities and limitations, activity tolerance and potential problems related to immobility.
+ Develop nursing outcomes and interventions related to activity, exercise and mobility problems.
+ Explain the functions and the physiology of sleep.
+ Identify the characteristics of NREM and REM sleep.
+ Identify the four stages of NREM sleep.
+ Describe variations in sleep patterns throughout the life span.
+ Identify factors that affect normal sleep.
+ Describe common sleep disorders.
+ Identify the components of a sleep pattern assessment.
+ Develop nursing diagnoses, outcomes and nursing interventions related to sleep problems.
+ Describe interventions that promote normal sleep.

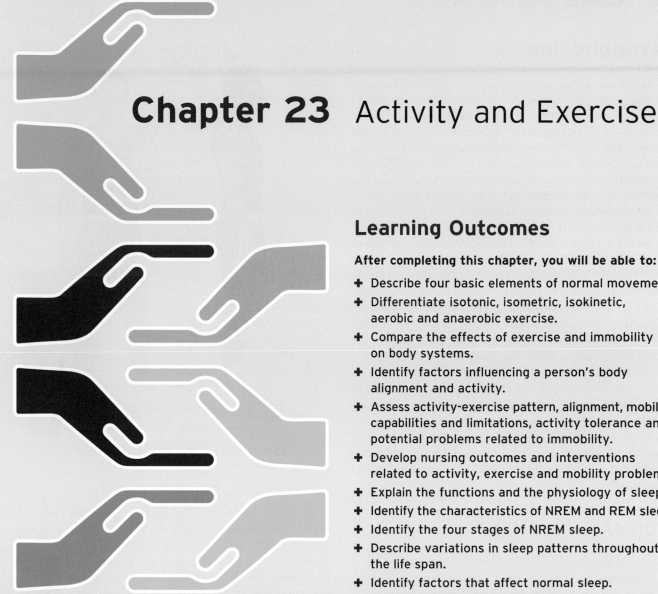

CASE STUDY

You are admitting Janet who is 72 years old and during her assessment you discuss her mobility and sleep patterns. Janet tells you that in the past 12 months her mobility has decreased and she has been having ever-increasing problems sleeping at night. She has tried a variety of over-the-counter medications to help her sleep with no effect. As you begin to assess Janet you discover a lot of her sleep problems relate to the frustration of not being as independent as she used to be.

As you progress through the assessment you explain to Janet how activity can affect normal sleep patterns and discuss a referral to the physiotherapy service. Janet agrees to this.

One week later when you evaluate Janet's care she states she feels more rested and is able to mobilise more independently with the aid of a walking frame.

INTRODUCTION

An **activity-exercise pattern** refers to a person's routine of exercise, activity, leisure and recreation. It includes (a) activities of daily living (ADLs) that require energy expenditure such as hygiene, cooking, shopping, eating, working and home maintenance, and (b) the type, quality and quantity of exercise, including sports (Gordon, 2002).

Mobility, the ability to move freely, easily, rhythmically and purposefully in the environment, is an essential part of living. People must move to protect themselves from trauma and to meet their basic needs. Mobility is vital to independence; a fully immobilised person is as vulnerable and dependent as an infant.

People often define their health and physical fitness by their activity because mental well-being and the effectiveness of body functioning depend largely on their mobility status. For example, when a person is upright, the lungs expand more easily, intestinal activity (peristalsis) is more effective and the kidneys are able to empty completely. In addition, motion is essential for proper functioning of bones and muscles.

The ability to move also influences self-esteem and body image. For most people, self-esteem depends on a sense of independence and a feeling of usefulness or being needed. People with mobility impairments may feel helpless and burdensome to others. Body image can be altered by paralysis, amputations or any motor impairment. The reaction of others to impaired mobility can also alter self-esteem and body image significantly.

NORMAL MOVEMENT

Normal movement and stability are the result of an intact musculoskeletal system, an intact nervous system and intact inner ear structures responsible for equilibrium.

Body movement requires coordinated muscle activity and neurological integration. It involves four basic elements: body alignment (posture), joint mobility, balance and coordinated movement.

Alignment and Posture

Proper body alignment and posture bring body parts into position in a manner that promotes optimal balance and maximal body function whether the patient is standing, sitting or lying down. A person maintains balance as long as the **line of gravity** (an imaginary vertical line drawn through the body's centre of gravity) passes through the **centre of gravity** (the point at which all of the body's mass is centred) and the **base of support** (the foundation on which the body rests). In humans, the usual line of gravity begins at the top of the head and falls between the shoulders, through the trunk, slightly anterior to the sacrum, and between the weight-bearing joints and base of support (see Figure 23-1). For a person in the upright position, the centre of gravity is located in the centre of the pelvis approximately midway between the umbilicus and the symphysis

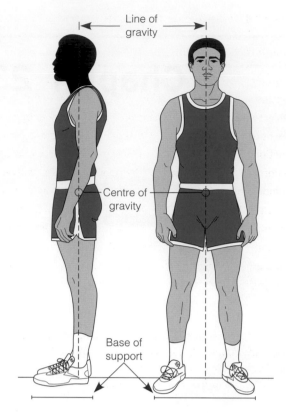

Figure 23-1 The centre of gravity and the line of gravity influence standing alignment.

pubis. For greatest balance and stability, a standing adult must centre body weight symmetrically along the line of gravity. Greater stability and balance are provided in a sitting or lying position than in a standing position. The feet of the chair or bed form a considerably wider base of support, the centre of gravity is lower and the line of gravity is less mobile.

When the body is well aligned, strain on the joints, muscles, tendons or ligaments is minimised and internal structures and organs are supported. People are usually unaware of the functions of the skeletal muscles that maintain body posture. These muscles function almost continuously, making tiny adjustments that enable an erect or seated posture despite the endless downward pull of gravity. The extensor muscles, often referred to as the *antigravity muscles*, carry the major load.

Proper body alignment enhances lung expansion and promotes efficient circulatory, renal and gastrointestinal functions. A person's posture is one criterion for assessing general health, physical fitness and attractiveness. Posture reflects the mood, self-esteem and personality of an individual.

Joint Mobility

Joints are the functional units of the musculoskeletal system. The bones of the skeleton articulate at the joints and most of the skeletal muscles attach to the two bones at the joint. These muscles are categorised according to the type of joint movement they produce on contraction. Muscles are therefore called

Table 23-1 Types of Joint Movements

Movement	Action
Flexion	Decreasing the angle of the joint (e.g. bending the elbow)
Extension	Increasing the angle of the joint (e.g. straightening the arm at the elbow)
Hyperextension	Further extension or straightening of a joint (e.g. bending the head backward)
Abduction	Movement of the bone away from the midline of the body
Adduction	Movement of the bone toward the midline of the body
Rotation	Movement of the bone around its central axis
Circumduction	Movement of the distal part of the bone in a circle while the proximal end remains fixed
Eversion	Turning the sole of the foot outward by moving the ankle joint
Inversion	Turning the sole of the foot inward by moving the ankle joint
Pronation	Moving the bones of the forearm so that the palm of the hand faces downward when held in front of the body
Supination	Moving the bones of the forearm so that the palm of the hand faces upward when held in front of the body

flexors, extensors, internal rotators and the like. The flexor muscles are stronger than the extensor muscles. Thus, when a person is inactive, the joints are pulled into a flexed (bent) position. If this tendency is not counteracted with exercise and position changes, the muscles permanently shorten, and the joint becomes fixed in a flexed position. Types of joint movement are shown in Table 23-1.

The **range of motion (ROM)** of a joint is the maximum movement that is possible for that joint. Joint range of motion varies from individual to individual and is determined by genetic makeup, developmental patterns, the presence or absence of disease and the amount of physical activity in which the person normally engages. Table 23-2 on page 598 shows the various joint movements and the usual ranges of motion.

Table 23-2 Selected Joint Movements

Body part - type of joint/movement	Normal range	Illustration
Neck - pivot joint		
Flexion. Move the head from the upright midline position forward, so that the chin rests on the chest (see Figure 23-2).	415° from midline	
Extension. Move the head from the flexed position to the upright position (Figure 23-2).	45° from midline	
Hyperextension. Move the head from the upright position back as far as possible (Figure 23-2).	45° from midline	**Figure 23-2**
Lateral flexion. Move the head laterally to the right and left shoulders (see Figure 23-3).	40° from midline	
		Figure 23-3
Rotation. Turn the face as far as possible to the right and left (see Figure 23-4).	70° from midline	
		Figure 23-4

Table 23-2 (continued)

Body part – type of joint/movement	Normal range	Illustration
Shoulder – ball-and-socket joint		
Flexion. Raise each arm from a position by the side forward and upward to a position beside the head (see Figure 23-5).	180° from the side	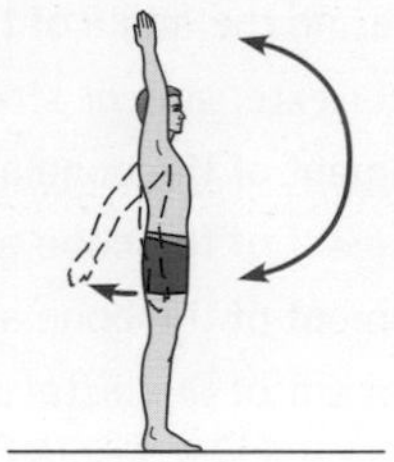
Extension. Move each arm from a vertical position beside the head forward and down to a resting position at the side of the body (Figure 23-5).	180° from vertical position beside the head	
Hyperextension. Move each arm from a resting side position to behind the body (Figure 23-5).	50° from side position	Figure 23-5
Abduction. Move each arm laterally from a resting position at the sides to a side position above the head, palm of the hand away from the head (see Figure 23-6).	180°	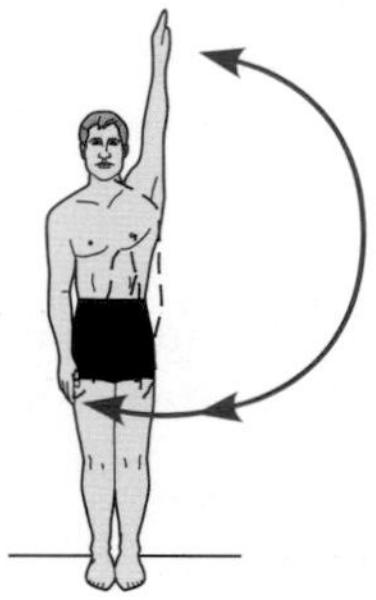
Adduction (anterior). Move each arm from a position at the sides across the front of the body as far as possible (see Figure 23-6). The elbow may be straight or bent.	50°	Figure 23-6
Circumduction. Move each arm forward, up, back and down in a full circle (see Figure 23-7).	360°	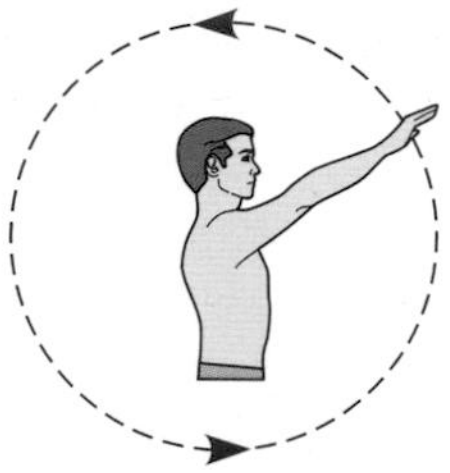 Figure 23-7
External rotation. With each arm held out to the side at shoulder level and the elbow bent to a right angle, fingers pointing down, move the arm upward so that the fingers point up (see Figure 23-8).	90°	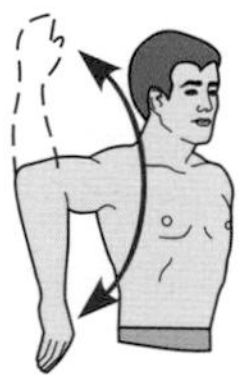
Internal rotation. With each arm held out to the side at shoulder level and the elbow bent to a right angle, fingers pointing up, bring the arm forward and down so that the fingers point down (Figure 23-8).	90°	Figure 23-8
Elbow – hinge joint		
Flexion. Bring each lower arm forward and upward so that the hand is at the shoulder (see Figure 23-9).	150°	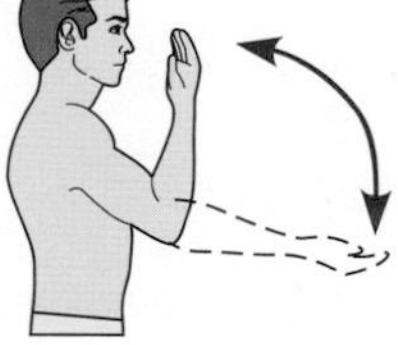
Extension. Bring each lower arm forward and downward, straightening the arm (Figure 23-9).	150°	Figure 23-9

Table 23-2 (*continued*)

Body part - type of joint/movement	Normal range	Illustration
Rotation for supination. Turn each hand and forearm so that the palm is facing upward (see Figure 23-10).	70° to 90°	
Rotation for pronation. Turn each hand and forearm so that the palm is facing downward (Figure 23-10).	70° to 90°	**Figure 23-10**
Wrist - condyloid joint		
Flexion. Bring the fingers of each hand toward the inner aspect of the forearm (see Figure 23-11).	80° to 90°	
Extension. Straighten each hand to the same plane as the arm (Figure 23-11).	80° to 90°	**Figure 23-11**
Hyperextension. Bend the fingers of each hand back as far as possible (see Figure 23-12).	70° to 90°	**Figure 23-12**
Radial flexion (abduction). Bend each wrist laterally toward the thumb side with hand supinated (see Figure 23-13).	0° to 20°	
Ulnar flexion (adduction). Bend each wrist laterally toward the fifth finger with the hand supinated (Figure 23-13).	30° to 50°	**Figure 23-13**
Hand and fingers: metacarpophalangeal joints - condyloid; interphalangeal joints - hinge		
Flexion. Make a fist with each hand (see Figure 23-14).	90°	
Extension. Straighten the fingers of each hand (Figure 23-14).	90°	**Figure 23-14**
Hyperextension. Bend the fingers of each hand back as far as possible (Figure 23-14).	30°	
Abduction. Spread the fingers of each hand apart (see Figure 23-15).	20°	
Adduction. Bring the fingers of each hand together (Figure 23-15).	20°	**Figure 23-15**
Thumb - saddle joint		
Flexion. Move each thumb across the palmar surface of the hand toward the fifth finger (see Figure 23-16).	90°	
Extension. Move each thumb away from the hand (Figure 23-16).	90°	**Figure 23-16**
Abduction. Extend each thumb laterally (see Figure 23-17).	30°	
Adduction. Move each thumb back to the hand (Figure 23-17).	30°	**Figure 23-17**
Opposition. Touch each thumb to the top of each finger of the same hand. The thumb joint movements involved are abduction, rotation and flexion (see Figure 23-18).		**Figure 23-18**

Table 23-2 (*continued*)

Body part - type of joint/movement	Normal range	Illustration
Hip - ball-and-socket joint		
Flexion. Move each leg forward and upward. The knee may be extended or flexed (see Figure 23-19).	Knee extended, 90°; knee flexed, 120°	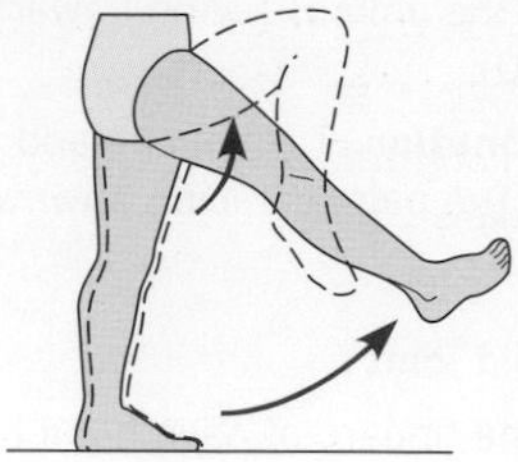 Figure 23-19
Extension. Move each leg back beside the other (see Figure 23-20).	90° to 120°	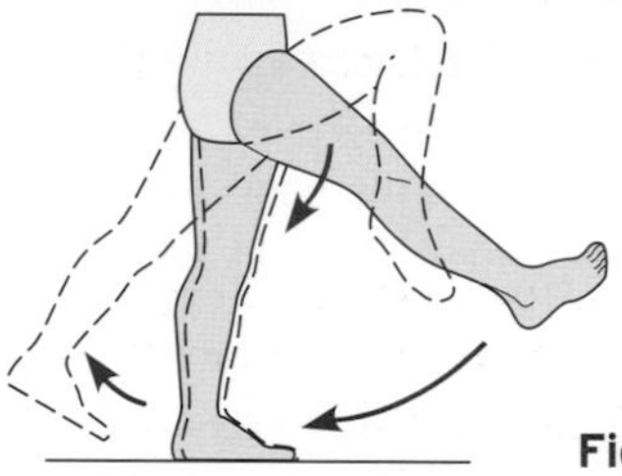
Hyperextension. Move each leg back behind the body (Figure 23-20).	30° to 50°	Figure 23-20
Abduction. Move each leg out to the side (see Figure 23-21).	45° to 50°	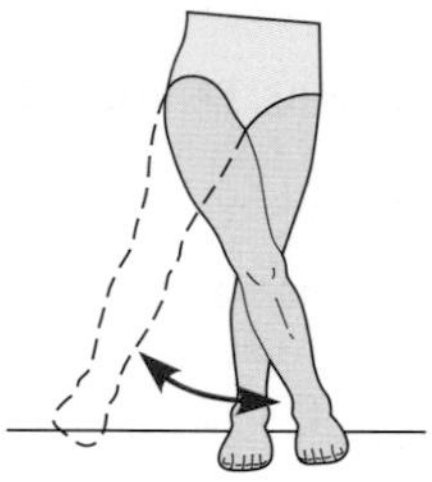
Adduction. Move each leg back to the other leg and beyond in front of it (Figure 23-21).	20° to 30° beyond other leg	Figure 23-21
Circumduction. Move each leg backward, up, to the side and down in a circle (see Figure 23-22).	360°	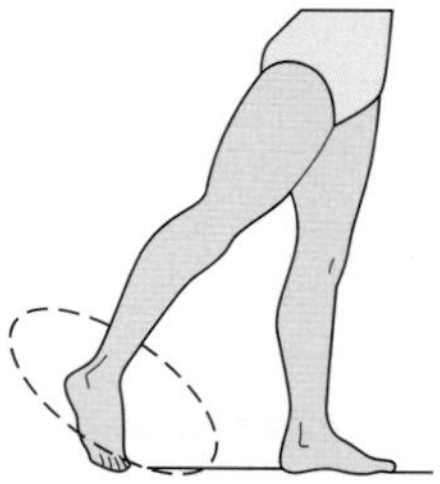 Figure 23-22
Internal rotation. Turn each foot and leg inward so that the toes point as far as possible toward the other leg (see Figure 23-23).	90°	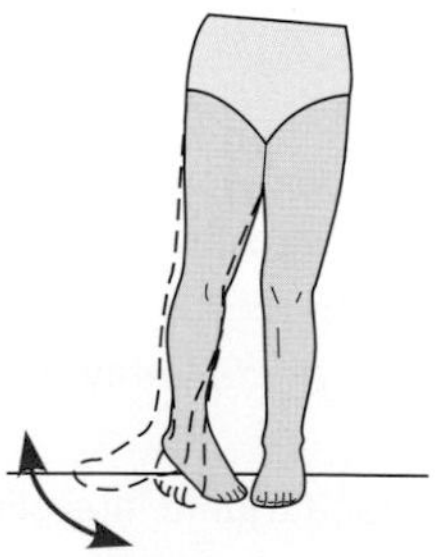
External rotation. Turn each foot and leg outward so that the toes point as far as possible away from the other leg (Figure 23-23).	90°	Figure 23-23
Knee - hinge joint		
Flexion. Bend each leg, bringing the heel toward the back of the thigh (see Figure 23-24).	120° to 130°	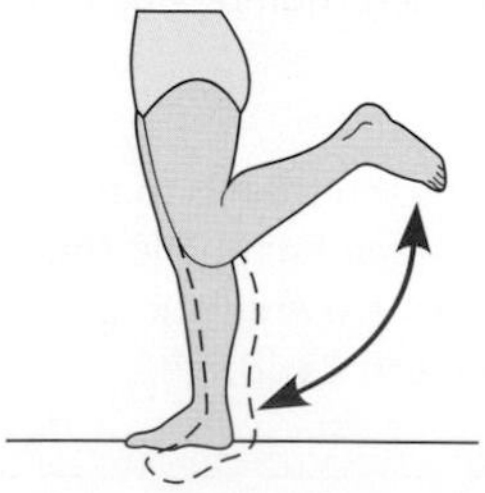
Extension. Straighten each leg, returning the foot to its position beside the other foot (Figure 23-24).	120° to 130°	Figure 23-24

Table 23-2 *(continued)*

Body part – type of joint/movement	Normal range	Illustration
Ankle – hinge joint		
Extension (plantar flexion). Point the toes of each foot downward (see Figure 23-25).	45° to 50°	
Flexion (dorsiflexion). Point the toes of each foot upward (Figure 23-25).	20°	**Figure 23-25**
Foot – gliding		
Eversion. Turn the sole of each foot laterally (see Figure 23-26).	5°	
Inversion. Turn the sole of each foot medially (Figure 23-26).	5°	**Figure 23-26**
Toes: interphalangeal joints – hinge; metatarsophalangeal joints – hinge; intertarsal joints – gliding		
Flexion. Curl the toe joints of each foot downward (see Figure 23-27).	35° to 60°	
Extension. Straighten the toes of each foot (Figure 23-27).	35° to 60°	**Figure 23-27**
Trunk – gliding joint		
Flexion. Bend the trunk toward the toes (see Figure 23-28).	70° to 90°	
Extension. Straighten the trunk from a flexed position (Figure 23-28).		
Hyperextension. Bend the trunk backward (Figure 23-28).	20° to 30°	**Figure 23-28**
Lateral flexion. Bend the trunk to the right and to the left (see Figure 23-29).	35° on each side	**Figure 23-29**
Rotation. Turn the upper part of the body from side to side (see Figure 23-30).	30° to 45°	**Figure 23-30**

Balance

The mechanisms involved in maintaining balance and posture are complex. Mechanisms of equilibrium (sense of balance) respond, frequently without our awareness, to various head movements. The equilibrium sense depends on informational inputs from the labyrinth (inner ear), vision (vestibulo-ocular input) and from stretch receptors of muscles and tendons (vestibulospinal input). The labyrinth consists of the cochlea, vestibule and semicircular canals. The cochlea is concerned with hearing and the vestibule and semicircular canals with equilibrium. Under normal conditions the equilibrium receptors in the semicircular canals and vestibule, collectively called the vestibular apparatus, send signals to the brain that initiate reflexes needed to make required changes in position. The receptors, hairlike cells, respond to displacement of the head in any direction. When the head moves, the fluid flow within the vestibule and semicircular canals stimulates sensory hair cells. Information from these balance receptors goes directly to reflex centres in the brain stem rather than to the cerebral cortex as with other special senses. This enables fast reflexive responses to body imbalance.

Coordinated Movement

Balanced, smooth, purposeful movement is the result of proper functioning of the cerebral cortex, cerebellum and basal ganglia. The cerebral cortex initiates voluntary motor activity, the cerebellum coordinates the motor activities of movement, and the basal ganglia maintain posture. The cerebral cortex operates movements, not muscles. The cortex, for example, may direct the arm to pick up a cup of coffee. The cerebellum, which operates below the level of consciousness, blends and coordinates the muscles involved in voluntary movement. It does not direct the movement but translates the 'instructions' from the cerebral cortex into detailed actions by the many different muscles in the hand, arm and shoulder. When a patient's cerebellum is injured, movements become clumsy, unsure and uncoordinated.

EXERCISE

Exercise and physical activity may be defined as:

+ **Physical activity** is bodily movement produced by skeletal muscles that requires energy expenditure and produces progressive health benefits.
+ **Exercise** is a type of physical activity defined as a planned, structured and repetitive bodily movement done to improve or maintain one or more components of physical fitness.

People participate in exercise programmes to decrease risk factors for cardiovascular disease and to increase their health and well-being. **Activity tolerance** is the type and amount of exercise or daily living activities an individual is able to perform without experiencing adverse effects.

TEACHING: WELLNESS CARE

Guidelines for Physical Activity

Frequency	Three times per week
Duration	Cumulative 30 minutes daily (can be divided throughout the day)
Intensity	'Moderate' intensity as measured by the talk test and perceived exertion scale
Type of exercise	Walking, biking and swimming are recommended for beginners and older adults. Activities that are more strenuous include jogging, running and skipping.
Safety	Outside of the home, use appropriate safety measures such as checking equipment for proper function, wearing a helmet and other protective gear, using reflective devices at night, carrying identification and emergency information.

Types of Exercise

Exercise involves the active contraction and relaxation of muscles. Exercises can be classified according to the type of muscle contraction (isotonic, isometric or isokinetic) and according to the source of energy (aerobic or anaerobic).

Isotonic (dynamic) exercises are those in which the muscle shortens to produce muscle contraction and active movement. Most physical conditioning exercises – running, walking, swimming, cycling and other such activities – are isotonic, as are activities of daily living (ADL) and active range of movement (ROM) exercises (those initiated by the individual). Examples of isotonic bed exercises are pushing or pulling against a stationary object, using a trapeze to lift the body off the bed, lifting the buttocks off the bed by pushing with the hands against the mattress, and pushing the body to a sitting position.

Isotonic exercises increase muscle tone, mass and strength, and maintain joint flexibility and circulation. During isotonic exercise, both heart rate and cardiac output quicken to increase blood flow to all parts of the body. Little or no change in blood pressure occurs.

Isometric (static or setting) exercises are those in which there is a change in muscle tension but there is no change in muscle length and no muscle or joint movement. These exercises involve exerting pressure against a solid object and are useful for strengthening abdominal, gluteal and quadriceps muscles used in ambulation; for maintaining strength in immobilised muscles in casts or traction; and for endurance training. Examples of isometric bed exercise would be extending the leg in a supine position, tensing the thigh muscles, and pressing the knee against the bed, holding it for several seconds. These are often called quadriceps (or quad) sets.

Isometric exercises produce a moderate increase in heart rate and cardiac output, but no appreciable increase in blood flow to other parts of the body.

Isokinetic (resistive) exercises involve muscle contraction or tension against resistance; thus, they can be either isotonic or isometric. During isokinetic exercises, the person moves (isotonic) or tenses (isometric) against resistance. Special machines or devices provide the resistance to the movement. These exercises are used in physical conditioning and are often done to build up certain muscle groups; for example, the pectorals (chest muscles) may be increased in size and strength by lifting weights.

Aerobic exercise is activity during which the amount of oxygen taken in the body is greater than that used to perform the activity. Aerobic exercises use large muscle groups, are performed continuously and are rhythmic in nature. Examples are walking, jogging, running, bicycling, dancing, cross-country skiing, skipping, rowing, swimming and skating. Aerobic exercises improve cardiovascular conditioning and physical fitness.

Intensity of exercise can be measured in two ways:

1. *Target heart rate.* With this system, the goal is to work up to and sustain a target heart rate during exercise, based on the person's age. To determine the target heart rate, first calculate the person's maximum heart rate by subtracting their current age in years from 220. Then obtain the target heart rate by taking 60% to 85% of the maximum. At least 60% of maximum heart rate is the recommended intensity. Because heart rates are so variable among individuals, the tests that follow are replacing this measure.

2. *Talk test.* This test is easier to implement and keeps most people at 60% of maximum heart rate or more. When exercising, the person should be able to carry on a conversation even with some laboured breathing. However, exercise intensity should be increased if the person can carry on with unlimited unlaboured discussion.

Anaerobic exercise involves activity in which the muscles cannot draw out enough oxygen from the bloodstream, and anaerobic pathways are used to provide additional energy for a short time. This type of exercise is used in endurance training for athletes.

Benefits of Exercise

Regular exercise is essential for healthy functioning of major body systems. The benefits of exercise on these systems follow.

Musculoskeletal System

The size, shape, tone and strength of muscles (including the heart muscle) are maintained with mild exercise and increased with strenuous exercise. With strenuous exercise, muscles **hypertrophy** (enlarge), and the efficiency of muscular contraction increases. Hypertrophy is commonly seen in the arm muscles of a tennis player, the leg muscles of a skater, and the arm and hand muscles of a plumber.

Exercise increases joint flexibility and range of motion. Bone density is maintained through weight-bearing. The stress of weight-bearing maintains a balance between osteoblasts (bone-building cells) and osteoclasts (bone-resorption and breakdown cells).

Cardiovascular System

Adequate exercise increases the heart rate, the strength of heart muscle contraction, and the blood supply to the heart and muscles. Cardiac output (the amount of blood pumped by the heart) increases as much as 30 l/min. Normal cardiac output is 5 l/min.

Respiratory System

Ventilation (air circulating into and out of the lungs) increases. In strenuous exercise, the intake of oxygen increases to as much as 20 times normal intake. Normal ventilation is about 5 or 6 l/min. Adequate exercise also prevents pooling of secretions in the bronchi and bronchioles, decreases breathing effort and improves diaphragmatic excursion.

Gastrointestinal System

Exercise improves the appetite and increases gastrointestinal tract tone, facilitating peristalsis.

Metabolic System

Exercise elevates the metabolic rate, thus increasing the production of body heat and waste products and calorie use. During strenuous exercise, the metabolic rate can increase to as much as 20 times the normal rate. Exercise increases the use of triglycerides and fatty acids, resulting in a reduced level of serum triglycerides and cholesterol. Exercise also enhances the effectiveness of insulin, lowering blood sugar. In diabetics, exercise can reduce their need for injecting supplemental insulin.

Urinary System

As adequate exercise promotes efficient blood flow, the body excretes wastes more effectively. In addition, stasis (stagnation) of urine in the bladder is usually prevented.

Psychoneurological System

Exercise produces a sense of well-being and improves tolerance to stress. It may also improve self-concept by reducing depression and improving one's body image. Energy level increases and quality of sleep is enhanced.

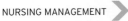
NURSING MANAGEMENT

FACTORS AFFECTING BODY ALIGNMENT AND ACTIVITY

A number of factors affect an individual's body alignment, mobility and daily activity level. These include growth and development, physical health, mental health, nutrition, personal values and attitudes, and certain external factors.

Growth and Development

A person's age and musculoskeletal and nervous system development affect posture, body proportions, body mass, body movements and reflexes. Newborn movements are reflexive and random. All extremities are generally flexed but can be passively moved through a full range of motion. The feet are usually inverted but can be passively everted. As the neurological system matures, control over movement progresses during the first year. Gross motor development precedes fine motor skills that is to say a child learns to walk before they can tie a shoe lace. Gross motor development occurs in a head-to-toe fashion, that is, progression from head control, to crawling, to pulling up to a standing position, to standing, and to walking, usually after the first birthday. Initially, walking involves a wide stance and unsteady gait, thus the term toddler. From ages 1–5 years, both gross and fine motor skills are refined. For example, pre-schoolers master riding a tricycle, dancing, running, jumping, using crayons to draw, fastening or using zippers, and brushing their teeth.

From 6–12 years, refinement of motor skills continues and exercise patterns for later life are generally determined. Many schools provide physical education and competitive sports programmes to enhance physical activity. Posture in school-age children is excellent, often the best during one's lifetime. In adolescence, growth spurts may result in awkwardness that can be manifested in posture. Postural habits formed during adolescence often persist into adulthood.

Adults between 20 and 40 years of age generally have few physical changes affecting mobility with the exception of pregnant women. Pregnancy alters centre of gravity, affects balance, and reduces exercise tolerance. As age advances, muscle tone and bone density decrease, joints lose flexibility, reaction time slows and bone mass decreases, particularly in women who have osteoporosis. **Osteoporosis** is a condition in which the bones become brittle and fragile due to calcium depletion. Osteoporosis is common in older women and primarily affects the weight-bearing joints of the lower extremities and the back, causing compression fractures of the vertebrae and hip fractures. All of these changes affect older adults' posture, gait and balance. Posture becomes forward leaning and stooped, which shifts the centre of gravity forward. To compensate for this shift, the knees flex slightly for support and the base of support is widened. Gait becomes wide based, short stepped and shuffling.

Physical Health

Mobility and activity tolerance are affected by any disorder that impairs the ability of the nervous system, musculoskeletal system, cardiovascular system, respiratory system and vestibular apparatus. Congenital problems such as hip dysplasia, spina bifida, cerebral palsy and the muscular dystrophies affect motor functioning. Disorders of the nervous system such as Parkinson's disease, multiple sclerosis, central nervous system tumours, cerebrovascular accidents (strokes), infectious processes (e.g. meningitis) and head and spinal cord injuries can leave muscle groups weakened, paralysed, **spastic** (with too much muscle tone) or **flaccid** (without muscle tone). Musculoskeletal disorders affecting mobility include strains, sprains, fractures, joint dislocations, amputations and joint replacements. Inner ear infections and dizziness can impair balance.

Many other acute and chronic illnesses that limit the supply of oxygen and nutrients needed for muscle contraction and movement can seriously affect activity tolerance. Examples include chronic obstructive lung disease, anaemia, congestive heart failure and angina.

Mental Health

Mental or affective disorders such as depression or chronic stress may affect a person's desire to move. The depressed person may lack enthusiasm for taking part in any activity and may even lack energy for usual hygiene practices. Lack of visible energy is seen in a slumped posture with head bowed. By contrast, happy, confident people usually stand erect. Chronic stress can deplete the body's energy reserves to the point that fatigue discourages the desire to exercise, even though exercise can energise the person and facilitate coping.

Nutrition

Both undernutrition and overnutrition can influence body alignment and mobility. Poorly nourished people may have muscle weakness and fatigue. Vitamin D deficiency causes bone deformity during growth. Inadequate calcium intake increases the risk of osteoporosis. Obesity can distort movement and can adversely affect posture and balance.

Personal Values and Attitudes

Whether people value regular exercise is often the result of family influences. In families that incorporate regular exercise in their daily routine or spend time together in activities, children learn to value physical activity. Sedentary families, on the other hand, participate in sports only as spectators, and this lifestyle is often transmitted to their children. Values about physical appearance also influence some people's participation in regular exercise. People who value a muscular build or physical attractiveness may participate in regular exercise programmes to produce the appearance they desire. Choice of physical activity or type of exercise is also influenced by values. Choices may be influenced by geographic location and cultural role expectations.

External Factors

Many external factors affect a person's mobility. Excessively high temperature and high humidity discourage activity, whereas comfortable temperature and humidity are conducive to activity. The availability of recreational facilities also influences activity; for example, lack of money may prohibit an individual from joining an exercise club or gymnasium. Neighbourhood safety promotes outdoor activity, whereas an unsafe environment discourages people from going outdoors. Adolescents, in particular, may spend many hours sitting at computers, watching television or playing video games rather than going outside to visit friends or to exercise.

Prescribed Limitations

Limitations to movement may be medically prescribed for some health problems. To promote healing, devices such as casts, braces, splints and traction are often used to immobilise body parts. Individuals who are short of breath may be advised not to walk up stairs. Bed rest may be the therapeutic choice for certain patients, for example, to relieve oedema, to reduce metabolic and oxygen needs, to promote tissue repair or to decrease pain.

The term **bed rest** varies in meaning to some extent. In some environments bed rest means strict confinement to bed or complete bed rest. Others may allow the patient to use a bedside commode or go to the bathroom. Nurses need to familiarise themselves with the meaning of bed rest in their practice setting.

EFFECTS OF IMMOBILITY

Individuals who have inactive lifestyles or who are faced with inactivity because of illness or injury are at risk for many problems that can affect major body systems. Whether immobility causes any problems often depends on the duration of the inactivity, the patient's health status and the patient's sensory awareness. The most obvious signs of prolonged immobility are often manifested in the musculoskeletal system. Individuals experience a significant decrease in muscular strength and agility whenever they do not maintain a moderate amount of physical activity. In addition, immobility adversely affects the cardiovascular, respiratory, metabolic, urinary and psychoneurological systems. Nurses need to understand these effects and encourage patient movement as much as possible. Early ambulation after illness or surgery is an essential measure to prevent complications. Potential effects of immobility on body systems follow.

Musculoskeletal System

+ *Disuse osteoporosis.* Without the stress of weight-bearing activity, the bones demineralise. They are depleted chiefly of calcium, which gives the bones strength and density. Regardless of the amount of calcium in a person's diet, the demineralisation process, known as *osteoporosis*, continues with immobility. The bones become spongy and may gradually deform and fracture easily.

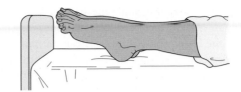

Figure 23-31 Plantar flexion contracture (foot drop).

+ *Disuse atrophy.* Unused muscles **atrophy** (decrease in size), losing most of their strength and normal function.
+ *Contractures.* When the muscle fibres are not able to shorten and lengthen, eventually a **contracture** (permanent shortening of the muscle) forms, limiting joint mobility. This process eventually involves the tendons, ligaments and joint capsules; it is irreversible except by surgical intervention. Joint deformities such as foot drop (see Figure 23-31) and external hip rotation occur when a stronger muscle dominates the opposite muscle.
+ *Stiffness and pain in the joints.* Without movement, the collagen (connective) tissues at the joint become **ankylosed** (permanently immobile). In addition, as the bones demineralise, excess calcium may deposit in the joints, contributing to stiffness and pain.

Cardiovascular System

+ *Diminished cardiac reserve.* Decreased mobility creates an imbalance in the autonomic nervous system, resulting in a preponderance of sympathetic activity over cholinergic activity that increases heart rate. Rapid heart rate reduces diastolic pressure, coronary blood flow and the capacity of the heart to respond to any metabolic demands above the basal levels. Because of this diminished cardiac reserve, the immobilised person may experience tachycardia with even minimal exertion.
+ *Increased use of the Valsalva manoeuvre.* The **Valsalva manoeuvre** refers to holding the breath and straining against a closed glottis. For example, patients tend to hold their breath when attempting to move up in a bed or sit on a bedpan. This builds up sufficient pressure on the large veins in the thorax to interfere with the return blood flow to the heart and coronary arteries. When the individual exhales and the glottis again opens, pressure is suddenly released and a surge of blood flows to the heart. Tachycardia and cardiac arrhythmias can result if the patient has cardiac disease.
+ *Orthostatic (postural) hypotension.* Orthostatic hypotension is a common result of immobilisation. Under normal conditions, sympathetic nervous system activity causes automatic vasoconstriction in the blood vessels in the lower half of the body when a mobile person changes from a horizontal to a vertical posture. Vasoconstriction prevents pooling of the blood in the legs and effectively maintains central blood pressure to ensure adequate perfusion of the heart and brain. During any prolonged immobility, this reflex becomes dormant. When the immobile person attempts to

sit or stand, this reconstricting mechanism fails to function properly in spite of increased adrenalin output. The blood pools in the lower extremities, and central blood pressure drops. Cerebral perfusion is seriously compromised, and the person feels dizzy or light headed and may even faint. This sequence is usually accompanied by a sudden and marked increase in heart rate, the body's effort to protect the brain from an inadequate blood supply.

+ *Venous vasodilation and stasis.* The skeletal muscles of an active person contract with each movement, compressing the blood vessels in those muscles and helping to pump the blood back to the heart against gravity. The tiny valves in the leg veins aid in venous return to the heart by preventing backward flow of blood and pooling. In an immobile person, the skeletal muscles do not contract sufficiently, and the muscles atrophy. The skeletal muscles can no longer assist in pumping blood back to the heart against gravity. Blood pools in the leg veins, causing vasodilatation and engorgement. The valves in the veins can no longer work effectively to prevent backward flow of blood and pooling (see Figure 23-32). This phenomenon is known as incompetent valves. As the blood continues to pool in the veins, its greater volume increases venous blood pressure, which can become much higher than that exerted by the tissues surrounding the vessel.

+ *Dependent oedema.* When the venous pressure is sufficiently great, some of the serous part of the blood is forced out of the blood vessel into the interstitial spaces surrounding the blood vessel, causing oedema. Oedema is most common in parts of the body positioned below the heart. Dependent oedema is most likely to occur around the sacrum or heels of a patient who sits up in bed or in the feet and lower legs of a patient who sits in a chair. Oedema further impedes

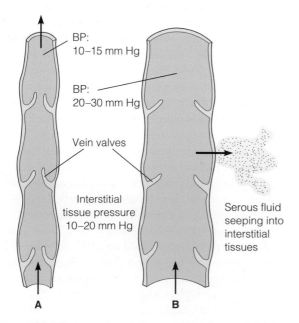

BP: 10–15 mm Hg

BP: 20–30 mm Hg

Vein valves

Interstitial tissue pressure 10–20 mm Hg

Serous fluid seeping into interstitial tissues

A   B

Figure 23-32 Leg veins: *A,* in a mobile person; *B,* in an immobile person.

venous return of blood to the heart, causing more pooling and more oedema. Oedematous tissue is uncomfortable and more susceptible to injury than normal tissue.

+ *Thrombus formation.* Three factors collectively predispose a patient to the formation of a **thrombophlebitis** (a clot that is loosely attached to an inflamed vein wall): impaired venous return to the heart, hypercoagulability of the blood, and injury to a vessel wall.

A **thrombus** (clot) is particularly dangerous if it breaks loose from the vein wall to enter the general circulation as an **embolus** (an object that has moved from its place of origin, causing obstruction to circulation elsewhere). Large emboli that enter the pulmonary circulation may occlude the vessels that nourish the lungs to cause an infarcted (dead) area of the lung. If the infarcted area is large, pulmonary function may be seriously compromised, or death may ensue. Emboli travelling to the coronary vessels or brain can produce a similarly dangerous outcome.

Respiratory System

+ *Decreased respiratory movement.* In a recumbent, immobile patient, ventilation of the lungs is passively altered. The body presses against the rigid bed and curtails chest movement. The abdominal organs push against the diaphragm, restricting lung movement and making it difficult to expand the lungs fully. An immobile recumbent person rarely sighs, partly because overall muscle atrophy also affects the respiratory muscles and partly because there is no stimulus of activity. Without these periodic stretching movements, the cartilaginous intercostal joints may become fixed in an expiratory phase of respiration, further limiting the potential for maximal ventilation. These changes produce shallow respirations and reduce **vital capacity** (the maximum amount of air that can be exhaled after a maximum inhalation).

+ *Pooling of respiratory secretions.* Secretions of the respiratory tract are normally expelled by changing positions or posture and by coughing. Inactivity allows secretions to pool by gravity (see Figure 23-33), interfering with the normal diffusion of oxygen and carbon dioxide in the alveoli. The ability to cough up secretions may also be hindered by loss of respiratory muscle tone, dehydration (which thickens secretions) or sedatives that depress the cough reflex. Poor oxygenation and retention of carbon dioxide in the blood can, if allowed to continue, predispose the person to respiratory acidosis, a potentially lethal disorder.

+ *Atelectasis.* When ventilation is decreased, pooled secretions may accumulate in a dependent area of a bronchiole and effectively block it. Because of changes in regional blood flow, bed rest decreases the amount of surfactant produced. (Surfactant enables the alveoli to remain open.) The combination of decreased surfactant and blockage of a bronchiole with mucus can cause atelectasis (the collapse of a lobe or of an entire lung) distal to the mucous blockage. Immobile elderly, post-operative patients are at greatest risk of atelectasis.

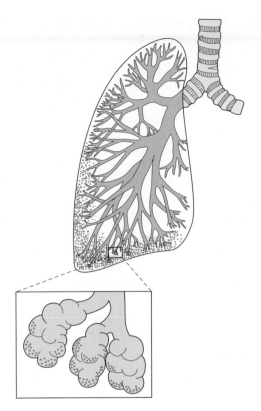

Figure 23-33 Pooling of secretions in the lungs of an immobile person.

+ *Hypostatic pneumonia.* Pooled secretions provide excellent media for bacterial growth. Under these conditions, a minor upper respiratory infection can evolve rapidly into a severe infection of the lower respiratory tract. Pneumonia caused by static respiratory secretions can severely impair oxygen–carbon dioxide exchange in the alveoli and is a fairly common cause of death among weakened, immobile persons, especially heavy smokers.

Metabolic System

+ *Decreased metabolic rate.* **Metabolism** refers to the sum of all the physical and chemical processes by which living substance is formed and maintained and by which energy is made available for use by the body. The **basal metabolic rate** is the minimal energy expended for the maintenance of these processes, expressed in calories per hour per square metre of body surface. In immobile patients, the basal metabolic rate and gastrointestinal motility and secretions of various digestive glands decrease as the energy requirements of the body decrease.

+ *Negative nitrogen balance.* In an active person, a balance exists between protein synthesis (**anabolism**) and protein breakdown (**catabolism**). Immobility creates a marked imbalance, and the catabolic processes exceed the anabolic processes. Catabolised muscle mass releases nitrogen. Over time, more nitrogen is excreted than is ingested, producing a negative nitrogen balance. The negative nitrogen balance represents a depletion of protein stores that are essential for building muscle tissue and for wound healing.

+ *Anorexia.* Loss of appetite (**anorexia**) occurs because of the decreased metabolic rate and the increased catabolism that accompany immobility. Reduced caloric intake is usually a response to the decreased energy requirements of the inactive person. If protein intake is reduced, the nitrogen imbalance may become more pronounced, sometimes so severely that malnutrition ensues.

+ *Negative calcium balance.* A negative calcium balance occurs as a direct result of immobility. Greater amounts of calcium are extracted from bone than can be replaced. The absence of weight-bearing and of stress on the musculoskeletal structures is the direct cause of the calcium loss from bones. Weight-bearing and stress are also required for calcium to be replaced in bone.

Urinary System

+ *Urinary stasis.* In a mobile person, gravity plays an important role in the emptying of the kidneys and the bladder. The shape and position of the kidneys and active kidney contractions are important in completely emptying the urine from the calyces, renal pelvis and ureters (see Figure 23-34, *A*). The shape and position of the urinary bladder (the detrusor muscle) and active bladder contractions are also important in achieving complete emptying (see Figure 23-35, *A* on page 608).

+ When the person remains in a horizontal position, gravity impedes the emptying of urine from the kidneys and the urinary bladder. To urinate, the person who is supine (in a back-lying position) must push upward, against gravity (Figures 23-34, *B* and 23-35, *B*). The renal pelvis may fill with urine before it is pushed into the ureters. Emptying is not as complete, and **urinary stasis** (stoppage or slowdown of flow) occurs after a few days of bed rest. Because of the overall decrease in muscle tone during immobilisation, including the tone of the detrusor muscle, bladder emptying is further compromised.

+ *Renal calculi.* In a mobile person, calcium in the urine remains dissolved because calcium and citric acid are balanced in an appropriately acid urine. With immobility and

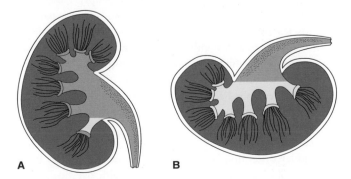

Figure 23-34 Pooling of urine in the kidney: *A*, The patient is in an upright position; *B*, the patient is in a back-lying position.

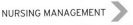

NURSING MANAGEMENT

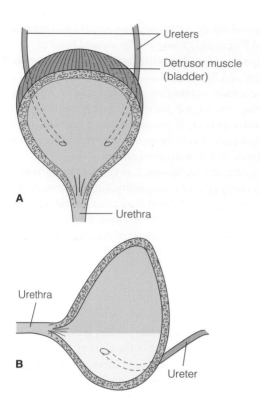

Figure 23-35 Pooling of urine in the urinary bladder: *A*, The patient is in an upright position; *B*, the patient is in a back-lying position.

the resulting excessive amounts of calcium in the urine, this balance is no longer maintained. The urine becomes more alkaline, and the calcium salts precipitate out as crystals to form renal **calculi** (stones). In an immobile person in a horizontal position, the renal pelvis filled with stagnant, alkaline urine is an ideal location for calculi to form. The stones usually develop in the renal pelvis and pass through the ureters into the bladder. As the stones pass along the long, narrow ureters, they cause extreme pain and bleeding and can sometimes obstruct the urinary tract.

+ *Urinary retention.* The immobile person may suffer from **urinary retention** (accumulation of urine in the bladder), bladder distention and, occasionally, **urinary incontinence** (involuntary urination). The decreased muscle tone of the urinary bladder inhibits its ability to empty completely, and the immobilised person is unable to relax the perineal muscles sufficiently to urinate. The discomfort of using a bedpan or urinal, the embarrassment and lack of privacy associated with this function, and the unnatural position for urination combine to make it difficult for the patient to relax the perineal muscles sufficiently to urinate while lying in bed.

When urination is not possible, the bladder gradually becomes distended with urine. The bladder may stretch excessively, eventually inhibiting the urge to void. When bladder distention is considerable, some involuntary urinary 'dribbling' may occur (retention with overflow). This does not relieve the urinary distention, because most of the stagnant urine remains in the bladder.

+ *Urinary infection.* Static urine provides an excellent medium for bacterial growth. The flushing action of normal, frequent urination is absent, and urinary distention often causes minute tears in the bladder mucosa, allowing infectious organisms to enter. The increased alkalinity of the urine caused by the hypercalcuria supports bacterial growth. The organism most commonly causing urinary tract infections is *Escherichia coli*, which normally resides in the colon. The normally sterile urinary tract may be contaminated by improper perineal care, the use of an indwelling urinary catheter or occasionally **urinary reflux** (backward flow). During reflux, contaminated urine from an overly distended bladder backs up into the renal pelvis to contaminate the kidney pelvis as well.

Gastrointestinal System

Constipation is a frequent problem for immobilised people because of decreased peristalsis and colon motility. The overall skeletal muscle weakness affects the abdominal and perineal muscles used in defecation. When the stool becomes very hard, more strength is required to expel it. The immobile person may lack this strength.

The bedfast person's unnatural and uncomfortable position on the bedpan does not facilitate elimination. The backward-leaning posture does not promote effective use of the muscles used in defecation. Some people are reluctant to use the bedpan in the presence of others. The embarrassment, lack of privacy, dependence on others to assist with the bedpan, and disruption of normal bowel habits may cause the individual to postpone or ignore the urge for elimination. Repeated postponement eventually suppresses the urge and weakens the defecation reflex.

Some persons may make excessive use of the Valsalva manoeuvre by straining at stool in an attempt to expel the hard stool. This effort dangerously increases intra-abdominal and intrathoracic pressures and places undue stress on the heart and circulatory system.

CLINICAL ANECDOTE

I have heard stories of patients becoming unconscious and even suffering a cardiac arrest when having their bowels open. Last month I was looking after an elderly lady admitted with constipation on a ward. She asked if she could use the toilet as she had been feeling 'constipated' and had been taking regular laxatives prior to being admitted to hospital. She felt these were now taking effect. I assisted her to the toilet and left her with a call alarm if she needed any assistance. After 15 minutes I went to check on her to find her unconscious.

After assessment she was diagnosed with a syncope episode probably as a result of Valsalva manoeuvre.

Sarah, second-year student nurse

Integumentary System

+ *Reduced skin turgor.* The skin can atrophy as a result of prolonged immobility. Shifts in body fluids between the fluid compartments can affect the consistency and health of the dermis and subcutaneous tissues in dependent parts of the body, eventually causing a gradual loss in skin elasticity.
+ *Skin breakdown.* Normal blood circulation relies on muscle activity. Immobility impedes circulation and diminishes the supply of nutrients to specific areas. As a result, skin breakdown and formation of pressure ulcers can occur.

Psychoneurological System

People who are unable to carry out the usual activities related to their roles (e.g. as breadwinner, husband, mother or athlete) become aware of an increased dependence on others. These factors lower the person's self-esteem. Frustration and the decrease in self-esteem may in turn provoke exaggerated emotional reactions. Emotional reactions vary considerably. Some individuals become apathetic and withdrawn, some regress and some become angry and aggressive.

Because the immobilised person's participation in life becomes much narrower and the variety of stimuli decreases, the person's perception of time intervals deteriorates. Problem-solving and decision-making abilities may deteriorate as a result of lack of intellectual stimulation and the stress of the illness and immobility. In addition, the loss of control over events can cause anxiety.

Immobility can impair the social and motor development of young children.

NURSING MANAGEMENT

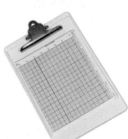

ASSESSING

Assessment relative to a patient's activity and exercise includes a patient history and a physical assessment of body alignment, gait, appearance and movement of joints, capabilities and limitations for movement, muscle mass and strength, activity tolerance, problems related to immobility and physical fitness. This physical assessment is usually completed by a physiotherapist.

The nurse collects information from the patient, from other nurses and from the patient's records. The examination and history are important sources of information about disabilities affecting the patient's mobility and activity status, such as contractures, oedema, pain in the extremities or generalised fatigue.

Patient History

An activity and exercise history is usually part of the comprehensive patient history and includes daily activity level, activity tolerance, type and frequency of exercise, factors affecting mobility and effects of immobility. If the individual indicates a recent pattern change or difficulties with mobility, a more detailed history is required. This detailed history should include the specific nature of the problem, when it first began and its frequency, its causes if known, how the problem affects daily living, what the patient is doing to cope with the problem, and whether these methods have been effective. Examples of interview questions to elicit this data are shown in the *Assessment interview*.

ASSESSMENT INTERVIEW

Activity and Exercise

Daily Activity Level
+ What activities do you carry out during a routine day?
+ Are you able to carry out the following tasks independently?
    (a) Eating
    (b) Dressing/grooming
    (c) Bathing
    (d) Toileting
    (e) Ambulating

    (f) Using a wheelchair
    (g) Transferring in and out of bed, bath and car
    (h) Cooking
    (i) House cleaning
    (j) Shopping
+ Where problems exist in your ability to carry out such tasks:
    (a) Would you rate yourself as partially or totally dependent?
    (b) How is the task achieved (by family, friend, agency or use of specialised equipment)?

Activity Tolerance

+ How much and what types of activities make you tired?
+ Do you ever experience dizziness, shortness of breath, marked increase in respiratory rate or other problems following mild or moderate activity?

Exercise

+ What type of exercise do you carry out to enhance your physical fitness?
+ What is the frequency and length of this exercise session?
+ Do you believe exercise is beneficial to your health? Explain.

Factors Affecting Mobility

+ Environmental factors. Do stairs, lack of railings or other assistive devices, or an unsafe neighbourhood impede your mobility or exercise regimen?
+ Health problems. Do any of the following health problems affect your muscle strength or endurance: heart disease, lung disease, stroke, cancer, neuromuscular problems, musculoskeletal problems, visual or mental impairments, trauma or pain?
+ Financial factors. Are your finances adequate to obtain equipment or other aids that you require to enhance your mobility?

Physical Examination

The physical examination is usually completed by a physiotherapist but in some clinical areas may be completed by a nurse practitioner. The assessment focuses on activity and exercise emphasises body alignment, gait, appearance and movement of joints, capabilities and limitations for movement, muscle mass and strength, and activity tolerance.

Body Alignment

Assessment of body alignment includes an inspection of the individual while they stand. The purpose of body alignment assessment is to identify

+ Normal developmental variations in posture
+ Posture and learning needs to maintain good posture
+ Factors contributing to poor posture, such as fatigue or low self-esteem
+ Muscle weakness or other motor impairments.

To assess alignment, the practitioner inspects the patient from lateral (see Figure 23-36, *A*), anterior and posterior perspectives. From the anterior and posterior views, the practitioner should observe whether

+ The shoulders and hips are level.
+ The toes point forward.
+ The spine is straight, not curved to either side.

The 'slumped' posture (Figure 23-36, *B*) is the most common problem that occurs when people stand. The neck is flexed far forward, the abdomen protrudes, the pelvis is thrust forward to create **lordosis** (an exaggerated inward curvature of the lumbar spine), and the knees are hyperextended. Low back pain and fatigue occur quickly in people with poor posture.

Gait

The characteristic pattern of a person's **gait** (walk) is assessed to determine the patient's mobility and risk for injury due to falling. Two phases of normal gait are stance and swing (see

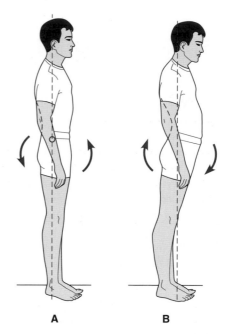

A   **B**

Figure 23-36 A standing person with *A*, good trunk alignment; *B*, poor trunk alignment. The arrows indicate the direction in which the pelvis is tilted.

Figure 23-37). When one leg is in the swing phase, the other is in the stance phase. In the *stance phase*, (a) the heel of one foot strikes the ground, and (b) body weight is spread over the ball of that foot while the other heel pushes off and leaves the ground. In the *swing phase*, the leg from behind moves in front of the body.

The practitioner assesses gait as the individual walks into the room or asks the individual to walk a distance of 10 metres down a hallway and observes for the following:

+ Head is erect, gaze is straight ahead and vertebral column is upright.
+ Heel strikes the ground before the toe.
+ Feet are dorsiflexed in the swing phase.

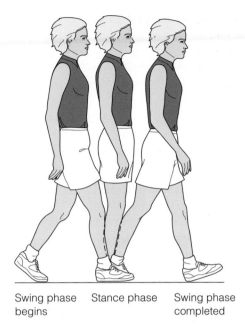

Swing phase   Stance phase   Swing phase
begins   completed

Figure 23-37 The stance and swing phases of a normal gait.

+ Arm opposite the swing-through foot moves forward at the same time.
+ Gait is smooth, coordinated and rhythmic, with even weight borne on each foot; it produces minimal body swing from side to side and directs movement straight ahead; and it starts and stops with ease.

The practitioner may also assess **pace** (the number of steps taken per minute). A normal walking pace is 70–100 steps per minute. The pace of an older person may slow to about 40 steps per minute.

The nurse should also note the individual for a prosthesis or assistive device, such as a walking stick or frame. For an individual who uses assistive aids, the practitioner assesses gait without the device and compares the assisted and unassisted gaits.

Appearance and Movement of Joints

Physical examination of the joints involves inspection, palpation, assessment of range of active motion, and if active motion is not possible, assessment of range of passive motion. The nurse should assess the following:

+ Any joint swelling or redness, which could indicate the presence of an injury or an inflammation.
+ Any deformity, such as a bony enlargement or contracture, and symmetry of involvement.
+ The muscle development associated with each joint and the relative size and symmetry of the muscles on each side of the body.
+ Any reported or palpable tenderness.
+ **Crepitation** (palpable or audible crackling or grating sensation produced by joint motion).

+ Increased temperature over the joint. Palpate the joint using the backs of the fingers and compare the temperature with that of the symmetric joint.
+ The degree of joint movement. Ask the patient to move selected body parts as shown in Table 23-2. If indicated, measure the extent of movement with a goniometer, a device that measures the angle of the joint in degrees.

Assessment of range of motion should not be unduly fatiguing, and the joint movements need to be performed smoothly, slowly and rhythmically. No joint should be forced. Uneven, jerky movement and forcing can injure the joint and its surrounding muscles and ligaments.

Capabilities and Limitations for Movement

The nurse needs to obtain data that may indicate hindrances or restrictions to the patient's movement and the need for assistance, including the following:

+ How the patient's illness influences the ability to move and whether the patient's health contraindicates any exertion, position or movement.
+ Encumbrances to movement, such as an intravenous line in place or a heavy cast.
+ Mental alertness and ability to follow directions. Check whether the patient is receiving medications that hinder the ability to walk safely. Narcotics, sedatives, tranquillisers and some antihistamines cause drowsiness, dizziness, weakness and orthostatic hypotension.
+ Balance and coordination.
+ Presence of orthostatic hypotension before transfers. Specifically, assess for any increase in pulse rate, marked fall in blood pressure, dizziness, lightheadedness and dimming of vision when the patient moves from a supine to a vertical posture.
+ Degree of comfort. People who have pain may not want to move and can require an analgesic before they are moved.
+ Vision. Is it adequate to prevent falls?

The nurse also assesses the amount of assistance the individual requires for the following:

+ Moving in the bed. In particular, observe for the amount of assistance the patient requires for turning:
  (a) From a supine position to a lateral position
  (b) From a lateral position on one side to a lateral position on the other
  (c) From a supine position to a sitting position in bed.
+ Rising from a lying position to a sitting position on the edge of the bed. Healthy people can normally rise without support from the arms.
+ Rising from a chair to a standing position. Normally this can be done without pushing with the arms.
+ Coordination and balance. Determine the patient's abilities to hold the body erect, to bear weight and keep balance in a standing position on both legs or only one, to take steps, and to push off from a chair or bed.

NURSING MANAGEMENT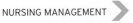

Muscle Mass and Strength

Before the patient undertakes a change in position or attempts to ambulate, it is essential that the nurse assesses the patient's strength and ability to move. Providing appropriate assistance lowers the risk of muscle strain and body injury to both the patient and nurse. Assessment of upper extremity strength is especially important for patients who use ambulation aids, such as walking frames and crutches.

Activity Tolerance

By determining an appropriate activity level for an individual, the nurse can predict whether the individual has the strength and endurance to participate in activities that require similar expenditures of energy. This assessment is useful in encouraging increasing independence in people who (a) have a cardiovascular or respiratory disability, (b) have been completely immobilised for a prolonged period, (c) have decreased muscle mass or a musculoskeletal disorder, (d) have experienced inadequate sleep, (e) have experienced pain or (f) are depressed, anxious or unmotivated.

The most useful measures in predicting activity tolerance are heart rate, strength and rhythm; respiratory rate, depth and rhythm; and blood pressure. These data are obtained at the following times:

+ Before the activity starts (baseline data), while the patient is at rest
+ During the activity
+ Immediately after the activity stops
+ Three minutes after the activity has stopped and the patient has rested.

The activity should be stopped immediately in the event of any physiological change indicating the activity is too strenuous or prolonged for the patient. These changes include the following:

+ Sudden facial pallor
+ Feelings of dizziness or weakness
+ Change in level of consciousness
+ Heart rate or respiratory rate that significantly exceeds baseline or pre-established levels
+ Change in heart or respiratory rhythm from regular to irregular
+ Weakening of the pulse
+ Dyspnoea, shortness of breath or chest pain
+ Diastolic blood pressure change of 10 mm Hg or more.

If, however, the patient tolerates the activity well, and if heart rate returns to baseline levels within five minutes after the activity ceases, the activity is considered safe. This activity, then, can serve as a standard for predicting the tolerance for similar activities.

Table 23-3 Assessing Problems of Immobility

Assessment	Problem
Musculoskeletal system	
Measure arm and leg circumferences	Decreased circumference due to decreased muscle mass
Palpate and observe body joints	Stiffness or pain in joints
Take goniometric measurements of joint ROM	Decreased joint ROM, joint contractures
Cardiovascular system	
Auscultate the heart	Increased heart rate
Measure blood pressure	Orthostatic hypotension
Palpate and observe sacrum, legs and feet	Peripheral dependent oedema, increased peripheral vein engorgement
Palpate peripheral	Weak peripheral pulses
Measure calf muscle circumferences	Oedema
Observe calf muscle for redness, tenderness and swelling	Thrombophlebitis
Respiratory system	
Observe chest movements	Asymmetric chest movements, dyspnoea
Auscultate chest	Diminished breath sounds, crackles, wheezes and increased respiratory rate
Metabolic system	
Measure height and weight	Weight loss due to muscle atrophy and loss of subcutaneous fat
Palpate skin	Generalised oedema due to low blood protein levels
Urinary system	
Measure fluid intake and output	Dehydration
Inspect urine	Cloudy, dark urine; high specific gravity
Palpate urinary bladder	Distended urinary bladder due to urinary retention
Gastrointestinal system	
Observe stool	Hard, dry, small stool
Auscultate bowel sounds	Decreased bowel sounds due to decreased intestinal motility
Integumentary system	
Inspect skin	Break in skin integrity

Problems Related to Immobility

When collecting data pertaining to the problems of immobility, the practitioner uses the assessment methods of inspection, palpation and auscultation; checks results of laboratory tests; and takes measurements, including body weight, fluid intake and fluid output. Specific techniques for assessing immobility problems and abnormal assessment findings related to the complications of immobility are listed in Table 23-3.

It is extremely important to obtain and record baseline assessment data soon after the individual first becomes immobile. These baseline data serve as the standard against which all data collected throughout the period of immobilisation are compared.

Because a major nursing responsibility is to prevent the complications of immobility, the nurse needs to identify patients at risk of developing such complications before problems arise. Individuals at risk include those who (a) are poorly nourished; (b) have decreased sensitivity to pain, temperature or pressure; (c) have existing cardiovascular, pulmonary or neuromuscular problems; and (d) have altered level of consciousness.

PLANNING

As part of planning, the nurse is responsible for identifying those patients who need assistance with body alignment and determining the degree of assistance they need. The nurse must be sensitive to the patient's need to function as independently as possible yet provide assistance when the patient needs it.

Most patients require some nursing guidance and assistance to learn about, achieve and maintain proper body mechanics. The nurse should also plan to teach patients applicable skills.

For example, a patient with a back injury needs to learn how to get out of bed safely and comfortably, a patient with an injured leg needs to learn how to transfer from bed to wheelchair safely, and a patient with a newly acquired walker needs to learn how to use it safely. Nurses often teach family members or caregivers safe moving, lifting and transfer techniques in the home setting (see Chapter 12).

The goals established for individuals will vary according to the diagnosis and defining characteristics related to each individual. Examples of overall goals for patients with actual or potential problems related to mobility or activity follow.

The patient will have:

+ Increased tolerance for physical activity.
+ Restored or improved capability to ambulate and/or participate in activities of daily living.
+ Absence of injury from falling or improper use of body mechanics.
+ Enhanced physical fitness.
+ Absence of any complications associated with immobility.
+ Improved social, emotional and intellectual well-being.

Planning for Home Care

Patients who have been hospitalised for activity or mobility problems often need continued care in the home. In preparation for discharge, the nurse needs to determine the patient's actual and potential health problems, strengths and resources. The *Community care considerations* describes the specific assessment data required before establishing a discharge plan for individuals with mobility or activity problems. A major aspect of discharge planning involves instructional needs of the patient and family.

COMMUNITY CARE CONSIDERATIONS

Mobility and Activity Problems

Patient and Environment

+ Capabilities or tolerance for required and desired activities: self-care (feeding, bathing, toileting, dressing, grooming, home maintenance, shopping, cooking); recreational activities
+ Mobility aids required: stick, walking frame, crutches, wheelchair, transfer boards
+ Equipment required if immobilised: special bed, side rails, pressure-reducing mattress
+ Current level of knowledge: body mechanics for use of mobility aids; specific exercises prescribed
+ Home mobility hazard appraisal: adequacy of lighting; presence of handrails; safety of pathways and stairs; congested areas; unanchored rugs, mats or electrical wires, and any other obstacles to safe movement; structural adjustments needed for wheelchair access

Family or Caregiver

+ Caregiver availability, skills and willingness: primary people able to assist patient with self-care, movement, shopping, and so on; physical and emotional status to assist with care; learning needs
+ Family role changes and coping: effect on financial status, parenting and spousal roles, social roles
+ Availability of caregiver support: other support people available for occasional duties such as shopping, transportation, housekeeping, cooking, budgeting, respite care

Community

+ Resources: availability and familiarity with sources of medical equipment, financial assistance, homemaker services, hygienic care; Meals on Wheels; spiritual counsellors and visitors; sources of respite for caregiver

TEACHING: COMMUNITY CARE

Activity and Exercise

Maintaining Musculoskeletal Function

+ Teach in conjunction with the physiotherapist the systematic performance of passive or assistive ROM exercises to maintain joint mobility.
+ As appropriate, demonstrate the proper way to perform isotonic, isometric or isokinetic exercises to maintain muscle mass and tone (collaborate with the physical therapist about these). Incorporate ADLs into exercise programme if appropriate.
+ Provide a written schedule for the type, frequency and duration of exercises; encourage the use of a progress graph or chart to facilitate adherence with the therapy.
+ Offer an ambulation schedule.
+ Instruct in the availability of assistive ambulatory devices and correct use of them.
+ Discuss pain control measures required before exercise.

Preventing Injury

+ Teach safe transfer and ambulation techniques.
+ Discuss safety measures to avoid falls (e.g. locking wheelchairs, wearing appropriate footwear, using rubber tips on crutches, keeping the environment

safe and using mechanical aids such as raised toilet seat, grab bars, urinal and bedpan or commode to facilitate toileting).
+ Teach the use of proper body mechanics.
+ Teach ways to prevent postural hypotension.

Managing Energy to Prevent Fatigue

+ Discuss activity and rest patterns and develop a plan as indicated; intersperse rest periods with activity periods.
+ Discuss ways to minimise fatigue such as performing activities more slowly and for shorter periods, resting more often and using more assistance as required.
+ Provide information about available resources to help with ADLs and home maintenance management.
+ Teach ways to increase energy (e.g. increasing intake of high-energy foods, ensuring adequate rest and sleep, controlling pain).
+ Teach techniques to monitor activity tolerance as appropriate.

Referrals

+ Provide appropriate information about accessing community resources: home care agencies, sources of equipment, and so on.

IMPLEMENTING

Nursing strategies to maintain or promote body alignment and mobility involve positioning patients appropriately, moving and handling patients, providing ROM exercises, ambulating patients with or without mechanical aids, and strategies to prevent the complications of immobility. Whenever positioning, moving, handling and ambulating patients, nurses must always use proper body mechanics to avoid musculoskeletal strain and injury (see Chapter 12).

Positioning Patients

Positioning a patient in good body alignment and changing the position regularly and systematically are essential aspects of nursing practice. Individuals who can move easily, automatically reposition themselves for comfort. Such people generally require minimal positioning assistance from nurses, other than guidance about ways to maintain body alignment and to exercise their joints. However, people who are weak, frail, in pain, paralysed or unconscious rely on nurses to provide or assist with position changes. For all patients, it is important to

assess the skin and provide skin care before and after a position change.

Any position, correct or incorrect, can be detrimental if maintained for a prolonged period. Frequent change of position helps to prevent muscle discomfort, undue pressure resulting in pressure ulcers, damage to superficial nerves and blood vessels, and contractures. Position changes also maintain muscle tone and stimulate postural reflexes.

When the individual is not able to move independently or assist with moving, the preferred method is to have two or more people move or turn the patient (see Chapter 12). Appropriate assistance reduces the risk of muscle strain and body injury to both the patient and nurse.

When positioning patients in bed, the nurse can do a number of things to ensure proper alignment and promote comfort and safety:

+ Make sure the mattress is firm and level yet has enough give to fill in and support natural body curvatures. A sagging mattress, a mattress that is too soft or an underfilled waterbed used over a prolonged period can contribute to the development of hip flexion contractures and low back strain and pain. Bed boards made of plywood and placed beneath a

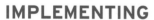

sagging mattress are increasingly recommended for individuals who have back problems or are prone to them. Some bed boards are hinged across the middle so that they will bend as the head of the bed is raised. It is particularly important in the home setting to inspect the mattress for support.

+ Ensure that the bed is clean and dry. Wrinkled or damp sheets increase the risk of pressure ulcer formation. Make sure extremities can move freely whenever possible. For example, the top bedclothes need to be loose enough for the patient to move the feet.

+ Place support devices in specified areas according to the patient's position. *Box 23-1* lists commonly used support devices. Use only those support devices needed to maintain alignment and to prevent stress on the individual's muscles and joints. If the person is capable of movement, too many devices limit mobility and increase the potential for muscle weakness and atrophy. Common alignment problems that can be corrected with support devices include the following:

   (a) Flexion of the neck
   (b) Internal rotation of the shoulder
   (c) Adduction of the shoulder
   (d) Flexion of the wrist
   (e) Anterior convexity of the lumbar spine
   (f) External rotation of the hips
   (g) Hyperextension of the knees
   (h) Plantar flexion of the ankle.

+ Avoid placing one body part, particularly one with bony prominences, directly on top of another body part. Excessive pressure can damage veins and predispose the patient to thrombus formation. Pressure against the popliteal space may damage nerves and blood vessels in this area.

+ Plan a systematic 24-hour schedule for position changes.

+ Sometimes a person who appears well aligned may be experiencing real discomfort. Both appearance, in relation to alignment criteria, and comfort are important in achieving effective alignment.

Fowler's Position

Fowler's position, or a semi-sitting position, is a bed position in which the head and trunk are raised 45–90 degrees. In **low-Fowler's** or **semi-Fowler's position** (see Figure 23-38), the head

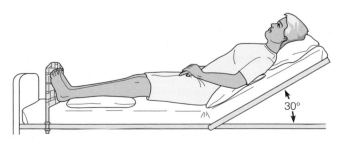

Figure 23-38 Low-Fowler's (semi-Fowler's) position (supported). Note that arm support is omitted in this instance. The amount of support depends on the needs of the individual patient.

> ### BOX 23-1 Support Devices
>
> + Pillows. Different sizes are available. Used for support or elevation of a body part (e.g. an arm). Specially designed dense pillows can be used to elevate the upper body.
> + Mattresses. There are two types of mattresses: ones that fit on the bed frame (e.g. standard bed mattress) and mattresses that fit on the standard bed mattress (e.g. egg crate mattress). Mattresses should be evenly supportive.
> + Bed boards. The boards are usually made of wood and are placed under the mattress to provide support.
> + Chair beds. These beds can be placed into the position of a chair for patients who cannot move from the bed but require a sitting position.
> + Foot boot. These are made of a variety of substances. They usually have a firm exterior and padding of foam to protect the skin. They provide support to the feet in a natural position and keep the weight of covers off the toes. Individuals who are able to sit may benefit from high-top shoes to maintain foot alignment.
> + Footboard. A flat panel often made of plastic or wood. It keeps the feet in dorsiflexion to prevent plantar flexion.

and trunk are raised 15–45 degrees; in **high-Fowler's position**, the head and trunk are raised 90 degrees (see Table 23-5 on page 616). In this position, the knees may or may not be flexed.

Fowler's position is the position of choice for people who have difficulty breathing and for some people with heart problems. When the patient is in this position, gravity pulls the diaphragm downward, allowing greater chest expansion and lung ventilation.

A common error nurses make when aligning patients in Fowler's position is placing an overly large pillow or more than one pillow behind the patient's head. This promotes the development of neck flexion contractures. If a patient desires several head pillows, the nurse should encourage the patient to rest without a pillow for several hours each day to extend the neck fully and counteract the effects of poor neck alignment.

Orthopnoeic Position

In the **orthopnoeic position**, the individual sits either in bed or on the side of the bed with an overbed table across the lap (see Figure 23-39 on page 616). This position facilitates respiration by allowing maximum chest expansion. It is particularly helpful to patients who have problems exhaling, because they can press the lower part of the chest against the edge of the overbed table.

Table 23-5 Fowler's Position

Unsupported position	Problem to be prevented	Corrective measure*
Bed-sitting position with upper part of body elevated 30–90° commencing at hips	Posterior flexion of lumbar curvature	Pillow at lower back (lumbar region) to support lumbar region
Head rests on bed surface	Hyperextension of neck	Pillows to support head, neck and upper back
Arms fall at sides	Shoulder muscle strain, possible dislocation of shoulders, oedema of hands and arms with flaccid paralysis, flexion contracture of the wrist	Pillow under forearms to eliminate pull on shoulder and assist venous blood flow from hands and lower arms
Legs lie flat and straight on lower bed surface	Hyperextension of knees	Small pillow under thighs to flex knees
Heels rest on bed surface	Pressure on heels	Pillow under lower legs
Feet are in plantar flexion	Plantar flexion of feet (foot drop)	Footboard to provide support for dorsal flexion

The amount of correction depends on the needs of the individual patient.

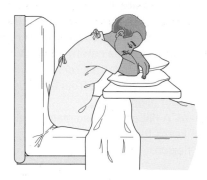

Figure 23-39 Orthopnoeic position.

Dorsal Recumbent Position

In the **dorsal recumbent** (back-lying) **position** (see Figure 23-40), the patient's head and shoulders are slightly elevated on a small pillow. In some areas, the terms *dorsal recumbent* and *supine* are used interchangeably; strictly speaking, however, in the **supine** or **dorsal position** the head and shoulders are not elevated. In both positions, the patient's forearms may be

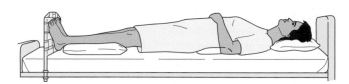

Figure 23-40 Dorsal recumbent position (supported).

elevated on pillows or placed at the patient's sides. Supports are similar in both positions, except for the head pillow (see Table 23-6). The dorsal recumbent position is used to provide comfort and to facilitate healing following certain procedures or anaesthetics (e.g. spinal).

Prone Position

In the **prone position**, the patient lies on the abdomen with the head turned to one side (see Figure 23-41). The hips are not flexed. Both children and adults often sleep in this position, sometimes with one or both arms flexed over their heads. This position has several advantages. It is the only bed position that

Table 23-6 Dorsal Recumbent Position

Unsupported position	Problem to be prevented	Corrective measure*
Head is flat on bed surface	Hyperextension of neck in thick-chested person	Pillow of suitable thickness under head and shoulders if necessary for alignment
Lumbar curvature of spine is apparent	Posterior flexion of lumbar curvature	Roll or small pillow under lumbar curvature
Legs may be externally rotated	External rotation of legs	Roll or sandbag placed laterally to trochanter of femur (optional)
Legs are extended	Hyperextension of knees	Small pillow under thigh to flex knee slightly
Feet assume plantar flexion position	Plantar flexion (foot drop)	Footboard or rolled pillow to support feet in dorsal flexion
Heels on bed surface	Pressure on heels	Pillow under lower legs

The amount of correction depends on the needs of the individual patient.

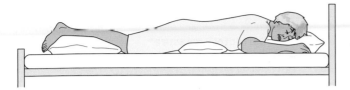

Figure 23-41 Prone position (supported).

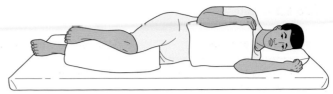

Figure 23-42 Lateral position (supported).

allows full extension of the hip and knee joints. When used periodically, the prone position helps to prevent flexion contractures of the hips and knees, thereby counteracting a problem caused by all other bed positions. The prone position also promotes drainage from the mouth and is especially useful for unconscious patients or those recovering from surgery of the mouth or throat (see Table 23-7).

The prone position poses some distinct disadvantages. The pull of gravity on the trunk produces a marked lordosis in most people, and the neck is rotated laterally to a significant degree. For this reason, the prone position may not be recommended for people with problems of the cervical or lumbar spine. This position also causes plantar flexion. Some patients with cardiac or respiratory problems find the prone position confining and suffocating because chest expansion is inhibited during respirations. The prone position should be used only when the patient's back is correctly aligned, only for short periods, and only for people with no evidence of spinal abnormalities.

Lateral Position

In the **lateral** (side-lying) **position** (see Figure 23-42), the person lies on one side of the body. Flexing the top hip and knee and placing this leg in front of the body creates a wider, triangular base of support and achieves greater stability. The greater the flexion of the top hip and knee, the greater the stability and balance in this position. This flexion reduces lordosis and promotes good back alignment. For this reason, the lateral position is good for resting and sleeping patients. The lateral position helps to relieve pressure on the sacrum and heels in people who sit for much of the day or who are confined to bed and rest in Fowler's

or dorsal recumbent positions much of the time. In the lateral position, most of the body's weight is borne by the lateral aspect of the lower scapula, the lateral aspect of the ilium and the greater trochanter of the femur. People who have sensory or motor deficits on one side of the body usually find that lying on the uninvolved side is more comfortable (see Table 23-8 on page 618).

Sims' Position

In **Sims'** (semiprone) **position** (see Figure 23-43), the individual assumes a posture halfway between the lateral and the prone positions. The lower arm is positioned behind the patient, and the upper arm is flexed at the shoulder and the elbow. Both legs

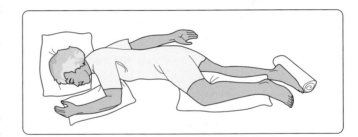

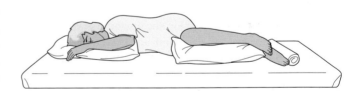

Figure 23-43 Sims' position (supported).

Table 23-7 Prone Position

Unsupported position	Problem to be prevented	Corrective measure*
Head is turned to side and neck is slightly flexed	Flexion or hyperextension of neck	Small pillow under head unless contraindicated because of promotion of mucous drainage from mouth
Body lies flat on abdomen accentuating lumbar curvature	Hyperextension of lumbar curvature; difficulty breathing; pressure on breasts (women); pressure on genitals (men)	Small pillow or roll under abdomen just below diaphragm
Toes rest on bed surface; feet are in plantar flexion	Plantar flexion of feet (foot drop)	Allow feet to fall naturally over end of mattress, or support lower legs on a pillow so that toes do not touch the bed

The amount of correction depends on the needs of the individual patient.

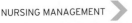

NURSING MANAGEMENT

Table 23-8 Lateral Position

Unsupported position	Problem to be prevented	Corrective measure*
Body is turned to side, both arms in front of body, weight resting primarily on lateral aspects of scapula and ilium	Lateral flexion and fatigue of sternocleidomastoid muscles	Pillow under head and neck to provide good alignment
Upper arm and shoulder are rotated internally and adducted	Internal rotation and adduction of shoulder and subsequent limited function; impaired chest expansion	Pillow under upper arm to place it in good alignment; lower arm should be flexed comfortably
Upper thigh and leg are rotated internally and adducted	Internal rotation and adduction of femur; twisting of the spine	Pillow under leg and thigh to place them in good alignment; shoulders and hips should be aligned

The amount of correction depends on the needs of the individual patient.

Table 23-9 Sims' (Semiprone) Position

Unsupported position	Problem to be prevented	Corrective measure*
Head rests on bed surface; weight is borne by lateral aspects of cranial and facial bones	Lateral flexion of neck	Pillow supports head, maintaining it in good alignment unless drainage from the mouth is required
Upper shoulder and arm are internally rotated	Internal rotation of shoulder and arm; pressure on chest, restricting expansion during breathing	Pillow under upper arm to prevent internal rotation
Upper leg and thigh are adducted and internally rotated	Internal rotation and adduction of hip and leg	Pillow under upper leg to support it in alignment
Feet assume plantar flexion	Foot drop	Sandbags to support feet in dorsal flexion

The amount of correction depends on the needs of the individual patient.

are flexed in front of the patient. The upper leg is more acutely flexed at both the hip and the knee than is the lower one.

Sims' position may be used for unconscious patients because it facilitates drainage from the mouth and prevents aspiration of fluids. It is also used for paralysed individuals because it reduces pressure over the sacrum and greater trochanter of the hip. It is often used for patients receiving enemas and occasionally for those undergoing examinations or treatments of the perineal area. Many people, especially pregnant women, find Sims' position comfortable for sleeping. People with sensory or motor deficits on one side of the body usually find that lying on the uninvolved side is more comfortable (see Table 23-9).

LIFESPAN CONSIDERATIONS

Positioning Patients

Infants

+ Position infants on their back for sleep, or side particularly after feeding.

Children

+ Carefully inspect the dependent skin surfaces of all infants and children confined to bed at least three times in each 24-hour period.

Older Adults

+ Decreased subcutaneous fat and thinning of the skin place elders at risk for skin breakdown.

Repositioning at least every two hours helps reduce pressure on bony prominences and avoid skin trauma.

+ In patients who have had cerebrovascular accidents (strokes), there is a risk of shoulder displacement on the paralysed side from improper moving or repositioning techniques. Use care when moving, positioning in bed and transferring. Pillows or foam devices are helpful to support the affected arm and shoulder and prevent injury.

NURSING MANAGEMENT

Providing Range of Movement (ROM) Exercises

When people are ill, they may need to perform ROM exercises until they can regain their normal activity levels. **Active ROM exercises** are isotonic exercises in which the individual moves each joint in the body through its complete range of movement, maximally stretching all muscle groups within each plane over the joint. These exercises maintain or increase muscle strength and endurance and help to maintain cardiorespiratory function in an immobilised individual. They also prevent deterioration of joint capsules, ankylosis and contractures.

Full ROM does not occur spontaneously in the immobilised individual who independently achieves ADLs, moves about in bed, transfers between bed and wheelchair or chair or ambulates a short distance, because only a few muscle groups are maximally stretched during these activities. Although the patient may successfully achieve some active ROM movements of the upper extremities while combing the hair, bathing and dressing, the immobilised patient is very unlikely to achieve any active ROM movements of the lower extremities when these are not used in the normal functions of standing and walking about. For this reason, most wheelchair and many ambulatory patients need active ROM exercises until they regain their normal activity levels.

At first, the nurse may need to teach the patient to perform the needed ROM exercises; eventually, the patient may be able to accomplish these independently. Instructions for the patient performing active ROM exercises are shown in the *Teaching: patient care.*

During **passive ROM exercises**, another person moves each of the patient's joints through its complete range of movement, maximally stretching all muscle groups within each plane over each joint. Because the individual does not contract the muscles, passive ROM exercises are of no value in maintaining muscle strength but are useful in maintaining joint flexibility. For this reason, passive ROM exercises should be performed only when the patient is unable to accomplish the movements actively.

Passive ROM exercises should be accomplished for each movement of the arms, legs and neck that the individual is unable to achieve actively. As with active ROM exercises, passive ROM exercises should be accomplished to the point of slight resistance, but not beyond, and never to the point of discomfort. The movements should be systematic, and the same sequence should be followed during each exercise session. Each exercise should consist of three repetitions, and the series of exercises should be done twice daily. Performing one series of exercises along with the bath is helpful. Passive ROM exercises are accomplished most effectively when the individual lies supine in bed. General guidelines for providing passive exercises are shown in the *Practice guidelines* on page 620.

During active-assistive ROM exercises, the patient uses a stronger, opposite arm or leg to move each of the joints of a limb incapable of active motion. The patient learns to support and move the weak arm or leg with the strong arm or leg as far as possible. Then the nurse continues the movement passively to its maximal degree. This activity increases active movement on the strong side of the patient's body and maintains joint flexibility on the weak side. Such exercise is especially useful for stroke victims who are hemiplegic (paralysed on one-half of the body).

Functional joint flexibility is also maintained in the performance of ADLs. The following are examples:

+ Eating, shaving, grooming and bathing exercise the elbow (flexion and extension) and shoulder (abduction).
+ Activities requiring fine motor skills, such as writing and eating, exercise the fingers (flexion, extension, adduction, abduction) and the thumb (opposition).
+ Walking exercises the shoulders (flexion, extension), hip (flexion, extension, hyperextension), knee (flexion, extension) and ankle (plantar flexion and dorsiflexion).
+ Reaching for articles exercises the shoulders (flexion, extension and perhaps slight abduction or adduction).
+ Dressing involves many joint movements.

Ambulating Patients

Ambulation (the act of walking) is a function that most people take for granted. However, when people are ill they are often confined to bed and are thus nonambulatory. The longer individuals are in bed, the more difficulty they have walking.

TEACHING: PATIENT CARE

Active ROM Exercises
+ Perform each ROM exercise as taught to the point of slight resistance, but not beyond, and never to the point of discomfort.
+ Perform the movements systematically, using the same sequence during each session.
+ Perform each exercise three times.
+ Perform each series of exercises twice daily.

Older Adults
+ For older adults, it is not essential to achieve full range of motion in all joints. Instead, emphasise achieving a sufficient range of motion to carry out ADLs, such as walking, dressing, combing hair, showering and preparing a meal.

PRACTICE GUIDELINES

Providing Passive ROM Exercises

+ Ensure that the individual understands the reason for doing ROM exercises.
+ If there is a possibility of hand swelling, make sure rings are removed.
+ Clothe the patient in a loose gown, and cover the body with a bath blanket.
+ Use correct body mechanics when providing ROM exercise to avoid muscle strain or injury to both yourself and the patient.
+ Position the bed at an appropriate height.
+ Expose only the limb being exercised to avoid embarrassing the patient.
+ Support the patient's limbs above and below the joint as needed to prevent muscle strain or injury (see Figure 23-44). This may also be done by cupping joints in the palm of your hand or cradling limbs along your forearm (see Figure 23-45). If a joint is painful (e.g. arthritic), support the limb in the muscular areas above and below the joint.
+ Use a firm, comfortable grip when handling the limb.
+ Move the body parts smoothly, slowly and rhythmically. Jerky movements cause discomfort and, possibly, injury. Fast movements can cause spasticity (sudden, prolonged involuntary muscle contraction) or rigidity (stiffness or inflexibility).
+ Avoid moving or forcing a body part beyond the existing range of motion. Muscle strain, pain and injury can result. This is particularly important for people with flaccid (limp) paralysis, whose muscles can be stretched and joints dislocated without their awareness.

+ If muscle spasticity occurs during movement, stop the movement temporarily, but continue to apply slow, gentle pressure on the part until the muscle relaxes; then proceed with the motion.
+ If a contracture is present, apply slow firm pressure, without causing pain, to stretch the muscle fibres.
+ If rigidity occurs, apply pressure against the rigidity and continue the exercise slowly.
+ Avoid hypertension of joints in older adults if joints are arthritic.
+ Use the exercises as an opportunity to also assess skin condition.

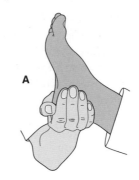

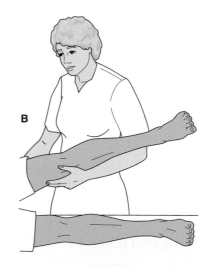

Figure 23-45 Holding limbs for support during passive exercise: *A*, cupping; *B*, cradling.

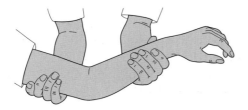

Figure 23-44 Supporting a limb above and below the joint for passive exercise.

Even one or two days of bed rest can make a person feel weak, unsteady and shaky when first getting out of bed. A patient who has had surgery, is elderly or has been immobilised for a longer time will feel more pronounced weakness. The potential problems of immobility are far less likely to occur when patients become ambulatory as soon as possible. The nurse can assist patients to prepare for ambulation by helping them become as independent as possible while in bed. Nurses should encourage individuals to perform ADLs, maintain good body alignment and carry out active ROM exercises to the maximum degree possible yet within the limitations imposed by their illness and recovery programme.

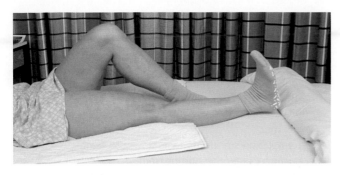

Figure 23-46 Tensing the quadriceps femoris muscles before ambulation.

Preambulatory Exercises

Individuals who have been in bed for long periods often need a plan of muscle tone exercises to strengthen the muscles used for walking before attempting to walk. One of the most important muscle groups is the quadriceps femoris, which extends the knee and flexes the thigh. This group is also important for elevating the legs, for example, for walking upstairs. These exercises are frequently called quadriceps drills or sets. To strengthen these muscles, the individual consciously tenses them, drawing the kneecap upward and inward. The patient pushes the popliteal space of the knee against the bed surface, relaxing the heels on the bed surface (see Figure 23-46). On the count of 1, the muscles are tensed; they are held during the counts of 2, 3, 4; and they are relaxed at the count of 5. The exercise should be done within the patient's tolerance, that is, without fatiguing the muscles. Carried out several times an hour during waking hours, this simple exercise significantly strengthens the muscles used for walking.

Assisting Patients to Ambulate

Patients who have been immobilised for even a few days may require assistance with ambulation. The amount of assistance will depend on the individual's condition, including age, health status and length of inactivity. Assistance may mean walking alongside the patient while providing physical support or providing instruction to the patient about the use of assistive devices such as a stick, walking frame or crutches.

Some individuals experience postural (orthostatic) hypotension on assuming a vertical position from a lying position and may need information about ways to control this problem (see *Teaching: patient care*). The individual may exhibit some or all of the following symptoms: pallor, diaphoresis, nausea, tachycardia and dizziness. If any of these are present, the patient should be assisted to a supine position in bed and closely assessed.

TEACHING: PATIENT CARE

Controlling Postural Hypotension

+ Rest with the head of the bed elevated 18-26 cm (8-12 inches). This position makes the position change on rising less severe.
+ Avoid sudden changes in position. Arise from bed in three stages:
  (a) Sit up in bed for one minute.
  (b) Sit on the side of the bed with legs dangling for one minute.
  (c) Stand with care, holding onto the edge of the bed or another nonmovable object for one minute.
+ Never bend down all the way to the floor or stand up too quickly after stooping.
+ Postpone activities such as shaving and hair grooming for at least one hour after rising.

+ Wear elastic stockings at night to inhibit venous pooling in the legs.
+ Be aware that the symptoms of hypotension are most severe at the following times:
  (a) 30-60 minutes after a heavy meal.
  (b) 1-2 hours after taking an antihypertension medication.
+ Get out of a hot bath very slowly, because high temperatures can lead to venous pooling.
+ Use a rocking chair to improve circulation in the lower extremities. Even mild leg conditioning can strengthen muscle tone and enhance circulation.
+ Refrain from any strenuous activity that results in holding the breath and bearing down. This Valsalva manoeuvere slows the heart rate, leading to subsequent lowering of blood pressure.

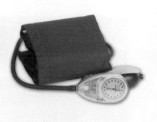

LIFESPAN CONSIDERATIONS

Assisting the Patient to Ambulate

Older Adults

+ Enquire how the patient has ambulated previously and modify assistance accordingly.

+ Take into account a decrease in speed, strength, resistance to fatigue, reaction time and coordination due to a decrease in nerve conduction.

+ Be cautious when using a transfer belt with a patient with osteoporosis. Too much pressure from the belt can increase the risk of vertebral compression fractures.

+ If assistive devices, such as a walker or walking stick are used, make sure patients are supervised in the beginning to learn the proper method of using them. Crutches may be much more difficult for older adults due to decreased upper body strength.

+ Be alert to signs of activity intolerance, especially in older adults with cardiac and lung problems.

+ Set small goals and increase slowly to build endurance, strength and flexibility.

+ Be aware of any fall risks the elder may have, such as:

  (a) Effects of medications
  (b) Neurological disorders
  (c) Environmental hazards
  (d) Orthostatic hypotension.

+ In older adults, the body's responses return to normal more slowly. For instance, an increase in heart rate from exercise may stay elevated for hours before returning to normal.

Using Mechanical Aids for Walking

Mechanical aids for ambulation include walking sticks, walking frames and crutches.

Walking Sticks

Two types of stick are used today: the standard straight-legged stick and the quad device, which has four feet and provides the most support (see Figure 23-47). Stick tips should have rubber caps to improve traction and prevent slipping. The standard length is 91 cm long; some aluminium sticks can be adjusted from 56–97 cm. The length should permit the elbow to be slightly flexed. Individuals may use either one or two sticks, depending on how much support they require.

Walking Frames

Walking frames are mechanical devices for ambulatory individuals who need more support than a stick provides. Walking frames come in many different shapes and sizes, with devices suited to individual needs. The standard type is made of polished aluminium. It has four legs with rubber tips and plastic hand grips (see Figure 23-48). Many walking frames have adjustable legs.

The standard frame needs to be picked up to be used. The patient therefore requires partial strength in both hands and wrists, strong elbow extensors and strong shoulder depressors. The individual also needs the ability to bear at least partial weight on both legs.

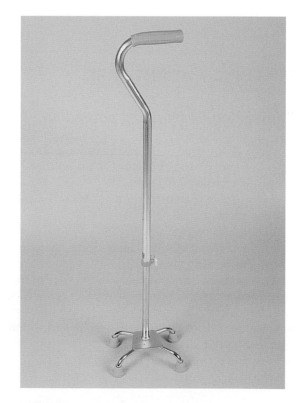

Figure 23-47 A quad device.

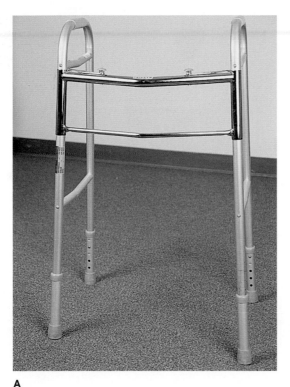

A

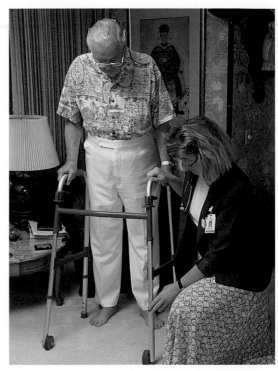

B

Figure 23-48 *A*, standard walker; *B*, two-wheeled walker.

TEACHING: PATIENT CARE

Using Walking Sticks
+ Hold the stick with the hand on the stronger side of the body to provide maximum support and appropriate body alignment when walking.
+ Position the tip of a standard stick (and the nearest tip of other stick) about 15 cm to the side and 15 cm in front of the near foot, so that the elbow is slightly flexed.

When Maximum Support is Required
+ Move the stick forward about 30 cm or a distance that is comfortable while the body weight is borne by both legs (see Figure 23-49, *A*).
+ Then move the affected (weak) leg forward to the stick while the weight is borne by the stick and stronger leg (see Figure 23-49, *B*).

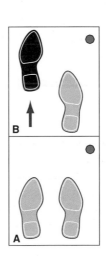

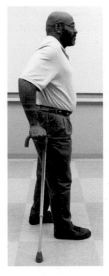

Figure 23-49 Steps involved in using a stick to provide maximum support.

+ Next, move the unaffected (stronger) leg forward ahead of the stick and weak leg while the weight is borne by the stick and weak leg.
+ Repeat the steps. This pattern of moving provides at least two points of support on the floor at all times.

As You Become Stronger and Require Less Support

+ Move the stick and weak leg forward at the same time, while the weight is borne by the stronger leg (see Figure 23-50, *A*).
+ Move the stronger leg forward, while the weight is borne by the stick and the weak leg (see Figure 23-50, *B*).

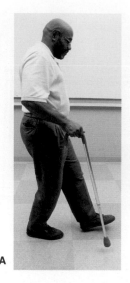
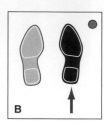

Figure 23-50 Steps involved in using a stick when less than maximum support is required.

TEACHING: PATIENT CARE

Using Walking Frames

When Maximum Support is Required

+ Move the walker ahead about 15 cm while your body weight is borne by both legs.
+ Then move the right foot up to the walker while your body weight is borne by the left leg and both arms.
+ Next, move the left foot up to the right foot while your body weight is borne by the right leg and both arms.

If One Leg is Weaker Than the Other

+ Move the walker and the weak leg ahead together about 15 cm while your weight is borne by the stronger leg.
+ Then move the stronger leg ahead while your weight is borne by the affected leg and both arms.

Four-wheeled and two-wheeled models of walkers (roller walkers) do not need to be picked up to be moved, but they are less stable than the standard walker is. They are used by patients who are too weak or unstable to pick up and move the walker with each step. Some roller walkers have a seat at the back so the patient can sit down to rest when desired. An adaptation of the standard and four-wheeled walker is one that has two tips and two wheels. This type provides more stability than the four-wheeled model yet still permits the patient to keep the walker in contact with the ground all the time. The patient tilts the walker toward the body, lifting the tips while the wheels remain on the ground, and then pushes the walker forward.

The nurse may need to adjust the height of a patient's walker so that the hand bar is just below the patient's waist and the patient's elbows are slightly flexed. This position helps the patient assume a more normal stance. A walker that is too low causes the patient to stoop; one that is too high makes the patient stretch and reach.

Crutches

Crutches may be a temporary need for some people and a permanent one for others. Sometimes individuals are discouraged when they attempt crutch walking. Patients confined to bed are often unaware of weakness that becomes apparent when they try to stand or walk. Patients realise that they can no longer take balance for granted when they must cope with the weight of a heavy cast or a paralysed limb. Frequently, progress may be slower than the patient anticipated. Encouragement from the nurse and the setting of realistic goals are especially important.

There are several kinds of crutches. The most frequently used are the underarm crutch, or axillary crutch with hand bars, and the Lofstrand crutch, which extends only to the forearm (see Figure 23-51). On the Lofstrand crutch, the metal cuff around the forearm and the metal bar stabilise the wrists and thus make walking safer and easier. The

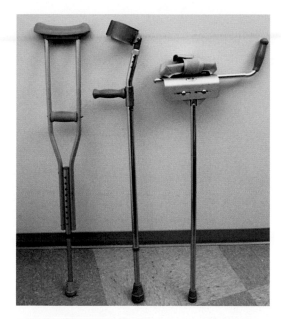

Figure 23-51 Types of crutches: axillary, Lofstrand and platform.

platform, or elbow extensor, crutch also has a cuff for the upper arm (Figure 23-51). All crutches require suction tips, usually made of rubber, which help to prevent slipping on a floor surface.

In crutch walking, the patient's weight is borne by the muscles of the shoulder girdle and the upper extremities. Before beginning crutch walking, exercises that strengthen the upper arms and hands are recommended.

Measuring Patients for Crutches

When nurses measure patients for axillary crutches, it is most important to obtain the correct length for the crutches and the correct placement of the hand piece. There are two methods of measuring crutch length:

1. The patient lies in a supine position and the nurse measures from the anterior fold of the axilla to the heel of the foot and adds 2.5 cm.
2. The patient stands erect and positions the crutch as shown in Figure 23-52 on page 626. The nurse makes sure the shoulder rest of the crutch is at least three finger widths, that is, 2.5–5 cm below the axilla.

To determine the correct placement of the hand bar:

1. The patient stands upright and supports the body weight by the hand grips of the crutches.
2. The nurse measures the angle of elbow flexion. It should be about 30 degrees. A goniometer may be used to verify the correct angle.

Crutch Gaits

The crutch gait is the gait a person assumes on crutches by alternating body weight on one or both legs and the crutches. Five standard crutch gaits are the four-point gait, three-point gait, two-point gait, swing-to gait and swing-through gait. The gait used depends on the following individual factors: (a) the ability to take steps, (b) the ability to bear weight and keep balance in a standing position on both legs or only one, and (c) the ability to hold the body erect.

TEACHING: PATIENT CARE

Using Crutches

+ Follow the plan of exercises developed for you to strengthen your arm muscles before beginning crutch walking.
+ Have a healthcare professional establish the correct length for your crutches and the correct placement of the handpieces. Crutches that are too long force your shoulders upward and make it difficult for you to push your body off the ground. Crutches that are too short will make you hunch over and develop an improper body stance.
+ The weight of your body should be borne by the arms rather than the axillae (armpits). Continual pressure on the axillae can injure the radial nerve and eventually cause crutch palsy, a weakness of the muscles of the forearm, wrist and hand.
+ Maintain an erect posture as much as possible to prevent strain on muscles and joints and to maintain balance.

+ Each step taken with crutches should be a comfortable distance for you. It is wise to start with a small rather than a large step.
+ Inspect the crutch tips regularly, and replace them if worn.
+ Keep the crutch tips dry and clean to maintain their surface friction. If the tips become wet, dry them well before use.
+ Wear a shoe with a low heel that grips the floor. Rubber soles decrease the chances of slipping. Adjust shoelaces so they cannot come untied or reach the floor where they might catch on the crutches. Consider shoes with alternate forms of closure (e.g. Velcro), especially if you cannot easily bend to tie laces. Slip-on shoes are acceptable only if they are snug and the heel does not come loose when the foot is bent.

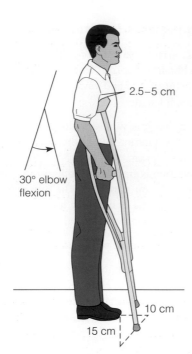

Figure 23-52 The standing position for measuring the correct length for crutches.

Patients also need instruction about how to get into and out of chairs and go up and down stairs safely. All of these crutch skills are best taught before the patient is discharged and preferably before the patient has surgery. This teaching is usually undertaken by a physiotherapist.

Crutch Stance (Tripod Position)

Before crutch walking is attempted, the patient needs to learn facts about posture and balance. The proper standing position with crutches is called the **tripod (triangle) position** (see Figure 23-53). The crutches are placed about 15 cm in front of the feet and out laterally about 15 cm, creating a wide base of support. The feet are slightly apart. A tall person requires a wider base than a short person does. Hips and knees are extended, the back is straight, and the head is held straight and high. There

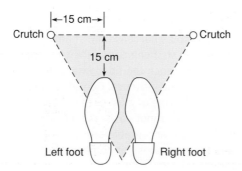

Figure 23-53 The tripod position.

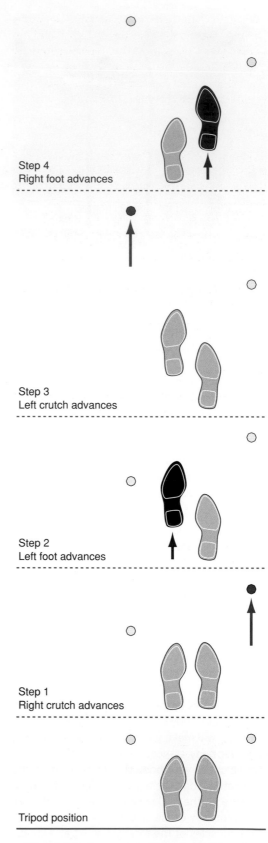

Step 4
Right foot advances

Step 3
Left crutch advances

Step 2
Left foot advances

Step 1
Right crutch advances

Tripod position

Figure 23-54 The four-point alternate crutch gait.

NURSING MANAGEMENT

should be no hunch to the shoulders and thus no weight borne by the axillae. The elbows are extended sufficiently to allow weight-bearing on the hands. If the patient is unsteady, the nurse places a walking belt around the patient's waist and grasps the belt from above, not from below. A fall can be prevented more effectively if the belt is held from above.

Four-point Alternate Gait

This is the most elementary and safest gait, providing at least three points of support at all times, but it requires coordination. Patients can use it when walking in crowds because it does not require much space. To use this gait, the patient needs to be able to bear weight on both legs (see Figure 23-54, reading from bottom to top). The nurse asks the patient to:

1. Move the right crutch ahead a suitable distance, such as 10–15 cm.
2. Move the left front foot forward, preferably to the level of the left crutch.
3. Move the left crutch forward.
4. Move the right foot forward.

Three-point Gait

To use this gait, the patient must be able to bear the entire body weight on the unaffected leg. The two crutches and the unaffected leg bear weight alternately (see Figure 23-55, reading from bottom to top). The nurse asks the patient to:

1. Move both crutches and the weaker leg forward.
2. Move the stronger leg forward.

Two-point Alternate Gait

This gait is faster than the four-point gait. It requires more balance because only two points support the body at one time; it also requires at least partial weight-bearing on each foot. In this gait, arm movements with the crutches are similar to the arm movements during normal walking (see Figure 23-56, reading from bottom to top). The nurse asks the patient to:

1. Move the left crutch and the right foot forward together.
2. Move the right crutch and the left foot ahead together.

Swing-to Gait

The swing gaits are used by patients with paralysis of the legs and hips. Prolonged use of these gaits results in atrophy of the unused muscles. The swing-to gait is the easier of these two gaits. The nurse asks the patient to:

1. Move both crutches ahead together (see Figure 23-57, A on page 628.
2. Lift body weight by the arms and swing to the crutches (see Figure 23-57, B).

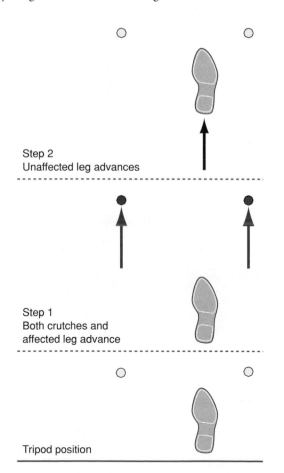

Step 2
Unaffected leg advances

Step 1
Both crutches and
affected leg advance

Tripod position

Figure 23-55 The three-point crutch gait.

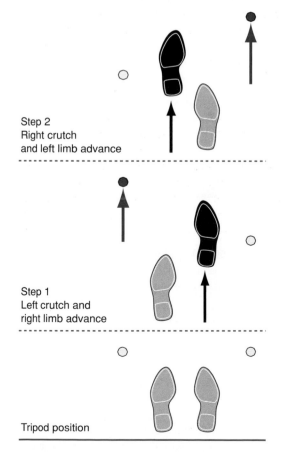

Step 2
Right crutch
and left limb advance

Step 1
Left crutch and
right limb advance

Tripod position

Figure 23-56 The two-point alternate crutch gait.

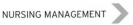

NURSING MANAGEMENT

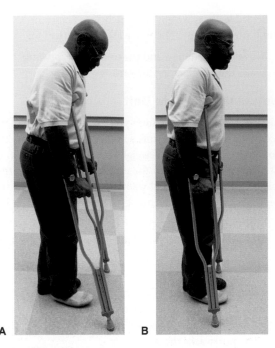

Figure 23-57 The swing-to crutch gait.

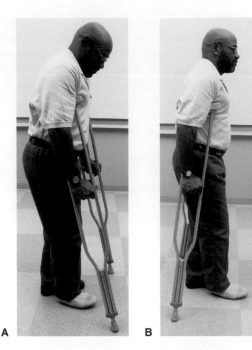

Figure 23-58 The swing-through crutch gait.

Swing-through Gait

This gait requires considerable skill, strength and coordination. The nurse asks the patient to:

1. Move both crutches forward together (see Figure 23-58, *A*).
2. Lift body weight by the arms and swing through and beyond the crutch (see Figure 23-58, *B*).

Getting into a Chair

Chairs that have armrests and are secure or braced against a wall are essential for patients using crutches. For this procedure, the nurse instructs the patient to:

1. Stand with the back of the unaffected leg centred against the chair. The chair helps support the patient during the next steps.
2. Transfer the crutches to the hand on the affected side and hold the crutches by the hand bars. The patient grasps the arm of the chair with the hand on the unaffected side (see Figure 23-59). This allows the patient to support the body weight on the arms and the unaffected leg.
3. Lean forward, flex the knees and hips, and lower into the chair.

Getting Out of a Chair

For this procedure, the nurse instructs the patient to:

1. Move forward to the edge of the chair and place the unaffected leg slightly under or at the edge of the chair. This position helps the patient stand up from the chair and achieve balance, since the unaffected leg is supported against the edge of the chair.
2. Grasp the crutches by the hand bars in the hand on the affected side, and grasp the arm of the chair by the hand on

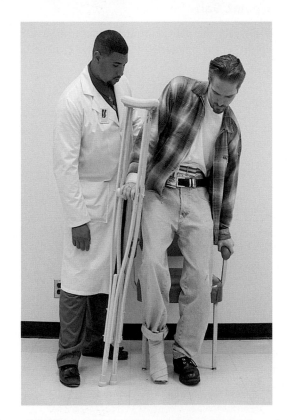

Figure 23-59 A patient using crutches getting into a chair.

the unaffected side. The body weight is placed on the crutches and the hand on the armrest to support the unaffected leg when the patient rises to stand.
3. Push down on the crutches and the chair armrest while elevating the body out of the chair.
4. Assume the tripod position before moving.

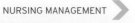

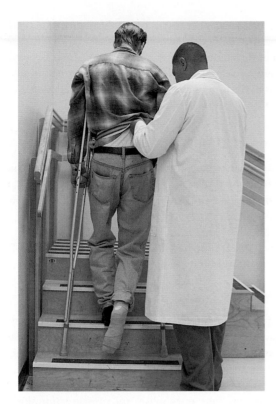

Figure 23-60 Climbing stairs: placing weight on the crutches while first moving the unaffected leg onto a step.

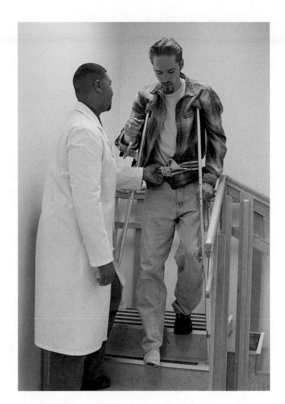

Figure 23-61 Descending stairs: moving the crutches and affected leg to the next step.

Going Up Stairs

For this procedure, the nurse stands behind the patient and slightly to the affected side if needed. The nurse instructs the patient to:

1. Assume the tripod position at the bottom of the stairs.
2. Transfer the body weight to the crutches and move the unaffected leg onto the step (see Figure 23-60).
3. Transfer the body weight to the unaffected leg on the step and move the crutches and affected leg up to the step. The affected leg is always supported by the crutches.
4. Repeat steps 2 and 3 until the patient reaches the top of the stairs.

Going Down Stairs

For this procedure, the nurse stands one step below the patient on the affected side if needed. The nurse instructs the patient to:

1. Assume the tripod position at the top of the stairs.
2. Shift the body weight to the unaffected leg, and move the crutches and affected leg down onto the next step (see Figure 23-61).
3. Transfer the body weight to the crutches, and move the unaffected leg to that step. The affected leg is always supported by the crutches.

4. Repeat steps 2 and 3 until the patient reaches the bottom of the stairs.

EVALUATING

The goals established during the planning phase are evaluated according to specific desired outcomes, also established in that phase.

If outcomes are not achieved, the nurse, patient and support person if appropriate need to explore the reasons before modifying the care plan. For example, the following questions may be considered if an immobilised patient fails to maintain muscle mass and tone and joint mobility:

+ Has the patient's physical or mental condition changed motivation to perform required exercise?
+ Were appropriate range-of-motion exercises implemented?
+ Was the patient encouraged to participate in self-care activities as much as possible?
+ Was the patient encouraged to make as many decisions as possible when developing a daily activity plan and to express concerns?
+ Did the nurse provide appropriate supervision and monitoring?
+ Was the patient's diet adequate to provide appropriate nourishment for energy requirements?

REST AND SLEEP

Rest and sleep are essential for health and important following any strenuous activities. People who are ill frequently require more rest and sleep than usual. Often, debilitated individuals expend excessive amounts of energy to regain health or perform the activities of daily living. As a result, such people experience increased and frequent fatigue and need extra rest and sleep. Rest restores a person's energy, allowing the individual to resume optimal functioning. When people are deprived of rest, they are often irritable, depressed and tired, and they may have poor control over their emotions. Providing a restful environment for patients is an important function of nurses.

The meaning of rest and the need for rest vary among individuals. **Rest** implies calmness, relaxation without emotional stress and freedom from anxiety. Therefore, rest does not always imply inactivity; in fact, some people find certain activities such as walking in fresh air restful. When rest is prescribed for a patient, both nurse and patient must know whether the patient is to be inactive and whether that inactivity involves the whole body or a body part (e.g. an arm).

Sleep is a basic human need; it is a universal biological process common to all people. Historically, sleep was considered a state of unconsciousness. More recently, **sleep** has come to be considered an altered state of consciousness in which the individual's perception of and reaction to the environment are decreased. Sleep is characterised by minimal physical activity, variable levels of consciousness, changes in the body's physiological processes and decreased responsiveness to external stimuli. Some environmental stimuli, such as a smoke detector alarm, will usually awaken a sleeper, whereas other noises will not. It appears that individuals respond to meaningful stimuli while sleeping and selectively disregard unmeaningful stimuli.

PHYSIOLOGY OF SLEEP

The cyclic nature of sleep is thought to be controlled by centres located in the lower part of the brain. These centres actively inhibit wakefulness, thus causing sleep.

Circadian Rhythms

Biorhythms (rhythmic biological clocks) exist in plants, animals and humans. In humans, these are controlled from within the body and synchronised with environmental factors, such as light and darkness, gravity and electromagnetic stimuli. The most familiar biorhythm is the circadian rhythm. The term circadian is from the Latin *circa dies*, meaning 'about a day'.

Sleep is a complex biological rhythm. When a person's biological clock coincides with sleepwake patterns, the person is said to be in **circadian synchronisation**; that is, the person is awake when the physiological and psychological rhythms are most active and is asleep when the physiological and psychological rhythms are most inactive.

Circadian regularity begins by the third week of life and may be inherited. Babies are awake most often in the early morning and the late afternoon. After four months of age, infants enter a 24-hour cycle in which they sleep mostly during the night. By the end of the fifth or sixth month, infants' sleep wake patterns are almost like those of adults.

Stages of Sleep

The **electroencephalogram (EEG)** provides a good picture of what occurs during sleep. Electrodes are placed on various parts of the sleeper's scalp. The electrodes transmit electric energy from the cerebral cortex to pens that record the brain waves on graph paper.

Two types of sleep have been identified: **NREM** (non-REM) **sleep** and **REM** (rapid eye movement) **sleep**.

NREM Sleep

NREM sleep is also referred to as slow-wave sleep because the brain waves of a sleeper are slower than the alpha and beta waves of a person who is awake or alert. Most sleep during a night is NREM sleep. It is a deep, restful sleep and brings a decrease in some physiological functions. Basically, all metabolic process including vital signs, metabolism and muscle action slow.

NREM sleep is divided into four stages. *Stage I* is the stage of very light sleep. During this stage, the person feels drowsy and relaxed, the eyes roll from side to side, and the heart and respiratory rates drop slightly. The sleeper can be readily awakened and this stage lasts only a few minutes.

Stage II is the stage of light sleep during which body processes continue to slow down. The eyes are generally still, the heart and respiratory rates decrease slightly, and body temperature falls. Stage II lasts only about 10–15 minutes but constitutes 40–45% of total sleep.

During *Stage III*, the heart and respiratory rates, as well as other body processes, slow further because of the domination of the parasympathetic nervous system. The sleeper becomes more difficult to arouse. The person is not disturbed by sensory stimuli, the skeletal muscles are very relaxed, reflexes are diminished and snoring may occur.

Stage IV signals deep sleep, called delta sleep. The sleeper's heart and respiratory rates drop 20–30% below those exhibited during waking hours. The sleeper is very relaxed, rarely moves and is difficult to arouse. Stage IV is thought to restore the body physically. During this stage, the eyes usually roll, and some dreaming occurs.

REM Sleep

REM sleep usually recurs about every 90 minutes and lasts 5–30 minutes. REM sleep is not as restful as NREM sleep, and most dreams take place during REM sleep. Furthermore, these dreams are usually remembered; that is, they are consolidated in the memory.

During REM sleep, the brain is highly active, and brain metabolism may increase as much as 20%. This type of sleep is also

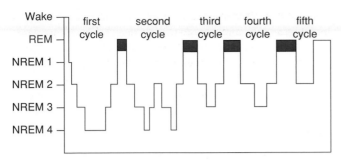

Figure 23-62 Time spent in REM and non-REM stages of sleep cycles.

called paradoxical sleep because it seems a paradox that sleep can take place simultaneously with this type of brain activity. In this phase, the sleeper may be difficult to arouse or may wake spontaneously, muscle tone is depressed, gastric secretions increase, and heart and respiratory rates often are irregular.

Sleep Cycles

During a sleep cycle, people pass through NREM and REM sleep, the complete cycle usually lasting about $1\frac{1}{2}$ hours in adults. In the first sleep cycle, a sleeper passes through all of the first three NREM stages in a total of about 20–30 minutes. Then, Stage IV may last about 30 minutes. After Stage IV NREM, the sleep passes back through Stages III and II over about 20 minutes. Thereafter, the first REM stage occurs, lasting about 10 minutes, completing the first sleep cycle. The usual sleeper experiences four to six cycles of sleep during 7–8 hours (see Figure 23-62). The sleeper who is awakened during any stage must begin anew at Stage I NREM sleep and proceed through all the stages to REM sleep.

The duration of NREM stages and REM sleep varies throughout the sleep period. As the night progresses, the sleeper becomes less tired and spends less time in Stages III and IV of NREM sleep. REM sleep increases and dreams tend to lengthen. If the sleeper is very tired, REM cycles are often short – for example, five minutes instead of 20 – during the early portion of sleep. Before sleep ends, periods of near wakefulness occur, and Stages I and II NREM sleep and REM sleep predominate.

FUNCTIONS OF SLEEP

The effects of sleep on the body are not completely understood. Sleep exerts physiological effects on both the nervous system and other body structures. Sleep in some way restores normal levels of activity and normal balance among parts of the nervous system. Sleep is also necessary for protein synthesis, which allows repair processes to occur.

The role of sleep in psychological well-being is best noticed by the deterioration in mental functioning related to sleep loss. Persons with inadequate amounts of sleep tend to become emotionally irritable, have poor concentration and experience difficulty making decisions.

NORMAL SLEEP PATTERNS AND REQUIREMENTS

It has been suggested that maintaining a regular sleep wake rhythm is more important than the number of hours actually slept. Some people, for example, can function well on as little as five hours of sleep each night. Re-establishing the sleep wake rhythm (e.g. after the disruption of surgery) is an important aspect of nursing.

Newborns

Newborns sleep 16–18 hours a day, usually divided into about seven sleep periods. NREM sleep is characterised by regular respirations, closed eyes and the absence of body and eye movements. REM sleep has rapid eye movements that are observable through closed lids, body movement and irregular respirations. Most of the sleep time is spent in Stages III and IV of NREM sleep. Nearly 50% of sleep is REM.

Infants

Some infants sleep as long as 22 hours a day, others 12–14 hours a day. About 20–30% of sleep is REM sleep. At first, infants awaken every three or four hours, eat and then go back to sleep. Periods of wakefulness gradually increase during the first months. By four months, most infants sleep through the night and establish a pattern of daytime naps that varies among individuals. They generally awaken early in the morning, however. At the end of the first year, an infant usually takes one or two naps per day and sleeps about 14 of every 24 hours.

About half of the infant's sleep time is spent in light sleep. During light sleep, the infant exhibits a great deal of activity, such as movement, gurgles and coughing. Parents need to ascertain that infants are truly awake before picking them up for feeding and changing. Many infants begin waking up again in the middle of the night between 5 and 9 months of age. For parents who find this behaviour a problem, the nurse needs to assess the infant's total sleep pattern and compare it with the parents' sleep schedule. Parents need reassurance that there is no one correct way to handle this situation. The best solution is one that provides a continuous healthy environment for both the infant and the parents.

Toddlers

The sleep requirements of toddlers decrease to 10–12 hours per day. About 20–30% is REM sleep. Most still need an afternoon nap, but the need for midmorning naps gradually decreases. The toddler's normal sleep wake cycle is usually established by age two or three. The toddler may exhibit a great deal of resistance to going to bed. Parents need assurance that if the child has had adequate attention from them during the day, maintaining a consistent approach with respect to bedtime will promote good sleep habits for the entire family. The child who awakens at night may be afraid of the dark or have experienced night terrors or nightmares.

Pre-schoolers

The pre-school child usually requires 11–12 hours of sleep per night, particularly if the child is in pre-school. Sleep needs fluctuate in relation to activity and growth spurts. Many children of this age dislike bedtime and resist by requesting another story, game or television programme. The four- to five-year-old may become restless and irritable if sleep requirements are not met. A nap or quiet time during the day may be needed to restore energy levels.

Children in this age group still require bedtime rituals. Parents can help children who resist bedtime by warning them that bedtime is approaching and by continuing to use the same firm and consistent approach suggested for the toddler. Pre-school children wake up frequently at night. REM sleep is still 20–30% higher than for adults; however, Stage I sleep is less.

School-age Children

The school-age child sleeps 8–12 hours a night without daytime naps. The eight-year-old requires at least 10 hours of sleep each night. As the child approaches 11 or 12 years of age, less sleep is required and bedtime may be as late as 10 p.m. The REM sleep of children at this age is reduced to about 20%. Although some children still experience night awakenings due to nightmares, this problem continues to decrease with age.

Adolescents

Most adolescents require 8–10 hours of sleep each night to prevent undue fatigue and susceptibility to infections. A change in sleep pattern is common in adolescence. Children who once were early risers begin to sleep late in the mornings and occasionally take afternoon naps. The reason for daytime sleeping is not fully understood, but it is possibly a result of physical maturity and reduced nocturnal sleep. Sleep at this age is about 20% REM.

During adolescence, boys begin to experience **nocturnal emissions** (orgasm and emission of semen during sleep), known as 'wet dreams', several times each month. Boys need to be informed about this normal development to prevent embarrassment and fear.

Young Adults

The sleep wake cycle is very important to young adults. They usually have an active lifestyle, and are thought to require 7–8 hours of sleep each night but may do well on less.

Middle-aged Adults

Middle-aged adults generally maintain the sleep pattern established at a younger age. They usually sleep 6–8 hours per night.

About 20% is REM sleep. The numbers of arousals from sleep increases and the amount of Stage IV sleep begins to decrease.

Older Adults

The older adult sleeps about six hours a night. About 20–25% is REM sleep. Stage IV sleep is markedly decreased and in some instances absent. The first REM period is longer. Many older adults awaken more often during the night and it often takes them longer to go back to sleep. Because of the change in Stage IV sleep, older people have less restorative sleep (see *Lifespan considerations*).

Some older adults may be said to have *Sundowner's syndrome*. Although not a sleep disorder directly, it refers to a confusional state that tends to appear at dusk (thus the name) and may happen because of a change in circadian rhythms (changes in the sleep wake cycle), decreased sensory stimulation at the end of the day, a mental condition such as Alzheimer's disease.

CLINICAL ANECDOTE

When I did my first set of night shifts on an elderly care unit I was amazed by the number of patients that developed acute confusion as soon as it became dark. The routine would be the same night after night: the visitors would leave, it would become dark and the pleasant elderly people would have a complete reversal of personality. They would shout, sing, scream or attempt to wander around all night. Almost as soon as it started to become light outside the pattern would change back to normal. I was amazed when I saw this for the first time after I had read of it. It was almost surreal.

Caroline, first-year student

FACTORS AFFECTING SLEEP

Both the quality and the quantity of sleep are affected by a number of factors. *Quality of sleep* refers to the individual's ability to stay asleep and to get appropriate amounts of REM and NREM sleep. *Quantity of sleep* is the total time the individual sleeps.

RESEARCH NOTE

Do People Really Need Eight Hours of Sleep?

Often, healthcare providers attempt to intervene with patients who report receiving less than eight hours of sleep each night on the unproved assumption that eight hours is the optimal amount.

Researchers examined this assumption by investigating the relationship between survival and length of sleep (Kripke *et al.*, 2002). After controlling for various other variables, data from more than one million adult subjects (collected for other purposes) showed that the best survival was in those who slept seven hours per night.

The worst survival was among those who slept for more than 8.5 hours or less than 3.5 or 4.5 hours each night. No relationship was found between reports of insomnia and mortality.

Implications

This very large study reassures both providers and patients that few if any health dangers are associated with sleeping between six and eight hours per night. The nurse should focus on the patient's subjective feelings of being rested and any other aspects of disturbed sleep that may exist rather than the exact length. Eight is not the magic number.

Note: From 'Mortality Associated with Sleep Duration and Insomnia,' by D.F. Kripke, L. Garfinkel, D.L. Wingard, M.R. Klauber, and M.R. Marler, 2002, *Archives of General Psychiatry*, 59(2), pp. 131-136.

Illness

Illness that causes pain or physical distress can result in sleep problems. People who are ill require more sleep than normal, and the normal rhythm of sleep and wakefulness is often disturbed. People deprived of REM sleep subsequently spend more sleep time than normal in this stage.

Respiratory conditions can disturb an individual's sleep. Shortness of breath often makes sleep difficult, and people who have nasal congestion or sinus drainage may have trouble breathing and hence may find it difficult to sleep.

People who have gastric or duodenal ulcers may find their sleep disturbed because of pain, often a result of the increased gastric secretions that occur during REM sleep.

LIFESPAN CONSIDERATIONS

Older Adults

The quality of sleep is often diminished in older adults. Some of the leading factors that often are influential in sleep disturbances are:

+ Side-effects of medications
+ Gastric reflux disease
+ Respiratory and circulatory disorders, which may cause breathing problems or discomfort
+ Pain from arthritis, increased stiffness, or impaired immobility
+ Nocturia
+ Depression
+ Loss of life partner and/or close friends
+ Disruptions of bedtime rituals/routines when a person is hospitalised or institutionalised
+ Confusion related to delirium or dementia.

Interventions to promote sleep and rest can help enhance the rejuvenation and renewal that sleep provides. Rituals and routines that become the rhythm of one's life and have been performed for years are often disrupted by being hospitalised or institutionalised. The following interventions can help promote sleep and rest is follows:

+ Maintain usual bedtime ritual, or develop a new one with the individual that will encourage relaxation or sleep, such as music, relaxation techniques and warm drinks.
+ Be sure their environment is warm and safe, especially if they get out of bed during the night.
+ Provide comfort measures, such as analgesics if indicated, and proper positioning.
+ Enhance the sense of safety and security by checking on patients frequently and making sure that the call bell is within reach.
+ If lack of sleep is caused by medications or certain health conditions, work on specific interventions related to these problems.
+ Evaluate the situation and find out what the rest and sleep disturbances mean to the patient. They may not perceive sleeplessness to be a serious problem, but will just do other activities and sleep when tired.

Certain endocrine disturbances can also affect sleep. Hyperthyroidism lengthens presleep time, making it difficult for a patient to fall asleep. Hypothyroidism, conversely, decreases Stage IV sleep. Women with low levels of oestrogen often report excessive fatigue. In addition, they may experience sleep disruptions due, in part, to the discomfort associated with hot flushes or night sweats that can occur with reduced oestrogen levels.

Elevated body temperatures can cause some reduction in Stages III and IV NREM sleep and REM sleep.

The need to urinate during the night also disrupts sleep, and people who awaken at night to urinate sometimes have difficulty getting back to sleep.

Environment

Environment can promote or hinder sleep. Any change – for example, noise in the environment – can inhibit sleep. The absence of usual stimuli or the presence of unfamiliar stimuli can prevent people from sleeping. Stage I sleep is the lightest and Stages III and IV the deepest; as a result, louder noises are needed to awaken a person in Stages III and IV. However, over time people can be habituated to a noise so that the level has less effect.

Discomfort from environmental temperature and lack of ventilation can affect sleep. Light levels can be another factor. A person accustomed to darkness while sleeping may find it difficult to sleep in the light.

Fatigue

It is thought that a person who is moderately fatigued usually has a restful sleep. Fatigue also affects a person's sleep pattern. The more tired the person is, the shorter the first period of paradoxical (REM) sleep. As the person rests, the REM periods become longer.

Lifestyle

A person who does shift work and changes shifts frequently must arrange activities to be ready to sleep at the right time. Moderate exercise usually is conducive to sleep, but excessive exercise can delay sleep. The person's ability to relax before retiring is an important factor affecting the ability to fall asleep.

Emotional Stress

Anxiety and depression frequently disturb sleep. A person preoccupied with personal problems may be unable to relax sufficiently to get to sleep. Anxiety increases the norepinephrine blood levels through stimulation of the sympathetic nervous system. This chemical change results in less Stage IV NREM and REM sleep and more stage changes and awakenings.

Stimulants and Alcohol

Caffeine-containing beverages act as stimulants of the central nervous system, thus interfering with sleep. People who drink an excessive amount of alcohol often find their sleep disturbed. Excessive alcohol disrupts REM sleep, although it may hasten the onset of sleep. While making up for lost REM sleep after some of the effects of the alcohol have worn off, people often experience nightmares. The alcohol-tolerant person may be unable to sleep well and become irritable as a result.

Diet

Weight loss has been associated with reduced total sleep time as well as broken sleep and earlier awakening. Weight gain, on the other hand, seems to be associated with an increase in total sleep time, less broken sleep and later waking. Dietary L-tryptophan – found, for example, in cheese and milk – may induce sleep, a fact that might explain why warm milk helps some people get to sleep.

Smoking

Nicotine has a stimulating effect on the body, and smokers often have more difficulty falling asleep than nonsmokers do. Smokers are usually easily aroused and often describe themselves as light sleepers. By refraining from smoking after the evening meal, the person usually sleeps better; moreover, many former smokers report that their sleeping patterns improved once they stopped smoking.

Motivation

The desire to stay awake can often overcome a person's fatigue. For example, a tired person can probably stay alert while attending an interesting concert. When a person is bored and is not motivated to stay awake, by contrast, sleep often readily ensues.

Medications

Some medications affect the quality of sleep. Hypnotics can interfere with Stages III and IV NREM sleep and suppress REM sleep. Beta-blockers have been known to cause insomnia and nightmares. Narcotics, such as Tramadol hydrochloride and morphine, are known to suppress REM sleep and to cause frequent awakenings and drowsiness. Tranquillisers interfere with REM sleep. Amphetamines and antidepressants decrease REM sleep abnormally. A patient withdrawing from any of these drugs gets much more REM sleep than usual and as a result may experience upsetting nightmares.

COMMON SLEEP DISORDERS

Knowledge of common sleep disorders helps nurses obtain and recognise pertinent data. Sleep disorders may be categorised as parasomnias, primary disorders and secondary disorders.

Parasomnias

A **parasomnia** is behaviour that may interfere with sleep or that occurs during sleep. The *International Classification of Sleep*

BOX 23-1 Parasomnias

+ *Bruxism.* Usually occurring during Stage II NREM sleep, this clenching and grinding of the teeth can eventually erode dental crowns and cause teeth to come loose.
+ *Nocturnal enuresis.* Bed-wetting during sleep can occur in children over three years old. More males than females are affected. It often occurs 1-2 hours after falling asleep, when rousing from NREM Stages III to IV.
+ *Nocturnal erections.* Nocturnal erections and emissions occur during REM sleep. They begin during adolescence and do not present a sleep problem.
+ *Periodic limb movements disorder (PLMD).* In this condition, the legs jerk twice or three times per minute during sleep and is most common among older adults. This kicking motion can wake the individual and result in poor sleep. The condition may be treated with medications such as those otherwise used for Parkinson's disease. PLMD differs from restless leg syndrome (RLS), which occurs whenever the person is at rest, not just at night when sleeping. RLS may occur during pregnancy or be due to other medical problems that can be treated.
+ *Sleeptalking.* Talking during sleep occurs during NREM sleep before REM sleep. It rarely presents a problem to the person unless it becomes troublesome to others.
+ *Somnambulism.* Somnambulism (sleepwalking) occurs during Stages III and IV of NREM sleep. It is episodic and usually occurs 1-2 hours after falling asleep. Sleepwalkers tend not to notice dangers (e.g. stairs) and often need to be protected from injury.

Disorders (American Sleep Disorders Association, 1997) subdivides parasomnias into arousal disorders (e.g. sleepwalking, sleep terrors), sleep wake transition disorders (e.g. sleep talking), parasomnias associated with REM sleep (e.g. nightmares) and others (e.g. bruxism). *Box 23-1* describes examples of parasomnias.

Primary Sleep Disorders

Primary sleep disorders are those in which the person's sleep problem is the main disorder. These disorders include insomnia, hypersomnia, narcolepsy, sleep apnoea and sleep deprivation.

Insomnia

Insomnia, the most common sleep disorder, is the inability to obtain an adequate amount or quality of sleep. People suffering from insomnia do not feel refreshed on arising. There are three types of insomnia:

1. Difficulty in falling asleep (initial insomnia)
2. Difficulty in staying asleep because of frequent or prolonged waking (intermittent or maintenance insomnia)
3. Early morning or premature waking (terminal insomnia).

Insomnia can result from physical discomfort but more often is a result of mental overstimulation due to anxiety. People who become habituated to drugs or who drink large quantities of alcohol are likely to have insomnia.

Treatment for insomnia frequently requires the patient to develop new behaviour patterns that induce sleep. The usefulness of sleeping medications is questionable. Such medications do not deal with the cause of the problem and their prolonged use can create drug dependencies.

Hypersomnia

Hypersomnia, the opposite of insomnia, is excessive sleep, particularly in the daytime. The afflicted person often sleeps until noon and takes many naps during the day. Hypersomnia can be caused by medical conditions, for example, central nervous system damage and certain kidney, liver or metabolic disorders, such as diabetic acidosis and hypothyroidism. In some instances, a person uses hypersomnia as a coping mechanism to avoid facing the responsibilities of the day.

Narcolepsy

Narcolepsy – from the Greek *narco*, meaning 'numbness' and *lepsis*, meaning 'seizure' – is a sudden wave of overwhelming sleepiness that occurs during the day, thus, it is referred to as a 'sleep attack'. Its cause is unknown, although it is believed to be a lack of the chemical hypocretin in the central nervous system that regulates sleep. Onset of symptoms tends to occur between ages 15 and 30. In narcoleptic attacks, sleep starts with the REM phase. Even though people who have narcolepsy sleep well at night, they nod off several times a day even when conversing with someone or driving a car. Narcolepsy historically has been controlled by central nervous system stimulants and antidepressants.

Sleep Apnoea

Sleep apnoea is the periodic cessation of breathing during sleep. This disorder needs to be assessed by a sleep expert, but it is often suspected when the person has loud snoring, frequent nocturnal awakenings, excessive daytime sleepiness, insomnia, morning headaches, intellectual deterioration, irritability or other personality changes, and physiological changes such as hypertension and cardiac arrhythmias. It is most frequent in men over 50 and in postmenopausal women.

The periods of apnoea, which last from 10 seconds to two minutes, occur during REM or NREM sleep. Frequency of episodes ranges from 50–600 per night. These apnoeic episodes drain the person of energy and lead to excessive daytime sleepiness.

Three common types of sleep apnoea are obstructive apnoea, central apnoea and mixed apnoea. Obstructive apnoea occurs when the structures of the pharynx or oral cavity block the flow of air. The person continues to try to breathe; that is, the chest and abdominal muscles move. The movements of the diaphragm become stronger and stronger until the obstruction is removed. Enlarged tonsils, a deviated nasal septum, nasal polyps and obesity predispose the individual to obstructive apnoea.

Central apnoea is thought to involve a defect in the respiratory centre of the brain. All actions involved in breathing, such as chest movement and airflow, cease. Patients who have brain stem injuries and muscular dystrophy, for example, often have central sleep apnoea. At this time, there is no available treatment. Mixed apnoea is a combination of central apnoea and obstructive apnoea.

An episode of sleep apnoea usually begins with snoring; thereafter, breathing ceases, followed by marked snorting as breathing resumes. Toward the end of each apnoeic episode, increased carbon dioxide levels in the blood cause the individual to wake.

Treatment for sleep apnoea can be directed at the cause of the apnoea. For example, enlarged tonsils may be removed. Other surgical procedures, including laser removal of excess tissue in the pharynx, reduce or eliminate snoring and may be effective in relieving the apnoea. In other cases, the use of a nasal continuous positive airway pressure (CPAP) device at night is effective in maintaining an open airway.

Sleep apnoea profoundly affects a person's work or school performance. In addition, prolonged sleep apnoea can cause a sharp rise in blood pressure and may lead to cardiac arrest. Over time, apnoeic episodes can cause cardiac arrhythmias, pulmonary hypertension and subsequent left-sided heart failure.

CLINICAL ALERT

Partners of patients with sleep apnoea may become aware of the problem because they hear snoring that stops during the apnoea period and then restarts. Surgical removal of tonsils or other tissue in the pharynx, if not the cause of the sleep apnoea, can actually worsen the situation by removing the snoring and, thus, the warning that apnoea is occurring.

Sleep Deprivation

A prolonged disturbance in amount, quality and consistency of sleep can lead to a syndrome referred to as **sleep deprivation**. This is not a sleep disorder in itself but a result of sleep disturbances. It produces a variety of physiological and behavioural symptoms, the severity of which depends on the degree of the deprivation. Two major types of sleep deprivation are REM deprivation and NREM deprivation. A combination of the two increases the severity of symptoms. Table 23-10 shows the causes and clinical signs of sleep deprivation.

Secondary Sleep Disorders

Secondary sleep disorders are sleep disturbances caused by other clinical conditions. They may be associated with mental, neurological or other conditions. Examples of conditions causing secondary sleep disorders include depression, alcoholism, dementia, Parkinsonism, thyroid dysfunction, chronic obstructive pulmonary disease and peptic ulcer disease.

Table 23-10 Types, Causes and Signs of Sleep Deprivation

Type	Causes	Clinical signs
REM deprivation	Alcohol, barbiturates, shift work, jet lag, extended ICU hospitalisation, morphine	Excitability, restlessness, irritability and increased sensitivity to pain Confusion and suspiciousness Emotional instability
NREM deprivation	All the above plus diazepam (Valium), flurazepam hydrochloride, hypothyroidism, depression, respiratory distress disorders, sleep apnoea and age (common in the elderly)	Withdrawal, apathy, hypo-responsiveness Feeling physically uncomfortable Lack of facial expression Speech deterioration Excessive sleepiness
Both REM and NREM deprivation	As above	Decreased reasoning ability (judgement) and ability to concentrate Inattentiveness Marked fatigue: blurred vision, itchy eyes, nausea, headache Difficulty performing activities of daily living Lack of memory, mental confusion, visual or auditory hallucinations, illusions

NURSING MANAGEMENT

ASSESSING

Assessment relative to a patient's sleep includes a sleep history, a sleep diary, a physical assessment and a review of diagnostic studies.

Sleep History

A brief general sleep history, which is usually part of the comprehensive patient history, is obtained for all patients on admission. This enables the nurse to incorporate the patient's needs and preferences in the plan of care. A general sleep history includes the following:

+ Usual sleeping pattern, specifically sleeping and waking times; hours of undisturbed sleep; quality of or satisfaction with sleep (e.g. effect on energy level for daily functioning); and time and duration of naps.
+ Bedtime rituals performed to help the person fall asleep (e.g. a glass of hot fluid, reading or other method of relaxing, and special equipment or positioning aids).
+ Use of sleep medication and other drugs. Sleep can be disturbed by a variety of drugs, such as stimulants or steroids, if they are taken close to bedtime. Hypnotics and sedating antidepressants may cause excessive daytime sleepiness.
+ Sleep environment (e.g. dark room, cool or warm temperature, noise level, night-light).
+ Recent changes in sleep patterns or difficulties in sleeping.

If the patient indicates a recent pattern change or difficulties in sleeping, a more detailed history is required. This detailed history should explore the exact nature of the problem and its cause, when it first began and its frequency, how it affects daily living, what the patient is doing to cope with the problem, and whether these methods have been effective. Questions the nurse might ask the patient with a sleeping disturbance are shown in the *Assessment interview*.

Sleep Diary

Sometimes patients with a sleeping problem can provide more precise information if they keep a written record of their sleep pattern and the habits associated with it. Such a sleep diary or log can be kept by patients who are sleeping at home and should be maintained for at least a week. A sleep diary may include all or selected aspects of the following information that pertain to the patient's specific problem:

+ Total number of sleep hours per day
+ Activities performed 2–3 hours before bedtime (type, duration and time)
+ Bedtime rituals (e.g. ingestion of food, fluid or medication) before going to bed
+ Time of (a) going to bed, (b) trying to fall asleep, (c) falling asleep (approximate), (d) any instances of waking up and duration of these periods and (e) waking up in the morning

ASSESSMENT INTERVIEW

Sleep Disturbances

+ How would you describe your sleeping problem? What changes have occurred in your sleeping pattern? How often does this happen?
+ Do you have difficulty falling asleep?
+ Do you wake up often during the night? If so, how often?
+ Do you wake up earlier in the morning than you would like and have difficulty falling back to sleep?
+ How do you feel when you wake up in the morning?
+ Do you sleep more than usual? If so, how often do you sleep?
+ Do you have periods of overwhelming tiredness? If so, when does this happen?
+ Have you ever suddenly fallen asleep in the middle of a daytime activity? If so, has any

muscle weakness or paralysis occurred?
+ Has anyone ever told you that you snore, walk in your sleep, talk in your sleep, or stop breathing for a while when sleeping?
+ What have you been doing to deal with this sleeping problem? Does it help?
+ What do you think might be causing this problem? Do you have any medical condition that might be causing you to sleep more (or less)? Are you receiving medications for an illness that might alter your sleeping pattern? Are you experiencing any stressful or upsetting events or conflicts that may be affecting your sleep?
+ How is your sleeping problem affecting you?

+ Any worries that the patient believes may affect sleep
+ Factors that the patient believes have a positive or negative effect on sleep.

Keeping such a diary may become stressful for some patients and further affect their sleep. The nurse needs to advise the patient to obtain the assistance of a bed partner in keeping the diary or to discontinue the diary if it presents a problem. When a diary is completed, the nurse and patient can develop flow charts or graphs that will assist in organising the data and identifying the specific problem.

Physical Assessment

Examination of the patient includes observation of the patient's facial appearance, behaviour and energy level. Darkened areas around the eyes, puffy eyelids, reddened conjunctiva, glazed or dull-appearing eyes and limited facial expression are indicative of sleep insufficiency. Behaviours such as irritability, restlessness, inattentiveness, slowed speech, slumped posture, hand tremor, yawning, rubbing the eyes, withdrawal, confusion and uncoordination are also suggestive of sleep problems. Lack of energy may be noted by observing whether the patient appears physically weak, lethargic or fatigued.

In addition, the nurse assesses whether the patient has a deviated nasal septum, enlarged neck or is obese. These findings may be associated with obstructive sleep apnoea or snoring.

Diagnostic Studies

Sleep is measured objectively in a sleep disorder laboratory by **polysomnography**: an electroencephalogram (EEG), electromyogram (EMG) and electro-oculogram (EOG) are recorded simultaneously. Electrodes are placed on the centre of the scalp to record brain waves (EEG), on the outer canthus of each eye to record eye movement (EOG) and on the chin muscles to record the structural electromyogram (EMG). The following may also be monitored, depending on findings of the initial interview: respiratory effort and airflow, ECG, leg movements and oxygen saturation. Oxygen saturation is determined by monitoring with a pulse oximeter, a light-sensitive electric cell that attaches to the ear or a finger. Oxygen saturation and ECG assessments are of particular importance if sleep apnoea is suspected. Through polysomnography, the patient's activity (movements, struggling, noisy respirations) during sleep can be assessed. Such activity of which the patient is unaware may be the cause of arousal during sleep.

PLANNING

The major goal for patients with sleep disturbances are to maintain (or develop) a sleeping pattern that provides sufficient energy for daily activities. Other goals may relate to enhancing the patient's feeling of well-being or improving the quality (as opposed to the quantity) of the patient's sleep. The nurse plans specific nursing interventions to reach the goal based on the aetiology of each nursing problem. These interventions may include reducing environmental distractions, promoting bedtime rituals, providing comfort measures, scheduling nursing care to provide for uninterrupted sleep periods, and teaching stress reduction, relaxation techniques or ways to develop good sleep habits.

IMPLEMENTING

Nursing interventions to enhance the quantity and quality of patients' sleep involve largely non-pharmacological measures. These involve health teaching about sleep habits, support of bedtime rituals, the provision of a restful environment, specific measures to promote comfort and relaxation, and essential considerations about the use of sleep medications.

For hospitalised patients, sleep problems are often related to the hospital environment or their illness. Assisting the patient to sleep in such instances can be challenging to a nurse, often involving scheduling activities, administering analgesics and providing a supportive environment. Explanations and a supportive relationship are essential for the fearful or anxious patient.

Patient Teaching

Healthy individuals need to learn the importance of rest and sleep in maintaining active and productive lifestyles. They need to learn (a) the conditions that promote sleep and those that interfere with sleep, (b) safe use of sleep medications, (c) effects of other prescribed medications on sleep, and (d) effects of their disease states on sleep. Patient teaching for promoting sleep is shown in *Teaching: wellness care*.

Supporting Bedtime Rituals

Most people are accustomed to bedtime rituals or pre-sleep routines that are conducive to comfort and relaxation. Altering or eliminating such routines can affect an individual's sleep. Common pre-bedtime activities of adults include an evening stroll, listening to music, watching television, taking a soothing bath and praying. Children, too, are socialised into pre-sleep routines such as a bedtime story, holding onto a favourite toy or blanket, and kissing everyone goodnight. Sleep is also usually preceded by hygienic routines, such as washing the face and hands (or bathing), brushing the teeth and voiding.

In institutional settings, nurses can provide similar bedtime rituals – assisting with a hand and face wash, hot drink, plumping of pillows and providing extra blankets as needed. Conversing about accomplishments of the day or enjoyable events such as visits from friends can also help to relax patients and bring peace of mind.

Creating a Restful Environment

All people need a sleeping environment with minimal noise, a comfortable room temperature, appropriate ventilation and

TEACHING: WELLNESS CARE

Promoting Rest and Sleep

Sleep Pattern
+ Establish a regular bedtime and wake-up time for all days of the week to prevent disruptions in your biological rhythm. Eliminate lengthy naps, or if a daytime nap is necessary, take it at the same time each day and limit the time to 30 minutes, preferably once a day.
+ Get adequate exercise during the day to reduce stress, but avoid excessive physical exertion two hours before bedtime.
+ Avoid dealing with office work or family problems before bedtime.
+ Establish a regular routine before sleep such as reading, listening to soft music, taking a warm bath or doing some other quiet activity you enjoy.
+ When you are unable to sleep, pursue some relaxing activity until you feel drowsy.
+ If you have trouble falling asleep, get up and pursue nonstrenuous activity until you feel sleepy.
+ Use the bed mainly for sleep, so that you associate it with sleep.

Environment
+ Ensure appropriate lighting, temperature and ventilation.
+ Keep noise to a minimum; block out extraneous noise as necessary with soft music.

Diet
+ Avoid heavy meals three hours before bedtime.
+ Avoid alcohol and caffeine-containing foods and beverages (coffee, tea, chocolate) at least four hours before bedtime. Caffeine can interfere with sleep and both caffeine and alcohol act as diuretics, creating the need to void during sleep time.
+ Decrease fluid intake 2–4 hours before sleep if necessary to avoid the need to use the bathroom during sleeping hours.
+ If a bedtime snack is necessary, consume only light carbohydrates or a milk drink. Heavy or spicy foods can cause gastrointestinal upsets that disturb sleep.

Medications
+ Use sleeping medications only as a last resort. Use over-the-counter medications sparingly because many contain antihistamines that cause daytime drowsiness.
+ Take analgesics before bedtime to relieve aches and pains.
+ Consult with your healthcare provider about adjusting other medications that may cause insomnia.

---

appropriate lighting. Although most people prefer a darkened environment, a low light source may provide comfort for children or those in a strange environment. Infants and children need a quiet room usually separate from the parents' room, a light or warm blanket as appropriate, and a location away from open windows or drafts.

Environmental distractions such as environmental noises and staff communication noise are particularly troublesome for hospitalised patients. Environmental noises include the sound, telephones and call lights/buzzers; doors closing; elevator chimes; furniture squeaking; and linen trolleys being wheeled through corridors. Staff communication is a major factor creating noise, particularly at staff change of shift.

To create a restful environment, the nurse needs to reduce environmental distractions, reduce sleep interruptions, ensure a safe environment and provide a room temperature that is satisfactory to the patient. Some interventions to reduce environmental distractions, especially noise, may be practised.

The environment must also be safe so that the patient can relax. People who are unaccustomed to narrow hospital beds may feel more secure with side rails.

Promoting Comfort and Relaxation

Comfort measures are essential to help the patient fall asleep and stay asleep, especially if the effects of the person's illness interfere with sleep. A concerned, caring attitude, along with the following interventions, can significantly promote patient comfort and sleep:

+ Provide loose-fitting nightwear.
+ Assist patients with hygienic routines.
+ Make sure the bed linen is smooth, clean and dry.
+ Assist or encourage the patient to void before bedtime.
+ Position dependent patients appropriately to aid muscle relaxation, and provide supportive devices to protect pressure areas.
+ Schedule medications, especially diuretics, to prevent nocturnal awakenings.
+ For patients who have pain, administer analgesics 30 minutes before sleep.
+ Listen to the patient's concerns and deal with problems as they arise.

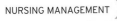

NURSING MANAGEMENT

Emotional stress obviously interferes with a person's ability to relax, rest and sleep, and inability to sleep further aggravates feelings of tension. Sleep rarely occurs until a person is relaxed. Relaxation techniques can be encouraged as part of the nightly routine. Slow, deep breathing for a few minutes followed by slow, rhythmic contraction and relaxation of muscles can alleviate tension and induce calm. Imagery, meditation and yoga can also be taught.

Enhancing Sleep with Medications

Sleep medications often prescribed on a prn (as-needed) basis for patients include the sedative-hypnotics, which induce sleep, and anti-anxiety drugs or tranquillisers, which decrease anxiety and tension. When prn sleep medications are prescribed in institutional settings, the nurse is responsible for making decisions with the patient about when to administer them. These medications should be administered only with complete knowledge of their actions and effects and only when indicated. Whenever possible, nonpharmacological interventions to induce and maintain sleep, discussed earlier, are the preferred interventions.

Both nurses and patients need to be aware of the actions, effects, and risks of the specific medication prescribed. Although medications vary in their activity and effects, considerations include the following:

+ Sedative-hypnotic medications produce a general central nervous system (CNS) depression and an unnatural sleep; REM or NREM sleep is altered to some extent and daytime drowsiness and a morning hangover effect may occur.
+ Antianxiety medications decrease levels of arousal by facilitating the action of neurons in the CNS that suppress responsiveness to stimulation. These medications are contraindicated in pregnant women because of their associated risk of congenital anomalies, and in nursing mothers because the medication is excreted in breast milk.
+ Sleep medications vary in their onset and duration of action and will impair waking function as long as they are chemically active. Some medication effects can last many hours beyond the time that the patient's perception of daytime drowsiness and impaired psychomotor skills have disappeared. Patients need to be cautioned about such effects and about driving or handling machinery while the drug is in their system.
+ Sleep medications affect REM sleep more than NREM sleep. Patients need to be informed that one or two nights of increased dreaming (REM rebound) are usual after the drug is discontinued.

+ Initial doses of medications should be low and increases added gradually, depending on the patient's response. Older adults, in particular, are susceptible to side-effects because of their metabolic changes; they need to be closely monitored for changes in mental alertness and coordination. Patients need to be instructed to take the smallest effective dose and then only for a few nights or intermittently as required.
+ Regular use of any sleep medication can lead to tolerance over time (e.g. four weeks) and rebound insomnia. In some instances, this may lead patients to increase the dosage. Patients must be cautioned about developing a pattern of drug dependency.
+ Abrupt cessation of barbiturate sedative-hypnotics can create withdrawal symptoms such as restlessness, tremors, weakness, insomnia, increased heart rate, seizures, convulsions and even death. Long-term users need to taper withdrawal by about 25–30% weekly.

EVALUATING

Using data collected during care and the desired outcomes developed during the planning stage as a guide, the nurse judges whether patient goals and outcomes have been achieved. Data collection may include (a) observations of the duration of the patient's sleep and the presence of signs of REM and NREM sleep and (b) questions about how the patient feels on awakening, or about the effectiveness of specific interventions such as the use of relaxation techniques, adherence to a consistent sleep wake cycle or the ingestion of milk products before bedtime.

If the desired outcomes are not achieved, the nurse, patient and support people if appropriate should explore the reasons, which may include answers to the following questions:

+ Were aetiological factors correctly identified?
+ Has the patient's physical condition or medication therapy changed?
+ Did the patient comply with instructions about establishing a regular sleep wake pattern?
+ Did the patient avoid ingesting caffeine?
+ Did the patient participate in stimulating daytime activities to avoid excessive daytime naps?
+ Were all possible measures taken to provide a restful environment for the patient?
+ Were bedtime rituals supported?
+ Were the comfort and relaxation measures effective?

CRITICAL REFLECTION

Let us revisit the case study on page 595. Now that you have read this chapter what methods can you use to assess individuals' mobility? What factors affect the ability of a person to sleep? How can patient positioning while sleeping affect long-term mobility?

CHAPTER HIGHLIGHTS

+ The ability to move freely, easily and purposefully in the environment is essential for people to meet their basic needs.
+ Purposeful coordinated movement of the body relies on the integrated functioning of the musculoskeletal system, the nervous system and the vestibular apparatus of the inner ear.
+ Body movement involves four basic elements: body alignment, joint mobility, balance and coordinated movement.
+ People maintain alignment and balance when the line of gravity passes through the centre of gravity and the base of support.
+ The broader the base of support and the lower the centre of gravity, the greater the stability and balance achieved.
+ Exercise is physical activity performed to maintain muscle tone and joint mobility, to enhance physiologic functioning of body systems and to improve physical fitness. Activity tolerance is the type and amount of exercise or daily living activities an individual is able to perform without experiencing adverse effects.
+ Exercise is classified as either isotonic, isometric or isokinetic and as either aerobic or anaerobic.
+ Many factors influence body alignment and activity. These include growth and development, physical health, mental health, personal values and attitudes, and prescribed limitations to movement.
+ Immobility affects almost every body organ and system adversely; complications also include psychosocial problems. Exercise, by contrast, provides many benefits to the same body organs and systems.
+ Problems of immobility include disuse osteoporosis and atrophy; contractures; diminished cardiac reserve; orthostatic hypotension; venous stasis, oedema and thrombus formation; decreased respiratory movement and pooling of secretions; decreased metabolic rate and negative nitrogen balance; urinary stasis, retention and infection; constipation; and varying emotional reactions.

+ The nurse has responsibilities (a) to prevent the complications of immobility and reduce the severity of any problems resulting from immobility and (b) to design exercise programmes for patients that promote wellness.
+ Assessment relative to a patient's activity and exercise includes a nursing assessment and physical examination of body alignment, gait, joint appearance and movement, capabilities and limitations for movement, muscle mass and strength, activity tolerance, and problems related to immobility.
+ An activity and exercise history includes daily activity level, activity tolerance, type and frequency of exercise, and factors affecting mobility.
+ Body mechanics is the efficient, coordinated and safe use of the body to move objects and carry out the activities of daily living.
+ Preambulatory exercises that strengthen the muscles for walking are essential for patients who have been immobilised for a prolonged period.
+ Sleep is a naturally occurring altered state of consciousness in which a person's perception and reaction to the environment are decreased.
+ Rest and sleep are restorative, protective and energy conserving.
+ The sleep cycle is controlled by specialised areas in the brain stem and is affected by the individual's circadian rhythm.
+ During a normal night's sleep, an adult has four to six sleep cycles, each with NREM (quiet sleep) and REM (rapid eye movement) sleep.
+ REM sleep recurs about every 90 minutes, is less restful than NREM sleep and is often associated with dreaming.
+ Many factors can affect sleep, including illness, environment, fatigue, lifestyle, emotional stress, stimulants and alcohol, diet, smoking, motivation and medications.

+ Common sleep disorders include parasomnias (such as bruxism, nocturnal enuresis, sleeptalking and somnambulism), insomnia, hypersomnia, narcolepsy, sleep apnoea and sleep deprivation.
+ Assessment of an individual's sleep includes obtaining a sleep history, reviewing a sleep diary, and conducting a physical examination to detect signs of sleep deprivation.

+ Nursing responsibilities to help patients sleep include (a) teaching patients ways to enhance sleep and rest, (b) supporting bedtime rituals, (c) creating a restful environment, (d) promoting comfort and relaxation, and (e) using prescribed sleep medications.
+ Nonpharmacological interventions to induce and maintain sleep are always the preferred interventions.

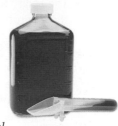

REFERENCES

American Sleep Disorders Association (1997) *The international classification of sleep disorders: Diagnostic and coding manual,* Lawrence, KS: Allen Press.

Gordon, M. (2002) *Manual of nursing diagnosis* (10th edn), St. Louis, MO: Mosby.

Kripke, D.F., Garfinkel, L., Wingard, D.L., Klauber, M.R. and Marler, M.R. (2002) 'Mortality associated with sleep duration and insomnia', *Archives of General Psychiatry,* 59(2), 131–136.

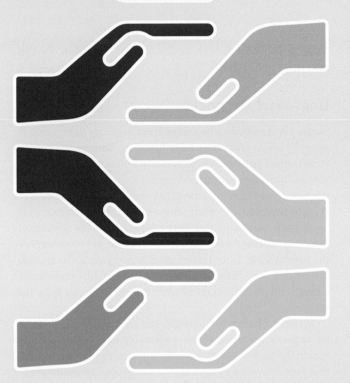

Chapter 24 Pre- and Post-operative Care

Learning Outcomes

After completing this chapter, you will be able to:

+ Describe the phases of surgery.

+ Discuss various types of surgery according to degree of urgency, degree of risk and purpose.

+ Identify essential aspects of pre-operative assessment.

+ Identify nursing responsibilities in planning pre- and post-operative nursing care.

+ Describe essential pre-operative teaching, including pain control, moving, leg exercises, and coughing and deep-breathing exercises.

+ Describe essential aspects of preparing a patient for surgery, including skin preparation.

+ Identify essential nursing assessments and interventions during the immediate post-anaesthetic phase.

+ Demonstrate ongoing nursing assessments, interventions and evaluation of the care provided to the post-operative patient.

+ Identify potential post-operative complications and describe nursing interventions to prevent them.

+ Describe appropriate wound care for a post-operative patient.

CASE STUDY

Mr Teng is a 77-year-old man with a history of chronic obstructive pulmonary disease (COPD). Currently his respiratory condition is being controlled with medications and he is free of infection. He has just been transferred to the recovery unit following a hernia repair performed under spinal anaesthesia. His blood pressure is 132/88, pulse 84, respirations 28 and tympanic temperature 36.5°C (97.8°F). He is awake and stable.

After reading this chapter you will be able to identify the factors that place Mr Teng at increased risk of complications during and after surgery and understand why he was given a spinal anaesthesia as opposed to a general anaesthesia.

INTRODUCTION

Mr Teng's decision to undergo a surgical procedure was probably not taken lightly as it can be a terrifying thought. But imagine the prospect of having surgery before the advent of modern anaesthesia and pain relief. Well, that is what faced people living in the Middle Ages. In those days surgery was a crude practice and not considered to be a skilled trade as it is today. Yet they still performed complex operations such as amputations, setting of broken bones and replacing dislocations. If the patient was lucky when undergoing these surgical procedures they were given opium as an anaesthetic which merely served to dull the pain.

You may think that surgery was only performed by trained physicians but this was not the case in the Middle Ages. In fact physicians, who were well educated, felt it was beneath them to actually perform surgery but chose to diagnose their patients by examining and treating the outside of the body. The forerunners of medicine and surgery were in fact barbers. The 'Barber Surgeons', as they became known, were extremely versatile and innovative characters acting not only as barbers but also as local doctors and dentists. The most well-known barber surgeon from the 16th century, Frenchman Ambroise Paré, is said to be the founder of modern surgery as he developed a number of surgical techniques that are still used today, in particular the ligating or tying off of blood vessels to control bleeding during surgery.

Despite these developments, death following surgery was extremely common, particularly for those undergoing amputations. In fact the most common cause of death post-surgery was infection and this remained so until the mid-19th century when the French chemist Louis Pasteur discovered that the death of body tissue was caused by bacteria in the air. Simultaneously, a Hungarian physician, Ignaz Semmelweiss demonstrated that the transmission of infectious diseases could be reduced by hand washing. With this knowledge, in 1865, Joseph Lister, a renowned British surgeon, developed antiseptic techniques, including the use of carbolic acid, to kill bacteria in his operating theatres.

Modern day surgery has benefited from these and other pioneers. In particular it has benefited from the development of effective anaesthesia in the 1840s. Ether and chloroform, the first anaesthetic agents to be used, helped to alleviate patient suffering. Effective anaesthesia meant that more intricate operations could be performed to the internal organs of the body. This both advanced knowledge of the human body and surgical techniques.

Today surgery is much more advanced and less traumatic for patients as a result of these developments. In fact, it has become a commonplace occurrence in hospitals with nearly seven million patients undergoing surgery each year in England alone (Hospital Episode Statistics, 2006). The types of surgery available to patients have become progressively more sophisticated over the past 20–30 years with the advent of less invasive techniques such as keyhole surgery and a number of different types of surgery are available. Advancing techniques, an increase in surgical workload and increasing pressure to reduce waiting lists has led to more and more minor operations being performed in community hospitals and general practitioner practices. This has obviously had an impact on nursing provision within these environments as there must be adequate care for patients undergoing surgery.

CLASSIFICATION OF SURGERY

Surgery is classified according to its purpose, whether it is urgent or not and the degree of risk associated with the surgery.

Purpose

Surgical procedures may be categorised according to their purpose (see *Box 24-1*).

Degree of Urgency

Surgery is classified by its urgency and necessity to preserve the patient's life, body part or body function. **Emergency surgery** is performed immediately to preserve function or the life of the patient. Surgeries to control internal haemorrhage or repair a fracture are examples of emergency surgeries. **Elective surgery** is performed when surgical intervention is the preferred treatment for a condition that is not imminently life threatening (but may ultimately threaten life or well-being) or to improve the patient's life. Examples of elective surgeries include cholecystectomy for chronic gallbladder disease, hip replacement surgery and plastic surgery procedures such as breast reduction surgery.

Mr Teng's hernia was probably not life-threatening therefore his surgery was elective. His surgeon would have probably wanted him in the peak of condition before operating on him to ensure that post-operative complications were kept to a minimum.

BOX 24-1 Purposes of Surgical Procedures

Diagnostic	Confirms or establishes a diagnosis; for example, biopsy of a mass in a breast.
Palliative	Relieves or reduces pain or symptoms of a disease; it does not cure; for example, resection of nerve roots.
Ablative	Removes a diseased body part; for example, removal of a gallbladder (cholecystectomy).
Constructive	Restores function or appearance that has been lost or reduced; for example, breast implant.
Transplant	Replaces malfunctioning structures; for example, hip replacement.

Degree of Risk

Surgery is also classified as major or minor according to the degree of risk to the patient. **Major surgery** involves a high degree of risk, for a variety of reasons: It may be complicated or prolonged, large losses of blood may occur, vital organs may be involved or post-operative complications may be likely. Examples are organ transplant, open heart surgery and removal of a kidney. In contrast, **minor surgery** normally involves little risk, produces few complications and is often performed in a 'day surgery'. Examples are breast biopsy, removal of tonsils and knee surgery.

The degree of risk involved in a surgical procedure is affected by the patient's age; general health, nutritional status, use of medications and mental status (see *Boxes 24-2* and *24-3*).

Although there may be different types of surgery each surgical procedure will have three distinct phases: pre-operative, intra-operative and post-operative. Together these make up the total management of a patient undergoing surgery.

BOX 24-2 Factors that Increase the Risk of Surgery

Age	Infants and older adults have greater surgical risks due to reduced physiological reserves and reduced ability to meet the demands placed on them during and after surgery.
General health	Any infection or underlying disease increases the risks associated with surgery for example chronic obstructive pulmonary disease (COPD) can be exacerbated by the effects of general anaesthesia and also predisposes the patient to post-operative chest infections. (See *Box 24-3* for other health problems that increase the risk of surgery.)
Nutritional status	Poor nutrition delays wound healing. Also obese patients are at increased risk of chest infections, wound infection and wound dehiscence (separating). Obese and underweight patients are both at increased risk of pressure ulcer development.
Medications	The regular use of certain medications can increase surgical risk: for example, anticoagulants such as warfarin often used to treat cardiac arrhythmias and deep vein thrombosis can lead to bleeding during and after surgery.
Mental status	A patient's ability to understand the purpose of or implications of surgery is important. For example children may become extremely distressed before and/or after surgery and patients with dementia may become unpredictable after anaesthesia.

BOX 24-3 Health Problems that Increase Surgical Risk

+ Malnutrition can lead to delayed wound healing, infection and reduced energy. Protein and vitamins are needed for wound healing; vitamin K is essential for blood clotting.
+ Obesity leads to hypertension, impaired cardiac function and impaired respiratory ventilation. Obese patients are also more likely to have delayed wound healing and wound infection because adipose tissue impedes blood circulation and its delivery of nutrients, antibodies and enzymes required for wound healing.
+ Cardiac conditions such as angina pectoris, recent myocardial infarction, hypertension and heart failure weaken the heart. Well-controlled cardiac problems generally pose minimal operative risk.
+ Blood coagulation disorders may lead to severe bleeding, haemorrhage and subsequent shock.
+ Upper respiratory tract infections or chronic obstructive lung diseases as in Mr Teng's case can adversely affect pulmonary function, especially when renal disease impairs regulation of the body's fluids and electrolytes, and excretion of drugs and other toxins.
+ Diabetes mellitus predisposes the patient to wound infection and delayed healing.
+ Liver disease (e.g. cirrhosis) impairs the liver's abilities to detoxify medications used during surgery, produce the prothrombin necessary for blood clotting, and metabolise nutrients essential for healing.
+ Uncontrolled neurological disease such as epilepsy may result in seizures during surgery or recovery.

The **pre-operative phase** begins when the decision to have surgery is made and ends when the patient is transferred to the operating table. The nursing activities associated with this phase include assessing the patient, identifying potential or actual health problems, planning specific care based on the individual's needs, and providing pre-operative teaching for the patient and their family and friends.

The **intra-operative phase** begins when the patient is transferred to the operating table and ends when the patient is admitted to the recovery unit. The nursing activities related to this phase include a variety of specialised procedures designed to create and maintain a safe therapeutic environment for the patient and the healthcare personnel.

The **post-operative phase** begins with the admission of the patient to the recovery unit and ends when healing is complete. During the post-operative phase, nursing activities include assessing the patient's physiological and psychological response to surgery, performing interventions to facilitate healing and prevent complications, teaching and providing support to the patient and their family and friends, and planning for their discharge. The goal is to assist the patient to achieve the most optimal health status possible following surgery.

Regardless of the type of surgery a patient is to undergo all will go through this process. What will differ is the length of each phase. For instance, a person who has been in a road traffic accident who requires emergency surgery will have a short pre-operative phase while a patient who has a chronic condition may have a longer pre-operative phase in order to ensure they are at their optimum health status before surgery.

PRE-OPERATIVE PHASE

Pre-operative care is the psychological and physical preparation of the patient for surgery and involves a number of nursing interventions. It must be said that the psychological preparation of the patient is equally as important as their physical preparation as inadequate psychological preparation and anxiety can have a negative impact on post-operative recovery (Kiecolt-Glaser *et al.*, 1998). In fact it has been found that the more anxious patients are, the more pain they experience post-operatively (Thomas *et al.*, 1995). Psychological preparation involves informing and obtaining written consent for the procedure and allaying any unnecessary fears that the patient may have.

Most hospitals have policies and protocols for the physical preparation of patients for surgery and usually involves:

+ A thorough assessment of the patient including the patient's surgical and anaesthetic background, risk factors such as impaired healing, drug or alcohol abuse, malnutrition.
+ Pre-operative investigations such as blood tests and x-rays.
+ Preparation of the patient such as improving nutritional

status, administration of bowel preparations to clear the bowels, skin preparation such as shaving.

The type of physical and psychological preparation required depends on a number of factors, such as the type of surgery and the individual patients. Regardless of the type of surgery and preparation required all patients will be required to give their consent to the procedure.

Informed Consent

Prior to any nursing, surgical or medical intervention, the patient should give their consent to the intervention. Indeed the Nursing and Midwifery Council (NMC, 2004) states that nurses have a professional responsibility to ensure that patients in their care consent to these interventions.

But what is **informed consent**. According to UK law patient's have the right to **self-determination** or the right to choose their own fate voluntarily, which basically means they have their own free will. The law also states that healthcare professionals have a duty to provide the patient with sufficient information in order for the patient to make informed choices.

In the clinical environment this means that the health professional needs to gain consent before continuing with the desired intervention. As far as surgical procedures are concerned, the surgeon is responsible for ensuring that valid consent is obtained from the patient, but the nurse may be involved in the clarification of certain aspects of the procedure. If it is not clear that the patient understands and consents to the surgery, the nurse should contact the surgeon before surgery proceeds.

Pre-operative informed consent should include:

+ nature and intention of the surgery;
+ name and qualifications of the person performing the surgery;
+ risks, including tissue damage, disfigurement or even death;
+ chances of success;
+ possible alternative measures;
+ the right of the patient to refuse consent or later withdraw consent.

Informed consent is only possible when the patient understands the information being provided, that is, speaks the language and is conscious, mentally competent and not sedated. As far as the treatment of children is concerned they may be able to give their consent to surgery depending on whether they have sufficient understanding and intelligence to be able to make up their own mind. This is known as the **Gillick principle** which stems from a judgment made in the House of Lords in 1985 which held that a doctor could lawfully prescribe contraception to a girl under the age of 16 without the consent of her parents. (See Chapter 3 for further details on informed consent and the Gillick principle.)

NURSING MANAGEMENT

ASSESSING

Pre-operative assessment should include the gathering of information from the patient, their medical and nursing notes to establish what their physical, psychological and social needs are both pre-operatively and post-operatively. The most essential pre-operative information that should be gathered is summarised in *Box 24-4*.

Physical Assessment

Pre-operatively, the nurse will perform a brief physical assessment. This will form baseline information that can be used to evaluate the patient post-operatively. For example, the nurse will assess the patient's mental status by recording their Glasgow Coma and establishing if they are orientated to time and place and have the ability to

---

BOX 24-4 Pre-operative Assessment

+ *Current health.* What is the patient's general health like at the present time? Does the patient have any chronic diseases, such as diabetes or asthma that may affect the patient's response to surgery or anaesthesia? Any physical limitations that may affect the patient's mobility or ability to communicate after surgery should be noted, as well as any prostheses such as hearing aids or contact lenses.

+ *Allergies.* Include allergies to prescription and non-prescription drugs, food allergies, and allergies to tape, latex, soaps or antiseptic agents. Some food allergies may indicate a potential reaction to drugs or substances used during surgery or diagnostic procedures; for example, an allergy to seafood alerts the nurse to a potential allergy to iodine-based dyes commonly used in radiological procedures.

+ *Medications.* List all current medications. It may be vital to maintain a blood level of some medications (e.g. anticonvulsants) throughout the surgical experience; others, such as anticoagulants or aspirin, increase the risks of surgery and anaesthesia and may need to be discontinued several days prior to surgery. It is important to include in the list any herbal remedies the patient currently takes as these can interact with some medications.

+ *Previous surgeries.* Previous surgery may influence the patient's physical and psychological responses to surgery or may reveal unexpected responses to anaesthesia.

+ *Activities of daily living.* The patient's abilities to meet their activities of daily living in order to establish a baseline for the recovery process (see Chapter 2 for ADLs).

+ *Mental status.* The patient's mental status and ability to understand and respond appropriately can affect the whole surgical process. Any developmental disabilities, mental illness, dementia or excessive anxiety need to be noted.

+ *Understanding of the surgical procedure and anaesthesia.* The patient should have a good understanding of the planned procedure and what to expect during and after surgery as well as the expected outcome of the procedure.

+ *Smoking.* Smokers may have more difficulty clearing respiratory secretions after surgery, increasing the risk of post-operative complications such as pneumonia and atelectasis (collapse of part of the lung).

+ *Alcohol and substance abuse.* Use of substances that affect the central nervous system, liver or other body systems can affect the patient's response to anaesthesia and surgery, and post-operative recovery.

+ *Coping mechanisms.* Patients who use appropriate coping mechanisms such as talking with the family may be better able to deal with the stress of surgery.

+ *Social support.* Determine the availability of family or other caregivers as they are important to the patient's recovery, particularly for the patient undergoing day surgery.

+ *Religious and cultural considerations.* Religion and culture can influence the patient's response to surgery; respecting religious and cultural beliefs and practices can reduce pre-operative anxiety and improve recovery.

Table 24-1 Routine Pre-operative Investigations and Tests

Test	Rationale
Full blood count (FBC)	Red blood cells (RBC), haemoglobin (Hb) and haematocrit (Hct) are important to the oxygen-carrying capacity of the blood; white blood cells (WBC) can indicate infection
Blood grouping and cross-matching	Determined in case blood transfusion is required during or after surgery
Serum electrolytes (sodium, potassium, calcium, magnesium, chloride, bicarbonate)	To evaluate fluid and electrolyte status
Fasting blood glucose	High levels may indicate undiagnosed diabetes mellitus
Blood urea nitrogen (BUN) and creatinine	To evaluate renal function
Alanine Aminotransferase (ALT), Aspartarte Aminotransferase (AST) and bilirubin	To evaluate liver function
Serum albumin and total protein	To evaluate nutritional status
Urinalysis	To determine urine composition and possible abnormal components (e.g. protein or glucose) or infection
Chest x-ray	To evaluate respiratory status and heart size
Electrocardiogram (ECG)	To identify pre-existing cardiac problems or disease

understand what is happening. This information will then be used to establish the patient's mental status and alertness after surgery. Also the nurse will perform respiratory and cardiovascular assessments not only provide baseline data for evaluating the patient's post-operative status but also may alert them to any underlying problem (e.g. a respiratory infection or irregular pulse rate) that may affect the patient's response to surgery and anaesthesia. Other systems (gastrointestinal, genitourinary and musculoskeletal) may also be examined to provide baseline data (see Chapter 24). However it is important to note that it is not only the nurse that will assess the patient pre-operatively, the patient will be assessed by the surgeon and the anaesthetist.

Pre-operative Investigations and Tests

It is usually the surgeon that orders specific investigations or test pre-operatively. However the National Institute for Health and Clinical Excellence (NICE, 2003) suggest which tests should be performed according to the patient's age, the type of surgery and whether the patient has any underlying health problems such as diabetes or ischaemic heart disease. If abnormalities are detected from these tests they may need to be treated prior to surgery.

These tests should be carried out and the results obtained and brought to the surgeon's attention prior to surgery. In addition to these routine tests, diagnostic tests directly related to the patient's disease are usually appropriate (e.g. gastroscopy to clarify the condition before gastric surgery).

PLANNING

The overall goal in the pre-operative period is to ensure that the patient is mentally and physically prepared for surgery. Planning should involve the patient and their family and friends. The

length of the pre-operative period affects pre-operative care and planning. When the patient is admitted several days before surgery, a nursing care plan is compiled during this period. However it is becoming more common for patients to attend pre-operative assessment clinics before or even on the day of surgery.

Planning for Discharge

For the surgical patient, discharge planning should begin on or before admission for the planned procedure. Early planning to meet the discharge needs of the patient is particularly important for the day-surgery patient who is to be discharged soon after recovering from anaesthesia. Care pathways are a useful way to plan care for surgical patients. Care pathways are structured multidisciplinary care plans that map the expected recovery of patient's undergoing specific procedures.

Discharge planning usually incorporates an assessment of the patient's and their family's resources for caring for the patient at home, including their financial status, and assesses the need for referral to other agencies (e.g. to the district nurse or social services). However, the extent of discharge planning will vary significantly for patients having different types of surgery.

IMPLEMENTING

One of the most important nursing interventions to prepare the patient for surgery is pre-operative teaching.

Pre-operative Teaching

Pre-operative teaching is a vital part of nursing care. Studies have shown that pre-operative teaching reduces patients' anxiety and post-operative complications and increases their satisfaction with the surgical experience (Krupat *et al.*, 2000). Good pre-operative teaching also facilitates the patient's return to work and other activities of daily living.

Pre-operative teaching involves:

+ Giving the patient information about what will happen to them and when, and what they will experience such as expected sensations and discomfort.
+ Psychosocial support to reduce anxiety.
+ Teaching patients ways of improving their recovery such as how to move, deep breathing and coughing exercises, how to splint incisions to ease pain when moving or coughing, and leg exercises to reduce the risk of clots forming in the veins in the legs (deep vein thrombosis – DVT). (*Procedure 24-1*

discusses teaching patients specific exercises to improve their recovery.)

If the patient is having day surgery, pre-operative teaching is often provided before the day of surgery in pre-admission or pre-assessment clinics, using some combination of videos and verbal and written instructions. Information may then be re-inforced on admission where any concerns that the patient or their family have may be discussed. This is particularly vital if the patient is a child, as both the child and the parents need to know what to expect and be able to express their concerns. Indeed some consider the parents as part of the team caring for the child and as such they should actively participate in as much of the care as possible.

PROCEDURE 24-1 Teaching Moving, Leg Exercises, Deep Breathing and Coughing

Surgery, although meant to benefit the patient, can cause serious complications post-operatively (see Table 24-2 on page 659). In order to prevent post-operative complications and aid the patient's recovery, the nurse needs to teach the patient techniques that will aid this process regardless of the type of surgery the patient has undergone.

Purposes

Moving

Following surgery most patients are encouraged to move early on in the recovery period: for example, patients who have undergone coronary artery bypass grafts (a treatment for coronary heart disease) are encouraged to sit out in a chair and walk around within 24 hours of surgery, to reduce the risk of post-operative complications.

Moving:

+ Maintains blood circulation and prevents the formation of clots (thrombi).
+ Stimulates respiratory function.
+ Increases gut motility.
+ Facilitates early mobilisation.

Leg Exercises

Intra-operatively and post-operatively patients usually have reduced mobility, which causes blood to pool in the veins in the legs (venous stasis) resulting in the formation of clots (deep vein thrombosis). Blood clots in the veins are a very serious complication as the clots can travel back to the heart and then to the lungs

(pulmonary emboli) resulting in serious illness or even death. Patients should therefore be encouraged to perform leg exercises to reduce the risk of blood clots forming.

Deep Breathing and Coughing

Chest infection is a common complication associated with surgery. If the patient is immobile or is not able to take deep breaths, the sputum that would normally be coughed up (expectorated) stays in the lungs and becomes the focus of infection. This can be prevented by encouraging the patient to perform deep breathing exercises. Following major surgery such as joint replacements or coronary artery bypass grafts, the physiotherapist may be involved in encouraging deep breathing and coughing exercises.

Deep breathing and coughing:

+ Facilitates lung expansion for patients with known respiratory (breathing) problems, thereby preventing collapse of the lung (atelectasis) and pneumonia.

Assessment

Assess

+ Vital signs
+ Discomfort/pain
+ Temperature and colour of feet and legs
+ Breath sounds
+ Presence of dyspnoea (shortness of breath) or cough

+ Learning needs of the patient
+ Anxiety level of the patient
+ Patient experience with previous surgeries and anaesthesia

Planning

Before beginning to teach moving, leg exercises, deep-breathing exercises and coughing, the nurse needs to determine:

+ The type of surgery
+ The time of the surgery
+ The name of the surgeon and their individual pre-operative orders

+ The hospital's protocols regarding pre-operative care.

Equipment

+ Pillow or rolled up towel
+ Teaching materials (e.g. videotape, written materials) if available.

Implementation

Preparation

Ensure that there is as little distraction as possible (e.g. TV, visitors) and that the patient is not in pain as this too can distract them. If appropriate the nurse can include the patient's family and friends if the patient so wishes.

Performance

1. Explain to the patient what you are going to do, why it is necessary and how they can cooperate. Discuss how the patient's participation in the exercises they are going to be taught pre-operatively will be helpful during the post-operative recovery.
2. Wash hands and observe appropriate infection control procedures.
3. Provide for patient privacy.
4. Show the patient ways to turn in bed and to get out of bed.
   - Patients with right-sided abdominal or chest incisions should be taught to get out of bed on the left side while patients with left-sided incisions should be taught to get out of bed on the right side. Rolling on the unaffected side will help them rise to a sitting position on the edge of the bed.
   - In order for the patient to sit up before getting out of bed the patient should be instructed to:
     (a) Bend their knees.
     (b) Splint the wound by holding a small pillow or rolled up towel against the incision.
     (c) Turn onto their unaffected side by pushing with their opposite foot.

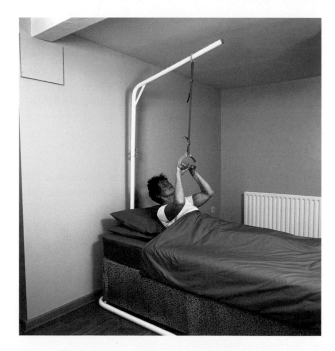

Figure 24-1 Monkey pole.

     (d) Come to a sitting position on the side of the bed by using the affected side's arm and hand to push down against the mattress and swinging the feet over the edge of the bed.
   - For patients with orthopaedic surgery (e.g. hip surgery), use special aids, such as a monkey pole (see Figure 24-1), to assist with movement.

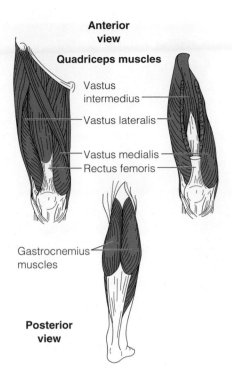

Figure 24-2 Leg muscles: anterior and posterior views.

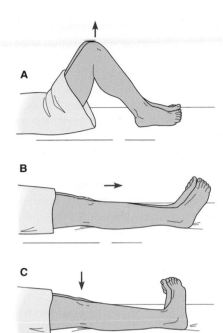

Figure 24-3 Flexing and extending the knees.

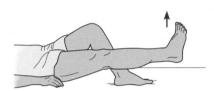

Figure 24-4 Raising and lowering the legs.

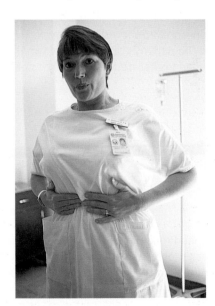

Figure 24-5 Demonstrating deep breathing.

5. Teach the patient the following three leg exercises:
- Alternate dorsiflexion and plantar flexion of the feet. This exercise is sometimes referred to as calf pumping, because it alternately contracts and relaxes the calf muscle (see Figure 24-2).
- Flex and extend the knees, and press the backs of the knees into the bed while dorsiflexing the feet (see Figure 24-3). Instruct patients who cannot raise their legs to do isometric exercises that contract and relax the muscles.
- Raise and lower the legs alternately from the surface of the bed. Flex the knee of the stable leg and extend the knee of the moving leg (see Figure 24-4). This exercise contracts and relaxes the quadriceps muscles.

6. Demonstrate deep-breathing (diaphragmatic) exercises as follows:
- Place your hands palms down on the border of your rib cage, and inhale slowly and evenly through the nose until the greatest chest expansion is achieved (Figure 24-5).
- Hold your breath for 2–3 seconds.
- Then exhale slowly through the mouth.
- Continue exhalation until maximum chest contraction has been achieved.

7. Help the patient perform deep-breathing exercises.
- Ask the patient to assume a sitting position.
- Place the palms of your hands on the border of the patient's rib cage to assess respiratory depth.
- Ask the patient to perform deep breathing, as described in step 6.

8. Instruct the patient to cough voluntarily after a few deep inhalations.

- Ask the patient to inhale deeply, hold the breath for a few seconds, and then cough once or twice.
- Ensure that the patient coughs deeply and does not just clear the throat.

9. If the incision is painful when the patient coughs, demonstrate techniques to splint the incision.
   - Show the patient how to support the incision by placing the palms of the hands on either side of the incision site or directly over the incision site, holding the palm of one hand over the other. Coughing uses the abdominal and other accessory respiratory muscles. Splinting the incision may reduce pain while coughing if the incision is near any of these muscles.
   - Show the patient how to splint the incision with clasped hands and a firmly rolled pillow or towel held against the patient's wound (see Figure 24-6).

10. Inform the patient about the expected frequency of these exercises.
    - Instruct the patient to start the exercises as soon after surgery as possible.
    - Encourage patients with abdominal or chest surgery to carry out deep breathing and coughing at least every two hours, taking a minimum of five breaths at each session. Note, however, that the number of breaths and frequency of deep breathing varies with the

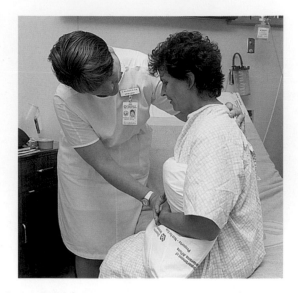

Figure 24-6 Splinting an incision with a pillow while coughing.

patient's condition. People who are susceptible to pulmonary problems may need deep-breathing exercises every hour. People with chronic respiratory disease may need special breathing exercises (e.g. pursed-lip breathing, abdominal breathing, exercises using various kinds of incentive spirometers). See Chapter 16.

11. Document the teaching and all assessments.

Evaluation

Conduct appropriate follow-up such as:

- Evaluate the patient's ability to perform the exercises and reiterate the teaching if needed.
- Ask the patient to verbally recap the key information given.

LIFESPAN CONSIDERATIONS

Pre-operative Teaching

Children

- Parents need to know what to expect and to be able to express their concerns.
- Separation from parents often is the child's greatest fear; the time of separation should be minimised and parents allowed to interact with the child both immediately preceding and following the surgery.
- Teaching of children should be appropriate for their age and development.
- Use simple terms to help the child understand (e.g. 'You will have a sore tummy').
- Play is an effective teaching tool with children; the child can put a bandage on an incision on a doll.

Older Adults

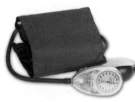

- Assess hearing ability to ensure the patient hears the necessary information.
- Assess short-term memory. Presenting one focused idea at a time and repeating or reinforcing information may be necessary.
- Older adults are at greater risk for post-operative complications, such as pneumonia. Reinforce moving and deep-breathing and coughing exercises.
- Assess potential post-operative needs. The patient may need to be referred to occupational therapy for equipment such as raised toilet seats.
- Assess the patient for risk of pressure ulcer development post-operatively.

Physical Preparation of the Patient

Pre-operative physical preparation of the patient ensures that they are in the best condition prior to surgery. This includes that the patient is adequately nourished and hydrated, that there are no elimination problems, that appropriate medication has been discontinued, that prostheses are removed or notified to the surgeon or anaesthetist and that there is appropriate preparation of the skin. Most hospitals utilise pre-operative checklists to ensure that all aspects of pre-operative care are addressed.

Nutrition and Fluids

Adequate hydration and nutrition promote healing. Nurses need to record any signs of malnutrition or fluid imbalance. If the patient is on intravenous fluids or on measured fluid intake, nurses must ensure that the fluids are carefully measured.

The order 'nil by mouth (NBM) from midnight' is a long-standing tradition as it was believed that anaesthetics depress gastrointestinal functioning and there was a danger that the patient could vomit and aspirate during the administration of a general anaesthetic. However the recent Royal College of Nursing (RCN, 2005) guidelines state that healthy adult and child patients can drink clear fluids up to two hours before surgery while solid foods including milk can be eaten up to six hours before surgery. According to this guideline higher risk patients should be assessed on an individual basis but could follow the same regimen as healthy patients.

> ### CLINICAL ALERT
>
> *To help the patient cope with thirst while NBM, the nurse can provide the patient with oral hygiene packs and mouth wash. The use of chewing gum and sweets should not be encouraged as these are classed as solid food.*

Elimination

Some surgery requires that the bowels or the bladder are empty. Therefore it is the nurses' responsibility to ensure that this preparation is carried out. Enemas may be administered or osmotic laxatives such as Picolax to empty the bowel while a urinary catheter could be ordered to ensure that the bladder remains empty. If the patient does not have a catheter, it is important to empty the bladder prior to receiving pre-operative medications as patients can be unsteady on their feet after taking medication such as diazepam or temazepam.

Medications

The anaesthetist or surgeon may temporarily discontinue routinely taken medications, such as aspirin, the day of surgery or a few days before surgery in order to prevent intra-operative and post-operative complications such as bleeding. In some settings pre-operative medications are given to patients for a number of reasons:

+ *sedatives and tranquillisers* such as diazepam (Valium) to reduce anxiety and ease anaesthetic induction;
+ *narcotic analgesics* such as morphine to sedate the patient and reduce the amount of anaesthetic required;
+ *anticholinergics* such as atropine to reduce oral and pulmonary secretions and prevent laryngospasm (closing of the larynx);
+ *histamine-receptor antihistamines* such as ranitidine (Zantac) to reduce gastric fluid volume and gastric acidity.

Pre-operative medications must be given at a scheduled time or when the operating theatre notifies the nurse to give the medication.

Rest and Sleep

Nurses should do everything to help the patient sleep the night before surgery as this helps the patient manage the stress of surgery and help healing. If the patient is having difficulty sleeping the surgeon may prescribe a sedative.

Prostheses

All prostheses (artificial body parts, such as partial or complete dentures, contact lenses, artificial eyes and artificial limbs) and eyeglasses, wigs and false eyelashes must be removed before surgery. Hearing aids are often left in place and the operating theatre staff notified.

As well as dentures the nurse should check if the patient has capped, crowned or loose teeth as these can become dislodged and aspirated during anaesthesia.

Skin Preparation

Some types of surgery require preparation of the skin pre-operatively. Often patients are asked to bathe or shower the evening or morning of surgery (or both) in a specific antiseptic solution (e.g. Hibiscrub). The purpose of this is to reduce the risk of wound infection post-operatively. Some hospitals and surgeons also ask for patients to shave the part of the body that is to be operated on before surgery, again to minimise the risk of infection. However this is a controversial subject as some research has shown that shaving actually increases the risk of infection rather than minimising it (Joanna Briggs Institute, 2003).

All nail polish and makeup should be removed prior to surgery so that the nail beds, skin and lips are visible for circulation to be assessed during and following surgery. Also any hair grips or pins should be removed from the hair as they may cause pressure ulcers while the patient is unconscious.

As part of the physical preparation of the patient pre-operatively, the patient may require the use of antiembolic stockings. This is particularly important for patients who will have long recovery periods or will have reduced mobility post-operatively. Antiembolic (elastic) stockings compress the veins of the legs and thereby facilitate the return of venous blood to the heart. This helps to prevent or reduce oedema (swelling) of the feet and lower legs and helps to reduce the formation of clots (deep vein thrombosis) in the lower legs. These stockings are frequently applied pre-operatively as well as post-operatively.

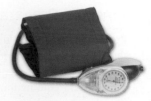

LIFESPAN CONSIDERATIONS

Antiembolic Stockings

Children
+ Antiembolic stockings are infrequently used on children.

Older Adults
+ As the elastic is quite strong in antiembolic stockings; the older adult may need assistance with putting on the stockings. Patients with arthritis may need to have another person put the stockings on for them.
+ Stockings should be removed once every 24 hours or more often if required, so that a thorough assessment can be made of legs and feet. Redness and skin breakdown on the heels can occur quickly and go undetected if not thoroughly assessed on a regular basis.

INTRA-OPERATIVE PHASE

The intra-operative nurse is a vital member of the surgical team, acting as the patient advocate, maintaining safety, and continually assessing the needs of the patient and the team. There are a number of nursing roles within the theatre, including anaesthetics, scrub and circulating nurses.

Anaesthetic Nurses

The anaesthetic nurse works closely with the anaesthetist, giving assistance from induction to the immediate recovery of the patient. The main functions of the anaesthetic nurse are outlined in *Box 24-5*.

Part of the role of the anaesthetic nurse is the induction of the patient using anaesthetics therefore the nurse needs to have a comprehensive knowledge of the types of anaesthetics used.

Types of Anaesthesia

There are two common types of anaesthesia, namely general and local. Generally anaesthetic agents are administered by an anaesthetist or nurse anaesthetist. **General anaesthesia** is the loss of all sensation and consciousness. Under general anaesthesia, protective reflexes such as cough and gag reflexes are lost. A general anaesthetic acts by blocking awareness centres in the brain so that amnesia (loss of memory), analgesia

---

BOX 24-5 Main Functions of the Anaesthetic Nurse

Provision of a Safe Environment:
+ Preparing equipment, medicines and fluids
+ Checking monitors and apparatus
+ Ensuring adequate stock
+ Ensuring a clean environment and equipment

Administrative Functions:
+ Arranging to send for the patient from the ward/clinic
+ Ensuring correct patient for correct procedure
+ Recording patient details in departmental records/database
+ Ensuring appropriate information accompanies the patient (case notes, results, forms, etc.)

Communication:
+ Providing the patient with an explanation and reassurance

+ Relaying information from the patient to the surgeon or anaesthetist
+ Providing a link to ensure colleagues are appropriately informed (ward, scrub team, recovery)

Practical Functions:
+ Assisting with induction of anaesthesia and airway management
+ Assisting with local anaesthetic blocks
+ Assisting with the positioning of the patient

Expertise:
+ Observing the patient's condition
+ Monitoring for any adverse effects of the anaesthesia
+ Monitoring for the maintenance of fluids and medications
+ Ensuring that safe systems of work are being employed at all times.

(insensibility to pain), hypnosis (artificial sleep) and relaxation (rendering a part of the body less tense) occur. General anaesthetics are usually administered by intravenous infusion or by inhalation of gases through a mask or through an endotracheal tube inserted into the trachea.

General anaesthesia has certain advantages such as the relatively easy regulation of the patient's respirations and cardiac function because the patient is unconscious and therefore is not anxious. General anaesthesia can be adjusted according to the patient's age, their physical status and the length and type of operation. The main disadvantage with general anaesthetic is that it depresses the respiratory function. This means that the patient is unable to maintain their own airway and cannot ventilate their lungs themselves. In order to maintain the patient's airway and provide ventilation to the patient the anaesthetist will usually introduce a tube into the patient's airway and attach this to a ventilator which helps to aerate the patient's lungs.

Patients are often fearful of general anaesthetic more than surgery, possibly as a result of the lack of control over their body and others. **Local anaesthesia** on the other hand only anaesthetises the local area (e.g. a hand) by temporarily interrupting the transmission of nerve impulses to and from that area or region. The patient loses sensation in an area of the body but remains conscious. Several techniques are used.

+ **Topical (surface) anaesthesia** is applied directly to the skin and mucous membranes, open skin surfaces, wounds and burns. The most commonly used topical agents are lidocaine (Xylocaine) and benzocaine. These are particularly useful for numbing a child's hand to introduce an intravenous catheter. However it is very important that the topical agent is given time to numb the area before proceeding.
+ **Local anaesthesia** (infiltration) is injected into a specific area and is used for minor surgical procedures such as suturing a small wound or performing a biopsy. Lidocaine 0.1% may be used for this purpose.
+ A **nerve block** is a technique in which the anaesthetic agent is injected into and around a nerve or small nerve group that supplies sensation to a small area of the body. Major blocks involve multiple nerves or a plexus (e.g. the brachial plexus anesthetises the arm); minor blocks involve a single nerve (e.g. a facial nerve).
+ An **intravenous block (Bier block)** is used most often for procedures involving the arm, wrist and hand. An occlusion tourniquet is applied to the extremity to prevent infiltration and absorption of the injected intravenous agent beyond the involved extremity.
+ **Spinal anaesthesia**, as in Mr Teng's case, requires a lumbar puncture through one of the interspaces between lumbar disc 2 (L_2) and the sacrum (S_1) and the introduction of an anaesthetic agent into the cerebrospinal fluid (CSF). Spinal anaesthesia is often categorised as a low, mid or high spinal. Low spinals (saddle or caudal blocks) are primarily used for surgeries involving the perineal or rectal areas. Mid spinals (below the level of the umbilicus – T_{10}) can be used for hernia repairs or appendectomies, and high spinals (reaching the nipple line – T_4) can be used for surgeries such as caesarean sections. Spinal anaesthesia is usually chosen as it reduces the effects on the respiratory system and recovery is much quicker than general anaesthesia.
+ **Epidural anaesthesia** is an injection of an anaesthetic agent into the epidural space, the area inside the spinal column but outside the dura mater.

Some types of surgery may require that the patient has conscious sedation as well as the local anaesthetic for patient comfort and safety. **Conscious sedation** refers to minimal depression of the level of consciousness in which the patient retains the ability to maintain a patent airway and respond appropriately to commands (Kost, 1999). Intravenous narcotics such as morphine or fentanyl (Sublimaze) and anti-anxiety agents such as diazepam (Valium) or midazolam (Versed) are commonly used to induce and maintain conscious sedation. Conscious sedation increases the patient's pain threshold and induces a degree of amnesia but allows for prompt reversal of its effects and a rapid return to normal activities of daily living. Procedures such as endoscopies, incision and drainage of abscesses, and even balloon angioplasty may be performed under conscious sedation.

As well as assisting the anaesthetist with the administration of anaesthesia the anaesthetic nurse may also assist in the intubation (the procedure for inserting a tube into the trachea of a patient who is not able to breathe) and ventilation (movement of oxygen and air into and out of a patient's lungs) of the patient. Nurse anaesthetists have a more extended role than anaesthetic nurses and may be able to cannulate (insert intravenous catheters) into patient, intubate patients and administer anaesthesia themselves.

Anaesthetic nurses however are only part of the theatre team of nurses. Surgery would not be able to take place if there were no scrub nurses or circulating nurses.

Scrub Nurses

The scrub nurse performs a vital function in any operation theatre, ensuring that all the appropriate instruments and equipment are available and sterile. The scrub nurse works closely with the surgeon and needs to have the knowledge and expertise to anticipate the instruments that are needed by the surgeon. They wear sterile gowns, gloves, caps, and so on. Their main responsibilities include draping the patient with sterile drapes and handling sterile instruments and supplies. They also account for used sponges, needles and instruments. In some surgical settings a surgeon does not close, that is, suture an incision, until the scrub nurse can account for all sponges and instruments. This precaution avoids leaving any surgical materials inside the patient.

Circulating Nurse

The circulating nurse, or 'runner' as they are colloquially called, assists the scrub nurses and surgeons by ensuring that the operating theatre is adequately stocked with supplies. They help position the patient for the operation and often position any needed equipment such as cameras or lighting.

NURSING MANAGEMENT

ASSESSING

On admission to theatre or surgical suite, the anaesthetic nurse confirms the patient's identity and assesses the patient's psychological and physical state. The nurse verifies the information on the pre-operative checklist and evaluates the patient's knowledge about the surgery and events to follow. The patient's response to pre-operative medications is assessed, as well as the placement and patency of any tubes such as IV lines, nasogastric tubes and urinary catheters.

Assessment continues throughout surgery, as the nurse and the anaesthetist continuously monitor the patient's vital signs (including blood pressure, heart rate, respiratory rate and temperature), ECG and oxygen saturation. Fluid intake and urinary output are monitored throughout surgery, and blood loss is estimated. Depending on the complexity of the surgery and the status of the patient other health parameters may be monitored such as haemoglobin and haematocrit (components of the blood), blood glucose and electrolytes within the blood. A more accurate way of monitoring the patient's oxygen and carbon dioxide levels can be achieved by taking regular arterial blood gases. Continual assessment is necessary to rapidly identify adverse responses to surgery or anaesthesia and intervene promptly to prevent complications.

PLANNING

The overall goals of care in the intra-operative period are to maintain the patient's safety and to maintain homoeostasis (stability). Examples of nursing activities to achieve these goals include the following:

+ Position the patient appropriately for surgery.
+ Perform pre-operative skin preparation.
+ Assist in preparing and maintaining the sterile field.
+ Open and dispense sterile supplies during surgery.
+ Provide medications and solutions for the sterile field.
+ Monitor and maintain a safe, aseptic environment.
+ Manage catheters, tubes, drains and specimens.
+ Perform sponge, sharp and instrument counts.
+ Document nursing care provided and the patient's response to interventions.

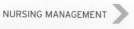

IMPLEMENTING

Surgical Skin Preparation

Even though the patient may have been asked to wash in antiseptic solution and shave appropriate parts of their body before surgery, while in theatre, the surgeon may insist that the skin be further prepared. This involves cleaning the surgical site with an antiseptic solution such as Betadine, which helps to reduce the risk of post-operative wound infection.

Positioning

Proper positioning of the patient during surgery is an important responsibility shared by the nurse, surgeon and anaesthetist. The ideal intra-operative patient position provides:

+ Optimal visualisation of and access to the surgical site
+ Optimal access for assessing and maintaining anaesthesia and vital functions (vital signs, respirations, cardiovascular function)
+ Protection of the patient from harm.

Positioning is performed after anaesthesia is induced and before surgical draping of the patient. The patient is manoeuvred into position in such a manner as to prevent shearing forces on the skin. The exact position for the patient depends on the operation; that is, the surgical approach. For example, a lithotomy position (lying on back with legs apart and feet supported in stirrups) is usually used for vaginal surgery.

Positions on the operating table are maintained by straps, and body prominences are frequently padded.

> **CLINICAL ALERT**
>
> *Be especially aware of the intra-operative position required for older adults as they are vulnerable to pressure ulcer formation. Check the appropriate pressure points of that surgical position on the patient.*

EVALUATING

This is performed by considering whether the goals set out in the planning stage have been met (e.g. maintain patient safety).

Documentation

Throughout the intra-operative phase the nurse documents patient care activities such as IV fluid infusions, positioning, gastric suction and urinary catheterisation.

POST-OPERATIVE PHASE

Nursing during the post-operative phase is especially important for the patient's recovery. Patients who have undergone surgery under general or local anaesthetic are at risk of compromise to their airway, breathing and circulation. Therefore it is important that post-operative patients are closely monitored.

Immediate Post-anaesthetic Phase

Recovery nurses have specialised skills to care for patients recovering from anaesthesia and surgery (see Figure 24-7). Once the patient is stabilised, they can be returned to the ward or unit from which they came from. It is the recovery nurse's role to stabilise the patient before transfer by continuously monitoring and treating them. Assessment of the patient in the immediate post-anaesthetic period is summarised in *Box 24-6* on page 658.

The return of the patient's reflexes, such as swallowing and gagging, usually indicates that the anaesthetic is wearing off. Recovery time from anaesthesia varies according to the type of anaesthetic used, its dosage and the patient's response to it. Nurses should arouse patients by calling them by name, and in

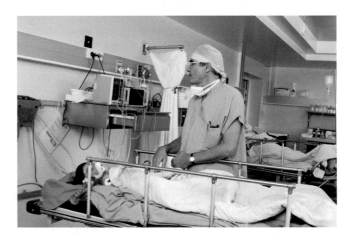

Figure 24-7 Recovery room nurse provides constant assessment and care for patients recovering from anaesthesia and surgery.

a normal tone of voice repeatedly telling them that the surgery is over and that they are in the recovery room.

Once the patient's condition is stabilised, they are returned to the ward or unit. However there are strict transfer criteria that the patient has to meet before they can be discharged from the recovery room.

The patient must:

+ Be conscious and oriented.
+ Be able to maintain a clear airway and deep breathe and cough freely.

 NURSING MANAGEMENT

BOX 24-6 Clinical Assessment

Immediate Post-anaesthetic Phase

+ Adequacy of airway
+ Oxygen saturation
+ Adequacy of ventilation
  - Respiratory rate, rhythm and depth
  - Use of accessory muscles
  - Breath sounds
+ Cardiovascular status
  - Heart rate and rhythm
  - Peripheral pulse amplitude and equality
  - Blood pressure
  - Capillary filling
+ Level of consciousness
  - Not responding
  - Arousable with verbal stimuli
  - Fully awake
  - Oriented to time, person and place
+ Presence of protective reflexes (e.g. gag, cough)

+ Activity, ability to move extremities
+ Skin colour (pink, pale, dusky, blotchy, cyanotic, jaundiced)
+ Fluid status
  - Intake and output
  - Status of IV infusions (type of fluid, rate, amount in container, patency of tubing)
  - Signs of dehydration or fluid overload
+ Condition of operative site
  - Status of dressing
  - Drainage (amount, type and colour)
+ Patency of and character and amount of drainage from catheters, tubes and drains
+ Discomfort (i.e. pain) (type, location and severity), nausea, vomiting
+ Safety (i.e. necessity for side rails, call bell within reach)

+ Have stable vital signs that are consistent with their pre-operative vital signs for at least 30 minutes.
+ Have active protective reflexes (e.g. gag, swallowing).
+ Be able to move their limbs.
+ Have adequate intake and urinary output (at least 30 ml/hr).
+ Have dry and intact dressings. Any drains that may be in place should not have excessive drainage for the type of operation.

Once the immediate recovery period is over and the patient is stable, they can be transferred back to the ward or unit. It is usual for the recovery nurse to inform the ward nurse that the patient is ready for collection from the recovery room. The ward nurse will then take over from the recovery nurse and ensure themselves that the patient is stable before transferring them back to the ward or unit. It is important to note that if the ward nurse feels that the patient does not meet the criteria for discharge they must voice this to the recovery nurse and delay transfer until they are happy with the patient's condition.

NURSING MANAGEMENT

ASSESSING

As soon as the patient returns to the nursing unit, the nurse conducts an initial assessment. Once the nurse has performed the initial assessment, the specific orders set out by the surgeon such as the intake of fluids and food, any intravenous solutions and medications that need to be administered, the position that they should be nursed in, and any further tests that may be required, need to be considered.

The nurse also checks the theatre notes to establish:

+ Operation performed
+ Presence and location of any drains
+ Anaesthetic used
+ Post-operative diagnosis

+ Estimated blood loss
+ Medications administered in the recovery room.

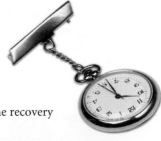

Many hospitals have post-operative protocols for regular assessment of patients. Some protocols require that assessments are made every 15 minutes until vital signs stabilise, every hour for the next four hours, then every four hours for the next two days. It is important that the assessments be made as often as the patient's condition requires. The nurse assesses the following:

+ *Level of consciousness.* Assess orientation to time, place and person. Most patients are fully conscious but drowsy when returned to their unit. Assess reaction to verbal stimuli and ability to move extremities.

+ *Vital signs.* Take the patient's vital signs (pulse, respiration, blood pressure and oxygen saturation level) every 15 minutes until stable or in accordance with the hospital's policy. These should be compared with the initial findings in the recovery room and with the patient's pre-operative vital signs. In addition, assess the patient's lung sounds and assess for signs of common circulatory problems such as post-operative hypotension, haemorrhage or shock. Hypovolaemia due to fluid losses during surgery is a common cause of post-operative hypotension. Haemorrhage can result from insecure ligation of blood vessels or disruption of sutures. Massive haemorrhage or cardiac insufficiency can lead to shock post-operatively. Common post-operative complications with their manifestations and preventive measures are listed in Table 24-2.

+ *Skin colour and temperature,* particularly that of the lips and nail beds. The colour of the lips and nail beds is an indicator of **tissue perfusion** (passage of blood through the vessels). Pale, cyanotic, cool and moist skin may be a sign of circulatory problems.

CLINICAL ALERT

Older adults may not show the classic signs of infection (e.g. fever, tachycardia, increased WBC) as the defence mechanisms of the body tend to reduce as a person ages (e.g. ageing reduces the number of antibodies produced). However infection in the older adult can cause them to become confused, disorientated and agitated as the brain tolerates infection less with ageing.

+ *Comfort.* Assess pain with the patient's vital signs and as needed between vital sign measurements. Assess the location and intensity of the pain. Do not assume that reported pain is incisional; other causes may include muscle strains, flatus and angina. Ask the patient to rate pain on a scale of 0–10, with 0 being no pain and 10 the worst pain imaginable. Evaluate the patient for objective indicators of pain: pallor, perspiration, muscle tension, and reluctance to

Table 24-2 Potential Post-operative Problems

Problem	Description	Cause	Clinical signs	Preventive interventions
Respiratory				
Pneumonia	Inflammation of the alveoli	Infection, toxins or irritants causing inflammatory process	Elevated temperature, cough, expectoration of blood-tinged or purulent sputum, dyspnoea, chest pain	Deep-breathing exercises and coughing, moving in bed, early ambulation
Infectious pneumonia	May be limited to one or more lobes (lobar) or occur as scattered patches throughout the lungs (bronchial); also can involve interstitial tissues of lungs	Common organisms include *Streptococcus pneumoniae*, *Haemophilus influenzae* and *Staphylococcus aureus*	Same as above	Same as above
Hypostatic pneumonia		Immobility and impaired ventilation result in atelectasis and promote growth of pathogens	Same as above	Same as above
Aspiration pneumonia	Inflammatory process caused by irritation of lung tissue by aspirated material, particularly hydrochloric acid (HCl) from the stomach	Aspiration of gastric contents, food or other substances; often related to loss of gag reflex	Same as above	Same as above
Atelectasis	A condition in which alveoli collapse and are not ventilated	Mucous plugs blocking bronchial passageways, inadequate lung expansion, analgesics, immobility	Dyspnoea, tachypnoea, tachycardia; diaphoresis, anxiety; pleural pain, decreased chest wall movement; dull or absent breath sounds; decreased oxygen saturation (SaO_2)	Deep-breathing exercises and coughing, moving in bed, early ambulation

NURSING MANAGEMENT

Table 24-2 (continued)

Problem	Description	Cause	Clinical signs	Preventive interventions
Pulmonary embolism	Blood clot that has moved to the lungs and blocks a pulmonary artery, thus obstructing blood flow to a portion of the lung	Stasis of venous blood from immobility, venous injury from fractures or during surgery, use of oral contraceptives high in oestrogen, pre-existing coagulation or circulatory disorder	Sudden chest pain, shortness of breath, cyanosis, shock (tachycardia, low blood pressure)	Turning, ambulation, antiembolic stockings, sequential compression devices
Circulatory				
Hypovolaemia	Inadequate circulating blood volume	Fluid deficit, haemorrhage	Tachycardia, decreased urine output, decreased blood pressure	Early detection of signs; fluid and/or blood replacement
Haemorrhage	Internal or external bleeding	Disruption of sutures, insecure ligation of blood vessels	Overt bleeding (dressings saturated with bright blood; bright, free-flowing blood in drains or chest tubes), increased pain, increasing abdominal girth, swelling or bruising around incision	Early detection of signs
Hypovolaemic shock	Inadequate tissue perfusion resulting from markedly reduced circulating blood volume	Severe hypovolaemia from fluid deficit or haemorrhage	Rapid weak pulse, dyspnoea, tachypnoea; restlessness and anxiety; urine output less than 30 ml/hr; decreased blood pressure; cool, clammy skin, thirst, pallor	Maintain blood volume through adequate fluid replacement, prevent haemorrhage; early detection of signs
Thrombophlebitis	Inflammation of the veins, usually of the legs and associated with a blood clot	Slowed venous blood flow due to immobility or prolonged sitting; trauma to vein, resulting in inflammation and increased blood coagulability	Aching, cramping pain; affected area is swollen, red and hot to touch; vein feels hard; discomfort in calf when foot is dorsiflexed or when patient walks (Homans' sign)	Early ambulation, leg exercises, antiembolic stockings, adequate fluid intake
Thrombus	Blood clot attached to wall of vein or artery (most commonly the leg veins)	As for thrombophlebitis for venous thrombi; disruption or inflammation of arterial wall for arterial thrombi	*Venous:* same as thrombophlebitis *Arterial:* pain and pallor of affected extremity; decreased or absent peripheral pulses	*Venous:* same as thrombophlebitis *Arterial:* maintain prescribed position; early detection of signs
Embolus	Foreign body or clot that has moved from its site of formation to another area of the body (e.g. the lungs, heart or brain).	Venous or arterial thrombus; broken intravenous catheter, fat or amniotic fluid	In venous system, usually becomes a pulmonary embolus (see pulmonary embolism); signs of arterial emboli may depend on the location	As for thrombophlebitis or thrombus; careful maintenance of IV catheters
Urinary				
Urinary retention	Inability to empty the bladder, with excessive accumulation of urine in the bladder	Depressed bladder muscle tone from narcotics and anaesthetics; handling of tissues during surgery on adjacent organs (rectum, vagina)	Fluid intake larger than output; inability to void or frequent voiding of small amounts, bladder distention, suprapubic discomfort, restlessness	Monitoring of fluid intake and output, interventions to facilitate voiding, urinary catheterisation as needed

Table 24-2 (Continued)

Problem	Description	Cause	Clinical signs	Preventive interventions
Urinary tract infection	Inflammation of the bladder, ureters or urethra	Immobilisation and limited fluid intake, instrumentation of the urinary tract	Burning sensation when voiding, urgency, cloudy urine, lower abdominal pain	Adequate fluid intake, early ambulation, aseptic straight catheterisation only as necessary, good perineal hygiene
Gastrointestinal				
Nausea and vomiting		Pain, abdominal distention, ingesting food or fluids before return of peristalsis, certain medications, anxiety	Complaints of feeling sick to the stomach, retching or gagging	IV fluids until peristalsis returns; then clear fluids, full fluids and regular diet; antiemetic drugs if ordered; analgesics for pain
Constipation	Infrequent or no stool passage for abnormal length of time (e.g. within 48 hours after solid diet started)	Lack of dietary roughage, analgesics (decreased intestinal motility), immobility	Absence of stool elimination, abdominal distention and discomfort	Adequate fluid intake, high-fibre diet, early ambulation
Tympanites	Retention of gases within the intestines	Slowed motility of the intestines due to handling of the bowel during surgery and the effects of anaesthesia	Obvious abdominal distention, abdominal discomfort (gas pains), absence of bowel sounds	Early ambulation; avoid using a straw, provide ice chips or water at room temperature
Post-operative ileus	Intestinal obstruction characterised by lack of peristaltic activity	Handling the bowel during surgery, anaesthesia, electrolyte imbalance, wound infection	Abdominal pain and distention; constipation; absent bowel sounds; vomiting	
Wound				
Wound infection	Inflammation and infection of incision or drain site	Poor aseptic technique; laboratory analysis of wound swab identifies causative micro-organism	Purulent exudate, redness, tenderness, elevated body temperature, wound odour	Keep wound clean and dry, use surgical aseptic technique when changing dressings
Wound dehiscence	Rupture or splitting open of a wound	Malnutrition (emaciation, obesity), poor circulation, excessive strain on suture line	Increased incision drainage, tissues underlying skin become visible along parts of the incision	Adequate nutrition, appropriate incisional support and avoidance of strain
Wound evisceration	Exposure of the internal organs and tissues through a wound	Same as for wound dehiscence	Opening of incision and visible protrusion of organs	Same as for wound dehiscence
Psychological				
Post-operative depression	Mental disorder characterised by altered mood	Weakness, surprise nature of emergency surgery, news of malignancy, severely altered body image, other personal matter; may be a physiologic response to some surgeries	Anorexia, tearfulness, loss of ambition, withdrawal, rejection of others, feelings of dejection, sleep disturbances (insomnia or excessive sleeping)	Adequate rest, physical activity, opportunity to express anger and other negative feelings

cough, move or ambulate. Determine when and what analgesics were last administered, and assess the patient for any side-effects of medication such as nausea and vomiting.

+ *Fluid balance.* Assess the type and amount of intravenous fluids, flow rate and infusion site. Monitor the patient's fluid intake and output. In addition to watching for shock, assess the patient for signs of circulatory overload and monitor serum electrolytes. Anaesthetics and surgery affect the hormones regulating fluid and electrolyte balance (aldosterone and ADH in particular), placing the patient at risk for decreased urine output and fluid and electrolyte imbalances.

+ *Dressing and bedclothes.* Inspect the patient's dressings and bedclothes underneath the patient. Excessive bloody drainage on dressings or on bedclothes, often appearing underneath the patient, can indicate haemorrhage. The amount of drainage on dressings is recorded by describing the diameter of the stains or by denoting the number and type of dressings saturated with drainage.

+ *Drains and tubes.* Determine colour, consistency and amount of drainage from all tubes and drains. All tubes should be patent, and tubes and suction equipment should be functioning. Drainage bags must be hanging properly.

Document the patient's time of arrival and all assessments. The frequency of assessment should be altered according to the patient's condition. If a patient is showing signs of deterioration, assessments may need to be performed much more regularly.

PLANNING

Post-operative care planning and discharge planning begin in the pre-operative phase when pre-operative teaching is implemented.

Planning for Discharge

In order to provide continuity of care for the surgical patient after discharge from the hospital, the nurse needs to consider what type of assistance the patient requires in the home setting according to their individual needs. Discharge planning for both the day-surgery patient and the patient who has been hospitalised for several days following surgery incorporates an assessment of the patient's ability to self-care and the family's abilities to support the patient's physical and psychological needs after discharge. The nurse may feel that the patient may require further assistance from the district nurse, social services or private care agencies. This is discussed fully with the patient and family and a package of care is established.

IMPLEMENTING

The main aim of post-operative care is prevention, early identification and treatment of post-operative complications,

in order for the patient to be safely discharged home. Some of the nursing interventions that promote recovery and prevent complications, in most cases, will have been introduced to the patient pre-operatively, such as deep-breathing and coughing exercises, leg exercises and moving (see *Procedure 24-1* on page 649). However, there are a number of other nursing interventions used to help the patient recover, including pain management, positioning, incentive spirometry, hydration, nutrition and wound care.

Pain Management

Pain is a natural response to injury and serves to alert us to the harm and initiate responses to minimise harm. Pain is both a sensory and emotional experience that can hinder a patient's recovery after surgery. In fact, surgical pain can be severely detrimental to the patient leading to tachycardia (heart rate over 100 beats per minute), shallow breathing, atelectasis (lung collapse), altered gas exchanged, immobility and immunosuppression (Van Keuren and Eland, 1997). Chapter 20 provides a more in-depth discussion of pain and pain management.

Pain is usually greatest 12–36 hours after surgery, decreasing after the second or third post-operative day. During the initial post-operative period, patient-controlled analgesia (PCA) or continuous analgesic administration through an intravenous or epidural catheter may be prescribed. The nurse monitors the infusion or amount of analgesic administered by PCA, assesses the patient's pain relief, and notifies the doctor or anaesthetist if the patient is experiencing unacceptable side-effects or inadequate pain relief. Analgesia that is prescribed as required (PRN) should be administered on a routine basis for the first 24–36 hours. Once the patient's pain is more controlled then routine pain relief need only be administered before moving or dressing changes.

Alongside pharmacological analgesia the nurse may implement other forms of pain relief. These include ensuring that the patient is warm and providing back rubs, position changes, diversional activities such as a book or television, and adjunctive measures such as imagery (using the person's imagination to relieve the pain).

Positioning

The positioning of the patient may be governed by the type of surgery the patient has undergone and the type of anaesthetic they have received. For instance, patients who have had a laminectomy (surgical removal of part of the vertebra in the spine) must be nursed on their back. In order for them to eat and drink the patient must have an appropriate bed that can be positioned so that the patient's back is not bent. Likewise patients who have had spinal anaesthetics usually lie flat for 8–12 hours. On the other hand an unconscious or semiconscious patient is placed on one side with the head slightly elevated, if possible, or in a position that allows fluids to drain from the mouth. If, however, there are no specific orders for the patient, they should be positioned so that they are comfortable.

Incentive Spirometry

Following surgery and a period of immobility sputum can collect in the lungs and lead to chest infection. Incentive spirometry is often used to encourage deep breathing following surgery to reduce the risk of chest infections. This device measures the flow of air inhaled through a mouthpiece (see Chapter 16). The patient is instructed to breathe in through the mouthpiece until a certain level is achieved (usually measured by a ball within an enclosed chamber). Inhalation and ventilation are enhanced using the incentive spirometer.

Hydration

Initially post-operatively hydration is usually maintained by intravenous infusions, in order to replace body fluids lost either before or during surgery. If oral intake of fluids is not contraindicated, it is wise for the nurse to only offer sips of water to the patient initially as large amounts of water can induce vomiting. If the patient is unable to take fluid orally it is important that the nurse provides mouth care and offers mouthwashes to the patient. Post-operative patients oftens complain of thirst and a dry sticky mouth. These symptoms are a sign of dehydration due to pre-operative fasting, medications and loss of body fluid.

If the patient is receiving intravenous fluids post-operatively it is important to measure the patient's fluid intake and output. Adequate hydration is important as it keeps the respiratory mucous membranes and secretions moist and maintains cardiovascular and renal function.

Nutrition

Depending on the extent of surgery and the organs involved, the patient may be allowed nothing by mouth for several days or may be able to resume oral intake when nausea is no longer present. If the surgeon states that the patient can have 'diet as tolerated', the nurse should begin by offering clear fluids. If the patient tolerates these with no nausea, the diet can often progress to full liquids and then to a regular diet, provided that gastrointestinal functioning is normal. Assess the return of peristalsis by auscultating the abdomen. Gurgling and rumbling sounds indicate peristalsis. Anaesthetic agents, narcotics, handling of the intestines during abdominal surgery, fasting and inactivity all inhibit peristalsis. Therefore, bowel sounds should be carefully assessed every 4–6 hours. Oral fluids and food are usually started after the return of peristalsis. It is important that the nurse documents the patient's food tolerance and the passage of flatus or abdominal distention.

Wound Care

Most patients return from surgery with a sutured wound covered by a dressing, although in some cases the wound may be left unsutured. Dressings are inspected regularly to ensure that they are clean, dry and intact. Excessive drainage may indicate haemorrhage, infection or an open wound.

When dressings are changed, the nurse assesses the wound for appearance, size, drainage, swelling, pain and the status of a drain or tubes. Details about these assessments are outlined in the *Practice guidelines*.

PRACTICE GUIDELINES

Assessing Surgical Wounds

Appearance
+ Inspect colour of wound and surrounding area and approximation of wound edges.

Size
+ Note size and location of dehiscence, if present.

Drainage
+ Observe location, colour, consistency, odour and degree of saturation of dressings. Note number of gauzes saturated or diameter of drainage on gauze.

Swelling
+ Observe the amount of swelling; minimal to moderate swelling is normal in early stages of wound healing.

Pain
+ Expect severe to moderate post-operative pain for 3-5 days; persistent severe pain or sudden onset of severe pain may indicate internal haemorrhaging or infection.

Drains or Tubes
+ Inspect drain security and placement, amount and character of drainage, and functioning of collecting apparatus, if present.

 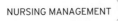

Because surgical incisions heal by primary intention (see Chapter 14), the nurse can expect the following signs of healing:

1. *Absence of bleeding and the appearance of a clot binding the wound edges.* The wound edges are well approximated and bound by fibrin in the clot within the first few hours after surgical closure.
2. *Inflammation (redness and swelling) at the wound edges for 1–3 days.*
3. *Reduction in inflammation when the clot diminishes,* as granulation tissue starts to bridge the area. The wound is bridged and closed within 7–10 days. Increased inflammation associated with fever and drainage is indicative of wound infection; the wound edges then appear brightly inflamed and swollen.
4. *Scar formation.* Collagen synthesis starts four days after injury and continues for six months or longer.
5. *Diminished scar size over a period of months or years.* An increase in scar size indicates keloid formation (excessive tissue forming on a scar).

CLINICAL ALERT

Assess the patient immediately if they report a 'giving' or 'popping' sensation in the incisional area. The patient may be experiencing dehiscence (splitting) or evisceration (contents of body cavity spilling out) of the wound.

Surgical Dressings

Dressings are applied to the incision while the patient is in theatre. If there are no signs of bleeding or excessive drainage on the dressing it should be left for at least 24 hours. Too many dressing changes can cool the wound, open the wound to micro-organisms and ultimately delay healing. However if there is drainage on the dressing the wound needs to be inspected to ensure that there are no signs of haemorrhage or infection. Cleaning a wound and applying a sterile dressing are detailed in *Procedure 24-2.*

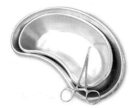

PROCEDURE 24-2 Cleaning a Sutured Wound and Applying a Sterile Dressing

Purposes

+ To promote wound healing by primary intention
+ To prevent infection
+ To assess the healing process
+ To protect the wound from mechanical trauma

Assessment

Assess

+ Patient allergies to wound cleaning agents
+ The appearance and size of the wound
+ The amount and character of exudates (liquid discharge)
+ Patient complaints of discomfort
+ The time of the last pain medication
+ Signs of systemic infection (e.g. elevated body temperature, diaphoresis, malaise, leukocytosis)

Planning

Before changing a dressing, determine any specific orders about the wound or dressing.

Equipment

+ Sterile dressing pack
+ Clean gloves
+ Sterile gloves
+ Sterile saline
+ Dressings
+ Surgical tape
+ Clinical waste bag

Implementation

Preparation

Prepare the patient and assemble the equipment.

+ If the patient is confused or restless then acquire assistance to change the dressing. The person might move and contaminate the sterile field or the wound.
+ Assist the patient to a comfortable position in which the wound can be readily exposed. Expose only the wound area, using a sheet to cover the rest of the patient. Undue exposure is physically and psychologically distressing to most people.
+ Place the clinical waste bag close to the wound. Placement of the bag within reach prevents the nurse from reaching across the sterile field and the wound and potentially contaminating these areas.

Performance

1. Explain to the patient what you are going to do, why it is necessary and how they can cooperate. Discuss how the results will be used in planning further care or treatments.
2. Wash hands and observe other appropriate infection control procedures.
3. Provide for patient privacy.
4. With clean gloves on loosen the dressing, holding down the skin and pulling the dressing gently but firmly toward the wound. Pressing down on the skin provides counter traction against the pulling motion. The dressing is pulled toward the incision to prevent strain on the sutures or wound.

5. Remove and dispose of soiled dressings in the clinical waste bag, remove gloves and wash hands.
6. Assess the location, type (colour, consistency) and odour of any wound drainage. Assess the wound, size, wound closure, signs of infection.
7. Set up the sterile supplies.
   - Open the sterile dressing pack, using aseptic technique.
   - Place the sterile towel beside the wound.
   - Open the sterile cleaning solution and pour it over the gauze sponges in the plastic container.
   - Put on sterile gloves.
8. Clean the wound, only if visibly soiled.
   - Clean the wound, using your gloved hands or forceps and gauze swabs moistened with cleaning solution.
   - Use the cleaning methods illustrated and described in Figure 24-8.
   - Use a separate swab for each stroke and discard each swab after use. This prevents the introduction of micro-organisms to other wound areas.
   - If a drain is present, clean it next, taking care to avoid reaching across the cleaned incision. Clean the skin around the drain site by swabbing in half or full circles from around the drain site outward, using separate swabs for each wipe (see Figure 24-8, C).

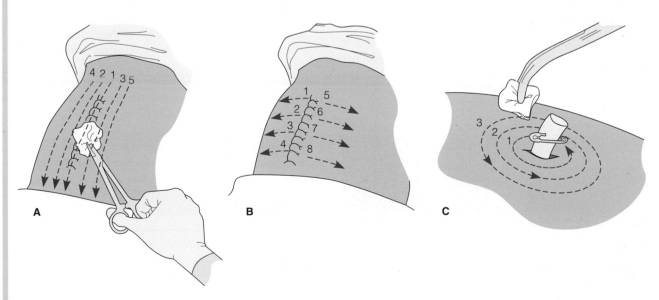

Figure 24-8 Methods of cleaning surgical wounds: *A*, cleaning the wound from top to bottom, starting at the centre; *B*, cleaning a wound outward from the incision; *C*, cleaning around a Penrose drain site. For all methods, a clean sterile swab is used for each stroke.

- Support and hold the drain erect with a sterile swab while cleaning around it. Clean as many times as necessary to remove the drainage.
- Dry the surrounding skin with dry gauze swabs as required. Do not dry the incision or wound itself. Moisture facilitates wound healing.
9. Apply dressings to the drain site and the incision (see Figure 24-9).
   - Remove gloves and dispose of all equipment used in the clinical waste.
10. Document the procedure and all nursing assessments.

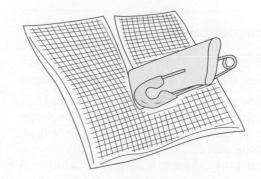

Figure 24-9 Pre-cut gauze in place around a drain.

Evaluation

+ Evaluate the choice of dressings by relating assessment to previous assessment of the wound.

+ Report any significant changes to a tissue viability nurse, wound care nurse or doctor.

Wound Drains and Suction

Surgical drains are inserted to permit the drainage of excessive serosanguineous (liquid light red) fluid and purulent material and to promote healing of underlying tissues. These drains may be inserted and sutured through the incision line, but they are most commonly inserted through stab wounds a few centimetres away from the incision line so that the incision itself may be kept dry. Without a drain, some wounds would heal on the surface and trap the discharge inside, and an abscess might form.

Drains vary in length and width. The length can be 25–22 cm, and the width 1.2–4 cm. If the drainage is minimal the surgeon may ask the nurse to remove the drain. The wound where the drain was will usually heal in a day or two.

A **suction drainage system** consists of a drain connected to either an electric suction or portable drainage suction (see Figure 24-10). The closed system reduces the possible entry of micro-organisms into the wound through the drain. The

drainage tubes are sutured in place and connected to a reservoir, this allows for accurate measurement of the drainage.

When emptying the container of the closed-wound drainage systems the nurse should adhere to universal precautions wearing gloves, apron and even goggles.

Sutures

A **suture** is a thread used to sew body tissues together. Sutures used to attach tissues beneath the skin are often made of an absorbable material that disappears in several days. Skin sutures, by contrast, are made of a variety of nonabsorbable materials, such as silk, cotton, linen, wire, nylon and Dacron (polyester fibre). Silver wire clips or staples are also available. Usually skin sutures are removed 7–10 days after surgery.

There are various methods of suturing. Skin sutures can be broadly categorised as either interrupted (each stitch is tied and knotted separately) or continuous (one thread runs in a series of stitches and is tied only at the beginning and at the end of the run). Common methods of suturing are illustrated in Figure 24-11.

Retention sutures are very large sutures used in addition to skin sutures for some incisions (see Figure 24-12). They attach underlying tissues of fat and muscle as well as skin and are used to support incisions in obese individuals or when healing may be prolonged. They are frequently left in place longer than skin sutures (14–21 days) but in some instances are removed at the same time as the skin sutures. To prevent these large sutures from irritating the incision, the surgeon may place rubber tubing over them or a roll of gauze under them extending down the incision line.

Usually the surgeon will inform the nurse when the sutures are to be removed. Sterile technique and special suture cutters are used in suture removal. Suture cutters have a short, curved blade that readily slides under the suture (see Figure 24-13).

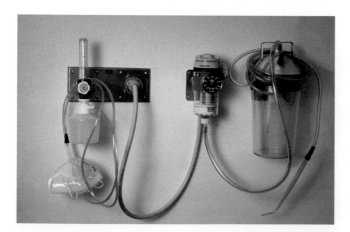

Figure 24-10 Suction drainage system.

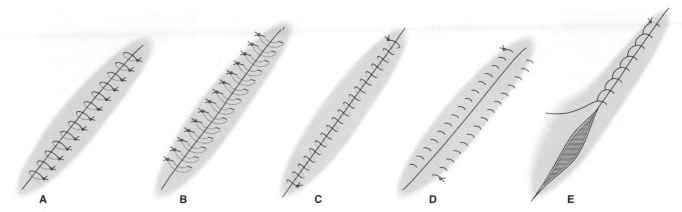

Figure 24-11 Common sutures: *A*, plain interrupted; *B*, mattress interrupted; *C*, plain continuous; *D*, mattress continuous; *E*, blanket continuous.

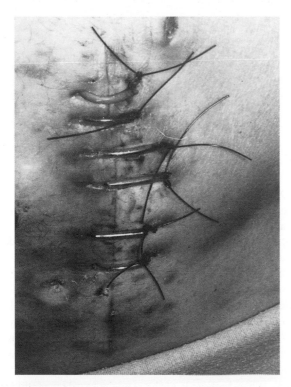

Figure 24-12 A surgical incision with retention sutures.

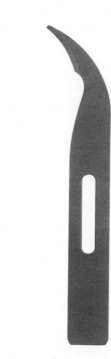

Figure 24-13 Suture or stitch cutters.

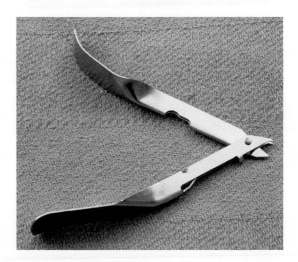

Figure 24-14 Staple remover.

Wire clips or staples are removed with a special instrument that squeezes the centre of the clip to remove it from the skin (see Figure 24-14). Guidelines for removing sutures and staples follow:

+ Before removing skin sutures, verify (a) the orders for suture removal (in many instances, only *alternate* interrupted sutures are removed one day, and the remaining sutures are removed a day or two later) and (b) whether a dressing is to be applied following the suture removal. Some surgeons prefer no dressing; others prefer small, light gauze dressing to prevent friction by clothing.
+ Inform the patient that suture removal may produce slight discomfort, such as a pulling or stinging sensation, but should not be painful.

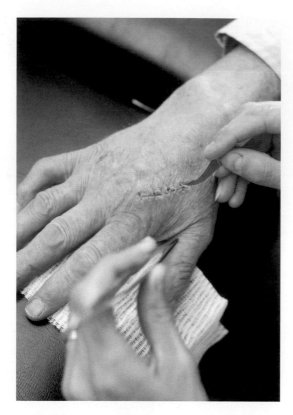

Figure 24-15 Removing a plain interrupted skin suture.

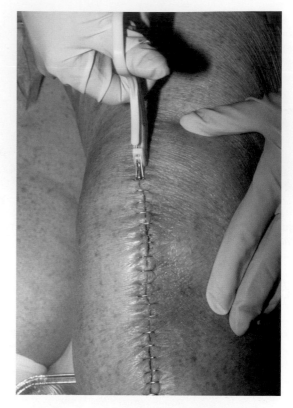

Figure 24-16 Removing surgical clips or staple.

+ Remove dressings and clean the incision if necessary.
+ Put on sterile gloves.
+ Remove plain interrupted sutures as follows:
  (a) Grasp the suture at the knot with a pair of forceps.
  (b) Place the curved tip of the suture cutter under the suture as close to the skin as possible, either on the side opposite the knot (see Figure 24-15) or directly under the knot. Cut the suture. Sutures are cut as close to the skin as possible on one side of the visible part because the suture material that is visible to the eye is in contact with resident bacteria of the skin and must not be pulled beneath the skin during removal. Suture material that is beneath the skin is considered free from bacteria.
  (c) With the forceps, pull the suture out in one piece. Inspect the suture carefully to make sure that all suture material is removed. Suture material left beneath the skin acts as a foreign body and causes inflammation.
+ Discard the suture onto a piece of sterile gauze or into a clinical waste bag, being careful not to contaminate the forceps tips.
+ Continue to remove alternate sutures, that is, the third, fifth, seventh, and so forth. Alternate sutures are removed first so that remaining sutures keep the skin edges in close approximation and prevent any dehiscence from becoming large.
+ If no dehiscence occurs, remove the remaining sutures. If dehiscence does occur, do not remove the remaining sutures, and report the dehiscence to the nurse in charge.
+ Reapply a dressing, if indicated.

+ Document the suture removal; number of sutures removed; appearance of the incision; application of a dressing, patient teaching; and patient tolerance of the procedure.
+ Remove staples as follows:
  (a) Remove dressings and clean the incision if necessary.
  (b) Place the lower tips of a sterile staple remover under the staple.
  (c) Squeeze the handles together until they are completely closed (see Figure 24-16). Pressing the handles together causes the staple to bend in the middle and pulls the edges of the staple out of the skin. Do not lift the staple remover when squeezing the handles.
  (d) When both ends of the staple are visible, gently move the staple away from the incision site.
  (e) Hold the staple remover over a disposable container, release the staple remover handles and release the staple.

EVALUATING

Using the goals developed during the planning stage, the nurse collects data to evaluate whether the identified goals and desired outcomes have been achieved. If the desired outcomes are not achieved, the nurse, patient and family need to explore the reasons before modifying the care plan. For example, if the outcome 'Pain control' is not met, questions to be considered include:

+ What is the patient's perception of the problem?
+ Does the patient understand how to use PCA (patient controlled analgesia)?

+ Is the prescribed analgesic dose adequate for the patient?
+ Is the patient allowing pain to become intense prior to requesting medication or using PCA (patient controlled analgesia)?

+ Where is the patient's pain? Could it be due to a problem unrelated to surgery (e.g. chronic arthritis, anginal pain)?
+ Is there evidence of a complication that could cause increased pain (an infection, abscess or haematoma)?

CRITICAL REFLECTION

Let us revisit the case study on page 643. Now that you have read the chapter you can explore the following questions. What factors place Mr Teng at increased risk for the development of complications during and after surgery? What preparations were taken during the pre-operative period in order to protect him from possible complications during and after his surgery? How will Mr Teng's post-operative assessments differ from a person who received general anaesthesia?

CHAPTER HIGHLIGHTS

+ Surgery is a unique experience that creates stress that requires the patient to make necessary physical and psychological changes.
+ There are three phases: pre-operative, intra-operative and post-operative.
+ Surgical procedures are categorised by degree of urgency, purpose and degree of risk.
+ Factors such as age, general health, nutritional status, medication use and mental status affect a patient's risk during surgery.
+ Patients must agree to surgery and sign an informed consent.
+ Pre-operative physical and psychological assessment can provide important information for planning pre-operative and post-operative care.
+ The overall goal of nursing care during the pre-operative phase is to prepare the patient mentally and physically for surgery.
+ Pre-operative teaching includes situational information and psychosocial support, the role of the patient, expected sensations and discomfort, and training for the post-operative period.
+ Pre-operative teaching should include moving, leg exercises and coughing and deep-breathing exercises. Many aspects of pre-operative teaching are intended to prevent post-operative complications.
+ Physical preparation includes the following areas: nutrition and fluids, elimination, rest, medications, care prostheses and skin preparation.
+ A pre-operative checklist provides a guide to and documentation of a patient's preparation before surgery.
+ Maintaining the patient's safety is the overall goal of nursing care during the intra-operative phase.

+ Anaesthesia may be general or local.
+ Positioning of the patient during surgery is important to reduce the risk of tissue and nerve damage.
+ Immediate post-anaesthetic care focuses on assessment and monitoring parameters to prevent complications from anaesthesia or surgery.
+ Initial and ongoing assessment of the post-operative patient includes level of consciousness, vital signs, oxygen saturation, skin colour and temperature, comfort, fluid balance, dressings, drains and tubes.
+ The overall goals of nursing care during the post-operative period are to promote comfort and healing, restore the highest possible level of wellness, and prevent associated risks such as infection or respiratory and cardiovascular complications.
+ Ongoing post-operative nursing interventions include (a) managing pain (see Chapter 21), (b) appropriate positioning, (c) encouraging incentive spirometry and deep-breathing and coughing exercises, (d) promoting leg exercises and early ambulation, (e) maintaining adequate hydration and nutritional status, (f) promoting urinary elimination, (g) continuing gastrointestinal suction and (h) providing wound care.
+ Aseptic technique (sterile technique) is used when changing dressings on surgical wounds to promote healing and reduce the risk of infection.
+ Sutures, wire clips or staples are used to approximate skin and underlying tissues after surgery. These are generally removed 7-10 days after surgery.

REFERENCES

Hospital Episode Statistics (2006) *Headline figures 2004–05*, London: Department of Health. Available from http://www.hesonline.nhs.uk/Ease/servlet/ContentServer?ID+1937&categoryID=193. (Accessed on 6 September 2006.)

Joanna Briggs Institute (2003) 'The impact of pre-operative hair removal on surgical site infection', *Best Practice*, 7(2), 1–6.

Kiecolt-Glaser, J.K., Page, G.G., Marucha, P.T., Maccallum, R.D. and Glaser, R. (1998) 'Psychological influences in surgical recovery', *American Psychologist*, 53, 1209–1218.

Kost, M. (1999) 'Conscious sedation: Guarding your patient against complications', *Nursing*, 29(4), 34–39.

Krupat, E., Fancey, M. and Cleary, P.D. (2000) 'Information and its impact on satisfaction among surgical patients', *Social Science and Medicine*, 51(12), 1817–1825.

NICE (2003) *Pre-operative tests: The use of routine pre-operative tests for elective surgery*, London: NICE.

NMC (2004) *The NMC Code of Professional Conduct: Standards for conduct, performance and ethics*, London: NMC.

RCN (2005) *Perioperative fasting in adults and children*, London: RCN.

Thomas, V.J., Health, M., Rose, D. and Flory, P. (1995) 'Psychological characteristics and the effectiveness of patient-controlled analgesia', *British Journal of Anaesthesia*, 74, 271–276.

Van Keuren, K. and Eland, J.A. (1997) 'Perioperative pain management in children', *Nursing Clinics of North America*, 32(1), 31–44.

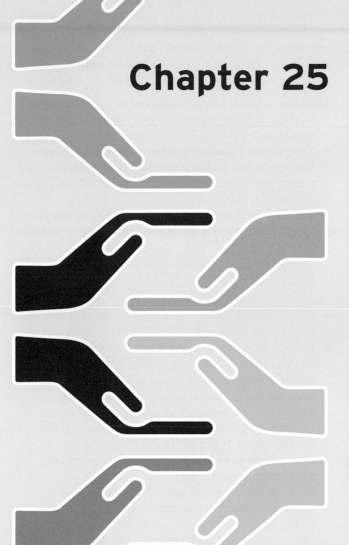

Chapter 25

Emergency Management of the Patient and Resuscitation

Learning Outcomes

After completing this chapter, you will be able to:

+ Discuss the history of resuscitation and emergency management of the sick patient.

+ Explain the initial actions to take with regard to managing a patient who is unwell or deteriorating.

+ Explain the term primary survey and associated actions.

+ Discuss adjuncts which may be used for airway management.

+ Describe the procedure of resuscitation for an infant, child and adult.

+ Discuss the reversible causes of and drugs used in cardiac arrest management.

CASE STUDY

You are a nurse working on an acute medicine ward. While checking the patient's vital signs in a six-bedded subward, you note Mrs G is having problems breathing and her skin and lips appear blue. As you approach her she suddenly slumps in the bed and is not moving.

You perform a primary survey, quickly checking for danger; assess her level or response, airway, breathing and circulation. You shout for help and a healthcare support worker comes to assist you looking for guidance and direction. Anxiety, emotion and feelings of the need to be professional all tug at your professionalism. The sequences of actions all come flooding back instinctively as you recall the emergency patient management training session you attended recently. The support worker goes and collects the resuscitation equipment on the ward and you work as a team, continuing basic life support until help arrives.

You breathe a sigh of relief as the medical emergency team arrive and take over with your assistance.

After reading this chapter you will be able to discuss the management of a patient who has suffered a cardiac arrest and the nurse's role in this procedure.

INTRODUCTION

Managing the acutely ill emergency patient is an aspect of clinical practice that most nurses dread. However a systematic approach to the management of such incidents eases the emotional panic the practitioner experiences. The systems used to assess such incidents have been researched extensively and have withstood the test of time.

Resuscitation of the patient is not a new concept, being described as far back as 3000 BC (see *Box 25-1*). The technique of closed chest cardiopulmonary resuscitation (CPR) in humans began in 1891. The early 1960s hailed the development of formal training for healthcare professionals and the public, and equipment being developed for education in CPR.

The International Liaison Committee on Resuscitation (ILCOR) was formed in 1992–93. Its sole purpose is to identify and review worldwide international science and knowledge relevant to CPR, as well as to offer consensus on treatment recommendations. The objectives of the ILCOR are to:

+ provide a forum for discussion and for coordination of all aspects of cardiopulmonary and cerebral resuscitation worldwide;
+ foster scientific research in areas of resuscitation where there is a lack of data or where there is controversy;
+ provide for dissemination of information on training and education in resuscitation;
+ provide a mechanism for collecting, reviewing and sharing international scientific data on resuscitation;

BOX 25-1 Brief History of CPR

+ 3000 BC - Mayan and Peruvian hieroglyphics show resuscitation by rectal fumigation.
+ 800 BC - The book of Kings in the Christian Bible describes Elijah breathing into a child's mouth with the child starting to breathe again.
+ AD 500-1500 - Various methods were used including flagellation with a whip, rolling over a barrel, external heating with warm ashes or burning excrement, and strapping the person to the back of a horse that runs around. All in an attempt to stimulate life.
+ 1530 - The bellows method was used, where a bellows from a fireplace blew hot air or smoke into the victim's mouth. This method was used for over 300 years and saw the development of the early bag valve mask devices.
+ 1543 - Andreas Versalius published *De Humanis Corporis Fabrica* describing blowing into a tube to resuscitate an animal.
+ 1700s - Various methods used including warming, rubbing, rectal insufflation with tobacco smoke, and bleeding. The method of using tobacco smoke was abandoned in 1811 after Benjamin Brodie demonstrated that four ounces of tobacco would kill a dog and one ounce would kill a cat.
+ 1770 - Inversion method used on a person who had drowned. The victim was hung by his feet with chest pressure to aid in expiration and pressure release to aid inspiration.
+ 1773 - Barrel method was introduced where the victim would be placed on top of a large wine barrel and rolled back and forth to force air in and out of the lungs.
+ 1774 - Royal Humane Society recommended the resuscitation of drowned victims by the application of warmth.

+ 1803 - Russian method: this involved packing the victim in ice to reduce the body's metabolism.
+ 1812 - Trotting horse method: each lifeguard station was equipped with a horse tied up. If a victim drowned they would be placed across the horse's back and the horse run up and down the beach.
+ 1861 - Silvester method was introduced and was performed by the rescuer pressing on the victim's back to get air in and out of the chest cavity.
+ 1900 - Open and closed chest compressions were performed during surgery.
+ 1903 - Schafer method was introduced where the victim was placed in a prone position to keep the airway open.
+ 1932 - Holger Neilson technique introduced; prone position hands under head, expire by pressing on chest, inspire by lifting elbows.
+ 1947 - first successful defibrillation performed.
+ 1949 - Efficacy of manual methods checked, Schafer replaced by Holger Neilson.
+ 1954 - Jude and Elam published a text on the physiology of resuscitation declaring oxygen would work well with resuscitation.
+ 1957 - Safar introduced the ABC method with mouth to mouth being declared as the most efficient.
+ 1958 - During a conference on anaesthesia a paper was presented by Safar. Laerdal heard about this and began development of the Resusci Anne doll as a training aid. Knickerbocker also rediscovered external chest compressions worked on dogs and re-tested on humans.
+ 1960 - First demo of Resusci Anne doll, and external chest compressions proved to be effective.
+ 1962 - Resus panel of Vienna established.
+ 1970s - Guidelines on CPR published, demonstrations performed and public education begun.

✦ produce, as appropriate, statements on specific issues related to resuscitation that reflect international consensus.

ILCOR meets twice each year, usually alternating between a venue in the USA and one elsewhere in the world. In collaboration with the American Heart Association (AHA), ILCOR produced the first International CPR Guidelines in 2000. Also in collaboration with the AHA, ILCOR coordinated an evidence-based review of resuscitation science, which culminated in the International Consensus on CPR and ECC (External Cardiac Compression) Science with Treatment Recommendations Conference in January 2005. The proceedings of this conference provided the material for regional resuscitation organisations, such as the European Resuscitation Council (ERC), on which to base their resuscitation guidelines.

This consensus and review of information draws upon the work of many member organisations with the aim of developing truly international best practice. At present, ILCOR comprises representatives of the American Heart Association (AHA), the European Resuscitation Council (ERC), the Heart and Stroke Foundation of Canada (HSFC), the Australian and New Zealand Committee on Resuscitation, the Resuscitation Councils of Southern Africa (RCSA) and the Inter American Heart Foundation (IAHF). The Resuscitation Council (UK), although not a direct member of ILCOR, works closely in association with the ERC and is represented in this manner.

The Resuscitation Council (UK) was formed in August 1981 by a group of medical practitioners from a variety of specialities who shared an interest in, and concern for, the subject of resuscitation. The objective of the council is to facilitate education of both lay and healthcare professional members of the population in the most effective methods of resuscitation appropriate to their needs.

To achieve its objective, the Resuscitation Council (UK) has the following aims:

✦ To encourage research into methods of resuscitation.
✦ To study resuscitation teaching techniques.
✦ To establish appropriate guidelines for resuscitation procedures.
✦ To promote the teaching of resuscitation as established in the guidelines.
✦ To establish and maintain standards for resuscitation.
✦ To foster good working relations between all organisations involved in resuscitation and to produce and publish training aids and other literature concerned with the organisation of resuscitation and its teaching.

Many practitioners question the need for the regular changes, stating they get confused by the frequent protocol variations that occur in resuscitation practice, the most recent being published in November 2005. Major guidance updates occur about once every five years with interim statements of new therapies that may significantly improve patient outcome. Work began on the new guidelines as early as 2003, when ILCOR established six working groups; basic life support, advanced cardiac life support, acute coronary syndromes,

paediatric life support, neonatal life support and a group to look at overlapping issues such as education. These working groups then established consensus documentation based on research and studies from ILCOR members. The current ERC and Resuscitation Council (UK) guidelines are based upon this consensus information and courses of instruction for healthcare professionals with regard to managing the sick patient have been adapted to reflect this guidance. A number of courses are delivered on behalf of the Resuscitation Council (UK) from standard syllabuses in order to improve patient outcome in resuscitation ranging from advanced cardiac life support of the adult, paediatric life support, neonatal life support and immediate life support. The courses cover basic life support, automatic external defibrillation and basic airway management (see *Box 25-2* on page 674).

A systematic approach to the sick patient is essential and can be based upon the ERC chain of survival system (see Figure 25-1 on page 676).

EARLY RECOGNITION OF THE SICK PATIENT TO PREVENT CARDIAC ARREST

Peberdy *et al.* (2003) suggested that fewer than 20% of adult patients having an in-hospital cardiac arrest survive to go home. A possible hypothesis suggested for this poor outcome is the failure of staff in clinical areas to recognise promptly the patient who is unwell or deteriorating. The approximate 20% of patients who survive to discharge tend to have had their cardiac arrests witnessed or monitored in critical care areas where immediate intervention is possible. In this instance the major heart rhythm tends to be ventricular fibrillation (VF), a random chaotic electrical heart rhythm or pulseless ventricular tachycardia (VT) where the heart is beating in excess of 200 beats per minute. Those patients who arrest in unmonitored ward areas tend to have a slow physiological deterioration where low levels of cellular oxygenation and organ blood perfusion are not recognised. When a cardiac arrest occurs in these circumstances the main heart rhythm tends to be **asystole** (absence of any electrical activity) or **pulseless electrical activity** (PEA) (electrics are present but the mechanics of the heart are not working). With these two rhythms the chance of a successful resuscitation and survival to discharge is extremely poor.

Therefore when considering vital signs the regular monitoring of patients and action upon detecting abnormal vital signs is essential. Frequently, abnormalities of airway, breathing and circulation are recognisable prior to the patient suffering a serious cardiac event. Lack of confidence and inappropriate use of oxygen therapy also affect patient survival. Factors that aid in patient survival include a systematic approach to the assessment of critically ill patients, good inter-professional communication and teamwork.

A patient who is deteriorating may display common physiological signs of failing respiratory, cardiovascular and neurological status. One rationale for monitoring a patient's vital signs

BOX 25-2 Courses offered via Resuscitation Council (UK)

+ **This Advanced Life Support Provider Course (ALSP)** is designed for healthcare professionals who would be expected to apply the skills taught as part of their clinical duties, or to teach them on a regular basis. Appropriate participants include doctors and nurses working in critical care areas (e.g. A&E, CCU, ICU, HDU, operating theatres, medical admissions units) or on the cardiac arrest/medical emergency team and paramedics. All applicants should hold a current clinical appointment and professional healthcare qualification. The curriculum reflects contemporary practice, and builds on the content of the Immediate Life Support Course.

+ **The ALS Recertification Course** is designed to refresh the theory and practical skills required to correctly manage cardiopulmonary arrest in adults from the time when arrest seems imminent, until the patient is transferred to an intensive care department or dies. Only those candidates who hold a valid ALS Provider certificate are eligible to attend the one day recertification course. (Certificates are valid for three years but candidates have an additional one year in which they may still attend a one-day recertification course.)

+ **The European Paediatric Life Support Provider Course (EPLSP)** is intended to provide training for multi-disciplinary healthcare professionals in the early recognition of the child in respiratory or circulatory failure and the development of the knowledge and core skills required to intervene to prevent further deterioration towards respiratory or cardiac arrest.

+ **ELS Recertification Course** is designed to refresh the theory and practical skills in the early recognition of the child in respiratory or circulatory failure and consolidate the knowledge and core skills required to intervene to prevent further

deterioration towards respiratory or cardiac arrest. Only those candidates who hold a valid EPLS Provider certificate are eligible to attend the one day recertification course. (Certificates are valid for three years but candidates have an additional one year in which they may still attend a one-day recertification course.)

+ **Immediate Life Support Provider Course (ILS)** has been developed in order to standardise much of the in-hospital training undertaken already by Resuscitation Officers. Its aim is to train healthcare personnel in basic life support (BLS), simple airway management and safe defibrillation (manual and/or AED), enabling them to manage patients in cardiac arrest until arrival of a cardiac arrest team and to participate as members of that team. The certification is valid for one year.

+ **Immediate Life Support Provider Recertification** is a half-day course revisiting the components of the ILS course and allows candidates to recertify and practise the core skills learnt as part of the original ILS course.

+ **Newborn Life Support Provider Course (NLSP).** The aim of the course is to give those responsible for initiating resuscitation at birth the background knowledge and skills to approach the management of a newborn infant during the first 10-20 minutes in a competent manner. The course concentrates on the importance of temperature control, practical airway management and ventilatory support. The certification is valid for three years.

+ **NLS Recertification Course.** The half-day NLS provider recertification course is designed to allow candidates the opportunity to be updated on any changes in management practice during lectures and to have the opportunity to practise the relevant skills during skill stations and scenarios.

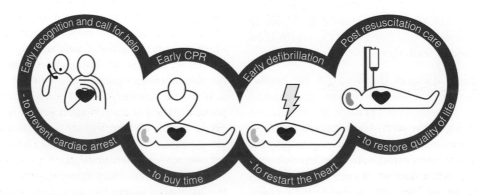

Figure 25-1 Chain of survival.

	4	2	1	0	1	2	4
Resp Rate per min	<10			10–14	15–20	21–29	>30
Altered Conscious level				Alert	Confused Or Agitated	Drowsy	Unresponsive Or To pain only
Heart rate per min	<50			50–90	91–110	111–129	>130
Systolic blood pressure (mmHg)	<90	90–110		110–150	150–200		>200
Age				<70	>70		

IF THE TOTAL SCORE FOR YOUR PATIENT >10?

Call Medical Emergency Team 2222

IS THE SCORE >7–10?

Fast bleep the Patients Team's SHO/SpR
AND FOLLOW PROCEDURES

IS THE SCORE >4–6?

1. Inform the Senior Nurse on the ward/Nurse Practitioner and
2. Inform the Patients Team or on call Team's SHO/HO and ask them to attend.
3. If unable to attend in <30 mins, call the SpR
4. After a further 30 mins the Patients SpR is unable to attend, then call the Consultant/on call Consultant.

IN THE MEANTIME
MONITOR – RR, O₂ Saturations BP, Pulse
OXYGEN – Administrate 100% oxygen score >7 40% score >4
VENOUS – Prepare Venflons. Blood bottles. Fluids
ECG – Have ready in case needed

Referral to the intensive Therapy Unit is at the discretion of clinical staff. Early referral is encouraged in appropriate patients with high scores or patients whose scores are not improving.

THIS SCORING SYSTEM MUST BE USED AS AN ADJUNCT TO CLINICAL EXPERIENCE AND PROFESSIONAL JUDGEMENT. IT DOES NOT REPLACE COMMON SENSE.

Figure 25-2 Patient at risk (PAR) scoring system.

on a routine basis would not only be to monitor the effectiveness of interventions but also to detect early enough patient deterioration. Harrison *et al.* (2005) noted that abnormal physiology is common on general wards, yet the important physiological observations of sick patients are recorded less frequently than is desirable for numerous reasons. The monitoring of respiratory rate is essential in being able to predict cardiorespiratory arrest, yet it is the least frequently and least accurately recorded vital sign.

Risk Scoring Systems and Other Indicators

In many clinical settings early warning or patient at risk scoring systems have been implemented and developed with the aim of preventing cardiac arrests from occurring. These systems have been developed over a number of years and McArthur-Rouse (2001) reviewed the literature relating to these scales. Although some scales have been in use for a number of years

it is only recently that these 'patient at risk' scales have been widely used in practice. The scales assign a points system to routine measurements of vital signs and deviation from the agreed normal range. The weighted score of one or more, or frequently the total score, alert clinical staff to the deterioration of a patient's condition and facilitate a protocol for the early management and intervention of key staff. An example of a patient at risk (PAR) scoring system is shown in Figure 25-2.

In addition to the use of patient at risk score systems other physiological signs and symptoms may be noted as a patient deteriorates, such as a narrowing of the patient's pulse pressure. This would manifest itself as the systolic and diastolic blood pressure figures become closer together: for example, a blood pressure of 140/90 mmHg would give relatively little cause for concern, whereas a blood pressure of 100/90 mmHg has a narrow pulse pressure of 10 mmHg, and the patient is at an increased risk of suffering a cardiac arrest.

The early recognition of a deteriorating child is also important. In children, cardiac arrest tends to be due more to low oxygen levels and low blood pressure than to actual heart disease. The commonest cardiac arrest rhythms children experience are pulseless electrical activity/asystole. In **pulseless electrical activity** the electrics of the heart are working but the mechanics of the heart beating are not. **Asystole** is the complete lack of electrical activity, with the heart not working at all. Again the key factor to preventing a child from sustaining an arrest is early recognition and correction of factors causing deterioration. Tume (2005) in a three-year review of emergency paediatric intensive care unit admissions from wards noted abnormalities in vital signs similar to those found in adults.

The key factors with a patient whose condition is deteriorating are to ensure help is summoned promptly to assess the patient. This may be a nurse practitioner, medical team responsible for the management of the patient or the **medical emergency/cardiac arrest team**. Prompt action and early recognition of a patient's condition deteriorating can save a life. Priestley *et al.* (2004) note that in the UK a system of critical care outreach has developed, which when utilised effectively may reduce ward deaths, post-operative adverse events, intensive care admissions/readmissions and increase survival. This outreach may also be in the form of the medical emergency team.

EARLY CARDIOPULMONARY RESUSCITATION (CPR)

When a patient suffers a cardiac arrest it is essential that prompt action is taken by staff within the clinical environment in order to maximise the chances of patient survival. Initially, this prompt action means systematically assessing the patient and recognising a cardiac arrest has occurred, and promptly summoning help. The Resuscitation Council (UK) has published a flow chart that should be followed for in-hospital patient resuscitation (see Figure 25-3).

The series of actions are both systematic and logical. Upon initially finding a collapsed/sick patient the nurse should shout for help while assessing the patient. Often simply pulling the 'emergency' buzzer is not sufficient as these tend to be frequently activated by false alarms and staff may ignore this call initially. Once the nurse has ensured help has been summoned then a check should be made for response and signs of life. When assessing a patient for response a three-point assessment plan should be used. Firstly, ask the patient a question, 'Hello are you alright?'; then give a command, 'Open your eyes!'; finally if there is no response from either of these assessments a painful stimulus should be used, such as a trapezius pinch, or tapping the patient's shoulders. The rationale for this three-point approach is to assess whether a patient is responding on a four-point level of consciousness **AVPU scale**.

+ Alert – spontaneous eye opening and awareness of surroundings.
+ Voice – responds to commands only.
+ Pain – responds only to painful stimulus.
+ Unresponsive – does not respond to voice or pain.

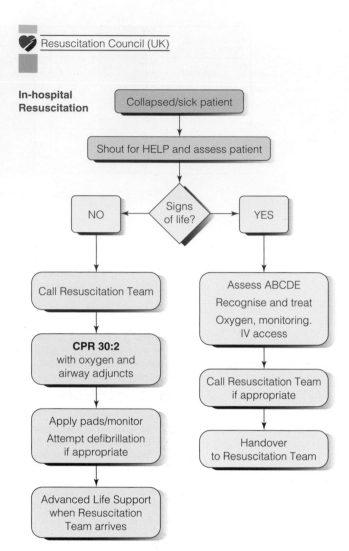

Figure 25-3 Flow chart for in-hospital resuscitation. (Based on guidelines for resuscitation published by the RC(UK) and ERC. While based on international consensus and science, these may not illustrate the guidance in other countries. The guidelines are revised every five years: the next revision is due in 2010.)

It is essential when assessing a patient's level of consciousness that only acceptable painful stimuli are used. To perform a trapezius pinch, a thumb should be placed above the patient's clavicle bone near the front side of the neck in the natural hollow and squeezed gently but firmly. This will put pressure upon the local nerve endings and cause discomfort to which an individual with no altered consciousness would react (see Figure 25-4). Other painful stimuli such as rubbing the sternum, pinching the finger tip, pressure on the forehead and eyeball should be avoided when assessing a patient as part of the resuscitation protocol as this may cause damage to underlying structures.

If a patient has no signs of response then it is essential to move on to an assessment of signs of life including a check of the airway, breathing and signs of circulation. As soon as it has been determined that a person is unresponsive then immediately help should be summoned if this has not already been done or no help has arrived from an earlier shout for help.

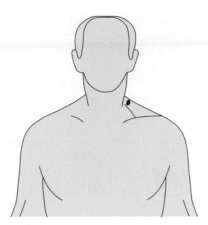

Figure 25-4 The pressure point used when performing a trapezius pinch.

Clearing the Airway of an Adult

As soon as it has been determined that the patient is unresponsive the airway should be checked. When an individual becomes unconscious the large muscular tongue falls to the back of the throat and potentially causes an airway obstruction. This can easily be corrected by opening the airway with manual techniques. Prior to opening the airway it is essential though to ensure that there are no other potential airway obstructions present. These could include loose or ill-fitting dentures, food stuff in the mouth (the person may have been eating at the time of their collapse) or even vomit.

The gold standard for clearing an airway in a clinical setting would be the use of suction equipment, as has been described in earlier chapters. However suction equipment may not always be readily available so manual techniques of airway clearance should be used, such as turning the head to the side and allowing any liquid to drain out. It is essential to remember that no finger sweeps into the mouth should be attempted to remove any airway obstructions. Potentially there is a risk that the patient may regain some degree of consciousness and bite on any fingers. If ill-fitting dentures need to be removed then this may be achieved by placing fingers around the dentures, but not between them, and removing them safely. Well-fitting dentures should always be left in place as they give shape to the patient's face and make other airway manoeuvres easier to perform.

Once it is verified the airway is clear then it should be opened in order to move the tongue from the back of the throat. This is achieved by simply placing one hand on the patient's forehead and two fingers on the bony part of the chin and tilting the head back (see Figure 25-5). It is essential to use minimal force to do this and caution should be exhibited with patients who may have neck or spinal problems, such as a fracture to the cervical spine or arthritis of the neck. In this instance a jaw thrust technique should be used (see Figure 25-6). This technique does not move the cervical spine but opens and maintains the airway. When the mandible (lower jaw) is pushed forward the tongue also comes forward out of the upper airway where it may be causing an obstruction.

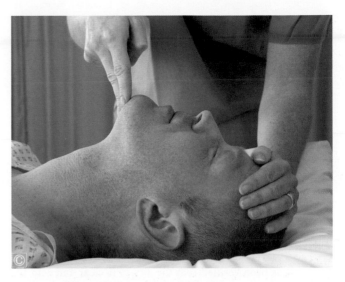

Figure 25-5 Opening the airway using head tilt chin lift technique.

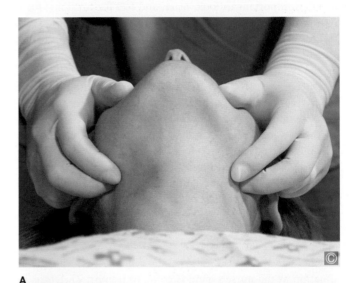

A

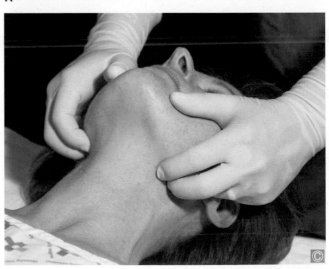

B

Figure 25-6 Jaw thrust.

Clearing the Airway of a Child or Baby

When opening the airway of a child or baby consideration must be given to the anatomical differences. The occiput is larger and when the head is in a neutral supine position it may cause buckling of the trachea as a child's airway is small and flexible. In order to prevent this the head should be maintained in the 'sniffing the morning air' position to reduce the risk of airway occlusion. This means the head is tilted back at a 45° plus angle. While maintaining the airway, caution must be taken not to press on soft tissues beneath the chin as this increases the risk of airway obstruction, so fingers should always remain on the mandible.

The Next Steps

Once it has been verified that the airway is clear and with the airway maintained in the open position, a check should be made as to whether the individual is breathing or not. To assess this it is important to look, listen and feel for breathing for a minimum of 10 seconds. Look for chest movement, listen and feel for breath on your face by placing your head close to the patient's mouth. The occasional (agonal) gasp of breath should be ignored as this may occur in the early stages of cardiac arrest.

Once it is verified that the patient has no breathing a check for circulation should be made for 10 seconds. This should be done by the nurse checking the carotid pulse at the neck *on the same side as the nurse.* They should not lean over the patient as this could result in either a hand being pushed down onto the neck, causing damage to underlying structures, or the appearance from a distance that you are strangling the patient. The carotid pulse is located by placing the first and second fingers over the carotid artery. The carotid artery location can be found approximately 2 cm either side of the trachea and requires only gentle pressure.

Checks for a carotid pulse can be difficult in an emergency situation as the nurse's hand is going to tremor. Therefore, as recommended by the Resuscitation Council (UK) in their 2005 guidelines, only those who are experienced should check for a pulse. Other signs and symptoms of circulation should be looked for including swallowing, eye flickering/blinking (visible when eyes are closed) and any movements.

If there is any doubt as to whether the patient is in cardiac arrest then basic life support/CPR should be initiated immediately and the cardiac arrest/medical emergency team called. If, however, the patient does have signs of breathing and circulation then they should be placed in the recovery position on their side to maintain their airway and high flow/concentration oxygen at 15 l/min delivered via non rebreathe mask. They need to be continually monitored.

Performing CPR

If there is suspicion the adult patient is in cardiac arrest then after performing the initial checks/primary survey the patient should first be given 30 chest compressions and then two

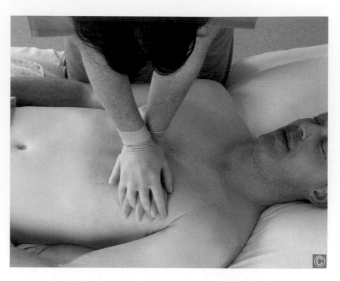

Figure 25-7 Hand position for chest compressions.

breaths. The chest compressions should be at an equivalent rate of 100 per minute, the hand position being in the middle of the lower sternum on the nipple line (based on an average male). One hand should be placed on the chest and then the other hand placed on top with the fingers interlocked. The fingers must be kept off the chest wall/ribs and pressure applied with the heel of the hand only directly onto the sternum. Arms should be kept straight and the pressure applied from the upper body. The compressions should be approximately one third of the chest depth which is 4–5 cm (see Figure 25-7).

Ventilations should be two every 30 compressions. To achieve effective ventilation there needs to be a good seal around the patient's mouth. In a healthcare environment appropriate equipment should be used to aid in the resuscitation attempt; this may include the use of a pocket resuscitation mask or a bag valve mask device. A pocket mask is simply a barrier device that may be used to assist with ventilating a patient's lungs while isolating the practitioner from any risk of infection (see Figure 25-8). Pocket masks can be used with supplemental oxygen at 15 l/min in order improve the oxygenation of the ventilation. There is approximately 21% oxygen in room air and 16% oxygen in expired air. By using supplemental oxygen when ventilating a patient with a pocket mask it is possible to give up to 40% oxygen concentration.

A bag valve mask device (BVM) may be used instead of a pocket mask in order to give a patient effective ventilation. This however requires two people to use the device: one to hold the mask in place and another to ventilate the patient (squeeze the bag). In some clinical areas where an experienced practitioner uses this skill on a regular basis they may be able effectively to ventilate a patient on their own with a BVM (see Figure 25-9). A bag valve mask device is literally a bag made from silicone or plastic of a set volume for adult, child or neonate lung volume. When squeezed, air is forced under pressure through a one-way valve and into the patient's lungs through the mask on their face. When a reservoir bag is connected to a BVM and the device connected to an oxygen supply at 15 l/min it is possible

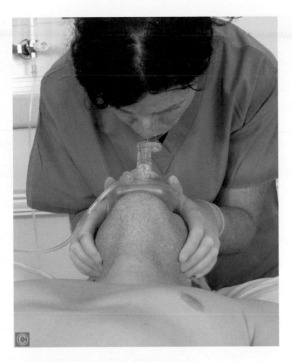

Figure 25-8 Using a pocket mask.

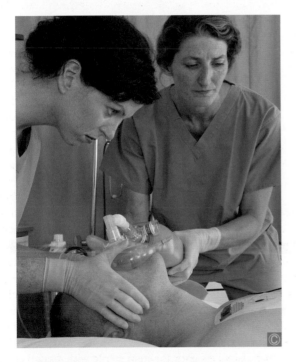

Figure 25-9 Using a bag valve mask device.

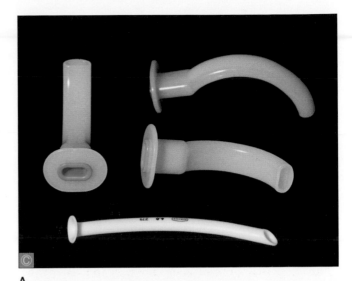

A

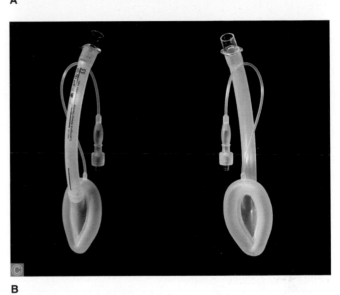

B

Figure 25-10 Oropharangeal airways, nasopharangeal airways and laryngeal mask airways.

to ventilate a patient with up to 80% plus oxygen. If used without a reservoir bag present and connected to high-flow oxygen then the patient can be given up to 40% oxygen and on room air alone, 21%. The effectiveness of ventilation when using a BVM is only as good as the technique used. This includes the depth of ventilation, the amount the bag is squeezed and the effectiveness of the airway maintenance (position of the head and seal with the mask).

In order to assist effective patient ventilation the patient's airway must be maintained effectively, if manual techniques are used then this may make ventilation a little more difficult. Simple airway adjuncts can effectively assist with airway management and may include oropharyngeal and nasopharyngeal airways (see Figure 25-10).

The most commonly used forms of airway are oropharyngeal (OPA). These are available as part of the standard equipment on a cardiac arrest trolley in a variety of sizes ranging from 000 for neonates to size 4 for large adults but the size guide is not a clinical method for selecting an appropriate OPA. The indication for use of an OPA on any patient is that the patient is unconscious and has no gag reflex when the airway is used. Firstly the airway must be sized appropriately from the corner of the mouth at the level of the incisor to the angle of the jaw, with the airway being held in the same position as it will be when inserted into the patient's mouth (see Figure 25-11).

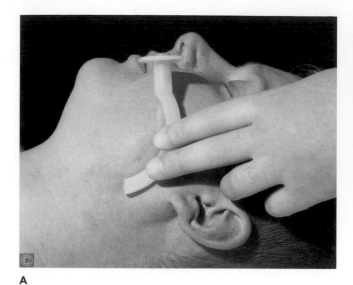

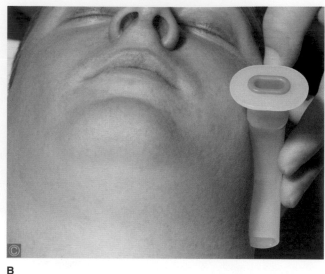

A

B

Figure 25-11 Sizing an oropharangeal airway.

If the patient is an adult then the airway should be inserted upside down and when one third of the way into the mouth be rotated so it sits flat and advanced until the flange rests on the lips. The principle of using an OPA is to maintain the airway by preventing the tongue from flopping to the back of the throat and causing an airway obstruction.

The principles of using an OPA on a child or infant are similar for the purposes of sizing. However differences do occur when the airway is inserted for a child or infant. Where the hard palate of the mouth has not developed, the OPA should be inserted the correct way up while a tongue depressor is used to hold the tongue flat. This is in order to prevent damage and trauma to the fragile under-developed hard palate (see Figure 25-12).

The use of nasopharyngeal airways (NPA) tends to be confined to specialist clinical areas. An NPA can often be an

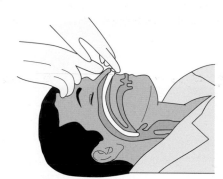

Figure 25-13 Inserting an nasopharangeal airway.
(Based on guidelines for resuscitation published by the RC(UK) and ERC. While based on international consensus and science, these may not illustrate the guidance in other countries. The guidelines are revised every five years; the next revision is due 2010.)

effective tool for airway management in a patient and is under-utilised in many clinical areas due to concerns regarding the contraindications. The contraindications for use of an NPA include, for a child or baby, the fractured base of skull, facial trauma, maxillofacial surgery or broken nose.

The NPA is sized from the corner of the right nostril to the angle of the patient's jaw and the length and diameter are sized according to the size of the patient's little finger (see Figure 25-13). Certain airways need to be prepared prior to use. Some manufacturers pack the item sterile with a safety pin to be placed through the end. This needs to be placed through the end of the airway near the flange in order to prevent the airway from going too far into the nostril (the safety pin only goes through the airway and not the patient's nostril).

Once sized, the airway is lubricated using a water-based lubricating jelly which is placed into the nostril in the angle of the airway. The NPA is gently rotated in order to facilitate its passage into the appropriate position. Once in place, the tip should rest at the top of the patient's airway thus facilitating a clearly maintained passage (see Figure 25-14).

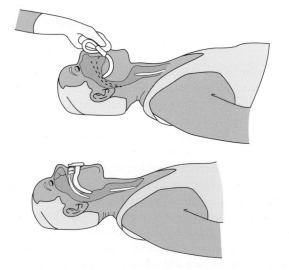

Figure 25-12 Inserting an oropharangeal airway.
(Based on guidelines for resuscitation published by the RC(UK) and ERC. While based on international consensus and science, these may not illustrate the guidance in other countries. The guidelines are revised every five years; the next revision is due 2010.)

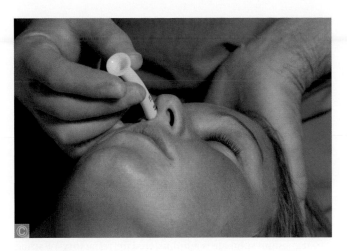

Figure 25-14 Inserting an nasopharangeal airway.

Variations Based Upon Age

For the purpose of these variations an infant is a child under one year, and a child is an individual between one year and the onset of puberty (see Figure 25-15).

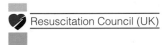
Resuscitation Council (UK)

Paediatric Basic Life Support
(Healthcare professionals with a duty to respond)

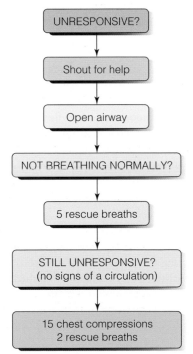

After 1 minute call resuscitation team then continue CPR

Figure 25-15 Paediatric basic life support flow chart.
(Based on guidelines for resuscitation published by the RC(UK) and ERC. While based on international consensus and science, these may not illustrate the guidance in other countries. The guidelines are revised every five years; the next revision is due 2010.)

Table 25-1 Variations Based Upon Age

	Child	Infant
Airway opening technique	Neutral position chin lift only	Head tilt chin lift
Position of hand for compressions	Lower third sternum One hand only	Lower third sternum Two fingers
Ratio of compressions to ventilations	15:2	15:2

If a child or infant is not breathing then five initial rescue breaths/ventilations should be given, each of which need to be effective enough for the chest to rise and fall. When performing the ventilations it should be noted whether there is any response, such as gagging or coughing, as this forms part of the circulation check. One minute of CPR should also be performed prior to calling the medical emergency/cardiac arrest team. Other variations are detailed in Table 25-1.

EARLY DEFIBRILLATION: TO RESTART THE HEART

As has already been discussed, often in adults who survive a cardiac arrest the primary rhythm in which they present is VF or pulseless VT. The only treatment for both of these rhythms is attempted defibrillation and with every one minute's delay the chance of patient survival decreases by 7–10%. Therefore it is essential that when a patient suffers a cardiac arrest the medical emergency/cardiac arrest team is summoned promptly and a defibrillator is brought to the patient's side. In an ideal world the first healthcare professional who responds to a cardiac arrest should be trained and authorised to use a defibrillator.

VF is a random chaotic electric heart rhythm that is incompatible with life. The heart is beating without any coordination and can often be described as quivering like a bag of worms. This lethal rhythm occurs when individual cells in the heart take over the pacemaker function simultaneously and prevent the sino-atrial node of the heart from coordinating activity. Likewise VT occurs when the heart is beating extremely fast and does not allow the atria and ventricles to fill and empty properly, thus preventing oxygenation of the body. If not treated promptly it can lead to death.

Simply, defibrillation gives a high-energy shock to the heart and may artificially 'reset' the pacemaker centres. This shock is delivered from two electrodes or paddles placed on the chest, one above the heart and one below. Paddles are placed on the right side of the chest in the midline below the right clavicle and the second in the midaxilla line at the level of the base of the heart on the lower ribs (see Figure 25-16 on page 682). When the heart is defibrillated all electrical activity stops

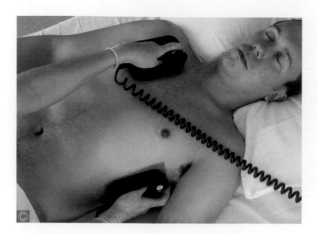

Figure 25-16 Defibrillator electrode positions.

instantaneously, which may be sufficient for the pacemaker centres to take control again. The sooner a patient who requires defibrillation receives a shock the better their chance of survival.

When a patient requires defibrillation this is treatment that is integral to the universal cardiac arrest treatment algorithm (see Figure 25-17). One shock is given and then two minutes of CPR are performed. During these two minutes if an appropriately trained healthcare professional or cardiac arrest team are present then drugs and interventions can be used in order to improve the outcome for the patient.

Commonly Used Drugs

Drugs that are used commonly during a cardiac arrest include epinephrine (adrenaline), atropine, amiodarone, magnesium sulphate, lidocaine (lignocaine), sodium bicarbonate and calcium chloride.

Adrenaline is the first-line cardiac arrest drug, given every 3–5 minutes during resuscitation in a dose of 1 mg (10 ml of 1 in 10,000) intravenously. It causes vasoconstriction, increased systemic vascular resistance and increases cerebral and coronary perfusion. It also increases myocardial excitability, when the myocardium is hypoxic or ischaemic.

Atropine is given for asystole or pulseless electrical activity with a rate less than 60 beats per minute. The dose is 3 mg and is given as a single intravenous dose. It works by blocking the activity of the vagus nerve on the SA and AV nodes, increasing sinus automaticity and facilitating AV node conduction.

Amiodarone is administered for refractory VF/VT, haemodynamically stable VT and other resistant tachyarrhythmias. Refractory VF/VT is said to occur after three to four shocks and is not corrected by defibrillation. In other words, if the patient does not revert from VF/VT after three shocks, or the patient has a fast heart rhythm that is not being corrected by other treatment options. If VF or pulseless VT persists after the first three shocks then amiodarone 300 mg is considered. If not pre-diluted, it must be diluted in 5% dextrose to 20 ml. The drug will crystallise if mixed with saline causing further problems. It should be given centrally but in an emergency can be given peripherally, and works by increasing the duration of the action potential in the atrial and ventricular myocardium.

Magnesium sulphate is administered for refractory VF when hypomagnesaemia is possible, or ventricular tachyarrhythmias when hypomagnesaemia is possible. The dose for refractory VF is 1 to 2 g (2–4 ml of 50% magnesium sulphate) peripherally over 1–2 minutes, followed by 2.5 g (5 ml of 50% magnesium sulphate) over 30 minutes.

Lignocaine can be administered for refractory VF/pulseless VT (when amiodarone is unavailable. The dose is 100 mg for VF/pulseless VT that persists after three shocks. Another 50 mg can be given if necessary.

Sodium bicarbonate is administered for severe metabolic acidosis and hyperkalaemia. The dose is 50 mmol (50 ml of 8.4% solution), where there is an acidosis or cardiac arrest associated with hyperkalaemia.

Calcium chloride may be administered for pulseless electrical activity caused by hyperkalaemia, hypocalcaemia or an overdose of calcium channel-blocking drugs. The dose is 10 ml of 10% calcium chloride repeated according to blood results.

When any drug is administered in a cardiac arrest the cannula that it is given through should always be flushed with a minimum of 20 ml of fluid. When amiodarone is administered it is important not to flush with saline or put saline through the same line as this will cause crystals to form in the cannula.

The potentially reversible causes of cardiac arrest tend to be summarised as the four H's and the four T's. If each of these can be excluded and treated then a successful resuscitation is possible. The four H's are:

+ Hypoxia, which is a low oxygen level, can be managed by ensuring the patient's airway is clear, and oxygen is being administered and ventilated into the lungs.

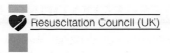

Adult Advanced Life Support Algorithm

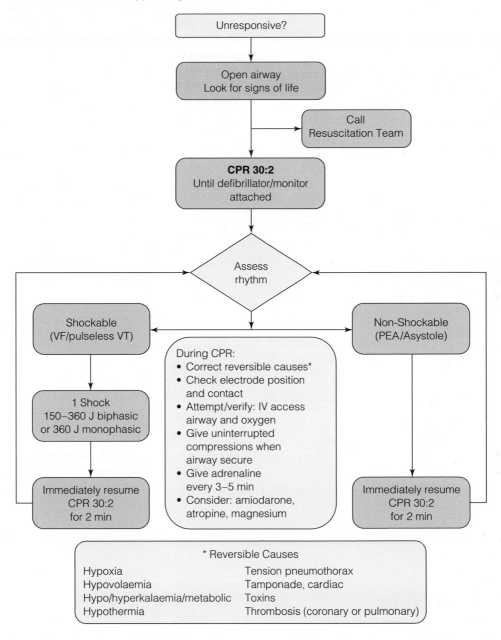

Figure 25-17 Adult advanced life support algorithm.
(Based on guidelines for resuscitation published by the RC(UK) and ERC. While based on international consensus and science, these may not illustrate the guidance in other countries. The guidelines are revised every five years; the next revision is due 2010.)

+ Hypovolaemia, or low-circulating volume, may be caused by dehydration or blood loss, this is managed by ensuring the patient receives appropriate amounts of intravenous fluids.
+ Hyper/hypokalaemia and metabolic disturbances, i.e. high or low potassium levels, may be excluded by checking the patient's potassium level from an arterial blood gas sample and administering appropriate treatment.

+ Hypothermia (low temperature) is managed by ensuring the patient's core temperature is near physiological normal.

The four T's are:

+ Tension pneumothorax, a collapsed lung, is managed by either placing a chest drain into the chest to allow the lung to reinflate or in an emergency, as a temporary measure, a large-bore intravenous cannula.

+ Tamponade is fluid in the pericardial sack surrounding the heart, which is preventing the heart from filling and emptying. This pressure is usually relieved by emergency surgery or aspiration of the fluid with a large needle by an experienced medical practitioner.

+ Toxic/therapeutic disturbances, such as drug therapy imbalances and toxicity.

+ Thrombo-embolic/mechanical obstruction are simply clots blocking the major cardiac blood vessels. This may be managed with the use of thrombolitic drugs.

POST-RESUSCITATION CARE

This should always be undertaken in a critical care environment such as an intensive care or coronary care unit where there is a high ratio of staff to patients. The airway may need to be managed with an adjunct such as an oral or nasal airway or even endotracheal intubation. Breathing will be supported by administering oxygen or the patient may be connected to a ventilator. Circulation function may be supported with the administration of medication to support cardiac output.

As a minimum, all surviving patients will have the investigations shown in *Box 25-3*.

BOX 25-3 Investigations for Surviving Patients

Full Blood Count
+ To check for anaemia
+ Baseline values
+ Rule out infection

Biochemistry Tests
+ Assess renal function
+ Check electrolyte levels (e.g. potassium and sodium)
+ Check blood glucose
+ Check cardiac enzymes to record amount of damage to the heart muscle
+ Record baseline values

12 Lead ECG
+ Record the baseline cardiac rhythm
+ Look for evidence of heart attack
+ Look for damage to the heart

Chest X-ray
+ Check the position of the trachea and any invasive monitoring equipment
+ Check for pulmonary oedema
+ Check for pulmonary aspiration
+ Exclude pneumothorax
+ Check size of heart
+ Check for any rib fractures from resuscitation

Arterial Blood Gas
+ Check for adequacy of ventilation
+ Check acid-base balance

CRITICAL REFLECTION

Let us revisit the case study on page 671. Now you have read this chapter, what airway adjuncts can be used in resuscitation? What is the ratio of compressions to ventilations for an adult, child and infant? What is the best way to ventilate a victim in cardiac arrest?

CHAPTER HIGHLIGHTS

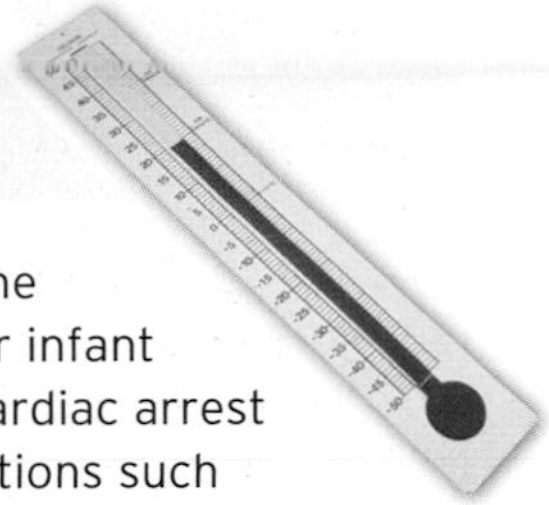

- A systematic approach to managing patient emergencies is essential.
- The history of resuscitation dates back to 3000 BC, with modern developments occurring from the 1960s onwards.
- Resuscitation guidelines change on a regular basis and are based upon current research, which is reviewed internationally. Most countries have their own resuscitation councils/committees who contribute toward this international review.
- Early recognition of the sick patient can prevent a cardiac arrest from occurring and various patient at risk (PAR) scoring systems have been developed to aid in this prevention strategy. Patient at risk scores use simple vital signs recordings to predict risk and require accurate, regular, vital signs recording.
- Prompt effective CPR following the algorithm for either adult, child or infant can improve the outcome from cardiac arrest and buy time for further interventions such as defibrillation or drug therapy to assist in improving patient outcome.
- Airway adjuncts and ventilation devices may also be used as part of the management of the patient being resuscitated.
- Several drugs are used to assist in managing the cardiac arrest patient and include the first-line drug, adrenaline, given once every two minutes of CPR.
- If the reversible causes summarised by the four H's and four T's can be excluded or treated then resuscitation may be successful if due to these.

REFERENCES

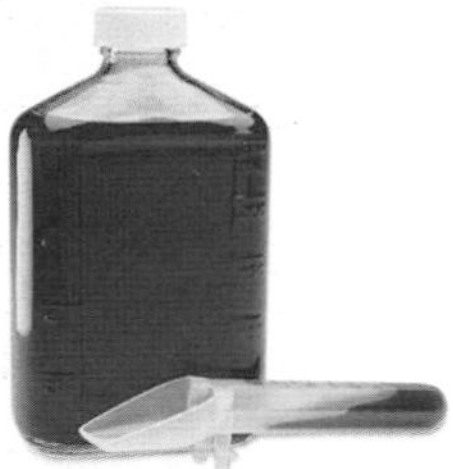

Harrison, G.A., Jacques, T.C., Kilborn, G. and McLaws, M.L. (2005) 'The prevalence of recordings of the signs of critical conditions and emergency responses in hospital wards – the SOCCER study', *Resuscitation*, 65, 149–157.

McArthur-Rouse, F. (2001) 'Critical care outreach services and early warning scoring systems: a review of the literature', *Journal of Advanced Nursing*, 36, 696–704.

Peberdy, M.A., Kaye, W., Ornato, J.P., Larkin, G.L., Nadkarni, V., Mancini, M.E., Berg, R.A. and Lane-Trultt, N.T. (2003) 'Cardiopulmonary resuscitation of adults in the hospital: a report of 14720 cardiac arrests from the National Registry of Cardiopulmonary Resuscitation', *Resuscitation*, 58, 297–308.

Priestley, G., Watson, W., Rashidian, A., Mozley, C., Russell, D., Wilson, J., Cope, J., Hart, S., Kay, D., Cowley, K. and Pateraki, J. (2004) 'Introducing Critical Care Outreach: A ward-randomised trial of phased introduction in a general hospital', *Intensive Care Medicine*, 30, 1398–1404.

The MERIT study investigators (2005) 'Introduction of the medical emergency team (MET) system: A cluster-randomise controlled trial', *Lancet*, 365, 2091–2097.

Tume, L. (2005) 'A three-year review of emergency PICU admissions from the ward in a specialist cardio-respiratory centre', *Care of the Critically Ill*, 21, 4–7.

Chapter 26

Physical Assessment and Diagnostic Testing

Learning Outcomes

After completing this chapter, you will be able to:

+ Identify the purposes of the physical health examination.

+ Explain the four methods of examining.

+ Explain the significance of selected physical findings.

+ Identify the steps in selected examination procedures.

+ Describe suggested sequencing to conduct a physical health examination in an orderly fashion.

+ Discuss variations in examination techniques appropriate for patients of different ages.

+ Discuss some diagnostic tests available.

CASE STUDY

You receive a call from ambulance control telling you that there has been a major road traffic collision (RTC) in the area and requesting a mobile medical team from your department. The nurse in charge delegates you, as a student nurse, to attend alongside an experienced accident and emergency (A&E) nurse, one other nurse, two doctors and an anaesthetist. On arrival at the scene, there is total carnage, bits of cars strewn across the road and injured people everywhere. A police officer calls you over to a woman. The woman is lying on the floor and complains of severe abdominal pain and you note that she is breathing rapidly 'because it hurts so much'. You and your mentor now have to decide how to assess this patient and prioritise the initial care that she needs.

After reading this chapter you will be able to prioritise the initial assessment of this patient. You will also be able to suggest possible investigations she would require once she arrives at hospital to aid in the diagnosis of this patient.

INTRODUCTION

Performing a comprehensive assessment of a patient requires the nurse to seek physical, psychological and sociological 'clues' as to the cause of a particular set of symptoms. Like a detective, the nurse needs to put all the pieces of the 'crime' together to establish the facts. The detective will examine the 'scene of the crime' (the patient's home environment, for example, do they live in a house/flat, do they have difficulty using the stairs, etc.), interview the 'victim of the crime' (the patient) and 'witnesses to the crime' (family members or friends) to establish the events that led up to the crime (past medical and patient history and signs and symptoms), and carry out finger printing and forensic tests (laboratory tests) to establish key data with regard to the crime. By ascertaining the facts or 'clues' the detective (nurse) can establish the cause of the 'crime' (disease/illness) and the 'motive' for it (why this disease/illness has developed).

This chapter will focus on the physical assessment and diagnostic testing that is required to diagnose a patient's condition. However, it is acknowledged that the full assessment of a patient requires more information that can be collected from a physical assessment and diagnostic testing. A full assessment requires exploration of the patient's past medical and patient history by questioning them and their significant others. It must also be acknowledged that in many areas some of the assessment skills described in this chapter may only be performed after further advanced post-registration training.

COMPLETE PHYSICAL ASSESSMENT

A physical assessment examination of a patient can come in a number of forms. For example, if a patient is admitted to a hospital with symptoms that are not specific, such as lethargy, weight-loss or nausea and vomiting, a complete physical assessment or examination may need to be carried out. Non-specific symptoms (mild or vague symptoms) can indicate the onset of serious conditions such as diabetes and cancer, so have to be assessed fully.

A complete physical assessment or examination of the patient is usually performed by a doctor but the nurse may be involved in some parts of the assessment process. A complete physical assessment requires a systematic examination of the patient from head-to-toe (see *Box 26-1* for the order of the head-to-toe assessment). However, if a patient is admitted to hospital with specific symptoms the nurse may only need to perform a part assessment of the particular body system or body area: for example, if a patient presents with chest pain the nurse may focus the examination on the patient's cardiovascular system or heart.

BOX 26-1 Head-to-Toe Framework

+ General assessment
+ Vital signs
+ Head
  - Hair, scalp, cranium, face
  - Eyes and vision
  - Ears and hearing
  - Nose and sinuses
  - Mouth and oropharynx
  - Cranial nerves
+ Neck
  - Muscles
  - Lymph nodes
  - Trachea
  - Thyroid gland
  - Carotid arteries
  - Neck veins
+ Upper extremities
  - Skin and nails
  - Muscle strength and tone
  - Joint range of motion
  - Brachial and radial pulses
  - Biceps tendon reflexes
  - Tendon reflexes
  - Sensation

+ Chest and back
  - Skin
  - Chest shape and size
  - Lungs
  - Heart
  - Spinal column
  - Breasts and axillae
+ Abdomen
  - Skin
  - Abdominal sounds
  - Specific organs (e.g. liver, bladder)
  - Femoral pulses
+ Genitals
  - Testicles
  - Vagina
  - Urethra
+ Anus and rectum
+ Lower extremities
  - Skin and toenails
  - Gait and balance
  - Joint range of motion
  - Popliteal, posterior tibial and pedal pulses
  - Tendon and plantar reflexes

Regardless of the type of assessment chosen, it is important that it is performed in a systematic and efficient manner that results in the fewest position changes for the patient as they may be in pain or have difficulty mobilising.

The purpose of a physical assessment is to:

+ obtain baseline information about the patient, that is information about the patient before treatment is commenced, such as recording their blood pressure;
+ add to, confirm or refute information obtained when questioning the patient or their family;
+ obtain information that will help establish a plan of care for the patient;
+ evaluate the care provided to the patient;
+ identify areas for health promotion and disease prevention.

Before performing a full or partial physical examination it is important to assemble the necessary tools needed. This will minimise the number of disruptions both for the patient and for the nurse. A range of tools may be required but the type and amount of tools required will depend on the type of examination performed, i.e. partial or full. *Box 26-2* provides a list of tools that may be required to perform a full physical assessment.

After assembling the equipment, the patient and environment needs to be prepared for the physical examination. When preparing the patient for a physical assessment the nurse should introduce themselves to the patient. This should be done, preferably, when the patient is dressed as this may help to decrease their anxieties when the nurse is assessing them. The nurse needs to keep in mind that the patient may find the whole process embarrassing and an invasion of privacy.

The nurse will need to explain the procedure to the patient and ascertain if there are any positions they may be uncomfortable in. For example, a breathless patient may be reluctant or unable to lie in a supine position (flat on their back) as this can exacerbate the breathlessness. The patient may need help with undressing or putting on a gown but the nurse should maintain the patient's privacy and dignity at all times.

As well as preparing the patient it is important to prepare the environment before starting the assessment. The time for the physical assessment should be convenient to both the patient and the nurse. The environment needs to be well lit and warm and the equipment should be organised for use.

The Four Primary Techniques

Preparation is the key to the efficient and effective examination but the nurse also needs to have a knowledge and understanding of the techniques used to examine a patient. There are four primary techniques used in the physical examination of a patient: inspection, palpation, percussion and auscultation. These techniques will be referred to throughout the chapter when discussing the assessment of particular parts of the body.

One of the first techniques the nurse may use when examining a patient is **inspection**. When inspecting the patient the nurse uses their visual (sight), olfactory (smell) and auditory (hearing) senses to observe normal and abnormal conditions. Visual examination can be performed either with the naked eye (e.g. when watching the chest rise and fall during respiration) or with the use of a lighted instrument such as an otoscope (used to view the ear).

Inspection is a valuable technique when assessing a patient and is often combined with other assessment techniques in order to gain a fuller picture of the patient's condition. The nurse may combine inspection with **palpation**, which is the examination of the body using the sense of touch. The pads of the fingers are used because their concentration of nerve endings makes them highly sensitive. Palpation can determine texture (e.g. of the hair); temperature (e.g. of a skin area); vibration (e.g. of a joint); position and size of organs or masses; distention (e.g. of the urinary bladder); pulsation; and the presence of pain upon pressure.

There are two types of palpation: light and deep. *Light* (superficial) *palpation* should always precede *deep palpation* because heavy pressure on the fingertips can dull the sense of touch. For light palpation, the nurse extends the dominant

BOX 26-2 Assessment Tools and Diagnostic Equipment

+ Gloves and apron
+ Stethoscope
+ Thermometer
+ Tape measure
+ Otoscope (for visualising the eardrum)
+ Percussion hammer
+ Wooden tongue depressors
+ Blood test tubes
+ Gauze swabs
+ Specimen pots
+ Lubricant gel

+ Sphygmomanometer (for blood pressure)
+ Oximeter (for oxygen saturation)
+ Metric ruler
+ Ophthalmoscope (to visualise interior of eye)
+ Pen torch
+ Weighing scales
+ Vaginal speculum
+ Vacutainer and needle
+ Adhesive tape and dressing
+ Electrocardiogram

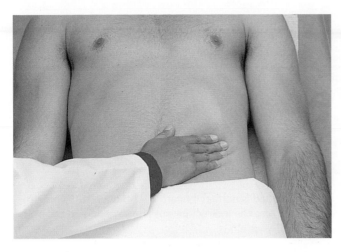

Figure 26-1 The position of the hand for light palpation.

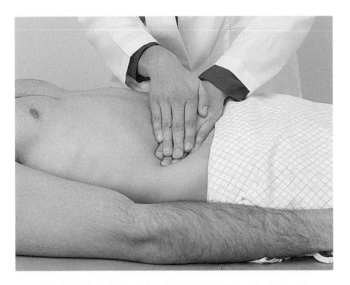

Figure 26-2 The position of the hands for deep bimanual palpation.

hand's fingers parallel to the skin surface and presses gently while moving the hand in a circle (see Figure 26-1). With light palpation, the skin is slightly depressed. If it is necessary to determine the details of a mass, the nurse presses lightly several times rather than holding the pressure.

Deep palpation is used to feel internal organs and masses and can be done with two hands (bimanually) or one hand (see Figure 26-2). Deep palpation is done with extreme caution because pressure can damage internal organs. It is usually not indicated in patients who have acute abdominal pain or pain that is not yet diagnosed.

The effectiveness of palpation depends largely on the patient's relaxation. Nurses can assist a patient to relax by positioning the patient comfortably and by ensuring that the patient's dignity and privacy are maintained at all time. It is important that while palpating the nurse should be sensitive to the patient's verbal and nonverbal communication that would indicate discomfort.

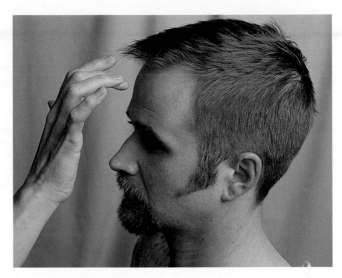

Figure 26-3 Direct percussion. Using one hand to strike the surface of the body.

The third technique used to examine a patient is **percussion**. This involves tapping or striking the body surface to elicit sounds that can be heard or vibrations that can be felt. There are two types of percussion: direct and indirect. Direct percussion is usually performed by tapping one or two fingers against a body part (see Figure 26-3). This is done to reveal tenderness in a particular part of the body. This technique is useful when assessing an adult's sinuses for tenderness.

Indirect percussion, on the other hand, is the striking of an object (e.g. a finger) held against the body area to be examined. In this technique, the middle finger of the nondominant hand is placed firmly on the patient's skin. The rest of the hand must be kept off the body surface. The tip of the middle finger of the other hand is then used to tap quickly and directly over the point where the other middle finger touches the body part (see Figure 26-4 on page 690). The nurse then listens to the sounds produced.

Percussion is used to determine the size and shape of internal organs. It indicates whether tissue is fluid filled, air filled or solid. Percussion elicits five types of sound (see Table 26-1 on page 690).

Usually the last technique used to examine a patient is **auscultation** or listening to sounds produced within the body. The nurse may use a stethoscope (indirect auscultation) to auscultate the body. The stethoscope transmits sounds from the body to the nurse's ears and is primarily used to listen to sounds from within the body, such as bowel sounds or valve sounds of the heart and blood pressure.

However nurses do not always need to use a stethoscope to listen to the sounds produced within the body. In fact they will often directly listen to the patient, for example if a patient has a wheezy chest on respiration the nurse may be able to auscultate these sounds without the help of a stethoscope.

Once the patient, environment and equipment have been prepared and a decision is made regarding the particular

Table 26-1 Percussion Sounds and Tones

Sound	Intensity	Pitch	Duration	Quality	Example of location
Flatness	Soft	High	Short	Extremely dull	This sound is normal if heard over bone or muscle. To hear this sound, use the indirect percussion method and tap your thigh.
Dullness	Medium	Medium	Moderate	Thudlike	This sound is normal if heard over the liver or heart. To hear this sound, use the indirect percussion method and tap just below your rib cage on the right-hand side of your abdomen. This is your liver.
Resonance	Loud	Low	Long	Hollow	This sound is normal if heard over the lungs. To hear this sound, use the indirect percussion method and tap over one of your lungs.
Hyperresonance	Very loud	Very low	Very long	Booming	This is an abnormal sound that indicates diseases such as chronic obstructive pulmonary disease.
Tympany	Loud	High	Moderate	Musical	Stomach filled with gas (air).

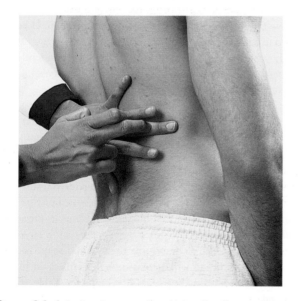

Figure 26-4 Indirect percussion. Using the finger of one hand to tap the finger of the other hand.

techniques that will be needed to examine the patient, the nurse then begins the physical examination/assessment. This usually starts with a general assessment of the patient before then going on to individual body parts and systems.

GENERAL ASSESSMENT

A general assessment involves a number of tasks including observation of the patient's general appearance and mental state, and measurement of baseline data such as vital signs, height and weight.

Appearance and Mental State

The general appearance and behaviour of an individual must be assessed bearing in mind the patient's culture, socioeconomic status, religion and current circumstances. For instance, it would be perfectly acceptable for a person who has recently been bereaved to appear depressed.

When assessing a patient's appearance and mental state, there are a number of questions the nurse needs to ask themselves.

+ Does the patient look their age?
+ Is the patient lean, stocky, obese or barrel chested?
+ Is the patient's face and body symmetrical?
+ Is the patient clean and appropriately dressed?
+ Does the patient appear ill, distressed or in pain?
+ Is the patient alert, agitated or confused?
+ Does the patient have coordination and good posture?
+ Is the patient's speech relaxed, clear, strong or does the patient sound stressed.

LIFESPAN CONSIDERATIONS

General Assessment

A general assessment involves the recording of baseline information such as height, weight and vital signs. When performing a general assessment on certain age groups the nurse needs to consider the following.

Infants

A general assessment of an infant will always involve measuring the child's length and weight. These can then be recorded on a centile chart and used to ascertain if the infant's growth is within normal limits. For children under the age of two, head circumference can also be used as an indicator or normal growth and development.

+ Measure height of children under age two in the supine position with knees fully extended.
+ Weigh without clothing.
+ Include measurement of head circumference until age two.

Children

A general assessment of a child will normally involve measuring the child's height and weight, again as an indicator of normal growth, but also because many of the drugs given to children are administered per kilogram of their body weight: for example, a child weighing 25 kg would receive considerably less of a drug than a child who weighs 40 kg. Therefore it is important that a child is weighed in their underwear rather than fully clothed.

Older Adult

A general assessment of an older adult will generally involve the collection of the same data as a younger adult however the nurse may need to consider the following:

+ Allow extra time for patients to answer questions.
+ Adapt questioning techniques as appropriate for patients with hearing or visual limitations.
+ Older adults with osteoporosis can lose several inches in height. Be sure to document height and ask if they are aware of becoming shorter in height.
+ When asking about weight loss, be specific about amount and time frame, for example, 'Have you lost more than five pounds in the last two months?'

CLINICAL ALERT

Ensure that you make yourself aware of local policies and procedures with regard to physical assessment, to ensure that you have the correct documentation and equipment.

Vital Signs

Vital signs are measured (a) to establish baseline data against which to compare future measurements and (b) to detect actual and potential health problems. See Chapter 15 for measurements of temperature, pulse, respirations, blood pressure and oxygen saturation. See Chapter 21 for pain assessment.

Height and Weight

Patient data such as height and weight are the key to evaluating their nutritional status, medication dosage calculations and assessing fluid loss and gain. Height and weight should be measured during the initial assessment of the patient so that any changes in weight can be determined. During the initial physical assessment the nurse needs to ascertain if there has been any significant unintentional weight gain or loss as this can be an indicator of a number of diseases/illnesses.

Height is measured using a measuring stick or wall chart. For the sake of accuracy the patient should remove their shoes and stand erect with their heels together. The measurement should be documented in metric measurements but as some patients find it difficult to understand metric units they may wish to have these measurements converted to imperial units.

Weight is usually measured when a patient is admitted and at regular intervals after admission, for example, each morning before breakfast. When accuracy is essential, the nurse should use the same scale each time (because every scale records slightly differently), take the measurements at the same time each day, and make sure the patient wears the same kind of clothing and no shoes. Patients who are wheelchair bound can be weighed on a special weighing scale made to accommodate the wheelchair (see Figure 26-5 on page 692) likewise patients who are bed bound can be weighed either by using a bed or trolley weighing scales (see Figure 26-6 on page 692), a weighing scale attached to a hoist (see Figure 26-7 on page 692) or using a bed that has an integral weighing scales.

The general assessment of the patient can in some circumstances include a number of initial diagnostic tests in order to establish further objective data about the patient's condition.

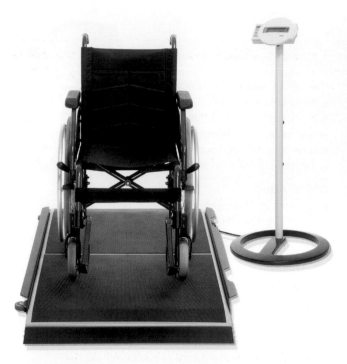

Figure 26-5 Wheelchair weighing scales.

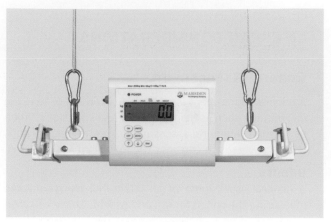

Figure 26-7 Hoist weighing scales.

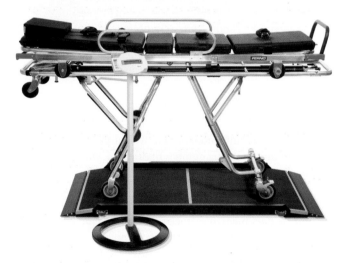

Figure 26-6 Trolley or bed scales.

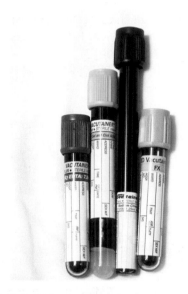

Figure 26-8 Full blood count tubes (purple lids); urea and electrolytes tube (yellow lids).

Diagnostic Testing as Part of the General Assessment

The most common initial diagnostic tests that are performed during a general assessment of the patient are full blood count (FBC), urea and electrolytes (U&E) and in some specific circumstances blood cultures.

Full Blood Count

This is a specific blood test that is usually taken from a vein but it can be collected from the capilliaries in babies. There is no specific patient preparation required for this test so it can

be taken randomly. However it needs to be collected in a specialised tube that contains an anticoagulant (K_2EDTA – Dipotassium ethylenediaminetetra-acetic acid), which prevents the blood from clotting and preserves the structure of the blood cells so that the different cells such as red blood cells and white blood cells can be distinguished from one another (see Figure 26-8).

The full blood count tests a number of blood components that can be associated with a number of conditions (see Table 26-2).

Urea and Electrolytes

This is one of the most frequently requested blood tests and is not one test but five tests performed simultaneously. The five tests are for sodium, potassium, bicarbonate, urea and creatinine which can establish if there any underlying conditions (see Table 26-3). Sodium, potassium and bicarbonate are

Table 26-2 Full Blood Count

Blood component	Normal range	Possible conditions associated with abnormal results
Red blood cell (RBC)	Males 4.5-6.5 × 10^{12}/l (4,500,000,000,000 to 6,500,000,000,000 red blood cells per litre of blood) Females 3.9-5.6 × 10^{12}/l (3,900,000,000,000 to 5,600,000,000,000 red blood cells per litre of blood	Low RBC = Anaemia, which is a collection of signs and symptoms that result in reduced oxygen delivery to tissues due to a decrease in red blood cells. The patient may complain of fatigue or short of breath. High RBC = Polycythaemia, which can be caused by low blood oxygen due to smoking or living at a high altitude or can be the result of other conditions.
Haemoglobin (Hb)	Males 13.5-17.5 g/dl (grams of haemoglobin per decilitre of blood) Females 11.5-15.5 g/dl (grams of haemoglobin per decilitre of blood)	Low Hb = Anaemia High Hb = Polycythaemia
Haematocrit or packed cell volume (PCV)	Males 40-52% of the blood is made up of red blood cells Females 36-48% of the blood is made up of red blood cells	Low PCV = Anaemia High PCV = Polycythaemia
Total white blood cell (leucocyte) count (WBC)	4.0-11.0 × 10^{9}/l (four to eleven thousand million white cells per litre of blood)	High WBC = Infection, Inflammation, significant tissue damage (e.g. large burn injury) or leukaemia which is a bone marrow cancer characterised by the prolific formation of immature white blood cells. Low WBC = some viral infections (mumps, influenza (flu), viral hepatitis or HIV), acute pancreatitis, appendicitis and Crohn's disease.

Table 26-3 Urea and Electrolyte

Blood component	Normal range	Possible conditions associated with abnormal results
Sodium (Na)	13.5-14.5 mmol/l (millimoles per litre is a standard SI unit to measure the amount of solute in a solution) which is equivalent to 31.05-33.35 milligrams of sodium per decilitre of blood.	Low Na = Diarrhoea and vomiting, profuse sweating or as the result of burns or haemorrhaging (excessive blood loss). High Na = Excess sodium replacement in an intravenous infusion or excess intake of salt or inadequate fluid intake.
Potassium (K)	3.5-5.2 mmol/l which is equivalent to 13.65-20.28 milligrams of potassium per decilitre of blood.	Low K = Chronic starvation for example anorexia nervosa, diuretic medication (water tablets, for example frusemide). High K = Acute renal failure or excessive potassium replacement.
Bicarbonate	22-28 mmol/l which is equivalent to 134.2-170.8 milligrams of bicarbonate per decilitre of blood.	Low bicarbonate = Diarrhoea, renal failure. High bicarbonate = Over-administration of bicarbonate, for example excessive use of antacids.
Urea	2.5-6.5 mmol/l which is equivalent to 15-39 milligrams of urea per decilitre of blood.	High urea = Renal failure, or diet rich in protein, chronic starvation. Low urea = Pregnancy as there is increased rate of urea excretion, liver disease.
Creatinine	55-105 μmol/l (micromoles per litre is a standard SI unit used to measure the amount of solute per litre of solvent) which is equivalent to 0.62-1.2 milligrams of creatinine per decilitre of blood.	Low creatinine = Pregnancy and any disease associated with significant decrease in muscle mass, for example muscular dystrophy as creatinine is produced by contracting muscle. High creatinine = Renal failure.

electrolytes (see Chapter 18). Like the full blood count test this does not require any specific patient preparation therefore it can be taken randomly: 5 ml of blood need to be collected in a specific blood tube (see Figure 26-8 on page 692).

Blood Culture

Blood cultures are usually performed if the doctor suspects that the patient's bloodstream has been invaded by bacteria (septicaemia). Normally blood is sterile (free from bacteria) and is kept this way by a number of defences such as the skin that acts as a physical barrier and white blood cells that fight infectious organisms. However, occasionally these defences are breached by bacteria and septicaemia develops. There are a number of factors that can cause septicaemia including:

+ Immunosuppression or compromised immunity, for example chemotherapy (chemical therapy or cytotoxic therapy), a treatment for cancer that acts by destroying cancerous cells. However normal cells can also be damaged or destroyed and as a result of this white blood cells may be damaged or destroyed, thereby reducing immunity.
+ An existing localised infection. Bacteria from the primary site (original infection) can invade the blood. The most common infections that develop into septicaemia are lower respiratory tract and urinary tract infections but bacteria can enter the body from any site of infection.
+ Virulence of the bacteria. Some strains of bacteria are less susceptible to the defences of the body and multiply more readily.
+ Invasive hospital procedures. Approximately 60% of patients who develop septicaemia acquire it from hospital (nosocomial) as a result of invasive procedures such as urinary catheterisation, intravenous catheterisation and surgical procedures.

The nurse or doctor will usually only take blood cultures if they suspect that the patient has septicaemia. Symptoms of septicaemia include:

+ a body temperature of more than 38°C;
+ rigors (shivering chills);
+ heart rate more than 100 beats per minute (tachycardia);
+ confusion or agitation.

Blood cultures should only be taken by nursing staff or doctors who have had specific training in the process as contamination of the blood can lead to inappropriate treatment of the patient. In many trusts only medical staff can actually perform blood cultures.

The blood must be collected into two specially designed blood culture bottles (see Figure 26-9). One of the bottles contains a culture medium (sterile liquid mixture of nutrients) with oxygen in the space above to test for aerobic organisms (oxygen breathing bacteria), while the other contains the same culture medium but instead of oxygen in the space there is a mixture of other gases to test for anaerobic organisms (bacteria that do not require oxygen to grow and reproduce).

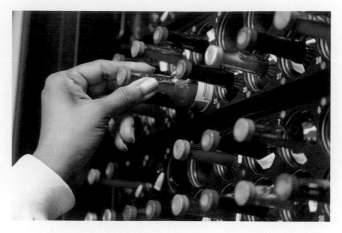

Figure 26-9 Blood culture bottles.

Although other blood tests are available, these are the most common that are performed during a general examination of the patient. Further, more specific, diagnostic tests will be discussed later in this chapter.

Once the nurse has completed the general assessment and initial diagnostic testing of the patient, ensuring that the data collected are documented accurately, the assessment of the individual body parts can begin. It is important that the nurse considers the signs and symptoms the patient has presented with and patient comfort when deciding which part of the body to assess first. Probably the easiest body part to assess first is the integument, which is made up of the skin, hair and nails.

THE SKIN, HAIR AND NAILS

Examination of the integument (outer covering of the body) usually begins with a generalised inspection of the skin, hair and nails followed by light palpation. When inspecting the integument the nurse must ensure there is a good source of light, such as indirect natural daylight.

Skin

When assessing the skin it is important to begin with an inspection of the skin's overall appearance. This will allow the nurse to identify areas that may need further investigation. These areas will need to be inspected more thoroughly and palpated, in order to identify changes in colour, texture, turgor (the ability of the skin to return to normal shape if pinched or pulled), moisture and temperature.

When assessing the colour of the skin, the nurse will look for areas of bruising, **pallor**, **cyanosis** and **erythema**. **Pallor** is the result of inadequate circulating blood or haemoglobin resulting in an ashen grey appearance. It may be difficult to determine in patients with dark skin, therefore it may be necessary to check the buccal mucosa (inside of the mouth), nail beds, palms of the patient's hands or soles of their feet.

Cyanosis, a bluish tinge, is caused by a lack of oxygen in the tissues and is most evident in the nail beds, lips and buccal mucosa. In dark-skinned patients, close inspection of the conjunctiva (the lining of the eyelids) and palms and soles may also show evidence of cyanosis. **Jaundice**, a yellowish tinge, is caused by an excess of bile products in the blood which may first be evident in the sclera (white, fibrous, protective layer) of the eyes and then in the mucous membranes and the skin. Nurses should take care not to confuse jaundice with the normal yellow pigmentation in the sclera of a dark-skinned or black patient. If jaundice is suspected, the posterior part of the hard palate should also be inspected for a yellowish colour tone. **Erythema** is a redness associated with a variety of rashes.

The nurse should note that dark-skinned patients have areas of lighter pigmentation, such as the palms, lips and nail beds. Likewise there may be localised areas of hyperpigmentation (increased pigmentation) which are normal and are the result of changes in the distribution of melanin (the dark pigment) in the skin. Some patients though suffer with conditions that cause hyperpigmentation such as birthmarks and hypopigmentation such as vitiligo (a chronic skin condition that causes loss of pigment in the skin resulting in irregular pale patches of skin).

Other localised colour changes may indicate a problem such as oedema or a localised infection. **Oedema** is the presence of excess fluid in the tissues below the skin or overhydration. When oedema is present in the skin the texture and turgor (elasticity) of the skin is also altered. An area of oedema appears swollen, shiny and taut, and tends to blanch the skin colour or, if accompanied by inflammation, may redden the skin. Generalised oedema is usually an indication of an impaired circulation through the veins caused by heart problems or abnormalities in the veins.

If a patient is dehydrated the skin turgor is also poor. The skin will usually have a dry texture and the skin will lose its elasticity. Skin turgor can be evaluated by gently squeezing the skin on the forearm or sternum (breastbone) between the thumb and the forefinger. Then release the skin. Normally the skin will spring back to its original shape but if it takes over 30 seconds to return to its original shape the skin has poor turgor.

The skin should be relatively dry to touch and excessively dry skin can appear red and scaly. On the other hand, overly moist skin, usually caused by excessive sweating, can irritate the skin particularly in skin folds (e.g. under the arms and breasts). This excessive moisture can be malodorous (smell unpleasant) and can indicate possible heart problems, fever or other diseases or disorders that increase the metabolic rate.

The temperature of the skin can also indicate different conditions: for example, generalised cool skin can indicate a lack of circulation as a result of shock or hypothyroidism (a disease caused by the insufficient production of the thyroid hormone that causes a range of symptoms such as weight gain and lethargy). On the other hand, localised cool skin can indicate impaired arterial circulation or reaction to a cold environment. Localised heat is usually the result of inflammation or infection to that part of the skin and should be assessed further; generalised heat is usually the result of systemic infection or fever.

As well as the above the nurse will assess the skin for alterations in a patient's normal skin appearance or skin lesion. Some skin lesions such as birthmarks, freckles and moles are normal. However, if the patient notes any changes to their mole such as an increase in size or change in colour this should be checked by a doctor as it may be skin cancer.

Skin lesions can be classified as either primary or secondary. Primary skin lesions are new changes that may be in response to some external or internal changes in the skin (see Figure 26-10 on page 696, *A–H*). Secondary skin lesions, on the other hand, are the result of changes to primary lesions: for example, a blister (primary lesion) may rupture and cause an erosion (secondary lesion). Nurses are responsible for describing skin lesions accurately in terms of location (e.g. face), distribution (i.e. body regions involved) and configuration (the arrangement or position of several lesions) as well as colour, shape, size, firmness, texture and characteristics of individual lesions.

> ## CLINICAL ALERT
>
> *If possible, and with the patient's consent, take a digital or instant photograph of significant skin lesions for the patient record. Include a measuring guide (ruler or tape) in the picture to demonstrate lesion size.*

As part of the assessment of the skin the nurse will also assess for any signs of the breakdown of the skin (e.g. pressure ulcers). The nurse will usually complete pressure ulcer risk assessment documentation to see if the patient is at risk of pressure ulcer development. Chapter 14 discusses this in further detail.

If there is a wound or breakage in the skin that the nurse suspects is infected a wound swab may be performed (see *Box 26-3* on page 697 for signs and symptoms of wound infection). A wound culture (or swab) consists of microscopic analysis of a specimen from a wound to confirm the existence of infection (see Figure 26-11 on page 697).

A wound swab should be taken using an aseptic technique (sterile technique). The wound should be exposed and a swab taken from the area that is suspected of being infected. The tip of the wound swab should touch nothing other than the wound. The specimen should be labelled immediately with the patient's details in order to prevent any confusion with other patients. The wound can then be dressed with appropriate wound dressings.

Once the microbiology department receives the swab they will culture the specimen and test for both anaerobic and aerobic organisms. If bacteria are isolated the microbiologist will then test the organisms to see if they are sensitive to any antibiotics. This is commonly termed culture and sensitivities (C&S).

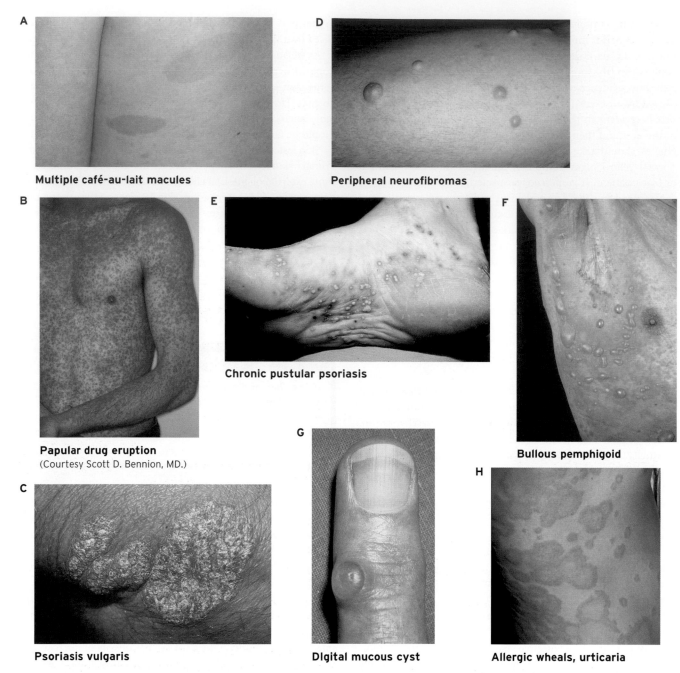

Figure 26-10 Primary skin lesions (*Note: (A–G)* from *Dermatology Secrets in Colour*, 2nd edn, by J.E. Fitzpatrick and J.L. Aeling, 2001, Philadelphia: Hanley and Belfus, Inc.; *(H)* Reprinted with permission from the American Academy of Dermatology. All rights reserved.)
A. Macule, Patch Flat, change in colour. Macules are 0.1–1 cm in size and are confined to one area. Examples: freckles, measles, petechiae, flat moles. Patches are larger than 1 cm and may have an irregular shape. Examples: port wine birthmark, vitiligo (white patches), rubella.
B. Papule Circumscribed, solid elevation of skin. Papules are less than 1 cm. Examples: warts, acne, pimples, elevated moles.
C. Plaque Plaques are larger than 1 cm. Examples: psoriasis, rubeola.
D. Nodule, Tumour Elevated, solid, hard mass that extends deeper into the dermis than a papule. Nodules have a circumscribed border and are 0.5–2 cm. Examples: squamous cell carcinoma, fibroma. Tumours are larger than 2 cm and may have an irregular border. Examples: malignant melanoma, haemangioma.
E. Pustule Vesicle or bulla filled with pus. Examples: acne vulgaris, impetigo.
F. Vesicle, Bulla A circumscribed, round or oval, thin translucent mass filled with serous fluid or blood. Vesicles are less than 0.5 cm. Examples: herpes simplex, early chicken pox, small burn blister. Bullae are larger than 0.5 cm. Examples: large blister, second-degree burn, herpes simplex.
G. Cyst A 1 cm or larger, elevated, encapsulated, fluid-filled or semi-solid mass arising from the subcutaneous tissue or dermis. Examples: sebaceous and epidermoid cysts, chalazion of the eyelid.
H. Wheal A reddened, localised collection of oedema fluid; irregular in shape. Size varies. Examples: hives, mosquito bites.
(Reprinted with permission from the American Academy of Dermatology. All rights reserved.)

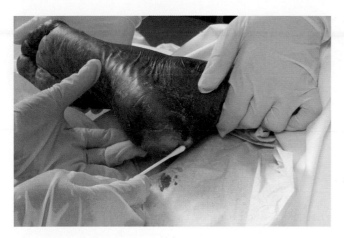

Figure 26-11 Wound swab.

BOX 26-3 Signs and Symptoms of Wound Infection

+ Inflammation
+ Malodorous or excessive wound exudate or pus
+ Fever
+ Necrotic or slough (dead tissue) (see Figure 26-12)
+ Pain

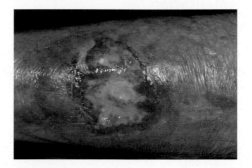

Figure 26-12 Sloughy wound.

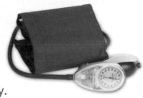

LIFESPAN CONSIDERATIONS

Assessing the Skin

Infants
+ Newborns may be jaundiced for several weeks after birth.
+ Newborns may have milia (whiteheads), small white nodules over the nose and face, and vernix caseosa (white cheesy, greasy material on the skin).
+ In dark-skinned races, areas of hyperpigmentation may be found in the sacral area (bottom of the spine).
+ If a rash is present, enquire in detail about immunisation history.
+ Assess skin turgor by pinching the skin on the abdomen.

Children
+ In dark-skinned races, areas of hyperpigmentation may be found in the sacral area.
+ As puberty approaches, skin may change in oiliness and acne may appear.

+ If a rash is present, enquire in detail about immunisation history.

Older Adults
+ The skin loses its elasticity and has poor skin turgor.
+ The skin appears thin and translucent because of loss of dermis and subcutaneous fat.
+ The skin is dry and flaky because sebaceous and sweat glands are less active. Dry skin is more prominent over the extremities.
+ Due to the normal loss of peripheral skin turgor in older adults, assess for hydration by checking skin turgor over the sternum or clavicle.
+ Flat tan to brown-coloured macules, referred to as *senile lentigines* or liver spots, are normally apparent on the back of the hand and other skin areas that are exposed to the sun.
+ Warty lesions with irregularly shaped borders and a scaly surface often occur on the face, shoulders and trunk. These benign lesions begin as yellowish to tan and progress to a dark brown or black.

Hair

Much of the information regarding the patient's hair can be collected by questioning the patient but in some circumstances the hair may need to be inspected.

Normal hair is flexible and evenly distributed but some conditions can cause problems, for example, patients with severe protein deficiency (kwashiorkor) may have faded, coarse and dry hair whereas hypothyroidism can cause very thin and brittle hair.

Procedure 26-1 on page 698 describes how to assess the hair.

PROCEDURE 26-1 Assessing the Hair

Planning

Equipment

+ Examination gloves

Implementation

Performance

1. Explain to the patient what you are going to do, why it is necessary and how they can cooperate. Discuss how the results will be used in planning further care or treatments.
2. Wash hands, apply gloves and observe other appropriate infection control procedures.
3. Provide for patient privacy.
4. Enquire if the patient has any history of the following: recent use of hair dyes, rinses or curling or straightening preparations; recent chemotherapy (if alopecia is present); presence of disease, such as hypothyroidism, which can be associated with dry, brittle hair.

Assessment	Normal findings	Deviations from normal
5. Inspect the evenness of growth over the scalp.	Evenly distributed hair	Patches of hair loss (i.e. alopecia)
6. Inspect hair thickness or thinness.	Thick hair	Very thin hair (e.g. in hypothyroidism)
7. Inspect hair texture and oiliness.	Silky, resilient hair	Brittle hair (e.g. hypothyroidism); excessively oily or dry hair
8. Note presence of infections or infestations by parting the hair in several areas, checking behind the ears and along the hairline at the neck.	No infection or infestation	Flaking, sores, lice, nits (louse eggs) and ringworm
9. Inspect amount of body hair.	Variable	Hirsutism (abnormal hairiness) in women

10. Document findings in the patient record using forms or checklists supplemented by narrative notes when appropriate.

Evaluation

+ Report significant deviations from normal to medical staff.

Nails

Assessing the nails is vital as they can be an indicator of general wellness and also can indicate if the patient is able to maintain their own hygiene or grooming. When assessing the nails the nurse should look at their colour, shape, thickness, consistency and contour. The parts of the nail are shown in Figure 26-13.

Firstly assess the colour of the nail. In light-skinned people the nail plate is usually pinkish in colour whereas darker-skinned

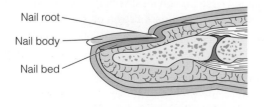
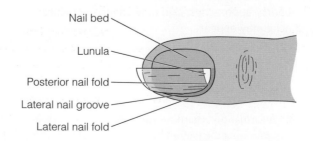

Figure 26-13 The parts of a nail.

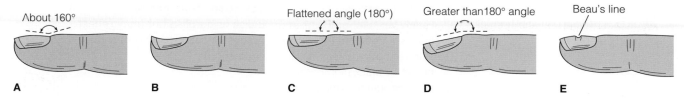

Figure 26-14 *A*, A normal nail, showing the convex shape and the nail plate angle of about 160 degrees; *B*, a spoon-shaped nail, which may be seen in patients with iron deficiency anaemia; *C*, early clubbing; *D*, late clubbing (may be caused by long-term oxygen lack); *E*, Beau's line on nail (may result from severe injury or illness).

people tend to have brown coloured nails. Any yellowing of the nail plate can be an indicator that the patient smokes.

The nail bed can be used to test the patient's peripheral circulation (amount of blood reaching the fingers or toes). Normal nail bed capillaries blanch when pressed but quickly turn pink or their usual colour when pressure is released. If the colour does not return within three seconds this could indicate problems with peripheral circulation.

When inspecting the nail, it is important to note that the angle between the nail and the nail bed is normally 160 degrees (see Figure 26-14, *A*). One nail abnormality is the spoon shape, in which the nail curves upward from the nail bed (see Figure 26-14, *B*). This condition, called koilonychia, may

be seen in patients with iron deficiency anaemia. **Clubbing** is a condition in which the angle between the nail and the nail bed is 180 degrees or greater (see Figure 26-14, *C* and *D*). Clubbing may be caused by a long-term lack of oxygen.

The texture of the nail is normally smooth but age, poor circulation and fungal infections can lead to thicker more brittle nails. However some conditions can lead to thin nails, for example, iron deficiency anaemia, which can also cause grooves in the nail, while Beau's lines are horizontal depressions in the nail that can result from injury to the nail or nail bed or illnesses such as diabetes (see Figure 26-14, *E*).

Procedure 26-2 describes how to assess the nails.

PROCEDURE 26-2 Assessing the Nails

Planning

Equipment

None

Implementation

Performance

1. Explain to the patient what you are going to do, why it is necessary and how they can cooperate. Discuss how the results will be used in planning further care or treatments.

2. Observe appropriate infection control procedures.

3. Provide for patient privacy.

4. Enquire if the patient has any history of the following: presence of diabetes mellitus, peripheral circulatory disease, previous injury or severe illness.

Assessment	Normal findings	Deviations from normal
5. Inspect fingernail plate shape to determine its curvature and angle.	Convex curvature; angle of nail plate about 160° (Figure 26-14, *A*)	Spoon nail (Figure 26-14, *B*); clubbing (180° or greater) (Figure 26-14, *C* and *D*)
6. Inspect fingernail and toenail texture.	Smooth texture	Excessive thickness or thinness or presence of grooves or furrows; Beau's lines (Figure 26-14, *E*)

Assessment	Normal findings	Deviations from normal
7. Inspect fingernail and toenail bed colour.	Highly vascular and pink in light-skinned patients; dark-skinned patients may have brown or black pigmentation in longitudinal streaks	Bluish or purplish tint (may reflect cyanosis); pallor (may reflect poor arterial circulation)
8. Inspect tissues surrounding nails.	Intact epidermis	Hangnails (triangular splits in the skin around the nail); paronychia (inflammation)
9. Perform capillary refill test. Press two or more nails between your thumb and index finger; look for blanching and return of pink colour to nail bed.	Prompt return of pink or usual colour (generally less than three seconds)	Delayed return of pink or usual colour (may indicate circulatory impairment)

10. Document findings in the patient record using forms or checklists supplemented by narrative notes when appropriate.

Evaluation

+ Perform a detailed follow-up examination of other individual systems based on findings that deviated from expected or normal for the patient. Relate findings to previous assessment data if available.

+ Report significant deviations from normal to medical staff.

Once examination of the integument is complete and the information documented, the nurse should move onto the next body part. It may be efficient at this point to assess the head as this will minimise the effort required by the patient to move.

THE HEAD

Assessment of the head includes inspection, palpation of the skull, face, eyes, ears, nose, sinuses, mouth and pharynx.

Skull and Face

The skull can be of variable size and shape according to the patient's age and body size. The skull is made up of a number of areas: frontal, parietal, occipital, mastoid process, mandible, maxilla and zygomatic (see Figure 26-15).

Facial changes can be the result of a number of disorders: for example, kidney or cardiac (heart) disease can cause oedema (swelling) of the eyelids while hyperthyroidism can cause protrusion of the eyeballs or **exophthalmoses**. Therefore it is

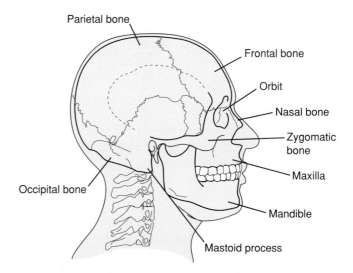

Figure 26-15 Bones of the head.

important to inspect the face for any abnormalities and relate these with the past medical history of the patient.

Procedure 26-3 describes how to assess the skull and face.

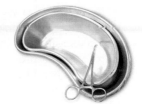

PROCEDURE 26-3 Assessing the Skull and Face

Planning

Equipment

None

Implementation

Performance

1. Explain to the patient what you are going to do, why it is necessary and how they can cooperate. Discuss how the results will be used in planning further care or treatments.
2. Observe appropriate infection control procedures.
3. Provide for patient privacy.
4. Enquire if the patient has any history of the following: any past problems with lumps or bumps, itching, scaling or dandruff; any history of loss of consciousness, dizziness, seizures, headache, facial pain or injury; when and how any lumps occurred; length of time any other problem existed; any known cause of problem; associated symptoms, treatment and recurrences.

Assessment	Normal findings	Deviations from normal
5. Inspect the skull for size, shape and symmetry.	Rounded and symmetrical, with frontal, parietal and occipital prominences; smooth skull contour	Lack of symmetry; increased skull size with more prominent nose and forehead; longer mandible (may indicate excessive growth hormone or increased bone thickness)
6. Using a gentle rotating motion with the fingertips palpate the skull for nodules or masses and depressions.	Smooth, uniform consistency; absence of nodules or masses	Sebaceous cysts; local deformities from trauma
7. Inspect the facial features (e.g. symmetry of structures and of the distribution of hair).	Symmetric or slightly asymmetric facial features are normal	Increased facial hair; thinning of eyebrows; pronounced asymmetric features
8. Inspect the eyes for oedema and hollowness.		Oedema; sunken eyes
9. Note symmetry of facial movements. Ask the patient to elevate the eyebrows, frown or lower the eyebrows, close the eyes tightly, puff the cheeks, and smile and show the teeth.	Symmetric facial movements	Asymmetric facial movements (e.g. eye on affected side cannot close completely); drooping of lower eyelid and mouth; involuntary facial movements (i.e. tics or tremors). Asymmetrical facial movements can be the result of a number of illnesses including cerebrovascular accidents (CVA or stroke) and facial nerve palsy (paralysis)

10. Document findings in the patient notes.

Evaluation

+ Perform a detailed follow-up examination of other systems based on findings that deviated from expected or normal for the patient. Relate findings to previous assessment data if available.

+ Report significant deviations from normal to medical staff.

If assessment of the skull and face identifies abnormalities the doctor or nurse practitioner may feel it necessary to do further investigations such as computed tomography (a CT scan). CT of the skull produces a series of cross-sectional images of the various brain layers (see Figure 26-16).

What does the CT mean? Basically the denser the tissue the whiter it will appear on the CT. Therefore, bone which is dense material appears white, brain matter will appear grey and areas that are filled with cerebrospinal fluid (normal fluid surrounding the brain) appear as black as they are the least dense.

CT scans can identify a number of abnormalities including tumours (lumps or masses), haematoma (collection of blood), cerebral atrophy (shrinking of the brain) and congenital anomalies such as hydrocephalus (excessive cerebrospinal fluid in the head).

CT scans are quite costly (between £350 and £500) and use x-rays, so are only performed if the practitioner feels that the patient clinically needs it.

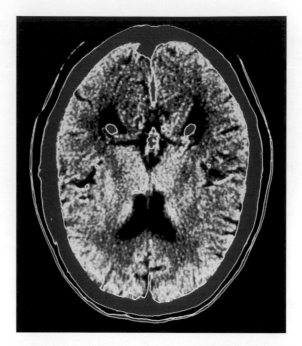

Figure 26-16 Computed tomography (CT) of head.

LIFESPAN CONSIDERATIONS

Assessing the Skull and Face

Infants

+ Most newborns' heads are shaped according to the method of delivery for the first week.

+ The posterior fontanel (soft spot) usually closes by eight weeks but the anterior fontanel may remain for up to 18 months.
+ Voluntary head control should be present by about six months of age.

The Eyes and Vision

Many people consider vision the most important sense because it allows them to interact freely with their environment. In order to maintain optimum vision a person will need to have their eyes examined by an ophthalmologist every two years or more often if there is a past medical history or family history of diabetes, hypertension or glaucoma.

Examination of the eyes includes assessment of **visual acuity** (the ability to distinguish details and shapes), ocular movement, **visual fields** (the area an individual can see when looking straight ahead), and external structures (see Figures 26-17 and 26-18).

Many people suffer with conditions that require them to wear eyeglasses or contact lenses for example **myopia** (short-sightedness), **hyperopia** (longsightedness) and **astigmatism** (an uneven curvature of the cornea). It is important to document in the patient's notes if the patient normally wears glasses or contact lenses and the reasons for wearing these. Testing visual

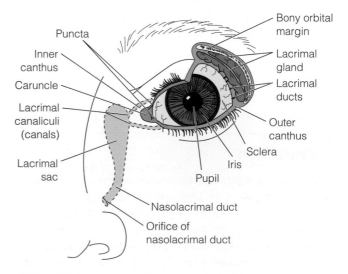

Figure 26-17 The external structures and lacrimal apparatus of the left eye.

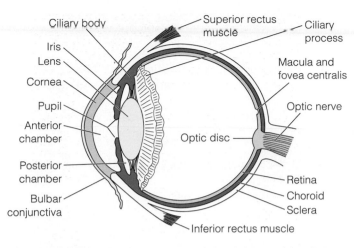

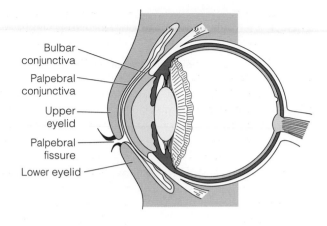

Figure 26-18 Anatomic structures of the right eye, lateral view.

BOX 26-4 Assessing Distance Vision

Distance vision is usually tested if there is some indication that a patient's distance vision is affected. The most common cause of problems with distance vision is astigmatism (irregularly shaped cornea), which causes problems with seeing objects in the distance or objects that are placed close to the eye. Astigmatism can be the result of a progressive disease called keratoconus where the normally round cornea thins into a cone shape. To assess distance vision:

+ Hold up an eye chart (see Figure 26-19) approximately 6 m from the patient.
+ Ask the patient to cover their right eye and read the eye chart.
+ Then do the same with the left eye covered
+ Finally, ask the patient to read the chart using both eyes.
+ Record the readings of each eye and both eyes, i.e. the smallest line from which the person is able to read one-half or more of the letters.

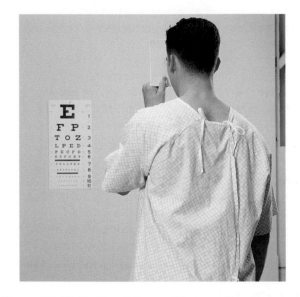

Figure 26-19 Testing distance vision.

---

acuity should be left to the expertise of an ophthalmologist but there are a couple of simple ways to determine whether a patient requires further investigation (see *Box 26-4* and *Box 26-5* on page 704).

The patient may also present with inflammatory visual problems, such as conjunctivitis (inflammation of the conjunctiva), hordeolum (sty – indicated by redness, swelling and tenderness of the hair follicle at the edge of the eyelid) and iritis (inflammation of the iris), that the nurse will need to document.

The patient could also be suffering from more serious conditions that affect visual acuity such as **cataracts** and **glaucoma**. A **cataract** is the clouding of the lens of the eye and tends to occur in those over 65 years old. These are frequently removed and replaced by a lens implant. Cataracts may

also occur in infants due to a malformation of the lens if the mother contracted rubella in the first trimester of pregnancy. **Glaucoma** on the other hand is the disturbance of the circulation of aqueous fluid, which causes an increase in pressure within the eye and is the most frequent cause of blindness in people over 40. However, if diagnosed early glaucoma can be controlled. Symptoms of glaucoma include blurred or foggy vision, loss of peripheral vision, difficulty focusing on close objects, difficulty adjusting to dark rooms and seeing rainbow-coloured rings around lights.

No assessment of the eyes would be complete without an inspection of the pupil of the eye. Pupils should be equal in size, round and appear black in colour. Pupils that are unequal usually indicate a problem with the eyes, for example, the patient may

BOX 26-5 Assessing Peripheral Visual Fields

Peripheral visual fields are usually assessed if there is some indication that a patient's peripheral vision is affected. There can be a number of causes for poor peripheral vision or tunnel vision including glaucoma (a group of diseases of the optic nerve that involves the loss of retinal cells) and alcoholism.

+ Sit directly in front of the patient and ask the patient to focus their gaze on your eyes.

+ Extend your arm out approximately 0.5 metre away from the left side of the patient's head and wiggle your fingers.
+ Tell the patient to focus their gaze on you as you gradually bring your wiggling fingers into their visual field.
+ Instruct the patient to tell you when they can see your fingers.
+ Repeat for the right side.

BOX 26-6 Assessing Pupil Reactions

Direct and Consensual Reaction to Light
+ Partially darken the room.
+ Ask the patient to look straight ahead.
+ Using a pen torch and approaching from the side, shine a light on the pupil.
+ Observe the response of the illuminated pupil. It should constrict (direct response).
+ Shine the light on the pupil again, and observe the response of the other pupil. It should also constrict (consensual response).
+ Pupil size and response should be documented (see Figure 26-20).

Reaction to Accommodation
+ Hold an object (a penlight or pencil) about 10 cm from the bridge of the patient's nose.
+ Ask the patient to look first at the top of the object and then at a distant object (e.g. the far wall) behind

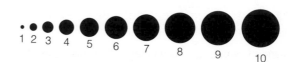

Figure 26-20 Variations in pupil diameters in millimetres.

the penlight. Alternate the gaze from the near to the far object.
+ Observe the pupil response. The pupils should constrict when looking at the near object and dilate when looking at the far object.
+ Next, move the penlight or pencil toward the patient's nose. The pupils should converge. To record normal assessment of the pupils, use the abbreviation PEARL (pupils equal and reacting to light).

have neurological damage, iritis or glaucoma. There are a number of assessment techniques used to examine the pupils (see *Box 26-6*).

The Ears and Hearing

Assessment of the ear includes direct inspection and palpation of the external ear, inspection of the remaining parts of the ear by an **otoscope**, followed by an assessment of the patient's hearing.

The ear is made up of the external ear, middle ear and inner ear (see Figure 26-21). The external ear includes the **pinna**, the skin and cartilage flap that focuses sound waves onto the **tympanic membrane** or eardrum. The external ear canal is curved and is about 2.5 cm long in the adult. It is covered with skin that has many fine hairs, glands and nerve endings. The glands secrete **cerumen** (earwax), which lubricates and protects the canal.

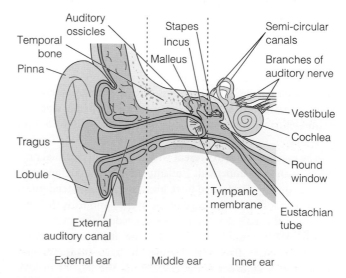

Figure 26-21 Anatomic structures of the external, middle and inner ear.

The curvature of the external ear canal differs with age. In the infant and toddler, the canal has an upward curvature. By age three, the ear canal assumes the more downward curvature of adulthood. This is important to know when using an otoscope to visualise the eardrum.

The middle ear is an air-filled cavity that starts at the tympanic membrane and contains three **ossicles** (bones of sound transmission): the **malleus** (hammer), which is the most easily seen, the **incus** (anvil) and the **stapes** (stirrups). The **Eustachian tube**, another part of the middle ear, connects the middle ear to the nasopharynx. The tube stabilises the air pressure between the external atmosphere and the middle ear, thus preventing rupture of the tympanic membrane and discomfort produced by marked pressure differences.

The inner ear contains the **cochlea**, a seashell-shaped structure essential for sound transmission and hearing, and the **vestibule** and **semicircular canals**, which contain the organs of equilibrium.

Sound is usually transmitted by air conduction which is carried to the eardrum and eventually to the auditory nerve and then the brain. Alternative sounds can be transmitted through the bones in the skull straight to the auditory nerve and then the brain.

Hearing tests are usually performed by audiologist but it is the nurse's responsibility to identify patients who may have problems with their hearing. Also it is important to note that some trusts have a policy that states nurses should not perform otoscopic examinations due to potential damage to the external ear. Despite this there are a number of techniques that the nurse can use to assess the patient's ears and hearing (see *Box 26-7*).

BOX 26-7 Assessment of the Ears and Hearing

+ Inspect the colour, size and position of the pinna (earlobe). The pinna should be the same colour as the face and of a similar size.
+ Palpate the pinna to test its texture, elasticity and areas of tenderness. The pinna should be mobile, firm and not tender.
+ Using either an otoscope or with the naked eye inspect the external ear canal for cerumen (ear wax), skin lesions, pus and blood. Any discharge should be documented.
+ If the trust policy allows, inspect the ear drum with an otoscope. The ear drum should be semi-transparent and a pearly grey colour (see Figure 26-22).
+ Assess the patient's response to normal speech. Document if there are any requests to repeat words or statements or if the patient leans towards the speaker.

+ Have the patient occlude one ear and out of the patient's sight place a ticking watch and document the response. Repeat for the other ear.

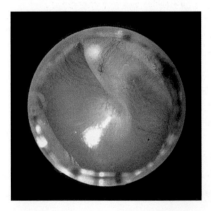

Figure 26-22 Normal tympanic membrane.

LIFESPAN CONSIDERATIONS

Assessing the Ears and Hearing

Infants
+ Assess overall hearing by ringing a bell from behind the infant or have the parent call the child's name to check for a response. At 3-4 months of age, the child will turn head and eyes toward the sound.

Children
+ To inspect the external canal and tympanic membrane in children less than three years old, pull the pinna down and back. Insert the otoscope only 0.5-1 cm.

Older Adults
+ The skin of the ear may appear dry and be less resilient because of the loss of connective tissue.
+ Increased coarse and wire-like hair growth may grow on the external ear.
+ The pinna increases in both width and length, and the earlobe elongates.
+ Earwax tends to be drier.
+ Generalised hearing loss tends to occur.

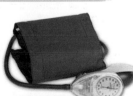

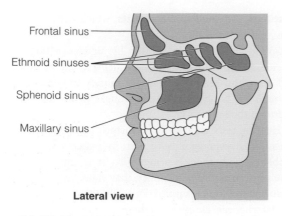
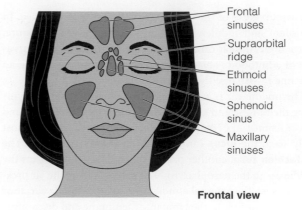

Lateral view

Frontal view

Figure 26-23 The facial sinuses.

Nose and Sinuses

The nasal passages can be easily inspected by the nurse with the naked eye and flashlight. However, in specialist environments such as an ear, nose and throat (ENT) department an otoscope can be used to facilitate examination of the nasal passages. In normal circumstances the assessment of the nose involves inspection and palpation of the external nose and inspection of the nasal passages.

Usually the nose is only inspected if there is a known injury to the nose or if the patient reports difficulty or abnormality in smell. If the patient complains about their sense of smell the nurse can quickly assess this sense by asking the patient to close their eyes and identify common smells such as coffee or mint.

Again if there is known injury to the face or if the patient complains of pain the nurse may need to inspect and palpate the facial sinuses (see Figure 26-23). If a facial fracture is suspected it is really important to use light palpation only as there is a risk that the injury could be made worse if deep palpation is used.

Procedure 26-4 describes how to assess the nose and sinuses.

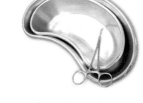

PROCEDURE 26-4 Assessing the Nose and Sinuses

Planning

Equipment

+ Gloves
+ Flashlight/penlight

Implementation

Performance

1. Explain to the patient what you are going to do, why it is necessary and how they can cooperate. Discuss how the results will be used in planning further care or treatments.
2. Observe appropriate infection control procedures.
3. Provide for patient privacy.

4. Enquire if the patient has any history of the following: allergies, difficulty breathing through the nose, sinus infections, injuries to nose or face, nosebleeds, any medications taken, any changes in sense of smell.
5. Position the patient comfortably, seated if possible.

Assessment	Normal findings	Deviations from normal
Nose		
6. Inspect the external nose for any deviations in shape, size or colour, and flaring or discharge from the nares (nostrils).	Symmetric and straight No discharge or flaring Uniform colour	Asymmetric – can indicate a deviated nasal septum. The nasal septum is the wall between the nostrils; if it is deviated to one side this can cause difficulty in breathing through the nose. Discharge from nares – this can be caused by the common cold, hay fever, nasal polyps (soft noncancerous growths that develop in the nasal passages as a result of chronic inflammation, cerebrospinal fluid (CSF) rhinorrhea following a head injury (the layers of the brain (meninges) are torn and CSF leaks down the nose). Localised areas of redness (inflammation caused by viruses such as the common cold or allergies) or presence of skin lesions (nasal polyps).
7. Lightly palpate the external nose to determine any areas of tenderness, masses and displacements of bone and cartilage.	Not tender; no lesions	Tenderness on palpation – as the result of inflammation or nasal polyps; presence of lesions (nasal polyps).
8. Determine patency of both nasal cavities. Ask the patient to close the mouth, occlude one nostril, and breathe through the opposite nostril. Repeat the procedure to assess patency of the opposite nostril.	Air moves freely as the patient breathes through the nostrils	Air movement is restricted in one or both nostrils possibly as the result of blockage of the nostril due to inflammation or nasal polyps, or deviation of the septum.
9. Inspect the nasal cavities using a flashlight.		
10. Observe for the presence of redness, swelling, growths and discharge.	Mucosa pink Clear, watery discharge No lesions	Mucosa red, oedematous – signs of inflammation Abnormal discharge (e.g. purulent) – see above Presence of lesions (e.g. polyps)
11. Inspect the nasal septum between the nasal chambers.	Nasal septum intact and in midline	Septum deviated to the right or to the left, which occurs naturally or as a result of nasal polyps.
Facial sinuses		
12. Palpate the maxillary and frontal sinuses for tenderness (see Figure 26-23).	Not tender	Tenderness in one or more sinuses which may indicate inflammation of the sinuses (sinusitis)
13. Document findings in the patient notes.		

Evaluation

+ Perform a detailed follow-up examination of other systems based on findings that deviated from expected or normal for the patient. Relate findings to previous assessment data if available.

+ Report significant deviations from normal to medical staff.

If the nurse suspects that there is presence of an infection in the nasal passages (see *Box 26-8* on page 708 for symptoms of infection in the nose), there may be a need to perform a swab of the nose. This requires the insertion of a swab through the nostril into the nasopharynx. This swab is then sent to the microbiology department for culture and sensitivity (C&S), the same as would be done for any culture (see Wound swab earlier in the chapter)

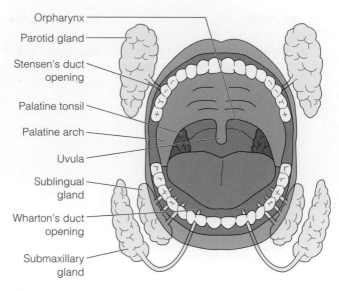

Figure 26-24 Anatomic structures of the mouth.

Following examination of the nose the next logical step to take is the examination of the mouth and oropharynx.

Mouth and Oropharynx

The mouth and pharynx are composed of a number of structures: lips, inner and buccal mucosa, the tongue and floor of the mouth, teeth and gums, hard and soft palate, uvula, salivary glands, tonsillar pillars and tonsils. Anatomic structures of the mouth are shown in Figure 26-24.

Saliva, a clear watery liquid that moistens the mouth and begins the digestion of starches, is emptied into the mouth through three pairs of salivary glands: the parotid, submandibular and sublingual glands. Too much or too little saliva can affect a person's oral health, for example insufficient saliva production can lead to dental cavities (caries).

Dental **caries** (cavities) is a problem most commonly associated with plaque, an invisible film made up of bacteria, saliva and epithelial cells. When plaque is unchecked, tartar (dental calculus) forms. **Tartar** is a visible, hard deposit of plaque and dead bacteria that forms at the gum lines. Also some patients may present with red, swollen gums otherwise known as

gingivitis. If left untreated this can lead to receding gum lines and loosened teeth.

Other problems nurses may see are **glossitis** (inflammation of the tongue), stomatitis (inflammation of the oral mucosa) and **parotitis** (inflammation of the parotid salivary gland). *Procedure 26-5* describes assessment of the mouth and oropharynx.

A detailed examination of the mouth and teeth are usually performed by an expert in this field such as a dentist. However there are a number of assessment techniques that the nurse can implement in order to identify those patients who need further investigation.

PROCEDURE 26-5 Assessing the Mouth and Oropharynx

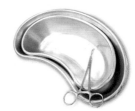

Planning

If possible, arrange for the patient to sit with the head against a firm surface such as a headrest or examination table. This makes it easier for the patient to hold the head still during the examination.

Equipment

+ Examination gloves
+ Tongue depressor
+ 2 × 2 gauze pads
+ Flashlight or penlight

Implementation

Performance

1. Explain to the patient what you are going to do, why it is necessary and how they can cooperate. Discuss how the results will be used in planning further care or treatments.
2. Observe appropriate infection control procedures.
3. Provide for patient privacy.

4. Enquire if the patient has any history of the following: routine pattern of dental care, last visit to dentist; length of time ulcers or other lesions have been present; any denture discomfort; any medications patient is receiving.
5. Position the patient comfortably, seated if possible.

Assessment	Normal findings	Deviations from normal
Lips and buccal mucosa		
6. Inspect the outer lips for symmetry of contour, colour and texture. Ask the patient to purse the lips as if to whistle.	Uniform pink colour (darker, e.g. bluish hue, in Mediterranean groups and dark-skinned patients) Soft, moist, smooth texture Symmetry of contour Ability to purse lips	Pallor; cyanosis Blisters; generalised or localised swelling. Inability to purse lips (indicative of facial nerve damage)
7. Inspect and palpate the inner lips and buccal mucosa for colour, moisture, texture and the presence of lesions.	Uniform pink colour (freckled brown pigmentation in dark-skinned patients) Moist, smooth, soft, glistening and elastic texture (drier oral mucosa in elderly due to decreased salivation)	Pallor. Excessive dryness Mucosal cysts; irritations from dentures; abrasions, ulcerations; nodules
Teeth and gums		
8. Inspect the teeth and gums while examining the inner lips and buccal mucosa.	32 adult teeth Smooth, white, shiny tooth enamel Pink gums (bluish or dark patches in dark-skinned patients) Moist, firm texture to gums No retraction of gums (pulling away from the teeth)	Missing teeth; ill-fitting dentures Brown or black discoloration of the enamel (may indicate staining or the presence of caries) Excessively red gums Spongy texture; bleeding; tenderness (may indicate periodontal disease) Receding, atrophied gums; swelling that partially covers the teeth
9. Inspect the dentures. Ask the patient to remove complete or partial dentures. Inspect their condition, noting in particular broken or worn areas.	Smooth, intact dentures	Ill-fitting dentures; irritated and excoriated area under dentures
Tongue/floor of the mouth		
10. Inspect the surface of the tongue for position, colour and texture. Ask the patient to protrude the tongue.	Central position Pink colour (some brown pigmentation on tongue borders in dark-skinned patients); moist; slightly rough; thin whitish coating Smooth, lateral margins; no lesions Raised papillae (taste buds)	Deviated from centre (may indicate damage to hypoglossal (12th cranial) nerve); excessive trembling Smooth red tongue (may indicate iron, vitamin B_{12} or vitamin B_3 deficiency) Dry, furry tongue (associated with fluid deficit) Nodes, ulcerations, discolorations (white or red areas); areas of tenderness
11. Inspect tongue movement. Ask the patient to roll the tongue upward and move it from side to side.	Moves freely; no tenderness	Restricted mobility
12. Inspect the base of the tongue and the mouth floor. Ask the patient to place the tip of the tongue against the roof of the mouth.	Smooth tongue base with prominent veins	Swelling, ulceration

Assessment	Normal findings	Deviations from normal
13. Palpate the tongue and floor of the mouth for any nodules, lumps or excoriated areas.	Smooth with no palpable nodules	Swelling, nodules
Salivary glands		
14. Inspect salivary duct openings for any swelling or redness. See Figure 26-24.	Same as colour of buccal mucosa and floor of mouth	Inflammation (redness and swelling)
Palates and uvula		
15. Inspect the hard and soft palate for colour, shape, texture and the presence of bony prominences. Ask the patient to open the mouth wide and tilt the head backward. Then, depress tongue with a tongue blade as necessary, and use a penlight for appropriate visualisation.	Light pink, smooth, soft palate Lighter pink hard palate, more irregular texture	Discoloration (e.g. jaundice or pallor) Palates the same colour Irritations Bony growths (exostoses) growing from the hard palate (torus palatinus which are bony noncancerous growths on the hard palate)
16. Inspect the uvula for position and mobility while examining the palates. To observe the uvula, ask the patient to say 'ah' so that the soft palate rises.	Positioned in midline of soft palate	Deviation to one side may be the result of cerebrovascular accident (CVA or stroke), peritonsilar abscess (such as quinsy which is an abscess (collection of pus) between the back of the tonsil and the wall of the throat), tumour or trauma.
Oropharynx and tonsils		
17. Inspect the oropharynx for colour and texture. Inspect one side at a time to avoid eliciting the gag reflex. To expose one side of the oropharynx, press a tongue blade against the tongue on the same side about halfway back while the patient tilts the head back and opens the mouth wide. Use a penlight for illumination, if needed.	Pink and smooth posterior wall	Reddened or oedematous (inflammation); presence of lesions, plaques or drainage
18. Inspect the tonsils (behind the fauces) for colour, discharge and size.	Pink and smooth No discharge Of normal size or not visible	Inflamed Presence of discharge Swollen
19. Elicit the gag reflex by pressing the posterior tongue with a tongue blade.	Present	Absent (may indicate problems with glossopharyngeal or vagus nerves)
20. Document findings in the patient notes.		

Evaluation

+ Perform a detailed follow-up examination of neurological and other systems based on findings that deviated from expected or normal for the patient. Relate findings to previous assessment data if available.

+ Report significant deviations from normal to medical staff.

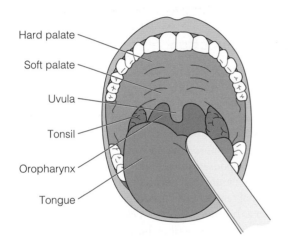

Hard palate
Soft palate
Uvula
Tonsil
Oropharynx
Tongue

Figure 26-25 Throat swab.

Like the nasal swab, a throat swab would be considered by the nurse or doctor if there were signs and symptoms of an infection. When taking a swab of the throat, the tonsillar areas need to be swabbed but it is important not to touch the tongue, cheeks or teeth with the swab as these areas can contaminate the swab and could result in inappropriate treatment of the patient (see Figure 26-25).

If during the examination of the head there is any suspicion that there may be neurological damage it is important that the nurse assesses the neurological system of the patient.

NEUROLOGICAL SYSTEM

A thorough neurological examination may take 1–3 hours; however, routine screening tests are usually done first. If the results of these tests raise questions, more extensive evaluations are made. Three major considerations determine the extent of a neurological exam: (a) the patient's main problems, (b) the patient's physical condition (i.e. level of consciousness and ability to ambulate), because many parts of the examination require movement and coordination of the extremities, and (c) the patient's willingness to participate and cooperate.

Examination of the neurological system includes assessment of (a) mental status including level of consciousness, (b) the cranial nerves, (c) reflexes, (d) motor function and (e) sensory function (see *Procedure 26-6* on page 712). Parts of the neurological assessment are performed throughout the health examination. For example, the nurse performs a large part of the mental status assessment during the taking of the history and when observing the patient's general appearance.

Mental Status

This usually begins when the nurse talks with the patient while taking a history. The nurse will pick up clues as to the patient's intellectual functions and emotional functions. If problems with use of language, memory, concentration or thought processes are noted during the patient history, a more extensive examination is required during neurological assessment. Major areas of mental status assessment include language, orientation, memory and attention span and calculation.

Level of Consciousness

Level of consciousness (LOC) is the earliest and most sensitive indicator of a change in a patient's neurological state. LOC can lie anywhere along a continuum from a state of alertness to coma. A fully alert patient responds to questions spontaneously; a comatose patient may not respond to verbal stimuli. The

Table 26-4 Levels of Consciousness: Glasgow Coma Scale

Faculty measured	Response	Score
Eye opening	Spontaneous	4
	To verbal command	3
	To pain	2
	No response	1
Motor response	To verbal command	6
	To localised pain	5
	Flexes and withdraws	4
	Flexes abnormally	3
	Extends abnormally	2
	No response	1
Verbal response	Oriented, converses	5
	Disoriented, converses	4
	Uses inappropriate words	3
	Makes incomprehensible sounds	2
	No response	1

Glasgow Coma Scale was originally developed to predict recovery from a head injury; however, it is used by many professionals to assess LOC. It tests in three major areas: eye response, motor response and verbal response. An assessment totalling 15 points indicates the patient is alert and completely oriented. A comatose patient scores 7 or less (see Table 26-4).

Cranial Nerves

Cranial nerves are nerves that emerge directly from the brain. There are 12 pairs of cranial nerves, some of which transmit information from the sensory organs (eye and ears) to the brain, others control muscles, or are attached to glands or organs such as the heart and lungs. The nurse needs to be aware of specific nerve functions and assessment methods for each cranial nerve to detect abnormalities (see Table 26-5 on page 721). In some cases, each nerve is assessed; in other cases only selected nerve functions are evaluated.

Reflexes

A **reflex** is an automatic response of the body to a stimulus. It is not voluntarily learned or conscious. Several reflexes are normally tested during the physical examination: (a) the biceps reflex, (b) the triceps reflex, (c) the brachioradialis reflex, (d) the patellar reflex, (e) the Achilles reflex and (f) the plantar (Babinski) reflex. (See *Procedure 26-6* for details of all these reflexes).

Motor Function

Neurological assessment of the motor system includes inspection of the muscles and testing muscle tone and strength (see *Procedure 26-6*). The nurse would be inspecting for any signs of muscle weakness that could indicate damage to the muscle itself or damage to the brain as the result of a cerebrovascular accident (CVA or stroke).

Sensory Function

Sensory functions include touch, pain, temperature, position and tactile discrimination. The first three are routinely tested. Generally, the face, arms, legs, hands and feet are tested for touch and pain, although all parts of the body can be tested. If the patient complains of numbness, peculiar sensations or paralysis, the nurse should check sensation more carefully. Abnormal responses to touch stimuli include loss of sensation (anaesthesia); more than normal sensation (hyperaesthesia); less than normal sensation (hypoaesthesia); or an abnormal sensation such as burning, pain or an electric shock (paraesthesia).

Procedure 26-6 describes how to assess the neurological system.

PROCEDURE 26-6 Assessing the Neurological System

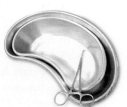

Planning

If possible, determine whether a screening or full neurological examination is indicated. This will impact preparation of the patient, equipment and timing.

Equipment (Depending on Components of Examination)

+ Percussion hammer

+ Tongue depressors (one broken diagonally for testing pain sensation)
+ Cotton wool to assess light-touch sensation

Implementation

Performance

1. Explain to the patient what you are going to do, why it is necessary and how they can cooperate. Discuss how the results will be used in planning further care or treatments.
2. Wash hands and observe appropriate infection control procedures.
3. Provide for patient privacy.
4. Enquire if the patient has any history of the following: presence of pain in the head, back or extremities, as well as onset and aggravating and alleviating factors; disorientation to time, place or person; speech disorder; any history of loss of consciousness, fainting, convulsions, trauma, tingling or numbness, tremors or tics, limping, paralysis, uncontrolled muscle movements, loss of memory, mood swings, or problems with smell, vision, taste, touch or hearing.

Language

5. Ask the patient to:
   - Point to common objects and ask the patient to name them.
   - Ask the patient to read some words and to match the printed and written words with pictures.
   - Ask the patient to respond to simple verbal and written commands (e.g. 'point to your toes' or 'raise your left arm').

Orientation

6. Determine the patient's orientation to *time, place* and *person* by tactful questioning. Ask the patient for their home address, time of day, date, day of the week, duration of illness and names of family members. More direct questioning may be necessary for some people (e.g. 'Where are you now?' 'What day is it today?').

Memory

7. Listen for lapses in memory. Ask the patient about difficulty with memory. If problems are apparent, three categories of memory are tested: immediate recall, recent memory and remote memory.
   To assess immediate recall:
   - Ask the patient to repeat a series of three digits, for example, 7-4-3, spoken slowly.
   - Gradually increase the number of digits, for example, 7-4-3-5, 7-4-3-5-6 and 7-4-3-5-6-7-2, until the patient fails to repeat the series correctly.
   - Start again with a series of three digits, but this time ask the patient to repeat them backward.

The average person can repeat a series of five to eight digits in sequence and four to six digits in reverse order.

To assess recent memory:

- Ask the patient to recall the recent events of the day, such as how the patient got to the clinic. This information must be validated, however.
- Ask the patient to recall information given early in the interview (e.g. the name of a doctor).
- Provide the patient with three facts to recall (e.g. a colour, an object, an address or a three-digit number), and ask the patient to repeat all three. Later in the interview, ask the patient to recall all three items.

To assess remote memory, ask the patient to describe a previous illness or surgery, e.g. five years ago, or a birthday or anniversary.

Attention span and calculation

8. Test the ability to concentrate or *attention span* by asking the patient to recite the alphabet or to count backward from 100. Test the ability to calculate by asking the patient to subtract 7 or 3 progressively from 100, i.e. 100, 93, 86, 79 or 100, 97, 94, 91 (referred to as *serial sevens* or *serial threes*). Normally, an adult can complete serial sevens test in about 90 seconds with three or fewer errors. Because educational level and language or cultural differences affect calculating ability, this test may be inappropriate for some people.

Level of consciousness

9. Apply the Glasgow Coma Scale: eye response, motor response and verbal response. An assessment totalling 15 points indicates the patient is alert and completely oriented. A comatosed patient would score 7 or less (see Table 26-5 on page 721).

Cranial nerves

10. For the specific functions and assessment methods of each cranial nerve, see Table 26-6 on page 723. The names and order of the cranial nerves can be recalled by a mnemonic device: 'On old Olympus's treeless top, a Finn and German viewed a hop.' The first letter of each word in the sentence is the same as the first letter of the name of the cranial nerve, in order. Test each nerve not already being evaluated in another component of the health assessment.

Reflexes

11. Test reflexes using a percussion hammer, comparing one side of the body with the other to evaluate the symmetry of response.

Biceps reflex

The biceps reflex tests the spinal cord level C-5, C-6.

+ Partially flex the patient's arm at the elbow, and rest the forearm over the thighs, placing the palm of the hand down.
+ Place the thumb of your nondominant hand horizontally over the biceps tendon.
+ Deliver a blow (slight downward thrust) with the percussion hammer to your thumb.
+ Observe the normal slight flexion of the elbow, and feel the bicep's contraction through your thumb (see Figure 26-26, A).

Triceps reflex

The triceps reflex tests the spinal cord level C-7, C-8.

+ Flex the patient's arm at the elbow, and support it in the palm of your nondominant hand.
+ Palpate the triceps tendon about 2-5 cm above the elbow.

+ Deliver a blow with the percussion hammer directly to the tendon (see Figure 26-26, B).
+ Observe the normal slight extension of the elbow.

Brachioradialis reflex

The brachioradialis reflex tests the spinal cord level C-3, C-6.

+ Rest the patient's arm in a relaxed position on your forearm or on the patient's own leg.
+ Deliver a blow with the percussion hammer directly on the radius 2-5 cm above the wrist or the styloid process (the bony prominence on the thumb side of the wrist) (see Figure 26-26, C).
+ Observe the normal flexion and supination of the forearm (movement of the arm into a palm up position). The fingers of the hand may also extend slightly.

Patellar reflex

The patellar reflex tests the spinal cord level L-2, L-3, L-4.

+ Ask the patient to sit on the edge of the examining table so that the legs hang freely.
+ Locate the patellar tendon directly below the patella (kneecap).

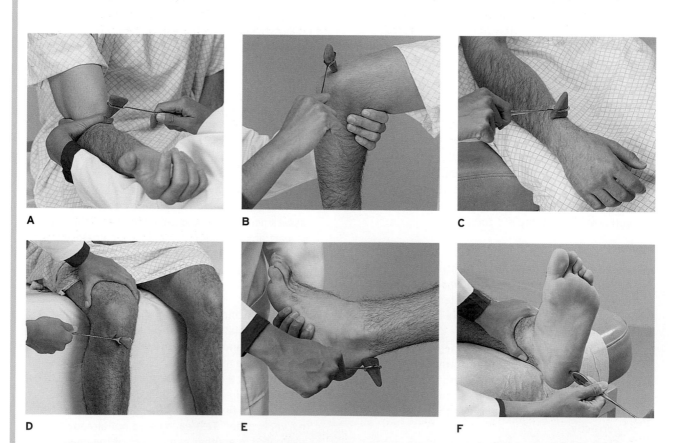

Figure 26-26 Testing reflexes: *A*, the biceps reflex; *B*, the triceps reflex; *C*, the brachioradialis reflex; *D*, the patellar reflex; *E*, the Achilles reflex; *F*, the plantar (Babinski) reflex.

+ Deliver a blow with the percussion hammer directly to the tendon (see Figure 26-26, *D*).
+ Observe the normal extension or kicking out of the leg as the quadriceps muscle contracts.
+ If no response occurs and you suspect the patient is not relaxed, ask the patient to interlock the fingers and pull. *This action often enhances relaxation so that a more accurate response is obtained.*

Achilles reflex

The Achilles reflex tests the spinal cord level S-1, S-2.

+ With the patient in the same position as for the patellar reflex, slightly raise the upper part of the foot towards the shin (dorsiflexion) while supporting the foot lightly in the hand.
+ Deliver a blow with the percussion hammer directly to the Achilles tendon just above the heel (see Figure 26-26, *E*).

+ Observe and feel the normal plantar flexion (downward jerk) of the foot.

Plantar (Babinski) reflex

The planter, or Babinski, reflex is superficial. It may be absent in adults without pathology or overridden by voluntary control.

+ Use a moderately sharp object, such as the handle of the percussion hammer, a key or the dull end of a pin or applicator stick.
+ Stroke the lateral border of the sole of the patient's foot, starting at the heel, continuing to the ball of the foot, and then proceeding across the ball of the foot toward the big toe (see Figure 26-26, *F*).
+ Observe the response. Normally, all five toes bend downward; this reaction is negative Babinski. In an abnormal Babinski response the toes spread outward and the big toe moves upward.

Motor function

Assessment	Normal findings	Deviations from normal
Walking gait		
12. Ask the patient to walk across the room and back, and assess the patient's gait.	Has upright posture and steady gait with opposing arm swing; walks unaided, maintaining balance	Has poor posture and unsteady, irregular, staggering gait with wide stance; bends legs only from hips; has rigid or no arm movements
Romberg test		
Ask the patient to stand with feet together and arms resting at the sides, first with eyes open, then closed. Stand close during this test *to prevent the patient from falling.*	*Negative Romberg:* may sway slightly but is able to maintain upright posture and foot stance	*Positive Romberg:* cannot maintain food stance; moves the feet apart to maintain stance. If patient cannot maintain balance with the eyes shut, patient may have sensory ataxia which is the loss of coordination when the eyes are closed. If balance cannot be maintained whether the eyes are open or shut, patient may have cerebellar ataxia (loss of coordination)
Standing on one foot with eyes closed		
Ask the patient to close the eyes and stand on one foot and then the other. Stand close to the patient during this test.	Maintains stance for at least five seconds	Cannot maintain stance for five seconds
Heel-toe walking		
Ask the patient to walk a straight line, placing the heel of one foot directly in front of the toes of the other foot.	Maintains heel-toe walking along a straight line (see Figure 26-27 on page 716)	Assumes a wider foot gait to stay upright

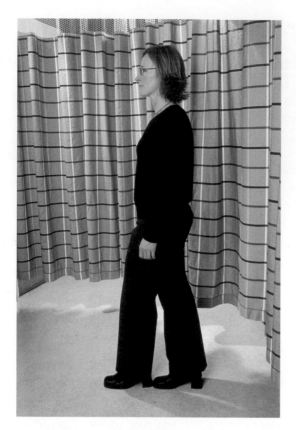

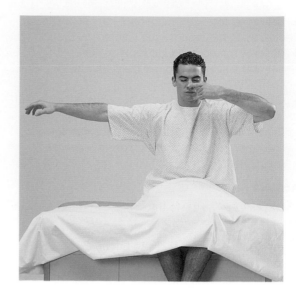

Figure 26-28 Finger-to-nose test.

Figure 26-27 Heel-toe walking test.

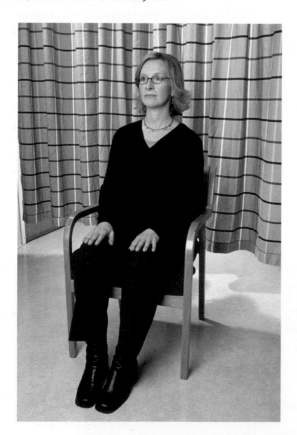

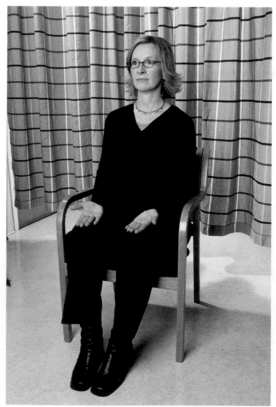

Figure 26-29 Alternating supination and pronation of hands-on-knees test.

Assessment	Normal findings	Deviations from normal
Toe or heel walking		
Ask the patient to walk several steps on the toes and then on the heels.	Able to walk several steps on toes or heels	Cannot maintain balance on toes or heels
Finger-to-nose test		
13. Ask the patient to abduct and extend the arms at shoulder height and rapidly touch the nose alternately with one index finger and then the other. The patient repeats the test with the eyes closed if the test is performed easily.	Repeatedly and rhythmically touches the nose (see Figure 26-28)	Misses the nose or gives lazy response which may indicate cerebellar disease (dysfunction of the cerebellum)
Alternating supination and pronation of hands on knees		
Ask the patient to pat both knees with the palms of both hands and then with the backs of the hands alternately at an ever-increasing rate.	Can alternately supinate and pronate hands at rapid pace (see Figure 26-29)	Performs with slow, clumsy movements and irregular timing; has difficulty alternating from supination to pronation which may indicate cerebellar disease (dysfunction of the cerebellum)
Finger to nose and to the nurse's finger		
Ask the patient to touch the nose and then your index finger, held at a distance at about 45 cm, at a rapid and increasing rate.	Performs with coordination and rapidity (see Figure 26-30 on page 718)	Misses the finger and moves slowly which may indicate cerebellar disease (dysfunction of the cerebellum)
Fingers to fingers		
Ask the patient to spread the arms broadly at shoulder height and then bring the fingers together at the midline, first with the eyes open and then closed, first slowly and then rapidly.	Performs with accuracy and rapidity (see Figure 26-31 on page 718)	Moves slowly and is unable to touch fingers consistently which may indicate cerebellar disease (dysfunction of the cerebellum)
Fingers to thumb (same hand)		
Ask the patient to touch each finger of one hand to the thumb of the same hand as rapidly as possible.	Rapidly touches each finger to thumb with each hand (see Figure 26-32 on page 718)	Cannot coordinate this fine discrete movement with either one or both hands which may indicate cerebellar disease (dysfunction of the cerebellum)
14. Fine motor tests for the lower extremities. Ask the patient to lie supine and to perform these tests.		
Heel down opposite shin		
Ask the patient to place the heel of one foot just below the opposite knee and run the heel down the shin to the foot. Repeat with the other foot. The patient may also use a sitting position for this test.	Demonstrates bilateral equal coordination (see Figure 26-33 on page 718)	Has tremors or is awkward; heel moves off shin which may indicate cerebellar disease (dysfunction of the cerebellum)
Toe or ball of foot to the nurse's finger		
Ask the patient to touch your finger with the large toe of each foot.	Moves smoothly, with coordination (see Figure 26-34 on page 718)	Misses your finger; cannot coordinate movement which may indicate cerebellar disease (dysfunction of the cerebellum)

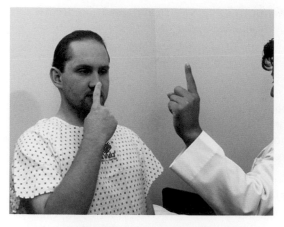

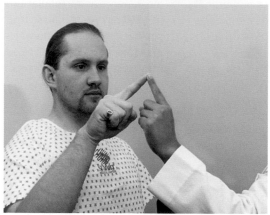

Figure 26-30 Finger to nose and to the nurse's finger test.

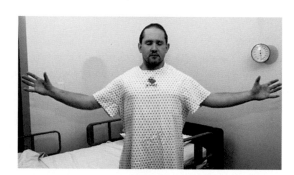

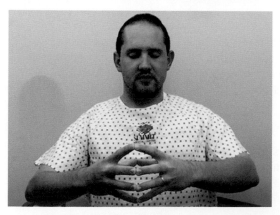

Figure 26-31 Fingers-to-fingers test.

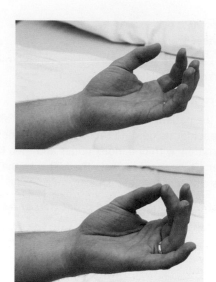

Figure 26-32 Fingers-to-thumb (same hand) test.

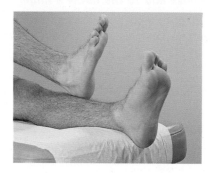

Figure 26-33 Heel down opposite shin test.

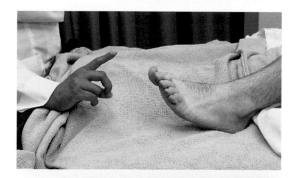

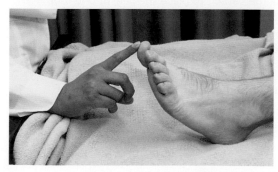

Figure 26-34 Toe or ball of foot to the nurse's finger test.

Assessment	Normal findings	Deviations from normal
15. Light-touch sensation Compare the light-touch sensation of symmetric areas of the body. *Sensitivity to touch varies among different skin areas.*	Light tickling or touch sensation	Anaesthesia (loss of bodily sensation), hyperaesthesia (increased sensitivity to stimulation, e.g. pain), hypoaesthesia (decreased sensitivity to stimulation, e.g. pain), and paraesthesia (sensation of burning, tingling or prickly)

- Ask the patient to close the eyes and to respond by saying 'yes' or 'now' whenever the patient feels the cotton wisp touching the skin.
- With a wisp of cotton, lightly touch one specific spot and then the same spot on the other side of the body.
- Test areas on the forehead, cheek, hand, lower arm, abdomen, foot and lower leg. Check a specific area of the limb first (i.e. the hand before the arm and the foot before the leg), *because the sensory nerve may be assumed to be intact if sensation is felt at its most peripheral part.*
- Ask the patient to point to the spot where the touch was felt. *This demonstrates whether the patient is able to determine tactile location (point localisation), i.e. can accurately perceive where the patient was touched.*
- If areas of sensory dysfunction are found, determine the boundaries of sensation by testing responses about every 2.5 cm in the area. Make a sketch of the sensory loss area for recording purposes.

Assessment	Normal findings	Deviations from normal
16. Pain Sensation Assess pain sensation as follows:	Able to discriminate 'sharp' and 'dull' sensations	Areas of reduced, heightened or absent sensation (map them out for recording purposes)

- Ask the patient to close the eyes and to say 'sharp', 'dull' or 'don't know'
  When the sharp or dull end of the broken tongue depressor is felt.
- Alternately, use the sharp and dull end of a sterile pin or needle to lightly prick designated anatomic areas at random (e.g. hand, forearm, foot, lower leg, abdomen). The face is not tested in this manner. *Alternating the sharp and dull ends of the instrument more accurately evaluates the patient's response.*
- Allow at least two seconds between each test to prevent summation effects of stimuli, i.e. several successive stimuli perceived as one stimulus.

Assessment	Normal findings	Deviations from normal
17. Temperature sensation Temperature sensation is not routinely tested if pain sensation is found to be within normal limits. If pain sensation is not normal or is absent, testing sensitivity to temperature may prove more reliable. • Touch skin areas with test tubes filled with hot or cold water. • Have the patient respond by say saying 'hot', 'cold' or 'don't know'.	Able to discriminate between 'hot' and 'cold' sensations	Areas of dulled or lost sensation (when sensations of pain are dulled, temperature sense is usually also impaired because distribution of these nerves over the body is similar)
18. Test if the patient has a sense of their position, posture or movement (kinaesthetic sensation) Commonly, the middle fingers and the large toes are tested for the kinaesthetic sensation (sense of position). • To test the fingers, support the patient's arm with one hand, and hold the patient's palm in the other. To test the toes, place the patient's heels on the examining table. • Ask the patient to close the eyes. • Grasp a middle finger or a big toe firmly between your thumb and index finger, and exert the same pressure on both sides of the finger or toe while moving it. • Move the finger or toe until it is up, down or straight out, and ask the patient to identify the position. • Use a series of brisk up-and-down movements before bringing the finger or toe suddenly to rest in one of the three positions.	Can readily determine the position of fingers and toes	Unable to determine the position of one or more fingers or toes. This may be due to cerebral problems or nerve problems
19. Tactile discrimination For all tests, the patient's eyes need to be closed.		

One- and two-point discrimination

Alternately stimulate the skin with two pins simultaneously and then with one pin. Ask whether the patient feels one or two pinpricks.	Perception varies widely in adults over different parts of the body	Unable to sense whether one or two areas of the skin are being stimulated by pressure. This can indicate a problem with the sensory nerves. For example a patient who has recently cut his finger may receive this test to see if there has been nerve damage

20. Document findings in the patient notes using appropriate tools supplemented by narrative notes.

Evaluation

+ Relate findings from previous assessment data.
+ Report significant abnormalities to the medical staff.

Table 26-5 Cranial Nerve Functions and Assessment Methods

Cranial nerve	Name	Type	Function	Assessment method
I	Olfactory	Sensory	Smell	Ask patient to close eyes and identify different mild aromas, such as coffee, vanilla, peanut butter, orange, lemon, lime, chocolate.
II	Optic	Sensory	Vision and visual fields	Ask patient to read Snellen chart (see Figure 26-19 on page 703).
III	Oculomotor	Motor	Movement of the eye, pupil and the ciliary muscles of the lens.	Assess pupil reaction to light. Assess the movement of each eye individually and then together.
IV	Trochlear	Motor	EOM; specifically, moves eyeball downward and laterally	Assess the movement of each eye individually and then together.
V	Trigeminal Ophthalmic branch	Sensory	Sensation of cornea, skin of face and nasal mucosa	While patient looks upward, lightly touch lateral sclera of eye to elicit blink reflex. To test light sensation, have patient close eyes, wipe a wisp of cotton over patient's forehead and paranasal sinuses. To test deep sensation, use alternating blunt and sharp ends of a safety pin over same areas.
	Maxillary branch	Sensory	Sensation of skin of face and anterior oral cavity (tongue and teeth)	Assess skin sensation as for ophthalmic branch above.
	Mandibular branch	Motor and sensory	Muscles of mastication; sensation of skin of face	Ask patient to clench teeth.
VI	Abducens	Motor	EOM; moves eyeball laterally	Assess directions of gaze.
VII	Facial	Motor and sensory	Facial expression; taste (anterior two-thirds of tongue)	Ask patient to smile, raise the eyebrows, frown, puff out cheeks, close eyes tightly. Ask patient to identify various tastes placed on tip and sides of tongue: sugar (sweet), salt, lemon juice (sour) and quinine (bitter); identify areas of taste.
VIII	Auditory Vestibular branch	Sensory	Equilibrium	Assessment methods are discussed with cerebellar functions (in next section).
	Cochlear branch	Sensory	Hearing	Assess patient's ability to hear spoken word and vibrations of tuning fork.
IX	Glossopharyngeal	Motor and sensory	Swallowing ability, tongue movement, taste (posterior tongue)	Apply tastes on posterior tongue for identification. Ask patient to move tongue from side to side and up and down.
X	Vagus	Motor and sensory	Sensation of pharynx and larynx; swallowing; vocal cord movement	Assessed with cranial nerve IX; assess patient's speech for hoarseness.
XI	Accessory	Motor	Head movement; shrugging of shoulders	Ask patient to shrug shoulders against resistance from your hands and turn head to side against resistance from your hand (repeat for other side).
XII	Hypoglossal	Motor	Protrusion of tongue; moves tongue up and down and side to side	Ask patient to protrude tongue at midline, then move it side to side.

LIFESPAN CONSIDERATIONS

Assessing the Neurological System

Infants

+ Reflexes commonly tested in newborns include the rooting reflex - when the baby's cheek is touched, the head turns toward that side; palmar grasp - the baby's fingers curl around an object; tonic neck reflex - when the baby is supine and the head is turned to one side, the arm and leg on that side extend while those on the opposite side flex (fencing position). Most of these disappear by six months of age.

Children

+ Present the procedures as games whenever possible.
+ Positive Babinski reflex is abnormal after the child ambulates or at age two.
+ Note the child's ability to understand and follow directions.
+ Assess immediate recall or recent memory by using names of cartoon characters. Normal recall in children is one less than age in years.
+ Assess for signs of hyperactivity or abnormally short attention span.

+ Should be able to walk backward by age two, balance on one foot for five seconds by age four, heel-toe walk by age five, and heel-toe walk backward by age six.
+ Romberg test is appropriate over age three.

Older Adults

+ A full neurological assessment can be lengthy. Conduct in several sessions if indicated and cease the tests if the patient is noticeably fatigued.
+ A decline in mental status is not a normal result of ageing. Changes are more the result of physical or psychological disorders (e.g. fever, fluid and electrolyte imbalances, medications). Acute, abrupt-onset mental status changes are usually caused by delirium. These changes are often reversible with treatment. Chronic subtle insidious mental health changes are usually caused by dementia and are usually irreversible.
+ Intelligence and learning ability are unaltered with age. Many factors, however, inhibit learning (e.g. anxiety, illness, pain, cultural barrier).
+ Short-term memory is often less efficient. Long-term memory is usually unaltered.
+ As a person ages, reflex responses may become less intense.

CLINICAL ANECDOTE

I honestly didn't realise how important assessing a patient's neurological status was until I went on placement last week. A lady was admitted via her GP after having a severe headache for over a week. She had deteriorated at home and had become quite confused. On admission we could not get much information from her as she was in so much pain and was quite agitated. The information we did have came from her husband and her GP. We checked her vital signs which appeared stable and her Glasgow Coma Scale was 12. We informed the doctors of our assessment and decided that we needed to keep a close eye on her by assessing her neurological status every half hour. The next time she was assessed her GCS had dropped to 10 so we informed the doctors immediately who decided to send her straight to theatre for investigation. It turned out that she had a subarachnoid haemorrhage and would have died if we had not picked up her deterioration.

Sarah Roberts, student nurse

NECK

Examination of the neck includes the muscles, lymph nodes, trachea, thyroid gland, carotid arteries and jugular veins (Figure 26-35).

One of the most common reasons for examining the neck is to assess the lymph nodes for size, shape, mobility and tenderness.

Lymph nodes occur throughout the body however chains of lymph nodes can be found in the neck, armpits and groin. Lymph nodes play an important part in a patient's immune system as lymph and lymph nodes contain lymphocytes and antibodies that fight off infection (see Table 26-6). As a result, if there is systemic or localised infection the lymph nodes can become swollen and tender. Also some forms of cancer, such as Hodgkin's

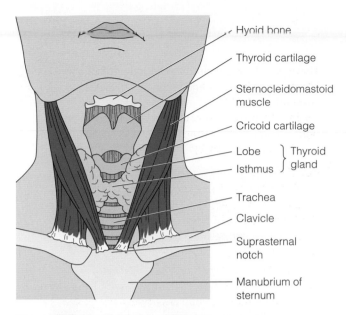

Figure 26-35 Structures of the neck.

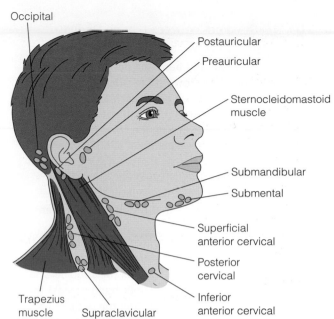

Figure 26-36 Lymph nodes of the neck.

Lymphoma, can increase the size of the lymph nodes but generally there is no tenderness when the nodes are palpated.

The neck has approximately 40 or so lymph nodes arranged individually or in chains (see Figure 26-36). Examination of the lymph nodes is usually done by palpating the neck with the finger pads of both hands. Both sides of the neck should be done at the same time so a comparison can be made (see *Box 26-9* on page 724).

As part of the examination of the neck the nurse may also wish to assess the thyroid gland which is situated under the skin

Table 26-6 Lymph Nodes of the Head and Neck

Node centre	Location	Part of the body drained of lymph
Head		
Occipital	At the posterior base of the skull	The occipital region of the scalp and the deep structures of the back of the neck
Postauricular (mastoid)	Behind the auricle of the ear or in front of the mastoid process	The parietal region of the head and part of the ear
Preauricular	In front of the tragus of the ear	The forehead and upper face
Floor of mouth		
Submandibular (submaxillary)	Along the medial border of the lower jaw, halfway between the angle of the jaw and the chin	The chin, upper lip, cheek, nose, teeth, eyelids, part of the tongue and the floor of the mouth
Submental	Behind the tip of the mandible in the midline, under the chin	The anterior third of the tongue, gums and floor of the mouth
Neck		
Superficial (anterior) cervical chain	Along the anterior to the sternocleidomastoid muscle	The skin and neck
Posterior cervical chain	Along the anterior aspect of the trapezius muscle	The posterior and lateral regions of the neck, occiput and mastoid
Deep cervical chain	Under the sternocleidomastoid muscle	The larynx, thyroid gland, trachea and upper part of the oesophagus
Supraclavicular	Above the clavicle, in the angle between the clavicle and the sternocleidomastoid muscle	The lateral regions of the neck and lungs

BOX 26-9 Palpating Neck Lymph Nodes

+ Face the patient and bend the patient's head forward slightly or toward the side being examined to relax the soft tissue and muscles.
+ Palpate the nodes using the pads of the fingers. Move the fingertips in a gentle rotating motion.
+ When examining the submental and submandibular nodes, place the fingertips under the mandible on the side nearest the palpating hand, and pull the skin and subcutaneous tissue laterally over the mandibular surface so that the tissue rolls over the nodes.
+ When palpating the supraclavicular nodes, have the patient bend the head forward to relax the tissues of the anterior neck and to relax the shoulders so that the clavicles drop. Use your hand nearest the side to be examined when facing the patient, i.e. your left hand for the patient's right nodes. Use your free hand to flex the patient's head forward if necessary. Hook your index and third fingers over the clavicle lateral to the sternocleidomastoid muscle (see Figure 26-37).
+ When palpating the anterior cervical nodes and posterior cervical nodes, move your fingertips slowly in a forward circular motion against the sternocleidomastoid and trapezius muscles, respectively.
+ To palpate the deep cervical nodes, bend or hook your fingers around the sternocleidomastoid muscle.

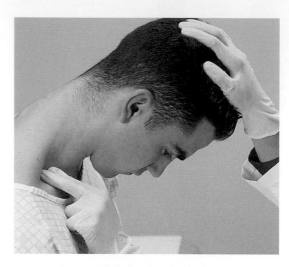

Figure 26-37 Palpating the supraclavicular lymph nodes.

below the Adam's apple or larynx. The thyroid gland makes hormones that regulate the metabolic rate within the body. Sometimes the thyroid gland can become enlarged from over-activity (as in Grave's disease) or from under-activity (as in hypothyroidism). An enlarged thyroid gland is often called a 'goiter'. Sometimes an inflammation of the thyroid gland (Hashimoto's disease) will cause enlargement of the gland.

Assessment of the neck involves examination of a number of structures including the upper airways therefore it would make sense for the nurse to extend this examination to the lungs and lower airways.

THORAX AND LUNGS

The respiratory system is made up of the airways, lungs, the bony thorax and respiratory muscles. Assessment of this system is critical to the immediate well-being of the patient as a compromised respiratory system can lead to a very sick patient. Changes in the respiratory system can come about slowly or quickly. In patients with chronic obstructive pulmonary disease (COPD), such as chronic bronchitis, emphysema and asthma, changes are frequently gradual.

Assessment of the thorax and lungs usually begins with an inspection of the chest shape and size as this can be an indicator of chronic respiratory problems such as emphysema.

Chest Shape and Size

In adults, the thorax is normally oval-shaped. Inspection of the chest shape can indicate underlying health problems (see Figure 26-38): for example, the disease rickets can cause a patient to have a pigeon chest (pectus carinatum) while a barrel chest is usually the result of chronic obstructive pulmonary disease (COPD).

Once the chest shape and size has been inspected and documented the nurse will need to establish if the patient's breath sounds are abnormal.

Breath Sounds

Abnormal breath sounds are the result of air passing through narrowed airways or airways filled with fluid or mucus, or when pleural linings are inflamed. Table 26-7 describes normal breath sounds. Abnormal sounds include crackles (referred to as rales or **crepitations**), gurgles, pleural friction rubs and wheezes (see Table 26-8 on page 726 for a description of these). Absence of breath sounds over some lung areas is also a significant finding and is usually associated with collapsed and surgically removed lobes.

Assessment of the lungs and thorax includes all methods of examination: inspection, palpation, percussion and auscultation. *Procedure 26-7* on page 726 describes how to assess the thorax and lungs.

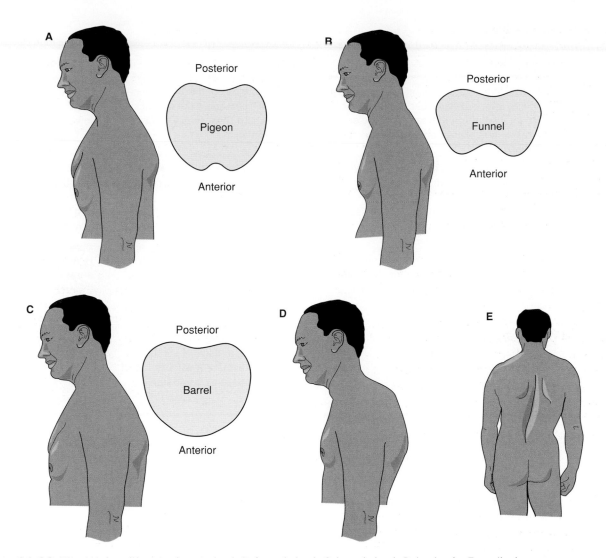

Figure 26-38 Chest deformities. *A*, pigeon chest; *B*, funnel chest; *C*, barrel chest; *D*, kyphosis; *E*, scoliosis.

Table 26-7 Normal Breath Sounds

Type	Description	Location
Vesicular	'Gentle sighing' or low pitched sounds.	Over peripheral lung; best heard at base of lungs
Broncho-vesicular	Moderate-pitched 'blowing' sounds created by air moving through larger airway (bronchi)	Between the scapulae and to the side of the breast bone or sternum at the first or second intercostals spaces.
Bronchial (tubular)	High-pitched, loud, 'harsh' sounds created by air moving through the trachea	Anteriorly over the trachea; not normally heard over lung tissue

Table 26-8 Abnormal Breath Sounds

Name	Description	Cause	Location
Crackles (rales)	Fine crackling sounds. Sound can be simulated by rolling a lock of hair near the ear. Best heard on inspiration but can be heard on both inspiration and expiration. May not be cleared by coughing.	Air passing through fluid or mucus in any air passage. Course crackles can indicate chest infection or pneumonia.	Most commonly heard in the bases of the lower lung lobes.
Gurgles (rhonchi)	Continuous, low-pitched, coarse, gurgling, harsh, louder sounds with a moaning or snoring quality. Best heard on expiration but can be heard on both inspiration and expiration. May be altered by coughing.	Air passing through narrowed air passages as a result of secretions, swelling, tumours.	Loud sounds can be heard over most lung areas but predominate over the trachea and bronchi.
Friction rub	Superficial grating or creaking sounds heard during inspiration and expiration. Not relieved by coughing.	Rubbing together of inflamed pleural surfaces. Can be a sign of pleural effusion (collection of fluid between the pleural membranes).	Heard most often in areas of greatest thoracic expansion (e.g. lower anterior and lateral chest).
Wheeze	Continuous, high-pitched, squeaky musical sounds. Best heard on expiration. Not usually altered by coughing.	Air passing through a constricted bronchus as a result of secretions, swelling, tumours. A wheeze heard on expiration is a classic sign of asthma.	Heard over all lung fields.

PROCEDURE 26-7 Assessing the Thorax and Lungs

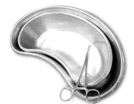

Planning

For efficiency, the nurse usually examines the back of the patient's chest first, then the front of the chest. When checking the back (posterior) or the side (lateral) of the chest the patient should be in a sitting position. However for examining the front (anterior) of the chest the patient can be in a sitting or lying position.

Equipment

+ Stethoscope

Implementation

Performance

1. Explain to the patient what you are going to do, why it is necessary and how they can cooperate. Discuss how the results will be used in planning further care or treatments.
2. Wash hands and observe appropriate infection control procedures.
3. Provide for patient privacy. In women, drape the anterior chest when it is not being examined.
4. Enquire if the patient has any history of the following: family history of illness, including cancer, allergies, tuberculosis; lifestyle habits such as smoking and occupational hazards (e.g. inhaling fumes); any medications being taken; current problems (e.g. swellings, coughs, wheezing and pain).

Assessment	Normal findings	Deviations from normal
5. Inspect the shape and symmetry of the thorax from posterior and lateral views. Compare one side of the chest with the other. Note masses or scars.	Both sides of the chest should be equal at rest and expand equally when the patient breathes in.	Barrel chest; chest asymmetric.
6. Inspect the muscles used in respiration.	When the patient inhales, the diaphragm should descend and the intercostals muscles should contract. This causes the abdomen to push out and the lower ribs to expand laterally. When the patient exhales the abdomen and ribs should return to their resting position.	Patients in respiratory distress will use accessory muscles in the neck and shoulders to help them expand their lungs.
7. Observe the patient's skin colour, face and fingers while breathing.	The patient's skin colour should be normal coloured for their type of skin. Nostrils and lips should be relaxed. Fingers should be of normal shape (see earlier in the chapter).	Any bluish tint to the skin or mucous membranes indicates cyanosis. In respiratory distress the patient may purse their lips and flare their nostrils while breathing. Clubbing of the fingers (thickening of the flesh under the nail causing the nail to curve downward instead of laying flat) can indicate long term hypoxia.
8. Count the patient's respiratory rate for one minute or longer if abnormalities are noted. Do not tell the patient what you are doing as this can affect the results. A trick is to pretend you are counting the person's pulse rate.	Adults normally breathe at a rate of between 12 and 20 breaths/minute. An infant's breathing rate may reach 40 breaths/minute. The respiratory pattern should be regular, even and coordinated with occasional sighs. The ratio of inspiration to expiration is 1:2.	See *Box 26-10* on page 728 for abnormal respiratory patterns.
9. Percuss the thorax (see Table 26-9 on page 728 for percussion sounds).	Percussion notes resonate, except over scapula. Lowest point of resonance is at the diaphragm.	Asymmetry in percussion. Areas of dullness or flatness over lung tissue (associated with consolidation of lung tissue or a mass).
10. Auscultate the chest using the flat-disc diaphragm of the stethoscope (best for transmitting the high-pitched breath sounds). • Use the systematic zigzag procedure used in percussion (see Figure 26-39). • Ask the patient to take slow, deep breaths through the mouth. Listen at each point to the breath sounds during a complete inspiration and expiration. • Compare findings at each point with the corresponding point on the opposite side of the chest.	Vesicular and bronchovesicular breath sounds (see Table 26-7). 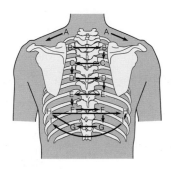 **Figure 26-39** Sequence for posterior chest percussion.	Abnormal breath sounds (e.g. crackles, rhonchi, wheeze, friction rub; see Table 26-8) Absence of breath sounds (associated with collapsed and surgically removed lung lobes).

Anterior thorax

11. Repeat steps 1-6 for the anterior thorax.

12. Document findings in the patient record using forms or checklists supplemented by narrative notes when appropriate.

Evaluation

+ Relate findings to previous assessment data if available. Report significant deviations from normal to the doctor.

BOX 26-10 Abnormal Respiratory Patterns

+ Tachypnoea	Shallow breathing with increased respiratory rate (>25 breaths per minute in adults, however it is difficult to define in children)
+ Bradypnoea	Decreased rate (<8 breaths per minute in adults)
+ Apnoea	Absence of breathing
+ Hyperpnoea	Deep, fast breathing
+ Kussmael's respirations	Rapid deep breating without pauses, breathing usually sounds laboured with deep breaths that resemble sighs.
+ Cheyne-Stokes respirations	Periods of apnea then tachypnoea. Usually indicates that the patient is towards the end of life.

Table 26-9 Percussion Sounds

Sound	Description	Clinical significance
Flat	Soft high pitched, extremely dull sounding	Usually indicates consolidation (lung tissue that is engorged with fluid) possibly due to an extensive pleural effusion (collection of fluid between the pleural membranes)
Dull	Thudlike	Usually indicates a solid area as in lobar pneumonia
Resonant	Low pitched, loud	Normal lung tissue
Hyperresonant	Very loud, lower pitched	Hyperinflated lung (e.g. pneumothorax or emphysema)
Tympanic	Loud, high pitched, drum-like	Air collection such as air in the intestines however it could indicate a large pneumothorax

---

LIFESPAN CONSIDERATIONS

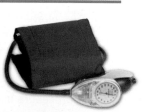

Assessing the Thorax and Lungs

Infants

+ The thorax is usually rounded.
+ Auscultated sounds will be louder and harsher.
+ Infants tend to breathe more abdominally than thoracically.

Children

+ Children tend to breathe more abdominally than thoracically up to age six.

Older Adults

+ The thoracic curvature may be accentuated because of osteoporosis and changes in cartilage, resulting in collapse of the vertebrae. This can also compromise and decrease normal respiratory effort.
+ Breathing rate and rhythm are unchanged at rest; the rate normally increases with exercise but may take longer to return to the pre-exercise rate.
+ Expiration may require the use of accessory muscles.
+ Cilia in the airways decrease in number and are less effective in removing mucus; older patients are therefore at greater risk for pulmonary infections.

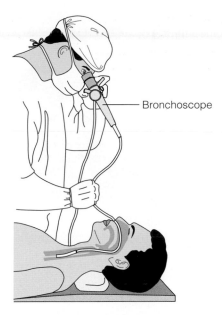

Figure 26-40 Bronchoscopy.

Diagnostic Testing of the Respiratory System

There are a number of diagnostic tests available to establish information regarding the respiratory system. The most common of these is the **sputum specimen** or culture which is a bacteriological examination of the sputum. **Sputum** is the mucus coughed up from the lungs and bronchi. The usual method of specimen collection is expectoration (coughing up and spitting out) of the sputum, however a specimen can also be acquired by suctioning the trachea or during a bronchoscopy. A sputum specimen or culture will usually inform the practitioner if an infection is present within the respiratory system and will only be performed if clinically indicated as the results will usually not be available for three days.

A **bronchoscopy** is the visualisation of the larynx, trachea and bronchi through a bronchoscope (see Figure 26-40). During a bronchoscopy the doctor can remove suspicious tissue, foreign bodies and suction sputum from the lower airways for analysis. A bronchoscopy can diagnose conditions such as cancer, tuberculosis and other infections. Bronchoscopies are usually only performed if the doctor thinks it is clinically indicated, for example if during the physical assessment of the respiratory system an abnormality is noted.

The findings of the assessment and any diagnostic testing ordered should be documented clearly before moving onto the next body system. As the respiratory system is closely linked to the cardiovascular system this is usually assessed next.

CARDIOVASCULAR AND PERIPHERAL VASCULAR SYSTEMS

Heart

In the average adult, most of the heart lies behind and to the left of the sternum. A small portion (the right atrium) extends to the right of the sternum. The apex (bottom) of the left ventricle actually touches the chest wall slightly below the left nipple. This point where the apex touches the anterior chest wall is known as the **point of maximal impulse (PMI)**.

Nurses assess the heart through observations (inspection), palpation and auscultation, usually in that sequence as auscultation is more meaningful when other data are obtained first. Heart examinations are usually performed while the patient is in a semi-recumbent position.

Inspecting the Heart

To begin assessment of the cardiovascular system, it is important to inspect the patient's general appearance, taking note of the patient's skin colour, the colour of the mucous membranes inside the eyes and mouth, checking for signs of clubbing of the fingers (thickening of the flesh under the nail causing the nail to curve downwards instead of laying flat) which can be a sign of long-term hypoxia (lack of oxygen in the tissues), or whether the patient is obese or if there are signs that the patient has lost a lot of body weight (e.g. loose clothing). Abnormalities in these findings may indicate a problem with the cardiovascular system.

Examine the **precordium**, the area of the chest overlying the heart, for the presence of abnormal pulsations or heaves. The term heave is a strong outward thrust of the chest wall and occurs when cardiac action is very forceful. It should be confirmed by palpation with the palm of the hand. Enlargement of the left ventricle produces a heave lateral to the apex, whereas enlargement of the right ventricle produces a heave at or near the sternum.

Palpating the Heart

The nurse may palpate for the apical pulse. This is found just below the left nipple (in the midclavicular line in the fifth intercostal space). In order to correctly assess the apical pulse, it is important to use one hand to assess the carotid pulse (which can be found alongside the windpipe or trachea in the neck) and the other hand to palpate the apical pulse. The apical pulse should roughly coincide with the carotid pulse.

Sometimes the apical pulse cannot be palpated and the nurse may have to use a stethoscope for accurate assessment. Assessment of the apical pulse is far more accurate than assessment of the radial pulse as it directly assesses the left ventricle. Assessment of the apical pulse may be used in infants and children or older adults when it is difficult to assess peripheral pulses (which are found in underneath the thumb on the underside of the wrist (radial artery) or in the inside of the elbow (brachial artery)).

Auscultating the Heart

The nurse can gain a lot of information about the heart through auscultation. However auscultation of the heart requires a stethoscope, a systematic approach and a lot of practice.

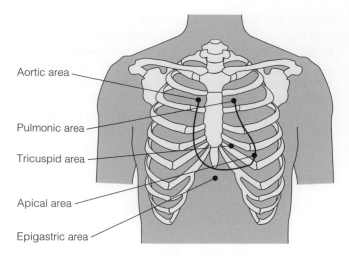

Figure 26-41 Anatomic sites of the precordium.

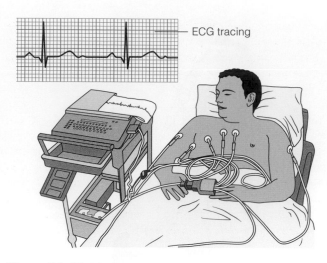

Figure 26-42 Electrocardiogram (ECG).

The first two heart sounds heard are produced by closure of the valves of the heart. The first heart sound, **S₁**, occurs when the atrioventricular (A-V) valves close causing a dull, low-pitched sound described as 'lub'. After the ventricles empty their blood into the aorta and pulmonary arteries, the semilunar valves close, producing the second heart sound, **S₂**, described as 'dub'. S₂ has a higher pitch than S₁ and is also shorter. These two sounds, S₁ and S₂ ('lub-dub'), occur within a second or less, depending on the heart rate. These heart sounds are audible anywhere in the precordium, but they are best heard over the aortic, pulmonic, tricuspid and apical areas (see Figure 26-41).

The inexperienced nurse may only recognise the 'lub-dub' sound however, the experienced nurse may perceive extra heart sounds (S₃ and S₄) during diastole (when the heart relaxes). Both sounds are low in pitch and heard best at the apical site, with the bell of the stethoscope, and with the patient lying on the left side. S₃ occurs early in diastole right after S₂ and sounds like 'lub-dub-*ee*' (S₁, S₂, S₃). It often disappears when the patient sits up. S₃ is normal in children and young adults. In older adults, it may indicate heart failure. It occurs near the very end of diastole just before S₁ and creates the sound of '*dee*-lub-dub' (S₄, S₁, S₂). S₄ is rarely heard in healthy young adults. S₄ may be heard in many older patients and can be a sign of hypertension.

Diagnostic Testing of the Heart

There are a number of tests available to aid the diagnosis of any heart conditions. The most common of these is the **electro-cardiograph (ECG)** which graphically records the electrical impulse of the heart through electrodes placed on the skin. These electrodes are connected to an amplifier and strip chart recorder. A normal (or standard) 12 lead ECG provides 12 different views of the heart by attaching 10 electrodes to the patient's skin. An electrode is attached to each of the patient's arms and legs, which are known as limb leads. These leads

produce six views of the patient's heart. While six other electrodes are attached to the patient's chest around the patient's heart producing another six views of the heart (see Figure 26-42).

An ECG can pick up a number of cardiac abnormalities including myocardial infarction (heart attack), arrhythmias, ischaemia, pericarditis and electrolyte abnormalities to name a few. It is quick to perform, noninvasive and relatively inexpensive. As a result of its effectiveness and efficiency ECG is a common diagnostic test that can be performed by nurses who have had training in the use of the machine. However, interpretation of the graphical records takes far more knowledge and experience therefore interpretation of ECG is usually the role of the experienced nurse or doctor.

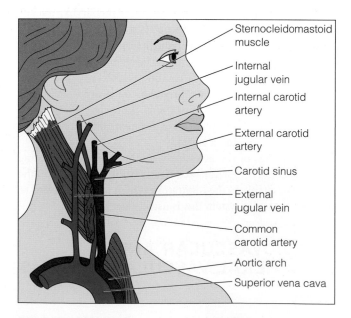

Figure 26-43 Arteries and veins of the right side of the neck.

A less common diagnostic procedure is echocardiography which is usually only performed if the patient's clinical condition warrants. An **echocardiogram** is a noninvasive test that uses ultrasound to visualise structures of the heart and to evaluate left ventricular function.

Central Vessels

The carotid arteries supply oxygenated blood to the head and neck (see Figure 26-43). Because they are the only source of blood to the brain, prolonged occlusion (blockage) of these arteries can result in serious brain damage.

The carotid artery can be auscultated for a bruit, and if a bruit is found, the carotid artery is then palpated for a thrill.

A **bruit** (a blowing or swishing sound) is created by turbulence of blood flow due either to a narrowed arterial lumen (space in the centre of an artery) (a common development in older people) or to a condition, such as anaemia or hyperthyroidism, which elevates cardiac output. A **thrill**, which frequently accompanies a bruit, is a vibrating sensation like the purring of a cat or water running through a hose. It, too, indicates turbulent blood flow due to arterial obstruction.

The jugular veins can also be assessed for pulsations and distention as these can indicate inadequacies in the right side of the heart. Raised jugular vein pressure (JVP) may indicate right sided heart failure.

Procedure 26-8 describes how to assess the heart and central vessels.

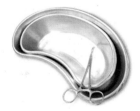

PROCEDURE 26-8 Assessing the Heart and Central Vessels

Planning

Heart examinations are usually performed while the patient is in a semi-recumbent position. The practitioner stands at the patient's right side, where palpation of the cardiac area is facilitated and optimal inspection allowed.

Equipment

+ Stethoscope

Implementation

Performance

1. Explain to the patient what you are going to do, why it is necessary and how they can cooperate. Discuss how the results will be used in planning further care or treatments.

2. Wash hands and observe appropriate infection control procedures.

3. Provide for patient privacy.

4. Enquire if the patient has any history of the following: family history of incidence and age of heart disease, high cholesterol levels, high blood pressure, stroke, obesity, congenital heart disease, arterial disease, hypertension and rheumatic fever; patient's past history of rheumatic fever, heart murmur, heart attack, varicosities or heart failure; present symptoms indicative of heart disease (e.g. fatigue, dyspnoea, orthopnea, oedema, cough, chest pain, palpitations, syncope, hypertension, wheezing, haemoptysis); presence of diseases that affect heart (e.g. obesity, diabetes, lung disease, endocrine disorders); lifestyle habits that are risk factors for cardiac disease (e.g. smoking, alcohol intake, eating and exercise patterns, areas and degree of stress perceived).

Assessment	Normal findings	Deviations from normal
5. Simultaneously inspect and palpate the precordium (the external surface of the body overlying the heart) for the presence of abnormal pulsations or heaves.	No pulsations	Pulsations which can indicate enlargement of the heart due to heart failure.

Assessment	Normal findings	Deviations from normal
6. Auscultate the heart	S$_1$: Usually heard at all sites Usually louder at apical area S$_2$: Usually heard at all sites Usually louder at base of heart Systole: silent interval; slightly shorter duration than diastole at normal heart rate (60–90 beats/min) Diastole: silent interval; slightly longer duration than systole at normal heart rates S$_3$ in children and young adults S$_4$ in many older adults	Increased or decreased intensity Varying intensity with different beats Increased intensity at aortic area Increased intensity at pulmonic area Sharp-sounding ejection clicks S$_3$ in older adults S$_4$ may be a sign of hypertension

Jugular veins

7. Inspect the jugular veins for distention while the patient is placed in a semi-Fowler's position (sitting up at a 30° to 45° angle), with the head supported on a small pillow.	Veins not visible (indicating right side of heart is functioning normally)	Veins visibly distended (indicating advanced cardiopulmonary disease)

8. Document findings in the patient record using forms or checklists supplemented by narrative notes when appropriate.

Evaluation

+ Perform a detailed follow-up examination based on findings that deviated from expected or normal for the patient. Relate findings to previous assessment data if available.

+ Report significant deviations from normal to medical staff.

BOX 26-11 Auscultating the Heart

+ Eliminate all sources of room noise. Heart sounds are of low intensity, and other noise hinders the nurse's ability to hear them.
+ Keep the patient in a supine position with head elevated 30° to 45°.

+ Use both the flat-disc diaphragm and the bell-shaped diaphragm to listen to all areas.
+ In every area of auscultation, distinguish both S$_1$ and S$_2$ sounds.
+ When auscultating, concentrate on one particular sound at a time in each area.

LIFESPAN CONSIDERATIONS

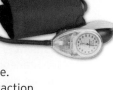

Assessing the Heart and Central Vessels

Children
+ Heart sounds are louder because of the thinner chest wall.
+ A third heart sound, best heard at the apex, is present in about one-third of all children.

Older Adults
+ If no disease is present, heart size remains the same size throughout life.
+ Cardiac output and strength of contraction decrease with age.
+ The heart rate returns to its resting rate more slowly after exertion than it did when the individual was younger.
+ S$_4$ heart sound is considered normal in older adults.

Peripheral Vascular System

Assessing the peripheral vascular system includes measuring the blood pressure, palpating peripheral pulses, and inspecting the skin and tissues to determine **perfusion** (blood supply to an area) to the extremities. Certain aspects of peripheral vascular assessment are often incorporated into other parts of the assessment procedure. For example, blood pressure is usually measured at the beginning of the physical examination (see the section on assessing blood pressure in Chapter 15).

Procedure 26-9 describes how to assess the peripheral vascular system.

PROCEDURE 26-9 Assessing the Peripheral Vascular System

Planning

Equipment

None

Implementation

Performance

1. Explain to the patient what you are going to do, why it is necessary and how they can cooperate. Discuss how the results will be used in planning further care or treatments.
2. Wash hands and observe appropriate infection control procedures.
3. Provide for patient privacy.
4. Enquire if the patient has any history of the following: past history of heart disorders, varicosities, arterial disease and hypertension; lifestyle habits such as exercise patterns, activity patterns and tolerance, smoking and use of alcohol.

Assessment	Normal findings	Deviations from normal
Peripheral pulses		
5. Palpate the peripheral pulses (except the carotid pulse) on both sides of the patient's body individually, simultaneously, and systematically to determine the symmetry of the pulses.	Pulses should be of the same intensity on both sides of the body	Pulses that are not the same on each side of the body may indicate impaired circulation. Absence of pulsation can indicates arterial spasm or occlusion. Decreased, weak, thready pulsations indicate impaired cardiac output (the amount of blood pumped out of the heart each minute). Increased pulse volume (may indicate hypertension, high cardiac output or circulatory overload).
Peripheral perfusion		
6. Inspect the skin of the hands and feet for colour, temperature, oedema and skin changes.	Skin colour pink	Cyanotic (venous insufficiency). Pallor that increases with limb elevation. Dusky red colour when limb is lowered (arterial insufficiency). Brown pigmentation around ankles (arterial or chronic venous insufficiency).
	Skin temperature not excessively warm or cold	Skin cool (arterial insufficiency).
	No oedema	Marked oedema (venous insufficiency).
	Skin texture resilient and moist	Mild oedema (arterial insufficiency). Skin thin and shiny or thick, waxy, shiny and fragile, with reduced hair and ulceration (venous or arterial insufficiency).
7. Assess the adequacy of arterial flow if arterial insufficiency is suspected (see *Box 26-12* on page 734).	Capillary refill test: immediate return of colour	Delayed return of colour (arterial insufficiency).

8. Document findings in the patient record using forms or checklists supplemented by narrative notes when appropriate.

Evaluation

+ Perform a detailed follow-up examination of the heart or central vessels, integument or other systems based on findings that deviated from expected or normal for the patient.

Relate findings to previous assessment data if available.

+ Report significant deviations from normal to medical staff.

BOX 26-12 Assessing the Adequacy of Arterial Blood Flow Capillary Refill Test

+ Squeeze the patient's fingernail and toenail between your fingers sufficiently to cause blanching.
+ Release the pressure, and observe how quickly normal colour returns. Colour normally returns immediately.

Diagnostic Tests of the Peripheral Vascular System

One of the most common diagnostic tests used to assess the peripheral vascular system is the **Doppler ultrasound** which can be performed in a hospital or community setting. This test evaluates the blood flow in the major blood vessels of the arms and legs. A handheld probe directs high-frequency sound waves to the artery or veins when held against the patient's skin. The sound wave strikes the red blood cells and is reflected back to the probe which then amplifies the sound waves to permit direct listening (see Figure 26-44). The Doppler ultrasound can detect a number of abnormalities including occlusion of the arteries and thrombi (clots).

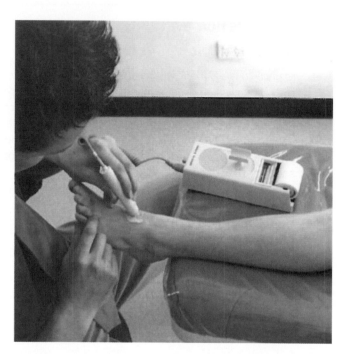

Figure 26-44 Doppler.

LIFESPAN CONSIDERATIONS

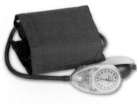

Assessing the Peripheral Vascular System

Infants

+ Palpation of the pulses in the lower extremities (particularly the femoral pulses) is essential to screen for coarctation (narrowing) of the aorta.

Older Adults

+ Peripheral vascular assessment should always include upper and lower extremities

temperature, colour, pulses, oedema, skin integrity and sensation. Any differences in symmetry of these findings should be noted.

+ Peripheral oedema is frequently observed and is most commonly the result of chronic venous insufficiency or low protein levels in the blood (hypoproteinaemia).

BREASTS AND AXILLAE

Examination of breast can be extremely stressful for the patient therefore the nurse must ensure that the patient's privacy and dignity are maintained throughout. Most people associate breast problems such as cancer with women but it is important to note that men are also at risk of developing breast cancer. Therefore the assessment of male patients should include an examination of the breast tissue. However the Royal College of Nursing (RCN) do not advise nurses to examine patients' breasts unless they have adequate training.

The majority of breast tumours can be found in the upper outer quadrant of the breast and in the projection of breast tissue into the axilla, called the *axillary tail of Spence* (see Figure 26-45).

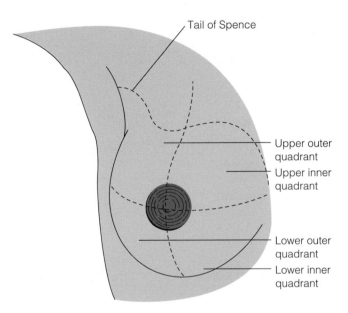

Figure 26-45 Four breast quadrants and the axillary tail of Spence.

Examination of the breast includes:

+ inspection of the size, symmetry and contour or shape of the patient's breasts;
+ inspection of the skin of the breast for localised discolorations or dimpling;
+ inspection of the areola area for size, shape, colour and symmetry;
+ inspection of the nipples for size, shape, position, colour, discharge and lesions;
+ palpation of the lymph nodes of the axilla and breast (see Figure 26-46);
+ palpation of the breast, areola and nipples for masses or tenderness.

Diagnostic Testing of the Breast

As part of the NHS Breast Screening Programme, all female patients between the ages of 50 and 70 are invited for breast screening or mammography. Mammography is used to screen and monitor breast cancer. It is a radiological technique that is very sensitive, having the ability to detect breast tumours or cysts that are not palpable.

Although the screening programme is aimed at 50- to 70-year-old females, mammography is available to those patients who may be symptomatic, for example, have felt a lump in their breast. The advice for these types of patients is to ensure that they are examined by their general practitioner who will refer them for further testing which could include mammography.

Following assessment of the breasts and axillae, the findings should be documented before proceeding to the next body area. For efficiency it is advisable that the nurse next assesses the abdomen of the patient.

ABDOMEN

In order for the nurse to accurately assess a patient's abdomen they must use a systematic method to locate the abdominal contents. A common method is to subdivide the abdomen into

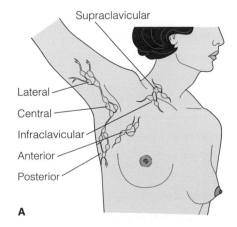
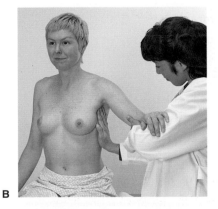

Figure 26-46 Location and palpation of the lymph nodes that drain the lateral breast. *A*, Lymph nodes; *B*, palpating the axilla.

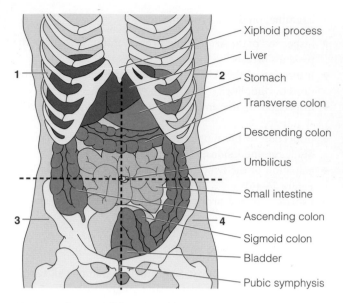

Xiphoid process
Liver
Stomach
Transverse colon
Descending colon
Umbilicus
Small intestine
Ascending colon
Sigmoid colon
Bladder
Pubic symphysis

Figure 26-47 The four abdominal quadrants and the underlying organs: *1*, right upper quadrant; *2*, left upper quadrant; *3*, right lower quadrant; *4*, left lower quadrant.

quadrants. To divide the abdomen into quadrants, the nurse imagines two lines: a vertical line from the xiphoid process (bottom of the breast bone) to the pubic symphysis (top of the pubic region), and a horizontal line across the umbilicus (see Figure 26-47). These quadrants are labelled right upper quadrant (*1*), left upper quadrant (*2*), right lower quadrant (*3*) and left lower quadrant (*4*). Specific organs or parts of organs lie in each abdominal quadrant (see *Box 26-13*).

Assessment of the abdomen involves all four methods of examination (inspection, auscultation, palpation and percussion). When assessing the abdomen, the nurse performs inspection first, followed by auscultation, percussion and/or palpation. Auscultation is done before palpation and percussion because palpation and percussion cause movement or stimulation of the bowel, which can increase bowel motility and thus heighten bowel sounds, creating false results. *Procedure 26-10* describes how to assess the abdomen.

BOX 26-13 Organs in the Four Abdominal Quadrants

Right upper quadrant
Liver
Gallbladder
Duodenum
Head of pancreas
Right adrenal gland
Upper lobe of right kidney
Hepatic flexure of colon
Section of ascending colon
Section of transverse colon

Left upper quadrant
Left lobe of liver
Stomach
Spleen
Upper lobe of left kidney
Pancreas
Left adrenal gland
Splenic flexure of colon
Section of transverse colon
Section of descending colon

Right lower quadrant
Lower lobe of right kidney
Caecum
Appendix
Section of ascending colon
Right ovary
Right fallopian tube
Right ureter
Right spermatic cord
Part of uterus

Left lower quadrant
Lower lobe of left kidney
Sigmoid colon
Section of descending colon
Left ovary
Left fallopian tube
Left ureter
Left spermatic cord
Part of uterus

PROCEDURE 26-10 Assessing the Abdomen

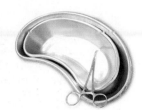

Planning

+ Ask the patient to urinate since an empty bladder makes the assessment more comfortable.
+ Ensure that the room is warm since the patient will be exposed.

Equipment

+ Examining light
+ Tape measure
+ Stethoscope

Implementation

Performance

1. Explain to the patient what you are going to do, why it is necessary and how they can cooperate. Discuss how the results will be used in planning further care or treatments.
2. Observe appropriate infection control procedures.
3. Provide for patient privacy.
4. Enquire if the patient has any history of the following: incidence of abdominal pain: its location, onset, sequence and chronology, its quality (description); its frequency; associated symptoms (e.g. nausea, vomiting, diarrhoea); bowel habits; incidence of constipation or diarrhoea (have patient describe what they mean by these terms); change in appetite, food intolerances and foods ingested in last 24 hours; specific signs and symptoms (e.g. heartburn, flatulence and/or belching, difficulty swallowing, haematemesis (vomiting blood), blood or mucus in stools, and aggravating and alleviating factors); previous problems and treatment (e.g. stomach ulcer, gallbladder surgery, history of jaundice).
5. Assist the patient to a supine position, with the arms placed comfortably at the sides. Place small pillows beneath the knees and the head to reduce tension in the abdominal muscles. Expose only the patient's abdomen from chest line to the pubic area to avoid chilling and shivering, which can tense the abdominal muscles.

Assessment	Normal findings	Deviations from normal
Inspection of the Abdomen		
6. Inspect the abdomen for skin integrity (refer to the discussion of skin assessment, earlier in this chapter).	Unblemished skin Uniform colour	Presence of rash or other lesions Tense, glistening skin (may indicate ascites (collection of fluid in the abdomen) or oedema (fluid in the tissue))
	Silver-white striae (stretch marks) or surgical scars	Purple striae (associated with Cushing's disease a hormonal disorder resulting in upper body obesity which makes the skin fragile and prone to bruising)
7. Inspect the abdomen for contour and symmetry:		
• Observe the abdominal contour while standing at the patient's side when the patient is supine.	Flat, rounded (convex) or scaphoid (concave)	Distended
• Ask the patient to take a deep breath and to hold it (_makes an enlarged liver or spleen more obvious_).	No evidence of enlargement of liver or spleen	Evidence of enlargement of liver or spleen
• Assess the symmetry of contour while standing at the foot of the bed.	Symmetric contour	Asymmetric contour (e.g. localised protrusions around umbilicus, inguinal ligaments or scars (possible hernia or tumour)

Assessment	Normal findings	Deviations from normal
• If distention is present, measure the abdominal girth by placing a tape around the abdomen at the level of the umbilicus (see Figure 26-48).		
8. Observe abdominal movements associated with respiration, peristalsis or aortic pulsations.	Symmetric movements caused by respiration. Visible peristalsis in very lean people. Aortic pulsations in thin persons at epigastric area (upper part of the abdomen)	Limited movement due to pain or disease process. Visible peristalsis in nonlean patients (with bowel obstruction). Marked aortic pulsations
Auscultation of the Abdomen		
9. Auscultate the abdomen for bowel sounds. The auscultation procedure is shown in *Box 26-14*.	Audible bowel sounds	Absent, hypoactive or hyperactive bowel sounds
Percussion of the Abdomen		
11. Percuss several areas in each of the four quadrants to determine presence of tympany (gas in stomach and intestines) and dullness (decrease, absence or flatness of resonance over solid masses or fluid). Use a systematic pattern (see Figure 26-49).	Tympany over the stomach and gas-filled bowels; dullness, especially over the liver and spleen, or a full bladder	Large dull areas (associated with presence of fluid or a tumour)
Percussion of the Liver		
12. Percuss the liver to determine its size. Listening for the sounds (see Table 26-9 on page 728) can determine the size of the liver. If percussing the liver the sound produced would be dull.	6–12 cm in the midclavicular line; 4–8 cm at the midsternal line	Enlarged size (associated with liver disease)
Palpation of the Abdomen		
13. Perform light palpation first to detect areas of tenderness and/or muscle guarding. Systematically explore all four quadrants. See *Box 26-15* on page 740 for palpation technique.	No tenderness; relaxed abdomen with smooth, consistent tension	Tenderness and hypersensitivity Superficial masses Localised areas of increased tension
14. Perform deep palpation over all four quadrants. See *Box 26-15* on page 740.	Tenderness may be present near xiphoid process, over caecum and over sigmoid colon	Generalised or localised areas of tenderness Mobile or fixed masses
Palpation of the Liver		
15. Palpate the liver to detect enlargement and tenderness.	May not be palpable Border feels smooth	Enlarged (abnormal finding, even if liver is smooth and not tender) Smooth but tender; nodular or hard
Palpation of the Bladder		
16. Palpate the area above the pubic symphysis if the patient's history indicates possible urinary retention (see Figure 26-50).	Not palpable	Distended and palpable as smooth, round, tense mass (indicates urinary retention)

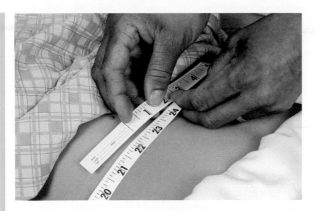

Figure 26-48 Measuring abdominal girth.

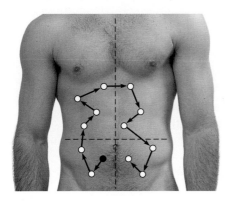

Figure 26-49 Systematic percussion sites for all four quadrants.

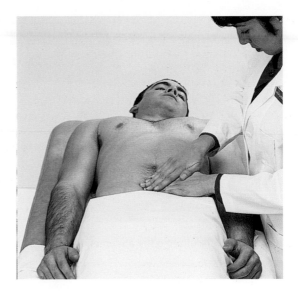

Figure 26-50 Palpating the bladder.

17. Document findings in the patient record using forms or checklists supplemented by narrative notes when appropriate.

Evaluation

+ Relate the findings of this examination to previous assessment data.

+ Report any significant abnormalities to the medical staff.

BOX 26-14 Auscultating the Abdomen

Warm the hands and the stethoscope diaphragms. Cold hands and a cold stethoscope may cause the patient to contract the abdominal muscles, and these contractions may be heard during auscultation.

For Bowel Sounds
+ Use the flat-disc diaphragm. Intestinal sounds are relatively high pitched and best accentuated by the flat-disc diaphragm. Light pressure with the stethoscope is adequate.
+ Ask when the patient last ate. Shortly after or long after eating, bowel sounds may normally increase. They are loudest when a meal is long overdue.
+ Place the flat-disc diaphragm of the stethoscope in each of the four quadrants of the abdomen over all of the auscultatory sites shown in Figure 26-51 on page 740.
+ Listen for active bowel sounds – irregular gurgling noises occurring about every 5–20 seconds. The duration of a single sound may range from less than a second to more than several seconds.

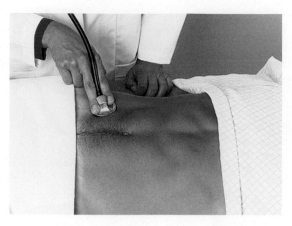

Figure 26-51 Auscultating the abdomen for bowel sounds.

+ Normal bowel sounds are described as audible. Alterations in sounds are described as absent, hypoactive, i.e. extremely soft and infrequent (e.g. one per minute), or hyperactive/increased, i.e. high-pitched, loud, rushing sounds that occur frequently (e.g. every three seconds). True absence of sounds (none heard in 3-5 minutes) indicates a cessation of intestinal motility. Hypoactive sounds indicate decreased motility and are usually associated with manipulation of the bowel during surgery, inflammation, paralytic ileus (paralysis of the bowel) or late bowel obstruction. Hyperactive sounds indicate increased intestinal motility and are usually associated with diarrhoea, an early bowel obstruction or the use of laxatives.

BOX 26-15 Palpating the Abdomen

Palpation is used to detect tenderness, the presence of masses or distention, and the outline and position of abdominal organs (e.g. the liver, spleen and kidneys).

Light Palpation
+ Hold the palm of your hand slightly above the patient's abdomen, with your fingers parallel to the abdomen.
+ Depress the abdominal wall lightly, about 1 cm or to the depth of the subcutaneous tissue, with the pads of your fingers (see Figure 26-52).
+ Move the finger pads in a slight circular motion.
+ Note areas of tenderness or superficial pain, masses and muscle guarding. To determine areas of tenderness, ask the patient to tell you about them and watch for changes in the patient's facial expressions.

Deep Palpation
+ Palpate sensitive areas last.
+ Use the bimanual method of palpation discussed earlier in this chapter.
+ Depress the abdominal wall about 4-5 cm (see Figure 26-53).
+ Note masses and the structure of underlying contents. If a mass is present, determine its size, location, mobility, contour, consistency and tenderness.
+ Check for rebound tenderness in areas where the patient complains of pain. With one hand, press slowly and deeply over the area indicated and then lift the hand quickly. If the patient does not complain of pain during the deep pressure but indicates pain at the release of the pressure, rebound tenderness is present. This can indicate peritoneal inflammation and should be reported to the medical staff immediately.

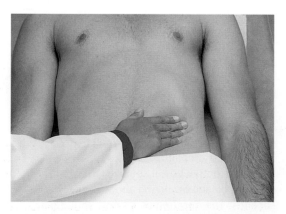

Figure 26-52 Light palpation of the abdomen.

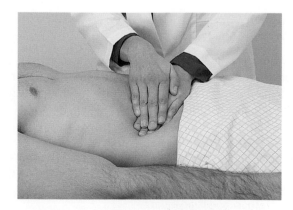

Figure 26-53 Deep palpation of the abdomen.

Diagnostic Testing of the Abdomen

Although a number of abdominal diagnostic tests exist the most commonly used one is the **abdominal ultrasound**. As with all ultrasound tests a transducer is placed on the skin of the abdomen which sends sound waves through the abdominal tissue. These waves are then reflected back to the transducer and converted to electrical impulses. These are then amplified and displayed on a screen. Abdominal ultrasound can evaluate organ size and structure and can differentiate between cysts and solid tumours.

LIFESPAN CONSIDERATIONS

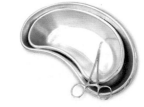

Assessing the Abdomen

Infants

+ The abdomen of the newborn and infant is round.

Children

+ Toddlers have a characteristic 'pot belly' appearance, which persists until about the fifth year.
+ Children may not be able to pinpoint areas of tenderness; by observing facial expressions the examiner can determine areas of maximum tenderness.
+ The liver is relatively larger than in adults. It can be palpated 1–2 cm below the right costal margin.

Older Adults

+ The rounded abdomens of older adults are due to an increase in adipose tissue and a decrease in muscle tone.
+ The abdominal wall is slacker and thinner, making palpation easier and more accurate than in younger patients.
+ Faecal incontinence may occur in confused or neurologically impaired older adults.
+ Many older adults wrongly believe that the absence of a daily bowel movement signifies constipation.
+ Decreased absorption of oral medications often occurs with ageing.

Following assessment of the abdomen it may be necessary to assess the musculoskeletal system but this will depend on the signs and symptoms that the patient presents with.

MUSCULOSKELETAL SYSTEM

The musculoskeletal system encompasses the muscles, bones and joints. However it may only be necessary to assess parts of this system depending on the needs and problems of the patient.

The nurse usually assesses the musculoskeletal system for muscle strength, tone, size and symmetry of muscle development, and twitches and tremors (an involuntary trembling of a limb or body part).

Bones are assessed for normal form. Joints are assessed for tenderness, swelling, thickening, crepitation (the sound of bone grating on bone), presence of nodules and range of motion. Body posture is assessed for normal standing and sitting positions.

Procedure 26-11 describes how to assess the musculoskeletal system.

PROCEDURE 26-11 Assessing the Musculoskeletal System

Implementation

Performance

1. Explain to the patient what you are going to do, why it is necessary and how they can cooperate. Discuss how the results will be used in planning further care or treatments.
2. Wash hands and observe appropriate infection control procedures.
3. Provide for patient privacy.
4. Enquire if the patient has any history of the following: presence of muscle pain: onset, location, character, associated phenomena (e.g. redness and swelling of joints), and aggravating and alleviating factors; any limitations to movement or inability to perform activities of daily living; previous sports injuries; any loss of function without pain.

Assessment	Normal findings	Deviations from normal
Muscles		
5. Inspect the muscles for size. Compare the muscles on one side of the body (e.g. of the arm, thigh and calf) to the same muscle on the other side. For any discrepancies, measure the muscles with a tape.	Equal size on both sides of body	Atrophy (a decrease in size) or hypertrophy (an increase in size)
6. Inspect the muscles and tendons for contractures (shortening).	No contractures	Malposition of body part (e.g. foot drop (foot flexed downward))
7. Inspect the muscles for twitches and tremors. Inspect any tremors of the hands and arms by having the patient hold the arms out in front of the body.	No twitches or tremors	Presence of twitches or tremor
8. Palpate muscles at rest to determine muscle tonicity (the normal condition of tension, or tone, of a muscle at rest).	Normally firm	Atonic (lacking tone)
9. Palpate muscles while the patient is active and passive for flaccidity, spasticity and smoothness of movement.	Smooth coordinated movements	Flaccidity (weakness or laxness) or spasticity (sudden involuntary muscle contraction)
10. Test muscle strength. See tests in _Box 26-16_. Compare the right side with the left side.	Equal strength on each body side	25% or less of normal strength
Bones		
11. Inspect the skeleton for normal structure and deformities.	No deformities	Bones misaligned
12. Palpate the bones to locate any areas of oedema or tenderness.	No tenderness or swelling	Presence of tenderness or swelling (may indicate fracture, neoplasms or osteoporosis)
Joints		
13. Inspect the joint for swelling. Palpate each joint for tenderness, smoothness of movement, swelling, crepitation and presence of nodules.	No swelling No tenderness, swelling, crepitation or nodules Joints move smoothly	One or more swollen joints Presence of tenderness, swelling, crepitation or nodules
14. Assess joint range of motion. Ask the patient to move selected body parts.	Varies to some degree in accordance with person's genetic makeup and degree of physical activity	Limited range of motion in one or more joints
15. Document findings in the patient record using forms or checklists supplemented by narrative notes when appropriate.		

Evaluation

✚ Relate the findings of this examination to previous assessment data.

✚ Report any significant abnormalities to the medical staff.

BOX 26-16 Testing Muscle Strength

Sternocleidomastoid (muscles in the neck) can be tested by asking the patient to turn their head to one side against the resistance of your hand.

Trapezius (muscles found running from the neck across the shoulder) can be tested by asking the patient to shrug their shoulders against the resistance of your hands.

Deltoid (the muscle that contours the top of the arm) can be tested by asking the patient to raise their arms in the air and resist your attempts to push the arms down again.

Biceps (the muscles that run along the front of the upper arm) can be tested by asking the patient to bend their arm at the elbow against resistance.

Triceps (the muscles that run along the back of the upper arm) can be tested by asking the patient to bend

their arm at the elbow and then attempt to straighten their arm against resistance.

Grip strength can be tested by asking the patient to grasp your fingers and resist your attempts to free your fingers.

Hip muscles can be tested by lying the patient down and asking them to raise their legs one at a time against resistance.

Quadriceps (the muscles of the top of the leg) can be tested by asking the patient to lie down and resist you trying to bend their knees.

Muscles of the ankles and feet can be tested by asking the patient to resist your attempts to bend the foot upwards and downwards.

Diagnostic Testing for the Musculoskeletal System

A universal investigation used to test the musculoskeletal system is the **x-ray**. A plain x-ray is a simple procedure that is noninvasive and entirely painless. It is done by a radiographer and involves placing the part of the body to be x-rayed in front of an x-ray plate. An x-ray beam is then directed at this area. It is important that during the procedure that the patient remains as still as possible. The information is then placed on a film or into a computer package for the appropriate healthcare professionals to interpret. X-ray interpretation should only be done by nurses and doctors who have the appropriate level of knowledge and expertise.

LIFESPAN CONSIDERATIONS

Assessing the Musculoskeletal System

Infants
+ Newborns naturally return their arms and legs to the foetal position when extended and released.
+ Check infants for developmental dysphasia of the hip (congenital dislocation) by examining for asymmetric gluteal folds, asymmetric abduction of the legs or apparent shortening of the femur.

Children
+ Should be able to sit without support by eight months of age.
+ Pronation of the feet, where the inner edge of the foot and the ankle are bent inwards, is

common in children between 12 and 30 months of age.
+ Genu varum (bowleg) is normal in children for one year after beginning to walk.

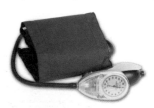

Older Adults
+ Muscle mass decreases progressively with age, but there are wide variations among different individuals.
+ The bones become more fragile and osteoporosis leads to a loss of total bone mass. As a result, elderly people are predisposed to fractures and compressed vertebrae.
+ In most elderly people, osteoarthritic changes in the joints can be observed.

The assessment of the musculoskeletal system is for most patients the final system to be assessed however for some patients further examinations may be required. For some patients there may be a need to examine their genitals depending on the clinical signs and symptoms that they present with.

FEMALE GENITALS AND INGUINAL AREA

Assessment of the female genitals and inguinal area are only performed if there is an indication for it. Firstly as it can cause anxiety in the patient and secondly assessment of this area of the body requires extensive knowledge and expertise so it is usually only performed by nurses who have had specific training. If there is an indication for the genitals and inguinal area to be examined the nurse should explain each part of the examination in advance and ensure that the patient's dignity and privacy are maintained at all times during the examination.

Assessment of the female genitals and reproductive tract includes:

+ inspection of the distribution of the pubic hair;
+ inspection of the skin of the pubic area for any signs of inflammation, swelling, lesions or parasites;
+ inspection of the urethral and vaginal orifice;
+ palpation of the inguinal lymph nodes (see Figure 26-54);
+ assessing the pelvic musculature;
+ inspection of the cervix and vagina using a speculum (which consists of two blades and an adjustable thumb screw, see Figure 26-55);
+ obtaining a cervical smear.

Diagnostic Testing of the Female Genitals

Probably the most common diagnostic test of the female genital area is the cervical smear or 'pap' test (short for papanicolaou the stain used to colour the smear). This is offered, as part of a UK programme, to every woman between the ages of 20 and 65 years every three to five years depending on the local area.

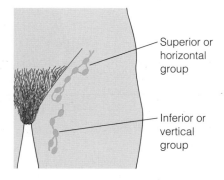

Figure 26-54 Lymph nodes of the groin area.

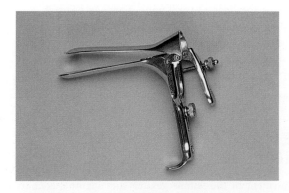

Figure 26-55 A vaginal speculum.

Currently around 80% of cervical smears are performed in primary care settings (in the community) usually by practice nurses who have had detailed training on the technique used. Training is crucial as inappropriate collection of cervical cells can potentially lead to incorrect treatment of the patient.

MALE GENITALS AND INGUINAL AREA

In adult men, complete examination should include assessment of the external genitals, the presence of any hernias and the prostate gland. As with women, nurses in some practice settings performing routine assessment of patients may assess only the external genitals as examination of the prostate gland requires expert knowledge.

The male reproductive and urinary systems (see Figure 26-56) share the urethra, which is the passageway for both urine and semen. Therefore, in physical assessment of the male these two systems are frequently assessed together.

Examination of the male genitals by a female practitioner is becoming increasingly common. Most male patients accept examination by a female, especially if she is emotionally comfortable herself about performing it and does so in a professional and competent manner. However, if the male patient is uncomfortable with a female nurse performing the examination they may request examination by a male practitioner.

All male patients should be screened for the presence of inguinal or femoral hernias (where soft tissue protrudes through a weak point in the groin). A **hernia** is a protrusion of the intestine through the inguinal wall. The loop of bowel may even extend down to the scrotum.

Cancer of the prostate gland is the most common cancer in adult men and occurs primarily in men over age 50. Examination of the prostate gland is performed with the examination of the rectum and anus (see later in the chapter).

Testicular cancer is much rarer than prostate cancer and occurs primarily in young men aged 15–35. Testicular cancer is most commonly found on the anterior and lateral surfaces

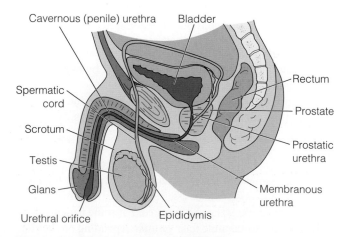

Figure 26-56 The male urogenital tract.

of the testes. Male patients are advised to examine their testicles monthly.

Examination of the male genitals and inguinal areas includes:

+ inspection of the distribution, amount and characteristics of pubic hair;
+ inspection of the penile shaft and glans for lesions, nodules, swellings or inflammation;
+ inspection of the urethral meatus for swelling, inflammation and discharge;
+ palpation of the penis to detect areas of tenderness;

+ inspection of the scrotum for appearance, general size and symmetry;
+ palpation of the scrotum to assess the status of the underlying testes, epididymis and spermatic cord;
+ inspection of both inguinal areas for any bulges while the patient is standing;
+ palpation of any hernias.

Examination of the prostate gland is complex and should only be performed by nursing staff who have undergone appropriate training.

LIFESPAN CONSIDERATIONS

Assessing the Male Genitals and Inguinal Area

Infants
+ The foreskin of the uncircumcised infant is normally tight the first two or three months of life and is not readily retractable.

Children
+ The scrotum is usually palpated to determine whether testes are descended.

Older Adults
+ The penis decreases in size with age; the size and firmness of the testes decrease.
+ Testosterone is produced in smaller amounts.
+ Seminal fluid is reduced in amount and viscosity.
+ Urinary frequency, nocturia, dribbling and problems with beginning and ending the stream are usually the result of prostatic enlargement.

CLINICAL ANECDOTES

I remember the first time I had to examine a male patient's genitals. I was a student nurse on my first placement and had had no healthcare experience before. I was apprehensive when my mentor said that we needed to check a patient who had recently had a transurethral resection of his prostate gland (TURP) (removal of the prostate gland through the urethra). The nightshift nurse stated that she felt that the urinary catheter that he had in place had eroded the urethral meatus. When I faced the patient I know I went red with embarrassment but I could not help it. I don't think the patient noticed because he was too embarrassed himself. Since then I haven't felt as embarrassed when examining a male patient's genitals.

Juliet Thomas, staff nurse

RECTUM AND ANUS

Like examination of the genitals, the rectum and anus are only examined if there is an indication to do so and by a nurse who has undergone appropriate training. Usual symptoms that would require the nurse to examine the rectum and anus are history of haemarrhoids, rectal pain or a family history of colorectal cancer.

Assessment of the rectum and anus includes:

+ inspection of the anus and surrounding tissue for colour, integrity and skin lesions;

+ palpation of the rectum for anal sphincter tonicity, masses and tenderness.

Diagnostic Testing for the Rectum and Anus

Although a number of tests are available to assess the gastrointestinal tract (GI), one of the more common tests is the **barium enema**. The GI tract does not show up well on plain x-rays. However if a barium (a soft white metal) is instilled into the tract the outline of the gut usually shows up well. X-ray films can then be taken with the patient in different positions for example supine or in a lateral position.

Barium enemas are indicated for patients who present with lower abdominal pain, blood pus or mucus in their stool, or if they have altered bowel habits, all of which could indicate some form of malignancy. However, malignancy is usually confirmed by endoscopic biopsy or colonoscopy.

Assessment of the rectum and anus is the final physical examination that will take place. An extensive examination that involves an assessment of all of the body systems is time consuming, so the nurse may perform the test over a number of hours or days as appropriate. This relies on the nurse using her clinical judgement to decide which parts of the assessment should be performed first. The nurse will base her decision on the patient's signs and symptoms and past medical history.

Physical assessment of the patient is important as it aids diagnosis. Some of the assessment procedures discussed in this chapter do require further training and could be considered advanced practice. However as a student nurse or newly qualified nurse you may need to refer to this chapter if you come across a full assessment of a patient to aid your understanding and develop your competence in this interesting area of nursing.

CRITICAL REFLECTION

Let us revisit the case study on page 686. Now that you have finished reading this chapter, reflect on how you would assess this patient, what you think are her initial needs and the possible diagnostic tests required to aid diagnosis.

CHAPTER HIGHLIGHTS

+ The health examination is conducted to assess the function and integrity of the patient's body parts.
+ The health examination may entail a complete head-to-toe assessment or individual assessment of a body system or body part.
+ The health assessment is conducted in a systematic manner that requires the fewest position changes for the patient.
+ Aspects of the physical assessment procedures should be incorporated in the assessment, intervention and evaluation phases of the nursing process.
+ Data obtained in the physical health examination supplement, confirm or refute data obtained during the patient history.
+ Patient history data help the nurse focus on specific aspects of the physical health examination.

+ Data obtained in the physical health examination help the nurse establish nursing diagnoses, plan the patient's care and evaluate the outcomes of nursing care.
+ Initial assessment findings provide baseline data about the patient's functional abilities against which subsequent assessment findings are compared.
+ Skills in inspection, palpation, percussion and auscultation are required for the physical health examination. These skills are used in that order throughout the examination except during abdominal assessment, when auscultation follows inspection and precedes percussion and palpation.
+ Knowledge of the normal structure and function of body parts and systems is an essential requisite to conducting physical assessment.

REFERENCE

Fitzpatrick, J.E. and Aeling, J.L. (2001) *Dermatology secrets in color* (2nd edn), Philadelphia: Hanley and Belfus, Inc.

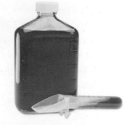

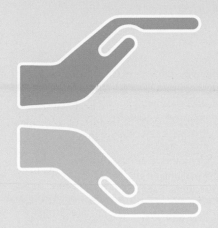
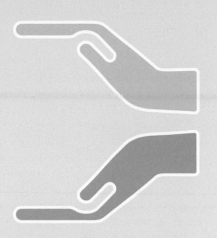

Index

Note: Figures and Tables are indicated by *italic page numbers*, and Boxes (Assessment Interview, Case Study, Clinical Alert, Critical Reflection, Procedure, etc.) by **emboldened numbers**. Alphabetical sort is word-by-word, ignoring prepositions as well as 'a', 'an' and 'the'.